NEUROPATHOLOGY

GREENFIELD'S NEUROPATHOLOGY

By

W. BLACKWOOD
M.B., Ch.B., F.R.C.S.E., F.R.C.P.E.
Professor of Neuropathology (Institute of Neurology)
University of London;
Hon. Consultant Pathologist,
The National Hospital for Nervous Diseases,
Queen Square, London

W. H. McMENEMEY
M.A., D.M., F.R.C.P.
Pathologist, Maida Vale Hospital for
Nervous Diseases, London

A. MEYER
M.D.
Emeritus Professor of Neuropathology,
University of London;
formerly at the Institute of Psychiatry,
Maudsley Hospital

R. M. NORMAN
M.D., F.R.C.P.
Research Consultant Neuropathologist
to the South Western Regional Hospital Board,
Burden Neuropathological Laboratory,
Frenchay Hospital, Bristol

DOROTHY S. RUSSELL
Sc.D., M.A., M.D., F.R.C.P., LL.D.
Late Director, Bernhard Baron Institute of Pathology,
London Hospital; Emeritus Professor of Morbid Anatomy,
University of London

LONDON
EDWARD ARNOLD (PUBLISHERS) LTD

First published 1958
Reprinted 1960
Second edition 1963
Reprinted 1965
Reprinted 1967
Reprinted 1969

SBN 7131 4044 5

Printed in Great Britain by
William Clowes and Sons, Limited, London and Beccles

PREFACE

Neuropathology was founded at the end of the last and the beginning of the present century by scientists of distinction among whom Franz Nissl and Santiago Ramon-y-Cajal were pre-eminent. The body of knowledge which they and many others, especially Charcot and his colleagues and pupils, have handed down is a precious heritage. Most of it has stood the test of the intervening years and, although modern technical advances have added many details, few fundamental errors have been discovered in the older work. Many of these early studies were remarkably complete and little has been added to some of them in more than half a century.

The pioneers of neuropathology were led on by the hope that the study of the diseased brain would lead to the interpretation of all disorders of action and conduct. Some, who found this quest unrewarding, were diverted to the more hopeful approach offered by psychopathology. But those who have followed the older discipline have been encouraged by seeing the return of a more organic conception of many disorders of behaviour. Each lobe of the brain has now its own symptomatology and the relation of hypothalamic, thalamic and rhinencephalic centres to emotion and emotional expression is becoming better understood. The pathology of the basal ganglia and brain stem has also been explored during the past fifty years, but physiological research has not yet clarified the relation between symptoms and lesions in that area of the brain.

Since many of the classical monographs of neuropathology are little known and few are available in the English language, more attention than usual is given in this book to the history of the subject and some sections are largely based on the original descriptions. To recall the names of the founders of neuropathology and the steps by which the science was built up has more than a pious interest since the principles of scientific advance remained unchanged.

The rapid progress of scientific technique is now challenging the older disciplines and not least histopathology. The advent of the electron microscope and of cytochemical and enzyme stains have called for a complete review of the older cytology which was based on the light microscope and traditional staining methods. Already knowledge of the structure of the neurone has been greatly extended and many of its changes under experimental conditions explored by these new techniques. Their application to human pathology has scarcely begun but offers an attractive field in which many advances are likely to be made in the near future. These new explorations must start from a base of existing knowledge and the provision of this is one of the objects of this book. In preserving and presenting in the English language what has been discovered by the established methods the authors hope not only to assist research but also to give the neurologist and psychiatrist that basis for diagnosis and logical treatment which only pathology can supply.

In a book compiled by several authors some overlapping and restatement have been unavoidable. In some places there may be difference of emphasis, but the editor considers this preferable to a dogmatic presentation of one view-point.

As the large subject of cerebral and spinal tumours is treated in a companion volume edited by Professor Dorothy S. Russell, it is omitted from this book.

The authors wish to express their gratitude to the Burden Trustees for financial assistance toward the illustration of Chapter 5. They are also greatly indebted to Professor Einarson and Drs. Frances D. Bosanquet, Martin Bodian, J. B. Brierley, J. B. Cavanagh, J. A. N. Corsellis, D. G. F. Harriman, W. Haymaker, Denis Leigh, T. McLardy, W. G. P. Mair, Wilder Penfield, Dorothy S. Russell, Sabina J. Strich and A. L. Woolf for permission to use illustrations, and to Mrs. Beck of the Institute of Psychiatry, and Mr. James Mills and Mr. Gordon Cox of the National Hospitals for Nervous Diseases for skilled photographic assistance.

Thanks are also due to the many friends in England and America who have given helpful advice and criticism.

J. G. GREENFIELD
A. MEYER
R. M. NORMAN
W. H. McMENEMEY
W. BLACKWOOD

PREFACE TO THE SECOND EDITION

Dr. Greenfield did not live to see the publication of the first edition of this book, which crystallises so much of his unrivalled experience at Queen Square. The loss of his guiding hand has been acutely felt in the preparation of this second edition but it has been the purpose of his original colleagues, now joined by Professor Dorothy Russell, to try to maintain the standards that he would have demanded.

Our chapters have been brought up to date, bearing in mind that this textbook is intended as a balanced account of the subject for senior students of neuropathology. The considerable amount of new information has been offset to some extent by the elimination of less important references and by some rearrangement of the subject matter to obviate undue repetition. Many new photographs have been added and a more useful index provided Mrs. Greenfield's help in preparing the latter is greatly appreciated.

The difficult task of revising Dr. Greenfield's own chapters has had to be faced, but so much of his fundamental teaching remains valid that in most instances only some amplification has been needed. In the section on demyelinating diseases, however, so many new observations have accumulated during the last five years that parts have had to be substantially rewritten in the interest of clarity and continuity of style.

The authors are greatly indebted to Drs. S. L. Palay, J. D. Robertson (Harvard), and A. L. Woolf (Birmingham) for permission to use illustrations.

R. M. NORMAN

CONTENTS

CHAPTER 1

GENERAL PATHOLOGY OF THE NERVE CELL AND NEUROGLIA

By J. G. Greenfield and A. Meyer

Introduction

The nervous system consists almost entirely of the cell bodies and processes of neurones. The science of neuropathology is therefore primarily concerned with the various methods by which neurones undergo degeneration and death. But since the neurones are fed by blood-vessels and are bound together by neuroglial and collagenous connective tissues, neuropathology must take account of changes in these tissues as also in the meningeal coverings of the brain and spinal cord. These may be more obvious than the changes in the neurones. For example, in inflammatory diseases, cellular proliferation may hide or mask the changes in the neurones which can only react by degeneration or death. It is true that in certain virus diseases the degenerative changes which the neurones undergo may be quite unusual and almost pathognomonic. But these changes are usually less evident than the 'inflammatory' and cellular proliferation and may need special staining methods for their demonstration. In many degenerative diseases also the overgrowth of astrocytes and proliferation of their fibres may be more striking than the disappearance of nerve cells or their axons. For this reason the term 'sclerosis' with various descriptive adjectives such as 'primary lateral', 'cortical' or 'lobar' has been given to processes which consist essentially in degeneration of certain neurones as a whole, and with the prefixes 'multiple', 'disseminated' or 'diffuse' to degenerations in which the myelin sheath is most affected. It was for a time thought that the neuroglial sclerosis in some of these diseases was primary and that the axons or myelin sheaths were strangled by the contraction of newly formed glial fibres. Similarly, before the virus etiology of poliomyelitis was discovered it was thought by some that the motor nerve cells were compressed and destroyed by the cellular exudate which invaded the ventral horns of the spinal cord. At the present time it is considered that the proliferation of neuroglial cells is almost always either a reaction to the degeneration of neurones or a concomitant reaction to the noxa to which this is due.

However much the study of the reactions of the vascular and conjunctival tissues may help towards our understanding of the pathogenesis of nervous diseases, it should never be allowed to supplant the study of the changes in the neurones themselves since it is to these that the symptoms of disease are due. This study has two chief objectives, first the *topography* of the lesion and secondly its *nature*. The relative importance of these two objectives varies in different conditions; when the nature of the process is evident the study of its topography may be more important and vice versa. But in most diseases the two objectives are complementary and both are essential.

In the early days of neuropathology the great French and German schools were distinguished by the emphasis laid on one or the other of these objectives. The French genius for anatomy was reflected in the School of Charcot for which the distribution of the lesions in relation to nuclei and tracts had special importance. When the lesion was focal, or confined to a special system or related group of systems, it could be correlated with the symptoms observed during life and thus provide evidence of the function of tracts or nuclei in the human brain. Such clinicopathological studies formed an important part of French neurological literature during the latter part of the nineteenth and the earlier part of the twentieth centuries. Many observations contributed in this way, for example on the sensory tracts and nuclei and on various aspects of mental activity, especially aphasia and apraxia, cannot, by their nature, be confirmed by animal experiment. Some have been confirmed by neurosurgery; others still await full confirmation; but the influence which studies of this kind have had on clinical neurology has been far reaching and profound.

On the other hand the German school of Weigert, Nissl and Alzheimer was specially interested in the alterations which the neurones and neuroglial cells underwent in disease and in the interpretation of these changes in relation to etiology and pathogenesis. The experimental studies of these scientists and of their pupils, especially Jakob and Spielmeyer, many of which were published in the Nissl-Alzheimer Arbeiten during the years 1904–20, form a wide and for the most part solid foundation for the structure of neuropathology. It was unfortunate that Alzheimer's work on the neuroglia was considerably invalidated by his failure to distinguish the different forms of cell included in this tissue. This distinction was later made in Madrid by Ramon-y-Cajal and his pupil del Rio Hortega, whose description and nomenclature is now universally accepted, although all do not entirely agree with their interpretations of the functions of these cells. This method of study has a less immediate relation to clinical neurology, but it is fundamental to the understanding of diseases of the nervous system. It is the object of present-day neuropathology to integrate these two disciplines, and while retaining the careful study of the topography of diseases, to seek to advance ever further knowledge of the pathology of the individual cells which constitute the nervous system.

This twofold quest of neuropathology imposes a heavy task on those who undertake it, since they must be not only pathologists but also anatomists and to some extent clinical neurologists and psychiatrists. A neuropathologist must know the history and details of the patient's illness before he makes his examination, otherwise he will often fail to examine some part of the nervous system. This applies most obviously to such outlying parts as the optic nerves and retina, the internal ear, and the dorsal root ganglia and peripheral nerves, but it happens too often that no examination is made of the spinal cord even in cases with signs of paraplegia or ataxia.

This combined aim of modern neuropathology has resulted in a technique which is far removed from the simpler methods in every day use for the other tissues of the body. In general, paraffin embedding is not so suitable for nervous tissues as either celloidin or frozen sections, owing to the greater shrinkage of the tissues and more complete removal of lipids during the process of embedding. Post-mordanting with mercury or chrome salts may reduce these disadvantages, but restricts the choice of staining methods. Very large paraffin sections are also less easily handled than celloidin sections of similar size. In some laboratories skill in dealing with large frozen sections had made their use the method of choice for many techniques. More general is the use of smaller frozen sections both as a preliminary to further examination and for special staining methods such as fat stains and silver impregnation. But celloidin embedding remains, in many laboratories, the most popular routine method. Its relative freedom from shrinkage and other artefacts, the greater retention of lipids, even without post-mordanting, and the wide range of staining processes available for celloidin sections offset the disadvantage of slowness and expense.

Not only does neuropathology demand a technique different from that of general pathology but it also uses a different language. This is largely inevitable in so far as it deals with quite different tissues. The nerve cell, nerve fibre, myelin sheath and neuroglial cell have characters of their own and undergo processes of degeneration which have no counterpart in other tissues. Therefore some terms used in general pathology such as 'cloudy swelling' and 'hyaline change' are inapplicable to changes in neurones. The term 'cloudy swelling' is often applied to the very characteristic changes in the cell body which follow section of the axon, but it would be equally applicable to Nissl's *acute swelling*, to the swollen cells of Pick's disease and of Lissauer's paresis, and to the distension of the nerve cell with lipid which occurs in the various cerebrospinal lipidoses. Such attempts to bring neuropathological terminology into line with the much less exact terminology of general pathology can only result in confusion. The old names 'central chromatolysis' and 'Wallerian degeneration' have, through long study, acquired a very precise meaning, and indicate a method of reaction to injury which is fairly well understood. The meaning of other terms used in neuropathology is less definite. For example the terms 'demyelination' and 'demyelinating disease' are often used for conditions in which the nerve fibre is damaged on its course through the white matter of the brain, although in some of these conditions the damage to the myelin may not be much more severe than that to the axons. It is often also convenient or even necessary to postulate, from what is seen by a general cell stain, changes which can only be fully proved by the use of special techniques. For example a phagocytic cell laden with the products of myelin katabolism may be recognised in a section stained by haematoxylin and eosin and the name 'fat granule cell', instead of the more descriptive term 'foamy cell', may be given to it, although the constitution of the granules can only be decided by the use of special stains for lipids. Similarly some forms of neuroglial cell can only be recognised by their nuclei when general cell stains are used, but the terms 'astrocytic proliferation', 'Alzheimer type of astrocyte' and 'hyperplasia' or 'multiplication of microglia' may be quite justified by such an examination alone.

Thus the value of special techniques in neuropathology is, for the most part, rather to make more evident and more definite what can be faintly discerned by more ordinary staining methods, than to discover structures or abnormalities which are otherwise invisible. In many cases, however, their use is obligatory. The extent and degree of demyelination, of damage to axons or neurofibrils, of nerve cells and of fibrous gliosis can only be judged by the use of special techniques, and such changes as neurofibrillary tangles in nerve cells and senile plaques are difficult to see without the use of silver impregnations. In this way some techniques come into routine use while others are reserved for special cases.

In the past neuropathology has suffered through being tied to too few special technical methods. For example, Nissl's stain has, in many laboratories, been the only cytological method in routine use, and details which are more easily visible by haematoxylin and eosin or other general stains have thereby been missed. In recent years there has been a trend in the opposite direction, and polychrome stains, and some special histochemical methods, such as those for amyloid and polysaccharides have proved to have a special value when applied to the nervous system.

The rapid growth of neurochemistry and the development of ultramicroscopes imposes a heavy task upon the neuropathologist who will be responsible for integrating these developments with established techniques. Since a single worker cannot hope to acquire expert knowledge in all these new fields, arrangements must be made to include trained specialists in the neuropathological laboratory. Many neuropathologists now appoint biochemists in their departments, where also the electron microscope is no longer an unfamiliar sight. Such teams will succeed, however, only to the extent that the specialists have a basic understanding of each other's provinces.

In a sense, the old-established techniques of neuropathology have always been histochemical, although often based more on empiricism than on scientific principles. Thus

Nissl's method is founded on the well-known affinity of acid proteins for basic dyes. Weigert's use of haematoxylin to stain myelin is not very different from Baker's stain for phosphatides, and the osmic acid techniques are based upon the reducing power of unsaturated fatty acids on osmium tetroxide. On the other hand, the various staining methods for glial fibres have been developed almost entirely from empirical observations by such masters as Carl Weigert and Frank B. Mallory. A similar empiricism appears to have guided the Spanish school as well as Golgi and Bielschowsky in their use of silver stains.

Modern histochemical techniques aim less at staining structural elements than at localising and making biochemical activities visible within the cells and their organelles. Numerous methods have been developed to visualise the activities of enzymes such as the cytochrome oxidases, dehydrogenases, specific and unspecific phosphatases, and cholinesterases, to quote only a few. Most of these techniques are still in their experimental stage, and their present limitations as well as their potentialities have been emphasised by workers experienced in this field (Roizin 1955; Potanos, Wolf and Cowen 1959; Feigin and Wolf 1955; Koelle 1955). Moreover, they usually require tissue near the living state, sectioning before fixation, freezing–drying techniques etc.: conditions which, with the exception of biopsies, are not obtainable in ordinary neuropathological work. This applies also to certain procedures which are not histochemical in a strict sense, but are, nevertheless, of considerable interest to neuropathology: such as, for example, differential centrifugation (introduced by Bensley and Hoerr, 1934) and the bold microchemical analyses on microdissected single neurones and glial cells which have been carried out by Lowry (1957) and Hydén and Pigon (1960).

Among the ultramicroscopes, Caspersson's ultraviolet histospectroscope, small angle X-ray diffraction and the electron microscope appear to be the most promising. Microscopy in ultraviolet light increases magnification to the extent, for example, which includes wavelengths of 2,600 Å, at which absorption of ribonucleic acids of the Nissl bodies takes place. X-ray diffraction gives valuable information of the atomic structure of molecules; although its data are not 'histological' in a narrow sense, it has nevertheless proved of considerable value in comparison with electron microscopic findings. On the other hand, the electron microscope is very much in the histological tradition: fixation, often by perfusion, is carried out in osmium tetroxide or potassium permanganate. 'Staining' with phosphotungstic acid increases the contrasts. After dehydration, the tissue is embedded in substances such as methacrylate or araldite and eventually cut by spccially constructed microtomes provided with glass knives which allow sectioning to the required thinness of approximatelo 0.1 μ. The resolving power is so high that useful magnification is possible up to × 1,000,000, though the most frequent magnification for nervous tissue is well below × 200,000. Even so, the prospect offered is stupendous and brings into the range of observation most of the larger and medium-sized molecules and viruses. As Roizin (1960) has pointed out, we are moving fast from the era of cellular pathology to that of molecular pathology. The very magnitude of this advance naturally evokes many initial difficulties and divergencies of interpretation and, although certain facts have been established (as will be described presently), it will be some time before the new ultramicroscopic as well as cytochemical developments become an assured province of neurohistology.

THE NEURONE

Normal histology

The neurone is the most complex cell in the body and the alterations which it may undergo in disease are similarly complex. These are manifested histologically by a number of alterations, in shape, staining reactions and even in structure, which cannot be interpreted without a more intimate knowledge of the composition of the neurone than we possess at present. Certain typical histological alterations have, however, been recognised for many years to be the results of certain forms of lesion or disease, and the metabolic changes which lead to some of these histological changes are beginning to be understood. These are essentially problems in histochemistry which may soon be clarified by the rapid advances which are taking place in this subject.

In the central nervous system the cell bodies or perikarya of the neurones are for the most part grouped either in layers, as in the cerebral and cerebellar cortex, or in irregular collections of similar cells termed 'nuclei'. In the brain and cerebellum there is a 'cortex' containing several layers of the bodies of nerve cells and a dense mass of their dendrites, and a 'white matter' which contains only nerve fibres. The cerebrum also contains large central nuclei of grey matter or basal ganglia. The cerebellum has basal nuclei in which its efferent fibres are relayed. In the spinal cord the 'grey matter' containing the nerve cells forms a central H-shaped column which is surrounded by white matter. In the brain stem grey and white matter are less separable, but various nuclei, such as the substantia gelatinosa of the medulla, the substantia nigra and the nuclei in the floor of the 4th centricle, consist chiefly of grey matter. Other nuclei, such as the nucleus subthalamicus, nucleus ruber and nuclei pontis, contain a larger admixture of myelinated fibres, whereas in others, especially the reticular formation the nerve cells are rather loosely scattered in a heavy network of myelinated fibres. Therefore in sections of the brain stem stained for myelin some nuclei are clearly outlined areas containing very little myelin, others are less clearly defined areas with some myelin staining, while yet others can scarcely be outlined at all.

It has been calculated that there are in the brain more than 20,000 million nerve cells. These are of varied form and size. The larger cells in the cerebral cortex and corpus striatum, and those which give rise to the motor nerves in the brain stem and spinal cord, are pyramidal in shape with their axons arising from the base of the cell. This shape is characteristic of efferent cells. The cells of the dorsal root ganglia and those of the mesencephalic root of the trigeminal nerve are spherical in shape; and in the secondary sensory nuclei of the brain stem and spinal cord and the thalamus a more or less oval shape is the rule. Other nerve cells vary between these two extremes, some being more multipolar, others having more rounded outlines.

Bipolar cells are found in the cochlear and vestibular ganglia, the olfactory organ and the retina. The fusiform cells described by Cajal in the auditory cortex are a special form. The shape of the Purkinje cells of the cerebellar cortex is also unusual. They may be described as flask-shaped. The spherical cell body gives off at one pole an axon and at the other a thicker process which breaks up into a frond of dendrites which spreads out across the lamella at right angles to its length.

The size of nerve cells varies with all gradations from very large to very small cells. The largest cells, the Betz cells in the 5th layer of the motor cortex, the large anterior horn cells in the cervical and lumbosacral enlargements of the spinal cord and the cells in the dorsal root ganglia, may measure 80μ in their greatest diameter. The smallest neurones, the granule cells in the cerebellar cortex, and in the retina and olfactory bulb, consist of little more than a rounded darkly staining nucleus, about 5μ in diameter, and an axon which runs for a comparatively short distance among neighbouring cells. Golgi divided neurones into two types. Neurones of his Type 1 have a long axon which passes into the white matter and extends for a considerable distance from the perikaryon. In Type 2 the axon does not leave the grey matter in which the nutrient cell body lies. These terms are only applicable to the largest and smallest cells, and there are many of intermediate type. In the brain stem particularly there are cells of all sizes, the axons of which run for very varied distances from the perikarya.

According to Hydén (1947) in the larger neurones the axon may have 1,000 times the bulk of the cell body and the nutrition of this large process must make great demands on the metabolism of the cell.

The neurone theory

According to the neurone theory which arose from the pioneer work of Cajal, His and Forel in 1889–91, each neurone is a separate cellular entity consisting of a perikaryon or cell body, dendrites or short processes which ramify in the neighbourhood of the cell body, and a longer or shorter axon which passes from the cell body to make contact by means of nerve endings of various kinds either with the dendrites or cell body of other neurones, or with muscle or other effector cells. The primary afferent neurones of the peripheral nerves differ from this general scheme in having no dendrites; they are connected, by nerve endings at one end of the axon, to the skin or a sensory end organ, and at the other end of the axon make synaptic connection with other neurones; their nutrient cell body lies at one side of the axon, on some part of its course, being attached to it by a short side process. Cajal postulated that the neurone is 'polarised' in the sense that the nervous impulse normally passes from the dendrites to the axon. In this sense he considered that in such receptor neurones as those of the olfactory organ, the retina and the internal ear, the peripheral processes represented the dendrites.

At the present time the neurone theory is accepted by most histologists. A few, however, consider that axons at their terminations blend with the cytoplasm of the cell with which they make contact (Boeke 1950). Others admit that in the sympathetic nervous system there are nerve plexuses in which the processes of different cells blend with one another. The old catenary theory, according to which the peripheral nerve fibre consists of a chain of internodal segments, joined together at the nodes of Ranvier and each nourished by a cell of Schwann, is no longer accepted for the axon, although it is probably true in a more limited sense for the myelin sheath.

Constitution and structure

The nerve cell is one of the very few types of cell in the human body which cannot be replaced if it is destroyed and which does not undergo cell division after the first few weeks of infancy. At the same time it has great metabolic activity, requiring a constant large supply of oxygen and glucose. No nerve cell in the central nervous system can tolerate absence of oxygen for much more than 15 minutes at the normal temperature of the body, and the more susceptible cells in the cerebral cortex cannot survive 5 minutes, or perhaps less, of complete arrest of the circulation. When the metabolic needs of cortical neurones are reduced by lowering the body temperature these times can be considerably exceeded, but the relation between body temperature and the time for which it is safe to stop the heart beating has not yet been fully worked out. Similarly if the level of blood sugar falls to 20 mg. per 100 ml. consciousness is lost and hypoglycaemia at this level for several hours usually entails the death of many neurones in the cerebral cortex. (Lawrence, Meyer and Nevin (1942) point out that low blood sugar estimations, if made by the usual laboratory techniques, may mean much lower true blood sugar values or even complete absence of blood sugar as other substances in the blood may have a reducing power equivalent to that of 20 mg. glucose per 100 ml. It is certain that when the blood sugar is estimated at 20 mg. per 100 ml. no trace of glucose may be found in the cerebrospinal fluid.)

These two characteristics, ability to survive for 100 years or more and great susceptibility to environmental and metabolic disturbances, are associated with an unusual toughness and density of cytoplasm and tenuity of cell membrane. De Renyi (1931) showed by microdissection that if a fresh unfixed frog's nerve cell were stretched until it tore into two halves, there was no escape of cytoplasm from the cell membrane; the torn edges remained irregular and when the two halves were again brought into apposition, the irregularities of one surface fitted more or less exactly into those of the other. The high density of nerve cells has enabled Chu (1954) to study isolated neurones, since they can be differentially sedimented by centrifugalising an emulsion of grey matter from the ventral horns of a rabbit's spinal cord in isotonic fluid with a specific gravity of 1,060. He found that nerve cell cytoplasm behaved like jelly in a bag. The consistency of this jelly was so viscid that no Brownian movement could be seen in it. This toughness may be associated with a high lipid content which is reckoned by Brante (1949) to be about 40 per cent. The lipids are chiefly ganglioside and lecithin. They are present not only in the mitochrondria and Golgi apparatus, but also more widely throughout the cytoplasm of nerve cells, especially in the neighbourhood of the axon hillock where they may become apparent as granules of 'lipochrome' or 'lipofuscin'.

The neurone contains in its cell body and processes various structures. About some of these, we know little. Others have been thoroughly studied and the changes which they may undergo in disease form the basis of neuropathology. As these changes can only be understood by comparison with the normal the various constituents of the nerve cell must first be shortly described.

Nucleus and nucleolus

The nucleus varies considerably in different types of nerve cell and in the same cell type in different mammalian species. The vesicular nucleus with large central nucleolus seen in larger nerve cells appears distinctive, but it contains the same chemical elements as other nuclei, although in different proportions. These are (1) *nucleoplasm* composed of weakly acidophilic protein. (2) *Chromatin* or desoxyribose nucleic acid (DNA) in granules of varying size and fine threads. These stain with basic aniline dyes and are Feulgen positive. (3) *True nucleolus*, which is spherical, more or less central and is composed of a mixture of ribosenucleic acid (RNA) and a basic (acidophilic) protein. It is amphiphilic and Feulgen negative. Its ribosenucleic acid content gives it the same staining and optical properties as Nissl granules, but in virtue of its basic protein it takes the red acid dye in mixtures of eosin, phloxin or acid fuchsin with dyes of more neutral character (Mann, Alzheimer's fuchsin light green, Mallory's and Masson's trichrome stains and their variants). With Unna-Pappenheim's methyl green-pyronin also it stains red while the chromatin stains green. (If the methyl green is impure, it may stain chromatin violet.) The nucleolus often contains one or more 'vacuoles'.

The proportions of chromatin and nucleolus vary considerably in neurones of different types, especially in relation to their size. In the large nerve cells the nucleolus is large and the chromatin is present in small amount being confined to very fine granules under the nuclear membrane and one or two larger paranucleolar granules. At the other extreme the cerebellar granule cells have a small central nucleolus which is covered and partly obscured by abundant chromatin granules. In general, as Olszewski (1947) points out, there is a positive correlation in man between the amount of Nissl substance and the size of nucleolus, and a negative correlation between the amounts of Nissl substance and nuclear chromatin. Most nerve cells have only one nucleolus, although two or more have been described in developing neurones.

In some of the larger nerve cells the chromatin, in addition to fine granules, may form a rounded or oval mass, 0·5–2μ in diameter, which usually lies close to, or in contact with, the nucleolus, but sometimes free in the nucleoplasm or in contact with the nuclear membrane. This *nucleolar satellite* has been shown by Barr and Bertram (1949) to be related to the sex chromosome and to be larger in the female than in the male in many nerve cells. In the human this sex difference can be well seen in the sympathetic ganglia and cerebral cortex but is not so distinct in Purkinje cells. They call this body the *sex chromatin*.

In the cat, which was chiefly studied by Barr and his associates, the sex chromatin most often lies against the nucleus (61 per cent) but may lie free in the nucleoplasm (15 per cent) or adjacent to the nuclear membrane (6 per cent). In the monkey the sex chromatin granule is most often seen in contact with the nuclear membrane. Lindsay and Barr (1955) distinguish the sex chromatin from the basophil clots described by Levi (1897) in rodents. These consist of two, three or more small reniform masses of chromatin which lie closely applied to the spherical nucleolus. These are well seen in Purkinje cells.

Cajal (1909) described an argyrophilic dot in the nucleoplasm of large nerve cells under the name *accessory body*. This has no relation to chromatin and its nature is not known (Lindsay and Barr 1955). Hydén (1950) also describes a less sharply defined, strongly acidophilic area in the neighbourhood of the nucleolus. He found it to contain basic protein along with small quantities of pentose nucleic acids. It can be seen in the larger nerve cells of the human nervous system when well stained with haematoxylin and eosin.

As Marinesco (1909) pointed out, the cells of the substantia nigra and locus coeruleus may normally contain, in the nucleoplasm, acidophilic bodies which become larger, more sharply defined and more numerous in old people. These bodies may be mistaken for intranuclear inclusions, the earlier stages of which they closely resemble, but they do not displace the nucleolus. Although usually single, two or three of such bodies may be seen lying on either side of, or around, the nucleolus.

The *electron microscope* shows the nucleus surrounded by a double membrane which exhibits deep folds, indentations and pores which apparently allow passage between nuclear and cytoplasmic material. The chromatin has a rosette-like arrangement, quite different from the basophilic material in the cytoplasm, while the nucleolus contains aggregates of extremely fine granules measuring 10–30 Å (Palay and Palade 1955; Luse 1956, Fernandez-Moran 1957, and others).

Nissl granules

This name is now in general use for the flakes of basophilic material in the cytoplasm of nerve cells and dendrites which were described by Nissl in 1894 (a). It is preferable to the term 'chromophilic substance' since in other cells such as those of the pituitary the term 'chromophilic' denotes acidophilic cells. The name 'tigroid substance' is now seldom used. It is convenient to use the terms hyperchromic and hypochromic for nerve cells which, although normal in all other respects, stain more or less intensely than normal with basic aniline dyes.

It was considered for many years that the appearance of Nissl granules, in fixed and stained sections, was largely an artefact of fixation and depended on the fixative used. The position was well stated by Einarson (1933) who considered Nissl material as 'truly existing during life, being present in a fluid or semi-fluid state, possibly not of a completely diffuse nature, but in localised concentrations in the cell body, finally being coagulated *post mortem* or by the fixatives employed and giving rise to the well-known histological "cell pictures"'. Nissl accepted no fixative, except alcohol, for his staining method, and warned workers not to accept the histological appearances which they found as more than 'equivalent pictures' of what was present during life. Thus for each change which occurred during life there was an 'equivalent' or corresponding change in the nerve cells after fixation. We now know that such warnings were scarcely necessary. Fixation may increase the sharpness of outline of Nissl granules, but it does not greatly alter either their form or distribution. Further, any good fixative suitable for nuclear stains may be used. With some fixatives there is more tendency to shrinkage than with others, and with some there may even be some swelling of the cell. With these exceptions the appearance of Nissl granules in well-stained sections of tissue may therefore be accepted with little reserve as that which was present at the time of death.

It is, however, necessary to distinguish the changes which may have resulted from the mode of death, such as toxaemia or hyperpyrexia, and those due to post-mortem autolysis, from those which are related to a chronic or subacute nervous disease. Certain well-defined changes in the nerve cell such as central or peripheral chromatolysis fortunately require some little time to develop and are never the result of agonal or post-mortem changes.

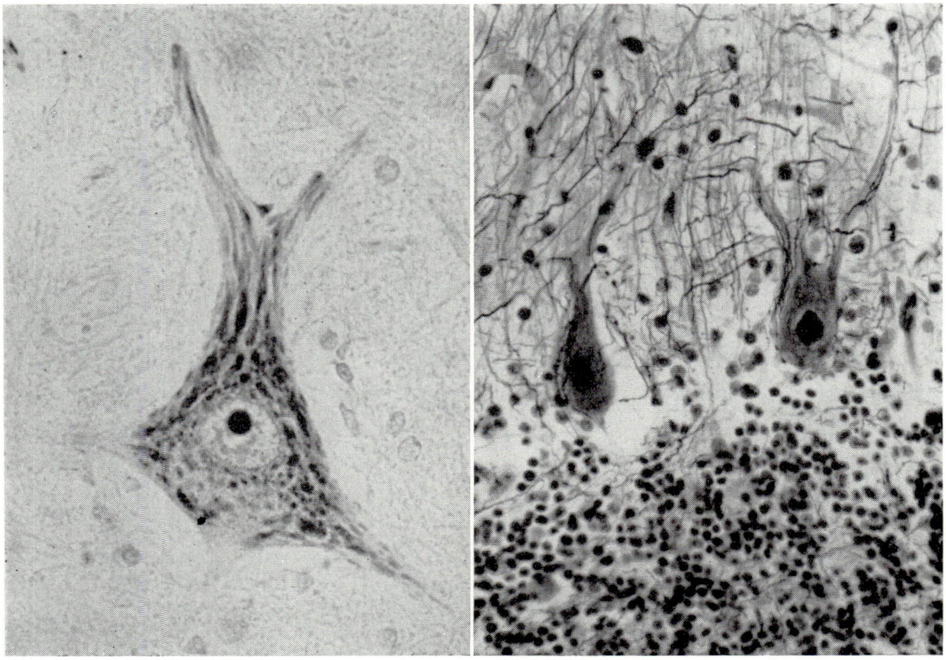

(*a*) (*b*)

FIG. 1.1. Normal nerve cells.

(*a*) Cell from ventral horn of lumbar cord. (Nissl ×550.) Note absence of Nissl granules in axon hillock. (*b*) Purkinje cells. Cerebellar cortex. (Bielschowsky ×400.) Basket fibres surround the cells and pass up the dendrites.

The amount of Nissl substance and the shape and position of the condensations or 'granules' varies in different types of nerve cell. Nissl (1894 b) distinguished three main types of nerve cells: *cytochrome* or granule cells; *karyochrome*, in which the nucleus is more deeply stained than the cytoplasm, and *somatochrome* in which the cytoplasm stained more darkly than the nucleus. These special terms are now rarely used, but it is important to realise that in the cells of some centres the basophilic granules have a special arrangement. For example the larger cells of the formatio reticularis have an onion-skin arrangement of Nissl granules in concentric layers round the nucleus which is usually eccentric (Olszewski and Baxter 1954). In the cells of Clarke's column and the nucleus of Clarke-Monakow (lateral cuneate nucleus) the Nissl granules are small and lie chiefly in the periphery of the cytoplasm, and the nucleus is eccentric, an appearance which resembles the early stages of 'central chromatolysis'.

The composition of Nissl granules has been studied in many ways. The early staining method of Nissl, who used basic aniline dyes, indicated that they contained an acid protein probably allied to nucleoprotein. Weimann (1925) photographed unfixed cells by ultra-violet light and obtained appearances very similar to those in fixed and stained cells, thus showing that Nissl granules exist in the living cell. The work of Caspersson (1940), who showed that ultra-violet light with a wavelength of about 2,570 Å was absorbed by purine and pyrimidine bases present in nucleic acid, was carried further by Hydén, who photographed Nissl granules with this light band and proved also, by the use of a pure ribonuclease, that they consisted of ribose-nucleoprotein. Gersh and Bodian (1943) and Hydén and Hartelius (1948) later adapted this technique to the quantitative study of Nissl substance in nerve cells.

Nicholson (1923–4) using the Prussian blue method and Macallum's haematoxylin, after treatment by acid, showed that Nissl granules contained masked iron, and this was further demonstrated by the technique of ashing sections by Scott (1933), Alexander and Myerson (1938) and Alexander (1938) who also revealed in them by this method a considerable amount of calcium. Their composition was further studied by Einarson (1933, 1935) who used gallamin blue and gallocyanin chrome alum. The latter method permits of quantitative studies, as does also the technique of Windle, Rhines and Rankin (1943) who use a very dilute, acid-buffered thionin after fixation in formol saline. Einarson found that the area of the Nissl bodies might under certain conditions be stained by acid dyes such as eosin or acid fuchsin and considered that there were in the Nissl body not only nucleoproteins but other basophilic and acidophilic proteins.

In the *electronmicroscopic picture*, the site of the Nissl bodies is formed by a delicate laminated system of cisternae (Fig. 1.17) to which, according to Palade (1956), the name 'endoplasmic reticulum' was given by Porter and Kallman in 1952. They are sometimes also referred to as α-cytomembranes (Mercer 1961). The cisternae are lined by deeply stained granules (ribosomes) chiefly compounded of ribonucleic acid and which are responsible for the basophilia of the Nissl bodies. These were first described by Palade (1955), and have been confirmed.

The granular endoplasmic reticulum is not specific for nerve cells; it is even more developed in the so-called ergoplasm of exocrine glandular cells. It is believed that the ribosomes and their equivalents subserve protein synthesis and that the cisternae are concerned with the transport of protein products and of the various enzymes involved in this process. The granular reticulum continues into dendrites and—to a lesser degree—throughout most of the length of axons. It is observed also in small nerve cells (for example, the cerebellar granules) which in light microscopy do not appear to have cytoplasmic chromatin, and there is an agranular reticulum (Palay and Palade 1955) believed to correspond to the Golgi apparatus of the cell.

Hyperchromic and hypochromic nerve cells

In experimental work on the lower mammals it is common to find that some nerve cells appear rather pale and rounded (hypochromic) and others darker and more polygonal (hyperchromic). These appearances may sometimes be seen also in human material. Considerable confusion has arisen from interpreting the dark 'hyperchromic' cells as diseased or abnormal. Cajal (1897) considered the hyperchromic cells of healthy animals as an histological expression of a state of inactivity in those cells, an opinion with which Einarson (1933) agreed. Miller (1949) who studied the mitochondria and Golgi apparatus in hyperchromic cells as well as the Nissl substance and nucleus, found the Golgi apparatus hypertrophied and the mitochondria more numerous than in normally staining cells. Such cells also gave a strong alkaline phosphatase reaction. He interpreted these results as indicating that hyperchromic cells were in a state of increased activity. In his material, which consisted of normal animals, shrinkage of nerve cells and a corkscrew appearance of dendrites was seen with certain fixatives and must therefore be considered as an artefact. Koenig, Groat and Windle (1945) found that swelling or shrinkage of nerve cells depended on the composition of the fixative and the method of fixation. They advise the use of intra-arterial injections with formol saline to which 2·4–4·6 per cent gum acacia is added according to the pressure employed in the injection.

Einarson has recently (1957, 1960) summarised his views on the functional significance of Nissl granules as follows: Chromoneutrality (after gallocyanin staining) indicates a resting state of the nerve cell; moderate chromophilia may point to initial activity, while extreme chromophilia suggests suppression of activity. Moderate chromophobia follows prolonged and increased activity; in extreme degree, it expresses severe stress and exhaustion. Extreme chromophobia may proceed to liquefaction, while the outcome of extreme chromophilia may be sclerosis and atrophy of the cell.

Relationship of Nissl substance to nucleus

The similarity in chemical composition of Nissl granules to most of the nucleoproteins of the nucleus led Einarson (1933) to consider that they might be derived from the nucleus, either during ontogenesis only, or both in the developing and adult nerve cell. Studying the response of motor nerve cells to prolonged electrical stimulation or to section of the axon, he found that, after the loss of Nissl granules which resulted from these procedures, there was first an increase in the amount of nucleoprotein round the nucleolus; this migrated to the periphery of the nucleus, especially in the region of the nuclear cap which became more prominent and was in these early stages partly intra- and partly extranuclear. Later it became entirely extranuclear and there was an accumulation of fine Nissl granules in its neighbourhood. As the Nissl substance increased the nuclear cap became less evident. These observations suggested that the Nissl substance was reformed after chromatolysis from the ribose nucleoprotein of the nucleus. Hydén (1950) accepted this derivation, but it is denied by Gersh and Bodian (1943).

Mitochondrial rodlets and granules have been studied in nerve cells by Cowdry (1912, 1914) by the supravital Janus green technique, by Bertrand and Bertrand and Hadzigeorgiou (1928) by infra-red photomicrography and by numerous workers with the phase contrast microscope. In normal cells they occupy the same position as Nissl granules, but Beams *et al.* (1952) by phase contrast microscopy found them also abundant in the axon hillock. They considered that highly refractile rodlets which they saw in the axon itself were probably also of this nature.

Mitochondria are easily identified in the *electron microscope* (Fig. 1.17–18) and have been clearly illustrated by Palay and Palade (1955) and many others. On the electronic screen they show a diffuse ground substance, surrounded by a double membrane the inner lamella of which forms the characteristic 'cristae'. Belt and Pease (1956), however, described 'tubules' instead of 'cristae', but the difference seems to be of functional degree, the cristae being formations at rest (Wilke 1959). Mitochondria occur throughout the cytoplasm, even between the cisternal lamellae of the endoplasmic reticulum, and extend into dendrites and—to a lesser degree—throughout the axon. They are particularly frequent near presynaptic membranes.

Mitochondria are known to be rapidly altered in many inflammatory, viral and toxic conditions (Choja 1936; Hurst 1929). In the early stages of neurone reaction to axon section, mitochondria have been reported to increase in number and size by Hartmann (1948) and Hudson and Hartmann (1961), while Barton and Causey (1958) found them degenerating in the superior cervical ganglion after section of its preganglionic fibres. Scholz and Hager (1959), in electron-microscopic studies on various types of hypoxia, observed swelling and mild vacuolation of the mitochondria at a stage when chromatolysis was already advanced. In later stages the mitochondria became vacuolic.

It has been shown by differential centrifugation, that many important biological processes such as those concerned with tissue respiration, phosphorylation, and the Krebs cycle take place almost exclusively in the mitochondria. Quastel (1957) found that snake venom lecithinase had an effect exclusively on mitochondrial enzymes, and Harman (1958) reported the same of certain bacterial toxins.

Neurofibrils. The neurofibrillary structures in the neurone were first revealed by Ehrlich (1886) with intravital methylene blue; and by Bethe (1898) by the use of toluidin blue: but their study in pathological material has been greatly aided by the reduced silver techniques of Cajal (1903) and Bielschowsky (1902, 1904), which were founded on the older techniques of Simarro (1900) and Fajerstajn (1901). Neurofibrils have not definitely been seen in an unfixed state in the vertebrate nervous system, but in living crustaceans (Kedrowski 1935) and other invertebrates they can be seen as fine threads which are in constant motion in the surrounding axoplasm. Their constancy in fixed material stained by silver impregnations, and the results of Ehrlich's intravital methylene blue technique, leave little doubt that they exist during life in a form which, if not similar, is readily changed by fixation to that which is demonstrated by these staining methods. At birth, neurofibrils—except for some precursory granules in Betz cells—are absent from the cerebral cortex, although they are fully developed in nerve cells of the spinal cord and brain stem (Conel 1939–59). The same author traced their development during the first 15 months of postnatal life: they appear first in the large cells of layers V and VI of the precentral cortex, to become generalised in later stages.

The neurofibrils in the cell body appear to be rather more resistant to many forms of injury than the Nissl granules and are often preserved when the latter have disappeared. They undergo less obvious changes in the chromatolysis which follows damage to the axon. In hibernating lizards (Tello 1904) and in mammals exposed to cold (Cajal 1904) they become clumped together into denser bundles.

Schmitt and Geren (1950), Fernandez-Moran (1952, 1957) and many others in studies with the *electron microscope* have found the axon to contain an irregular loose skein of fine filaments, with a smooth outline, which run without branching or joining other filaments for considerable distances. They vary from 100 to 200 Å in thickness. The number of filaments in an axon varies greatly. In the larger axons there may be several thousands, whereas in others there are relatively few. That the filaments seen in thin sections of nerves represented preformed structures was shown by ultracentrifugalisation of pieces of spinal cord before fixation. This displaced the filaments but did not disintegrate them as it would have done had they been originally discontinuous.

Axon and axoplasma

The behaviour of the axon in regeneration and minor conditions of pressure or constriction suggests that it is formed of a firmer outer gel layer and a more liquid inner core. It is considered that the core is always under some pressure, which is normally restrained by the outer layer; this pressure may be continuous or pulsatile. Weiss (1943) and Weiss and Hiscoe (1948) showed that an axon becomes swollen proximal to a constriction, suggesting that under normal conditions there may be some transport of material from the cell body to the periphery of the axon. Young (1950) considers that some fluid may be constantly passing out of the axon into the surroundings. As is well known, when an axon is cut new sprouts are quickly extruded from the cut end, and proceed to advance along interfaces or surfaces for considerable distances.

Some silver impregnation methods (e.g. Gros-Bielschowsky) stain the axon up to its finest branches without staining the nerve cell or dendrites, indicating that it contains an argyrophilic substance other than neurofibrils. In general the axon stains with neutral dyes such as anilin blue and remains unstained with haematoxylin unless it is diseased. It is very subject to shrinkage by fixation, especially with the more slowly acting fixatives; under such conditions fluid passes out of the axon into the surrounding myelin sheath causing swelling of the myelin at the expense of the axon (De Renyi 1929).

On leaving the cell body the axon is at first unmyelinated for a distance which may correspond roughly to the length of the perikaryon. It narrows slightly before entering the myelin sheath and expands again after entering the sheath. In the peripheral nerves it is slightly thinned at each node of Ranvier in the living state, but its protoplasm appears to be more condensed at this point than along the internodal segment, so that it does not shrink so much during fixation with the slower fixatives. Thus in fixed preparations the axon may be rather thicker at the node of Ranvier than elsewhere.

In the electron microscope the axon is seen surrounded by a membrane (axolemma) which participates in myelination.

Dendrites

All nerve cells within the central nervous system have one or more dendritic processes. No true dendrites are seen in the peripheral nervous system of vertebrates, although attention has already been drawn to Cajal's view that sensory nerve endings were functionally analogous. The number of dendrites varies greatly. Anterior horn cells in the spinal cord have from 3 to 20 (Chu 1954) and cortical pyramids also have many. Their length may be 20 times the width of the cell body, and they branch freely. The dendrites of Purkinje cells arise as one or two thick processes at the pole of the cell opposite to the axon, and these branch fanwise in a plane at right angles to the long axis of the folium. Cortical neurones have very few or no dendrites at birth, and the increase in the number and length of these is part of the process of maturation which takes place during the first few months of extra-uterine life (Conel).

Dendrites contain neurofibrils throughout their length and Nissl granules at least in their more proximal parts, although the endoplasmic reticulum extends further towards the periphery. Cajal described numerous fine club-shaped spicules, known also as thorns, globules and gemmules, which stand out from the dendrite throughout its length, except near its base. They are stained both by Ehrlich's methylene blue and Golgi's silver chromate techniques. They are best seen in cortical pyramidal cells and in Purkinje cells. Cajal considered the late appearance of these projections to indicate the maturity of the neurone, and that they may help to collect nervous impulses (i.e. to act as postsynaptic structures). Conel also observed their increase in calibre and number during early postnatal development; he admits, however, that their involvement in synaptic activity is not yet established beyond doubt. Gray (1961) described and illustrated the electronmicroscopic appearance of dendritic spines: these can be seen arising from dendrites, and to all appearances are postsynaptic structures, as Cajal had already suggested. They consist of two sacks which may be intercommunicating, with a band of considerable electronic density between them. Dendritic tubules have not yet been found to continue into the spine.

Nerve endings

In the central nervous system it is common to find that the larger axons, for example those arising from the pyramidal cells of the cerebral cortex and the Purkinje cells of the cerebellar cortex, give off one or more collateral fibres soon after leaving their cell of origin. Similarly the large axons which enter the spinal cord by the dorsal roots branch as soon as they enter the cord. Thereafter the fibres may run for long distances, either in the fibre tracts of the central nervous system or in peripheral nerves, without giving off any branches. Near their termination they divide into a greater or smaller number of branches and as these approach their termination they lose their myelin sheath and may break up into a number of fine terminal twigs, which enter the peripheral end-organ or make synaptic connection with the cell bodies or dendrites of other neurones.

In the central nervous system many axons make contact of this kind by means of ring-like endings which are usually called *boutons terminaux*. These can be stained by the more specific silver impregnations for axons. On the large nerve cells of the ventral horns of the spinal cord many such endings are seen both on the cell body and the dendrites. The pyramidal cells of the cerebral cortex have fewer, and the neurones of the corpus geniculatum externum may have only one small ring applied to the cell body (Glees and le Gros Clark 1941). With other nerve cells, for example those of the nucleus caudatus (Glees 1944), synaptic contact may be made by fine axonal ramifications without boutons. The ring endings degenerate when the axon which terminates in them is cut (Hoff and Hoff 1934, Foerster and Gagel 1934, Fedorow 1935). They are therefore dependent for their nutrition on the nerve cell from which the axon arises. At the same time it is well known that, when pyramidal cells undergo ischaemic degeneration, small triangular or oval basophilic granules may appear on the surface of the cell body or near the base of the dendrites. This appearance, usually called *incrustation of the Golgi network*, is not visible with silver impregnation methods which stain boutons and appears to depend on an alteration of the proteins in the area of the synapse. Thus both the neurone which forms the boutons and that to which the boutons are attached appear to take part in this synaptic structure.

The synaptic structures have aroused great interest among *electronmicroscopists* (De Robertis 1956, 1958; Wickoff and Young 1956; Palay 1956, 1958; Gray 1961, among others). Presynaptic and postsynaptic areas are well defined by membranes and are also separated by an intersynaptic space. Thus, the neurone theory has found yet another confirmation. Presynaptic terminals (for example, boutons terminaux) contain microvesicles together with numerous mitochondria (Fig. 1.18); microvesicles are absent, however, in the postsynaptic area. Microvesicles were first described by de Robertis and Bennett, in 1954. They occur in especially dense clusters near the densest (and probably most active) parts of the synaptic membranes. They are spherical or oval in shape with a limiting membrane 40–50 Å thick and a size varying between 200–650 Å. It has been suggested that they represent the quantal unit of transmitter substance: They have, in fact, been observed to increase both in number and in size after electrical stimulation and to disappear when the terminal degenerates (de Robertis 1958).

The *neuromuscular junction* is similar in structure (Fig. 1.19): the motor endings contain numerous synaptic vesicles and some mitochondria in intimate connection with the axolemma facing the muscle. The postsynaptic (sub-neural) structure is a groove (synaptic gutter) formed by the sarcoplasm and covering sarcolemma of the muscle. The bottom of the gutter shows a complex infolding of the sarcolemma dividing the sarcoplasm into numerous vertical lamellae. While synaptic vesicles are absent, larger vacuoles for which de Harven and Coers (1961) propose the name 'postsynaptic vacuoles' have been described. Mitochondria are very numerous near the synaptic cleft. Granules (aposynaptic granules) are also present, but their nature is still obscure.

The synaptic cleft, and the primary as well as the secondary infoldings, are filled with material of the same electron density as the functional membranes. The exact localisation of acetylcholinesterase activity has not yet definitely been established with the electron microscope; Couteaux (1958) postulates its site of action in the subneural sarcolemma, and its possible relation to the aposynaptic granules has also been tentatively discussed.

Birks, Katz and Miledi (1959) described honeycomb-like masses of agglutinated microvesicles and swollen mitochondria in the presynaptic motor ending which were seen from the third day following section of the axon. Subsequently the terminals were ingested by Schwann cells.

Certain aberrations such as multiplication, elongation and collateral sprouting of nerve terminals which had been revealed by intravital staining in cases of myasthenia gravis, myopathy etc. (*vide* Coers and Woolf 1959), have not yet been confirmed on the electronic screen. Coers and de Harven (1962), Bickerstaff *et al.* (1960) and Woolf (1962) advocate restraint in interpretation until such time as the considerable range of normal electronmicroscopic findings can be assessed more accurately.

Myelin sheath

According to Duncan (1934) all axons in the central and peripheral nervous systems of vertebrates with a diameter greater than 1μ are surrounded by a myelin sheath. This rule does not apply to the autonomic nervous system which, except for white rami communicantes, is unmyelinated. The thickness of this sheath varies and does not always bear the same relation to the thickness of the axon. De Renyi (1929) found that in the average peripheral nerve fibre the axon was 7 times the thickness of the myelin sheath. Arnell (1936) in unfixed peripheral nerves found the relative areas of myelin sheath to axon to average 1:3·5 with variations from 1:1 to 1:6. In other words the relation of the diameter of the axon to the thickness of the myelin sheath varies from 5:1 to 25:1. This ratio is fairly well preserved when nervous tissue is fixed directly in osmic acid, but with slower fixatives, as has been seen, the myelin sheath swells at the expense of the axon. In formalin fixed tissue, therefore, the myelin sheaths look thicker than they should.

The lipid of the myelin sheath is a complex substance containing cerebrosides (glycosphingoside), sphingomyelin (phosphosphingoside) and cholesterol. According to observations in polarised light (Schmidt 1936) and small angle X-ray diffraction (Schmitt *et al.* 1935), the lipid molecules are orientated radially in double concentric layers separated by a layer of denatured protein between each pair. This protein has long been identified with neurokeratin, but Le Baron and Folch-Pi (1956) and Folch-Pi *et al.* (1959) have suggested a trypsin resistant lipoprotein. In their opinion, neurokeratin is an artefact derived from the trypsin resistant protein fraction. The total thickness of these three layers has been calculated to be about 170–186 Å which would allow over 100 such repeating periods in a myelin sheath of 2μ thickness. X-ray diffraction studies have added more detail to the concept of this fundamental repeating unit, and both Finean (1961a) and Robertson (1961) have correlated these findings with those observed on the electronic screen.

Myelin is anisotropic. In cross-sections of nerve fibres, under crossed Nicol prisms, the sheath is interrupted along the line of polarisation and at right angles to this. The appearance of a thick myelin sheath or a globule of myelin under these optical conditions therefore resembles a bright Maltese cross. Thinner sheaths form a bright circle broken into 4 quadrants. In longitudinal sections the sheath is anisotropic in the plane of polarisation.

Sperry and Waelsch (1950) have produced evidence that myelin, and even the unsaponifiable lipids which it contains, are synthetised in the brain and not carried there in a preformed state by the blood stream. In the newborn infant myelin is almost entirely absent in the cerebrum, but increases gradually during the first months and more rapidly between the 3rd and 13th month of extra-uterine life. Thereafter there is a constant increase of myelin in relation to the lipids contained in the nerve cells and axons, until the brain reaches its full adult size at the age of 10–12 years when the proportion becomes the same as in the adult brain (Brante 1949). This increase in size of the white matter in relation to the grey characterises the growth of the brain during childhood. Sperry and Waelsch also showed that in adult rats about 10 per cent of brain lipids are replaced each week; more recently Davison, Dobbing, Morgan and Payling-Wright (1959) have shown, however, that radioactive cholesterol injected into 17-day-old rabbits was still detectable in the cerebral white matter for a period of up to 365 days.

The myelin sheath begins shortly after the axon leaves the cell body and is continued up to the terminal branches, which may carry a fine myelin sheath for part of their extent but are thereafter unmyelinated. Both in the peripheral and central nervous systems it is broken at intervals by constrictions or nodes. In peripheral nerves these have long been known as the nodes of Ranvier, which occur at regular intervals along the nerve fibre. Cajal (1909) described similar nodes on the nerve fibres of the central nervous system and these have been confirmed by Bielschowsky (1928) and more recently by numerous authors. Hess and Young (1949) found that the internodal distance in the rabbit's spinal cord bore a direct relationship to the thickness of the fibre, being, as a general rule, rather over 100 times its diameter. Bodian (1951), while agreeing with this in principle, finds that the ratio may be considerably greater and in the thicker fibres may be up to 300 times the fibre diameter. Collateral branches are given off only at these nodes, and in the cortex the nerve fibre may be naked for a considerable distance at these points (Chang 1952).

Sheath of Schwann or neurolemma* (*Neurilema of American literature*)

This sheath was described by Schwann in 1839 but its nature was not fully understood until it was examined by the electron microscope. Cajal was always careful to speak of the cell of Schwann as distinct from the sheath of Schwann, but electron microscopy has shown no such distinction.

Ranvier (1878) thought that the sheath of Schwann was composed of a series of segments each of which was joined to its neighbours at the node of Ranvier by cement substance similar to that which unites endothelial cells. This view has been restated uncritically by many writers since his time, although Nageotte (1932) considered that both on the unmyelinated fibres of the sympathetic system and in the regeneration of myelinated nerves, the sheath of Schwann appeared to be a syncytium. De Renyi (1929) showed that if the endoneurium and cement substance were dissected off a living nerve fibre in the frog, the neurolemma could easily be separated from the axon at the node by injecting fluid under the sheath and then appeared as an uninterrupted membrane. Further, if the injection was made with sufficient pressure to rupture the sheath, the break did not occur at the ring round the node where the junction between two cells was supposed to take place. The neurolemma behaved, in fact, as a tenuous but firm sheath continuous over the nodes, as well as in the internodal segments. Cajal described the neurolemma as resisting weak acids and alkalis, and staining reagents. It is in fact not easily stained and no good differential stain has been devised for it, but it can be stained by alum-haematoxylin, or by iron haematoxylin after fixation in Fleming's fluid (Nageotte 1932).

The *nucleus of Schwann* lies between this sheath and the myelin, flattened to some extent by this position, so that in tangential sections of a nerve fibre it appears elongated. When viewed from the surface it is somewhat quadrangular with rounded corners, its length, in the direction of the fibre, being rather greater than its width. It is vesicular with numerous fine chromatin granules scattered through it. In the cytoplasm at either pole of the nucleus fine lipid granules may be seen with appropriate staining. Some of these, which take a metachromatic stain with thionin or toluidin blue, were called π granules by Reich who supposed

* The name neurolemma is derived from the Greek words *neuron* and *lemma* (husk). The old spelling should therefore be retained. Recent American writers, deriving the name from *neuron* and *eilema* (sheath), spell it *neurilema*. This is justifiable but an unnecessary break with tradition. The spelling *neurilemma* has no justification and is confusing as in French this name is sometimes used for the sheath of Henle.

that they consisted of 'protagon'. Their metachromasia and staining with Schiff's leucofuchsine method indicate that they contain glycolipid. Other granules which stain by Marchi's method are known as Elzholz granules (μ granules of Reich). They may consist of phospholipid. Variations in the number of both types of granule have been attributed to disease. While there is no doubt that Elzholz granules increase in size and are more widely distributed in the earlier stages of Wallerian degeneration, there is also little doubt that both forms of lipid granule are normal constituents of the cell of Schwann. Differences in technique, as with other lipid granules, may produce very different pictures, and false impressions are easily gained by the use of unfamiliar techniques, since nerves which are suspected of abnormality are more frequently examined than those which are known to be normal.

Electron microscopy shows the sheath of Schwann as a compact, finely granular double membrane, about 200 Å thick, adhering closely to the myelin and covering the internodes completely. It is continuous with the protoplasm of the Schwann cells. Fine collagen and elastin fibres, attached to its outer surface, constitute the sheath of Henle (Fernandez-Moran 1950–2). The latter sheath is easily stained by silver methods for reticulin (Laidlaw 1930). At the nodes of Ranvier it forms a circular ring which ensnares the neurolemma and there is an excess of argentophilic material in this situation. The term *cement substance* for this material has been seen to be a misnomer.

Before the advent of the electron microscope unmyelinated C fibres were believed to be completely enclosed within the Schwann cell cytoplasm. Gasser (1955) showed this to be incorrect and demonstrated that the axons, which at first are outside the Schwann cells, are engulfed and completely surrounded by the Schwann cell membranes. Even if eventually they come to rest at some depth within the cytoplasm of the cell, they are still attached to the surface by a double layer of enfolding membranes which Gasser has called the *mesaxon*.

The laminated appearance of myelin was first noted on the electronic screen by Fernandez-Moran (1950) and confirmed at higher magnification by the same author (1954) and by Sjöstrand (1953). The individual lamellae have a thickness of 120 Å and consist of two dense lines with a light zone between, which, in turn, may be divided by a thinner and less dense intraperiod line.

Geren's (1954) studies in chick embryos proved to be a landmark insofar as she was able to show that, during myelination, the mesaxons (i.e. the enfolding Schwann cell membranes) became elongated and formed spirals around the axon and its membranes. From this she concluded that the myelin sheath might consist of elongated and closely-packed Schwann cell membranes. This hypothesis has been confirmed by Robertson (1955) and many others. The last-named author has elaborated what he calls the Unit membrane theory, distinguishing an outer and an inner mesaxon (Figs. 1.20–21). Compared with the width of the unit (170–185 Å) as measured by X-ray diffraction, the electron microscope reveals a smaller space, due to shrinkage, measuring only 120 Å.

Owing to greater complexity of the tissue, the development of the myelin sheath in the central nervous system is more difficult to analyse, as Luse had already noticed in 1956. Finean (1961 b) has little doubt, however, that the process of myelination fundamentally follows that of peripheral nerves (*vide* also page 55).

The constant appearance of fine reticulin fibres on the surface of Schwann cells in electron micrographs, and the growth of reticulin fibres in cultures of Schwann cells from neurofibromas by Murray and Stout (1942), appear to prove that the Schwann cell can form reticulin. At the same time it forms myelin when it encloses axons of any but the smallest size.

It was shown by Ross Harrison (1910, 1924) that in the frog embryo the cells destined to form the sheath of Schwann migrated from the neural crests. If these were removed at an early stage of development, the axons of peripheral nerves remained for a considerable time naked of neurolemma. This origin from the same group of cells as forms the dorsal root ganglia has, for many years, been put forward as proof that the sheath of Schwann could not form connective tissue fibres. It was and still is considered by many as the neuroglia of the peripheral nervous system, but more recent work (Horstadius 1950), which has shown that many kinds of tissue including leptomeninges and membranous bone may be derived from the neural crest, has weakened this argument.

So far as is known remyelination does not occur in the central nervous system except when new nerve fibres come into relation with connective tissue, as around blood vessels. It appears to result from a combined action by axon and Schwann cell, and it has been suggested that both contribute to the lipids which constitute myelin. If the trophic influence of either is withdrawn myelin breaks down into its constituent lipids which are then removed by phagocytes. In Wallerian degeneration this follows the degeneration of the axon; with local pressure and in poisoning by lead and diphtheria toxin it appears to result from damage to the cell of Schwann.

Ground substance (*Nissl's Grey*)

Nissl recognised that the nerve cells, with their axons and dendrites and the neuroglia cells and their processes, did not fill all the substance of the grey matter which, however, in sections stained by eosin had a remarkably homogeneous composition. Nissl called the substance which filled the interstices between the fibres simply 'grey substance' (grau), and considered it to be an extracellular protein-rich substance. Little attention has been paid to this conception of recent years, but some authors refer to the ground substance as the seat of origin of senile plaques (Bouman 1934).

The cerebral cortex contains a higher water content than white matter (cortex 83 per cent, white matter 70 per cent of wet weight). The percentages of sodium and chloride are also higher than in white matter and much higher than in muscle. When calculated from the chloride values the extracellular volume is about 30 per cent and if calculated from the sodium values still higher, but both these substances may be to some extent intracellular (Holmes and Tower 1955). The specific gravity of cerebral cortex is approximately 1,040 but that of nerve cells is considerably higher, since they can be differentially sedimented by centrifugalisation in solutions with a specific gravity of 1,060 (Chu 1954). Either the neuroglial cells and their processes account for this difference or there must be a considerable amount of extracellular fluid with a specific gravity below 1,040.

Bok (1940) and Renes (1940) on reconstructing the nerve fibre pattern in small areas of cerebral cortex between nerve cells found it to be full of spherical spaces of regular size and arrangement, through which no nerve fibres ran. The distance from the centre of one of these to the centre of another was about 5·5μ. Nerve fibres in crossing never approximated to one another more closely than 1·9μ, and it appeared probable that this distance was related to the distance between the spherical chambers. The nerve fibres themselves did not run in straight lines but with fairly regular undulations, as though bending round these empty chambers. Bok likens the structure of the cortex to a froth in which the nerve fibres lie in the protoplasm surrounding spherical chambers, or it might be considered as an emulsion in which the nerve (fibres lie in the continuous phase and the fluid chambers form the dispersed phase. Bok (1960 has obtained support for this theory by examining sections of fresh cerebral cortex by phase-contrast microscopy by which the fluid-filled chambers stand out owing to their lower refraction and are seen to contain nearly always a mitochondrium. De Robertis *et al.* (1960) made the plausible suggestion that the vacuoles with their mitochondria represent swollen pieces of astrocytic cytoplasm, an interpretation which was not accepted, however, by Bok.

The majority of *electronmicroscopists* (among them Maynard *et al.* 1957; Hager 1961) believe that the cortex is almost completely filled by the branching processes of neuroglial and oligodendroglial cells, axons and dendrites. There is, therefore, no place for an independent ground substance in the sense of Nissl, even if small amounts of intercellular fluid be present within the very narrow interspaces between membranes—of up to a width of 200 Å, according to Hager. The cytoplasm of glial cells and processes, particularly that of the astroglia, appears of low density in the electron microscope and contains only sparse organelles. It seems probable that the low specific gravity of this cytoplasm may account to a large extent for the difference in specific gravity between neurones and the cortex as a whole.

Hess (1953, 1955), on the other hand, has, on the evidence of a clearly intercellular positive PAS reaction, postulated the existence of a mucopolysaccharide-containing ground substance. The same author (1958) concedes, however, that in very thin sections, PAS and sulphation metachromatic reactions are faint, suggesting that the intercellular spaces are very small and may consist only of the infinitesimal interval between two membranes. There is, thus, a considerable rapproachment between his more recent view and the electronmicroscopic findings.

PATHOLOGY OF THE NEURONE

Reaction of the neurone to injury of its axon, and other causes of exhaustion

(*Axonal reaction, Gudden's atrophy and trans-synaptic degeneration*)

Injury to the axon produces rather different reactions in the cell body in different types of nerve cell. In general the larger motor and sensory neurones react to section of the axon by attempted regrowth. This is associated with changes in the cell body which are described under the name of *central chromatolysis* or *axonal reaction*. This reaction, which is seen in typical form in the cells of the motor nuclei of the cranial nerves, was used by the pioneers of neuro-anatomy to map out the nuclei which give rise to different nerves or to different parts of such nerves as the oculomotor and vagoglossopharyngeal. Many of the nerve cells, which give rise to tracts which begin and end within the central nervous system, go on from this stage of reaction to atrophy and eventual disappearance (Gudden's atrophy). This biphasic reaction is well seen in the dorsomedian nucleus of the thalamus after frontal lobectomy or leucotomy (Meyer, Beck and McLardy 1947), in the corpus geniculatum externum after lesions of the optic radiations or calcarine cortex (Putnam and Putnam 1926), and in the inferior olives after lesions of the cerebellar cortex (Stewart and Holmes 1908, Brodal 1940). As in each of these instances the nerve cells which react are those from which the damaged fibres originate, an area-to-area relationship can be mapped out between the cerebral or cerebellar cortex and the nuclei which project to them. Gudden's atrophy is associated with shrinkage of the cell body, loss of Nissl granules, and dedifferentiation in the nucleus. Some nerve cells, such as those of the retina, show no stage of reaction to injury of their axon, but undergo atrophy from the first.

In certain nuclei, a similar atrophy of nerve cells may follow damage to the axons which make synaptic connection with them. This was called by Foix, Chavany and Hillemand (1926) *trans-synaptic atrophy* or *degeneration*. It is best known, and has been most studied, in the nerve cells of the corpus geniculatum externum after lesions of the retina, optic nerves or optic tracts (Fig. 1.2) and in the inferior olives after lesions of the central tegmental tract. In the former case the cells undergo simple atrophy similar to the later stages of their reaction to lesions of the optic radiations. The neurones of the inferior olive, on the other hand, undergo an initial irregular hypertrophy, often associated with vacuolation of their cytoplasm, during the first few months after the lesion (Fig. 1.3). Later the nerve cells atrophy and disappear. This trans-synaptic degeneration seems to occur most commonly after lesions of tracts which form the chief, or the only, afferent link to the neurones in question. But it may probably also occur, although much more slowly, in nerve cells which make synaptic or other functional connection with neurones which have degenerated or been destroyed. For example degeneration has been observed in the optic nerves and tracts after long-standing lesions of the optic radiations

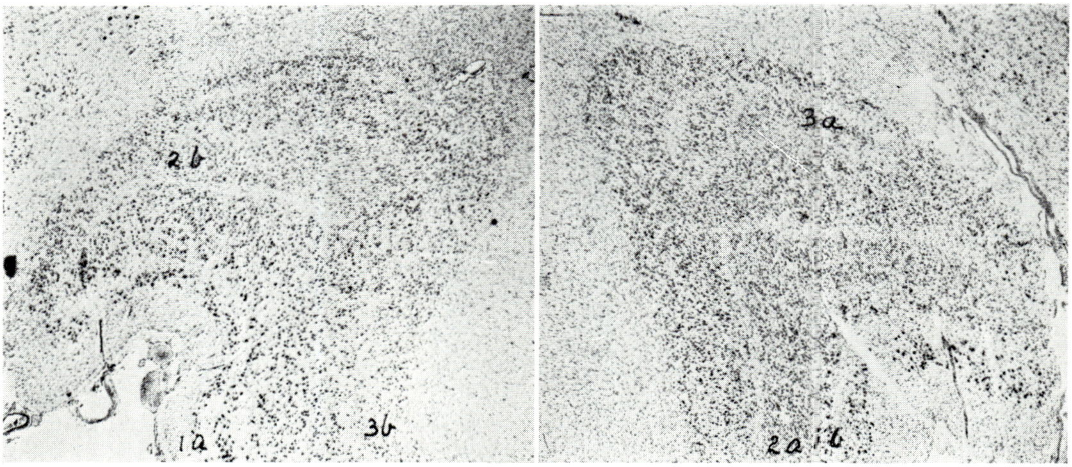

(*a*) (*b*)

FIG. 1.2. Trans-synaptic atrophy of external geniculate body resulting from the loss of the right eye. (*a*) Left side. Atrophy of layers 1*a*, 2*b* and 3*b*. (*b*) Right side. Atrophy of layers 1*b*, 2*a* and 3*a*.

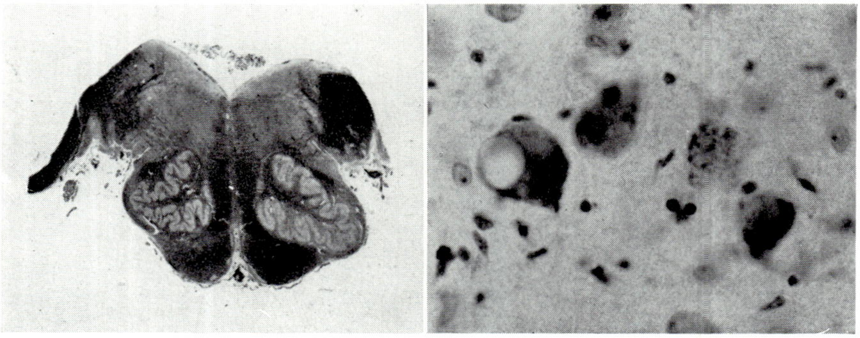

(*a*) (*b*)

FIG. 1.3. Swelling of the inferior olive and vacuolar degeneration of its neurones resulting from a lesion of the olivocerebellar fibres in the cerebellum. The appearances are similar to those seen after a lesion of the central tegmental tract.

or calcarine cortex (Niessl von Meyendorf 1934). A 'retrograde' trans-synaptic degeneration of this character is the most reasonable explanation for the degeneration of the inferior olives which follows destruction of the Purkinje cells by heat stroke and has also been accepted by many authors as the explanation of the olivary degeneration which accompanies cerebellar cortical degeneration of the familial type described by Holmes (1907) as well as in similar cases of isolated character (Marie, Foix and Alajouanin 1922).

Whether 'chain degenerations', that is successive degenerations of tracts which have synaptic connection with each other, may form the basis of certain systemic degenerations is a disputed question. It is certain that in Friedreich's ataxia degeneration of the medial fillet may follow degeneration of the dorsal columns of the cord. The association of cerebellar cortical degeneration with degeneration of the olives and nuclei pontis in olivopontocerebellar atrophy has also been explained on this basis.

Central chromatolysis (*Axonal reaction*)

The term *chromatolysis*, meaning loss of stainable substance, is frequently used at the present time for any form of neuronal degeneration in which Nissl granules are no longer stained by basic aniline dyes. When used in this way the word covers almost every form of lesion and ceases to have any special meaning. In classical neuropathology the name chromatolysis was applied to certain definite changes in the cell body in which loss of Nissl granules may be incomplete. The best known of these is *central chromatolysis* or *axonal reaction* (Fig. 1.4).

This reaction of the nerve cell to a lesion of its axon is seen typically in the large motor cells of the ventral horns of the spinal cord and in the motor nuclei of the brain stem, after section of the nerves which arise in them. It is most severe when the axon is sectioned or torn across near to its cell of origin. It begins within 48 hours after division of the nerve and reaches its maximum after 15–20 days. During this period the cell body becomes more rounded and swells to some extent and the Nissl granules in the neighbourhood of the nucleus become smaller and powdery and eventually disappear. The nucleus also swells and becomes eccentric moving away from the axon hillock and often coming to lie against the margin of the cell. In the later stages it may become oval or reniform. The typical appearances in the later stages are shown in Fig. 1.4*b*. At this stage the cell has a rather rounded contour and is somewhat enlarged, the nucleus is also enlarged and lies eccentrically and there is a zone of rather small Nissl granules near the cell margin; the centre of the cell contains no Nissl granules. From this stage the cell may either degenerate and disappear, or may gradually recover. If the latter, the Nissl substance is gradually re-formed, probably by the nucleus, and may eventually be present in larger amounts than normal (stage of hyperchromasia). The cell body shrinks, its outline between the dendrites becomes again concave, and the nucleus returns to its original situation. This is a slow process which may take as much as 80 days. Thus after section of a motor nerve close to the brain stem or spinal cord the process of reaction in the cell body covers a period of 100 days or more.

The cells of the dorsal root ganglia react in a similar manner to lesions of the peripheral nerves, but show much slighter changes after section of the proximal process. Section of the dorsal roots may cause some reaction in a few cells, but lesions of the cord involving the dorsal columns produce no change in these cells. No alteration of shape can, of course, be seen in these spherical cells but the disappearance of Nissl granules from the central zone of the cell, the more powdery appearance in the peripheral granules and the eccentricity of the nucleus are similar to those seen in motor cells. In these cells the reaction is said to be more rapid, but Penfield (1920), after cutting the sciatic nerve of the cat, found chromatolysis at its height on the 16th day.

Barr and his associates (1951) showed that, after prolonged electrical stimulation or crushing of the hypoglossal nerve in cats, the cells of the hypoglossal nucleus responded much more rapidly. In such experiments depletion of Nissl material was visible on the 1st day and became maximal by the 2nd or 3rd day. Nissl substance was restored by the 6th day, appearing first on the outer surface of the nuclear membrane as a nuclear cap or hood, and gradually accumulating near the nucleus. These changes were associated with slight swelling and vacuolation of the nucleolus which continued until the stage of full restoration of Nissl

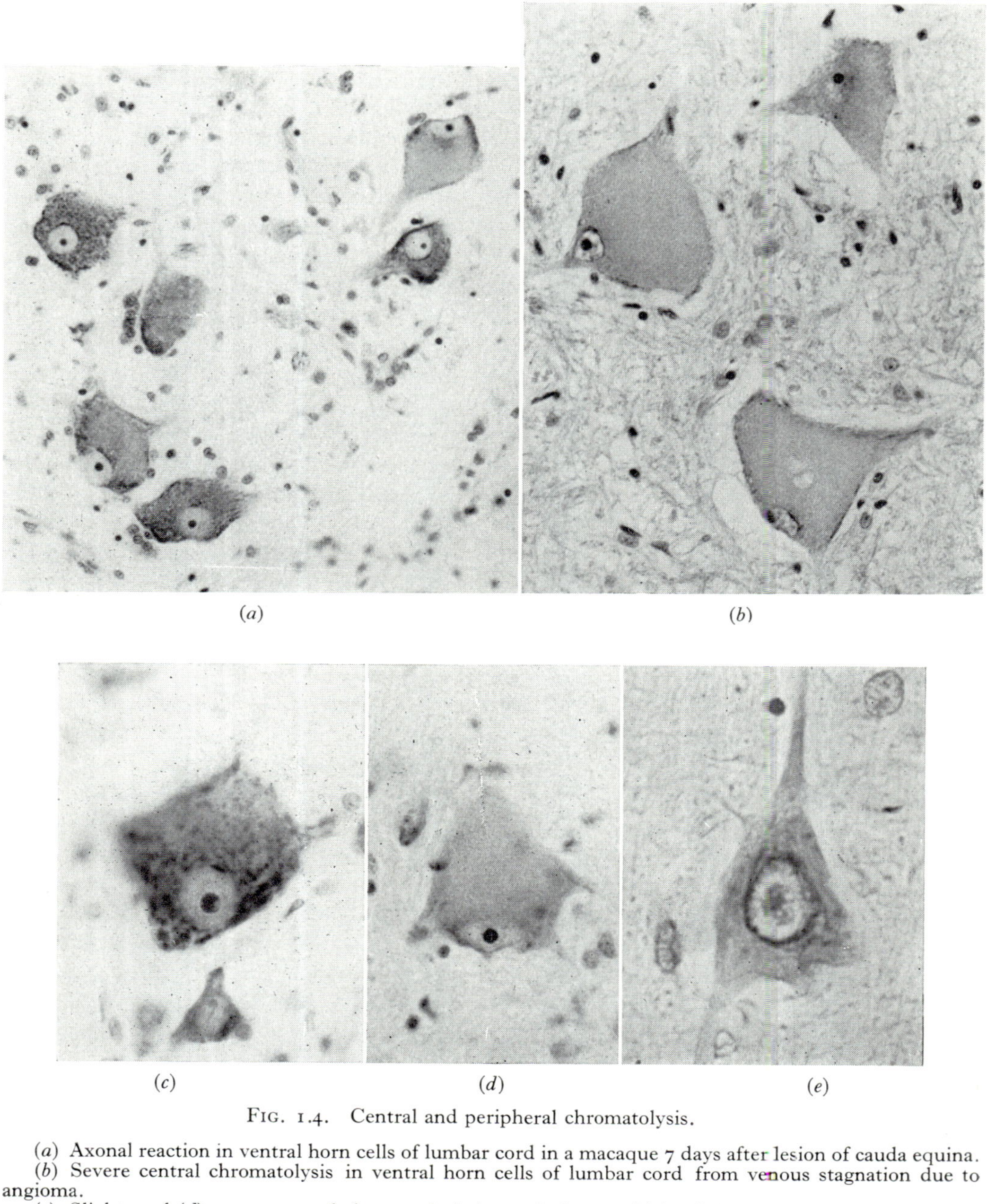

FIG. 1.4. Central and peripheral chromatolysis.

(*a*) Axonal reaction in ventral horn cells of lumbar cord in a macaque 7 days after lesion of cauda equina.
(*b*) Severe central chromatolysis in ventral horn cells of lumbar cord from venous stagnation due to angioma.
(*c*) Slight, and (*d*) severe central chromatolysis in cortical pyramidal cells in pellagra.
(*e*) Peripheral chromatolysis in a case dying in severe epileptic attack. (By the kindness of Prof. L. Einarson.)
(*a*, *b*, *c*, *d*, Thionin; *e*, Gallocyanin chromalum.)

substance. At the same time the sex chromatin in female cats tended to move away from the nucleolus towards the nucleolar membrane but did not reach this and gradually returned to the nucleolus after Nissl substance was restored. After section of the hypoglossal nerve there was a similar movement of the sex chromatin away from and towards the nucleolus and this was followed by a second similar movement during the stage of hyperchromasia.

A similar reaction to section or injury of the axon is seen in the cells of origin of certain intrinsic tracts in the brain stem and spinal cord. It has been most studied in the Betz cells of the motor cortex and in the cells of Clarke's column. However, in these situations recovery does not usually occur, and after a time the cells degenerate further and disappear. Meyer, Beck and McLardy (1947) found that some of the cells which remained in the dorsomedial nucleus of the thalamus 4 months after prefrontal leucotomy were shrunken and deeply stained; this may represent a stage of partial recovery in these cells.

Axonal reaction similar to that seen in the cells of the dorsal root ganglia is also seen in the autonomic system. Section of the cervical sympathetic nerve produces swelling, chromatolysis and eccentricity of the nucleus in cervical sympathetic ganglia below it, and resection of the hypogastric plexus may cause typical chromatolysis in the cells of the intermediolateral column in the lumbosacral segments of the cord.

This reaction to axonal injury is considered by Hydén to represent an exhaustion of the nucleo-proteins of the cell body. This exhaustion may result from overwork or from attempts to regenerate the severed part of the axon. It has been seen that, in the peripheral nerves, a very large amount of axonal cytoplasm may have to be re-formed, a process which entails an enormous metabolic effort on the part of the cell body.

Various stages of the reaction are also seen after simple exhaustion of the nerve cell; for example, it was found by Holmes (1903) in the motor cells of the spinal cord of the frog after strychnine convulsions; and by Hydén (1950) in the cells of Deiter's nucleus after repeated and prolonged rotation. The similar appearances, in Betz cells and other large neurones in pellagra, may be similarly interpreted as due to the exhaustion of nucleoprotein reserves by metabolic requirements.

It is doubtful whether prolonged partial deprivation of blood may produce a similar reaction in the cell body. While it is commonly seen in the anterior horn cells of the lumbar cord in cases of subacute phlebitis of the meningeal veins ('subacute necrotic myelitis') it is possible that in these cases the axon is damaged in its passage through the anterior columns, which commonly show evidence of ischaemia (Fig. 1.4*b*). Apart from this disease, central chromatolysis is not usually seen in ischaemic lesions. It is so characteristic of lesions of the axon that Adolf Meyer (1902) called the reaction of the pyramidal cells of the cerebral cortex in pellagra *central neuritis*. In general it is an unusual finding in neuropathology and one which in most cases suggests an axonal lesion rather than direct damage to the nerve cell. It may, however, be found in typical form in certain virus infections of the nervous system such as poliomyelitis (Einarson 1949) and subacute inclusion body encephalitis (Brain *et al.* 1948). In poliomyelitis it may appear as early as 3 days after the onset of paralysis. In these diseases it may go on to complete destruction of the nerve cell or, according to Bodian (1949), may be a reversible change.

Penfield (1920), who studied in cats the reaction of the cells in the anterior horns and dorsal root ganglia after section of the sciatic nerve and the cells of Clarke's column after section of the spinal cord, showed that the *Golgi apparatus* reacts to section of the axon in a similar manner to the Nissl granules. It becomes displaced from its normal perinuclear position to the periphery of the cell ('retispersion') and may become broken up to some extent ('retisolution'). This reaction occurs more rapidly than that of the Nissl granules in afferent cells, but not in motor cells. In the neurones of the dorsal root ganglia it had reached its peak 7 days after section of the sciatic nerve and in the cells of Clarke's column 'the Goigi reticulum was close against the periphery of the cell, except where some remained about the nucleus'

4 days after section of the spinal cord. Retispersion of moderate degree could also be made out in the dorsal root ganglion cells 17 days after section of the dorsal roots, and seemed to be rather more common and definite than chromatolysis after such a lesion.

The intracellular neurofibrils show a rather less intense reaction. There is, in the early stages, some loosening of the network of neurofibrils in the central part of the cell, and this may later break up and disappear. The more peripheral neurofibrils and those in the dendrites react only when chromatolysis is intense. In the stage of repair the neurofibrils are reconstituted and eventually fill the cell, although for a time they may appear less numerous than normal.

Electronmicroscopic investigations of central chromatolysis have so far been sparse. Eleven days after sectioning the vagal nerve, Evans and Gray (1961) described a peripheral shift of the nucleus and the complete disappearance not only of the ribosomes, but, surprisingly, also of the cisternae and membranes of the granular endoplasmic reticulum. In their place numerous neurofilaments, coarser than normal, were seen in araldite embedded specimens. The agranular reticulum (Golgi apparatus) was normal. After 25 days, while the granular reticulum remained depleted, only few neurofilaments had survived. The most striking change was now in the agranular reticulum. Swarms of small dark vesicles were seen to be budded off from the normal flattened cisternae of this structure. The authors suggest that they may play a part in the resynthesis of the granular endoplasmic reticulum. Changes in the mitochondria were not mentioned.

Peripheral chromatolysis

Peripheral chromatolysis is, in some respects, the antithesis of central chromatolysis. It is most often seen in human pathology as a change affecting the motor nerve cells in the anterior horns of the spinal cord in cases of progressive muscular atrophy. In such cases it appears to be a stage in the degenerative process, or, perhaps more accurately, in the fight for survival. Nerve cells showing peripheral chromatolysis are usually smaller and more rounded than normal. The dendrites and the peripheral zone of the cell contain no Nissl granules, but a darkly staining mass of these is collected round the nucleus, which is usually in or near the centre of the cell and contains rather more chromatin than that of normal cells. Einarson (1945) and Einarson and Lorentzen (1946) have shown that cells showing some degree of peripheral chromatolysis are found in normal dorsal root ganglia and especially in sympathetic ganglia, in which their numbers increase on mild stimulation, but diminish with progressively longer stimulation giving place to cells showing central chromatolysis. In the dorsal root ganglion cells, peripheral chromatolysis is not uncommonly seen as a late stage of reaction to lesions or sections of the peripheral nerves. According to Einarson, peripheral chromatolysis, when seen as an early reaction to noxious agents, is a stage towards cell death, but when it occurs as a late reaction it appears to be a stage in the process of recovery, and indicates an active restoration of Nissl substance from the nucleus (Fig. 1.4*e*).

Wallerian degeneration (*Secondary degeneration*)

Waller in 1850 showed that when an axon is severed its peripheral segment, being separated from the nutrient cell body, quickly disintegrates and disappears. Along with this the myelin covering this segment undergoes a slower breakdown into simpler lipids which are eventually removed. This process has been extensively studied in peripheral nerves (Cajal 1927, Nageotte 1932) and by a few workers in the tracts of the spinal cord (Cajal 1927, Jakob 1912, Hurst 1925). Owing to the absence of a sheath of Schwann in the central nervous system the process, as seen in the spinal cord, differs to some extent from that in peripheral nerves, although it is essentially the same in both situations.

(*a*) When a *nerve fibre in a peripheral nerve* is cut across or damaged in such a way as to cause local destruction of the axon the peripheral part of the axon and myelin sheath undergo a regular series of changes. Within the first few days the axon shrinks in diameter, at first becoming moniliform or varicose. Within 48 hours the neurofibrils disappear and the structure becomes more granular. The axon then breaks up into fragments which shrink and become wavy and contorted. The first breaks tend to occur near the nodes but soon further breaks occur, often at first opposite the nucleus of Schwann and later throughout the fibre, resulting in numerous small segments which eventually become oval. The myelin sheath reacts at the same time. Even before there are any breaks in the axon, the myelin shrinks back from the nodes of Ranvier so that what was a narrow constriction becomes a length of thin unmyelinated fibre. The myelin sheath in each internodal segment then breaks up into shorter lengths. When these breaks coincide with breaks in the axon, the myelin at the line of severance comes together by the action of surface tension (Nageotte) to form a hollow ellipse or oval which contains a fragment of axon. Cajal found that breaks in the myelin might at first occur independently of breaks in the axon, but eventually, usually within 10 days in small animals, the myelin sheath is converted into an irregular series of ellipsoids or ovoids each of which contains some plasma and a fragment of axon. Cajal has called them *digestive chambers* as the axon gradually disappears in them apparently without any process of phagocytosis.

After the first few days an increasing number of globules and granules of lipid appear outside the ellipsoids and ovoids but still within the sheath of Schwann. These become progressively more sudanophilic and stain by the Marchi technique which usually begins to show definite evidence of degeneration 10 days after the original injury. The digestive chambers become progressively more rounded, becoming ovoids and spheres, but their walls retain the properties of myelin (Noback and Montague 1952). Between 20 and 40 days from the date of the damage to the axon the globules and granules of lipid become more numerous, while the ovoids and spheres of myelin diminish in number and eventually disappear. Up to this time birefringence is present not only in the myelin but in many of the lipid granules. Thereafter cholesterol and cholesterol esters diminish and disappear and the lipid progressively assumes the characters of neutral fat.

The earlier stages of this process of disintegration of the axon and myelin sheath appear to be independent of cellular action, as they take place *in vitro* if the nerve is kept in warm Locke's solution. They appear to depend on enzyme action as they cease when the nerve is heated to 47° C (Nageotte). In the living body they are associated with cellular activity both by the sheath of Schwann and by wandering phagocytes.

About the 4th day (Cajal) the nuclei of Schwann undergo mitotic division and the protoplasm surrounding them increases in bulk. According to Young (1942) it divides into long tapering cells, but others consider that it remains as a syncytal rod of cytoplasm containing numerous nuclei. At a still earlier stage the nodes of Ranvier have disappeared and the sheath of Schwann in this position has lost its constrictions, becoming cylindrical or even showing fusiform swellings. Within the following days the contents of the sheath of Schwann have become a core of protoplasm containing numerous Schwann nuclei and nuclei of histiocytic cells, as well as ellipsoids and spheres of myelin and droplets of lipid. As the latter disappear the protoplasm, within the sheath of Schwann, continues to increase, and the cylinder or *band fibre* thus formed may attain a thickness of 10μ, though usually it is less than this. This protoplasm is very liable to shrink under conditions of fixation and embedding and is therefore not easily studied unless special precautions are taken.

In the thinner nerve fibres the process of breakdown into simpler fatty droplets and the eventual disappearance of these may take place without the action of phagocytes. In the larger nerve fibres, on the other hand, histiocytes and probably also polymorphonuclear leucocytes (Cajal) penetrate the sheath of Schwann at an early stage and engulf the lipid granules. They appear to hasten the processes of lipid katabolism as they are soon filled with sudanophilic granules and become typical *fat granule cells*. In this condition they leave the sheath of Schwann and either they themselves or other fat containing cells are found free in the tissue spaces of the nerve. The process of lipid katabolism and removal in human peripheral nerves takes several weeks. The band fibre which is formed by the syncytium of Schwann may remain in much the same condition for many months, during which it is ready to receive any new neurites which may reach it from the proximal cut end of the axon, but unless it is thus re-innervated it gradually becomes encroached on by thickening of the connective tissue of the endoneurium.

(*b*) Nerve fibres *within the central nervous system* undergo Wallerian degeneration, according to Cajal, at a rate which is proportional to their thickness. In young animals, in which he studied the phenomena, the largest axons show varicosities as early as 30 hours from the time of severance from the nerve cell. In 4–8 days they become broken up into shorter oval or spherical fragments which progressively disintegrate and disappear. In medium-sized myelinated fibres the axon is still in the varicose or beaded state at the end of a week and breaks up from the 14th to the 15th day onwards. In fine fibres the process is even slower, and many show little change during the first 10 days. Changes in the myelin sheath occur along with these changes in the axon. As the latter becomes varicose irregular fusiform swellings also appear along the course of the myelin sheath, which soon breaks at the constrictions and forms a series of ellipsoids enclosing fragments of axon. These are again broken or shrink into shorter ovoid or spherical plasmatic chambers containing balls of axon. Breakdown of the myelin into simpler lipids occurs at the same time, and according to Jakob lipids which stain by Marchi's method begin to appear about the 4th day. Lorrain-Smith and Mair, using a modified myelin stain, also found the earliest evidence of myelin katabolism on the 4th day, but in human pathology the process is a comparatively slow one, and it is not usual to find much evidence of Marchi degeneration before the 10th day, and ovoids and spherules of unchanged myelin may be present 6 weeks after a necrotic lesion affecting the proximal part of the nerve fibre. At this stage considerable free cholesterol is present as well as phosphatides, cerebrosides, fatty acids and neutral fat (Hurst 1925). By 3 months most or all of the myelin has broken down into simpler lipids and neutral fat, and some is in process of removal by phagocytic cells. After 6 months most of the lipid has become neutral fat and much has been removed from the area occupied by the degenerated tract. These times naturally vary with the age of the patient and with the calibre of the fibres composing the degenerated tract. It is however a general rule that the interval, between the occurrence of a tract lesion and the death of the patient, which is most favourable for tracing Marchi degeneration is from 3 to 6 weeks or rather longer, and that disappearance of myelin in a tract, as seen by the Weigert method, is not very evident under 2 months from the time of the lesion.

The process of myelin katabolism is more easily followed by the use of Sudan IV on frozen sections, combined with a polarising microscope. The normal chrome or terra-cotta staining of myelin, associated with a Maltese-cross anisotropism, may still be seen in ovoids and balls of myelin for several weeks after Wallerian degeneration has begun in the tract or fibre system; cholesterol does not take up the dye and when viewed under crossed Nicol prisms appears as colourless anisotropic crystals; the other lipids assume an increasingly red colour as their composition approaches that of neutral fat, and at the same time they lose their anisotropic character.

The *chemical* changes accompanying Wallerian degeneration have been much investigated since the pioneer studies of Mott and Halliburton. This work has been reviewed by Rossiter (1961) who, with his collaborators, had made substantial earlier contributions. During the first (approximately the pre-Marchi) stage little change in the concentration and chemical reactions of the myelin lipids (i.e. non-esterified cholesterol, sphingomyelin and cerebrosides) is observed; the resting oxygen consumption falls and there is gradual loss of important enzymes such as true cholinesterase, choline acetylase, alkaline phosphatase, the thiamine containing and several other coenzymes. Stage 2 exposes the chemical degradation and the cellular proliferation. The myelin lipids disappear, cholesterol esters increase. It has been suggested that osmium tetroxide reacts (in the Marchi stain) with a mucopolysaccharide containing breakdown product of myelin (Wolman 1957), but this has been rejected by Wolfgram and Rose (1958) and by Adams (1958) who identified the lipid as cholesterol oleate. Accompanying the cellular reaction the content of nucleic acids, total protein, pseudo cholinesterase, acid phosphatase and 5-nucleotidase sharply increases. This increase of acid phosphatase was first demonstrated by Bodian (1947), who used Gomori's histochemical reaction. His findings in degenerating fibres (and their cell bodies) have been repeatedly confirmed. The enzyme 5-nucleotidase, normally found in white matter (Naidoo and Pratt 1954), participates in catalysing the liberation of inorganic phosphates from degraded myelin lipids. During stage 3 (characterised mainly by the formation of fibrosis), collagen increases, while nucleic acids and the enzymes active during the second stage, gradually return to normal levels.

Only few *electronmicroscopic* investigations in degenerating nerves are available, so far. They include work by Terry and Harkins (1959) in mice; Causey and Barton (1961) in rabbits; Webster *et al.* (1961) in guinea pigs experimentally inflicted with diphtheritic neuritis, and by Finean and Woolf (1962) in a biopsy of a patient, suffering from the Guillain-Barré syndrome. Although interpretation was often difficult (because of artefacts to which large fibres are particularly prone), all investigators reported definitive changes either in axons or in myelin spirals or in both. In the case of Finean and Woolf, the axis cylinders had almost completely disappeared in places, and the fragmentation of the myelin sheaths was tentatively considered to be secondary to physical stresses during the—*in vivo*—removal of the axonal debris.

The cellular reaction to Wallerian degeneration in the central nervous system differs from that in peripheral nerves in the absence of the sheath of Schwann. To what extent the interfascicular oligodendroglia undertakes similar functions to those of the cells of Schwann is not yet decided. It seems probable that these cells are related in some way to the nutrition of myelin and they seem to react fairly early to the degeneration of myelin sheaths. But the chief cellular agents in the breakdown and removal of myelin are the microglia which exercise in the central nervous system the functions of the wandering histiocytes. The first reacting cells in Wallerian degeneration were called *myeloclasts* by Jakob, who considered them to be derived from microglia. Cramer and Alpers (1932) however derive them from oligodendroglia. These are small cells with a rather ragged cell body and small irregularly rounded nucleus. They appear after the 4th day both between fibres and also, very characteristically, in the plasmatic spaces within distended myelin sheaths. They increase in numbers during the next two weeks and their cytoplasm becomes more granular, containing fine fatty droplets, but they appear to be transitory and their nuclei are often pyknotic or have undergone karyorrhexis. As the myelin breaks down into simpler lipids, microglial phagocytes seem able to absorb larger amounts of fatty granules without showing degenerative changes in the nucleus. It is indeed not unusual to see fat-laden microglial cells undergoing mitosis. But it seems probable that relays of microglial cells engulf the lipid granules and eventually migrate with them to the walls of the blood vessels where they are seen from 3 months onwards filling the adventitial or

Virchow-Robin spaces. Jakob called these *granule cells*, and divided them under the letters α, β and γ according to the size and nature of the fatty droplets. This distinction is somewhat schematic and it is not easy to distinguish the earlier intracellular products of myelin katabolism from neutral fat without special staining methods. It seems probable that these cells contribute to the process of katabolism, but this may also occur in acellular areas, for example in the centre of an ischaemic softening, although it is probable that in the absence of cellular enzymes the process takes place more slowly. Cajal considered that leucocytes played a part in the early stages, but in human pathology these cells are very rarely seen in Wallerian degeneration.

Another type of cellular reaction was described by Jakob. About the 4th day larger phagocytic cells appear and engulf fragments of axon and globules of myelin and other lipids. Later these cells may become multinucleated. They were called *myelophages* by Jakob who derived them from the interfascicular oligodendroglia. They are much less numerous than the lipid phagocytes derived from microglia.

The astrocytes also react to the breakdown of the nerve fibre and myelin sheath by enlargement of both cell body and nucleus. This appears at a rather later stage than the reactions already described and proceeds at a slower tempo. Although fine lipid droplets may be seen along their margins it is unlikely that they take any active part in the katabolism of myelin.

Degeneration of boutons terminaux, which is an essential part of Wallerian degeneration, has been studied both in the living animal and in stained preparations of experimental and post-mortem tissue. In the latter it is a valuable aid to anatomical research. Fedorow (1935), who studied the boutons of the vagus terminals in the living frog's heart, found that their appearance varied with the acidity or alkalinity of the fluids in which they were bathed. When the fluid was hypotonic or slightly acid the boutons became more sharply defined and refractile (gelatinisation), whereas if the fluid were made hypertonic or slightly alkaline they swelled, becoming more rounded and transparent. Gelatinisation was also seen after prolonged electrical stimulation of the vagus and as a passing phase following vagal section. Hoff and Hoff (1934), Foerster and Gagel (1934) and Glees and le Gros Clark (1941) have used degenerative changes in the boutons terminaux to indicate the termination of fibre tracts. Swelling and thickening of these nerve endings can be seen as early as 24 hours after lesions of the axons, and after 3 days they become 'enlarged granular masses which are readily distinguished from normal terminals' (Hoff and Hoff). Disintegration of the boutons occurs within the next few days. The study of these nerve endings may therefore be used to localise the termination of degenerating fibres in cases in which death occurs within 4 days of a lesion, that is at a stage when the degeneration of the myelin sheath is too early for the Marchi reaction.

Simple atrophy

Simple atrophy seems to be the best name to describe the effects of those disturbances of the metabolism of the neurone which lead to its gradual degeneration and death. Simple atrophy is the basis of many systemic degenerations, both hereditary, such as Friedreich's ataxia, or isolated, such as some cases of olivopontocerebellar degeneration. Many forms of peripheral neuropathy, especially those due to vitamin deficiency (Aring *et al.* 1941), show a similar pathogenesis. These have been studied experimentally by many workers among whom Bertrand *et al.* (1934), Swank (1940) and Swank and Prados (1942) have given full histological descriptions. Triorthocresyl phosphate, which in man and domestic fowls causes degeneration of the long tracts of the spinal cord as well as of the peripheral nerves, seems to affect the nerve fibres in a similar manner (Cavanagh 1954).

Simple atrophy has certain definite characteristics: Fibres of larger diameter are affected before those of medium and smaller size; the nerve fibre is affected more at its periphery than near the nerve cell, and the cell body often shrinks and becomes sclerotic without showing the chromatolysis of axonal reaction. To these general rules there may, of course, be exceptions.

The fact that in hereditary and other systemic atrophies the more distal part of the nerve fibre suffers before the part nearer to the nerve cell was recognised by many of the earlier workers, especially in olivopontocerebellar degeneration. It is easily demonstrable in the more acute cerebellar degenerations in which the long tracts of the spinal cord also undergo degeneration. In such cases the pyramidal tracts at the level of the medulla may show no evidence of myelin katabolism, but on passing down the spinal cord they contain progressively more sudanophilic and Marchi-staining lipids (Greenfield 1934). When the atrophic process is slow and the patient dies many years after the onset of symptoms, there may be little or no evidence of the katabolic processes which the nerve fibres have undergone. The tempo of degeneration is so slow that the products of the breakdown of myelin and axon are removed almost as quickly as they are formed, and sudanophilic lipids are very scanty. Nor does one see in such cases the beaded or fusiform swellings of the myelin sheath which are a very characteristic appearance in the early stages of Wallerian degeneration in the central nervous system. However, when Purkinje cells undergo simple atrophy their axons often end in the granular layer in a globular or fusiform swelling to which the name *torpedo* is usually given. This end-swelling is often seen to lie just distal to a recurrent collateral branch. It appears to have the characters of a retraction bulb. In the more chronic and slighter forms of simple atrophy in peripheral nerves, such as those seen in pellagra, the evidence that the nerve fibres are damaged is given more by the disappearance of the larger axons and myelin sheaths than by obvious katabolic changes in them (Aring *et al.* 1941), but in other more acute cases of peripheral neuropathy katabolic changes, similar to those described in Wallerian degeneration, may be seen, especially in the more distal parts of the nerves. When the process is severe and continues for some weeks it may result in death of the whole neurone. In peripheral neuropathy this is associated especially with loss of nerve cells in the dorsal root ganglia and secondary degeneration of the dorsal columns of the cord. Less often there is destruction of the motor neurones of the ventral horns.

Nissl's types of degeneration of the cell body

While central and peripheral chromatolysis and simple atrophy are characteristic reactions of the perikaryon to physiological stresses such as overwork, loss of function, or interference with metabolism owing to absence of vitamins, a number of other forms of degeneration were recognised in classical neuropathology as being the results of abnormal environmental conditions such as loss of oxygen supply, high temperatures and endogenous or exogenous toxins or chemical poisons. It is convenient to group these into (1) those in which the cell body swells and (2) those in which it shrinks. These types of cell change, although separated by Nissl on the grounds of appearance, have been found to be for the most part transition forms. The less severe may pass into the more severe, and the end result of all may be the death and disappearance of the neurone. Although each tends to have its own aetiology there is nothing pathognomonic in any of these types of cell degeneration except probably that seen in the earlier stages of severe anoxia.

Degeneration with swelling of the cell body

(*a*) *Nissl's acute cell disease* (*Spielmeyer's acute swelling*). In this form of degeneration the cell body and its processes swell and stain palely and more diffusely than normal. There is solution of Nissl substance along with pale staining of areas which do not normally stain with basic dyes. The dendrites and proximal part of the axon may also stain palely and diffusely. The nucleus swells, staining in a similar manner, and showing little evidence of chromatin except in the nucleolus which is intact. Sometimes a few fine chromatin granules may be seen in the nucleus but no chromatin lies in relation to the nuclear membrane which is sharply outlined. In spite of the loss of Nissl granules the neurofibrils are well preserved.

It is probable that this is in most instances a reversible change, but it may go on to more severe destruction of the neurone, and probably, at least in cases of heat stroke, to shrinkage. It is rather rare and when found tends to be spread widely over the nervous system. It occurs in general infections and intoxications such as typhoid fever and scarlatina. Bielschowsky (1932) found it especially in cases dying in hyperpyrexia (Fig. 1.5*a*). A similar change has been produced experimentally in animals by hyperthermia, and it may be found in cases of heat stroke which are fatal in the early stages (Malamud, Haymaker and Custer 1946).

(*b*) *Nissl's severe cell disease* (*Spielmeyer's liquefaction*). Neither of these names is sufficiently descriptive of a rather characteristic degeneration which usually goes on to the destruction and

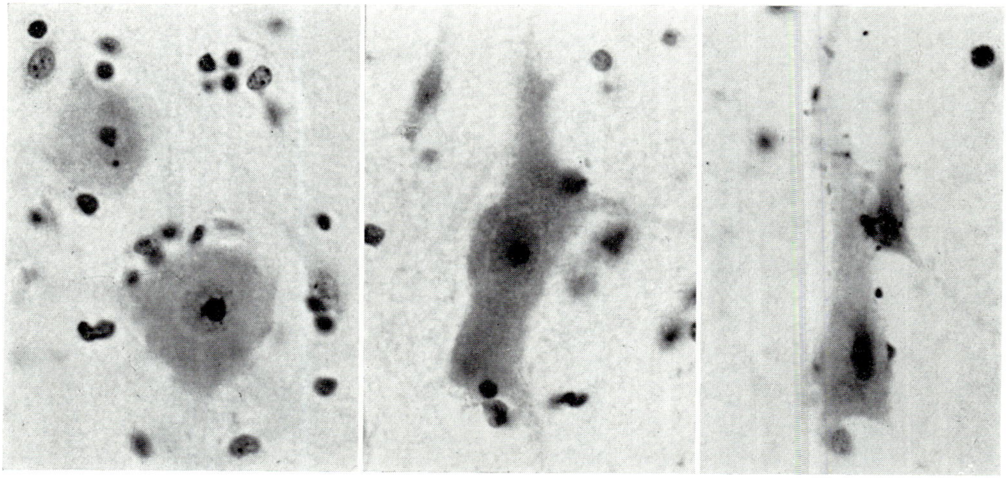

(*a*) (*b*) (*c*)

FIG. 1.5. Degenerations in cortical nerve cells.

(*a*) Hyperthermia before death. (*b*) Moderate ischaemia resulting from thrombosis of the internal carotid artery. (*c*) Severe ischaemia with incrustation of the Golgi network. (Thionin.)

disappearance of the nerve cell. In this form, along with the disappearance of Nissl granules, there appear in the swollen cell body, and especially in the bases of the dendrites, irregular basophilic rings and granules. The nucleus shrinks and stains more darkly than normal, often appearing finely granular, or diffusely hyperchromic. The nucleolus tends to become eccentric. As the process continues some of the dendrites disappear and the margins of the cell seem to melt away, sometimes leaving the basophilic ringlets and granules *in situ*. The axon and the base of the cell are usually more resistant and may even stain more darkly than normal at this stage. Sometimes vacuoles appear in the cytoplasm. In this form of degeneration the neurofibrils disappear early, especially in the cell body, but they may be preserved for a time in the axon and some of the dendrites. In association with this form of cell degeneration there is often an increase in the number of satellite cells which may appear to pass into the cell body.

Like his *acute cell disease*, Nissl's *severe cell disease* occurs in diffuse diseases of the brain such as the more acute forms of general paralysis, and in focal encephalitis and delirium. In animals it may be produced by subacute lead poisoning and severe hyperpyrexia. Spielmeyer groups along with this form of degeneration 'granular degeneration' in which, instead of little rings, more compact closely set granules staining intensely with basic anilin dyes appear throughout the cytoplasm and in the cell processes. Later the margins of the cell become ragged or eroded into bays. The nuclear changes in this form are similar to those seen in Nissl's severe cell disease. Spielmeyer considered this a slighter and more subacute form of degeneration which does not necessarily go on to the destruction of the nerve cell, and may remain in this stage for a long time. He found it especially in toxic psychoses such as delirium tremens, and the acute stages of Korsakow's psychosis.

Degeneration with shrinkage of the cell body

(*c*) *Ischaemic change* (Fig. 1.5*b* and *c*). This common form of degeneration is seen in early foci of softening resulting from vascular occlusions. The cell body shrinks becoming more angular and, in the pyramidal cells of the cortex, triangular. The cytoplasm rapidly loses its Nissl granules and becomes acidophilic. With haematoxylin and eosin it stains diffusely pink, but remains entirely or almost unstained with basic anilin dyes. The cell shrinks from its surroundings and, especially in paraffin sections, appears to be surrounded by a clear space, an appearance which has sometimes been confused with oedema of the cortex; but it may be associated with oedema, that is an increase in water content of the cortical tissues, due to increased permeability of ischaemic capillary walls (Byrom 1954). The nucleus also shrinks, becoming triangular in pyramidal cells, and stains darkly and diffusely. Owing to this the nucleolus may not easily be recognised. Nerve cells showing this change are not infrequently surrounded by small triangular or oval basophilic bodies which probably represent the points of attachment of boutons terminaux. This appearance is often called *incrustation of the Golgi network* (Fig. 1.5*c*). These bodies, which may be seen on the proximal part of the dendrites as well as on the cell body, stain best with basic anilin dyes but may sometimes be visible in sections stained with haematoxylin.

This incrustation is curiously haphazard in its distribution. In some cases and some areas almost every nerve cell is affected. In other cases, or in other areas of the same case, none are seen, although the ischaemic change in the neurones is otherwise similar. Areas which differ in this respect may be so close to one another as to be included in the same low power field. It is tempting to assume that the appearance of incrustation may depend on lesions both to the neurones round which it is seen and to the axons which make synaptic relations with them, but of this there is so far no evidence.

Ischaemic cell change is found usually in cases of circulatory arrest with survival of 14–15 hours, although it has been reported after considerably shorter survival periods (Scholz and Boellaard 1959; Steegman 1961).

It seems unlikely that nerve cells can recover from the ischaemic cell change as thus described, and it must be considered to be a stage in the disintegration of the cell. While it is commonly seen on the margins of areas of cortical infarction, or within them if they are small or recent, more severe alterations are also common. In these the cell body has disintegrated, leaving only a few small tags round a shrunken nucleus, which may either appear full of chromatin granules or be diffusely and darkly stained. This more severe kind of change may also be seen in or near areas of contused cortex in cases of head injury, or it may affect most of the pyramidal cells of the cortex in patients who survive an arrest of the heart beat lasting for more than 5 minutes (Fig. 1.6).

(*d*) *Homogenising cell change*. Spielmeyer (1922) described in Purkinje cells a type of cell change which closely resembles the ischaemic form and indeed may, under certain conditions, be a variant of this. Spielmeyer found it especially in certain fevers (typhus, typhoid, gas gangrene) and therefore considered that it was not necessarily due to ischaemia. However, he himself and later authors (Bielschowsky 1932, Wertham 1934) found that it may occur along with the classical ischaemic change in cases of circulatory disturbance. We have found it in Purkinje cells in a case of temporary cardiac arrest for 10 minutes which survived for 46 hours (Fig. 1.6*b* and *c*). Lawrence, Meyer and Nevin (1942), who described it both in Purkinje cells and pyramidal cells of the cerebral cortex in fatal cases of hypoglycaemia, did not see it when

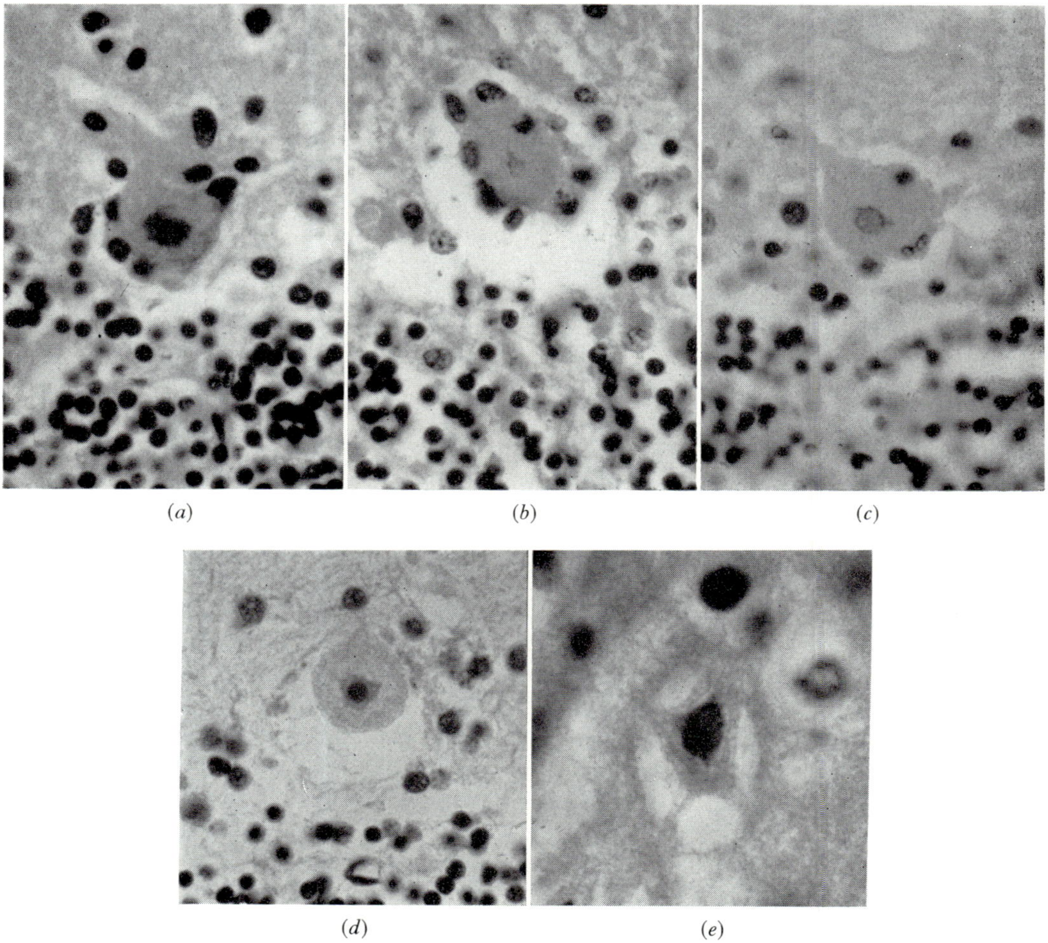

(*a*) (*b*) (*c*)

(*d*) (*e*)

FIG. 1.6. Changes in neurones after anoxia of short duration.

(*a*) Purkinje cells; 24 hours survival after 11 minutes of cardiac arrest.
(*b*) and (*c*) Purkinje cells; 46 hours' survival after 8 minutes of cardiac arrest, showing homogenising change. (Nissl ×550.)
(*d*) Purkinje cell 40 hours after high-altitude hypoxia. (Nissl ×550. By the courtesy of Dr. Webb Haymaker.)
(*e*) Cortical nerve cell; 100 hours' survival after 6 minutes of cardiac arrest.

death occurred within a few hours of the onset of coma. Haymaker has found it in a case of hypoxia surviving for 40 hours. It appears to be caused by less severe or less prolonged anoxia and to make its appearance at a rather later stage than the ischaemic changes which have already been described.

In this homogenising degeneration the cell body becomes pale, opalescent and eosinophilic. With anilin dyes it may be unstained or appear yellowish and more highly refractile than normal, or the cytoplasm may appear foamy or granular. The nuclear changes are the most characteristic part of this type of degeneration. The nucleus shrinks, the nuclear membrane disappears and the fine granules of chromatin become clumped close together sometimes in a triangular or pyriform group, round the spherical nucleolus; this stains less deeply than normal with basic anilin dyes and haematoxylin and therefore appears more eosinophilic. It may also appear swollen, but in the writer's (J.G.G.) opinion this is a false impression, given by the shrinkage of nucleus and cell body around a nucleolus which retains its normal size. These nuclear changes are so severe that recovery of the cell seems unlikely. Purkinje cells which show homogenising degeneration are often surrounded by satellite cells which may appear to pass a short distance into the cell body or there may be neuronophagy of the dendrites by microglial cells giving the appearance to which Spielmeyer gave the name 'glial shrubbery' (gliastrauchwerk). Mitoses are often seen among these proliferating microglial cells. The disappearance of cortical neurones which was found by Lawrence *et al.* (1942) in their more long-standing cases of hypoglycaemic coma also suggests that the usual termination of homogenising degeneration is the disintegration of the neurone, although this may take longer than after the more acute forms of ischaemic atrophy.

In cases of cardiac arrest the degree of damage which the neurones suffer depends on their intrinsic vulnerability seeing that all are equally deprived of oxygen. It is known both from observation and experiment that, *at normal body temperature*, all the neurones of the cerebral cortex, with the possible exception of Betz cells, are irreparably damaged if the heart beat is arrested for 5 or 6 minutes. (If the body temperature is lowered to abnormal levels these times are considerably increased.) The cells of the basal ganglia will survive arrest for periods up to 10 minutes with only minor alterations. The Purkinje cells of the cerebellum are only slightly less vulnerable than neurones of the cerebral cortex, whereas the granules of the cerebellar cortex are much less vulnerable (Fig. 1.6). The motor cells of the spinal cord and apparently also those of the brain stem can remain alive and recover after complete arrest of the circulation for periods up to 15 minutes (Tureen 1936). Certainly after cardiac arrest for 11 minutes neurones of this type may show very little alteration in staining reactions, and the fact that patients can survive, although unconscious, for several days after such a catastrophe shows that their lower nervous centres are still active.

Tureen's experiments are of special interest in that he studied the ischaemic changes compatible with restitution to normal appearances. When the blood supply to the large motor cells of the cat's lumbar cord was cut off by clamping the aorta for 15 minutes, all the nerve cells were affected to a greater or less degree. About 7 hours after the period of ischaemia there was loss of Nissl granules and the cytoplasm appeared finely granular but diffusely stained. Most of the nuclei were normal but some stained darkly and had become eccentric. At a rather later stage, about 36 hours after the experiment, when all traces of paralysis had passed off, the neurones stained deeply in their perikaryon, dendrites and nucleus but showed no Nissl granules. Reparative changes in the neurones appeared after about 72 hours with a gradual reappearance of Nissl granules, and normal appearances were restored by the 6th or 7th day. The earlier changes were found, by the technique of ashing sections, to be associated with a progressive increase in the mineral content, both of the nucleus and cell body, which attained its maximum in about 36 hours and persisted for 6 weeks or longer.

These experiments were confirmed and extended by Krogh (1945) who clamped the aorta of rabbits through the abdominal wall for various periods and thereafter used Einarson's gallocyanin stain. In rabbits whose aorta had been clamped for 20 minutes he described a change, seen about 24 hours after the experiment, in which the Nissl granules had become a dust-like powder, most condensed at the periphery of the cell, and the nucleus had coarser chromatin granules than normal and lay eccentrically. This appearance has some of the characters of Nissl's acute swelling and some of those of axonal reaction. When the aorta was clamped for longer periods, all stages of vacuolation and disintegration of the cytoplasm and pyknosis of the nucleus were seen. In these acute experiments Krogh did not produce sclerotic nerve cells.

(*e*) *Nissl's chronic cell degeneration.* This is a condition in which the cell shrinks and stains as a whole more deeply than normal and the areas between the Nissl granules also become stained with basic dyes. The cell margins become concave between the bases of the dendrites where the outline is more sharply angular than normal. The nucleus stains darkly and, shrinking with the cell body, may become triangular with a relatively large nucleolus. The dendrites also stain darkly and the apical dendrite often appears twisted like a corkscrew. In this form of degeneration the neurofibrils may become clumped together in some places and disappear in others. This degenerative form must be distinguished from simple hyperchromia, in which also the cell may be rather small, but is otherwise healthy. Spielmeyer, however, considered that hyperchromia may go on to Nissl's chronic change. This may go further to the stage of sclerosis in which the various constituents of the cell are scarcely recognisable in a darkly stained shrunken mass of finely granular cytoplasm.

Shrinkage and sclerosis are most commonly seen in the larger neurones of the deeper cortical layers in chronic conditions, for example in general paralysis and in some cases of chronic ischaemia. Changes of this kind were found by Morrison (1946) in the cortex of dogs which had been repeatedly exposed to atmospheres deficient in oxygen for 3–4 hours daily. They may therefore be produced by simple anoxia of insufficient intensity to lead to the rapid death of the neurone, especially if the anoxic effects are prolonged. Rand and Courville (1946), however, found sclerotic neurones at the margins of traumatic cortical haemorrhages within a few hours of the injury. In heat stroke Malamud *et al.* (1946) found early sclerotic changes in a case dying 18 hours after the onset of the condition, and they were commonly found in cases with longer survival. The Purkinje cells of the cerebellum are profoundly affected in this condition, being either swollen or pyknotic and tending to disappear (Freeman and Dumoff 1944, Krainer 1949). In contrast to what is seen in the two forms of nerve cell degeneration with swelling of the cell body it is common to see isolated sclerotic nerve cells surrounded by others which are either normal or show very slight change.

Binucleated and multinucleated nerve cells

It is generally accepted that once the neurone has passed from the neuroblast stage to that of the more mature nerve cell it becomes incapable of further division. In the human brain little if any multiplication of neurones appears to occur after the first month of extra-uterine life, although migration and maturation of neurones is not completed at this time either in the cerebral or cerebellar cortex. This early cell division occurs by mitosis but amitotic division may also occur.

Experimental work by Mondino (1885–6) showed that mitosis of nerve cells may occur in the neighbourhood of stab wounds of the brain in guinea-pigs. His observations were repeated and confirmed in young dogs by Coen (1888). Levi (1896) caused nuclear division in nerve cells by cauterising the cortex of guinea-pigs and others have used chemical irritants with similar effect. It is thus well established that the neurones of young animals may react to a variety of injuries by nuclear division. There is no evidence that this goes on to division of the cell body or axon and this seems unlikely in a nerve cell which is approaching or has reached maturity.

In human disease it has long been recognised that binucleated nerve cells may be found in many nervous disorders of childhood especially those of congenital origin, such as idiocy, megalencephaly and tuberose sclerosis. They also occur in the Werdnig-Hoffmann type of infantile muscular atrophy (Greenfield and Stern 1927). Binucleated Purkinje cells in general paralysis were for a time thought to indicate that the disease was due to congenital syphilis, but they have also been found in acquired syphilis, both in general paralysis and in the meningovascular form. Binucleated cells of the substantia nigra were found by Trétiakoff (1919) in a case of pseudobulbar palsy resulting from a tuberculoma of the thalamus and midbrain, as well as in cases of Parkinsonism. Greenfield and Bosanquet (1953) confirmed their presence in this nucleus in three cases of post-encephalitic Parkinsonism.

As long ago as 1863 Tigges had found binucleated nerve cells at the margin of cortical wounds, and this was confirmed by Jolly (1870), Ceccherinelli (1874) and Popoff (1875), and more recently by Gaupp (1933). Rand and Courville (1946) found binucleated nerve cells in the cortex of 16 cases of brain trauma, dying at intervals of 10 days to many years after the injury. In their material multinucleation was seen almost exclusively in degenerated neurones which had lost their Nissl granules, and they concluded that nuclear division was a stage in the disintegration of the nerve cell, and that it might take place at a considerable interval after the injury. But in the writer's experience binucleated nerve cells, in syphilitic and post-encephalitic cases, may contain normal Nissl granules and show no evidence of degeneration. It is however possible that on the margin of cortical wounds, nerve cells which have undergone nuclear division may be unable to reform the Nissl granules which they lost at the time of the injury. Nuclear division in nerve cells is therefore an indication of previous injury by disease or mechanical trauma, but does not throw any light either on the nature or the date of the lesion.

Haematin pigment in nerve cells

In haemorrhagic areas in the cortex, and less commonly elsewhere in the central nervous system, neurones containing small granules or rods or quadrangular black or dark-brown crystals are often seen. In some cases the neurones are the only cells in a haemorrhagic area to show these inclusions. In other cases they are seen also in microglial and endothelial cells and in polymorphonuclear leucocytes. These crystals resemble melanin in disappearing under treatment with hydrogen peroxide, but they may be distinguished from melanin both in being easily dissolved in alkalis, such as 50 per cent ammonia or 5 per cent caustic soda as well as in ammonium sulphide, and in being brightly anisotropic (Fig. 1.7). The latter characteristic is the most valuable distinguishing mark as it can be used on any section. They are insoluble in the cold in weak acids and in fat solvents and are in fact identical in composition with formol haemoglobin pigment, and with the pigment granules of malarial parasites. Although derived from haemoglobin they do not give a Prussian blue reaction unless very strong acids are used to unmask the iron they contain. It is not known in what form this pigment exists during life, or whether crystals with the characters described above may be found in alcohol fixed brains (apart from cerebral malaria) as up to the present they have only been seen when formalin has been used in the fixing fluid. They may therefore result from an alteration by formalin of haemoglobin which has been absorbed from the neighbouring haemorrhage by the nerve cells in the vicinity. Rand and Courville (1946), who found this pigment in the neurones in contused areas of cortex in cases dying from a few hours to 3½ days after head injury, consider that the nerve cells take up haemoglobin during life and that this is then agglutinated into smaller collections in the cytoplasm of the neurone. In a case dying 14 days after a head injury they found golden-yellow inclusion particles in the nerve cells in the neighbourhood of a cortical contusion and considered that the processes of disintegration of haemoglobin might be continued within the cytoplasm of the nerve cells. Our own experience confirms the early appearance of this pigment in nerve cells in cases of cortical contusion, but we have not seen crystals or granules corresponding to later breakdown products of haemoglobin.

Rand and Courville's observation, however, suggests that the intravital absorption of haemoglobin from neighbouring haemorrhage may be the forerunner of the iron-incrustation or ferrugination of nerve cells which is commonly seen in old areas of infarction. They did not consider that all nerve cells which contained pigment granules of this nature were degenerated, although some showed obvious changes and some were ghost cells. In the writer's (J.G.G.) experienceso me degree of ischaemic change is the rule in neurones containing haematin granules.

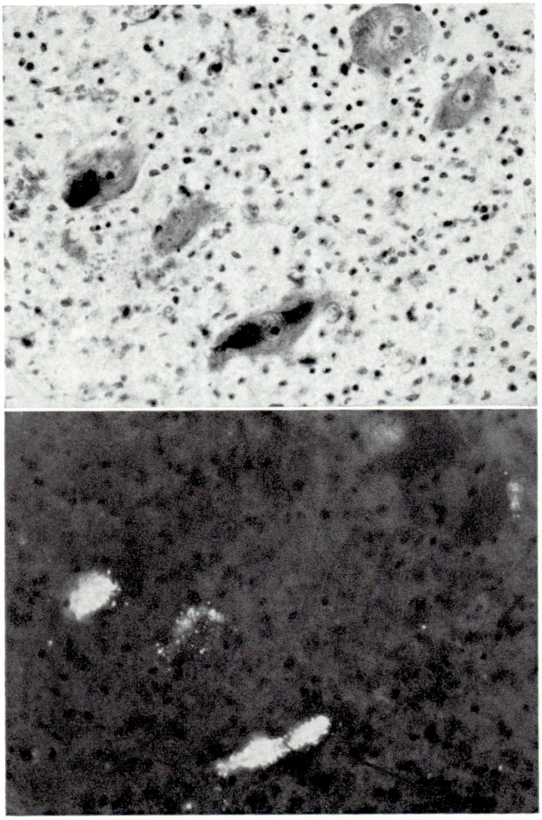

FIG. 1.7. Haematin pigment in nerve cells. An area of the cerebral cortex near small haemorrhages. The dark haematin granules in (*a*) appear bright under crossed Nicol prisms in (*b*).

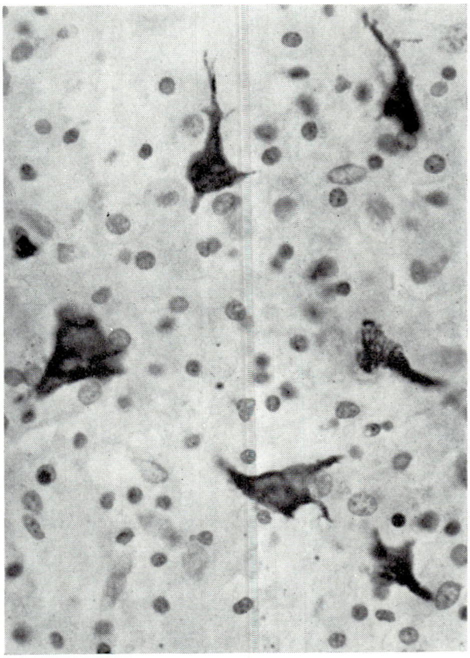

FIG. 1.8. Incrustation (ferrugination) of nerve cells in an old ischaemic area of cortex. (Haematoxylin van Gieson.)

Ferrugination or iron incrustation of nerve cells

Haematoxophilic granules replacing dead nerve cells are commonly seen in areas of old infarction. These granules may only depict the triangular shape of the cell body, or they may extend as thin strands for considerable distances in the lines of the dendrites. Usually there is no evidence of any protoplasm in relation to these granules, and they can only be considered as nerve cells in the sense that the position previously occupied by the neurone is now occupied more or less completely by haematoxophilic granules (Fig. 1.8). With Prussian blue staining they are seen to consist largely of iron. It is uncertain whether they also contain calcium as their staining reactions with haematoxylin would suggest. Why nerve cells dying from ischaemia are sometimes, but by no means always, replaced by these granules is quite unknown. The iron in them is too abundant to be accounted for by that present in their Nissl granules, and the suggestion that this appearance may result when neurones have absorbed haemoglobin from a neighbouring haemorrhage has at least this measure of support.

Types of neuronal degeneration related to certain forms of organic disease of the nervous system

Certain types of degeneration in nerve cells are recognised as occurring so constantly and characteristically in special forms of organic nervous disease as to be almost pathognomonic of that disease. In these diseases the diagnosis cannot be made unless the typical change is found in a considerable number of nerve cells, but the reverse is not always true since certain types of cell change occur in several different conditions. For example Alzheimer's neurofibrillary change is found in two groups of diseases which bear no known relationship to one another, and amyloid inclusions are not confined to cases of familial myoclonus epilepsy. The pathogenesis of all these types of cell change is still obscure, although in some the biochemical alteration in the cell is known. They are not, so far as is known, due to general causes such as toxaemia, infection or malnutrition.

Alzheimer's fibrillary degeneration

Alzheimer (1907), in the form of presenile dementia to which Kraepelin later gave the name of *Alzheimer's disease*, described a change in the cortical neurones. This consisted of argentophilic impregnation and apparent thickening and later contortion of fibrillary structures within

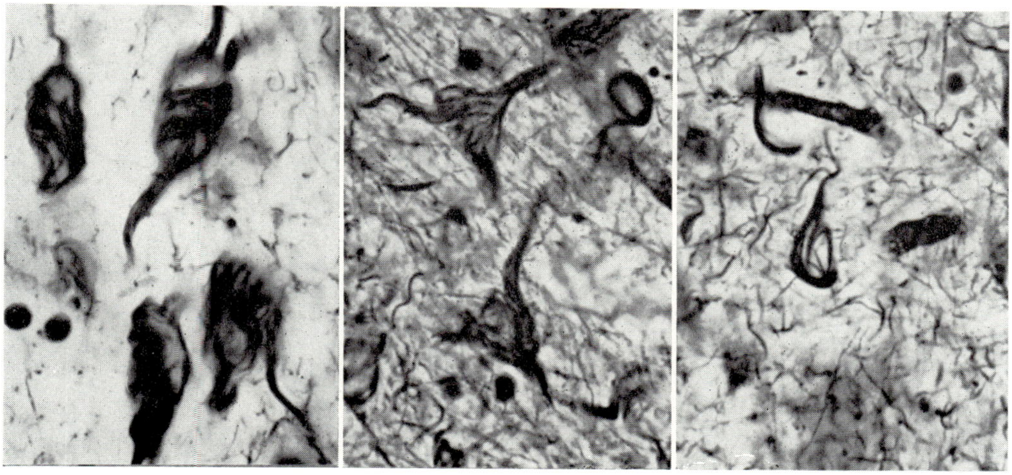

(*a*) (*b*) (*c*)

FIG. 1.9. Neurofibrillary change in presenile dementia (Alzheimer's disease). (Bielschowsky ×600.)
(*a*) From pyramidal layer of cornu Ammonis. (*b*) From hippocampal gyrus. (*c*) From temporal cortex.

the cytoplasm of nerve cells. In the early stages silver impregnation shows a darkly stained thick band often passing round, under or on the cell membrane, from the apical dendrite to the base. Later other similar bands appear either joining the proximal ends of the dendrites, or lying parallel to the original band on one side of the cell, or forming a basket-work round it. Sometimes the cell outline bulges from the contortion of these bands. In still later stages the nucleus and cytoplasm of the cell fail to stain and the cell appears as a hollow triangle formed by darkly stained single or double lines, or as a basket-work of fibres which curve round parallel to one another, often giving the appearance of a spool of thick thread or shaped like a torch (Fig. 1.9). The triangular type is most common in the frontal and temporal cortex and the spool and torch forms in the pyramidal cells of the hippocampus. Or a more intricate waving of argentophilic fibres may fill the cell body. With silver impregnation these fibres may stain darkly or may take a sepia colour. Cells which stain lightly in this way may form groups, especially in the hippocampus, or they may be interspersed with cells in which the fibres stain more darkly. As a rule the open triangles stain darkly and the spool-like forms palely, but this depends on the technique employed. With cell stains such as haematoxylin and eosin or with the basic anilin dyes, as in Nissl's method, the change is less easily recognised. The part of the cell containing thick fibres has lost its Nissl granules and may form a colourless area or a bulge on the side of the cell; or one half of the cell may fail to stain while the other contains the nucleus and some chromophilic granules. These appearances may at first sight suggest chromatolysis, but there is an increased refractility along the line of the thickened fibres which is not seen in chromatolytic cells. This alteration of refractility may be the only evidence, with these staining methods of cells which have reached the last stages of degeneration, in which the

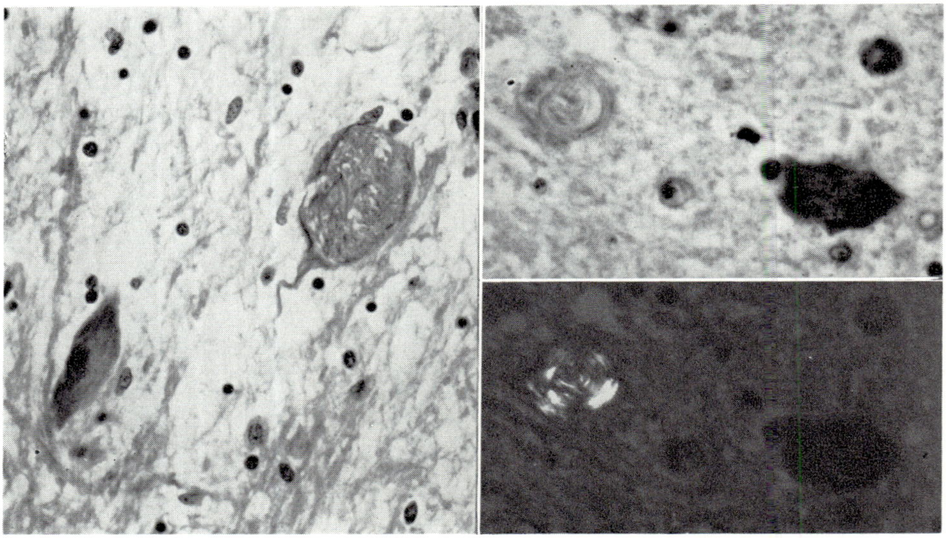

(*a*) (*b*)

FIG. 1.10. Neurofibrillary change in midbrain in post-encephalitic Parkinsonism.
(*a*) Haematoxylin-van Gieson. (*b*) Congo red (the lower half is the same field viewed through crossed Nicol prisms).

nucleus and other basophilic structures are lost and nothing remains except the fibrils. With Congo red the fibrillar structures stain rather more deeply than the remainder of the cell, although they usually appear pink rather than red. When stained in this way, the fibres become birefringent (anisotropic) along the line of their run (Fig. 1.10*b*).

Alzheimer regarded this change as an alteration in the neurofibrils themselves, resembling to some extent the clumping and thickening of the neurofibrillar network in hibernating animals (Tello 1904). Bielschowsky (1932) and Divry (1934) opposed this view for different reasons. For Bielschowsky the position of some of the threads, the frequent presence also of flakes or granules of similarly argentophilic material and the convoluted skeins of fibrils which are sometimes seen seemed to bear little relationship to the arrangement of neurofibrils found in normal nerve cells. Divry's objection was based on his discovery that much of the material forming the thick argentophil fibres in Alzheimer cells had the staining and optical properties of amyloid.

It was therefore in agreement with the teaching of general pathology that the material was deposited in the first place on the surface of the cell from the circulating fluids, and the early appearance of the fibres appeared to him consonant with this view. But there seems little doubt that in later stages argyrophilic fibres may also be found more deeply in the cytoplasm of the cell. The demonstration that the argentophilic material in Alzheimer cells as well as the central core of the senile plaques, with which they are commonly associated, consists of amyloid or a closely similar material, is of great importance from the point of view of pathogenesis and may also throw light on the etiology of this form of neuronal degeneration.

Although Alzheimer's fibrillary degeneration of nerve cells is most commonly seen in the form of presenile dementia which he described, it may also be found, especially in the hippocampus, in cases of senile dementia and occasionally in other conditions. It was observed by Fenyes (1932) and Hallervorden (1933) in nerve cells of the brain stem which were damaged by encephalitis lethargica, and by Malamud, Haymaker and Pinkerton (1950) and Corsellis (1951) in cortical nerve cells in long-standing cases of subacute encephalitis in a child and a young adult. The special characteristics of this change, as seen in the pigmented cells of the brain stem in post-encephalitic Parkinsonism, have been described by Greenfield and Bosanquet (1953). In the earlier stages the change is recognisable, in Nissl stained sections, by the orientation of the melanin granules at the apex or at one side of the cell in rows, with clear, highly refractile lines between them. Later one side or half of the cell might become filled with these refractile lines. In the later stages of fibrillary degeneration the cells may be triangular, rounded, fusiform or torch-shaped. When they have lost all basophilic structure they may still be recognisable in Nissl sections from the presence of a few melanin granules among the convoluted fibres (Fig. 1.10).

The view that Alzheimer's fibrillar change in nerve cells may be related to the thickening of the neurofibrils described in rabies by Achucarro (1910) is strongly opposed by Divry, but its occurrence in the more chronic forms of encephalitis is suggestive of some similarity in pathogenesis. In these diseases it appears to be a primary change in the nerve cell rather than the result of alteration in the chemistry of the body fluids. On the other hand in Alzheimer's disease the occurrence of amyloid also in the core of senile plaques and in the walls of blood-vessels in the cortex may be evidence of a more general metabolic dyscrasia. This question will be discussed later, but it may be said at present that there is no evidence that Alzheimer's disease bears any close relationship to generalised (para-) amyloidosis.

Granulovacuolar degeneration

The name *coarsely granular degeneration* was given by Simchowicz (1911) to an appearance which he found only in the pyramidal cells of the hippocampus in severe cases of senile dementia. It is common in this situation in Alzheimer's disease and may be seen also in Pick's disease. It consists in the appearance in the cytoplasm or the base of the dendrites of small vacuoles, measuring up to 5μ in diameter, each of which contains in its centre a small haematoxophilic or argyrophilic granule measuring from 0·5 to 1·5μ (Fig. 1.11*a*). These granules are not well stained by Nissl's method. With Lendrum's phloxin tartrazine stain, which demonstrates them brilliantly, they take a reddish tinge as well as the darker colour of the haematoxylin. They seem therefore to be to some extent acidophilic. Little otherwise is known as to the nature of this form of degeneration; there is no evidence of lipid in the vacuole. The affected cells are otherwise degenerated, having no Nissl granules in the vicinity of the granulovacuolar areas, and often having an eccentric nucleus. The restriction of granulovacuolar degeneration to forms of senile dementia and almost entirely to one group of cells gives it a special interest.

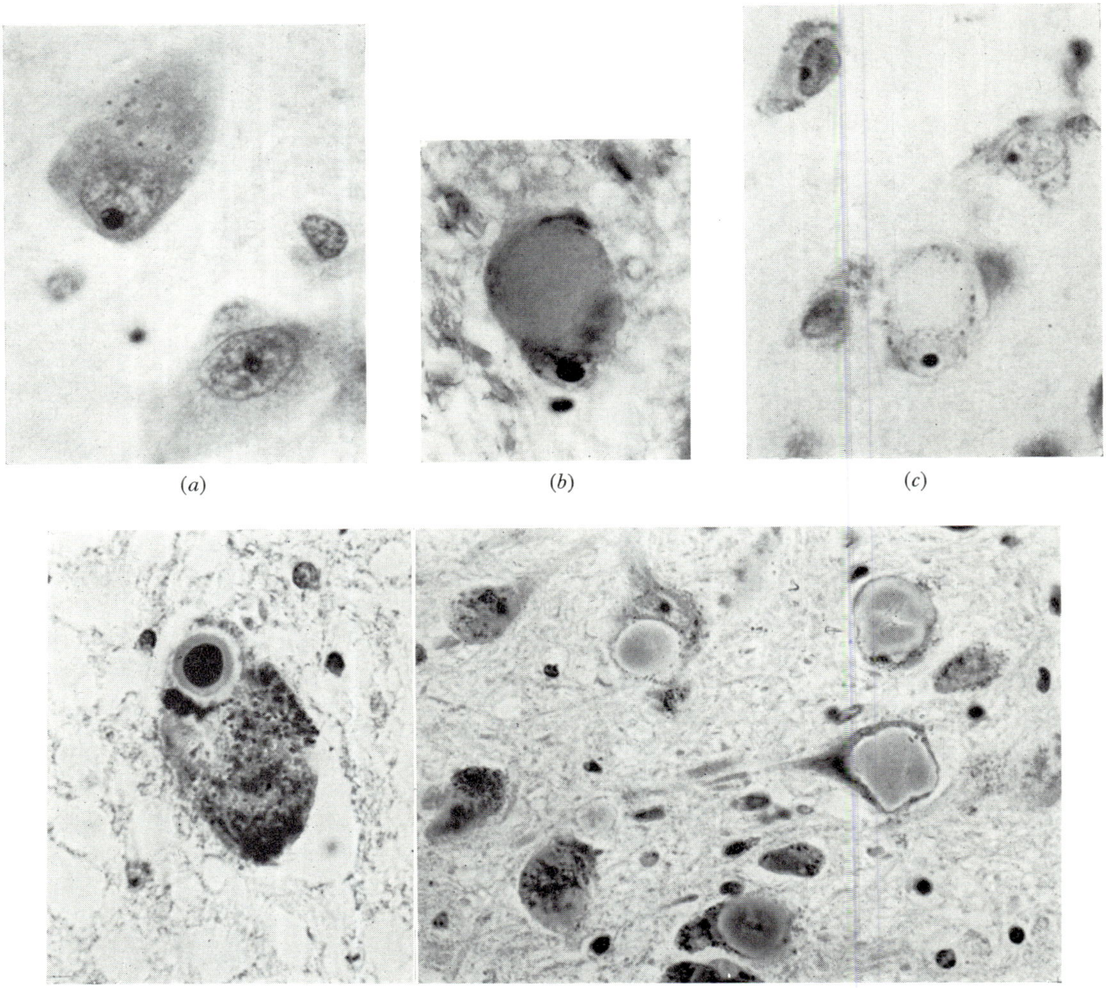

FIG. 1.11. Types of neuronal degeneration related to special diseases.

(*a*) Granulovacuolar degeneration in the pyramidal cells of the Cornu Ammonis (Lendrum's phloxin-tartrazine stain). Pick's disease.
(*b*) and (*c*) *Pick's disease*. Swollen nerve cells from frontal cortex. (*b*, phosphotungstic acid haematoxylin, *c*, Nissl.)
(*d*) *Paralysis agitans*. A Lewy's concentric inclusion in cell of locus coeruleus. (Giemsa ×800.)
(*e*) Lafora's amyloid inclusions in a case of familial myoclonus epilepsy. (H. and E. ×550. By the courtesy of Dr. D. G. F. Harriman.)

Swelling and argyrophilic inclusions in Pick's disease

While various forms of degeneration may be seen in the cortical neurones, the peculiar type of cell swelling which is seen in this disease deserves a special description. It is characterised by the accumulation close to the nucleus either on its basal or apical side of weakly acidophilic protein material which soon displaces the nucleus towards the cell membrane and may compress it, making it appear reniform. Later the cells enlarge, sometimes very considerably, and appear rounded or pyriform. With Nissl's method the swollen area of the cell remains colourless or stains a diffuse pale blue with a matt appearance, but Nissl granules may still be seen at the sides of the nucleus or at the apex of the cell. However, it is less easy to recognise this form of cell change with Nissl's method than with more diffuse stains such as haematoxylin-van Gieson or Mallory's phosphotungstic acid haematoxylin (Fig. 11*b* and *c*). With the latter stain especially the affected cells stand out as pale oval areas in the diffusely stained background. This appearance, combined as it often is with fibrous gliosis of the cortex, is very distinctive and may be of special diagnostic value in early cases in which the cortical and subcortical atrophy is still too slight for the diagnosis of Pick's disease to be made on macroscopic appearances alone.

Although a larger proportion of small than of large cortical cells is usually affected, individual large pyramidal cells in the 5th and 6th layers may be severely blown out, measuring up to 60μ by 45μ in diameter. In such cells the nucleus is at one pole of the cell and the nucleolus also is often eccentric, lying against the nuclear membrane. A few fine granules of chromatin may be present in the nucleus which has a fine sharply defined outline. With anilin stains the swollen cytoplasm appears matt rather than finely granular, as individual granules cannot be seen in it even with oil immersion objectives; but a few highly refractile granules which may stain with Nissl's method can often be seen near the cell margin. The tissue surrounding these distended cells may appear to be stretched forming a highly refractile ring round the body of the neurone.

With Bielschowksy's silver impregnation the swollen part of the cytoplasm in some of these cells may contain a globular, homogeneous, sharply outlined mass which stains with varying intensity, or the entire cytoplasm of the base of the cell may appear to consist of homogeneous argyrophilic material. In either case some intact neurofibrils may be seen at the periphery of the cell.

This form of cell degeneration may be found in a large proportion of the cells in the deeper cortical layers in areas which show the earlier stages of atrophy and sclerosis. Although most typically seen in these cortical neurones, it may also be found in the basal ganglia and in the pigmented cells of the brain stem. Williams (1935), while distinguishing it from the central chromatolysis which follows injury of the axon, considered that it only occurred when there was a lesion of the axon near its cell of origin. However, Cajal could not produce it experimentally by subcortical lesions.

The globular argyrophilic masses seen in this form of degeneration are often called inclusions, but they are less hyaline than the inclusions of paralysis agitans and show no such concentric structure as is seen both in these and in Lafora's amyloid inclusions. They do not appear to contain any lipid and indeed are entirely neutral in their staining reactions except for a varying degree of argyrophilia.

Nerve cells which in many ways resemble those of Pick's disease but in which the swollen areas are not argyrophilic are often present in cases of Lissauer's type of paretic dementia.

Concentric hyaline inclusions and their relation to paralysis agitans

This seems to be the most descriptive name for the bodies which are commonly found in the pigmented cells of the substantia nigra and locus coeruleus in cases of Parkinson's disease. They were first described in this disease by F. H. Lewy (1912) who found them especially in the nucleus basalis of the substantia innominata. Lafora (1913), who found them in the oculomotor, facial and vagal nuclei, called them *hyaline bodies*. They were first seen in the substantia nigra by Trétiakoff (1919) who called them Lewy bodies, and since that time they have been found to be almost constantly present in idiopathic paralysis agitans, although some writers have confused them with cytoplasmic vacuoles. They are rounded, acidophilic bodies which are always surrounded by a paler zone and often contain a sharply outlined, more refractile and more strongly acidophilic core. They may be single or multiple. Lafora found and pictured 12 in a nerve cell of the oculomotor nucleus, but this number is uncommon. When present in pigmented cells they tend to lie among the melanin granules which are displaced by them. Or they may lie on the cell margin and sometimes appear to be free in the tissues either owing to some artefact of sectioning or to the death of the nerve cell. With trichrome stains such as the Mallory or Masson technique or Heidenhain's Azan, they stain with the more neutral dye and only the central core, when it is present, takes the red acid dye. We have obtained very bright staining of the central core with Lendrum's phloxin-tartrazine method for virus inclusions (Greenfield and Bosanquet 1953). The core stains deep pink or purple by Giemsa's stain (Fig. 1.11*d*). With van Gieson's counterstain also the central core may stain with acid fuchsin, but this reaction is less certain. With eosin the whole body stains pink with a paler outer rim and a deeper red central core, but this stain does not demonstrate the bodies as well as the trichrome methods. These staining reactions, and their failure to stain by any method for amyloid, distinguish hyaline bodies from Lafora's amyloid inclusions which may show a similarly concentric structure.

The fact that later workers on paralysis agitans did not use the trichrome stains employed by Laforà and Trétiakoff, but were content with Nissl's stain and silver impregnation, may account for the lack of attention which was paid to this form of degeneration of nerve cells in paralysis agitans during the twenty-five years following Lewy's description. These bodies are most easily found, in idiopathic paralysis agitans, in the pigmented cells of the locus coeruleus, where a large proportion of the bodies contain a central core. They are also found in the substantia nigra, and less constantly in the pigmented cells of the dorsal vagal nucleus, the oculomotor nucleus and the substantia innominata.

Similar bodies have been described in the substantia nigra in cases of status pigmentosus (Hallervorden-Spatz disease) by Helfand (1935) and van Bogaert (1939). Their descriptions do not make it clear whether or not these bodies were identical with those found in paralysis agitans. Beheim-Schwarzbach (1952) also found them in the locus coeruleus in the brains of senile dements, aged 76–100, who showed no signs of Parkinsonism and in one centenarian whose intelligence was normal. It is therefore clear that this form of degeneration, although found with remarkable constancy in paralysis agitans, is not confined to this disease. It is not, however, a common senile change (Hassler 1937, Greenfield and Bosanquet 1953). Its pathogenesis is quite obscure. It is always associated with some other form of degeneration in the neurones in which it occurs, but this may be no more than the earlier stages of central chromatolysis.

In Parkinsonism degeneration with hyaline inclusions may be found in some pigmented neurones and fibrillary change in others. This is seen in post-encephalitic Parkinsonism (Hallervorden 1933, 1935) and also apparently in idiopathic cases, but in the writer's (J.G.G.) experience the cells showing fibrillary changes are much less numerous than those showing hyaline inclusions.

Lafora's amyloid inclusions

In a case of myoclonus epilepsy Lafora (1911) described intracytoplasmic concentric rounded inclusions in neurones of the cerebral cortex, basal ganglia, brain stem and spinal cord (Fig. 1.11*e*). The staining reactions of these bodies resembled those of corpora amylacea. Similar bodies were found in the globus pallidus by Bielschowsky (1913) in a case of double athetosis associated with status marmoratus of the lenticular nucleus. Westphal (1919) and Westphal and Sioli (1920) made a fuller study of these inclusions in a case of progressive myoclonus epilepsy and they have since then been reported in 10 further cases of this character, in which they have been present in large numbers, especially in the thalamus, substantia nigra and nucleus dentatus. In cases with progressive mental deterioration they are also present in the cerebral cortex. Davison and Keschner (1940) describe them as being of two types, homogeneous and concentric. The homogeneous bodies are separated from the other contents of the cell body by a narrow capsule of unstainable material; some of them have a central core which may be cruciform or stellate in shape. The concentric bodies have a central deeply stained core with concentric paler zones around this, or with darker radial striae in the pale outer zone. They vary greatly in size from 1μ up to 20μ (Harriman and Millar 1955) or 3–35μ (Davison and Keshner 1940) and there may be 4–5 bodies in a nerve cell. Lafora (1911) pictured a cell of the vagal nucleus containing one large and seven small inclusions, but so large a number is unusual. They may be found in axons or dendrites or apparently free in the tissues; the latter appearance may indicate the death and disappearance of the nerve cell in which they formed. In paraffin sections they may appear to be broken across, or to show central radial fissures, but this may be an artefact. Their presence in a nerve cell does not appear necessarily to entail degeneration and death of the cell, as Nissl granules are often normally present in the surrounding cytoplasm.

Harriman and Millar (1955) made a careful histochemical study of these bodies in a typical case of Unverricht's syndrome and found them to contain an acid mucopolysaccharide. They are readily distinguished from the Lewy inclusions of paralysis agitans in being basophilic with all stains, in giving γ metachromasia with methyl violet and toluidin blue, and in staining with the P.A.S. method for 1–2 glycol groupings after extraction with solvents for lipid, hyaluronic acid and glycogen. They found similar amyloid material in the muscle cells of the heart and in liver cells but none elsewhere in the body.

Lafora noted that the core might take the eosin stain with Mann's methyl blue eosin method after phosphomolybdic acid. Both the intraneuronal bodies and those found by Harriman and Millar in heart muscle and liver cells differ from amyloid as commonly seen in tissues in being basophilic and in failing to stain with Congo red or to show anisotropism after this stain.

Lipidosis of neurones

Accumulation of lipochrome or lipofuscin is common in senile neurones and may also occur in wasting disease. Neurones of different types and different systems have different tendencies to accumulate pigment. For example the larger pyramids of the cerebral cortex and the motor nerve cells of the ventral horns of the spinal cord very commonly contain a collection of lipochrome granules near the axon hillock, and the olivary and dentate nucleus and the external geniculate body in the adult always contain large accumulations of these granules, which may occupy about half the cell body. On the other hand the Purkinje cells normally contain none. Pathological accumulations of lipochrome are therefore not always easily distinguished from the normal, especially in the cerebral cortex. In certain forms of senile dementia many of the cortical nerve cells appear to consist of little except lipochrome granules, but this may be due rather to shrinkage and atrophy of the other constituents of the cell leaving the relatively resistant lipochrome in possession. Some writers consider that there is an alteration in the character of the lipid in such cases, but modern cytochemical methods have not yet been used to decide this question.

There is, however, a group of diseases which are characterised by the accumulation in neurones throughout the nervous system of lipid which is pathological both in its amount and often also in its character. For these diseases the term *cerebrospinal lipidoses* is most apt. The earliest described and best known form is *amaurotic family idiocy* (Waren Tay 1881, Sachs 1887) which usually manifests itself before the end of the first year of life. A later form occurring in childhood was described by Batten (1903), H. Vogt (1905), Spielmeyer (1905) and

Bielschowksy (1913). This differs from the earlier form especially in the type of retinal degeneration, but also in its special incidence on the granule and basket cells of the cerebellar cortex. Cases occurring in later life with or without retinal changes have also been described (Kufs 1928, Greenfield 1951). Closely related to these diseases are the cases of Niemann-Pick's and Gaucher's diseases in which the neurones of the central nervous system accumulate the abnormal lipid.

In all these diseases the neurones throughout the nervous system become filled and distended in varying degree with a lipid or lipoproteid material which is closely related to lipofuscin. Its composition and staining reactions vary in different forms of disease and probably also to some extent in different age groups. In pyramidal neurones it always fills and distends first the base of the cell pushing the Nissl granules and nucleus towards the apex of the cell and separating the neurofibrils. It may also accumulate in the dendrites or even the proximal part of the axon. In Purkinje cells it masses both at the points of bifurcation of dendrites, producing an antler-like appearance, and also as balls of larger or smaller size towards the termination of the dendrites near the surface of the molecular layer. The small granule and basket cells of the cerebellar cortex appear to tolerate this lipid accumulation poorly and to disappear rather than become distended. The larger cells also may burst (Bird 1948) and disappear and the enclosed granules of lipid may be broken down into simpler fatty substances by microglial cells.

These changes and their distribution in different forms of disease will be more fully dealt with in a later chapter. It may, however, be said here that the accumulation of lipid up to a certain amount does not appear to be inconsistent with the continued life of the cell. For example in amaurotic family idiocy the fibre tracts derived from lipid-laden cells (e.g. optic nerves and tracts) may remain myelinated for a considerable time and the Wallerian degeneration which is seen in them is probably to be related to the disappearance of nerve cells rather than to the lipidosis of those that remain. On the other hand the tendency to epilepsy and myoclonus which is seen in this group of disease may be related to the degenerated state of the nerve cells.

Ischaemic degeneration and necrosis of nerve fibres

The nerve fibre is probably less sensitive than the nerve cell to anoxia from loss of blood supply, but when completely deprived of oxygen for a sufficient time it undergoes necrosis. Less experimental study has been devoted to the effects of anoxia in the nerve fibre than to those in the nerve cell, but some experiments by Denny-Brown and others indicate the pathogenesis of anoxia in peripheral nerve fibres. In the central nervous system the softening of the white matter which results from arterial obstruction is well known but the effects of partial venous stagnation are less well recognised.

(1) *Acute ischaemic necrosis* is seen in the white matter of the brain and spinal cord as an almost immediate sequel of arterial embolism or thrombosis. It is associated with swelling and diminished consistency of the white matter, which is most evident when one of the larger arteries to the cerebral hemispheres is blocked. The microscopical changes are not at first evident, but after 24 hours there is progressive failure of the myelin in anaemic areas to stain with haematoxylin; this is not associated with distension of myelin sheaths, nor at first with obvious axonal changes. During the next few days these tissues gradually undergo granular disintegration. Within a week sudanophilic lipids appear and become engulfed in migrating histiocytes, at least in the outer zones of the necrotic area. In the more central parts there may be no living cells and the processes of myelin katabolism take place rather slowly, but in a period varying from a few weeks to some months the dead tissue disappears more or less completely from the necrotic area leaving a cavity which is filled with tissue fluids.

(2) In less completely anaemic areas and round the margin of necrotic areas the appearances are rather different. Here the first microscopical evidence of damage to the tissues is the formation of numerous small lacunae which result from irregular fusiform or moniliform distensions of the myelin sheaths. Many contain greatly swollen axons which may fill the myelin sheaths or may be separated from them by a clear zone. Although considerably thinned the myelin surrounding these lacunae still retains its normal staining and optical properties, at least for some days. The degree of distension of myelin sheaths is considerably greater than that of Wallerian degeneration. It closely resembles what is seen in subacute combined degeneration of the spinal cord, but in this disease axonal swellings are less in evidence. This lacunar appearance of the white matter, with swollen axons filling many of the spaces, is seen characteristically in the lateral columns of the spinal cord, when paraplegia results from deposits of malignant tumour in the epidural space, or when the spinal arteries or veins are obstructed or thrombosed for other reasons. The pathogenesis of this lacunar type of degeneration is not understood, but certain features of the reaction of peripheral nerve fibres to ischaemia grouped by Denny-Brown *et al.* (1944 a and b) under the heading of *oedema* simulate it closely. The contrast between the lacunar peripheral zone and the more solid necrotic core of an infarcted area indicates that the swelling of axon and myelin sheaths requires a certain flow of blood. It is evidence of a partial ischaemia or of a more complete anaemia of short duration and may not, under favourable conditions, go on to the complete destruction of the nerve fibres in the area.

(3) The slighter degrees of ischaemic anoxia in the central nervous system, such as may result from thrombosis or severe stasis in the veins or venous sinuses, have been studied in experimental occlusions of the sagittal sinus by Putnam (1935) and Woolf (1954). Their effects may be quite slow in appearing, especially when the stasis is incomplete. Both Putnam and Woolf found scarring of the white matter in the neighbourhood of the occluded part of the sagittal sinus after 3 months or more. Earlier effects were rarely seen. Putnam considered that the myelin was more damaged than the axons, but in Woolf's experiments both were affected over the same area. The demyelination was often incomplete and graded in severity from the margin to the centre of the scarred area. Similar ill-defined areas of partial loss of myelin may be seen in human cases both of venous thrombosis and of malignant hypertension associated with sclerosis of cerebral arterioles.

The ischaemic lesions in *peripheral nerves* will be discussed in the chapter on trauma, since they are closely related to mechanical injury.

NEUROGLIA AND MICROGLIA

The spongioblasts of the developing nervous system differentiate into three main types of cell, *astrocytes*, *oligodendroglia* and *ependymal* cells. It seems unlikely that oligodendrocytes can change into astrocytes or vice versa after the cells have reached their mature form, although in tumours some metaplasia of oligodendrocytic into astrocytic forms may probably occur. Nor does it seem likely that ependymal cells may alter into astrocytes except in tumour formation.

In addition to these essentially neural forms of supporting and lining tissue it will be convenient to describe here the microglia which was for long confused with the true neuroglia but is now considered as histiocytic in origin and function.

Astrocytes

Astrocytes were divided into *protoplasmic* and *fibrous* forms by Kölliker (1889–96) and Lloyd Andriezen (1893). As these names imply, the fibrous is distinguished from the protoplasmic form chiefly by the presence in the cell body and processes of fine firm fibres which were recognised by Ranvier (1883) from their high refractility and were differentially stained and thoroughly studied by Weigert (1895). The name *Ranvier-Weigert fibres* is therefore sometimes used. There now seems little doubt that astrocytes are single cells and do not form a reticular syncytium such as Held (1903) and Jakob (1927) described. In both types small, rounded or oval, argyrophilic dots called gliosomes lie near the surface of the cell body and processes. Although they are under the cell membrane (Fig. 1.12) they appear in fixed and stained preparations to be raised above the surface of the processes, as though lying on it. They have the same staining reactions as mitochondria and with the electron microscope have been identified as such. The processes of astrocytes run for a considerable distance into the surrounding tissues, branching freely. In fibrous astrocytes they are longer and branching is less frequent and takes place at a more acute angle than in protoplasmic astrocytes, in which the numerous branches, coming off at a wide angle, give a mossy appearance to the tissue. These differences help to distinguish fibrous from protoplasmic astrocytes in sections stained by gold-mercury or silver impregnation. With ordinary cell stains such as haematoxylin and eosin, the processes of normal astrocytes cannot be distinguished from the background of nervous tissue. They may be impregnated differentially by Cajal's gold mercuric-chloride or del Rio Hortega's silver carbonate technique. One or more of the processes, usually thicker than the others, make contact with the wall of a blood vessel by means of a conical *foot-plate*. This is most easily seen in the cerebral cortex round the smaller blood vessels. Similar more elongated foot-plates are seen attached to the pia mater both in the brain and cerebellum. These foot-plates appear to be a kind of cement substance. It has been suggested that those round capillaries form a filter for the tissue fluids which escape from the capillaries, thus preventing certain dyes such as trypan blue and other chemical substances from passing into the nervous tissue (Held's membrana limitans). There is indeed some evidence that the cerebral capillaries are almost covered by astrocytic foot-plates (*vide* page 236).

Neuroglial fibres. Under the light microscope their outline is straight and sharply defined. They are normally extremely fine and are only visible with high magnification. Their high refractility makes them visible when unstained under phase-contrast illumination. They have much the same staining reactions as fibrin. Weigert's method and its derivatives (Holzer, Victoria blue) demonstrate them beautifully, but do not show the cytoplasm of the astrocytes. Mallory's phosphotungstic acid haematoxylin also stains them differentially and has the advantage of being a more generally useful tissue stain. Its chief disadvantage is that it stains myelin a similar purple colour. With Mallory's connective tissue stain and its derivatives (Masson's tri-chrome, Heidenhain's Azan) after suitable fixation they stain red against the blue of the cytoplasm. With Mallory's methods and in good silver impregnations the fibres can be seen to lie in the protoplasm of the processes and cell body, sweeping past the nucleus from one process to another. Several fibres may lie in the thicker expansions, especially in the foot-plate processes, in which a few may pass through the foot-plate to become interwoven with the collagen fibres of the vessel wall or meninges (Ingleby 1925, Weigert 1895).

The identification of the various types of glia by the *electron microscope* has been slower than of other structures; even now rigid criteria are lacking (Gray 1959, 1961). The majority of workers, however (for example Schultz *et al.* 1957; Farquahr *et al.* 1957; De Robertis *et al.* 1958), describe the cytoplasm of astrocytes and their processes as watery, of low electron density, with sparse, occasionally elongated mitochondria and few laminated membranes of granular reticulum. Protoplasmic astrocytes, according to Schultz *et al.* have beaded margins which fit tightly into neighbouring structures, while the outline of the processes of fibrous astrocytes seems to be smooth. The end-feet show a similar watery cytoplasm. The nucleus is also of low density, with clumps of chromatin, usually near the border.

Fibrils have been observed and illustrated by Luse (1956) and Gray, but their presence in normal astrocytes is considered doubtful by other workers.

It has been suggested (de Robertis *et al.* 1960; Shimoda 1961; Dempsey 1961; Niessing *et al.* 1962 and Ule 1962) that astrocytes and, perhaps, also oligodendrocytes and their processes, are

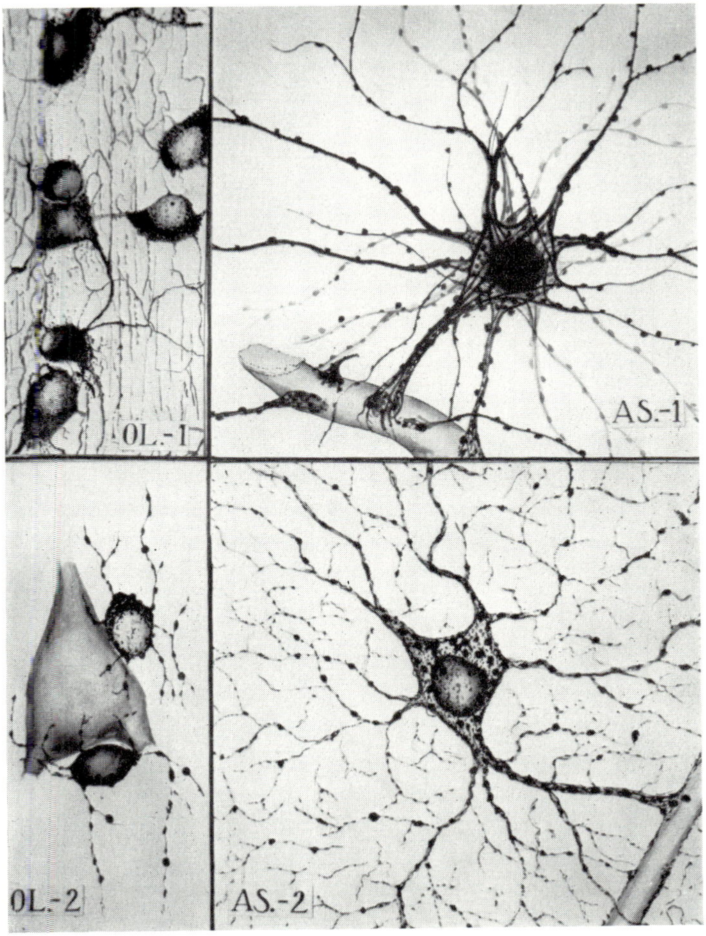

FIG. 1.12. Types of neuroglial cell.

AS.-1. Fibrous astrocyte. AS.-2. Protoplasmic astrocyte. OL.-1. Interfascicular oligodendroglia. OL.-2. Satellite oligodendrocytes. (By the kindness of Dr. Wilder Penfield.)

concerned with the transport of watery solutions from the blood to the nervous parenchyma. In oedema of the brain the fluid is assumed to be contained mainly in the processes and in the cytoplasm of glial cells. If confirmed, this would throw interesting new light on the genesis of retrogressive glial change, such as clasmatodendrosis and swelling of the oligodendroglia.

Fibrous astrocytes are present throughout the central nervous system, except in certain areas of grey matter in which only the protoplasmic type of astrocyte is normally found except for a few fibrous astrocytes round the larger vessels. These areas are (1) the deeper layers of the cerebral cortex, (2) the striatum and (3) the granular layer of the cerebellum. In the cortex a very few fibres are normally present in the 2nd and 6th layers and practically none in the

3rd, 4th and 5th layers. In the nucleus caudatus there is a fairly dense layer under the ependyma, but few or none elsewhere and none are usually found in the putamen. The globus pallidus contains fibrous astrocytes in the bundles of myelinated nerve fibres which traverse it and round the large vessels. Apart from this neuroglial fibres are not normally found here in young subjects but are less uncommon in senile brains. The substantia gelatinosa Rolandi is also very poor in neuroglial fibres (Weigert 1895). In many other nuclei in which fibrous astrocytes are present there are probably also astrocytes of protoplasmic type. In the sub-ependymal tissue, especially round the iter of Sylvius, the 4th ventricle and the central canal of the spinal cord, there is a specially thick feltwork of neuroglial fibres, and a thinner, but fairly dense, layer of tangential fibres is also present in the subpial layer of the brain and spinal cord. A similar layer may be seen round the larger blood vessels within the brain since their peri-adventitial sheath may be considered as an invagination of pia mater. These surface and perivascular layers tend to become thicker in the senile nervous system. Throughout the brain stem, and especially in the medulla, neuroglial fibres form a closer network than in the white matter of the brain and cerebellum. This may be associated with the movements and alterations of alignment which take place in the medulla. In the medullary olives the neuroglial feltwork is normally more dense than in any other part of the brain stem except under the floor of the 4th ventricle (Weigert). For this reason apparent neuroglial sclerosis of this nucleus cannot be accepted as pathological unless associated with degeneration of its cells and fibres.

The *cerebellar astrocytes* deserve special mention. As in other parts of the brain those in the white matter are of the fibrous type, but in the granular layer only protoplasmic astrocytes can be found. In the molecular layer two types of astrocyte have been described, (1) *Bergmann cells* or *Golgi's epithelial cells* and (2) *Feathered cells of Fañanas* (1916). But it is doubtful whether there is any real difference between these and some authors prefer to consider all the astrocytes in this layer as Fañanas cells. It is probable that the differences in appearance which have been described are partly due to variations in staining methods, since in many preparations only one type can be demonstrated, and partly to minor variations in one or another character of the cells. In both types the nuclei, which resemble those of other astrocyte types, usually lie either in the same zone as the Purkinje cells, or immediately superficial to this.

In the Bergmann cells, as often described and as seen by Weigert's or other stains for neuroglial fibres, a single process arises on the superficial side of the cell body and very soon branches, giving off a few fine parallel fibres which run straight to the pial surface. Penfield (1932) likens these branches to the prongs of a fork. They make contact with the pia mater by fine footplates. A few turn at right angles under the pia and run for a short distance parallel to the surface forming a rudimentary sub-pial layer. Weigert gave the credit for the first description of these cells to Deiters. When well stained by the metallic impregnations of Golgi, Cajal or Hortega, leaf-like sprouts can be seen on the proximal parts of the processes.

These astrocytes of the molecular layer, as well as the protoplasmic astrocytes of the granular layer, readily form fibres under pathological conditions. In most cases of cerebellar cortical sclerosis the majority of the neuroglial fibres in the molecular layer remain orientated perpendicular to the surface, but in congenital syphilis there is often a more disorderly arrangement.

Neuroglial fibres readily undergo autolysis and it is often impossible to stain them when the post-mortem has been delayed for more than 24 hours after death. Indeed for good demonstration of these fibres the brain should be well fixed as early as possible.

Reactions of astrocytes to disease or injury

Astrocytes are less vulnerable than nerve cells and fibres but are much more easily damaged than connective tissue. They react to all noxae which damage neurones by changes which may be regressive or progressive. These reactions may go on to necrosis and disintegration of the cells or may lead to the formation of new fibrous processes resulting in a glial scar or a more diffuse fibrous gliosis. Transition stages in which astrocytes remain for a considerable time without either undergoing dissolution or forming fibres are also recognised, at least in protoplasmic astrocytes. Apart from this the reactions of fibrous and protoplasmic astrocytes are to a great extent similar, since protoplasmic astrocytes in their progressive reactions tend to develop Ranvier-Weigert fibres, at least in some of their expansions.

Few investigations have been made into the stimuli which cause astrocytes to react. Those of Penfield (1927), and Penfield and Buckley (1928) though planned for a different purpose, are instructive. They showed that if the brain were punctured by a sterile blunt instrument the wound became filled with a core of fibrous tissue, derived from the meninges, and to this was attached a feltwork of new neuroglial fibres; if on the other hand the puncture were made with a cork borer with a sharp edge, which cleanly removed a cylinder of brain tissue, there was no connective tissue scarring and very little neuroglial reaction. It appeared from these experiments that the presence of necrotic brain tissue stimulated the formation both of fibrous tissue and of neuroglial fibres. Rand and Courville (1932), from the study of brain injuries, consider that gliosis occurs only as the result of tissue destruction and that 'the intensity of the glial reaction in the zone of proliferation is in direct proportion to the proximity of the reacting cells to the injury'. The neuroglial sclerosis, which follows degeneration of a tract or the demyelination of a plaque of disseminated sclerosis, is well explained by this theory. But there is evidence that neuroglial hyperplasia may be stimulated by other factors. Oedema and minor degrees of ischaemia are constantly associated with swelling of the cell bodies of astrocytes, which goes on to the formation of new neuroglial fibres. This begins quite early. The swelling of the cell body often appears within a week of an incomplete arterial occlusion. Syphilis, in general paralysis and chronic meningovascular syphilis, leads to the outgrowth of pads of neuroglial fibres through breaks in the ependyma and pia mater into the ventricular and the subarachnoid spaces, and some forms of virus encephalitis, especially subacute inclusion (sclerosing) encephalitis, are associated with a proliferation of astrocytes, both in the cortex and white matter, which appears to be out of proportion to the amount of neuronal destruction.

Regressive changes in astrocytes are often seen within the first few days in an ischaemic or traumatised area, and may be followed for longer periods in the neighbourhood of a focus of sepsis such as an abscess. The cell body swells and becomes visible at one side of the nucleus. Its outline is at first rounded but later becomes irregular. The processes break off and become disintegrated into a granular detritus to which the name 'filling bodies' (füllkörperchen) was given by Alzheimer (1910). To this loss of processes Cajal gave the name *clasmatodendrosis* (breaking up of branches). Lipid granules of varying size appear in these swollen cell bodies. The nucleus meanwhile becomes pyknotic and irregular and eventually disappears and the cytoplasm undergoes dissolution. If these changes take place rapidly there is little swelling of the cell body, but if more slowly it continues to enlarge for a time.

These swollen, irregularly shaped cells were called by Alzheimer *amoeboid neuroglial cells.* The name is descriptive of their appearance but conveys a suggestion that they can migrate through the tissues. Of this there is no evidence, and indeed it seems very unlikely that a dying cell should have such powers. The name is therefore misleading and should be dropped from the vocabulary of neuropathology.

In addition to the causes of astrocytic degeneration already mentioned, Alzheimer (1910) found this change in acute delirium, general paralysis, status epilepticus, cerebral syphilis, uraemia and diabetic coma, as well as experimentally in acute and subacute intoxications. It is commonly seen in very oedematous areas, but is not a necessary accompaniment of oedema.

It may occur as a post-mortem change but is most likely to be found post-mortem when death has resulted from an acute toxic process (Jakob 1927).

Under conditions which are less unfavourable to the brain tissue the astrocytes undergo progressive changes. In these the cell body enlarges without losing its processes. The nucleus also enlarges, stains more darkly and often divides amitotically, giving rise either to two daughter cells or to a large binucleated cell. When mildly unfavourable conditions persist for some time, as for example in an area of oedema round a cerebral abscess, the cell body may continue to enlarge up to 25μ or more. Large reniform or irregular nuclei may be seen in such cells. At this stage the cell body may lose its processes and become rounded and the nucleus may break up into fragments probably heralding the death of the cell. Although some such cells suggest an early stage in mitotic division it is probable that mitosis of astrocytes does not occur apart from tumours (Penfield 1932). Certainly small astrocytes in mitosis or the later phases of mitosis in swollen astrocytes are never seen.

These regressive changes may, however, be followed by recovery, with the formation of new fibre-containing processes. It seems probable that the giant astrocytes which are often seen in the scars of slowly progressive lesions, such as *diffuse sclerosis* of the white matter or in the neighbourhood of a tuberculoma, result from a long-continued reaction of this kind.

In areas involved in moderate degrees of ischaemia or subacute encephalitis, and in the oedematous white matter surrounding cerebral tumours, less severe degrees of swelling of the cell bodies of the astrocytes are commonly seen. It is characteristic of this swelling that it affects all the astrocytes in an area in almost equal degree with transitions to less or greater degrees at the margins of the area. It results in irregularly rounded cells with angular projections from which the processes arise. The cytoplasm is usually homogeneous, but may contain a few granules or vacuoles near its margin. Its outline is more clearly defined than in cells undergoing clasmatodendrosis. Swollen cells arising from fibrous astrocytes do not usually contain any fibres in their cell body, though these usually remain intact in the processes. The nucleus, which may be slightly enlarged, lies on one side of the cell, usually on that furthest from the chief processes. Occasionally two nuclei are present at opposite poles of the cell but mitoses are not seen. The names *swollen-bodied* and *plump astrocytes* are given to these cells.* Although swollen-bodied cells may arise from protoplasmic as well as from fibrous astrocytes, the absence of fibres from the cell body in both cases does not justify the use of the term *protoplasmic* as a general description of cells which have undergone this change.

The degree of swelling may vary greatly. In the slightest and earliest stages a small rounded or irregular cell body no larger than the nucleus may appear at one side of this. Enlargement to diameters of 15μ are common and are often accompanied by the formation of new fibres. From this stage, under favourable circumstances, the cell body gradually shrinks. At the same time, either by the extension of new processes from the cell body or by more frequent branching, new fibrous expansions are formed and increase the density of the glial feltwork. This process of gliosis after the formation of swollen-bodied astrocytes is usually associated with a moderate increase in astrocyte nuclei, but this is much less evident than the increase of neuroglial fibres.

The protoplasmic astrocytes of the cortex, however, often show more nuclear division than formation of new fibres (Fig. 1.14*a*). This is especially seen in some cases of subacute encephalitis and in the earlier stages of cortical atrophy. In these conditions we see numerous pairs of nuclei lying close together in the same cell or in closely apposed cells which are often mirror images of one another. Groups of four nuclei belonging to recently divided cells are

* The German term *gemästet* literally means *fattened*, and is sometimes translated as 'gemistocytic' in English writings (Penfield).

also not uncommon, and even larger groups may be seen. In dividing, astrocytes appear to share the expansions and if two foot-plate processes are present one goes to each cell. In this way the nuclei come to be near the inner, apposed margin of the cells and the expansions to come off from their outer margin (Fig. 1.13*c*).

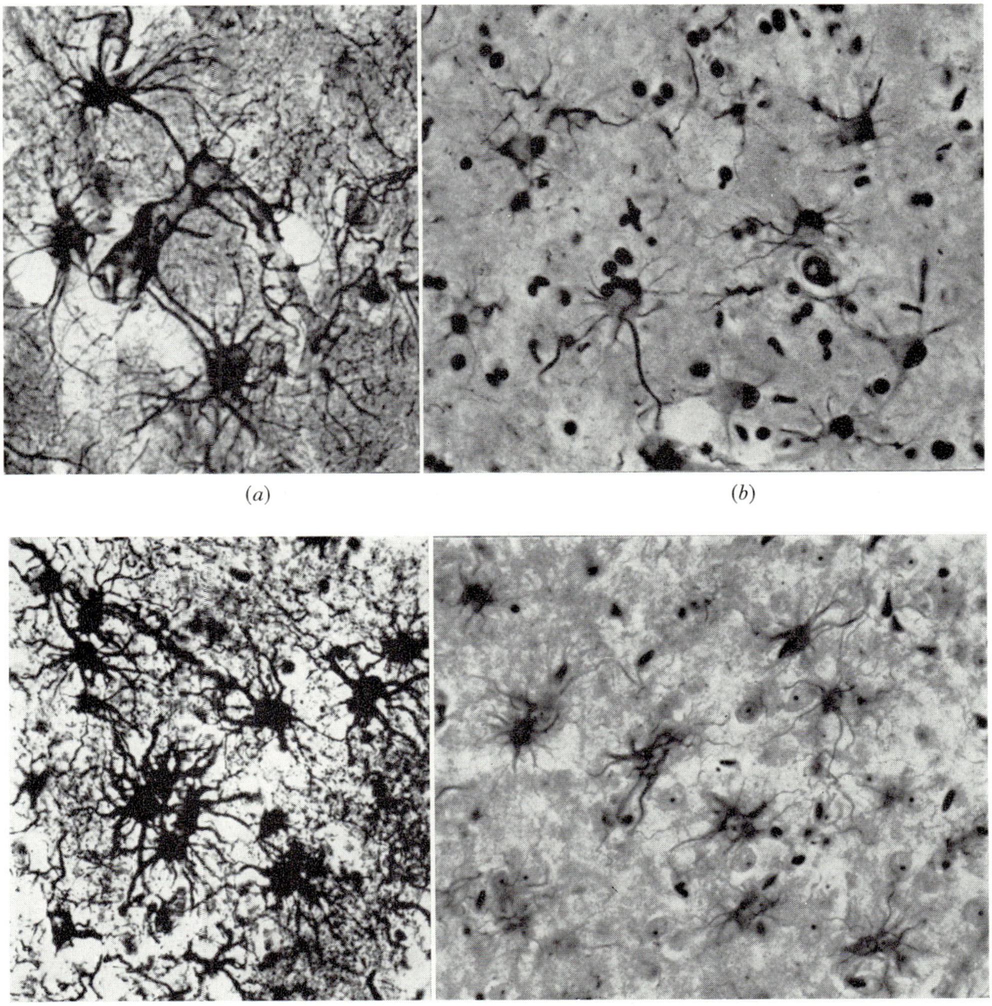

(*a*) (*b*)

(*c*) (*d*)

FIG. 1.13. Reactions of protoplasmic astrocytes.

(*a*) and (*b*) Cortical astrocytes in general paresis showing moderate hypertrophy. (*a*) Cajal's gold sublimate, ×450. (*b*) Silver carbonate, ×350.

(*c*) Cortical astrocytes in subacute encephalitis showing division into 4 daughter cells. (Cajal's gold sublimate.)

(*d*) Astrocytes in putamen in presenile chorea showing formation of fibres. (Mallory's phosphotungstic acid haematoxylin.)

This nuclear increase may not be associated with definite enlargement of the cell body especially in the slighter degrees of cortical atrophy, but in more acute processes some swelling both of the cell body and processes is usually present. Early formation of neuroglial fibres, especially in the foot-plate processes, may be seen in these recently divided cells. In the later stages of cortical atrophy with sclerosis closely set groups of astrocyte nuclei are less often seen, although there is a definite increase in the number of astrocyte nuclei, and it seems probable that the cells move apart from one another after division, as fibres form in their processes.

Wallerian degeneration of nerve fibres is constantly associated with fibrous gliosis. Swelling of the cell body is less evident in this process, but some rather diffuse increase of the protoplasm round the nucleus and the proximal parts of the processes is commonly seen in the astrocytes lying in a degenerating tract during the stage of myelin katabolism. The nucleus may become rather larger or more elongated and occasional cells have double nuclei, but the increase in the number of astrocyte nuclei is slight.

In simple atrophy of tracts, such as occurs in Friedreich's ataxia and other system diseases, an increase in the number of neuroglial fibres occurs and eventually leads to dense sclerosis in the area of the degenerated tracts, but the stages by which this occurs are usually too slow to be traceable. When the atrophy is more rapid some swelling of the cell body similar to that seen in Wallerian degeneration may be seen. The end result of all progressive neuroglial reaction is return of the cell body to its former insignificance and increase of neuroglial fibres, or *neuroglial sclerosis*.

The pattern of the newly formed neuroglial feltwork varies with environmental factors. In areas where there is preservation of some nerve fibres or axons, as when two or more tracts, only one of which is degenerated, lie in the same area, or in the plaques of disseminated sclerosis, the intact nerve fibres govern the orientation of neuroglial fibres. The name *isomorphous gliosis* is given to this pattern in which the previous arrangement of neuroglial fibres is preserved. On the other hand, when a tract is uniformly degenerated, or when there is gradual replacement of degenerating white matter by neuroglial tissue, the arrangement is more random. Neuroglial fibres which are attached to the connective tissue of meninges or blood-vessels run perpendicularly to them but elsewhere the pattern is quite irregular (*Anisomorphous gliosis*). Whorls of glial fibres are not uncommon in long-standing degenerations in the dorsal columns in tabes and Friedreich's ataxia. Penfield (1927) and del Rio Hortega and Penfield (1928) showed that, when collagenous tissue is formed in wounds of the brain, the neighbouring astrocytes become attached to it by strong processes, which appear to be pulled on by the later contraction of the collagen. In this way elongated or *piloid astrocytes* (Penfield 1932) may be formed. It is not uncommon in cortical scars to see a number of such cells lying parallel to one another in palisade arrangement above a layer of connective tissue.

Alzheimer types of neuroglial cell

Hösslin and Alzheimer (1912) described two unusual types of neuroglial cell in cases of hepatolenticular degeneration. In Type I the nucleus is large and stains darkly often showing a nucleolus which is basophilic with Nissl's stain. The cell body which is also large passes out into irregular blunt processes in which basophilic or greenish-yellow granules may be seen. With Nissl's stain these granules may be the only evidence of cytoplasm, and may roughly indicate the shape of the processes. In Type II the nucleus is swollen with a clearly defined nuclear membrane which may show infoldings. It contains little chromatin and one or two basophilic well-defined nucleoli (Fig. 1.14). These nuclei thus come to resemble those of small nerve cells. The cell body is usually invisible with most staining methods but a few fine greenish granules may be seen round the nucleus with Nissl's stain. Sometimes these nuclei are folded over so as to give a false impression of being double. No neuroglial fibres can be seen in relation to either type of neuroglial cell, and it is generally agreed that they arise from the protoplasmic astrocytes although, in Wilson's disease, they are commonly found in nuclei such as the substantia nigra and nucleus dentatus which contain many fibrous astrocytes.

These types of cell are constantly seen in cases of hepatolenticular degeneration and hepatic encephalopathy. While cells corresponding to Alzheimer's Type II are much the more common, transition forms between these and Type I are also frequently seen. They occur not only in the striatum but in other nuclei of the basal ganglia, pons and midbrain and in the cerebral cortex and the dentate nucleus and cortex of the cerebellum. They may be grouped close together suggesting recent division. In size they vary considerably, the largest nuclei measure up to 25μ in their longer diameter, but in some cases no nuclei larger than 15μ are seen. It is not always possible to be certain when a neuroglial nucleus acquires the characters of an Alzheimer nucleus of Type II. Rather large pale nuclei are commonly seen in the cerebral cortex in a variety of pathological conditions, such as general paralysis, and are often described as being those of Alzheimer cells, but the very large ballooned nuclei of Type II and cells of Alzheimer Type I are rarely found in these conditions. In hepatolenticular degeneration the smaller nuclei belonging to Type II cells are scarcely larger than those of normal astrocytes. There is, however, something rather characteristic in the distribution of the chromatin in these nuclei which draws attention to this abnormality and encourages the search for larger and more typical nuclei. The presence of granules round these nuclei varies not only from cell to cell but from case to case. They are of themselves no more characteristic of hepatolenticular degeneration than the nuclei. However, the association of large, ballooned, often infolded, nuclei with greenish-yellow granules in the surrounding cytoplasm, which is common in hepatolenticular degeneration, is rarely seen in other conditions.

Adams and Foley (1953) found ballooned, sometimes lobulated astrocyte nuclei corresponding to Alzheimer Type II in the cortex, basal ganglia, brain stem and cerebellum of 36 cases dying in hepatic coma. They were most numerous when the coma was prolonged. They may also be very abundant and widespread in long-standing cases of hepatic cirrhosis which show evidence of involvement of the nervous system such as attacks of coma, dementia, rigidity and tremor, but none of the biochemical features of Wilson's disease (Greenfield, 1953–4) (Fig. 1.14*f*).

Oligodendroglia

The credit for differentiating oligodendroglia from the other forms of supporting cell in the central nervous system must be given to del Rio Hortega, who in 1921 separated them from the neuroglia. Ford Robertson (1899, 1900), who had, much earlier, stained the interfascicular glia by a platinum method, called them mesoglial cells, but his description was inadequate and did not lead to general recognition of this cell type. Hortega's work was confirmed by Penfield (1924), and his nomenclature has become generally accepted.

On the electronic screen, the nuclei of oligodendroglial cells are denser than those of a neurone. According to de Robertis *et al.* (1958), they contain blocks of chromatin of a filamentous structure, similar to those found in chromosomes. They are separated from the cytoplasm by a double membrane. The cytoplasm is far denser than that of astrocytes and contains a moderate amount of endoplasmic reticulum lined by RNA granules, and of mitochondria. Their processes have been illustrated by Schultz *et al.* (1957) as passing between myelinated axons.

Hydén and Pigon were able to submit microdissected fresh nerve cells and their oligodendroglial satellites in Deiter's nucleus to separate microchemical analysis. They found that the two types of cells responded differently and often inversely to stimulation or hypoxia.

Lumsden and Pomerat (1951) observed pulsatile activity in normal oligodendrocytes, grown in culture. Such rhythmic activity has been previously seen by Canti, Bland and Russell

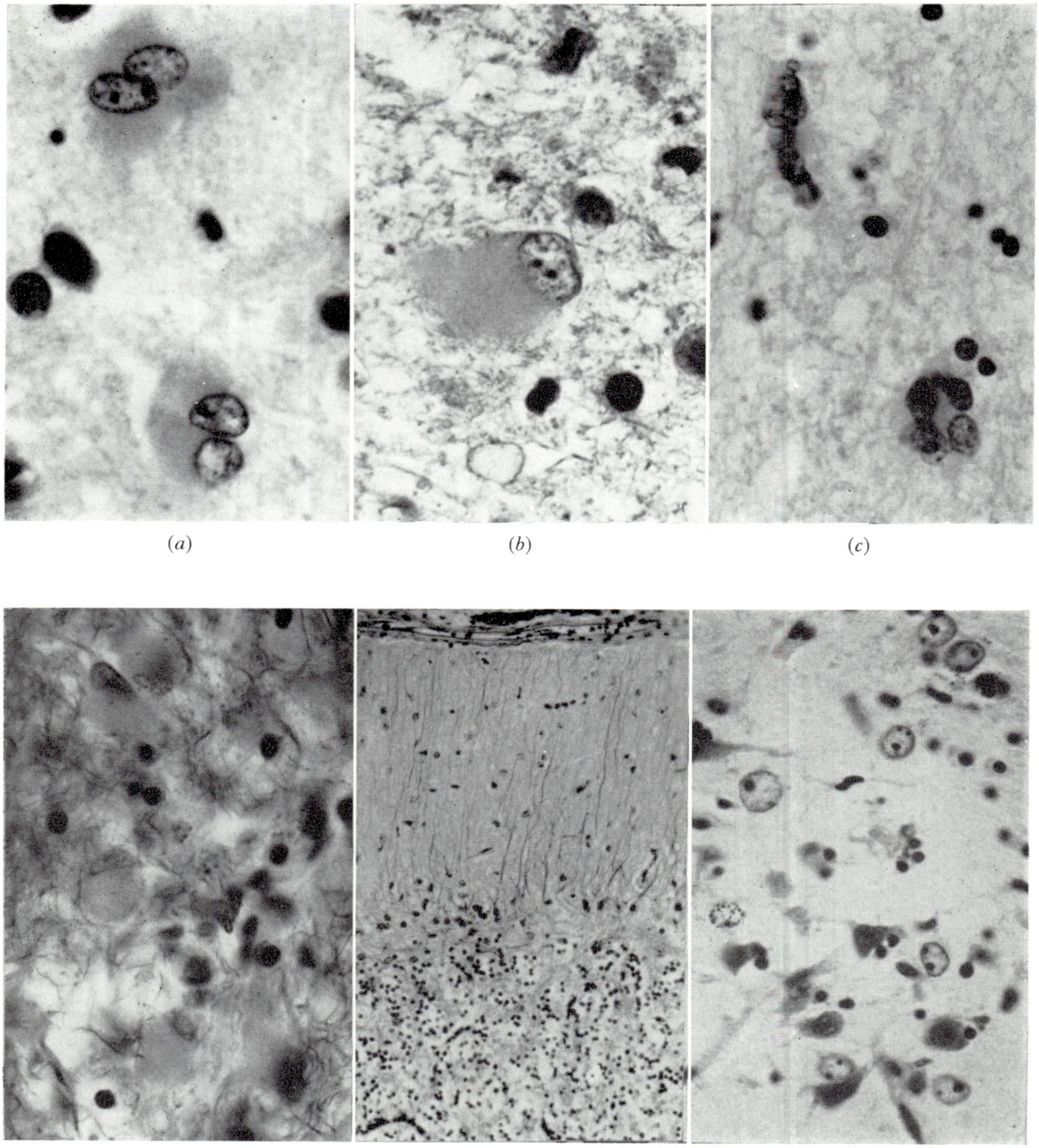

(*a*) (*b*) (*c*)

(*d*) (*e*) (*f*)

FIG. 1.14. Astrocytic reactions.

(*a*) Binucleated swollen-bodied cortical astrocytes. (*b*) Large fibre-forming astrocyte in white matter. (Mallory's phosphotungstic acid haematoxylin.) (*c*) Irregular multinucleation of astrocytes in white matter in area of oedema round a cerebral abscess. (*d*) Swelling of astrocytes and fibre formation in diffuse sclerosis (P.T.A.H.) (*e*) Isomorphous gliosis in cerebellar cortex in carcinomatous cerebellar degeneration (P.T.A.H.) (*f*) Swelling of nuclei of astrocytes in putamen in a case of hepatic encephalopathy. (Nissl.)

(1937) in outgrowths from cultures of an oligodendroglioma. However, as the authors are well aware, the occurrence of such movements *in vitro* does not imply that they are also present under normal living conditions.

Oligodendroglia appear as *perineuronal satellites* in the grey matter and as *interfascicular glia* in the white matter. A few occur as perivascular satellites. In all three types the nucleus is small, of the same size and appearance as that of a lymphocyte with abundant closely set chromatin granules. The cell body, which is small and irregularly rounded or oblong, gives off a few protoplasmic expansions some of which, in the satellite cells, wrap themselves round the cell body of a neurone while others end free. In the interfascicular cells they pass, often for considerable distances, along the surface of myelinated fibres. These expansions branch less often and less regularly than those of astrocytes and do not join connective tissue by foot-plates, but like astrocytes they contain gliosomes (mitochondria).

The *interfascicular oligodendroglia* are by far the most numerous cell in the white matter where they lie in rows of closely apposed nuclei, often as many as 20–40 in number (Penfield, 1932) between the myelinated fibres. Their close apposition makes it impossible to tell whether they normally multiply during life, but there is no obvious difference in their numbers at different ages. Lewis and Swank (1953) have shown experimentally that those in the neighbourhood of vessels may respond by proliferation and hypertrophy to mild ischaemia. Under these conditions no mitoses are seen. It seems probable that they may also respond by increase in numbers to other mild noxious stimuli, but of this there is so far no conclusive evidence.

Perineuronal satellites. Del Rio Hortega considered the perineuronal oligodendroglia to be analogous to the capsule cells of the dorsal root ganglia. They are common round the medium-sized pyramidal cells of the cortex and the large cells of the basal ganglia. They are not normally seen in relation to Purkinje cells and are rare round the large motor cells of the anterior horns of the cord, the motor nuclei of the brain stem and the precentral gyrus. It seems probable that they multiply in many forms of neuronal degeneration and the term *satellitosis of nerve cells* is often used, but it is difficult to tell whether the satellites round a particular neurone are in excess. Certainly six or more such cells are not infrequently seen round a single neurone under what appear to be normal conditions.

The relation of oligodendroglia to myelin

Del Rio Hortega (1928) considered that the interfascicular oligodendroglia held a relationship to myelin in the central nervous system similar to that of the Schwann cells in peripheral nerves. This view was supported by developmental evidence, since oligodendroglia are first differentiated in a tract or area of the central nervous system when myelination begins there. They then multiply rapidly and become arranged in rows between the nerve fibres. Further support is given to this view by the observation of Berliner (1931) that oligodendroglia are present among the myelinated nerve fibres of the rabbit's retina but are absent in retinae in which there is no myelin. They are not found in old standing plaques of disseminated sclerosis, and in some forms of diffuse sclerosis of the cerebral white matter they disappear before demyelination is evident (Greenfield 1933). Their relation to myelin is therefore definite but whether they are essential to the formation or nutrition of the myelin sheaths in the central nervous system is not known.

The *electron microscope* has so far not supplied unequivocal evidence of this relationship. De Robertis *et al.* (1958) found axons in different stages of myelination within the cytoplasm of oligodendrocytes, while Bunge *et al.* (1961) consider the myelin reforming cells in the spinal cord are not oligodendrocytes, but astrocytes. Maturana (1960) and Peters (1960), working with optic nerves of tadpoles and rats, and Périer and de Harven (1961) with mammalian cerebellar tissue, tentatively suggest that the external layer of myelin opens into a small cytoplasmic loop which may be the external mesaxon, and may be related to a glial process. Whether this belongs to astrocytes or oligodendrocytes is not yet established, but indirect electronmicroscopic evidence (relative density of cytoplasm and frequency of vesicular structures) seems to favour the oligodendrocyte as the myelin forming cell (Peters).

Acute swelling of the oligodendroglia

Penfield and Cone (1926) described, under the name *acute swelling*, a degenerative change in oligodendroglia which consisted in a rapid hypertrophy of the cytoplasm followed by swelling and vacuolation of the cell body and accumulation in it of unstainable fluid. This is usually associated with pyknotic changes in the nucleus. It may go on to the dissolution of the cell or the cell may recover and return to normal, at least from the earlier stages of the process. Penfield and Cone found this form of degeneration in a great variety of morbid conditions affecting the brain, both in post-mortem and biopsy material. It might appear as early as 6 hours in an area of cerebral embolism. It could be produced experimentally by guanidine poisoning and by the intravenous injection of water, and it was commonly found when death had occurred after prolonged coma. They considered that minor degrees might occur in post-mortem autolysis, and when slight before death it might increase *post mortem*, but more severe degrees were evidence that it had occurred during life.

Acute swelling of oligodendroglia may be associated with the appearance in the cell body of material which gives many of the staining reactions of mucin, and is probably a glycolipid. This material is not always present in swollen oligodendroglial cells and to what extent its demonstration depends on special techniques of fixation and embedding is not yet decided. It is commonly found in oligodendroglial cells in cases of diffuse sclerosis of the brain (Bailey and Schaltenbrand 1927) and also in oligodendroglial tumours in which it may accumulate between the cells (Bailey and Bucy 1929). Grynfeltt (1923), who found greatly distended cells filled with similar material in cases of senile dementia, used the term *mucocytes* to describe them. He considered that by dissolution of these swollen cells masses of mucinoid material could be set free in the tissues in which they tended to migrate to the walls of the ventricles. The lipid nature of this material was proved by Marion Smith (1949) by its solubility in lipase, but she was unable to confirm its origin in oligodendroglial cells. All that can be said at present is that under various conditions, many of which are associated with some degree of demyelination, swollen oligodendrocytes are found to contain a glycolipid resembling cerebroside, and that a similar material may be found in oligodendrogliomas.

Ependyma

The ventricles, iter of Sylvius and central canal of the cord, except at the area postrema of the 4th ventricle, are covered by ependymal cells which normally lie side by side in palisade formation. Their nuclei, which are oval and rather longer and more darkly stained than astrocyte nuclei, are arranged in a regular line. The inner, or ventricular, part of the cell body is cylindrical ending on a flat surface to which cilia are attached. Under these is a line of very small oval bodies named *blepharoplasts* (Greek for 'eyelash fixatives'), which are oriented in the long axis of the cells; they are well stained by phosphotungstic acid haematoxylin after Zenker fixation. The outer part of the cell consists of one, two or more tapering processes containing fine fibrils which pass into and merge with the underlying nervous tissues.

During life ependymal cells react little to disease processes. Under normal conditions they gradually lose their cilia, but those which line the ventricles and iter of Sylvius remain as an unbroken line. The central canal of the cord is usually encroached on, often during childhood, by ingrowth of neuroglial fibres and its ependymal cells remain in or near the same position, and appear as irregular groups of oval, darkly staining nuclei. These have been interpreted as proliferations in reaction to disease. While it is probable that there is some increase in the number of nuclei, the great variation in the normal makes any such interpretation apt to be fallacious.

The most common reaction of the ependymal surfaces to inflammation or irritation is *granular ependymitis*. In general paresis this is characteristically seen in the floor of the 4th ventricle, near the foramen of Monro and, in severe cases, also in the walls of the frontal horns of the lateral ventricle. It may also follow any inflammation of the ventricles, especially mild attacks of meningococcal meningitis. The appearance, which is best seen on oblique illumination, has been likened to coarse ground glass, but is usually more obviously granular than this.

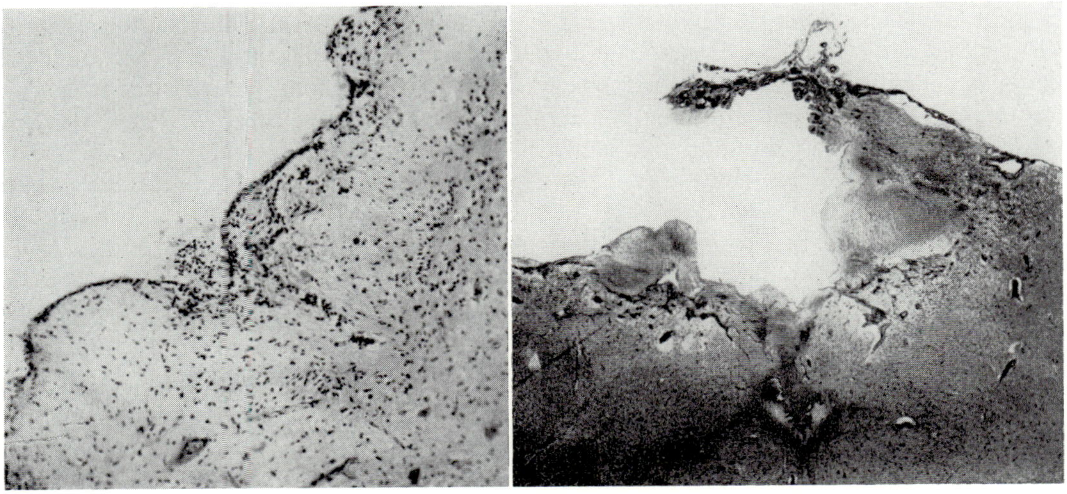

(*a*) (*b*)

FIG. 1.15. Ependymitis.

(*a*) Granular ependymitis in the 4th ventricle in a case of general paresis. (*b*) Neuroglial outgrowth filling the V of the 4th ventricle in chronic cerebrospinal syphilis.

Under the microscope the granulations appear as small hillocks of neuroglial fibres, which may be partly or entirely covered by ependymal cells or may have a broken line of ependymal nuclei at their base and one or two similar nuclei at higher levels (Fig. 1.15*a*). There is usually little evidence of proliferation or reaction by the ependymal cells and the name is therefore more applicable to naked eye than to microscopic appearances. A slight degree of granular ependymitis in the roof of the 4th ventricle near its upper end is so common that it cannot be considered abnormal.

In chronic meningovascular syphilis the whole of the ependyma on the floor of the 4th venticle is often covered with a pad of neuroglial fibres (Fig. 1.15*b*). In this case instead of being smooth and glistening the ventricular surface has a dull matt appearance and the median raphe is less clearly marked than normal.

In hydrocephalus the line of the ependyma in the ventricles is broken by the stretching of their walls. Usually rows of ependymal cells alternate with gaps in which none are seen. In subacute and chronic cases these gaps are filled by neuroglial fibres which form cushions elevated slightly above the line of the ependymal cells. There is no evidence that the ependyma proliferates in an attempt to cover these bared areas.

Microglia

The separation by del Rio Hortega (1919) of the microglia from the group of small cells in the central nervous system, which Cajal (1913) had called the *third element*, was an important turning point in the history of neuropathology. Earlier studies of the neuroglia had left opinion divided as to whether phagocytosis in the central nervous system was undertaken by wandering histiocytes arising in the vessel walls, or by cells of neuroglial origin. The demonstration by del Rio Hortega that the microglia, although normally present in the tissues of the central nervous system, was of mesoblastic origin and had many of the characters and potentialities of histiocytes elsewhere in the body, provided a simple answer to the question of phagocytosis. The name Hortega cells, which is often used in German literature, is therefore well justified, although his own name, *microglia*, is preferable. Del Rio Hortega found that microglial cells invaded the central nervous system from the meninges during the later stages of embryonic development when the vascularisation of the central nervous system was at its height. At this time large numbers of small cells with short irregular processes can be seen in those areas of white matter which are in contact with the meninges, especially at the base of the brain and round the brain stem.

From these foci the microglia migrate throughout the central nervous system and eventually become most abundant in the grey matter. In their resting stage they develop two or more thin processes with fine lateral projections which can be stained by special silver impregnation techniques but are not visible with ordinary tissue stains. In the grey matter they may lie free as bipolar or multipolar cells or may be perineuronal or perivascular satellites. In the white matter most of them occur round the vessels. The nucleus remains small and hyperchromic, and its shape is related to the number of cell processes. In bipolar cells it is elongated, and when three or more processes are present it may be irregularly triangular or polyhedral. Only rarely is it as evenly spherical as the nucleus of an oligodendrocyte and it is rather more hyperchromic. These characteristics usually make it possible to distinguish microglial from oligodendroglial nuclei with general tissue stains. In the *electron microscope* the microglia is characterised by the extreme overall density of its nucleus and cytoplasm, often making their delineation difficult. The angular branching processes retain this density. Moderate amounts of granular and agranular reticulum and of mitochondria are enclosed within the cytoplasm. Strongly osmophilic clumps may originate from digested material (Luse 1956; Schultz *et al.* 1957). Microglial cells react rapidly to noxious stimuli by hyperplasia and multiplacation by mitosis. They are actively phagocytic. As they are less vulnerable than neuroglial cells, they may remain active in areas where both the neurones and neuroglia have undergone necrosis and they are often seen, laden with lipid granules, in and around such partially necrotic areas. The reactions of the microglia may be classified as (*a*) *proliferation*, (*b*) *hypertrophy*, (*c*) *phagocytosis of lipid*, (*d*) *neuronophagy* and *dendrophagocytosis*.

(*a*) *Proliferation* of microglia is seen in many forms of acute and subacute encephalitis, as well as in the neighbourhood of softenings. It may be diffuse in an area, giving an appearance of increased cellularity, but where the reaction is less intense it may be quite local, either in the neighbourhood of vessels or independently of these. In this way clumps of microglial cells or *glial stars* may be formed. These often contain 10 or 20 small closely set microglial nuclei. These *glial stars* or *knots* are common in encephalomyelitis. They occur chiefly in the grey matter but may also be seen in the white matter both in the brain and spinal cord. While it is impossible to be certain that some of those in the grey matter are not related to dead nerve cells this is less likely in the white matter. Small glial knots may also be seen in the white columns of the cord in what appear to be purely degenerative conditions. Therefore, although they are very characteristic of the response to virus infection, they are not always evidence of inflammation. In typhus fever the characteristic perivascular nodules are, in the central nervous system, formed largely of microglial cells, although histiocytes from the vessel walls also take part in the process. It is often difficult or impossible to be certain whether cells which proliferate in the immediate neighbourhood of vessels, for example in post-infectious encephalomyelitis, are of microglial or vascular origin. In some the nuclei are too large to be characteristic of microglia, whereas in others hyperchromic nuclei of irregular shape may belong to either type of cell.

(*b*) *Hypertrophy* of microglial cells is seen most characteristically in the cerebral cortex in general paralysis (paretic dementia) but is also found in other forms of subacute encephalitis. The processes enlarge both in length and to a less extent in width. They may lose some of their lateral spines but do not otherwise change their form. The nucleus also enlarges. A very characteristic appearance is given by the bipolar microglial cells which normally lie radially orientated in the cerebral cortex. In these cells the nucleus becomes more elongated and the processes may become stainable by Nissl's method for some distance from its poles. With silver technique they may be seen to run for long distances perpendicular to the surface with little branching (Fig. 1.16*a*). To cells of this kind Nissl gave the name *rod cells* (Stäbchenzellen). In general paralysis their processes may contain fine granules which give the Prussian blue and Turnbull's blue reactions for iron. When the multipolar cells hypertrophy, their nuclei become more lobulated and may assume very irregular shapes though the lobules are never so separate as in polymorphonuclear leucocytes (Fig. 1.16*a*). Asteroid or long curved, sometimes horseshoe shaped, nuclei are not uncommon. This process of simple hypertrophy is often associated with some increase in numbers, but this is not so evident as in more acutely destructive lesions. It is probable that the hypertrophied cells may revert to a more normal size, since rod cells and other hypertropic forms may not be present in the cortex in cured cases of general paralysis.

(*c*) When microglial cells take on the *phagocytosis of lipids* the cell body enlarges and the processes become shorter and thicker. This process may go on until the cell becomes spherical, but in the earlier stages, or when degenerating myelin is less abundant as in the cerebral or cerebellar cortex, phagocytosis of lipid may occur in processes which still extend some distance from the cell body (Fig. 1.16*c*, *d*). Indeed fine lipid droplets may be found in typical rod cells. The reaction of microglia to the breakdown of nervous tissue is fairly rapid. It has been seen that, in Wallerian degeneration of tracts in the central nervous system, cells of microglial origin may invade the tubes of myelin about 4 days after the lesion. Rand and Courville (1932) in cases of cerebral trauma found reacting forms of microglia within a few hours of the accident, and rounded lipid phagocytes after 3 or 4 days. They noted that only amitotic division was seen during the first 2 or 3 days after an injury, but mitotic division was present in later stages. Even cells which are already charged with lipid granules may undergo mitosis during the first few days of a necrotic lesion.

The migratory activity of microglial cells was emphasised by del Rio Hortega (1932), who saw the accumulation of phagocytes in an area of necrosis as partly a multiplication of the cells already in the area and partly an invasion from outside. From the experiments of Wells and Carmichael (1930) and Costero (1930) it is clear that microglial cells have migratory powers in tissue culture, and it is probable that some potentialities of this kind are retained by the resting

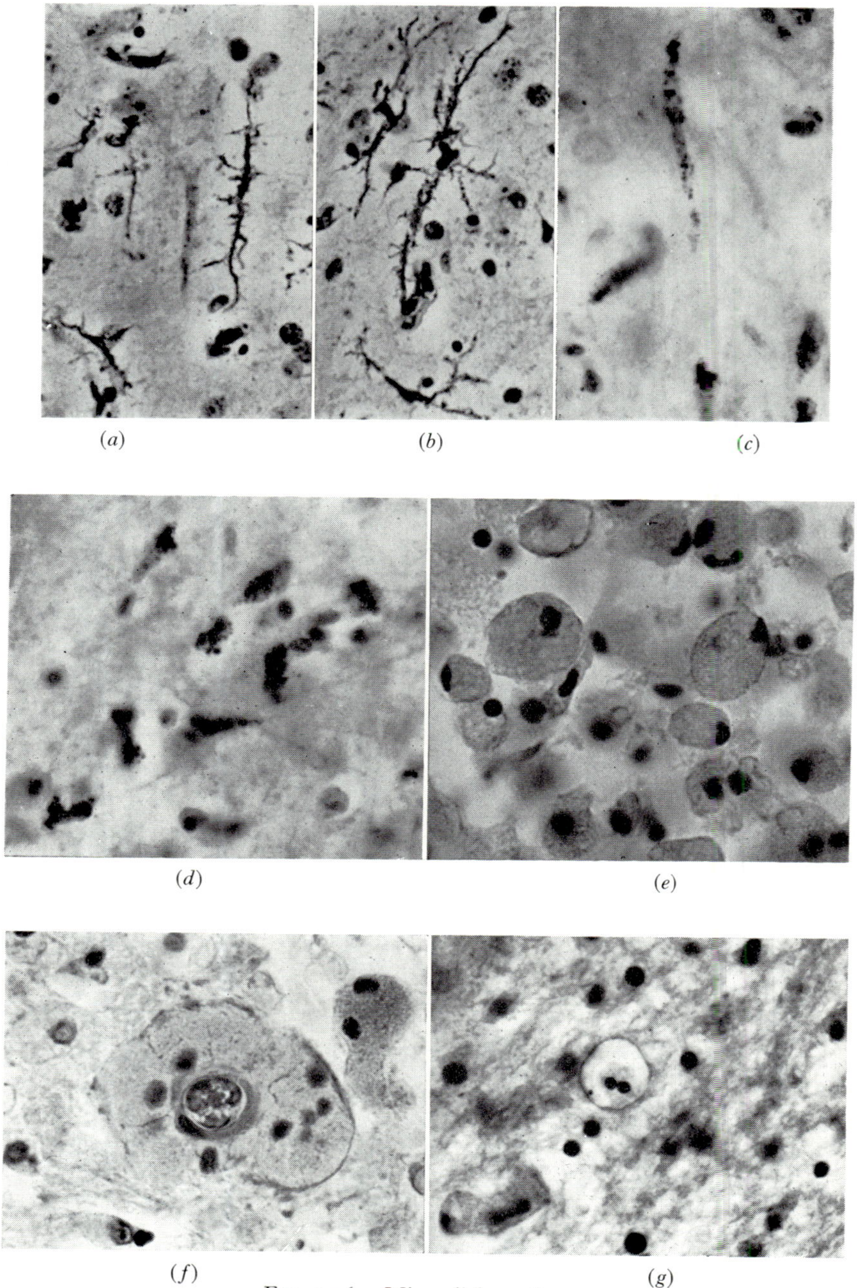

FIG. 1.16. Microglial reactions.

(*a*) and (*b*) Cerebral cortex in general paresis showing early enlargement of microglia; (*a*) rod cell, (*b*) triradiate cell. (Silver carbonate, ×400.)

(*c*) and (*d*) Cerebral cortex in subacute encephalitis; (*c*) rod cell filled with small lipid granules, (*d*) thickening and shortening of processes as lipid granules are absorbed. (Scharlach R. haemalum.)

(*e*) and (*f*) Focus of softening in spinal cord; (*e*) large lipid phagocytes, (*f*) collection of lipid phagocytes in Virchow-Robin space of small vessel. (Iron haematoxylin van Gieson, ×550.)

(*g*) Myeloclast in swollen myelin sheath in oedematous area of subcortical white matter.

microglia, and may be stimulated by chemiotactic influences arising in the necrotic nervous tissue. Their powers of migration are probably comparable to those of histiocytes in other tissues of the body. After ingestion of lipid they appear to be very inert and remain in the same area for many weeks in most cases. Eventually they find their way, either by slow migration or owing to the flow of tissue fluids, to the walls of the blood vessels where fat granule cells accumulate

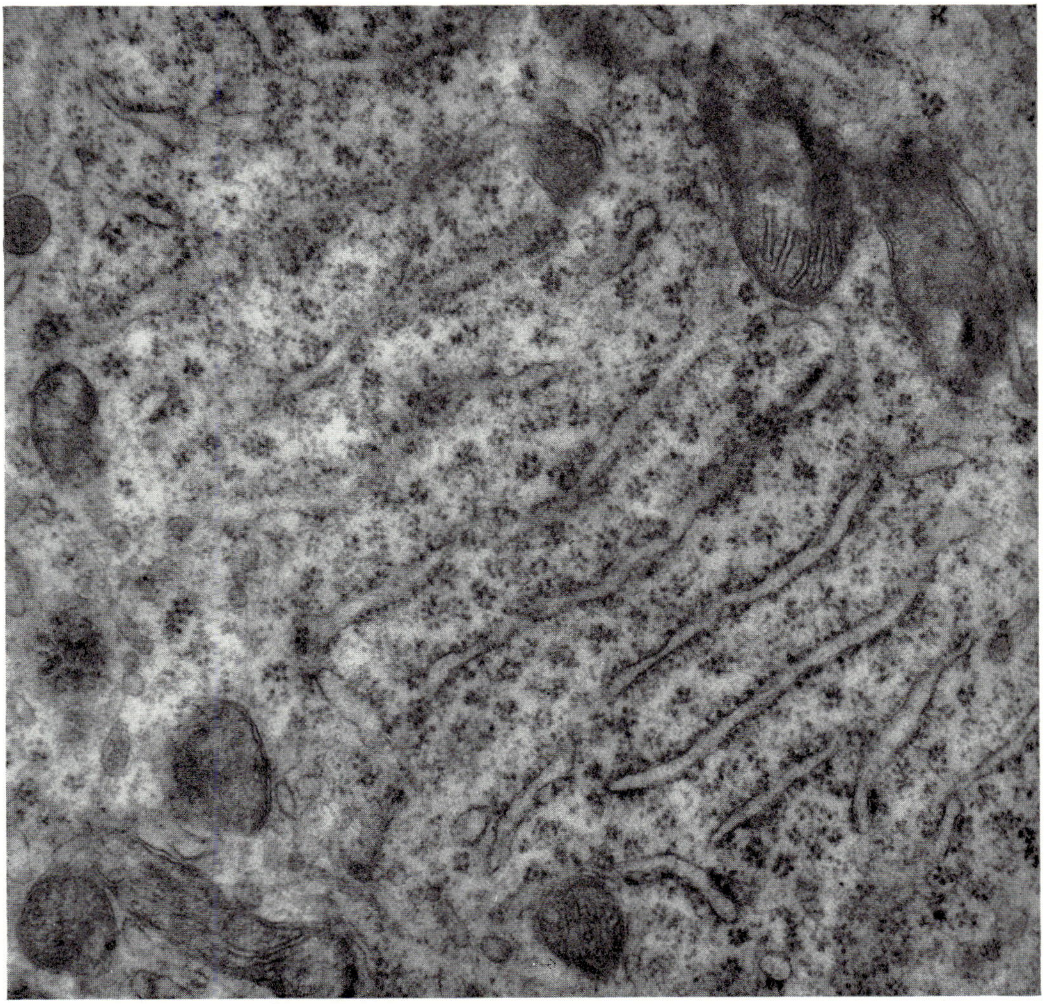

FIG. 1.17. Purkinje cell in the rat's cerebellum showing a Nissl body with mitochondria of varying size, the channels of the endoplasmic reticulum and the dense granules lining these or lying in clusters between. (×44,000.) (Reproduced from a forthcoming (1962) edition of Maximow and Bloom's Textbook of Histology, Saunders, Philadelphia, by kindness of Professor S. L. Palay.)

both round and within the perivascular (Virchow-Robin) spaces (Fig. 1.16*g*). These cells may not be the same as those which undertook the earlier stages of lipid katabolism. There may well be, as earlier German studies suggested, relays of lipid phagocytes, and histiocytic cells in the Virchow-Robin spaces may undertake the latest stages of the process. Nuclei of lipid phagocytes of microglial origin tend to retain the same shape as in the original cell (Fig. 1.16*e*).

Thus elongated or triangular nuclei are common in rounded granule cells, especially in the earlier stages, and should not be considered as evidence of pyknotic degeneration.

The nomenclature of lipid phagocytes in the central nervous system has never been very satisfactory. There are many objections to the old term *compound granular corpuscle*. The French omit the meaningless word 'compound' and call them 'corps granuleux', but this indicates neither that they are nucleated

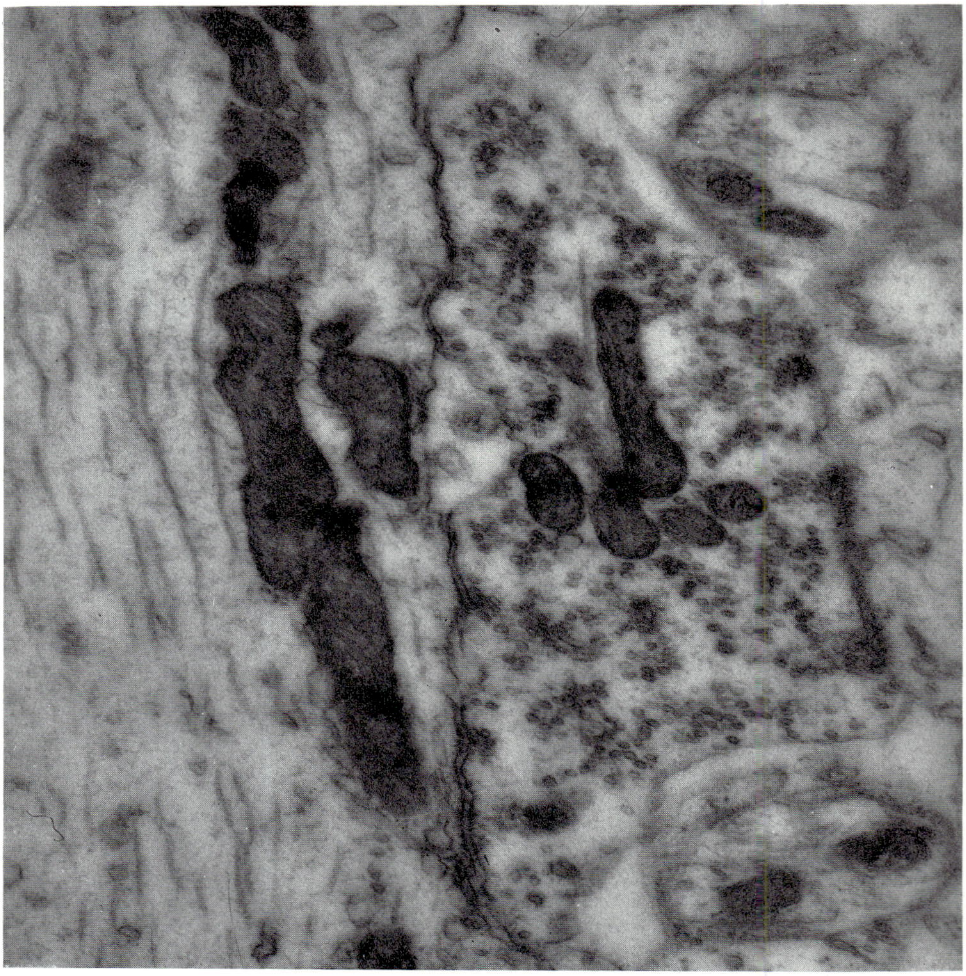

FIG. 1.18. Abducens nucleus of the rat. A terminal bouton (centre) containing mitochondria and numerous microvesicles; separated by a double membrane from dendrite (left) which shows mitochondria and endoplasmic reticulum. (×40,000.) (Reproduced from *J. Biophys. Biochem. Cytol.* 1956, **2** (suppl.), 193, fig. 2, by kindness of Professor S. L. Palay.)

cells nor that their contents are of lipid character. Jakob's 'granule cell' is scarcely more informative. The term *fat granule cell* is applicable to the later stages of myelin katabolism, but may be misleading in the earlier stages. *Foamy cell*, which is used in general pathology, is perhaps rather too indefinite, and *lattice cell*, though a literal translation of the German *Gitterzell* has no obvious meaning to the uninitiated. The term *lipid phagocyte* would seem to be exact and unobjectionable, but has not yet received general acceptance.

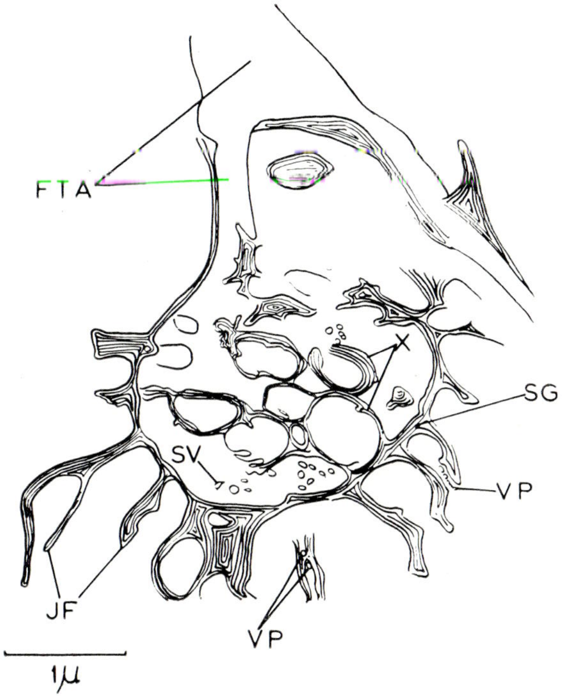

FIG. 1.19. Drawing from an electron micrograph of a myasthenic end plate, showing synaptic vesicles (SV), the synaptic grooves (SG) and the junctional folds (JF) in the muscle surface membrane. The structures labelled X may be degenerated mitochondria, but these and other changes are not considered specific of myasthenia. (Reproduced from *Brain* 1960, **83,** 638, fig. 10*a*, by kindness of Dr. A. L. Woolf.)

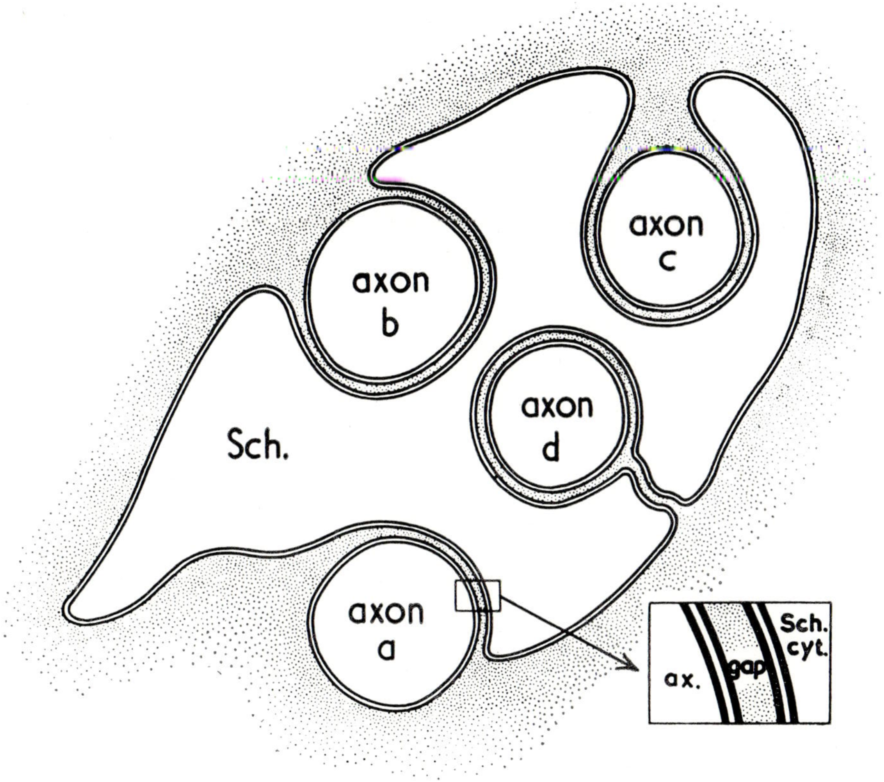

FIG. 1.20. Diagram showing a Schwann cell with 4 associated axons in different stages of envelopment. Only axon *d* is sufficiently deeply embedded to have a complete mesaxon formed by the enveloping double Schwann cell membranes. Robertson's 'Unit' (shown also enlarged) consists of the (double) membranes of both axon and cell. (Reproduced from text fig. 7.2 in 'Electronmicroscopy in Anatomy' London 1961, by kindness of Professor J. D. Robertson.)

In discussing Wallerian degeneration reference was made to Jakob's three forms of rounded lipid-containing cell which he called *granule cells* α, β and γ. Type α granule cells contain fine droplets of lipid; the β type both finer and coarser granules, while the γ type represents the last stage and contains only coarse granules, most of which have the characters of neutral fat. It is often impossible in embedded sections to be certain what stage of lipid katabolism has been reached by the contents of a cell, but the size of the droplets and their staining reactions with iron haematoxylin or phosphotungstic acid haematoxylin may be distinguishing features.

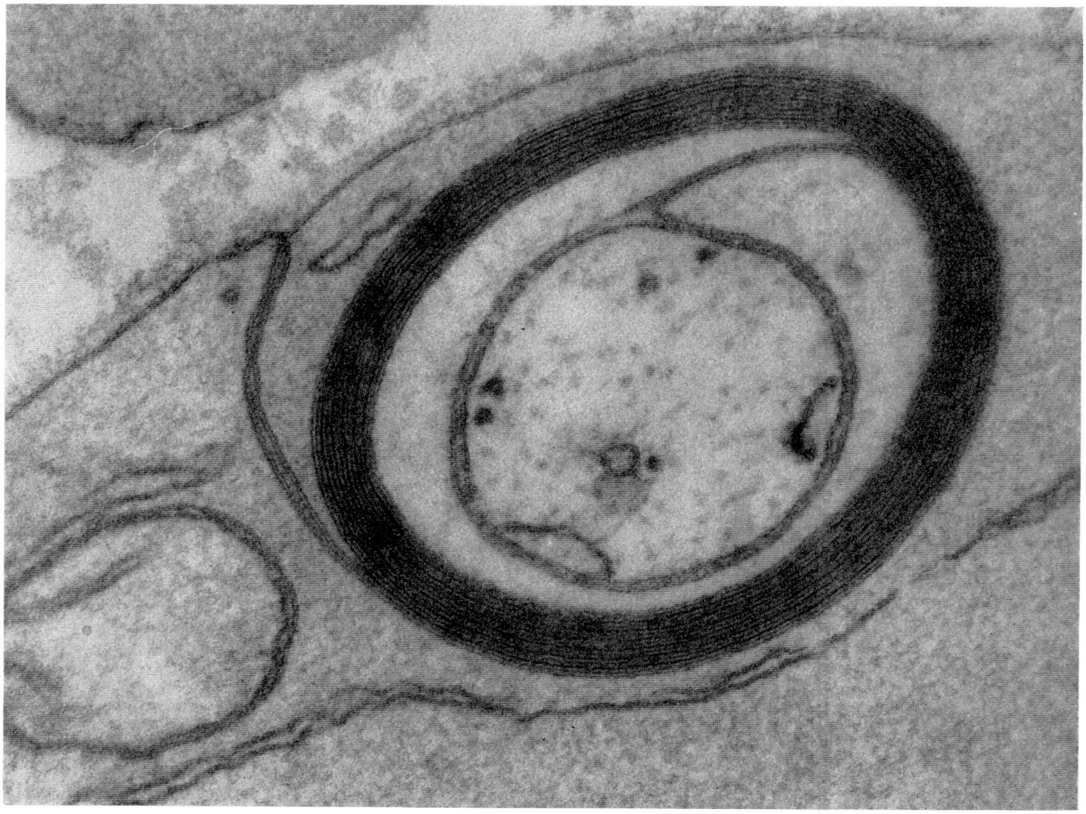

FIG. 1.21. Schwann cell of the giant nerve of the crayfish, with a myelinated axon embedded in it. The laminated structure of the myelin, and both the outer and inner mesaxons are clearly demonstrated. (×24,000.) (Reproduced from *Ann. New York Acad. Sc.*, 1961, **94**, 350, fig. 9, by kindness of Professor J. D. Robertson.)

Some newer staining methods, such as periodic acid-leucofuchsin (Schiff) or Lendrum's phloxin-tartrazine, although not designed for this purpose, are also of some value in distinguishing the more complex from the simpler lipids.

(*d*) *Neuronophagy*. When nerve cells undergo rapid death it is common to find their cell body and proximal dendrites invaded by phagocytic cells. When the necrotic process is very acute, as in the anterior horn cells in poliomyelitis, the earliest invading cells may be polymorphonuclear leucocytes, but in later stages the great majority of the phagocytes appear to be derived from the microglia. It is characteristic of poliomyelitis to see groups of twenty or more of these cells, indicating the positions of dead motor neurones. When the necrosis of nerve cells is less acute than in poliomyelitis the phagocytis cells are less numerous and often form a ring round the cell body or invade it at a few places only. For this process the term *neuronophagy*, which was given by classical writers, is apt and descriptive. True neuronophagy by microglial cells must be distinguished from satellitosis, which is mainly a reaction of oligodendroglia. In the former case the nerve cell is undergoing dissolution, while in the latter case it shows much less evidence of degeneration. Neuronophagy is specially common in all forms of encephalomyelitis which affect the grey matter, and it may be that the manner of death of the neurone has a special chemiotactic attraction for microglial cells. It is less common when neurones die as the result of anoxia or direct trauma, although it may be seen in both these conditions. For example in the anoxaemic condition of the lower spinal cord called *subacute necrotic myelitis* by Foix and Alajouanine (1926) neuronophagy of anterior horn cells is not uncommon.

Neuronophagy may be seen in the white matter in childhood involving nerve cells which have failed to reach the cortex in their developmental migration. A very characteristic appearance may be seen in the neuronophagy of Purkinje cells. Here the microglial phagocytes are grouped not only round the cell body but also along the dendrites in the molecular layer where the normal paucity of nuclei makes their increase very obvious. A shrub-like arrangement of cell bodies and short processes is thus formed to which Spielmeyer gave the name Gliastrauchwerk (glial shrub formation). This was first described in typhus fever, but is also seen, affecting few or many Purkinje cells, in some forms of virus encephalitis and also in non-inflammatory processes, for example in the cerebellar degeneration associated with carcinoma.

The microglia may calcify in conditions such as the Sturge-Weber syndrome, Fahr's disease and certain forms of encephalitis (Alexander and Norman, 1960). In the Sturge-Weber syndrome these calcified cells are frequently found in or near areas of neuronal cortical destruction and below areas of massive calcification, and they may stand out with the clarity of a silver impregnation. Other microglial cells are seen to be more coarsely incrusted and their branches to be ending in small balls of calcified material. These may be precursors of 'free' concretions. In contrast, neurones rarely calcify in the Sturge-Weber syndrome.

REFERENCES

The Neurone

Achucarro, N. (1910) *Nissl Alzheimer Arbeiten*, **3**, 143.
Adams, C. W. M. (1958) *J. Neurochem.*, **2**, 178.
Alexander, L. (1938) *Brain* **61**, 52.
Alexander, L. and Myerson, A. (1938) *Arch. Neurol. Psychiat.* (Chicago), **39**, 131.
Alzheimer, A. (1907) *Centralbl. f. Nervenheilk.*, **30**, 177.
Andriezen, W. L. (1893) *Brit. Med. J.*, ii, 227.
Aring, C. D., Bean, W. B., Roseman, E., Rosenbaum, M. and Spies, T. D. (1941) *Arch. Neurol. Psychiat.* (Chicago), **45**, 772.
Arnell, N. (1936) *Acta Psychiat. Neurol.*, **11**, 5.
le Baron, F. N. and Folch-Pi, J. (1956) *J. Neurochem*, **1**, 101.
Barr, M. L. and Bertram, L. F. (1949) *Nature*, **163**, 676.
Barr, M. L., Bertram, L. F. and Lindsay, H. D. (1950) *Anat. Rec.*, **107**, 283.
Barr, M. L. and Bertram, E. G. (1951) *J. Anat.*, **85**, 171.
Barton, A. A. and Causey, G. (1958) *J. Anat.*, **92**, 399.
Batten, F. E. (1903) *Trans. Ophthal. Soc. U.K.*, **23**, 386.
Beams, H. W., van Breemen, V. L., Newfang, D. M. and Evans, T.C. (1952) *J. Comp. Neurol.*, **96**, 249.
Beheim-Schwarzbach, D. (1952) *J. nerv. ment. Dis.*, **116**, 619.
Belt, W. D. and Pease, D. C. (1956) *J. Biophys. Biochem. Cytology*, **2**, 369.
Bensley, R. R. and Hoerr, N. L. (1934) *Anat. Rec.*, **60**, 251, 449.
Bertrand, I. and Hadzigeorgiou, G. (1928) *Ann. de Med.*, **24**, 119.

Bertrand, I., Liber, A. F. and Randoin, L. (1934) *Arch. d'anatom. microscop.* **30** 297.

Bethe, A. (1898) *Arch. f. Mikr. Anat.*, **51**, 382.

Bickerstaff, E. R., Evans, J. V. and Woolf, A. L. (1960) *Brain*, **83**, 638.

Bielschowsky, M. (1902) *Neurol. Centralbl.*, **21**, 579; (1904) ibid., **23**, 387; (1913) *Dtsch. Z. Nerverheilk.*, **50**, 7; (1928) in *Handbuch der Mikroskop. Anat. des Menschen*, W. von Möllendorff, **4**, 97, J. Springer, Berlin; (1932) in Penfield's *Cytology and Cellular Pathology of the Nervous System*, p. 147, Hoeber, New York.

Bird, A. (1948) *Brain*, **71**, 434.

Birks, R., Katz, B. and Miledi, R. (1959) *J. Physiol.*, **146**, 45.

Bodian, D. (1947) *Symp. Soc. Exp., Biol.*, **1**, 163 (1949) *Poliomyelitis*, p. 62, Pitman Medical, London; (1951) *J. Comp. Neurol.*, **94**, 475.

Boeke, J. (1950) In Weiss, P. *Genetic Neurology*, pp. 78–92, University of Chicago Press.

Bok, S. T. (1940) *Proc. Neder. Akad. van Wetenschappen*, **43**, 1191 (1960) In *Structure and Function of the Cerebral Cortex*, edited by Tower, D. B. and Schade, J., Amsterdam.

Bouman, L. (1934) *Brain*, **57**, 128.

Brain, W. R., Greenfield, J. G. and Russell, D. S. (1948) *Brain*, **71**, 365.

Brante, G. (1949) *Acta Physiol. Scand.*, **18**, Suppl. 63.

Brodal, A. (1940) *Z. ges. Neurol. Psychiat.*, **169**, 1.

Byrom, F. B. (1954) *Lancet*, (ii), 201.

Cajal, S. R. y. (1897) *Rev. trimest. micrograph. Madrid*, **2**, 29; (1903) *Trab. Lab. Invest. Biol.*, Madrid, **2**, 129; (1904) ibid., **3**, 9; (1909) *Histologie du Système Nerveux de l'homme et des vertébres*, Maloine, Paris; (1927–8) *Degeneration and regeneration of the Nervous System*, Oxford.

Calzavara, E. and Bertrand, I. (1927) *Ann. de l'Anatomie Pathol.*, **4**, 461.

Caspersson, T. (1940) *J. Roy. Micro. Soc.*, **60**, 8.

Causey, G. and Barton, A. A. (1961) In *Cytology of Nervous Tissue*, Proc. Anat. Soc., London.

Cavanagh, J. B. (1954) *J. Neurol. Neurosurg. and Psychiat.*, **17**, 163.

Ceccherinelli, A. (1874) *Med. Jahrbuch.*, p. 343.

Chang, H. T. (1952) *Cold Spring Harbour Symposia*, **17** 189.

Choja, N. (1936) *Mitt. med. Akad. Kioto*, **17**, 900; ibid., **18**, 322, 793, 1714.

Chu, L. W. (1954) *J. Comp. Neurol.*, **100**, 381.

Coen, E. (1888). Ziegler's *Beitrag z. path. Anat. u. Physiol.*, **2**, 103.

Coers, C. and de Harven, E. (1962) *Proc. 4th Int. Congr. Neuropath.*, **2**, 7.

Coers, C. and Woolf, A. L. (1959) *The Innervation of Muscle*, Oxford.

Conel, J. R. (1939–59) *The Postnatal Development of the Human Cerebral Cortex*, 6 Vols., Cambridge (Mass.).

Corsellis, J. A. N. (1951) *J. ment. Sc.*, **97**, 570.

Couteaux, R. (1958) *Exper. Cell. Research, Suppl.*, **5**, 294.

Cowdry, E. V. (1912) *Int. Mschr. Anat. Physiol.*, **29**, 443; (1914) *Amer. J. Anat.*, **17**, 1.

Cramer, F. and Alpers, B. J. (1932) *Arch. Pathol.*, **13**, 23.

Crouch, Y. F. and Barr, M. L. (1954) *J. Neuropath.*, **13**, 353.

Davison, A. N., Dobbin, J., Morgan, R. S. and Payling Wright, G. (1959) *Lancet*, (i) 658.

Davison, C. and Keschner, M. (1940) *Arch. Neurol. Psychiat.* (Chicago), **43**, 524.

Dempsey, E. W. (1961) In *Chemical Pathology of the Nervous System*, ed. Folch-Pi, J., New York, London.

Denny-Brown, D. and Brenner, G. (1944 a) *Arch. Neurol. Psychiat.* (Chicago), **51**, 1; (1944 b) *J. Neurol. Neurosurg. and Psychiat.*, **7**, 76.

Divry, P. (1934) *J. Belge. Neurol. Psychiat.*, **34**, 197.

Duncan, D. (1934) *J. Comp. Neurol.*, **60**, 437.

Ehrlich, P. (1886) *Dtsch. Med. Wschr.*, **12**, 49.

Einarson, L. (1933) *Amer. J. Anat.*, **53**, 141; (1935) *J. Comp. Neurol.*, **61**, 101; (1945) *Acta Jutlandica*, **17**; (1949) *Acta Orthopaed. Scand.*, **19**, 27; (1957 in *Metabolism of the Nervous System*, ed. Richter D. London; (1960) in *Modern Scientific Aspects of Neurology*, ed. Cumings, J. N. London.

Einarson, L. and Lorentzen, K. A. (1946) *Acta Jutlandica*, **18**.

Evans, D. H. L. and Gray, E. G. (1961) In *Cytology of Nervous Tissue*, Proc. Anat. Soc., p. 71, London.

Fajerstajn. (1901) *Neur. Centralbl.*, **20**, 98.

Farquhar, M. J. and Hartmann, J. F. (1957) *J. Neuropath.*, **16**, 18.

Fedorow, B. G. (1935) *Trab. lab. Invest. Biol.*, Madrid, **30**, 403.

Feigin, I. and Wolf, A. (1955) *J. Neuropath.*, **14**, 11.

Fenyes, I. (1932) *Arch. Psychiat. Nervenkr.*, **96**, 700.
Fernandez-Moran, H. (1950) *Exper. Cell. Research*, **1**, 143, 309; (1952) *Exper. Cell. Research*, **3**, 282. (1954) *Progr. Biophys.*, **4**, 112; (1957) In *Metabolism of the Nervous System*, ed. Richter, D., London;
Finean, J. B. (1961 a) In *Electron Microscopy in Anatomy*, ed. Boyd, J. D. *et al.*, London; (1961 b) *Proc. Roy. Soc. Med.*, **54**, 19.
Finean, J. B. and Woolf, A. L. (1962) *J. Neuropath.*, **21**, 105.
Foerster, O. and Gagel, O. (1934) *Z. mikro-anat. Forschung*, **36**, 567.
Foix, C., Chavany, J. A. and Hillemand, P. (1926) *Rev. Neurol.*, (i), 942.
Folch-Pi, J., Casals, J., Pope, A., Meath, J. A., le Baron, F. N. and Lees, M. (1959) In *Biology of Myelin*, ed. Korey, S. R., New York.
Freeman, W. and Dumoff, E. (1944) *Arch. Neurol. Psychiat.* (Chicago), **51**, 67.
Gasser, H. S. (1955) *J. gen. Physiol.*, **38**, 709.
Gaupp, R. (1933) *Z. ges. Neurol. Psychiat.*, **149**, 122.
Geren, B. B. (1954) *Exper. Cell Research*, **7**, 558.
Gersh, I. and Bodian, D. (1943) *J. Cell. Comp. Physiol.*, **21**, 253.
Glees, P. (1944) *J. Anat.*, **78**, 47.
Glees, P. and Le Gros Clark, W. E. (1941) ibid., **75**, 295.
Gray, E. G. (1961) In *Electron Microscopy in Anatomy*, ed. Boyd, J. D. *et al.*, London.
Greenfield, J. G. (1934) *Brain*, **57**, 161; (1951) *Proc. Roy. Soc. Med.*, **44**, 686.
Greenfield, J. G. and Bosanquet, F. D. (1953) *J. Neurol. Neurosurg. Psychiat.*, **16**, 213.
Greenfield, J. G. and Stern, R. O. (1927) *Brain*, **50**, 652.
Gudden, B. (1870) *Arch. Psychiat. Nervenkr.*, **2**, 693.
Hager, H. (1961) *Acta. Neuropath.*, **1**, 9.
Hallervorden, J. (1933) *Klin. Wschr.*, **12**, 692; (1935) *Dtsch. Z. Nervenheilk.*, **136**, 68.
Harman, J. W. (1958) *J. Clin. Path.*, **11**, 495.
Harriman, D. G. F. and Millar, J. H. D. (1955) *Brain*, **78**, 325.
Harrison, R. G. (1910) *J. exper. Zool.*, **9**, 787; (1924) *J. Comp. Neurol.*, **31**, 125.
Hartmann, J. F. (1948) *Anat. Record*, **100**, 49.
de Harven, E. and Coers, C. (1961) In *Electron Microscopy in Anatomy*, ed. Boyd, J. D. *et al.*, London.
Hassler, R. (1937) *J. Psychol. Neurol.*, **48**, 1, 387.
Helfand, M. (1935) *J. nerv. ment. Dis.*, **81**, 662.
Hess, A. J. (1953) *J. Compar. Neurol.*, **98**, 69; (1955) *J. Compar. Neurol.*, **102**, 65; (1958) *J. Anat.*, **92**, 298.
Hess, H. and Young, J. Z. (1949) *Nature*, **164**, 490.
Hoff, E. C. and Hoff, H. E. (1934) *Brain*, **57**, 454.
Holmes, G. (1903) *Z. allg. Physiol.*, **2**, 502; (1907) *Brain*, **30**, 466.
Holmes, J. H. and Tower, D. B. (1955) In *Neuro-chemistry*, edited by Elliott, Page and Quastel, C. C. Thomas, Springfield.
Horstadius, S. (1950) *The Neural Crest*, Oxford Univ. Press.
Hudson, G. and Hartmann, J. F. (1961) *Z. Zellforsch.*, **54**, 147.
Hurst, E. W. (1925) *Brain*, **48**, 1; (1929) *J. Path. Bact.*, **32**, 457.
Hydén, H. (1947) *Cold Spring Harbor Symposia Quant. Biol.*, **12**, 104; (1950) In Weiss P. *Genetic Neurology*, p. 177, Chicago Univ. Press.
Hydén, H. and Hartelius, H. (1948) *Acta psychiat. et neurol.*, **48**, Suppl.
Hydén, H. and Pigon, A. (1960) *J. Neurochem.*, **6**, 157.
Jakob, A. (1912) *Nissl-Alzheimer Arbeiten*, **5**.
Jolly. (1870) *Studien aus dem Institut f. experimentelle Pathologie in Wien.*
Kedrowski, B. (1935) *Arch. mikr. Anat.*, **31**, 451.
Koelle, B. (1955) *J. Neuropath.*, **14**, 24.
Koenig, H., Groat, R. A. and Windle, W. F. (1945) *Stain Technology*, **20**, 13.
Krainer, L. (1949) *Arch. Neurol. Psychiat.* (Chicago), **51**, 441.
Krogh, E. (1945) *Acta Jutlandica*, 17, Suppl.
Kufs, H. (1928) *Z. ges. Neurol. Psychiat.*, **117**, 753.
Lafora, G. R. (1911) Virchows *Arch. Path. Anat.*, **205**, 295; (1913) *Trab. lab. Invest. biol. Univ. Madrid*, **11**, 29, 43.
Laidlaw, G. F. (1930) *Amer. J. Path.*, **6**, 435.
Lawrence, R. D., Meyer, A. and Nevin, S. (1942) *Quart. J. Med.*, **35**, 181.
Levi, G. (1896) *Rivista patologia nerv. ment.*, **1**, 385; (1897) ibid., **2**, 193, 244.

Lewy, F. H. (1912) *Handbuch der Neurologie*, Lewandowsky, **3**, 920.
Lindsay, H. A. and Barr, M. L. (1955) *J. Anat.*, **89**, 47.
Lorrain-Smith, J. and Mair, W. (1909) *J. Path. Bact.*, **13**, 14.
Lowry, O. H. (1957) In *Metabolism of the Nervous System*, ed. Richter, D., London.
Luse, S. A. (1956) *J. Biophys. and Biochem. Cytology*, **2**, 531, 777.
Malamud, N., Haymaker, W. and Custer, R. P. (1946) *The Military Surgeon*, **99**, 397.
Malamud, N., Haymaker, W. and Pinkerton, H. (1950) *Amer. J. Path.*, **26**, 133.
Marie, P., Foix, C. and Alajouanine, T. (1922) *Rev. Neurol.*, **38**, 849, 1082.
Marinesco, G. (1909) *La Cellule Nerveuse*. Doin, Paris.
Maynard, E. A., Schultz, R. and Pease, D. C. (1957) *Amer. J. Anat.*, **100**, 409.
Mercer, E. H. (1961) *Proc. Roy. Soc. Med.*, **54**, 1057.
Meyer, A. (1901) *Brain*, **24**, 47.
Meyer, A., Beck, E. and McLardy, T. (1947) *Brain*, **70**, 18.
Miller, R. A. (1949) *Amer. J. Anat.*, **84**, 201.
von Monakow, C. (1882) *Arch. Psychiat. Nervenkr.*, **12**, 141; (1883) ibid., **14** 699; (1885) ibid., **16**, 151, 319.
Mondino, C. (1885–6) cited by Rand and Courville, 1947.
Morrison, L. R. (1946) *Arch. Neurol. Psychiat.* (Chicago), **55**, 1.
Murray, M. R. and Stout, A. P. (1942) *Amer. J. Path.*, **18**, 585.
Nageotte, J. (1932) W. Penfield's *Cytology and Cellular Pathology of the Nervous System*, p. 189, Hoeber, New York.
Naidoo, D. and Pratt, O. E. (1954) *Enzymologia*, **16**, 298.
Nicholson, F. M. (1923–4) *J. Comp. Neurol.*, **36**, 37.
Niessl von Meyendorf. (1934) *Rev. Neurol.* (i), 1024.
Nissl, F. (1894 a) *Centralbl. f. Nervenheilk.*, **17**, 337; (1894 b) *Neurol. Centralbl.*, **13**, 781.
Noback, C. R. and Montague, W. (1952) *J. comp. Neurol.*, **97**, 211.
Olszewski, J. (1947) *Biol. Zentralbl.*, **66**, 265.
Olszewski, J. and Baxter, D. (1954) *Cyto-architecture of the Human Brain Stem*, Karger, Basel.
Palade, G. E. (1955) *J. Biophys. Biochem. Cytol.*, **1**, 59; (1956) *Ibid.*, **2**, (Suppl.) 85.
Palay, S. L. and Palade, G. E. (1955) *J. Biophys. Biochem. Cytol.*, **1**, 69.
Palay, S. L. (1956) *Ibid.*, **2**, (Suppl.) 193; (1958) *Exper. Cell Research, Suppl.* **5**, 275.
Penfield, W. (1920) *Brain*, **43**, 290.
Popoff, L. (1875) *Virchow's Arch.*, **63**, 421.
Potanos, J. N., Wolf, A. and Cowen, D. (1959) *J. Neuropath.*, **18**, 627.
Putnam, T. J. (1926) *Arch. Neurol. Psychiat.* (Chicago), **16**, 566, 683.
Putnam, T. J. and Putnam, I. K. (1926) *Arch. Neurol. Psychiat.* (Chicago), **16**, 1.
Putnam, T. J. (1935) *Arch. Neur. Psychiat.* (Chicago), **33**, 929.
Quastel, J. H. (1957) In *Metabolism of the Nervous System*, ed. Richter, D., London.
Rand, C. W. and Courville, C. B. (1946) *Arch. Neur. Psychiat.* (Chicago), **55**, 79.
Ranvier, L. (1878) *Leçons sur l'histologie du système nerveux*, Paris.
Renes, R. C. (1940) *Over de vezelrykdom in de hersenschors* (Thesis) Leiden.
de Renyi, G. S. (1929) *J. comp. Neurol.*, **47**, 405; **48**, 293, 441; (1931) ibid., **53**, 497.
de Robertis, E. (1956) *J. Biophys. Biochem. Cytol.*, **2**, 503; (1958) *Exper. Cell Research, Suppl.* **5**, 347.
de Robertis, E. and Benett, H. S. D. (1954) *Fed. Proceed.*, **13**, 35.
de Robertis, E. Gerschenfeld, H. M. and Wald, F. (1960) In *Structure and Function of the Cerebral Cortex*, edited by Tower, D. B. and Schade, J., Amsterdam.
Robertson, J. D. (1955) *J. Biophys. Biochem. Cytol.*, **1**, 271; (1961) In *Electron Microscopy in Anatomy*, ed. Boyd, J. D. *et al.*, London.
Roizin, L. (1955) *J. Neuropath.*, **14**, 46; (1960) *Ibid.*, **19**, 591.
Rossiter, R. J. (1961) In *Chemical Pathology of the Nervous System*, ed. Folch-Pi, J., New York, London.
Sachs, B. (1887) *J. nerv. ment. Dis.*, **14**, 541.
Schmidt, W. J. (1936) *Z. Zellforsch.*, **23**, 657.
Schmitt, F. O., Bear, R. S. and Clark, G. L. (1935) *Radiology*, **25**, 131.
Schmitt, F. O. and Geren, B. B. (1950) *J. exper. Med.*, **91**, 499.
Scholz, W., Boellaard, J. W. and Hager, H. (1959) *Toxity Changes in the Central Nervous System, Oxygen Deficiency and its Influence on the Central Nervous System.* Technical Report Contr. AF61 pp. 514–945, U.S.A.F.
Scholz, W. and Boellaard, J. W. (1959) In Scholz, Boellaard and Hager.

Scholz, W. and Hager, H. (1959) In Scholz, Boellaard & Hager.
Schwann, T. (1839) *Mikroscopische Untersuchungen*, p. 174, Berlin.
Scott, G. H. (1933) *Anat. Record*, **53**, 243.
Simarro, L. (1900) *Rev. ibero–Amer. Cien. méd.*, **4**, 332.
Simchowicz, T. (1911) *Nissl Alzheimer Arbeiten*, **4**, 267.
Sjöstrand, F. S. (1953) *Experientia*, **9**, 68.
Sperry, W. M. and Waelsch, H. (1950) in *Multiple Sclerosis and the demyelinating diseases, Proc. Ass. Res. Nerv. Ment. Dis.*, **18**, 255, **28**.
Spielmeyer, W. (1905) *Arch. Psychiat. Nervenkr.*, **40**, 1038. (1905) *Neur. Centralbl.*, **24**, 51.
Spielmeyer, W. (1922) *Histopathologie des Nervensystems*, Springer, Berlin.
Steegman, A. T. (1961) *Rept. 7th Int. Congr. Neurol.*, p. 197.
Stewart, T. G. and Holmes, G. (1908) *Brain*, **31**, 125.
Swank, R. L. (1940) *J. exper. Med.*, **71**, 683.
Swank, R. L. and Prados, M. (1942) *Arch. Neur. Psychiat.* (Chicago), **47**, 97.
Tay, W. (1881) *Trans. Ophthal. Soc. U.K.*, London, **1**, 56.
Tello, F. (1904) *Trab. lab. invest. biol.*, Madrid, **3**, 113.
Terry, R. D. and Harkin, J. C. (1959) In *The Biology of Myelin*, ed. Korey, S. R., New York.
Tigges, W. (1863) *Allg. Z. Psychiat.*, **20**, 317.
Trétiakoff, C. (1919) *Contribution à l'étude de l'anatomie pathologique du Locus Niger de Soemmerring* Thèse de Paris.
Tureen, L. L. (1936) *Arch. Neurol. Psychiat.* (Chicago), **35**, 789.
van Bogaert, L. (1939) *Rev. Neurol.*, **72**, 448.
Vogt, H. (1905) *Mschr. Psychiat. Neurol.*, **18**, 164.
Waller, A. V. (1850) *Philos. Trans.*, **140**, 423.
Webster, H., de F., Spiro, D., Waksman, B. and Adams, R. D. (1961) *J. Neuropath.*, **20**, 5
Weimann, W. (1925) *Z. Neurol. Psychiat.*, **98**, 347.
Weiss, P. (1943) *Arch. Surg.*, **46**, 525.
Weiss, P. and Hiscoe, H. (1948) *J. exper. Zool.*, **107**, 315.
Wertham, F. and Wertham, F. L. (1934) *The Brain as an Organ*, New York.
Westphal, A. (1919) *Arch. Psychiat. Nervenkr.*, **60**, 769.
Westphal, A. and Sioli, F. (1921) *Ibid.* **62**, 1.
Wilke, G. (1959) *Fortschr. Neurol. Psychiat.*, **27**, 557.
Williams, H. W. (1935) *Arch. Neurol. Psychiat.* (Chicago), **34**, 508.
Windle, W. F., Rhines, R. and Rankin. J. (1943) *Stain Technology*, **18**, 77.
Wolfgram, F. and Rose, A. S. (1958) *Neurology*, **8**, 839.
Wolman, M. (1957) *Exper. Cell. Research*, **12**, 231.
Woolf, A. L. (1954) *J. Path. Bacter.*, **67**, 1; (1962) *Proc. 4th Int. Congr. Neuropath.*, **2**, 18.
Wykoff, R. G. W. and Young, J. Z. (1956) *Proc. Roy. Soc. (B)*, **144**, 440.
Young, J. Z. (1942) *Physiol. Reviews*, **22**, 318; (1945) *Nature*, **156**, 132; (1950) in Weiss, P. *Genetic Neurology*; pp. 92–102, Chicago.

The Neuroglia and Microglia

Adams, R. D. and Foley, J. M. (1953) in *Metabolic and Toxic Diseases of the Nervous System, Proc. Ass. Res. Nerv. Ment. Dis.*, **32**, Chapter 11.
Alexander, G. L. and Norman, R. M. (1960) *The Sturge-Weber Syndrome*, Bristol.
Alzheimer, A. (1910) *Nissl Alzheimer Arbeiten*, **3**, 401.
Andriezen, W. L. (1893) *Brit. Med. J.* (ii), 227.
Bailey, P. and Bucy, P. C. (1929) *J. Path. Bact.*, **32**, 735.
Bailey, P. and Schaltenbrand, G. (1927) *Dtsch. Z. Nervenheilk.*, **97**, 231.
Berliner, M. L. (1931) *Arch. Ophthal.*, **6**, 740.
Bunge, M. B., Bunge, R. P. and Ris, H. (1961) *J. Biophys. Biochem. Cytol.*, **10**, 67.
Cajal, S. Ramon y. (1913) *Trab. lab. invest. biol.*, Madrid, **11**, 254.
Canti, R. G., Bland, J. O. W. and Russell, D. S. (1937) *Proc. Ass. Res. Nerv. Ment. Dis.*, **16**, 1.
Costero, I. (1930) *Bol. Soc. Esp. Hist. Nat.*, **30**.
Dempsey, E. W. (1961) In *Chemical Pathology of the Nervous System*, ed. Folch-Pi, J., New York, London.

Fañanas, J. (1916) *Trab. lab. invest. biol. Madrid.*, **14**, 163.
Farquhar, M. J. and Hartmann, J. F. (1957) *J. Neuropath.*, **16**, 18.
Foix, C. and Alajouanine, T. (1926) *Rev. Neurol.* (ii), 1.
Gray, E. G. (1959) *J. Biophys. Biochem. Cytol.*, **6**, 121; (1961) In *Electron Microscopy in Anatomy*, ed. Boyd, J. D. *et al.*, London.
Greenfield, J. G. (1933) *J. Neurol. Psychopath.*, **13**, 289 and Volume Jubilaire de Marinesco Bucarest; (1953–4) *Proc. Roy. Soc. Med.*, **47**, 150.
Grynfeltt, E. (1923) *C.R. Soc. de Biol.*, Paris, **89**, 1264.
Held, H. (1903) *Abhandl. d. mathem. physikel. Klasse d. kgl. Sachs. Gesellsch. d. Wissensch.*
Hösslin, C. von and Alzheimer, A. (1912) *Z. Neurol. Psychiat.*, **8**, 183.
Ingleby, H. (1925) *J. Roy. Microscop. Soc.*, 423.
Jakob, A. (1927) *Normale und Pathologische Anatomie und Histologie des Grosshirns*, Deuticke, Leipzig.
Kölliker, A. (1889–96) *Handb. d. Gewebelehre des Menschen*, 6th Edition, Leipzig.
Lewis, R. C. and Swank, R. L. (1953) *J. Neuropathol.* **12**, 57.
Lumsden, C. E. and Pomerat, C. M. (1951) *Exper. Cell Research*, **2**, 103.
Luse, S. A. (1956) *J. Biophys. Biochem. Cytol.*, **2**, 531.
Maturana, H. R. (1960) *J. Biophys. Biochem. Cytol.*, **7**, 107.
Niessing, K. and Vogell, W. (1962) *Proc. 4th Int. Congr. Neuropath.*, **2**, 112.
Opalski, A. (1930) *Z. ges. Neurol. Psychiat.*, **124**, 420.
Penfield, W. (1924) *Brain*, **47**, 430; (1927) *Brain*, **50**, 499; (1928) *Arch. Neurol. Psychiat.* (Chicago), **20**, 1; (1932) in *The Neuroglia* in Penfield's *Cytology and Cellular Pathology of the Nervous System*, **2**, p. 423.
Penfield, W. and Buckley, W. (1928) *Arch. Neurol. Psychiat.* (Chicago), **20**, 1.
Penfield, W. and Cone, W. (1926) *Arch. Neurol. Psychiat.* (Chicago), **16**, 130.
Périer, O. and de Harven, E. (1961) In *Cytology of Nervous Tissue*, Proc. Anat. Soc., p. 78, London.
Peters, A. (1960) *J. Biophys. Biochem. Cytol.*, **8**, 431.
Rand, C. W. and Courville, C. B. (1932) *Arch. Neurol. Psychiat.* (Chicago), **27**, 605.
Ranvier, L. (1883) *Arch. de Physiol.*, 3rd series, **1**, 177.
del Rio-Hortega, P. (1919) *Bol. de la Soc. esp. de Biol.*, **9**, 154; (1928) *Mem. Real Soc. Esp. Hist. nat.*, **14**, 7.
del Rio-Hortega, P. (1932) in Penfield's *Cytology and Cellular Pathology of the Nervous System*, **2**, 483.
del Rio-Hortega, P. and Penfield, W. (1928) *Arch. Neurol. Psychiat.* (Chicago), **19**, 180.
de Robertis, E., Gerschenfeld, H. M. and Wald, F. (1958) *J. Biophys. Biochem. Cytol.*, **4**, 651; (1960) In *Structure and Function of the Cerebral Cortex*, edited by Tower, D. B. and Schade, J., Amsterdam.
Robertson, W. Ford. (1899) *Scottish Med. surg. J.*, **4**, 23; (1900) *J. ment. Sc.*, p. 724.
Schultz, R., Maynard, E. A. and Pease, D. C. (1957) *Amer. J. Anat.*, **100**, 369.
Shimoda, A. (1961) *Dtsch. Z. Nervenheilk*, **183**, 78.
Smith, M. C. (1949) *J. Neurol. Neurosurg. Psychiat.*, **12**, 100.
Ule, G. (1962) *Proc. 4th Int. Congr. Neuropath.* **2**, 118.
Weigert, C. (1895) *Festschrift zum fünfzigjährigen Jubiläum des ärztlichen Vereins zu Frankfurt a/Main.*
Wells, A. Q. and Carmichael, E. A. (1930) *Brain*, **53**, 1.

CHAPTER 2

VASCULAR DISEASE OF THE CENTRAL NERVOUS SYSTEM

By W. Blackwood

APPLIED ANATOMY AND PHYSIOLOGY

Arterial blood supply

The brain is supplied with blood through the internal carotid and vertebral arteries. There is an anastomosis between these sources of supply in the arteries of the circle of Willis. The potential efficiency of this anastomosis can be judged from one of our cases in which sufficient blood reached the brain through only one internal carotid artery, the other three arteries being closed by atherosclerosis. From the circle of Willis the arterial distribution may be simplified by considering it to consist of (1) paramedian vessels perforating the base of the brain to supply structures near the mid-line, (2) short circumferential vessels supplying the thalamus, lentiform nuclei and other basal ganglia, and (3) long circumferential branches, the anterior, middle and posterior cerebral arteries, supplying principally the cortex and underlying white matter.

There is evidence of anastomosis between the anterior, middle and posterior cerebral arteries, at arterial level in the pia-arachnoid (Vander Eecken and Adams 1953) and at capillary level within the cerebral tissue; but this anastomosis is of only limited value. Following obstruction of one of the main cerebral arteries, or of one of its major branches, the anastomosis is only sufficient to take over part of the bed of supply of the obstructed artery. The amount taken over depends, *inter alia*, upon the blood pressure in the anastomosing vessels. When this is high a considerable amount of tissue, in the theoretical field of supply of the occluded artery, may survive. When, however, the diastolic pressure is low, as in ulcerative endocarditis, the region of necrosis will be considerably larger. Such necrosis affects not only the cortex but also the underlying white matter. In the frontal and occipital lobes the region of necrosis is somewhat wedge-shaped and extends almost as far as the ventricular wall.

The brain stem and cerebellum are also supplied with blood on the basis of (1) paramedian branches from the basilar artery, (2) short circumferential branches and (3) long circumferential arteries such as the superior, anterior and posterior inferior cerebellar arteries. There are anastomoses between surface branches of these last three paired arteries across the midline and with each other; and also between branches of the superior cerebellar and posterior cerebral arteries. These surface anastomoses, although abundant, are however only occasionally sufficient to supply all the cerebellar cortex if one or more of the arteries, or pairs of arteries, is obstructed by disease. Atkinson (1949) found that coloured gelatin injected into the anterior inferior cerebellar artery always stained the cerebellar distribution of the artery, but did not spread into the territory of adjacent arteries. In the pons the paramedian arteries, which supply the ventromedial portion of the brain stem, do not anastomose significantly with each other across the midline, or with the other arteries supplying the brain stem.

The ventrolateral portions of midbrain and pons are supplied by the short circumferential arteries, but there is disagreement about the blood supply of the tegmentum, as revealed both by injection techniques and by infarction following vascular occlusion. Foix and Hillemand (1926) decided that the tegmentum of the midbrain is supplied by the superior cerebellar arteries and that the tegmentum of the pons is supplied by the short circumferential arteries. Kubik and Adams (1946) agreed that the tegmentum of the pons is supplied by the short circumferential arteries but considered that there is a varying contribution by the paramedian and long circumferential arteries. Atkinson (1949) found, however, that the lateral parts of the tegmentum of the pons are supplied by the anterior inferior cerebellar arteries whilst Biemond (1951) considered that the superior cerebellar arteries supply the tegmentum of both midbrain and pons.

Spinal cord. In the embryo the arterial supply of the spinal cord is upon a segmental basis. Each segment is supplied by a pair of anterior and a pair of posterior radicular arteries. Each radicular artery gives off an ascending and a descending branch which anastomose with the corresponding branches belonging to adjacent segments. With the passage of time many of the radicular arteries become rudimentary or disappear, but the anastomotic channels increase in calibre and importance, so that the end result is one large anterior anastomotic channel, or anterior spinal artery, and two small posterior anastomotic channels, or posterior spinal arteries.

The anterior spinal artery extends the whole length of the spinal cord. It supplies almost all the white and grey matter of the cord, except the posterior white columns which are supplied by the two posterior spinal arteries. The anterior spinal artery is formed superiorly by the spinal branches of the vertebral arteries and the blood flow is in a cranial to caudal direction. The stream is maintained over the length of the cord by the contributions of the infrequent radicular arteries. These appear to pour their blood into the anterior spinal artery in a predominantly caudal direction and thus supply the territory below their point of junction with the cord.

The posterior spinal arteries communicate inferiorly with the anterior spinal artery and superiorly with spinal branches of the vertebral arteries. The blood flow in the posterior spinal arteries appears to be in a cranial direction over the lower part of the cord and in a caudal direction in the cervical region (Bolton 1939).

The radicular arteries, which reach the cord along the anterior and posterior nerve roots, are branches of the lateral spinal arteries, which are branches of spinal arteries. In relation to the upper half of the spinal cord these come from the supra-aortic intercostals (branches of the ascending cervical and costovertebral arteries): in relation to the lower half of the cord they come from the posterior divisions of the aortic intercostals, lumbar, iliolumbar and lateral sacral arteries (Tureen 1937). There are about 8 anterior radicular arteries and about 8–16 smaller posterior radicular arteries. There is a constant anterior artery at C.6 or 7 and a large anterior artery at Th.10 or L.1 or L.2. The cervical and lumbosacral regions of the cord are well supplied, but the intervening thoracic cord is poorly supplied (Tureen 1937, Suh and Alexander 1939).

For some unknown reason certain kinds of vascular disease affect the vessels of the spinal cord less than those of the brain. Atherosclerosis is very rare and hypertensive arterial and arteriolar changes are much less severe in the cord than in the brain of the same patient.

Venous drainage

Brain. In contrast to the arteries, the surface veins of the brain have abundant anastomoses of large calibre. The ill effects of localised venous obstruction are therefore slight. Obstruction of portions of the superior sagittal sinus may cause only slight parasagittal infarction. Very much more serious is concomitant thrombosis of adjacent veins which obstructs the collateral circulation. The veins of the brain drain into the dural venous sinuses and through them into the internal jugular veins. The dural venous sinuses also communicate with the vascular channels in the diploe of the bones of the skull and these channels communicate with extracranial veins. Fracture of the skull can thus initiate retrograde thrombosis. In addition there are emissary veins which connect the dural venous sinuses with extracranial veins. The cavernous sinuses are connected via the ophthalmic veins with the facial veins, via emissary veins passing through foramen ovale and the carotid canal with the pterygoid and pharyngeal venous plexuses, and via the basilar venous sinuses with the spinal veins. The lateral venous sinuses are connected via mastoid emissary veins with the occipital veins, and the superior sagittal sinus is connected with extracranial posterior parietal veins via the parietal emissary veins. All these venous communications are potential pathways for the intracranial spread of extracranial pyogenic infection.

Spinal cord. The surface veins of the spinal cord are more numerous on the dorsal aspect of the cord, especially in the lumbosacral region. After the cord has been removed they are an anatomical guide to the dorsum of the cord, just as the anterior spinal artery is an indication of the ventral aspect. Thrombophlebitis of spinal veins is rare but serious (*vide infra*).

The spinal veins drain, via the radicular veins, to the paravertebral and intravertebral plexuses, which in turn communicate with the pelvic plexuses. There are about 38 radicular veins and they are fairly evenly distributed over the length of the cord.

Histology

The capillaries of the central nervous system are similar histologically to those elsewhere in the body except that they have no envelope of reticulin fibres (see p. 235). They are lined by flattened, polygonal, endothelial cells joined together by cement substance and covered by the expanded foot-plates of the astrocytes. The prolongations of the subarachnoid space, called the Virchow-Robin spaces, exist in relation to arteries and arterioles, veins and venules, but not to the capillaries.

The arterioles and *small arteries* are lined by endothelial cells surrounded by a well-developed internal elastic lamina. The media is composed of fibrous tissue and of plain muscle. The amount of muscle is much less than in vessels of similar calibre elsewhere in the body, so that in vessels as large as 70μ it is often difficult to find any muscle at all, the media being entirely fibrous. With age the muscle disappears and the elastica is reduced in amount (Baker 1937).

The larger arteries (Fig. 2.44) also have walls which are thinner than those of arteries in the rest of the body. The internal elastic lamina is well developed but both the muscular coat and the adventitia are thin. There is no external elastic lamina.

The venules and veins are lined by endothelial cells. The walls, which are thinner than those of most veins elsewhere in the body, are composed chiefly of fibrous tissue. Smooth muscle is not present and there is very little elastic tissue. There are no valves in the veins of the brain but they have been seen in relation to the spinal veins (Suh and Alexander 1939).

The walls of the *venous sinuses* are composed of dense fibrous tissue lined by endothelial cells.

OCCLUSION OF CERTAIN ARTERIES OF THE BRAIN AND SPINAL CORD

The arteries of the central nervous system have a fairly constant anatomical distribution, and occlusion of an artery, or of one or more of its larger branches, produces a relatively constant disorder of function. Full consideration of the anatomical distribution of the arteries and of the clinico-pathological correlation of the lesions is outside the scope of this book. For further information the literature referred to under each artery should be consulted. Additional anatomical publications are Beevor (1908), Stopford (1916, 1917), Abbie (1934). Adams (1943) gives a detailed list of the arterial distribution to the cerebellum. Critchley and Schuster (1933) and Atkinson (1949) describe the branches of the basilar artery. The clinical syndromes resulting from arterial occlusion have been reviewed by Tichy (1949) and by Kiloh (1953).

Usually the arterial occlusion has been secondary to atherosclerosis, sometimes to syphilis, less often to embolism, or to mechanical or surgical trauma. In patients with atherosclerosis or syphilis, which are generalised arterial diseases, the occlusion of the named artery is only the most obvious lesion: there are often many other small lesions elsewhere in the brain or spinal cord. Generalised arterial disease also modifies the opening up of collateral pathways. In cases due to embolism it is always possible that other emboli have occluded small vessels elsewhere, and in cases of mechanical trauma, or where the arteries have been clipped or cauterised by the surgeon, the ill effects of the arterial occlusion are seldom the only pathological process present. For all these reasons it is unlikely, in man, that the obvious arterial lesion is the only one present. It is therefore unwise to state that, in man, ischaemic destruction of a certain region is the cause of a certain disability of function. The study of a number of cases, however, reveals that there is a sufficiently close correlation, between a major lesion in the distribution of a certain artery and certain clinical findings, to make the investigation of this subject worth while. In patients who survive for an adequate length of time, a study of the secondary degenerations is of importance. Apart from surgical ablation or destruction of tissue, which in many parts of the brain is too dangerous or is not indicated, localised arterial obstruction is one of the few disease processes which has enabled us to make satisfactory observations on the course of fibre pathways, on secondary degenerations and on the anatomical basis of disordered functions.

Anterior cerebral artery

The principal field of supply of the anterior cerebral artery is the cortex and the underlying white matter (to a depth of about 25 mm.) on the medial aspect, and a 25-mm. broad strip on the superior part of the convexity of the frontal and parietal lobes as far back usually as the parieto-occipital fissure, also the genu and anterior four-fifths of the corpus callosum. Through the recurrent artery of Heubner, which leaves it early in its course and passes through the anterior perforated substance, it supplies the lower part of the head of the caudate, the lower part of the frontal pole of the putamen, the frontal pole of the globus pallidus and the portion of the anterior limb of the internal capsule lying between them.

The disturbance of function varies with the portion of the artery which is occluded. If the distal field of supply, which includes the paracentral lobule, is obstructed, there is crural monoplegia with sensory disturbance of a cortical type (Critchley 1930). In atheromatous cases this may be bilateral and cause spastic paraplegia.

Middle cerebral artery

The principal field of supply of this artery includes the lateral part of the orbital surface of the frontal lobe, the temporal pole, the insula and all the convexity of the cerebral hemisphere, except the strip supplied by the anterior cerebral artery and a part posteriorly, including the occipital pole, supplied by the posterior cerebral artery. It supplies the underlying white matter (which includes the superior half of both limbs of the internal capsule and the optic radiation, where it lies lateral to the occipital horn of the lateral ventricle). In addition the middle cerebral artery supplies the caudate (except for the inferior portion of its head, and its tail), the putamen (except for the lower part of its frontal pole) and the lateral part of the globus pallidus.

Our records show that this artery is more often obstructed than any other cerebral artery, the obstruction being either of the main trunk or of some of its branches. If the main artery is suddenly obstructed, as it commonly is by embolism, the region of infarction may correspond closely with the principal field of supply. Associated with this lesion there is severe hemiplegia (most severe in the arm), sensory disturbance of the cortical type, profound aphasia (if the dominant hemisphere is involved), sometimes hemianopia which is not always complete (Foix and Levy 1927) and disturbance of vestibular function (Carmichael, Dix and Hallpike 1956).

Anterior choroidal artery

The principal field of supply of the anterior choroidal artery is the pyriform cortex, the posteromedial border of the anterior commissure, part of the head and most of the tail of the caudate nucleus, the posteromedial part of the amygdaloid nucleus, the medial part of the globus pallidus, the lateral part of the lateral geniculate body, the middle third of the cerebral peduncle, the subthalamic region, the posterior two-thirds of the posterior limb of the internal capsule, the beginning of the optic radiation, the antero-inferior parts of the fascia dentata and hippocampus (including the uncus) and the choroid plexus.

Proven cases of occlusion of the anterior choroidal artery are rare (Abbie 1933). The infarcts were found in the distal portion of the distribution of the artery, and caused constant destruction of the retrolenticular portion of the internal capsule, part of the optic radiation and part of the globus pallidus, with inconstant damage to the cerebral peduncle, lateral part of the lateral geniculate body, the head of the caudate, optic tract, anterior commissure and amygdaloid nucleus. In association with this infarction there were hemiplegia, hemianaesthesia and hemianopia.

Earle *et al.* (1953) have postulated that the sclerotic lesions of the uncus, hippocampus and inferior temporal gyrus, which are often found in people with temporal lobe epilepsy, are the result of compression, during birth, of arteries and their branches against the free edge of the tentorium cerebelli. Of these they consider that the anterior choroidal artery and its branches are the most important.

Posterior cerebral artery

Although in the human, in the majority of cases, this artery is anatomically a branch of the basilar artery, it is morphologically a continuation of the posterior communicating artery and therefore a branch of the carotid artery (Abbie 1934, Williams 1936). This concept clarifies the distribution of the posterior communicating artery and the posterior cerebral artery to the basal ganglia.

The principal field of supply of the posterior cerebral artery is the inferior surface of the hemisphere behind the temporal pole, the medial surface of the occipital lobe, the lateral surface of the hemisphere in the region of the occipital pole, and the underlying white matter which, on the medial aspect of the occipital lobe, is narrow. It also supplies the mammillary body, the subthalamic nucleus, the posterior half of the thalamus including the geniculate bodies, the posterior two-thirds of the cerebral peduncle, the substantia nigra, red nucleus and the superior cerebellar peduncle.

Occlusion by atherosclerosis and thrombosis, or secondary to vertebral-basilar obstruction, or to pressure against the free edge of the tentorium cerebelli by a supratentorial space-occupying lesion, commonly obstructs the peripheral branches of the artery which supply the visual cortex. Occasionally the main stem of the artery is occluded, and this causes infarction in the major portion of its anatomical distribution. Because of the collateral circulation through the anterior choroidal artery, the subthalamic nucleus and the lateral geniculate body are not destroyed; because of the collateral circulation through the middle cerebral artery, the posterior portion of the calcarine cortex, where the macula is represented (Holmes 1934), is spared.

In association with the infarction there are numerous syndromes (Foix and Masson 1923) according to the portion of the artery which is occluded. If the whole artery is occluded there will be homonymous hemianopia with macular sparing, hemiparesis and disturbance of sensation. If the lesions are on the side of the dominant hemisphere there will be alexia.

Superior cerebellar artery

The principal field of supply of this artery is the dorsolateral portion of the upper part of the brain stem (midbrain and cranial part of the pons), the superior cerebellar peduncle, the roof nuclei of the 4th ventricle, part of the dentate nucleus and part of the cortex of the superior part of the cerebellar hemisphere. Exactly how much of the tegmentum of the midbrain and pons is supplied by this artery remains uncertain.

Occlusion of this artery is rare. It has been reported with atherosclerosis by Guillain *et al.* (1928) and by Russell (1931), with atherosclerosis and syphilis by Davison *et al.* (1935) and as the result of an embolus by Freeman and Jaffe (1941).

The infarction may involve the dorsolateral midbrain and pons, including the caudal portion of the mesencephalic root of the 5th nerve, the central tegmental tract, the lateral part of the medial lemniscus, and the lateral lemniscus; the superior cerebellar peduncle, the roof nuclei of the 4th ventricle, part of the dentate nucleus and the adjacent part of the superior surface of the cerebellum. Secondary degeneration may be seen in the contralateral red nucleus and the ipsilateral inferior olivary nucleus. In association with the infarction there may be ipsilateral signs of cerebellar dysfunction, ipsilateral involuntary movements especially of the upper extremity, together with contralateral loss of appreciation of pain and temperature over the whole body.

Anterior inferior cerebellar artery

The principal field of supply of this artery is the lateral portion of the tegmentum of the middle portion of the brain stem (the caudal part of the pons and the cranial part of the medulla), the inferior part of the middle cerebellar peduncle, the inferior cerebellar peduncle, the flocculus and adjacent cerebellar hemisphere.

Damage to this artery is considered by Atkinson (1949) to be the principal cause of death following operative removal of an acoustic neurofibroma. Proven cases of occlusion of this artery, secondary to atherosclerosis, are extremely rare. Two cases have been published, one by Goodhart and Davison (1936, case 6) and one by Adams (1943). In Goodhart and Davison's case the infarction was confined to the cerebellar cortex. In Adams's case the flocculus, the biventral and the superior and inferior semilunar lobules of the cerebellum were infarcted, and in the brain stem the lesion extended from the level of the mid-pons to the middle of the inferior olive. The structures involved were the caudal portion of the middle cerebellar peduncle, the inferior cerebellar peduncle, the rostral part of the spinal nucleus and tract of the 5th nerve, the 7th nerve, the 8th nerve, the ventral and dorsal cochlear nuclei, the lateral portion of the spinal vestibular nucleus and the ventral spinocerebellar tract: most of the adjacent lateral spinothalamic tract was spared. There was secondary degeneration of nerve cells in the 7th nerve nucleus, contralateral pontile and inferior olivary nuclei. In association with the infarction the patient showed ipsilateral cerebellar dysfunction, loss of pain and temperature and diminished light touch sensibility over the face, paralysis of the muscles of the face, deafness, Horner's syndrome, together with contralateral incomplete loss of pain and temperature sensibility over the body.

Posterior inferior cerebellar artery

This artery supplies a wedge of tissue in the medulla which extends vertically from just above the level of the cuneate and gracile nuclei to the upper limit of the medulla. On the surface the wedge extends from just posterior to the inferior olivary nucleus dorsally to include the inferior cerebellar peduncle. Centrally the apex of the wedge reaches the tegmentum in its lateral part. The artery also supplies part of the inferior surface of the cerebellar hemisphere and part of the dentate nucleus.

Ischaemic lesions occur more frequently in the distribution of this artery than of any other cerebellar artery. These are usually the result of atheroma with superadded thrombotic occlusion, which often commences in the vertebral artery (Fisher *et al.* 1961 (see also p. 94)). An infrequent cause is syphilis and embolism is rare. The principal lesion is a retro-olivary softening in the medulla. Infarction of the cerebellum is usually slight because of the free anastomosis with other cerebellar arteries. Spillane (1937) had a case with involvement of the dentate nucleus.

The lesion in the medulla has been described by Foix *et al.* (1925), Merritt and Finland (1930), Goodhart and Davison (1936), Smyth (1939) and Levine *et al.* (1949). It consists of an infarct which involves almost all the field of supply with the exception of the tegmentum. The structures involved are the descending nucleus and tract of the 5th nerve, some of the internal arcuate fibres, the spinal vestibular nucleus and tract or fibres passing from it to the medial longitudinal fasciculus, the nucleus ambiguus and fibres emerging from the dorsal motor nucleus of the 9th and 10th nerves, autonomic fibre pathways, the lateral spinothalamic and spinocerebellar tracts, olivo-cerebellar fibres as they pass to the inferior cerebellar peduncle, and the ventral part of the inferior cerebellar peduncle. The facial nucleus is occasionally involved.

Foix *et al.* considered that this lesion was not due to occlusion of the posterior inferior cerebellar artery, but to occlusion of a different artery, the artery of the lateral fissure, a branch of the basilar artery. Other investigators have not been able to confirm this opinion: Goodhart and Davison considered that the artery of the lateral fissure was not normally present.

Clinically the condition usually comes on suddenly, with dizziness, falling towards the side of the lesion, nystagmus, difficulty in swallowing, homolateral Horner's syndrome, ataxia and loss of appreciation of pain and temperature over the ipsilateral face and contralateral body.

Anterior spinal artery

This artery, which usually arises by the fusion of a branch from each vertebral artery, supplies the anterior and median regions of the lower medulla, in which the following structures are present: the pyramids and pyramidal decussations, the medial lemnisci, the medial longitudinal fasciculi, the caudal portions of the hypoglossal and dorsal vagal nuclei, the nucleus and tractus solitarius on each side (at the level of the decussation), the lateral spinothalamic and ventral spinocerebellar tracts (Gower's tracts), the olivocerebellar fibres as they cross the midline, part of the inferior olivary nuclei and the internal and ventral external arcuate fibres and nuclei. In the spinal cord this artery supplies all parts except the greater part of the posterior white columns and the dorsal part of the posterior grey columns.

Proven cases of occlusion of the anterior spinal artery in the medulla are few. Davison (1937 and 1944) had 5 cases with occlusion of the medullary portion of the artery (in 2 cases both branches of origin). The structures which were damaged were the pyramids, the medial lemnisci, the medial longitudinal fasciculi and the ventral part of the inferior olivary nuclei (3 cases). The hypoglossal nuclei and nerves were not affected.

In association with the infarct the patient shows contralateral or bilateral pyramidal tract involvement, sensory disturbance referable to the posterior columns, and sometimes urinary and faecal incontinence.

Occlusion of the spinal part of the anterior spinal artery is usually confined either to its cranial (cervical) or to its caudal (thoraco-lumbo-sacral) portion. The diagnosis of occlusion of the cervical portion of the artery is quite often made clinically, upon the basis of paraplegia, wasting of the muscles of the hands and subjective sensory disturbances in the distal portions of the upper limbs; but reports of cases which have been confirmed by post-mortem examination are few. Grinker and Guy's case (1927) was secondary to probable temporary dislocation of the 5th cervical vertebra in a boy of 15. There was thrombosis of the anterior spinal artery at this level with softening of the 4th, 5th and 6th cervical segments in the field of distribution of the artery. In Spiller's case (1909) the lesion extended from C.4 to Th.3 and was due to syphilitic arteritis. It was most extensive at Th.1 where it involved the whole of the distribution of the artery. This patient showed paraplegia, weakness, wasting and flaccidity of both upper limbs, incontinence of urine and faeces, impairment of temperature and pain sensation as high as the 1st or 2nd rib and in both upper limbs, but no loss to touch (posterior grey horns and most of posterior white columns intact). Dislocation of the odontoid process can produce ischaemic necrosis of the upper cervical cord; in one of our cases (unpublished) the major portion of the necrosis was in the field of, and was probably due to compression of, the anterior spinal artery. Mair and Druckman (1953) considered that the changes which occur in the spinal cord, in association with protrusion of cervical intervertebral discs, are secondary to compression of the anterior spinal artery and its branches.

Proven cases of occlusion of the caudal portion of the anterior spinal artery are also few. They were reviewed by Zeitlin and Lichtenstein (1936). All were due to syphilis. Their own case, which was due to arteriosclerosis, was unusual, in that the extent of the lesion was in the middle segments of the cord from C.5 to Th.10, being maximal at Th.7 where it involved all the distribution of the artery.

TYPES OF VASCULAR DISEASE

Amongst the principal functions associated with the blood-vessels of the central nervous system are: (1) Conveyance of oxygen to the tissues and carrying away of carbon dioxide. This exchange takes place at capillary level. (2) Conveyance of glucose and other metabolites to the tissues. (3) Removal of waste products, both those soluble in tissue fluids and those carried by phagocytes. (4) Regulation of tissue fluids with regard to water and acid-base level. (5) Regulation of temperature. (6) Production and absorption of cerebrospinal fluid. (7) Taking part in the work of the blood brain barrier.

When considering vascular disease one may therefore consider:

(1) *Abnormalities of the circulating blood whereby these functions cannot be carried out.* The blood may be abnormal in respect of the quantity of haemoglobin or the ability of the haemoglobin to carry oxygen: as in the anaemias, or in carbon monoxide poisoning. This is termed

anaemic hypoxaemia or *anaemic anoxaemia* in relation to the blood, and *anaemic hypoxia* or *anaemic anoxia* in relation to the oxygen available to the tissues. The haemoglobin may be sufficient but it may be unsaturated with oxygen as in drowning, asphyxia and in high-altitude sickness. The terms then used are *anoxic anoxaemia* and *anoxic anoxia.* The blood may be deficient in glucose as in hypoglycaemic coma; it may be too hot as in heat stroke. These abnormalities are dealt with in other sections of the book.

(2) *Disease processes whereby healthy blood does not circulate properly through the blood vessels* (ischaemia and stagnant anoxia). It is with such conditions that this chapter is largely concerned. The blood may not circulate through the whole central nervous system because of arrest or impairment of cardiac action; or part of the central nervous system because of embolism or thrombosis. The blood may be impeded by disease of the vessel wall. In addition, disease of the vessel may result in haemorrhage. Most of the disease processes considered in this chapter fit into one or other or both of the categories of *obstructive lesions* or *haemorrhagic lesions.*

Obstructive lesions

Interference with the supply of blood reaching a portion of the nervous system can be expected to cause damage which lies somewhere between the extremes of temporary impairment of function and death of the tissue.

The type of cell and tissue which dies and the extent of the necrosis depend largely upon the relative vulnerability of the cells and tissues, the rate of reduction of blood flow, and the type of vessel which is obstructed.

Relative vulnerability of cells and tissues. Nerve cells and their processes and oligodendroglia are the most vulnerable, astrocytes are more resistant, whilst microglia and capillaries survive longest under such conditions. Nerve cells in different regions of the brain are not equally damaged by ischaemia. From 3 to 8 minutes of ischaemia is sufficient to kill nerve cells in the cerebral cortex. The Purkinje cells of the cerebellum are almost as vulnerable. The granule cells of the cerebellum and the nerve cells of the brain stem are much more resistant. In the cerebral cortex itself there is a difference in vulnerability of the different layers. Layers 3 and 4 are particularly sensitive to ischaemia, which may destroy only these layers, giving rise to laminar necrosis.

The rate of reduction of blood flow below a critical level is most important in relation to the collateral or anastomotic circulation. If the blood flow through an artery is gradually reduced, as by atherosclerosis, then there is often sufficient time for the anastomotic vessels to dilate and compensate. If, however, the obstruction is sudden, as by an embolus, then much of the tissue dies before an adequate anastomotic circulation is established.

Type of vessel affected. The effects of vascular obstruction vary with the type of vessel which is principally involved. The obstruction may be in relation to a major artery or at arteriolar or capillary level or in relation to veins or dural venous sinuses.

The smallest cortical lesions, on the arterial side of the circulation, which are histologically recognisable, are those due to an impaired circulation through the smaller cortical arteries and arterioles. Sometimes the process is confined to the distribution of single arterioles, and the anoxia is of such a degree that the only cells which die are the nerve cells. In the early state the lesion is visible histologically (Fig. 2.1), in Nissl preparations, as a perivascular *region of pallor* running down at right angles to the surface of the cortex (Spielmeyer's *erbleichung*). The nerve cells are still present but they are smaller than normal, the cytoplasm stains poorly with basic dyes and the nuclei are small and darkly stained; in haematoxylin-eosin preparations the cytoplasm is eosinophilic. This picture soon changes to one of increased cellularity, due to the presence of numerous rod-shaped microglia. The final stage is one of tissue shrinkage and perivascular fibrous gliosis. Such regions of cortical pallor and scarring are found in patients with atherosclerosis and with hypertensive arteriolosclerosis.

Granular atrophy of the cortex has a similar anatomical basis and probably results from more severe focal anoxia. At post-mortem, after removal of the arachnoid, the affected surface of the brain resembles the surface of a kidney with 'granular atrophy' (Fig. 2.2). The condition, which is rare, is often bilaterally symmetrical. Pentschew (1933) found that it was usually limited to the middle frontal gyrus and to the parieto-occipital convolutions. Lindenberg and Spatz (1939), in one group of their cases of thrombo-angiitis obliterans, found a sickle-shaped zone of granular atrophy on the convexity of each cerebral hemisphere, stretching from

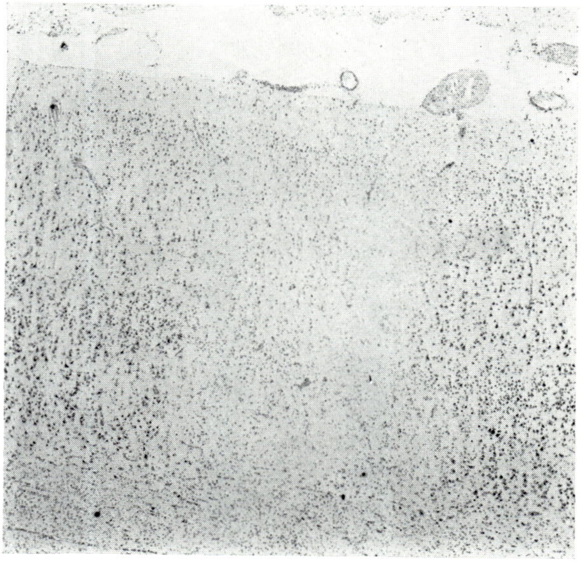

FIG. 2.1. *Region of pallor* in the cortex, situated near the temporal pole at the periphery of the distribution of the middle cerebral artery, in a patient with thrombosis of the middle cerebral artery on the same side. Note that the pial vessels appear healthy at this level. (Celloidin, Nissl, ×30.)

the frontal pole upwards towards the vertex and then down to the occipital pole. Sometimes it was also present on the inferior surface of the hemisphere, running from the occipital to the temporal pole. Lindenberg pointed out that this distribution corresponds with the border zone between the cortical fields of the anterior, middle and posterior cerebral arteries.

Microscopically, the multiple depressions in the cortex correspond with regions of softening and coarse fibrous gliosis which run in at right angles to the cortex (Fig. 2.3). Hyaline degeneration may affect the small intracerebral arterioles, but the cause of the cortical lesions probably lies at a more proximal site in the arterial tree, at the level of the arterioles and small arteries in the pia-arachnoid. Narrowing of these vessels by hypertensive arterio- and arteriolosclerosis, by syphilitic endarteritis, by atherosclerosis or by thrombo-angiitis obliterans has been reported in cases with granular atrophy. Pentschew found that it may occur as a sequel of carbon monoxide poisoning.

Granular atrophy of the brain is almost invariably associated with granular atrophy of the kidneys. Pentschew noted this association in 9 out of the 11 cases, and Lindenberg and Spatz in all 7 of the cases in which the kidneys were examined.

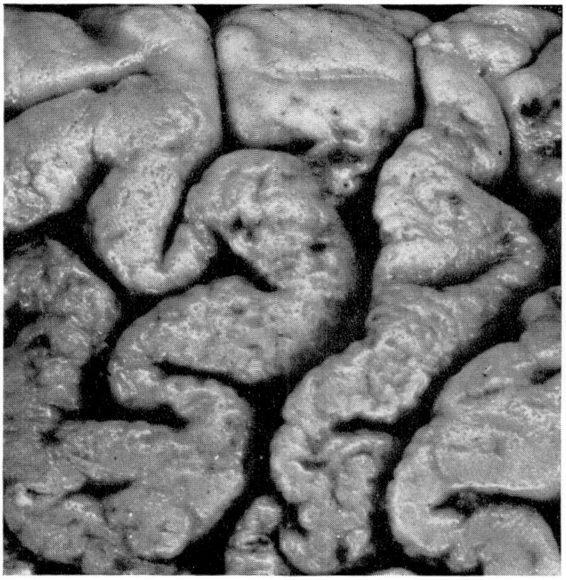

2.2

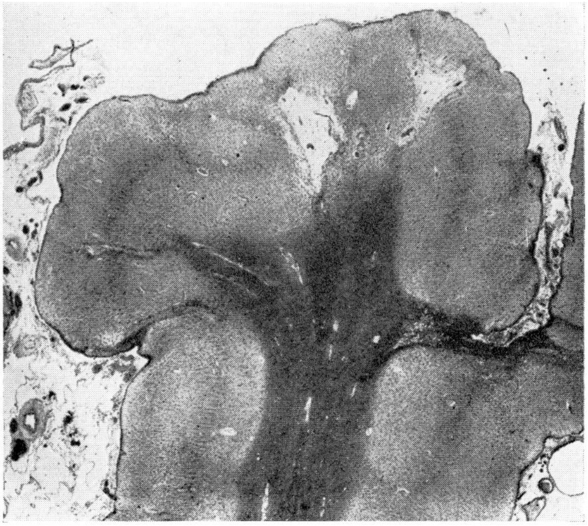

2.3

FIG. 2.2. Granular atrophy of the cortex. Lateral aspect of the left cerebral hemisphere after removal of the leptomeninges. Note the numerous depressions of the surface.

FIG. 2.3. Region of granular atrophy from the same case as the previous figure, from a man of 37 with chronic-endarteritis of uncertain type. Note the thickened and narrowed arteries in the leptomeninges and the numerous depressions in the cortex which are associated with the softenings and scars which run in at right angles to the surface. (Celloidin, phosphotungstic acid haematoxylin, ×9.)

INFARCTION

When a large artery, such as one of the named arteries of a cerebral hemisphere, is obstructed, especially if the obstruction is rapid as by an embolus, the region affected is usually an extensive zone of cortex and a considerable depth of the underlying white matter. The earliest change which is visible to the naked eye is one of swelling of both grey and white matter. The grey matter is congested, either diffusely or in a patchy fashion and it is often stippled with petechial haemorrhages. This is called *haemorrhagic infarction* (Figs. 2.4 and 2.5). The white matter looks pale and, in the early stages, may be difficult to distinguish from the normal. This appearance is called pale infarction or more accurately *ischaemic necrosis*. The swelling which accompanies these changes is considerable. In the case of a large infarct, it may constitute a 'space occupying lesion' and produce secondary vascular lesions in the region of the midbrain (*vide infra*).

Changes in the grey matter

In the early stages, microscopical examination of the infarcted grey matter reveals a state of widespread tissue damage. At the centre of a large infarct this may consist of coagulative necrosis of all elements. In small infarcts and at the periphery of large infarcts the damage is less severe and the appearances are those of disintegration of nerve cells, myelin sheaths and

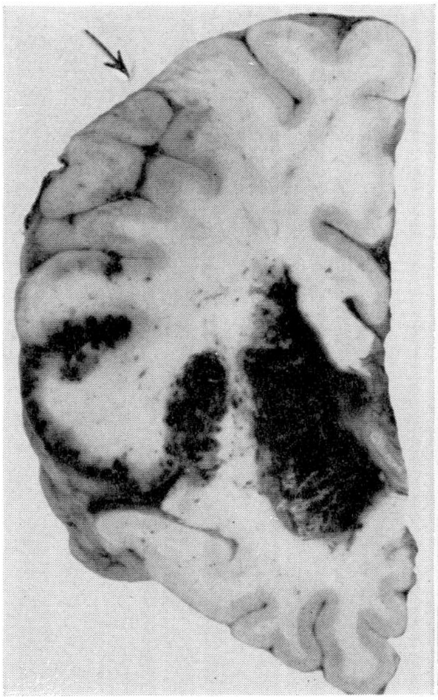

2.4

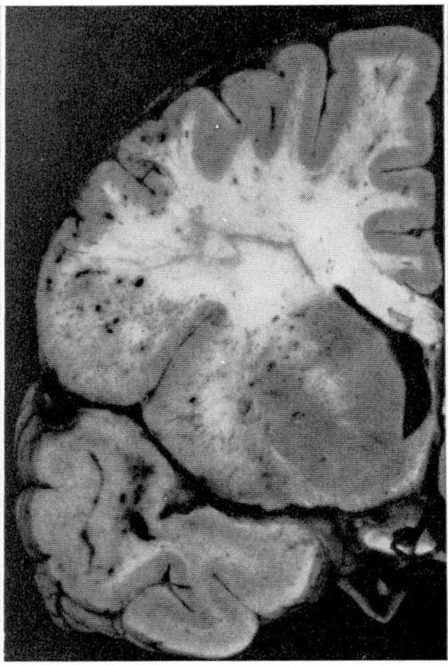

2.6

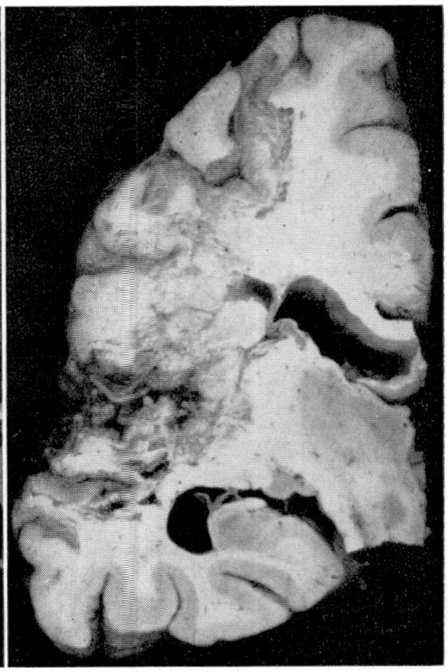

2.8

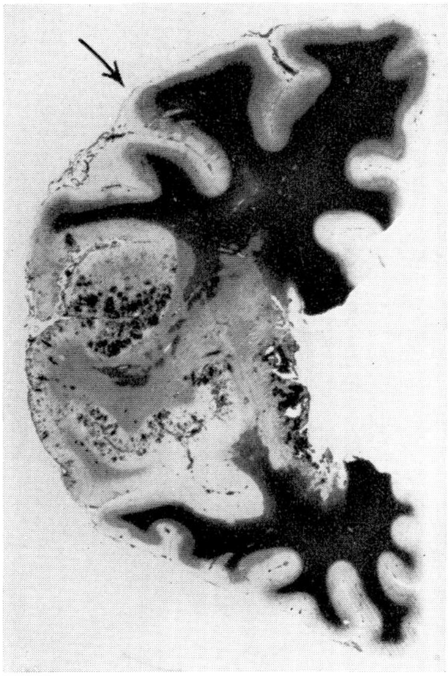

2.5

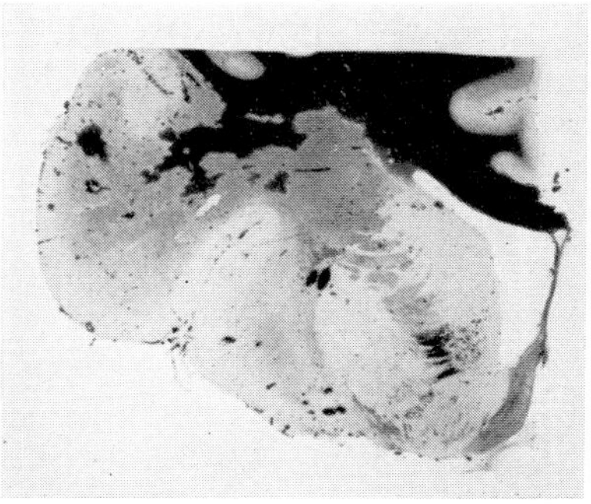

2.7

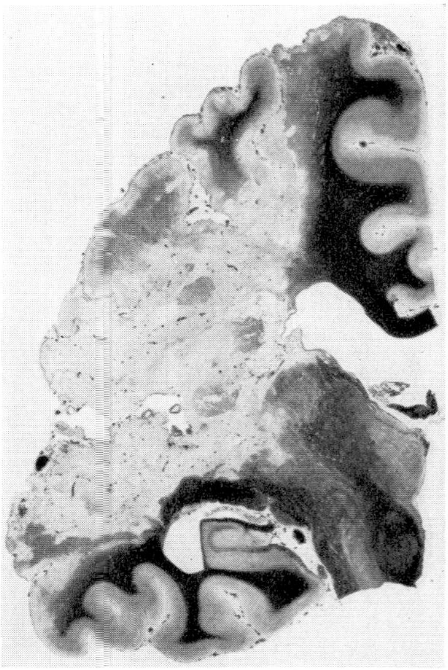

2.9

FIG. 2.4. Coronal section, frontal lobe, atherosclerotic carotid artery (same case as Figs. 2.17 and 2.18). In the lower part of the picture is recent, embolic, haemorrhagic infarction of the cortex. The underlying white matter is also necrotic, although this is not clearly visible. This part of the brain is swollen and the line of demarcation between cortex and white matter is ill-defined (see also Figs. 2.10 and 2.12). In the upper part of the picture (arrow) is an older lesion, of about 6 weeks' duration (see also Figs. 2.13 and 2.14).

FIG. 2.5. Myelin preparation of Fig. 2.4. Note the sharp edge to the necrotic white matter, which does not stain. In some places only the subcortical U-fibres are necrotic, in other places the deep white matter is damaged. Note the older lesions (arrow).

FIG. 2.6. Embolic occlusion of middle cerebral artery, of 3 weeks' duration, from thrombus overlying atherosclerotic myocardial infarct of left ventricle. The necrotic grey matter, which is friable, is not clearly defined from the white matter. In the centrum semi-ovale the edge of the necrotic white matter is clearly visible. The infero-medial half of the corpus striatum (supplied by the recurrent artery of Heubner) is not necrotic.

FIG. 2.7. Myelin preparation of middle part of Fig. 2.6. Note the sharp edge to the necrotic white matter.

FIG. 2.8. Old infarct (clinically 5 months), due to atherosclerotic carotid artery occlusion. The products of tissue destruction have been largely removed, leaving cystic spaces. Note that the edge of the infarct, which goes down to the ventricular wall, is clearly defined. The hemisphere is shrunken, the ventricle dilated. Middle cerebral artery distribution.

FIG. 2.9. Myelin preparation of Fig. 2.8 showing well-defined margin of the infarct corresponding with that seen in previous figure. (Celloidin, Loyez.)

oligodendroglia, varying degrees of damage to astrocytes, survival of microglia and blood-vessels, with pericapillary and perivenular haemorrhages. Often the small blood-vessels are filled by neutrophil polymorph leucocytes which can also be seen in the surrounding disintegrating parenchyma (Fig. 2.10), sometimes in large numbers. This is evidence that blood is flowing in this region. Many of these polymorphonuclear leucocytes pass, in the perivascular spaces, to the subarachnoid space and may be found in the cerebrospinal fluid on lumbar puncture (Cone and Barrera, 1931).

After 4 or 5 days, under usual circumstances, the polymorph leucocytic infiltration has been replaced by an infiltration of mononuclear phagocytes, many of which are already ingesting the sudanophilic and crystalline anisotropic products of neuronal and myelin disintegration. At this stage the endothelial cells of the capillaries show both hypertrophy and hyperplasia (Figs. 2.11 and 2.12); mitotic figures can sometimes be seen in them. The number of capillaries appears to be increased, although it is difficult to know whether this increase is real. The red blood corpuscles disintegrate and material staining positively with Prussian blue can be seen in phagocytes. To the naked eye, from about this stage onwards, a haemorrhagic infarct will look brown because of the blood pigments. At the margin of old haemorrhagic infarcts of the grey matter it is not uncommon to find small structures with the shape of shrunken nerve cells, which stain strongly with Prussian blue. These are called ferruginated nerve cells (*vide* Chapter 1).

The process of tissue breakdown and phagocytosis and removal continues (Figs. 2.6, 2.13 and 2.14). Cystic spaces filled with fluid replace the parenchyma (Figs. 2.8 and 2.9). Repair is effected by the astrocytes at the margins of the lesion. They show both hypertrophy and hyperplasia and lay down astrocytic fibres. The bodies of many of the astrocytes are swollen with an abundance of hyaline eosinophilic cytoplasm; some are binucleated (Figs. 2.15 and 2.16). After some months the picture is one of large or small cystic spaces, containing fluid and variable numbers of fat granule cells, bordered by astrocytes and astrocytic fibres. In many of the spaces run small healthy looking blood-vessels. It is the blood-vessels which first receive the benefit of the circulating blood after the opening up of the collateral circulation; their survival must be ascribed to this and perhaps to a relatively greater capacity to withstand anoxia.

The margin between an old infarct and the adjacent grey matter is sharply defined. The subpial margin of an infarct is usually composed of layer I of the cortex in which there is much astrocytic gliosis. Sometimes, however, the ischaemia has been so prolonged or severe that even this layer is absent. The wall is then formed of pia mater, from which a small number of delicate collagen fibrils pass towards the surviving blood-vessels at the margin of the cyst.

In large infarcts some central portions of the grey matter may, from the first, show coagulative necrosis (Fig. 2.17). Even when the collateral circulation opens up, the blood does not circulate through the capillaries of this central portion and everything within this zone dies. Disintegration and phagocytosis of this dead material proceeds from the periphery. Here the end stage is that of a large cavity filled only with clear fluid. This process, although it may occur in the cerebral cortex, is more commonly seen in the caudate and putamen (Fig. 2.23).

Changes in the white matter

In the white matter, the process, from the first, is one of coagulative necrosis without haemorrhage (so called pale infarct). In passing it should be mentioned that a similar process is found in infarction of the brain stem. In the first few days it may be very difficult to see a pale infarct with the naked eye (Figs. 2.4 and 2.5), but within about 24 hours it becomes visible in stained preparations by the poor staining of the myelin. The tissue swells, the nuclei of oligodendroglia and astrocytes disappear and Pickworth preparations show empty capillaries.

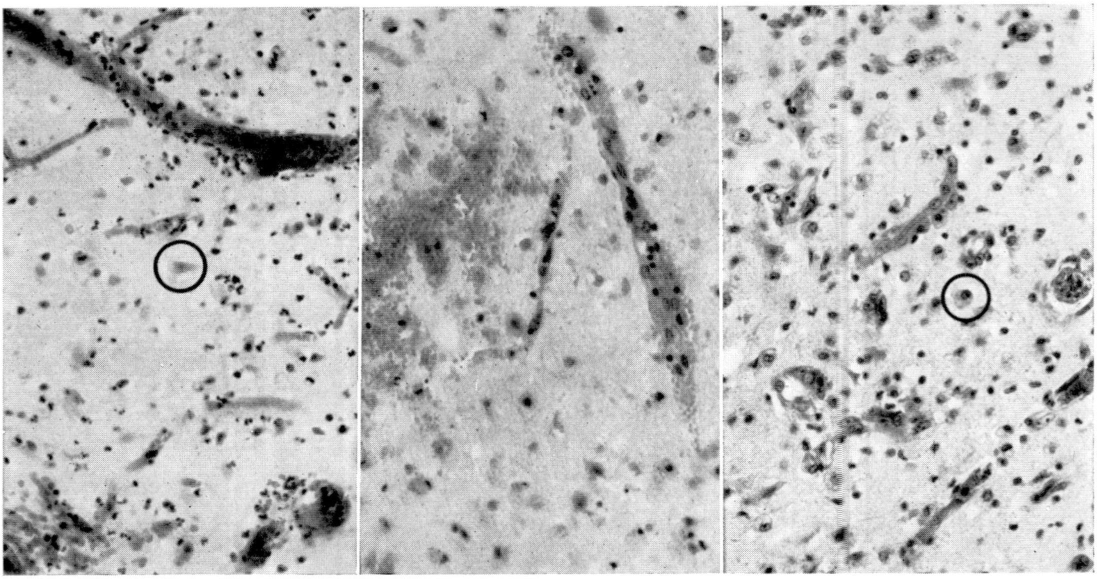

2.10 2.11 2.12

FIGS. 2.10, 2.11 and 2.12. Recent infarction of grey matter showing (2.10) polymorphonuclear leucocytes migrating from the dilated blood-vessels into the necrotic parenchyma. The circle encloses a dead nerve cell; (2.11) hyperplasia of the capillary endothelium and diapedetic haemorrhage; (2.12) at a later stage, capillary endothelial hyperplasia and the appearance of phagocytes distended with products of tissue disintegration (circle). (Celloidin, haematoxylin van Gieson, × 195.)

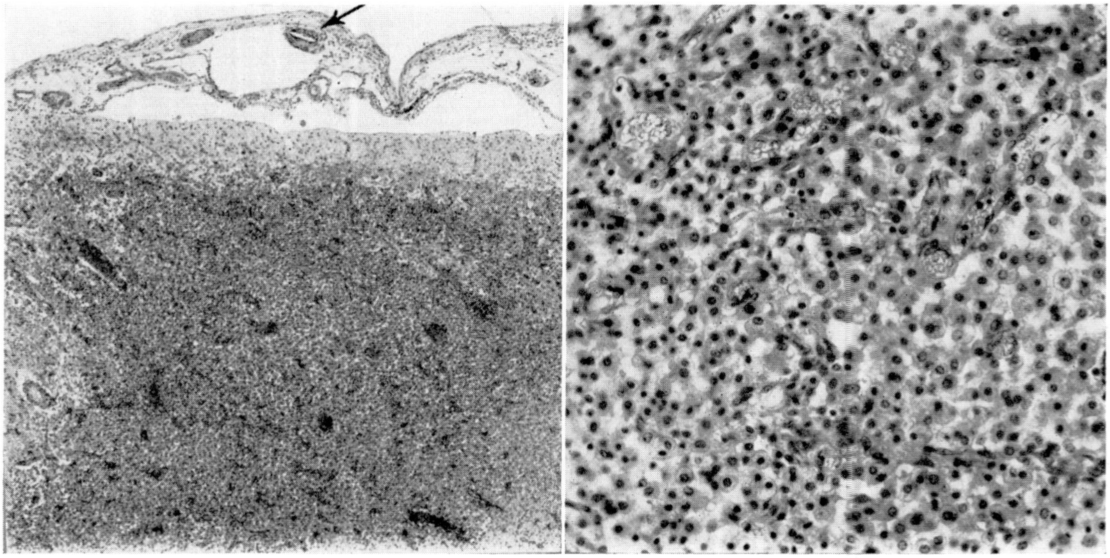

2.13 2.14

FIGS. 2.13 and 2.14. Portion of older (6-week) cortical infarct in Fig. 2.4 showing recanalised cortical artery (arrow) and disintegration of all but layer I of the cortex. The necrotic tissue has broken down and has been replaced by innumerable distended phagocytes. Blood appears to be circulating through the numerous capillaries which are dilated. They still show endothelial hyperplasia. (Celloidin, haematoxylin van Gieson, × 34 and × 195.)

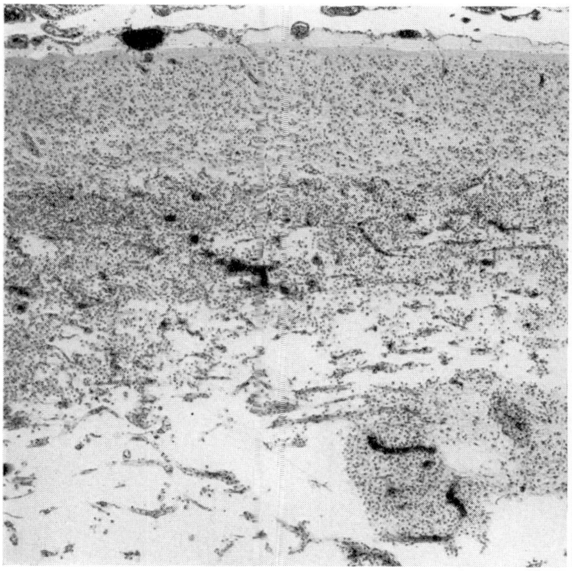

2.15

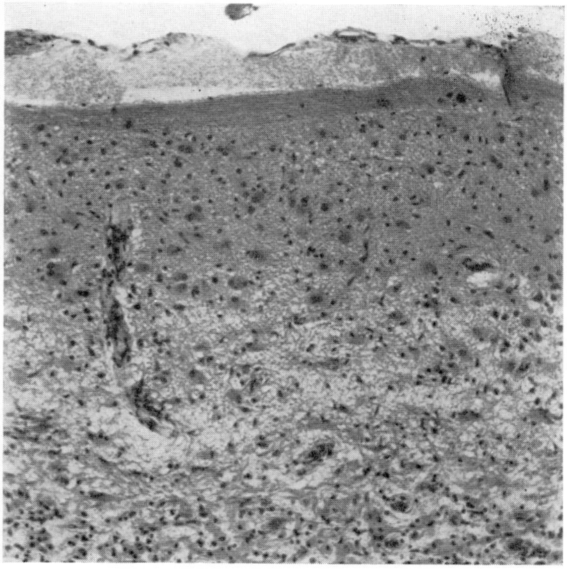

2.16

FIG. 2.15. Cerebral infarct, clinically 6 weeks' duration. The superficial layers of the cortex have survived. The rest of the cortex and the underlying white matter are largely replaced by spaces filled with fluid and traversed by blood vessels. Groups of phagocytes are also present. (Celloidin, haematoxylin and eosin, ×30.)

FIG. 2.16. Higher power of upper part of previous figure. Astrocytic hypertrophy and hyperplasia are visible in the superficial layers of the cortex. Some astrocytes are binucleated. (Haematoxylin and eosin, ×150.)

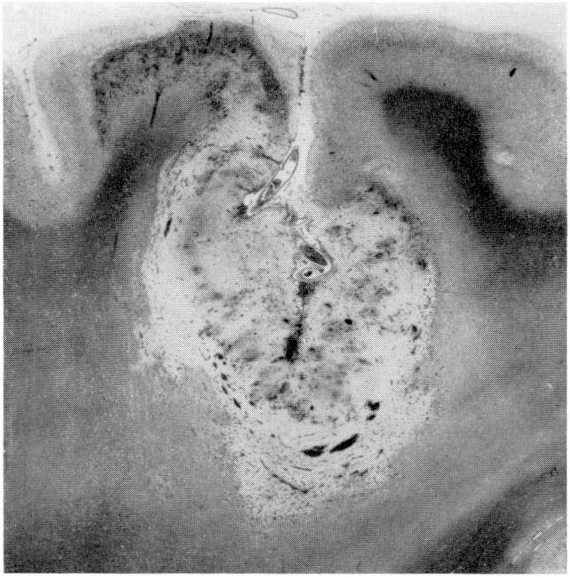

FIG. 2.17. Isolated embolic cerebral infarct, 3 weeks' duration, same case as Figs. 2.6 and 2.7. The central portion of the infarct shows coagulative necrosis. At the periphery there is cellular reaction, which is more marked in the grey matter. Organising thrombus is visible in the cortical arteriole within the sulcus. (Celloidin, haematoxylin van Gieson, ×4.)

Only at the periphery of the lesion is there any sign of reaction. Here the axons are swollen and the myelin sheaths are ballooned (Fig. 2.18). Between the thin rim of distended myelin and the axon there is a space which does not stain: presumably it contained fluid. The axons degenerate and disappear and then the distended myelin sheaths begin to disintegrate. Occasional cells are seen within them, either small mononuclear cells with rounded hyperchromatic nuclei or compound granular corpuscles. Reactionary changes take place in the adjacent blood-vessels. The larger vessels are distended with blood and the capillaries show endothelial hyperplasia. The myelin sheaths now disintegrate completely, sudanophilic lipid and anisotropic elongated crystalline material appear and are ingested by mononuclear phago-

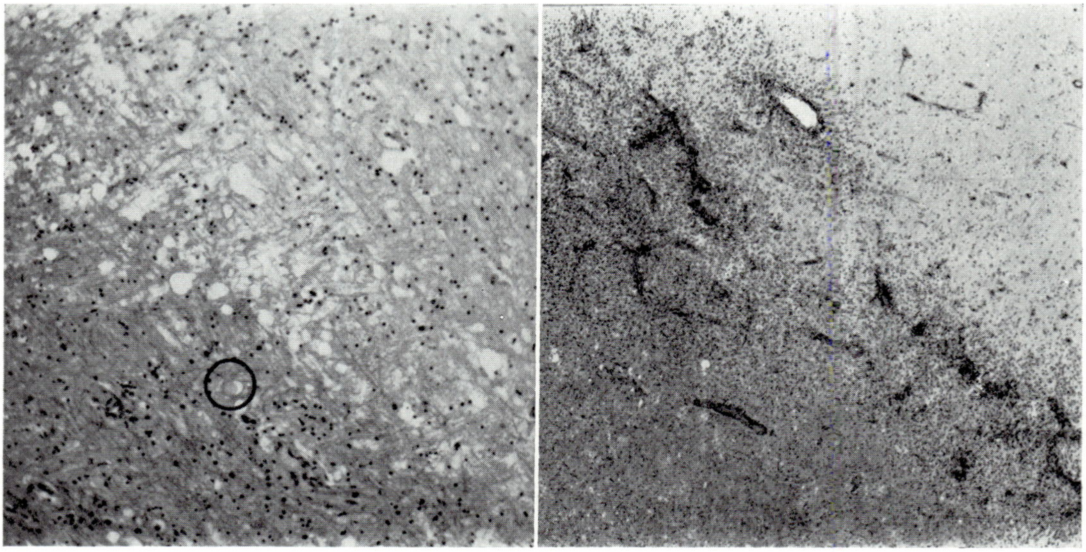

2.18 2.19

FIGS. 2.18 and 2.19. Edge of an infarct of the white matter

Fig. 2.18 was clinically of 5 days' duration (same case as Fig. 2.11). The infarcted white matter, upper right-hand side of picture, shows coagulative necrosis and stains poorly. At the margin of the lesion the myelin sheaths are distended and sometimes contain a swollen axon (circle). (Celloidin, haematoxylin van Gieson, × 100.)

Fig. 2.19 was clinically of 3 weeks' duration (same case as Figs. 2.6, 2.7 and 2.17). The infarcted white matter, upper right-hand side of picture, shows coagulative necrosis and stains poorly. At the margin of the lesion numerous phagocytes can be seen, particularly around the dilated blood-vessels. (Celloidin, haematoxylin van Gieson, × 28.)

cytes. Lymphocyte-like cells appear in the perivascular spaces. Gradually the phagocytes, distended with lipid, become less numerous in the parenchyma, more numerous in the perivascular spaces. Astrocytes show hypertrophy and hyperplasia and lay down astrocytic fibres.

The process of disintegration gradually spreads into the central zone of coagulative necrosis (Fig. 2.19) and the macroscopical appearance is one of a mass of slightly granular yellowish material separated by a narrow ragged cavity, from the surrounding healthy looking nervous tissue. Blood never returns to this central zone; the capillaries and the astrocytes die, in addition to the nerve fibres and oligodendroglia, so that there are no local cells to multiply and effect repair. Astrocytes from the periphery do not grow into this region to any appreciable extent and the end result is a cystic space filled with clear fluid.

Explanation of morphological changes

The process which underlies haemorrhagic infarction of the grey matter is considered to be as follows. Immediately after obstruction of the artery, blood ceases to flow through its arterioles and capillaries. The tissue around its capillaries ceases to receive oxygen, katabolic products accumulate and cellular damage commences in nerve cells, oligodendroglia, astrocytes, microglia and capillary walls, in that order of vulnerability. The next event is an opening up of the anastomotic vessels at the periphery of the ischaemic zone, and there is experimental evidence, Meyer *et al.* (1954), that this is dependent upon local metabolic factors, of which CO_2 appears to be relatively unimportant. If the blood pressure in the surrounding arterial fields is not low, blood will flow in through the anastomotic vessels and there will be a return of the circulation of blood through the capillary network.

These capillaries are not, however, quite normal. Sometimes the duration of ischaemia has been so short that they are only unduly distensible, in which case the result will be one of marked congestion. More often, however, the duration of ischaemia has been such that, not only are the walls unduly distensible, but also they are so damaged that they are unduly permeable to plasma and red blood corpuscles. The result will be congestion, swelling of the tissue from leakage of plasma and also petechial haemorrhages from diapedesis of red blood corpuscles. This is a red or haemorrhagic infarction.

A factor of great importance is the pressure of the blood in the arterial fields surrounding the ischaemic zone. It has been shown experimentally in the monkey (Meyer *et al.* 1954) that the anastomotic circulation does not become established if the systemic blood pressure falls below 60 mm. Hg. The same factor appears to operate in the human. In one of our cases the surgeon was forced, at operation for a suprasellar tumour, to ligate the anterior cerebral artery and the recurrent artery of Heubner. Following the operation the systemic blood pressure remained low. At post-mortem examination, 10 days later, the infarction in the grey matter in the distribution of the clipped arteries was pale, an indication that blood had not entered in any appreciable quantity through the anastomotic circulation.

The pallor, congestion or haemorrhagic nature of the infarct in the grey matter will be directly related to the amount of blood re-entering parts or the whole of the devitalised capillary bed. This blood may enter at various places, in varying amounts, through the anastomotic circulation. It may however also re-enter through the original artery if the obstruction is relieved, as by disintegration of the original embolus, the particles of which pass onwards to block only some of the branches of the original artery. Fisher and Adams (1951) consider that this is the main factor in the production of the mottled pale and haemorrhagic infarcts which are so commonly seen in the grey matter in cerebral embolism. They suggest that blockage of an artery by an embolus causes pale infarction in the tissues supplied by that artery. Later, due to fragmentation of the embolic material, and possibly to relaxation of local vascular spasm, the embolus moves from its original position into more distal branches. This exposes the necrotic tissue to the full force of the arterial blood pressure with resulting haemorrhage from damaged capillaries. Parts of the brain supplied by arteries which are still occluded remain anaemic.

Whilst we would agree that this happens in some cases, it is not necessarily the only explanation of the mixture of pale and haemorrhagic infarcts of the grey matter which are often found after sudden obstruction of a large artery. Not all parts of the initially anaemic region are equidistant from the anastomotic vessels. The parts which are very close will receive the greatest quantity of blood after the shortest interval of time and may indeed suffer no permanent damage. Further from the source of returning blood there is a zone where plasma and red blood corpuscles will leak from the damaged capillaries. This region will be haemorrhagic to the naked eye and under the microscope the vessels will be engorged. This histological appearance is not, however, a proof that the blood was circulating. The walls of many capillaries are so damaged and so much plasma has leaked away that the red blood corpuscles within both large and small vessels are stranded, clumped or conglutinated into slowly moving or immovable masses—a state of *pre-stasis* or *stasis*. This pre-stasis or stasis will impede or obstruct the return of blood to distal portions of the capillary bed and to parts which are, in any case, the farthest from the anastomotic vessels. For both these reasons the infarct in the distal portion is likely to remain pale.

Whilst infarction of cortical grey matter, when due to acute arterial obstruction, is often congested or haemorrhagic, the infarction in the underlying white matter is always pale. This appearance is probably due in part to the less dense and therefore less visibly prominent capillary meshwork in the white matter; and in part to the fact that the vessels which supply the white matter have fewer anastomoses and are more in the nature of 'end arteries', so that less blood will return to the white matter when the anastomotic circulation opens up. In the grey matter there are very numerous capillary anastomoses.

Upon the role of *spasm* in relation to infarction it is difficult to be dogmatic. From experimental work upon animals it is known that the plain muscle in the wall of an artery or arteriole goes into contraction or spasm if it is stretched. This response occurs if the intravascular pressure is raised above the normal, irrespective of whether the pressure is raised from the arterial side (Byrom 1954) or from the venous side (Denny-Brown *et al.* 1956). It is also the probable explanation of the spasm which can follow the manipulation of a cerebral artery. It is known that arteriolar spasm can follow the impaction of needle-like emboli made of crushed glass wool in the cerebral arteries of the dog (Villaret and Cachera 1939). It is thus possible that, in man, when an embolus impacts in a cerebral vessel, there is transient overdistension of the vessel wall and transient localised or even propagated spasm.

ARTERIAL EMBOLISM

The circulation of the blood through the brain and spinal cord may be impeded by emboli, which may be solitary or multiple. According to their size they become impacted in arteries, arterioles or capillaries. The blood flow is arrested suddenly, so that the ischaemic effects are not mitigated by the previous establishment of a collateral circulation. If emboli reach the brain through the internal carotid artery they usually become impacted in the distribution of the middle cerebral artery. When they come from the heart, they lodge as often in the left cerebral hemisphere as in the right (Jones 1910). The chief types of embolus are blood clot (either bland or infected), fat and gas (air or nitrogen).

Blood clot (bland)

These emboli usually originate from thrombi in the auricular appendages of the heart in patients with auricular fibrillation, from thrombi overlying myocardial infarcts, from thrombosed internal carotid or vertebral or basilar arteries. Cortical infarcts produced by these emboli are usually haemorrhagic; the question of fragmentation of the embolus has already been discussed (p. 87). Infarcts in the basal ganglia are usually pale, but sometimes they are very haemorrhagic (Fig. 2.21) and when this occurs there is usually reason to believe that the embolus has first occluded the striate arteries and then moved on down the middle cerebral artery.

Blood clot (infected)

These emboli usually originate in pulmonary suppuration or bacterial endocarditis or pyaemia. According to their size and virulence they may give rise to brain purpura, suppurative encephalitis or myelitis, abscess or mycotic aneurysm.

Fat embolism

Following fractures (especially of long bones) or trauma to subcutaneous tissues or to fatty viscera, innumerable small globules of fat may appear in the bloodstream. These fatty emboli are held up at capillary level, particularly in the lungs, kidneys and central nervous system. The symptoms of cerebral fat embolism do not immediately follow the trauma: there is usually an interval of time (average 3–6 days). Widespread involvement is shown by headache, fatigue and sleepiness progressing to stupor, coma and death. Hemiplegia and ocular palsy can occur. Strauss (1933) found that the prognosis was bad. In his series, of 89 cases, 70 died: 12 on the 1st day, 17 on the 2nd day, 19 on the 3rd day, 13 on the 4th day and 9 between the 6th and 11th day. In patients with multiple injuries, including damage to the brain, the possibility of associated fat embolism should always be considered.

In patients who die within the first 3 or 4 days, the white matter of the brain is diffusely studded with petechial haemorrhages, one type of cerebral purpura. Microscopically these are pericapillary, ring, and ball haemorrhages. Numerous fat globules are visible in these capillaries. Sometimes the capillary walls show focal necrosis. Around some capillaries there are zones of myelin pallor; around others the parenchyma is necrotic and infiltrated by numerous polymorphonuclear leucocytes. In the grey matter fat globules are equally numerous, but haemorrhages and tissue damage are not visible. The reason why the haemorrhages are confined to the white matter is probably dependent upon the capillary network. In the grey matter the capillaries are individually short, anastomoses are frequent. Should one segment of capillary be blocked, enough oxygen can usually diffuse out from the closely adjacent capillaries to keep alive the obstructed capillaries and the surrounding tissue. In the white matter the capillaries are long, anastomoses are few and the wall of the blocked capillary is rendered anoxic; the endothelial cells become less firmly bound together, or die, and red blood corpuscles and plasma leak out.

In patients who survive for several days changes may be found in the grey matter. In a case surviving 6½ days (Neubürger 1925) there were miliary foci of necrosis. These were chiefly in the deeper layers of the cortex. Nerve cells had disappeared but glial cells were numerous. Glial shrubs were present in the molecular layer of the cerebellum from which Purkinje cells had disappeared. Fat globules were present in the capillaries both in the lesions and also in vessels in normal regions.

In a case surviving 12 days Winkelman (1942) found small softenings of various ages in the deeper layers of the cortex, in the white matter especially of the frontal lobes, and in the brain stem especially in the pons. The oldest lesions were full of compound granular cells and the capillaries were prominent.

Air embolism

Air may enter the circulation during abortion, following trauma or operation on the lungs, during artificial pneumothorax, from suicidal or surgical damage to the veins of the neck, and during neurosurgical operations on the cervical region with the patient in the sitting position. If the volume of air is small there may be little change in the condition of the patient. If the quantity of air is large, it will rapidly be mixed with the blood in the heart to produce a frothy fluid, which will then be pumped into the coronary arteries and systemic circulation. The patient will immediately become pale, then cyanotic; coma, convulsions, hemiplegia and blindness may develop with great rapidity. Death occurs in 15–50 per cent of cases (Hamilton and Rothstein 1935), probably from ventricular fibrillation due to obstruction of the coronary arteries by air bubbles. The prognosis in air embolism is, however, much better than in fat embolism. If the patient can survive the first 10–15 minutes the danger has largely passed (Hiller 1936). Severe paralysis and blindness may completely disappear within hours or days, although mental disturbance may persist.

Post-mortem examination of patients with suspected air embolism must be carried out with care. Taylor (1952) recommends X-raying the intact body, when large collections of air will easily be seen. Before the rest of the body is disturbed the pericardial sac should be filled with water and the right ventricle should be incised under water. Air will then bubble out. If there is any possibility of gas having been formed by anaerobic bacilli such as *B. Welchii*, the blood should be cultured. If the amount of air has been large, frothy blood will be present in the right side of the heart and air will be visible in the veins. More gas bubbles than usual will be seen in the cerebral veins.

In patients who die within a few minutes the only abnormality is the excess of air in the veins. There are no haemorrhages and no microscopical abnormalities in the brain.

In Neubürger's patient (1925), who survived for 55 hours, there were small, perivascular, cortical foci of ischaemic neuronal damage. The nerve cells had pale eosinophilic cytoplasm and disintegrating nuclei (the appearances are similar to those seen after temporary recovery from cardiac arrest). In addition to the perivascular distribution of the lesions there was also a laminar pattern of neuronal damage. Lhermitte and Barrelet (1934) in a patient who died of pneumonia some weeks after air embolism, found marked changes in the cortex but none in the white matter. There was spongy transformation of the molecular and external granular layers of the cerebral cortex and scattered, small, irregularly shaped foci from which all the nerve cells and glial cells had disappeared; some of these foci contained the remains of a blood vessel, in others there was a vessel filled with blood but with a necrotic wall. Chromatolysis was present in some of the cortical layers, especially the 6th. In one part of the parietal cortex, the nerve cells of the 2nd and 3rd layers had completely disappeared, with replacement by glial cells including rod cells.

Nitrogen embolism. (*Decompression sickness*)

When a person has been living for some time in air which is at a pressure greater than the normal atmospheric and then the pressure is rapidly diminished, he often suffers from sensory and motor disturbances of a transient or permanent nature. Sometimes he dies within an hour or two. At post-mortem, in patients who have survived for only a short time, the central nervous system is intensely congested and there may be haemorrhages. In patients who have survived for a longer period, there may be regions of softening. These lesions are commoner in the thoracic portion of the spinal cord than elsewhere. Haymaker (1957), whose article should be consulted by all those more deeply interested in the subject, considers that the involvement of the spinal cord is due to embolism by bubbles of nitrogen which appear in the bloodstream after the reduction in atmospheric pressure, together with embarrassment of the spino-vertebral venous circulation by gas bubbles arising in the epidural and/or retroperitoneal fat. Decompression sickness was first noticed in underwater divers and workers in caissons (Caisson disease). It has now to be taken into consideration in high-altitude flyers who may suddenly find themselves in a subnormal atmospheric pressure.

STENOSIS AND OCCLUSION OF THE INTERNAL CAROTID AND VERTEBRAL SYSTEMS

It has long been known, forgotten by the majority, and re-emphasised (Gowers 1893, Chiari 1905, Hunt 1914, Hultquist 1942 and Fisher 1951) that ischaemic lesions of the brain, in particular infarction in the distribution of the middle cerebral artery, may be secondary to disease of the internal carotid arteries in the neck. For example, Hunt pointed out that the main artery of the neck should always come under suspicion when, at post-mortem, such a focus of softening is found in association with a healthy-looking circle of Willis or with no demonstrable occlusion of the middle cerebral artery. Hutchinson and Yates (1956, 1957, 1961) have emphasised the importance of concomitant consideration and investigation of the vertebral arteries, in the neck as well as within the skull. When a disease process, such as atherosclerosis, affects one of these four main arteries it is likely to have affected the others to a varying degree. For purposes of discussion, stenosis and occlusion of the internal carotid system will be separated from stenosis and occlusion of the vertebral-basilar system, but they should not be so considered in relation to the patient.

Stenosis and occlusion of the internal carotid artery

During recent years an increasing amount of attention has been paid to thrombosis of the internal carotid artery In the living, diagnosis has been made much easier by arteriography; and at post-mortem the relative frequency of atherosclerotic narrowing, pointed out by Chiari (1905), has been re-emphasised by Hultquist (1942) who, in 1300 unselected autopsies between 1938–41, found macroscopical thrombosis of a carotid artery in 38 cases. It was twice as frequent in men as in women and, although found in young persons, was commonest in the age groups 50–70 (men), 60–80 (women).

In all cases of apparent embolism or thrombosis of the middle cerebral artery an examination of the internal carotid arteries should be carried out; for it is in relation to the middle cerebral artery that disease of the internal carotid artery is most likely to give rise to complications.

Changes in the artery. Whilst giant-celled arteritis has been seen and thrombo-angiitis obliterans has been reported, the usual cause of obstruction of the internal carotid artery is atherosclerosis with superimposed thrombus (Figs. 2.20 and 2.22). This thrombus is often partly organised. The narrowing frequently commences just distal to the origin of the artery or less often in the sigmoid portion of the artery. The obstruction is often incomplete and from the old thrombus a tongue of recent thrombus may extend cranially within the lumen of the artery. Sometimes the obstruction is complete. Then the proximal part of the thrombus, which is older, is partly red and partly grey in colour. It is a laminated thrombus, for it has formed in flowing blood. Distal to this level the artery often contains red thrombus, formed from stagnant blood, which frequently fills the lumen as far as the origin of a branch of the artery, where laminated thrombus may once more be found. This branch may be the ophthalmic artery, but in some cases the thrombus may extend as far as, or into, the commencement of the middle and anterior cerebral arteries. Carotid artery obstruction may occur bilaterally (Frøvig 1946) but is commoner unilaterally, being as frequent on the left as on the right.

Changes in the brain (Figs. 2.21 and 2.23). The brain may show extensive softening, involving either the major part of the distribution of the middle cerebral artery or the peripheral portion of this territory, or small focal softenings particularly in the internal capsule. The softening is seldom of the same age in all regions, some being old and some recent: in the grey matter portions are haemorrhagic, portions are pale. In addition foci of softening are some-

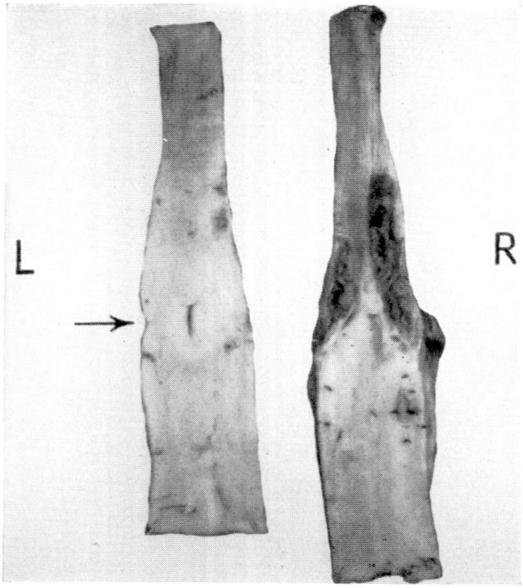

2.20

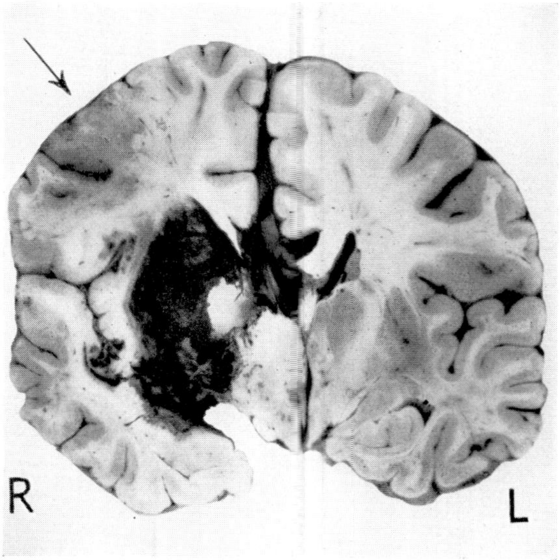

2.21

FIG. 2.20. Carotid arteries from the neck of a man aged 61. The common and internal carotid arteries have been opened up. The arrow indicates the site of origin of the internal carotid artery. Note that, on the left, there is atherosclerotic intimal thickening in this region, and that on the right, antemortem thrombus is adherent to this region and extends up the internal carotid artery.

FIG. 2.21. Same case as Fig. 2.20 showing recent infarction of cortex and basal ganglia (the hole on the medial aspect is artefact). Small thrombi, probably embolic from the internal carotid, were found in adjacent arteries. The exact age of this infarct is not certain but clinically it was within 7 days of death. Older infarction (clinically 6 weeks) is visible in the region of the arrow. No history of previous cerebral disease. Same case as Figs. 2.4, 2.5, 2.10, 2.12, 2.13 and 2.14.

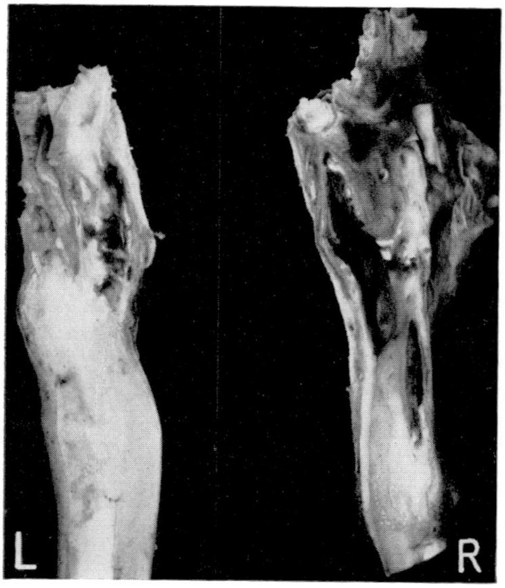

2.22

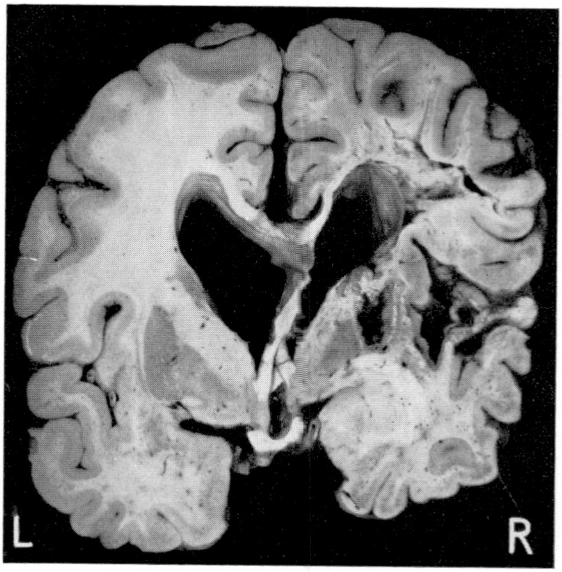

2.23

FIG. 2.22. Carotid arteries from the neck of a man, aged 62, with left hemiplegia of 18 months' duration. Both common carotid arteries showed a ring of calcification and atheroma at their points of bifurcation. On the left side the internal carotid, which has been opened up, is atheromatous with adherent thrombus. On the right side, about 1 inch above its origin, the internal carotid is almost completely occluded by old pale thrombus. Below this, recent reddish thrombus extends downwards into the lumen of the common carotid artery.

FIG. 2.23. Brain from same case as Fig. 2.22. On the right side there is old infarction, with cystic replacement of grey and white matter, including the putamen and internal capsule. The hemisphere is shrunken, the ventricles show compensatory dilatation.

times found in the distribution of the anterior or posterior cerebral arteries. Although the softenings are predominantly on the side of the thrombosed artery, they may be found on the opposite side, which has an apparently or relatively healthy carotid artery.

It may be possible to find obstructive lesions in the cerebral arteries related to the softenings. When the thrombosis extends into the middle cerebral artery the cause of the recent infarction is obvious. In some cases of long duration many branches of the middle cerebral artery are extensively occupied by old organised thrombus and appear pale, solid and threadlike (Fig. 2.8). But in other cases it may not be possible to find any macroscopical obstruction to the middle cerebral artery or to its larger branches. It may even be difficult or impossible to find any microscopical obstruction, although it cannot be said with certainty whether there is any organic obstruction until the whole vascular tree has been examined in serial sections.

When an obstruction is found it may be partial, complete or recanalised, concentric or eccentric, recent or old. If recent it may take the form of a partly coiled, partly organised, thrombus, with only slight attachment to the adjacent, otherwise healthy, vessel wall; an appearance compatible with an impacted embolus. The evidence of embolism is not, however, always definite and, especially when the obstruction is older and organised, it may not be possible to say whether it was originally embolic or locally thrombotic. In older lesions the internal elastic lamina and the media of the artery usually appear healthy, whilst the lumen is obstructed to a varying degree by cellular fibrous tissue in which, at some levels, long cholesterol crystals may be found. Sometimes, in the same microscopical section, healthy, patent, leptomeningeal arteries are found close to those with organic obstruction.

Clinically the condition may (1) be without symptoms or signs; (2) reveal itself by episodic attacks of transient motor or sensory impairment with considerable or complete recovery; (3) show gradual development of hemiplegia; (4) give rise to sudden permanent hemiplegia. Transient attacks of blindness are not uncommon. A full explanation of the clinical and arteriographic or post-mortem findings is not always easy. There is little doubt that some of the lesions are due to the spread of thrombus up into one or more of the branches of the circle of Willis. Some of the lesions appear to be embolic in nature, from detached portions of the thrombus in the internal carotid artery or its branches. Subsequent fragmentation and disimpaction of such emboli may explain the transitory character of some attacks. Pale friable emboli, probably composed mostly of platelets and a few polymorph leucocytes, have been seen with the ophthalmoscope passing along the retinal arteries during attacks of blindness (Fisher 1959, Russell 1961, McBrien *et al.* 1963). Alternatively such recurrent cerebro-vascular episodes may be the result of failure of the collateral circulation (Symonds 1955, Denny-Brown 1960).

When one internal carotid artery is obstructed, the blood flow to the ipsilateral hemisphere is assisted or taken over by a collateral circulation originating in (1) the contra-lateral internal carotid artery, which sends its blood across the midline via the anterior communicating artery, and (2) the ipsilateral external carotid artery, which, through branches of the facial artery and the superficial temporal artery, anastomoses with the dorsal nasal, frontal and supra-orbital branches of the ophthalmic artery. The direction of the blood flow in the ophthalmic artery is reversed so that the blood enters rather than leaves the internal carotid artery distal to its sigmoid portion. A collateral circulation may also originate in (3) the basilar artery from which the blood may pass anteriorly via the posterior communicating artery. These arteries have then to supply not only their original territory but also part or whole of the threatened cerebral hemisphere and possibly the optic nerve. Sometimes this collateral circulation is inadequate. This may be due to an incomplete circle of Willis or because of narrowness of calibre, from developmental causes or disease, of the arteries forming the circle. There will then be immediate irreversible ischaemic damage to the cerebral hemisphere. Often, however, the collateral circulation is, at first, adequate, or at least sufficient to prevent serious damage with permanent clinical symptoms and signs. With the passage of time, however, the diseased carotid artery will become further obstructed, the sources of collateral supply will themselves become narrowed by atherosclerosis, and the circulation through the vessels of the threatened cerebral hemisphere and the optic nerve will reach a precarious state. Such a circulation may easily be reduced below the critical level by such factors as a temporary fall in blood pressure or blood volume. This will produce temporary local ischaemia with reversible or irreversible clinical effects.

Stenosis and occlusion of the basilar-vertebral system

The basilar artery is formed inferiorly by the confluence of the two vertebral arteries. At its upper end it usually divides into two posterior cerebral arteries. All these arteries and their branches, including the extracranial portions of the vertebral arteries, should be considered or investigated *in toto* in any case where ischaemic lesions in the hind brain and occipital regions are suspected, or in cases where the contribution of this tree to the blood flow in the circle of Willis is under consideration (Hutchinson and Yates 1956).

Narrowing or occlusion may affect only the extracranial portions of the vertebral arteries and, in cases with concomitant narrowing of the internal carotid arteries, there may be cerebellar softenings. Sometimes the narrowing or obstruction extends into, or is only noticed in, the intracranial portions of the tree, in particular in the basilar artery (Kubik and Adams 1946, Biemond 1951).

This obstruction is usually atherosclerotic in origin but may be embolic or syphilitic.

Ischaemic lesions are most often found in the distribution of the short paramedian branches of the basilar artery (Fig. 2.24). Such infarcts may, in part, be unilateral and they are pale. Infarcts are less commonly present in the cerebellar cortex, or in the distribution of the short circumferential arteries of the brain stem, or in the distribution of the posterior cerebral arteries. The tegmentum of the pons is very seldom involved and then usually only in part. (See also Applied anatomy, p. 72.) As in the case of the internal carotid artery the ischaemic lesions may result from one or more factors, including local organic obstruction of the nutrient artery, secondary embolism and insufficiency of the collateral circulation.

NEUROLOGICAL COMPLICATIONS OF DISSECTING ANEURYSM OF THE AORTA

A dissecting aneurysm of the aorta is characterised by massive and extensive haemorrhage into the media of the aorta. This haemorrhage may extend out along the media of the innominate, carotid or femoral arteries, narrowing the lumen and impairing the blood flow. It may surround, stretch or even tear apart the intercostal and lumbar arteries and obliterate their lumen. Thrombosis may occur in the narrowed arteries.

In 45 out of 317 cases of dissecting aneurysm studied by Shennan (1934) there were neurological complications, due to ischaemia of nervous tissue, which may be divided into three groups (Weisman and Adams 1944).

(1) *With ischaemic necrosis of peripheral nerves:* this is the commonest neurological complication and is usually associated with extension of the haemorrhage out into the subclavian or iliac arteries, causing impairment of blood supply to the nerves of the limbs.

(2) *With ischaemic necrosis of the brain:* this is the least common complication. It is usually associated with extension of the dissection into the innominate or carotid arteries. The effects are similar to occlusion of the carotid artery, which has already been considered.

(3) *With ischaemic necrosis of the spinal cord:* the portion of the cord which is constantly and most severely damaged is the mid- and lower-thoracic region, normally supplied by intercostal arteries which are almost invariably damaged by the aneurysm. The upper part of the cord, which derives its blood supply from the vertebral arteries and the supra-aortic intercostals, is seldom involved. The lumbosacral portion of the cord, which is supplied by the lumbar, ilio-lumbar and lateral sacral arteries, is sometimes damaged when the aneurysmal dissection has been extensive.

The ischaemic necrosis always involves the grey matter and the adjacent white matter. The white matter at the periphery of the cord is often spared but, in severe cases, the whole cross-section of the cord may be necrotic at some levels (Kalischer 1914, Weisman and Adams 1944, Thompson 1956).

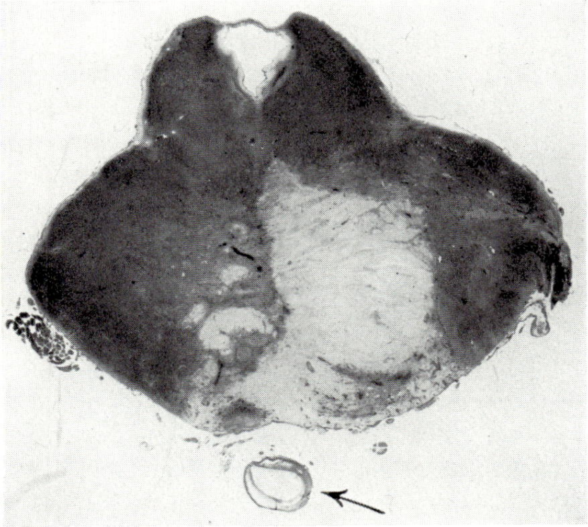

FIG. 2.24. Basilar artery occlusion of 7 weeks' duration. At this level of the pons the basilar artery (arrow) is atherosclerotilc and contains antemortem thrombus. Pale staining foci of coagulative necrosis, with peripheral organisation, are present in the distribution of the paramedian arteries. On the right side their complete field appears to be involved. Note the midline watershed and the relative escape of the tegmentum. (Celloidin, haematoxylin van Gieson, ×2.)

THROMBOSIS OF THE VEINS AND DURAL SINUSES OF THE BRAIN

Thrombosis of a dural venous sinus may occur alone or may be associated with thrombosis of the veins which drain into it or the veins alone may be involved. The thrombus may be (1) *Primary*, local and not infected and probably due to a defect in the circulating blood; or (2) *Secondary* to pyogenic infection, either local or remote, in which case the thrombus may or may not be purulent.

Primary thrombosis

This may complicate malnutrition, dehydration, infectious fevers, tuberculosis, heart disease, usually with right heart failure (Barnett and Hyland 1953), the post-operative state (excluding intracranial operations), head injury, cerebral arterial occlusion, intracerebral haemorrhage, leukaemia, polycythemia rubra vera and may occur in puerperal women and following abortion. The superior longitudinal sinus is the most commonly involved sinus, with possible extension of the clot into the lateral sinus.

The causes of primary thrombosis are not certain. In some of the associated conditions there is an alteration in the physical state of the blood: it may be more viscous and the circulation may be slow. In the superior longitudinal sinus there may be some significance in the fact that the venous blood enters against the blood stream. In the puerperal period there is an increase in plasma fibrinogen (Plass and Matthew 1926) and both then and following surgical operations there is an increase both in the number and the adhesiveness of the platelets (Wright 1942), which commences on the 4th day and is maximal on the 10th day.

The possibility of retrograde venous embolism must be considered. There is known to be anatomical continuity, in the human, between the utero-vaginal veins, the vertebral veins, the intracranial veins and the dural venous sinuses (Batson 1940). It is possible that, during periods of high intra-abdominal pressure, a small embolus might pass from the pelvic veins into the intracranial veins and dural venous sinuses by this route and there form a nidus for a larger thrombus (Martin 1941). Such an embolus could easily originate in one of the thrombosed vessels which are normally to be found in the pelvis following parturition or abortion.

Bland thrombosis confined to a portion of a venous sinus does not necessarily cause much obstruction to the venous drainage of the brain, because, especially over the cortex, there is an abundant anastomotic arrangement of the veins which lead into the sinus. Thus the blood can often find a new pathway and avoid the obstructed segment of the sinus. Extensive thrombosis of a sinus is, however, a danger to life. Thrombosis of the superior sagittal sinus, together with short portions of the lateral sinus, can produce coma and death. We have seen two such cases, in children, who died 9–10 days after the onset of the clinical signs, which were principally those of raised intracranial pressure. At post-mortem the surface veins were engorged, the brains were swollen and showed gyral flattening. Neither haemorrhage nor infarction was visible externally or on section. Microscopically there was extensive ischaemic damage to the cerebral cortex. The nerve cells were either shrunken, with pale staining cytoplasm and triangular dark staining nuclei, or had disappeared. There was vacuolar swelling of the cytoplasm of the oligodendroglia, and the capillary endothelial cells were swollen.

When both the sinus and considerable lengths of associated veins are obstructed by thrombus, there is serious interference with venous drainage. The affected portion of cortex and underlying white matter becomes congested, swollen, oedematous, and the site of numerous haemorrhages (Figs. 2.25 and 2.26). In venous infarction there are petechial or larger haemorrhages in the white matter and a relatively large amount of blood soon finds its way into the overlying subarachnoid space: two features which distinguish an infarct due to venous obstruction from one due to arterial obstruction. To the naked eye recently thrombosed sinuses and veins are distended by hard clot, mostly bluish in colour but with some flecks of pale material. The necrotic cortex and white matter disintegrate rapidly and are absorbed by the body in the usual fashion so that later the lesion is shrunken, cystic and brownish-yellow in colour (Bailey and Hass 1937). Thrombus in sinuses and veins is rapidly organised and recanalised and it may indeed be difficult to see with the naked eye or even to prove histologically that it was ever there.

Secondary thrombosis

This is most often found as a complication of pyogenic infection, either local or remote. Of local infections the commoner are those of the frontal air sinuses (superior longitudinal sinus), and of the mastoid air spaces or the middle ear (lateral sinus). Secondary thrombosis may also be a sequel to subdural abscess, or to pyogenic infection of the face, especially in the region of the eyes, nose, cheeks and the upper jaw, or to pyogenic infection of ethmoidal or sphenoidal air sinuses (cavernous sinus). The thrombus may spread to the sinus along the veins which drain into it, or sinus thrombosis may arise secondary to inflammation of the wall of the sinus when closely adjacent to a purulent process. The thrombus may not, apparently, be infected: or it may be septic, in which case it is liable to fragment and be carried away in the blood stream to the heart and lungs, giving rise to pyaemia and abscesses.

Superior longitudinal sinus thrombosis

This is usually not septic, except when associated with subdural abscess. This is the sinus usually found thrombosed in primary thrombosis and in puerperal women. The thrombus often extends into the lateral sinus.

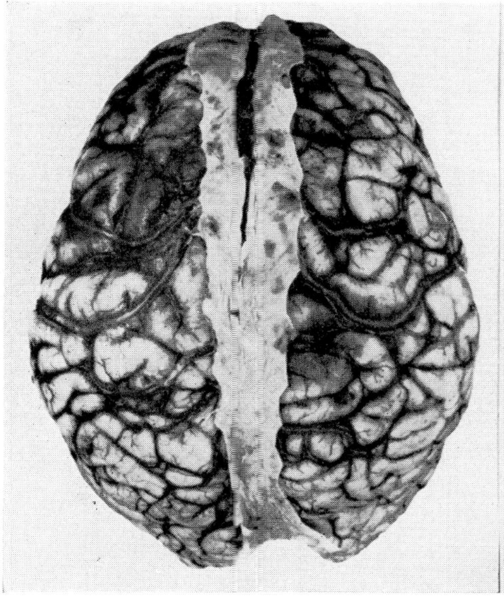

2.25

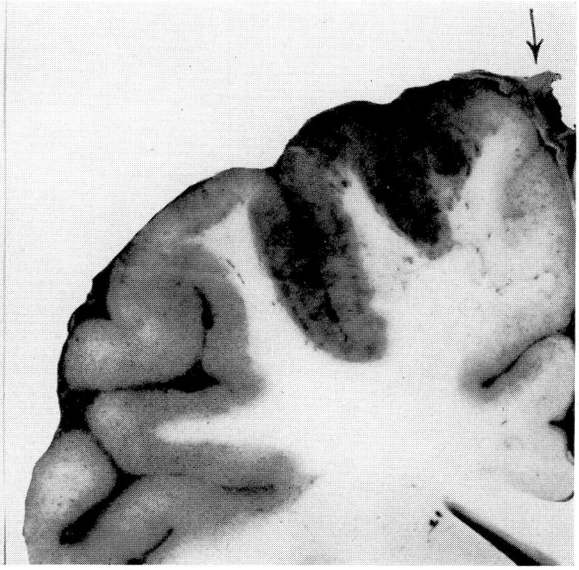

2.26

FIG. 2.25. Thrombosis of the superior sagittal sinus, and thrombophlebitis of the cortical veins which are distended by partly pale, partly dark thrombus. Note the marked perivenular subarachnoid haemorrhage. Clinically 3 days' duration. Puerperal woman with breast abscess.

FIG. 2.26. Same case as Fig. 2.25. Coronal section of brain showing thrombus in the superior sagittal sinus (arrow), with swelling and gross haemorrhagic streaking of the cortex and the underlying white matter.

Lateral sinus thrombosis

This commonly occurs secondary to otitis media and mastoiditis. It may or may not be septic. If there is no communication between the right and left lateral sinuses at the torcular, thrombosis of the left lateral sinus may obstruct the venous return from the basal ganglia via the great vein of Galen and straight sinus, with resulting infarction of the basal ganglia.

Otitic hydrocephalus

Rarely, patients with otitis media develop weakness of the lateral rectus muscle of one or both eyes and intermittent headache, from which they usually recover. There is papilloedema and the pressure of the lumbar cerebrospinal fluid is raised, but there is no appreciable increase of cells or protein. The ventricles of the brain are not increased in size: indeed, in early cases, they may be smaller than normal. Thrombosis of a lateral sinus has always been demonstrated in the few cases which have been examined *post mortem*. Foley (1955) considered that the obstructed sinus should be the major lateral sinus, or that the thrombus should extend to involve the torcular, thereby severely impeding the venous return from the brain. Symonds (1956), in a critical examination of the cases which have been examined *post mortem*, found that in 3 cases a lateral sinus, the torcular and the posterior part of the superior sagittal sinus were all obstructed; and that in 2 other cases the reports mentioned obstruction of one lateral sinus but gave no details of the findings in the torcular region; in particular it was not possible to judge whether the obstructed sinus was the major lateral sinus. He concluded that the venous obstruction caused cerebral oedema and swelling of the brain, which would account for the intracranial hypertension without ventricular dilatation. He considered that the 6th cranial nerves were damaged by the presence of blood clot in the inferior petrosal sinuses. Further careful post-mortem studies are necessary in this condition, particular attention being paid to the extent of the thrombus, the pattern of anastomosis at the torcular and the condition of the inferior petrosal sinus.

Cavernous sinus thrombosis

Cavernous sinus thrombosis, commonly accompanied by thrombosis of associated veins and venous sinuses, is usually secondary to pyogenic infection of the central half of the face or of the underlying bones and soft tissues. The thrombus usually becomes infected and, in untreated cases, purulent leptomeningitis is generally present at the time of death. The facial and ophthalmic veins are often obstructed and there is oedema of the soft tissues of the orbit, with proptosis. Haemorrhages are found in the retina. It has been suggested that the paralysis, of the 6th or less commonly the 3rd and 4th cranial nerves which may occur, is a pressure palsy produced by the hard swollen clot (Rich, quoted by Symonds 1952). Secondary infarction of the pituitary has been reported in a purulent case (Weisman 1944).

Thrombosis of internal cerebral veins

This, in the child, may be primary in the veins, or secondary to thrombosis of the dural sinuses (see section on lateral sinus thrombosis). It may arise with or without pyogenic infection. The usual result is a haemorrhagic infarct in part or the whole of the field of distribution of the veins, which includes the septum pellucidum, the corpus striatum, the thalamus, the ventral portion of the corpus callosum, the medial aspect of the occipital lobe and the superomedial surface of the cerebellum on each side (Ehlers and Courville 1936).

SPINAL THROMBOPHLEBITIS

(*Subacute necrotic myelitis*)

This rare condition, first described by Foix and Alajouanine (1926) under the title of subacute necrotic myelitis, is considered by Antoni (1952) and Mair and Folkerts (1953) to be due to subacute thrombophlebitis of spinal veins, especially at the lower levels of the cord. It may be associated with cavitation of the cord which is not easily distinguished from syringomyelia (Lhermitte *et al.* 1931).

It is more frequent in men and has been reported at ages from 23 to 61. Clinically it takes the form of progressive paralysis of both upper and lower motor neurone type, with a variable amount of sensory loss sometimes not affecting pain or temperature sensation. The level of involvement is from about the lower dorsal region downwards and the duration of the disease varies from 6 months to 4 years. The protein in the cerebrospinal fluid is raised; the cells are either not increased or moderately increased in number.

Morbid anatomy. If the lower spinal cord has been exposed at operation during life, the surface vessels of the spinal cord, in the lumbosacral region, have been seen to be prominent, dilated, varicose and thickened. This has also been seen at post-mortem. In some cases, however, it has been difficult to see any definite abnormality of the surface veins. The veins on the anterior aspect of the cord should be particularly examined for they are usually more severely involved. Gross surface angiomatosis, such as is seen in vascular malformations, is

2.28

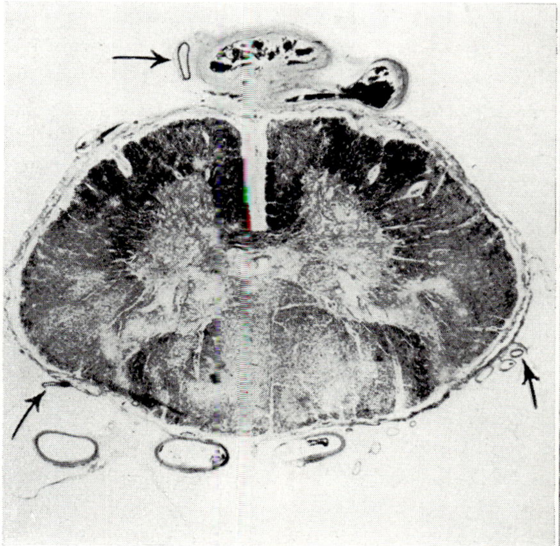

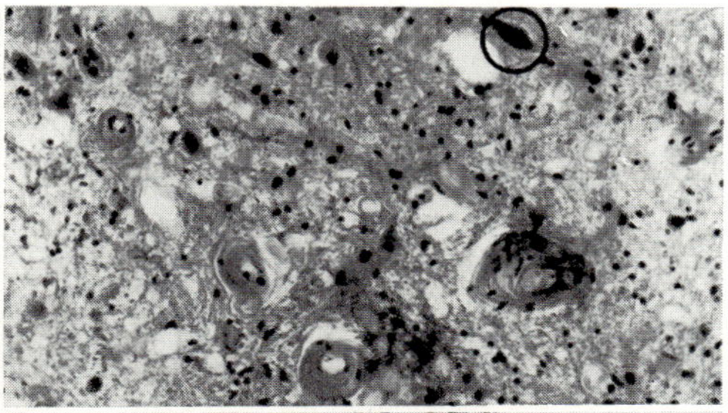

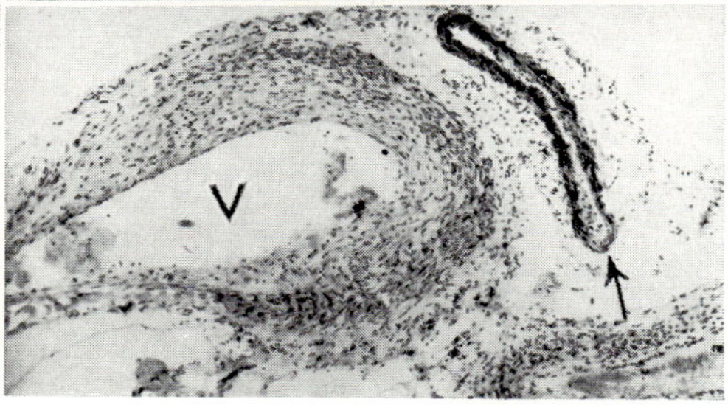

2.27

2.29

FIG. 2.27. Spinal thrombophlebitis. First lumbar segment, myelin preparation. Note the enlarged and thickened leptomeningeal veins. The arteries (arrows) appear healthy. There is extensive degeneration of the white matter. (Weigert-Pal, ×7.)

FIG. 2.28. Part of the anterior grey horn, same case as Fig. 2.27, showing marked hyaline fibrous thickening of the small vessels. The parenchyma is damaged but some nerve cells (circle) are still present. (Celloidin, haematoxylin van Gieson, ×155.)

FIG. 2.29. Anterior spinal vessels, same case as Fig. 2.27, different level, showing healthy artery (arrow) and enlarged veins, one (V) with intimal fibrous thickening. (Celloidin, haematoxylin van Gieson, ×64.)

not found. The leptomeninges are thickened and opaque; the spinal cord is soft and diminished in size.

Histological findings. The extent of severe spinal cord involvement has been from about the mid-dorsal region downwards. Above this level there is secondary ascending degeneration, predominantly in the posterior white columns. At the levels of severe involvement the appearances are those of extensive degeneration or necrosis of the white matter of the cord (Fig. 2.27) The lesions are poorly demarcated and usually severe. There is a variable degree of involvement of the grey matter, which may be slight, or severe with necrosis of the anterior horns. Phagocytic and astrocytic response varies from case to case. The smaller blood-vessels within the affected regions show fibrous mural thickening, sometimes with hyaline degeneration

(Fig. 2.28). These vessels are more numerous and more prominent in the grey matter. The surface veins are also strikingly abnormal. Owing in part to their tortuosity they appear, in ordinary transverse sections of the cord, to be more numerous than usual. Some are dilated; many have walls greatly thickened by concentric intimal layers of fibrous tissue, but the lumen is noticeably large (Fig. 2.29). Some show evidence of organisation and recanalisation of old thrombus. In Mair and Folkerts' case thrombophlebitis affected the anterior spinal vein as high as the cervical segments and in its upper part it was recent. In the cases of Foix and Alajouanine and that of Lhermitte *et al.*, the arteries were affected by medial thickening.

In Minea's case (1932) one optic nerve showed pathological changes similar to those seen in the cord.

Pathogenesis. This is at present unknown. We consider the condition to be due to thrombosis of the superficial veins of the spinal cord, with secondary tortuosity and dilatation of these veins. The venous anastomoses in the lower part of the cord are not adequate to deal with extensive obstruction and there are secondary changes in the intramedullary vessels of the cord and in the parenchyma.

Why thrombophlebitis should develop in these veins is unknown. Some of the reported cases have suffered from albuminuria or lead colic or auricular fibrillation or phlebitis of the legs or fever. Thrombosis of the left renal vein and inferior vena cava was found in one of the few cases in which a complete post-mortem has been performed (Greenfield and Turner 1939). Cases of spinal thrombophlebitis may be difficult to recognise both clinically and *post mortem*, but there is a great need for further clinical and post-mortem investigation, especially with regard to the state of the cerebral and pelvic venous plexuses.

Spinal thrombophlebitis should not be confused with spinal angiomatosis in which the primary condition is one of very numerous thin walled vessels both on the surface of the cord and within its substance.

VASCULAR LESIONS ASSOCIATED WITH SUPRATENTORIAL SPACE-OCCUPYING LESIONS

Patients with a rapidly expanding, unilateral or predominantly unilateral, space-occupying lesion, such as intracranial haemorrhage, neoplasm, abscess or cerebral œdema associated with other pathological process, often show clinical evidence of derangement of function at the upper level of the brain stem. If the pressure is not relieved the patient will die and *post mortem* one or more of the following may be found.

(1) *Injury to 3rd cranial nerves.* The 3rd cranial nerve, particularly on the side of the space-occupying lesion, as it passes between the posterior cerebral and superior cerebellar arteries, is flattened and may show haemorrhage within its substance (Fig. 2.30). The appearances suggest that the nerve has been held tight against one of the arteries.

(2) *Temporal or incisural herniation.* A portion of the uncus or hippocampal gyrus will have herniated through the incisura tentorii (Fig. 2.30). This incisural herniation is much more important than any tonsillar herniation which may also be present (Jefferson 1938). Among other effects the herniation compresses the aqueduct and causes supratentorial obstructive hydrocephalus (Smyth and Henderson 1938). When the space-occupying lesion is large and situated in the temporal region it is not uncommon to find that a wedge of uncus has intruded itself between the midbrain and the posterior cerebral artery (Fig. 2.31) (Allison and Morrison 1941).

(3) *Anteroposterior elongation of the midbrain.* As a result of the temporal herniation, the incisura tentorii contains both a portion of the hippocampus and the upper part of the brain

stem, which is secondarily deformed and elongated anteroposteriorly (Johnson and Yates 1956) (Fig. 2.30).

(4) *Damage to the contralateral cerebral peduncle.* Also as a result of the temporal herniation the cerebral peduncle, on the side opposite to the space-occupying lesion, is pressed against, indented by, and damaged by the free edge of the tentorium cerebelli (Kernohan and Woltman 1929) (Fig. 2.31).

(5) *Vascular lesions in the rostral portion of the brain stem.* In the midbrain and rostral portion of the pons, especially in the paracentral and lateral tegmental regions, there may be florid haemorrhages (Figs. 2.30 and 2.35). In addition, or in less severe cases as the only lesions, there may be sharply delimited foci of ischaemic necrosis. Patients with these vascular lesions usually die within 12–72 hours, so that the haemorrhagic lesions are easily seen, but the ischaemic lesions will not be visible to the naked eye. Microscopically, however, in the ischaemic lesions, the myelin sheaths stain poorly with haematoxylin and, at the periphery of the lesion, the myelin sheaths are ballooned and the axons often swollen (Fig. 2.32). Such appearances are similar to those found shortly after thrombosis of the basilar artery. When the patient is saved from rapid death by surgical relief of the supratentorial pressure, and death occurs later, small old regions of necrosis may be found in the brain stem (Wolman 1953).

There are two schools of thought with regard to the nature of the haemorrhages. Scheinker (1945), concentrating attention on the haemorrhage in the tegmental region, considered it venous in origin. Whilst not denying that some of the haemorrhages in this region may be venous, we would agree with Moore and Stern (1938) that the majority, and especially the paracentral haemorrhages, are related to capillaries and arterioles, and occur both into the sheaths of the arterioles and into the surrounding parenchyma (Fig. 2.33). This view is supported by the post-mortem injection experiments of Johnson and Yates (1956).

(6) *Vascular lesions in the occipital and temporal lobes.* A region of haemorrhagic infarction of the cortex and a thin belt of ischaemic necrosis in the underlying white matter are often seen on the medial and inferior aspects of the ipsilateral temporal and occipital lobes. Rarely the condition is bilateral. The lesion is often confined to the distribution of the calcarine branches of the posterior cerebral artery. It commences anteriorly at the margin of the indentation made in the temporal cortex by the free edge of the tentorium cerebelli, and it fans out posteriorly. All authors agree that it is due to obstruction of the posterior cerebral artery or its branches. Examination of the same region, in less florid cases where little or no change is to be seen with the naked eye, will often show, in frozen or celloidin sections, the changes of shrinkage and 'incrustation of the Golgi network' in the nerve cells. Such changes are known to occur as a result of anoxia.

(7) *Vascular lesions in the thalamus.* Small capillary and arteriolar haemorrhages, usually ipsilateral, are occasionally found in the posterior part of the thalamus, in regions in the distribution of the posterior cerebral artery.

Pathogenesis. The problem is one of explaining the occurrence of ischaemic and haemorrhagic lesions in the rostral portion of the brain stem (within the distribution of the paramedian and short circumferential branches of the basilar, superior cerebellar and posterior cerebral arteries), in the occipital and temporal lobes and the thalamus (within the distribution of the cortical and perforating branches of the posterior cerebral artery), and in the 3rd cranial nerves. Blackwood and Dott (1952, unpublished) consider that all these lesions can usually be explained by a study of the displacements of nervous tissue and arteries which occur in the region of the incisura tentorii.

As a supratentorial space-occupying lesion increases in bulk the volume of the supratentorial contents of the skull increases. In the adult the skull cannot expand to accommodate it, and

2.32

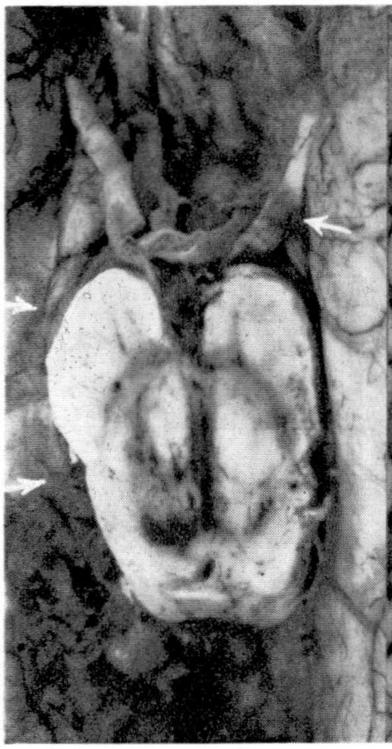

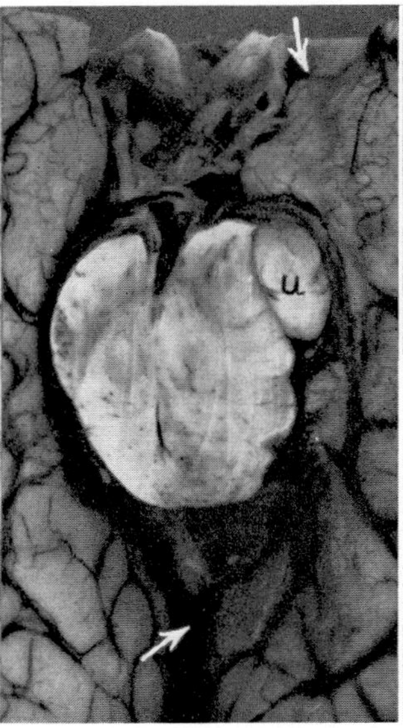

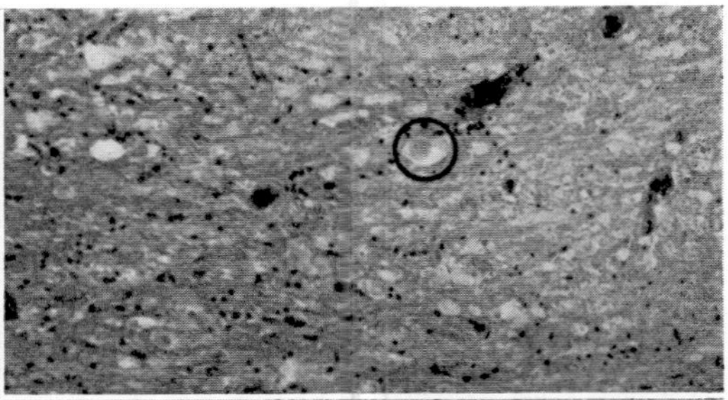

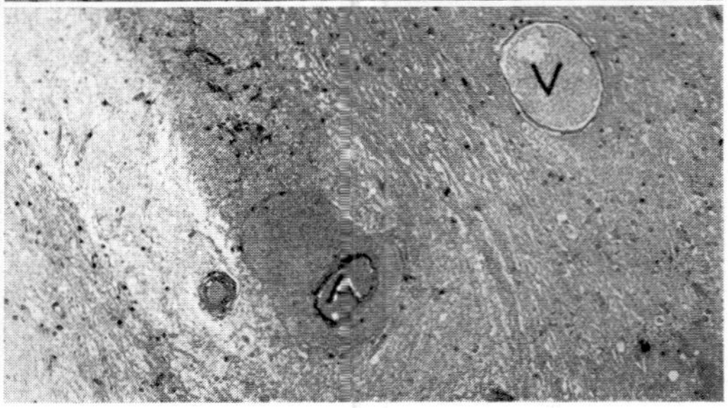

2.30 2.31 2.33

FIG. 2.30. Base of brain from below, right temporal glioblastoma. The 3rd nerves, as they lie caudal to the posterior cerebral arteries, are flattened and haemorrhage has occurred into them: this is more apparent on the right side of the picture (arrow). Temporal herniation is visible on the left side of the picture: arrows indicate the groove formed by the free edge of the tentorium cerebelli. On the right side of the picture there are petechial haemorrhages in the cerebral peduncle which was so soft that it was lacerated *post mortem*. Florid paramedian haemorrhages are visible in the midbrain. Note the paramedian arteries running posteriorly from the cranial end of the basilar artery and the distortion of the aqueduct (the side of the tumour is on the left of the picture).

FIG. 2.31. Base of brain from below, left temporal glioblastoma. Arrows indicate the line of the free edge of the tentorium cerebelli. A wedge of uncus (U) has intruded itself between the midbrain and the posterior cerebral artery. Note the concavity of the cerebral peduncle on the side of the tumour, the displacement of midline midbrain structures away from the side of the tumour, the narrowing and anteroposterior elongation of the aqueduct, and the bruising of the cerebral peduncle on side opposite to the tumour.

FIG. 2.32. Edge of ischaemic lesion in rostral pons, case of bilateral frontal glioblastoma. Ischaemic necrosis affects the tissue on the top right of the picture. At the junction of this and the healthier tissue is a swollen axon within a ballooned myelin sheath (circle). Compare with Fig. 2.18. (Celloidin, haematoxylin van Gieson, × 100.)

FIG. 2.33. Brain stem haemorrhage into the parenchyma and the sheath of an arteriole (A), which is recognised by its internal elastic lamina. A dilated venule (V) is also visible. (Paraffin, haematoxylin eosin, × 64.)

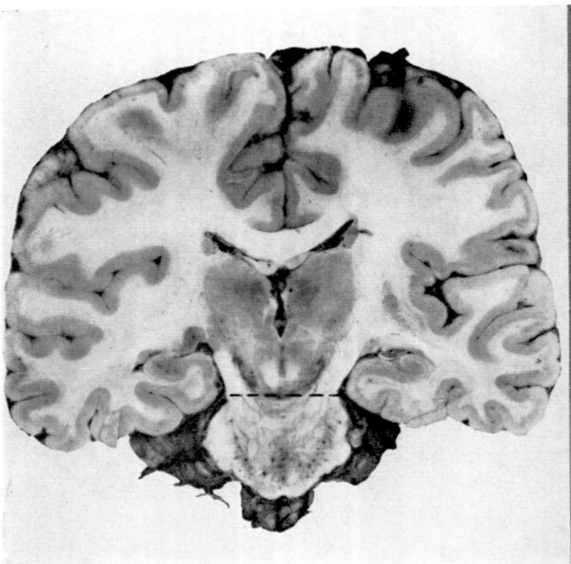

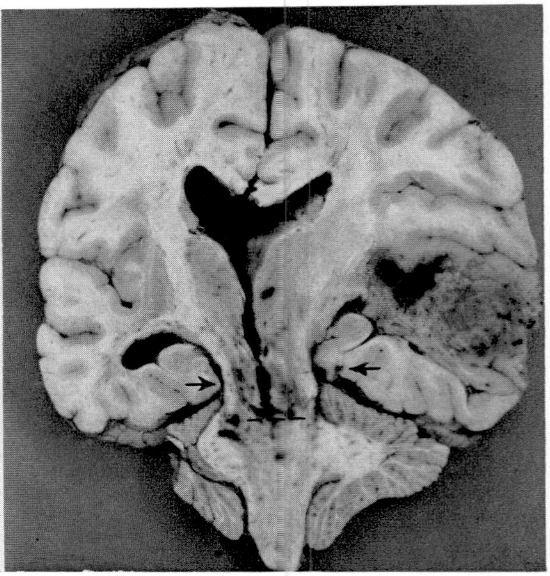

2.34 2.35

FIG. 2.34. Normal brain, fixed *in situ*. The dotted line indicates the level of the free edge of the tentorium cerebelli. Note that this line passes through the lowest part of the substantia nigra.

FIG. 2.35. Temporal glioblastoma. Coronal section similar to previous figure. Arrows indicate the level of the free edge of the tentorium cerebelli. A dotted line indicates the level of the lowest part of the substantia nigra. This is seen to be a considerable distance caudal to the level of the tentorial aperture.

the dura of the tentorium cerebelli is so well supported by the falx cerebri and by its peripheral attachments that it can only be pushed caudally to a very limited extent. The only aperture of any size in this bony and membranous box is the incisura tentorii and through this aperture the soft brain gradually herniates. The first structure to pass caudally is the midbrain (Figs. 2.34 and 2.35). Post-mortem fixation of brains *in situ* has revealed that the *caudal displacement* may be so marked that the whole midbrain passes below the level of the incisura tentorii. The mobility of the arteries of the circle of Willis and their branches is such that they can follow the displaced brain for a short distance. The circle of Willis is, however, anchored anteriorly to the skull by the internal carotid arteries (Fig. 2.36) and a point will be reached when the posterior communicating arteries and the supporting arachnoid will stretch no further. The caudal movement of the rostral portion of the basilar artery will then be arrested and, as the brain stem continues to be displaced, its paramedian and short circumferential branches will come under tension.

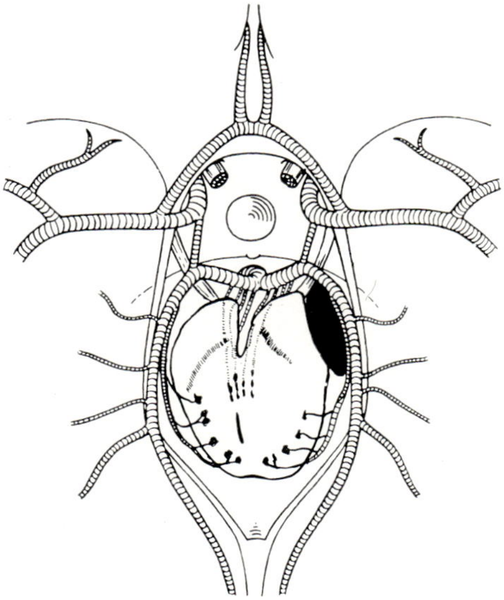

FIG. 2.36. Diagram to illustrate the mechanism of vascular lesions of the rostral brain stem in cases with an intruded wedge of uncus. Compare with Fig. 2.31. Note the anteroposterior elongation of the midbrain and its lateral displacement relative to the basilar artery, which is relatively fixed in relation to the skull and the free edge of the tentorium cerebelli. The midbrain is also displaced caudally (not shown). Abnormal tension develops in the paramedian and short circumferential arteries, with ischaemic or haemorrhagic lesions. The posterior cerebral artery, or its branches, may be compressed between the temporal lobe above it and the free edge of the tentorium cerebelli below it.

The posterior cerebral arteries also act as anchors for the basilar artery. Both temporal lobes are pressed firmly down on, and are often grooved by, the free edges of the tentorium cerebelli. The laterally placed branches of the posterior cerebral arteries become hooked over these edges and fixed. This prevents any further movement of the posterior cerebral arteries and, through them, limits the caudal movement of the rostral end of the basilar artery. In addition to being under tension, some of the branches of the posterior cerebral arteries are markedly kinked by the free edges of the tentorium cerebelli and the blood flow through these vessels is impeded, with consequent ischaemic or haemorrhagic necrosis in their distribution. The calcarine branches are most commonly affected.

Many supratentorial space-occupying lesions are predominantly or wholly unilateral, so that there is a greater degree of temporal herniation on one side than on the other and there is *lateral displacement of the caudal portion of the brain stem*. Such lateral displacement of the midbrain and pons is not only relative to the skull and incisura tentorii, but also relative to the branches of the circle of Willis and of the rostral end of the basilar artery. This factor increases the likelihood of tension in these branches. If in addition a wedge of uncus is intruded between the posterior cerebral artery and the brain stem, the distortion of cerebral tissue relative to the blood-vessels is increased.

With temporal herniation, either bilaterally symmetrical or asymmetrical, the upper part of the brain stem is elongated anteroposteriorly (Johnson and Yates 1956) and there is relative displacement of nervous tissue and the blood-vessels within its substance.

Thus there are several factors which cause abnormal tension in the arteries and arterioles in question. Such tension on elastic tubes will cause reduction in calibre of the lumen and this, together with any local vasospasm which may occur, will reduce the blood flow to the capillaries and produce ischaemic necrosis. Variations in the degree of tension, the factor of venous obstruction, and in some cases actual tearing or avulsion of arterioles, may be the basis of the haemorrhagic nature of some of the lesions.

Like the circle of Willis the 3rd cranial nerve is anchored anteriorly where it pierces the dura to reach the region of the cavernous sinus. The anterior part of the extramedullary portion of the nerve is pushed down on to the clivus by the herniated hippocampus and it may be flattened or bruised in this region. Nearer the midbrain, the caudally displaced posterior cerebral artery presses down upon the upper surface of the nerve. After leaving the midbrain the nerve has to pass round the postero-inferior and inferior aspect of the artery which flattens it and interferes with its local blood supply.

OEDEMA IN THE CENTRAL NERVOUS SYSTEM

Organismal infection, recent ischaemic necrosis, traumatic lacerations, and other inflammatory conditions (in the broad sense of the words) of the brain or spinal cord, are often accompanied by localised oedema. More extensive oedema is commonly found in the white matter around abscesses, recent massive haemorrhage, and tumours (Fig. 2.37) especially the metastases of carcinoma, some gliomata and around meningiomata (Greenfield 1939).

This extensive oedema does not affect grey matter and it noticeably spares the long fibre tracts such as the internal capsules, the corpus callosum and the optic radiations. While confined to the white matter it usually spares the subcortical arcuate fibres. It is most noticeable when it affects the centrum semi-ovale of the cerebral hemispheres (Fig. 2.38) or the deep white matter of the cerebellar hemispheres. It rarely spreads from one cerebral hemisphere to another. The margin of the oedematous change is not clear cut, either macroscopically or microscopically, and in this it differs from, and may be distinguished from, ischaemic necrosis of white matter, which has a sharply defined edge.

In the early stages of oedema the affected white matter is swollen, soft and has a damp appearance on cut section. It may be yellowish in colour. Since it occupies more volume than healthy white matter it acts as a space-occupying lesion causing flattening of the overlying gyri and distortion of the ventricular system. Within oedematous brain there is gradual destruction of axons and myelin sheaths, with a moderate amount of astrocytic gliosis. Oedema may be present for many months or years around a very slowly growing meningioma, in which case the destruction predominates and small or even large cavities may develop (Figs. 2.42 and 2.43).

In oedema of short duration (Figs. 2.39–2.41) and varying in severity from case to case, the myelinated fibres are less closely packed than normal and show degenerative changes. Some myelin sheaths are irregularly swollen, beaded, or have broken down into globules or granules. The axons are also widely separated and show irregular swellings. They may show end bulbs, a sign of loss of continuity. In general they are less severely affected than the myelin sheaths.

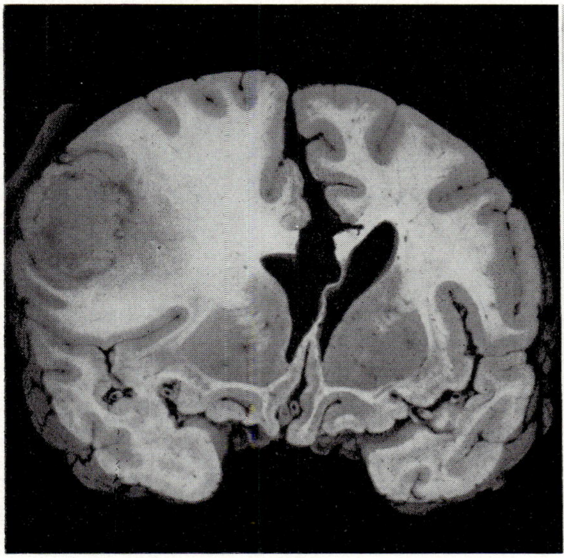

2.37

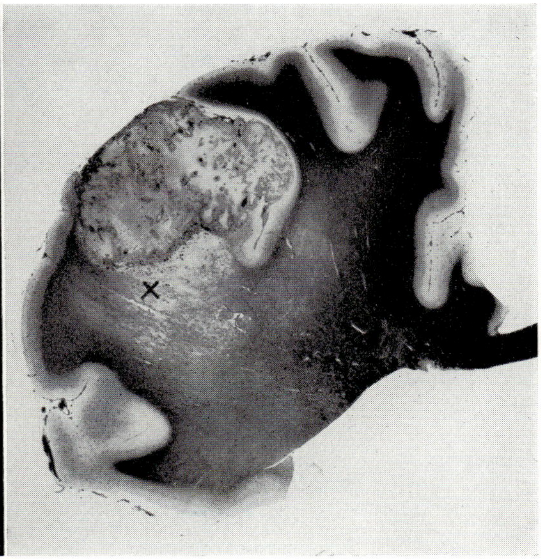

2.38

FIG. 2.37. Oedema associated with a frontal meningioma. Note the swelling of the white matter, but not the grey matter, adjacent to the tumour. The ventricles are displaced, and subfalcine herniation is visible on the side of the tumour.

FIG. 2.38. Oedema associated with a metastatic bronchial carcinoma, situated in a position similar to that of the tumour in Fig. 2.37. Myelin preparation. Note the pallor of the white matter adjacent to the tumour. This pallor is most marked close to the tumour, tends not to affect the U-fibres on the medial aspect of the tumour, has an indefinite edge, and extends further within the lateral white matter of the hemisphere than it does towards the corpus callosum.

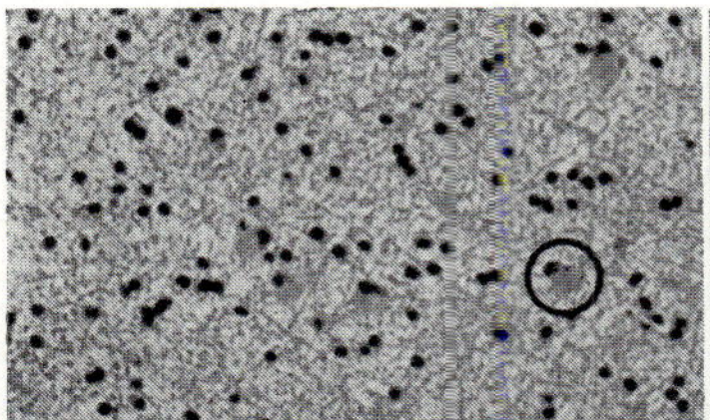

2.39

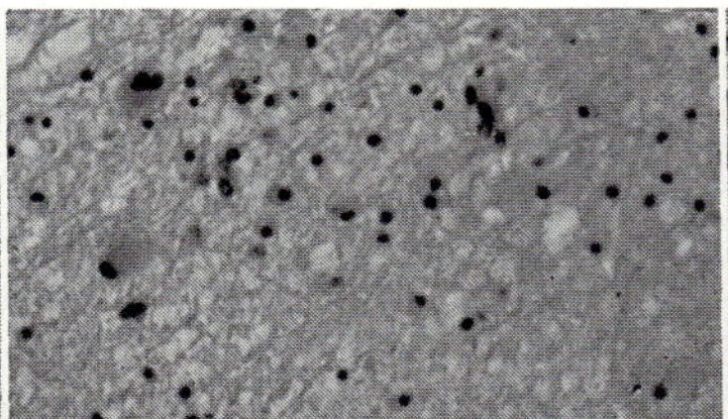

2.40

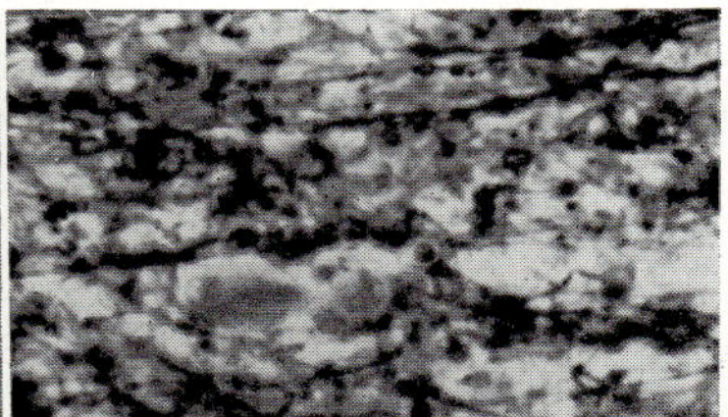

2.41

FIG. 2.39. Oedematous white matter from the region of the X in Fig. 2.38. Note the separation of the myelinated nerve fibres, the increase in cytoplasm of the astrocytes (circle), the large number of oligodendroglial nuclei, and the absence of any visible abnormality of the small blood vessels (arrow). (Celloidin, haematoxylin van Gieson, × 145.)

FIG. 2.40. Oedematous white matter close to a metastatic carcinoma. Note the swelling of the cytoplasm of the astrocytes which are sometimes binucleated, the separation of the myelinated nerve fibres and the numerous oligodendroglial nuclei. (Celloidin, haematoxylin van Gieson, × 145.)

FIG. 2.41. Oedematous white matter close to a secondary carcinoma, myelin preparation. The fibres are separated and often beaded. Two astrocytes with swollen cytoplasm are present near the centre of the picture. (Celloidin, Loyez, × 300.)

This damage to myelin and axons, which may be quite severe, is accompanied by a noticeably slight reaction on the part of the microglia and fat phagocytes. Seldom can any interstitial fluid be demonstrated. When it is present it is acidophilic in nature and occupies ovoid spaces. In acute severe cases the astrocytes show swelling of their cytoplasm and degenerative changes: in cases of longer duration and less severity the astrocytes are increased in number, have swollen cytoplasm and lay down astrocytic fibres. Oligodendroglial nuclei are not noticeably affected and blood vessels appear healthy. Changes in the grey matter are very slight but may include swelling of nerve cells.

By chemical examination of oedematous brain, Stewart-Wallace (1939) found that there was an increased fluid content, restricted to the portions of the brain which were microscopically oedematous. There was an increase of water, and also of sodium, chloride and potassium, in the same relative proportions as would be the case if the added fluid was a serum filtrate. This suggests that in cerebral oedema, as in oedema elsewhere, there is an increase in the interstitial fluid and that this is derived from the blood. Cumings (1961), examining water soluble proteins and enzymes extracted from oedematous white matter, found that there was an increase of

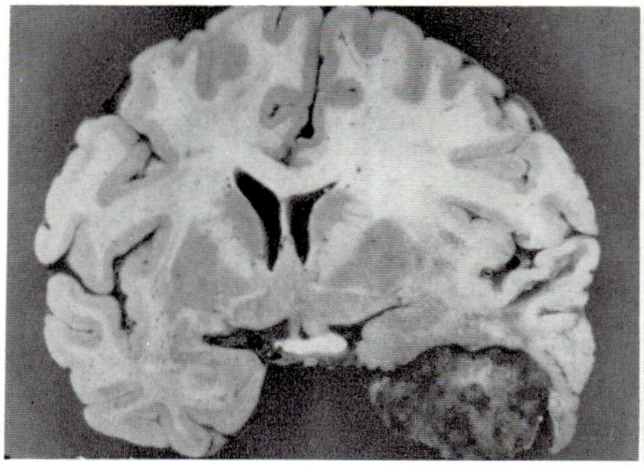

2.42

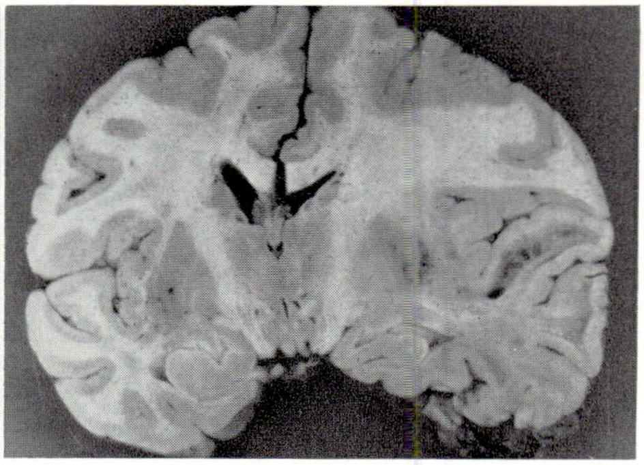

2.43

FIGS. 2.42 and 2.43. Patient with slow growing right temporal meningioma, no surgical treatment. Note the extensive cystic replacement of the white matter of the temporal lobe and insular region. Note the sparing of the grey matter, except immediately overlying the tumour. The most likely cause of these changes is considered to be oedema of long duration.

albumin but no gross alteration of the enzyme content—evidence in favour of the fluid being interstitial (extracellular) and not the result of breakdown of cells.

In *oedema of long standing* the degenerative process affects most of the tissue. Smaller or larger spaces are found, filled with clear fluid and separated by delicate astrocytic and vascular tissue. Few phagocytes are present (Figs. 2.42 and 2.43).

Pathogenesis. In addition to the interstitial fluid described above, there is also destruction of white matter. The interstitial fluid must come from vessels in some region of the oedematous white matter. Since, however, the oedema is most severe close to the causative lesion, it is reasonable to suppose that most of the fluid comes from vessels which are either close to or even within the causative lesion. Such leakage from damaged vessels may be due to one or more causes. It may be secondary to venous compression (as by a meningioma), to thrombosis (as in a malignant glioma), to damage by toxic metabolites (as in an abscess), or to anoxia (infarct or massive haemorrhage).

Once the fluid has left the vessels it will tend to diffuse. There is experimental evidence in the cat and rabbit (Bertrand 1952) that injected fluid will diffuse rapidly, in a widespread fashion, in the cerebral white matter but not in grey matter. In the experimental animal it tends to pass towards the walls of the lateral ventricle and towards the internal cerebral vein and its branches, where it is absorbed. It is noticeable in his diagrams that the fluid did not diffuse across the corpus callosum. He found also that diffusion ceased at the periphery of the white matter and in grey matter, because here also the fluid was absorbed. The distribution of injected fluid and of cerebral oedema are thus very similar. There is therefore support for the concept that, in cerebral oedema, excessive fluid leaks from the capillaries close to the causative lesion and diffuses widely towards the absorbing veins and venules, which are found in the walls of the ventricles, at the periphery of the white matter and in the grey matter itself. It may also be postulated that the excess of interstitial fluid interferes with the normal passage of oxygen from the capillaries to the nerve fibres, which will therefore gradually degenerate.

An alternative view, that the swelling in cerebral oedema is the result of an excess of intracellular fluid, is also worthy of consideration. In 1957 Magee *et al.* produced experimental cerebral 'oedema' with triethyl tin compounds; in 1958 Klatzo *et al* produced it by the application of cold to the exposed pia; in 1959 and 1960 Torack *et al.*, using similar techniques, examined brains with the electron microscope and suggested that the initial process, in experimental 'oedema' of the white matter, was an accumulation of fluid, not in the perivascular and intercellular spaces which they considered to be almost non-existent, but in the swollen perivascular processes of glial cells with clear cytoplasm. Whether these were oligodendroglia or astrocytes is still a matter of debate.

Portions of human cerebral tissue, obtained during neurosurgical procedures from regions close to intracranial tumours have been examined with the electron microscope by Torack *et al.* (1960) and changes were found similar to those seen in experimental triethyl tin 'oedema'. In some regions the cell membranes of the clear glial cells had ruptured but there was no accumulation of extracellular fluid. They drew attention to the fact that electronmicroscopic studies were lacking on the enlarged, soft and wet deep white matter which is considered typical of cerebral oedema.

BRAIN SWELLING

In 1905 Reichardt published his findings of swelling and increase in weight of the brain substance, in cases of epileptic and paralytic attacks and of catatonia, where no other abnormality of the brain was visible to the naked eye. He found a similar change in some brains with a disproportionately small cerebral tumour. Such brains showed flattened gyri and on section, before fixation, were very firm and dry. Since that time a similar naked-eye appearance has been seen in the brains of persons dying with uraemia and various infections and intoxications.

Provided that the term 'brain swelling' is used in this restricted macroscopical sense there is no difficulty in distinguishing it, macroscopically, from the soft wet enlargement of the white matter which is seen around cerebral tumours, etc., to which the term 'oedema' is given.

Difficulty does, however, arise when an attempt is made to distinguish them histologically, or to prove that they are two different processes. Histological examination of regions of macroscopical 'brain swelling' may not show any appreciable change (Jaburek 1936), or may show changes which many authors would find difficulty in distinguishing clearly from those described above in the less severe forms of oedema. Zülch (1954), however, believes that the two conditions can be distinguished morphologically.

In cases of trauma, tumour or abscess some authors consider that brain swelling and brain oedema can both be present at the same time in the same brain; and there is a further subdivision of opinion as to whether, in such cases, they can be separated microscopically, and whether cerebral oedema is but a more severe degree of the same process which may give rise to cerebral swelling.

ATHEROSCLEROSIS

Atherosclerosis in general

This is a disease process which most commonly affects the largest arteries of the brain. The main stems and branches of the anterior, middle and posterior cerebral arteries are often affected, less commonly the cerebellar arteries and the small arteries of the cerebral hemispheres including the perforating arteries to the basal ganglia. The spinal arteries are very seldom affected.

The changes seen in the cerebral arteries in atherosclerosis are similar to those seen in the rest of the body. To the naked eye there are initially eccentric patches of yellowish opacity of the vessel wall and the calibre of the vessel may be increased. Especially is this noticeable in the basilar artery which becomes dilated, elongated and tortuous.

The earliest lesions in atheroma and the true aetiology are still matters of debate. It is a condition which is more frequently seen with advancing years, although it can occur in the young. It tends to start around the origin of branches of arteries, indicative of a mechanical factor. Duguid (1948) considers that the initial lesion is a deposit of fibrin on the internal surface of the artery, that the endothelium grows over the surface of the fibrinous deposit, which becomes organised, and that red blood corpuscles, entangled in the fibrinous deposit, break down and liberate fatty material.

The other school of thought favours the concept that fatty material from the blood is deposited in the wall of the vessel, a concept which appeared to receive support from the atheroma-like lesions which can occur in rabbits fed on a rich cholesterol diet, and from the finding of a higher incidence of atheroma in people living on a diet rich in fat compared to people living on a low fat diet. Fullerton (1955) has shown that a high fat intake, which produces lipaemia, also produces a marked shortening of the clotting time of the blood. This must, at least, predispose to local intravascular clotting. The 'thrombotic' theory and the 'dietetic' theory may not therefore be as widely separated as was originally supposed. Whatever the initial lesion the subsequent progress of the disease appears to be largely one of repeated thrombosis upon the surface of the initial plaque. The deposited thrombus becomes organised, elastic tissue is formed within it and endothelium spreads from the edges over its free surface (Fig. 2.45). Regions of fresh or old haemorrhage may be found in the depths of an old plaque. Crystalline esters of cholesterol may also be present and sometimes these excite a foreign body giant cell reaction. Deep to the plaque the media degenerates and undergoes fatty change. The muscularis and internal elastic membrane are weakened and the vessel wall itself dilates, although the lumen may be narrowed by the plaque.

The process of thrombosis upon the surface of the plaque may reduce the blood flow through the artery to such an extent that some or all of the tissues within its bed of supply can no longer live and there is a region of ischaemic necrosis. Fortunately atherosclerosis is, as a rule, a slow process, so that anastomotic adjustments have time to develop. It is often difficult to differentiate, histologically, between atherosclerosis, organised local thrombosis and a healed embolism. For example a solitary patch of atheroma at the first main point of branching of a middle cerebral artery should always suggest the possibility of carotid artery thrombosis on the same side with previous embolism and subsequent organisation.

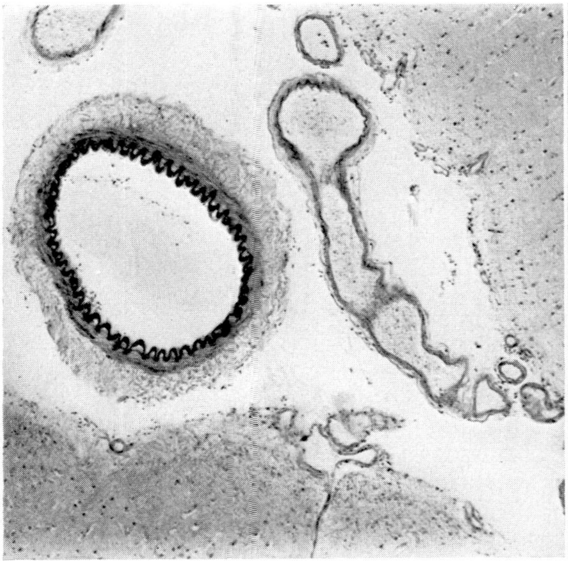

2.44

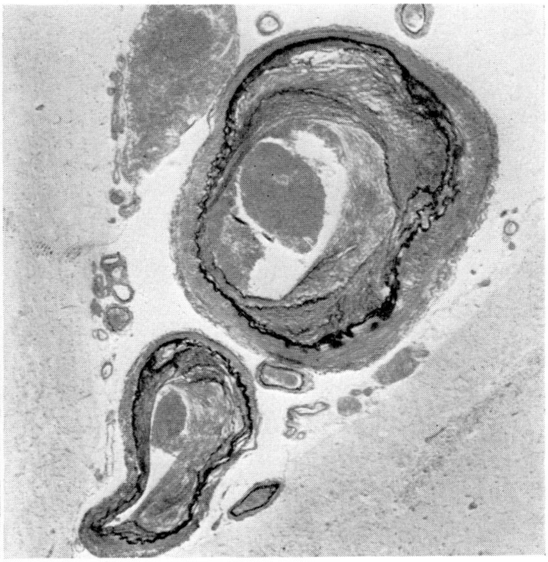

2.45

FIG. 2.44. *Normal* arteries and arterioles lying in a sulcus of the brain. Note the internal elastic lamina, the dark staining muscularis, no external elastic lamina, small amount of adventitia. (Celloidin, Weigert's elastic van Gieson, ×64.)

FIG. 2.45. *Atherosclerosis.* Cortical arteries and arterioles from a patient with marked atherosclerosis but without hypertension. Note that the abnormalities are in the arteries, which are eccentrically narrowed. The elastica is reduplicated. In places the media is thin. (Celloidin, Weigert's elastic van Gieson, ×24. Courtesy of Dr. W. G. P. Mair.)

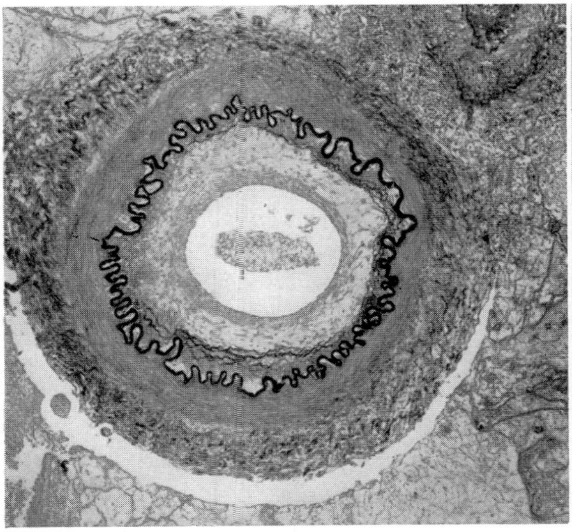

2.46

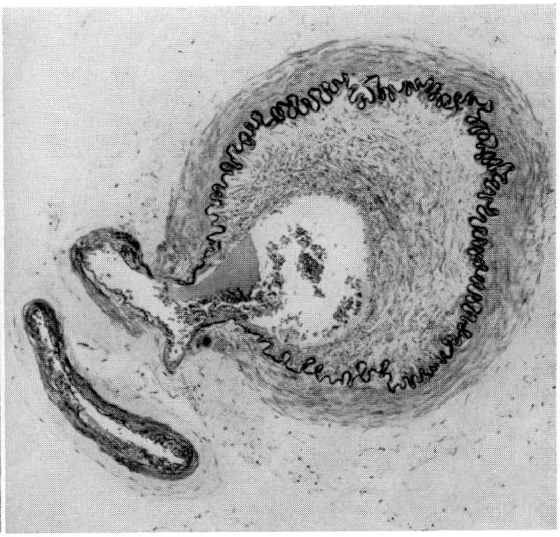

2.47

FIG. 2.46. *Endarteritis obliterans.* Artery at the base of the brain, pneumococcal leptomeningitis, treated sulpha drugs, one month's duration. Fibrinous exudate is present round the vessel which shows a thickened adventitia, an intact internal elastic membrane, and concentric intimal thickening. Fine elastic fibres are visible in the depths of the intimal thickening. An adjacent artery, in the upper right-hand side of the picture, shows necrosis and cellular infiltration of its wall. (Paraffin, Weigert's elastic van Gieson, ×57.)

FIG. 2.47. *Thrombo-angiitis obliterans.* Branch of the anterior cerebral artery. The lumen is narrowed by loosely packed cellular fibrous tissue. The internal elastic lamina and media are intact. There are no changes in the adventitia or leptomeninges. A healthy portion of artery lies close to the diseased one. (Paraffin, Weigert's elastic van Gieson, ×77. Courtesy of Prof. D. S. Russell.)

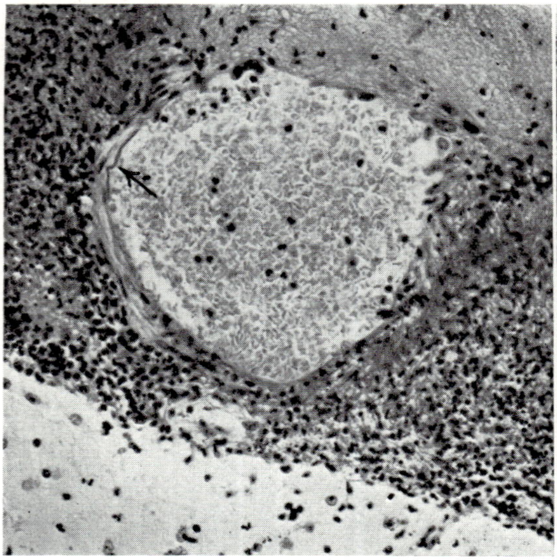

2.48

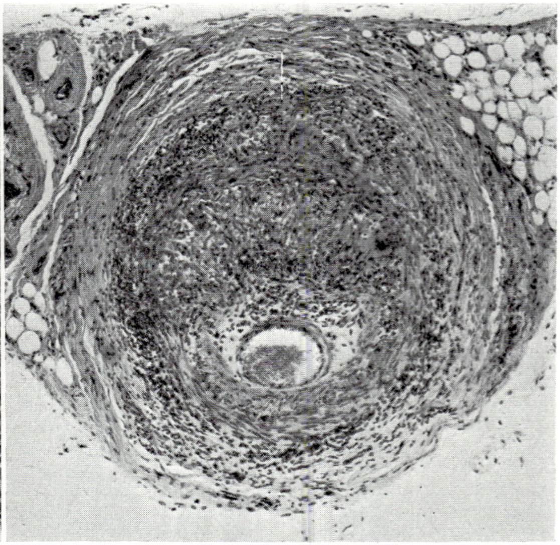

2.49

FIG. 2.48. *Polyarteritis nodosa.* Small leptomeningeal artery which is dilated. Only a small portion of the internal elastic lamina is visible (arrow) and most of the muscularis is destroyed. Polymorphonuclear leucocytes infiltrate the outer coats of the artery and the adjacent leptomeninges. (Celloidin, haematoxylin van Gieson, ×75.)

FIG. 2.49. *Giant-celled arteritis.* Ciliary artery of eye, showing intimal proliferation and cellular infiltration, including multinucleated giant cells close to the irregularly damaged internal elastic lamina. There is mononuclear infiltration of the media and, to a lesser extent, of the adventitia. (Celloidin, haematoxylin van Gieson, ×64.)

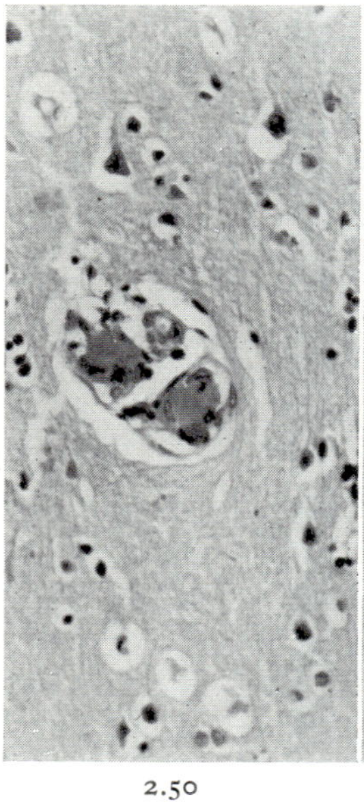

2.50

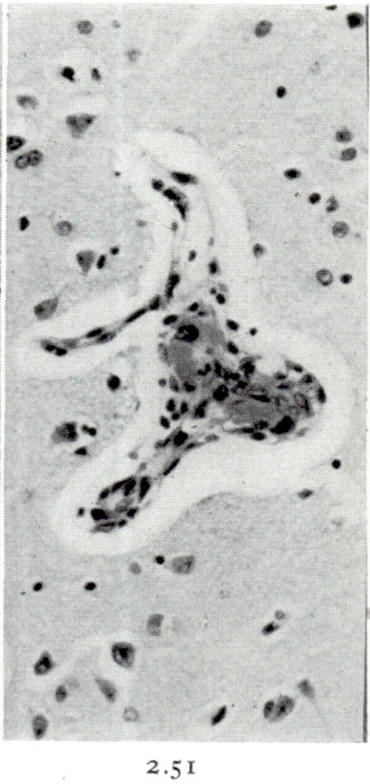

2.51

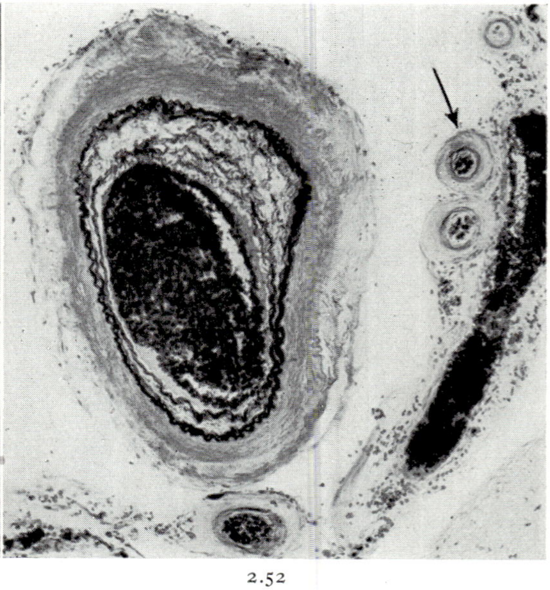

2.52

FIGS. 2.50 and 51. *Thrombotic micro-angiopathy.* Hyaline eosinophilic thrombus obstructs the dilated lumen at the arteriolocapillary junction zone. There is endothelial hyperplasia. The adjacent grey matter of the brain does not show any noticeable abnormality (apart from artefact due to shrinkage). (Paraffin, haematoxylin and eosin, ×200. Courtesy of Prof. Symmers.)

FIG. 2.52. *Hypertensive vascular disease.* Arteries and arterioles in a cerebral sulcus (Patient aged 51, B.P. 190/125, heart weight 470 g., same case as Figs. 2.58–2.62). The artery shows hypertrophy of the media, adventitial fibrosis and eccentric splitting and reduplication of the elastic lamina. The arterioles (arrow) show an increase in the thickness of the media and adventitia. (Celloidin, Weigert's elastic, ×100.)

Effects of atherosclerosis on the brain

If atherosclerosis is widespread, and almost certainly if the process is of many years duration, the brain will be atrophic. The ventricles will be dilated and the sulci widened. Foci of softening may be present in the cortex. These may be large or small and are usually of various ages. Small, irregularly shaped softenings are frequently present in the anterior part of the pons, less frequently in the centrum semi-ovale and in the basal grey nuclei. Microscopically these lesions are usually full of fat granule cells and are always close to a diseased artery or arteriole. These small softenings are quite different from 'état criblé' or 'état lacunaire' which are also found in senile arteriosclerotic brains (Bertrand 1923). The term 'état lacunaire' (of Pierre Marie) is usually applied to multiple, clearly visible, cavities with irregular contours in the basal grey nuclei; whilst the term 'état criblé' (of Vogt) is applied to similar cavities in the centrum semi-ovale and in other richly myelinated regions. Within each cavity there is an artery or an arteriole. Microscopical examination reveals that the cavity is a greatly dilated perivascular space and that the dilatation is secondary to irregular rarefaction and disintegration of the nervous parenchyma which surrounded the vessel. The artery or arteriole always looks healthy and the cavity contains very few cells. This condition therefore differs from a small softening in respect of its sites of election, state of the associated blood vessel and cell content within the cavity.

A lesser degree of this condition is sometimes present. The perivascular spaces are not dilated but, in the parenchyma which surrounds the vessel, the myelin sheaths are thin, pale and sinuous. When this change is widespread throughout the basal grey nuclei it is called 'état pré-criblé'. It may be seen less frequently in the centrum semi-ovale and the deep white matter of the gyri. It thus appears that the initial process is one of slow disintegration of the cerebral parenchyma around blood-vessels which are healthy in that particular region. Neither type of cavity should be confused with the numerous smooth walled, gas-filled cavities, which may be found in a brain which has been the site of post-mortem putrefaction and invasion by gas forming organisms. Around such cavities there is, of course, no cellular reaction.

ENDARTERITIS OBLITERANS

In meningovascular syphilis, in tuberculous leptomeningitis and in subacute or chronic pyogenic leptomeningitis when the arteries lie for a long time in tuberculous or purulent exudate, it is not uncommon to find thickening of the arterial wall (Fig. 2.46). The lumen of the artery is reduced in size because the intact endothelium is raised up, in a concentric or eccentric fashion, from the internal elastic lamina by a cellular infiltrate. This may at first be composed of mononuclear cells. In syphilis plasma cells are usually present and eosinophil leucocytes are common. At a later stage, or from the beginning, this cellular infiltrate may be replaced by fibroblasts and collagen with fine elastic fibrils lying internal to the internal elastic lamina, which itself remains intact. The media either appears intact or shows slight inflammatory cell infiltration or slight fibrosis. The adventitia is thickened, either by inflammatory cells or by fibrous tissue.

This condition is called endarteritis obliterans. It shows a stage, or stages, in the reaction of the arteries to infection of the body by more than one type of bacteria. Of itself it is neither diagnostic of any one of the infections named nor is it the only change produced in arteries by these organisms. It is therefore not a specific disease entity and the term should always be qualified by an adjective indicating its cause, if known.

In our opinion the most probable cause of most of the lesions described above is an irritant acting on the arteries from without. A process which is almost certainly due to an externally acting irritant is the paraplegia which may occur as a delayed sequel of *spinal anaesthesia*. In addition to fibrous thickening, and obliteration of the fluid spaces, of the pia-arachnoid, extending as far cranially as the base of the brain, these cases often show marked changes in the arteries and less severe changes in the veins.

In Brain and Russell's (1937) patient paralysis came on a month after the anaesthetic, and death occurred $3\frac{1}{2}$ months later. At post-mortem there was an endophlebitis and a necrotising pan-arteritis of the pial arteries and perforating arterioles of the lumbar region with extensive softening of the grey and white matter of the spinal cord.

In the cases of Greenfield *et al.* (1955) paralysis came on about 7, 8 and 24 weeks after the anaesthetic and death occurred about 5, 1 and 1 week later. At post-mortem the vascular changes were strictly limited to the lower thoracic and lumbo-sacral segments of the cord, and were confined to the leptomeningeal vessels. The usual change in the arteries consisted of adventitial fibrosis, collagenous replacement of the muscle of the media, stretching and breakage or thickening or reduplication of the elastica, and fibrous thickening (usually concentric) of the intima. One small artery showed coagulative necrosis; evidence of thrombosis was present in only one small artery. The walls of the veins were partially or wholly replaced by fibrous tissue. Haematogenous cellular infiltration was noticeably absent. It was considered that these changes were caused either by the anaesthetic material or by some contaminant introduced along with it. Whether the toxic action was direct or hyperallergic in nature remained undecided.

In order to test the possibility of the condition being due to a contaminant, Hurst (1955) injected a number of detergents and antiseptics in considerable dilution intracisternally into monkeys. He found that many of these substances, although of quite dissimilar chemical type, damaged superficial nervous structures, produced cellular proliferation and fibrosis in the pia-arachnoid, and caused necrosis of the media and often of the adventitia of the leptomeningeal arteries with subsequent intimal thickening. The end result was therefore similar to that described in man by Greenfield *et al.* Hurst considered that the experimental lesions were due to the direct irritative action of the chemicals tested; he did not find any evidence of a hyperallergic reaction. He was careful, however, to point out that his experiments did not prove that a contaminant was the cause of the post-anaesthetic changes in man.

THROMBO-ANGIITIS OBLITERANS

(*Winiwarter-Buerger's disease*)

This is a disease of the arteries and veins, of unknown aetiology, characteristically affecting the limbs of young males who are heavy smokers. In the limb vessels the histological changes are different from those in any other disease process. In the early stages there is acute inflammation of the wall and perivascular tissues of both artery and vein, with polymorphonuclear lymphocytic infiltration. Thrombosis is present within the vessel and is subsequently organised and recanalised. At the edge of the thrombus Buerger saw miliary foci not unlike tubercles. In the subacute and chronic stages there is medial and adventitial fibrosis involving and binding together both the artery and its accompanying vein. The internal elastic lamina is not particularly damaged. The lumen of both artery and vein contains organising thrombus which may be extensively recanalised. The vasa vasorum are prominent and may afford a local collateral pathway.

The disease process can affect vessels other than the limb vessels. When the cerebral vessels are affected the process is confined to the arteries and very rarely involves the veins. This feature may be due to the anatomical fact that the cerebral arteries and veins do not lie as close to each other as do the vessels of the limbs. Involvement of the spinal arteries is extremely rare (Eicke 1957).

In the brain there are two types of distribution: (1) widespread, focal, cortical lesions and (2) in both cerebral hemispheres symmetrically, in the peripheral part of the cortical distribution of the anterior, middle and posterior cerebral arteries, and sometimes in the retinal arteries (Lindenberg and Spatz 1939). The smaller arteries in the subarachnoid space are those particularly affected. The process involves considerable lengths of artery at a time and, in the chronic stage, they are shrunken, white and worm like. Healthy arteries are found close to those which are diseased. The underlying cortex shows many small zones of ischaemic necrosis giving a macroscopical appearance of granular atrophy.

Microscopically, in the central nervous system, the changes are confined to the lumen and to the endothelial and subendothelial layers of the intima; the internal elastic lamina and media are intact. Within the lumen there may or may not be a thrombus, varying in age from recent to old and recanalised. The endothelium is always affected. In the absence of thrombosis, in the early stages the endothelial cells are swollen and proliferated. In the later stages there is concentric or eccentric narrowing of the lumen by a ring of loosely packed, cellular, fibrous tissue, covered by endothelium (Fig. 2.47). When thrombosis is also present, the thrombotic and intimal proliferative processes are intermingled. Lymphocytic infiltration of the intimal tissues may be visible; occasionally polymorphonuclear leucocytes are present. The lesions vary in apparent age from place to place.

Histologically, the intact media and internal elastic lamina are sufficient to distinguish the condition from polyarteritis nodosa and giant-celled arteritis. Atherosclerosis, even if associated with hypertension, can be distinguished because atherosclerosis almost always affects the large vessels at the base of the brain, which are not involved in thrombo-angiitis obliterans; also when atheroma affects the cortical arteries it does so over short segments, not long distances; and in atherosclerosis the elastica and sometimes the media are damaged. Heubner's arteritis (endarteritis obliterans), whether due to syphilis or post-meningitic, can usually be diagnosed upon the basis of the clinical history, serological changes, widespread cerebral distribution and the histological changes in the media, adventitia and the leptomeninges. The principal difficulty is to distinguish a case of thrombo-angiitis obliterans from a case in which there have been multiple cerebral emboli. Spatz (1935), writing of his own cases, said that, on a purely histological basis, it would be very difficult to distinguish between what he saw and an embolic process (based for example on an endocarditis affecting the aortic valves). When only the brain is available for study then the bilateral symmetrical distribution may be suggestive but cannot exclude embolism or local thrombosis. Such a source of emboli or cause of possible local thrombosis may be present in thrombosed carotid arteries, a condition which is usually due to atherosclerosis. It seems doubtful whether the diagnosis of thrombo-angiitis obliterans can properly be made without a full post-mortem examination, including examination of the vessels of the limbs.

In view of the doubtful nature of many of the reported cases, we would agree with Adams and Michelson (1952) that a diagnosis of thrombo-angiitis obliterans should not be made, except in the event of (1) an acute inflammatory reaction in cerebral arteries, particularly an obliterating endarteritis with epithelioid and giant cells in the thrombus or intima and with relative sparing of the media (thereby distinguishing it from giant celled arteritis), or (2) obliteration of long stretches of brain arteries in non-atherosclerotic, non-syphilitic patients, with cortical necrosis at the periphery of the field of distribution of the middle cerebral artery, or (3) occlusion of cerebral arteries due to a non-specific endarteritis obliterans in cases with the characteristic findings of thrombo-angiitis obliterans in the limbs.

Of the cases published in English it is doubtful if any will satisfy these criteria. This does not, however, mean that we believe that cases of cerebral thrombo-angiitis do not exist for we have recently had the opportunity of examining a case of Prof. D. S. Russell's which satisfied the third criterion. The patient (P.M. 32/1953)* was a man of 46 with undoubted thrombo-angiitis obliterans of the vessels of the legs, without aortic endocarditis or carotid obstruction, in whom there was subacute endarteritis obliterans of the branches of the anterior cerebral arteries (Fig. 2.47). In addition, in the gall bladder and the kidneys, some small arteries showed the histological changes of polyarteritis nodosa: an association of thrombo-angiitis obliterans with polyarteritis nodosa which was also noticed by Jäger (1932).

POLYARTERITIS NODOSA

This is an acute and subacute disease of medium and small sized arteries, especially those of the kidney, liver and splanchnic region. Clinical involvement of voluntary muscle and peripheral nerve is quite frequent (Miller and Daley 1946). Clinical involvement of the central nervous system is considered to be less common, although it was found to be as high as 20 per cent by Foster and Malamud (1941) in their review of 300 cases. In their own case, which came to post-mortem examination, the arteries of the brain were extensively involved histologically, but this in our experience is rare. When present it is usually widespread but focal, so that a muscle biopsy in a suspected case should be cut at several levels. Recent, healing and healed lesions can often be found fairly close together. Hypertension and secondary left sided cardiac hypertrophy are common. Clinical recovery occurs in at least 50 per cent of cases (Miller and Daley 1946) and this has been confirmed histologically.

The primary pathological lession appears to be subendothelial oedema followed by fibrinoid or hyaline necrosis of the media, destruction of the internal elastic lamina and infiltration of all coats by inflammatory cells. These changes may involve only part of the arterial wall, as seen on cross-section. The cellular infiltration is most abundant in the adventitia (Fig. 2.48). It is composed of neutrophil polymorphonuclear leucocytes, lymphocytes, large mononuclear cells, and a variable number of eosinophil leucocytes which are often present in large numbers. Failure to demonstrate eosinophil leucocytes does not exclude a diagnosis of polyarteritis nodosa. The damage to the vessel coats may include the lining endothelium and secondary thrombus may occlude the vessel. Sometimes the damage to the vessel is so severe that nodular dilatation, aneurysm formation (rare) or rupture may occur. The walls of the arteries of the central nervous system are so thin that, in the few cases in which they are affected, rupture and haemorrhage are common.

In the healing or healed stage the arteries show a concentric or eccentric subendothelial fibrous deposit. The internal elastic lamina is partially or wholly fragmented, or destroyed. Part or all of the media is replaced by fibrous tissue and there is slight fibrous thickening of the adventitia.

Lesions of the small nutrient arteries of peripheral nerves are very frequent in cases of peri-arteritis nodosa. Gruber (1926) and Arkin (1930) found lesions of this kind in 20 per cent and Lovshin and Kernohan (1948) in 50 per cent of their cases, but in the latter series many of the lesions produced no clinical signs. Although symptomatology may indicate a lesion of a single nerve the disease more often affects many nerves in an asymmetrical manner. Kernohan and Woltman (1938) describe it as a *mononeuritis multiplex*. More rarely it appears in the guise of symmetrical paralysis of the muscles supplied by the sciatic nerves and may suggest the

* This case is being prepared for publication by L. J. Rubinstein.

diagnosis of polyneuritis. The paralysis may come on abruptly or more slowly; it may improve to some extent, even permanently (Marcus 1933), but often remains severe or progresses. The lesions are most common in the largest nerves such as the sciatic and brachial plexus (Lovshin and Kernohan) and consist of localised areas of infarction related to necrotic and thrombosed arteries and arterioles. Some nerves may be intact at the level where the arterial lesion is most severe but are degenerated more peripherally. Less often degenerative changes are seen in a nerve whose arteries appear healthy. The nerve fibres show all degrees of degeneration or frank necrosis, entailing Wallerian degeneration of the distal part of the nerve fibre. Subperineurial and interfascicular oedema is sometimes seen but inflammatory infiltration is usually confined to the immediate neighbourhood of the affected arteries in which the lesions differ in no respect from those found in other organs of the body.

Pathogenesis. Polyarteritis nodosa may follow organismal infection (especially streptococcal infection), drug intoxications and serum sickness. In such cases there is clinical evidence that it is a hypersensitivity reaction. This view was supported experimentally by Rich and Gregory (1943) who found the lesions of polyarteritis nodosa in rabbits in which they had established a condition analogous to serum sickness in man. In the human cases it appears that the antigen may vary from case to case but the antigen-antibody reaction remains histologically similar.

Polyarteritis nodosa may also occur spontaneously, under circumstances where its allergic basis is less certain. Zeek *et al.* (1948) considered that the necrotising panarteritis which is associated clinically with hypersensitivity differs in its morphology and distribution from spontaneous polyarteritis nodosa occurring without clinical evidence of hypersensitivity. They found that in spontaneous polyarteritis nodosa the lesions were related to the bifurcation of muscular arteries near their site of entrance into viscera, that pre-necrotic, necrotic and healing stages were all found at one time in the same patient and that the lungs and spleen were not involved: in hypersensitivity angiitis they found that the larger arteries were not involved, the condition affected venules, arterioles and small arteries, that the lesions were all of the necrotic type, and that the lungs and spleen were involved.

GIANT-CELLED ARTERITIS

This subacute inflammatory disease of arteries usually occurs in people over the age of 55 years. It often involves the superficial temporal arteries, which become swollen, tender, tortuous and nodular; pulsation is usually diminished or lost and the artery becomes reduced in size and hard. The disease is not limited to the temporal arteries. Nearly all the larger arteries in the body, from the aorta downwards, have been found to be involved in an irregular and focal manner. Of the medium and smaller sized arteries which may be affected, those of particular importance are the coronary arteries and the ophthalmic artery and its branches, including the ciliary arteries and the central artery of the retina (Crompton 1959). About 25 per cent of patients become blind in one or both eyes. The arteries of the brain are less often, and those of the spinal cord very rarely, involved. Two cases with involvement of the small meningeal and intracerebral vessels were published by McCormick and Neubürger (1958).

The affected arteries are not diseased throughout their length but in segments. The vessel wall is thickened and the lumen is eccentrically reduced in calibre. It may be blocked by recent thrombus, but this is an uncommon feature and a point of distinction from Buerger's disease.

Histologically, between the endothelium and the internal elastic lamina, there is a zone of intimal proliferation which can often, in the active stage of the disease, be divided into two zones,

(1) a thicker inner zone composed of loosely packed, cellular, fibrous tissue with a mucoid intercellular substance, and (2) a thinner outer zone of vascular granulomatous tissue infiltrated by a variable, but usually small, number of large and small mononuclear cells, plasma cells, and a few neutrophil polymorphonuclear leucocytes. Eosinophil leucocytes are very rare, a point of distinction from polyarteritis nodosa.

The internal elastic lamina and the media are always severely damaged, but in an irregular fashion. The internal elastic lamina stains poorly for elastic tissue and is fragmented. The media is infiltrated by small and large mononuclear cells, some of 'epithelioid' type. Giant cells, of foreign body type (10–100μ diameter), are almost invariably present, either in the media close to the damaged internal elastic lamina, or in the external portion of the intimal proliferation (Fig. 2.49). Sometimes the histological relationship of a fragment of elastica and a giant cell supports the view that the elastica is undergoing phagocytosis. A lesser degree of inflammatory cell infiltration is often present in the adventitia and giant cells may be found here (Harrison 1948, Heptinstall *et al.* 1954).

Pathogenesis. This is at present unknown.

THROMBOTIC MICRO-ANGIOPATHY

(*Thrombocytic acro-angiothrombosis*)

This is a rare disease, first described by Moschowitz (1925), with the clinical features of fever, purpura, haemolytic anaemia and thrombocytopenia, together with various neurological disorders such as hemiplegia, convulsions and coma. It runs a rapid course and death occurs within a few days or weeks. It is rather more common in adolescents and young adults than in older persons.

At post-mortem there are no specific changes visible to the naked eye, but microscopically, widespread in many organs including the brain, there is thrombosis of the smaller blood vessels. The region affected is the arteriolo-capillary junction zone, where there is an increased cellularity of the vessel wall and obstruction of the lumen by granular or hyaline, eosinophilic, thrombus (Figs. 2.50 and 2.51), which may be undergoing organisation. The exact nature of the thrombus is not certain. It has been generally considered that the staining qualities were those of platelets but Stuart *et al.* (1956) have put forward evidence that the thrombi stain more like fibrin. Because of the doubtful nature of the thrombi, Symmers (1952) has proposed that the disease should be called thrombotic micro-angiopathy rather than by any title which implies platelet thrombi.

In the brain the lesions are almost confined to the grey matter (Adams *et al.* 1948) and consist of (1) Hyperplasia of endothelial, and probably of adventitial, cells of terminal arterioles and capillaries, with increase in the total diameter of the vessels. Sometimes the vessel wall is necrotic. (2) Occlusion of these vessels by acidophilic thrombi. (3) Foci of nerve cell damage and, in some regions, proliferation of glia. There is, however, a striking disparity between the marked involvement of the vessels and the slight change in the surrounding brain. (4) Occasional petechial haemorrhages.

The aetiology is unknown. The possibility that hypersensitivity can sometimes play a part is suggested by Symmers' (1956) case of thrombotic micro-angiopathy associated with acute haemorrhagic leucoencephalitis and sensitivity to oxophenarsine.

THE CENTRAL NERVOUS SYSTEM IN RHEUMATIC FEVER

Patients who die in the acute stage of rheumatic fever were always found by Costero (1949) to have swollen oedematous brains in which, microscopically, the perivascular spaces were dilated, the capillaries showed fibrous sclerosis, there were recent and old diapedetic haemorrhages, regions of cellular devastation and foci of softening. Widespread reactive change was present in the microglia. Winkelman and Eckel (1932) had previously reported swelling and proliferation of the endothelial cells of cortical arterioles and capillaries, with thickening and hyalinization of their walls. Whilst none of these changes is specific for rheumatic fever, Costero considered them to be more important than heart failure as a cause of death. One of Winkleman's cases had vegetative endocarditis and a large temporal softening.

Specific lesions, such as the acute necrotic arteritis described in other bodily organs by von Glahn and Pappenheimer (1926), or Aschoff bodies, have not been reported; although Costero, in 6 children out of his 107 cases, found, in the brain stem, occasional nodules of branched microglia which he thought were a hyperergic response comparable to the Aschoff body; and von Santha (1932) saw fibrinous infiltration of the vessel wall.

Following rheumatic fever, or in patients with recurrent attacks, psychiatric or neurological symptoms may arise. In such cases post-mortem examination may show (Bruetsch 1942 and 1949) either:—

(1) Widespread obliterative arteritis of the small meningeal and cortical vessels, with proliferation of the endothelial cells, subendothelial fibrosis, and sometimes fibrous thickening of the media; numerous small secondary softenings are present in the brain. A similar change may occur in larger arteries with large secondary softenings. Kernohan (1942) considered that these arterial changes resemble local proliferation, *in situ*, of the endothelial cells rather than those secondary to emboli from the diseased heart. Taken by themselves the histological appearances in the brain may bear a close resemblance to syphilitic arteritis, or to thrombo-angiitis obliterans, from which they should be separated by an examination of the rest of the body; or

(2) Cerebral embolism, which occurs most often in patients with mitral stenosis in whom auricular thrombi are disturbed by auricular fibrillation; or

(3) Uncommonly, rheumatic meningo-encephalitis, with perivascular and diffuse round cell infiltration throughout the grey and white matter of the brain.

These changes are also non-specific and by themselves they are not diagnostic of rheumatic infection. Aschoff bodies and acute necrotic arteritis have not been reported.

With the exception of Costero's microglial nodules, most of the lesions in the central nervous system, in both the acute and chronic phases of rheumatic infection, are either directly due to the associated disease of the heart, or are non-specific changes which are found in other toxi-infective conditions. Some of the lesions are undoubtedly due to embolism, some may be due to local thrombosis or anoxia, all of which can be attributed to disease of the heart, especially to endocarditis or to auricular fibrillation or to cardiac insufficiency. Other findings, such as the vascular endothelial proliferation, are also seen in typhoid, toxaemia or pregnancy, erysipelas, Hodgkin's disease and chronic tuberculosis (Winkelman and Eckel 1929) but here also cardiac insufficiency cannot be entirely excluded.

Rheumatic chorea

The pathology and pathogenesis of chorea in rheumatic infection are still in the stage of investigation (Greenfield and Wolfsohn 1922, Buchanan *et al.* 1942). The histological findings in the central nervous system vary from case to case and include cellular infiltration of the brain (perivascular and throughout its substance), loss of nerve cells from the cortex, basal ganglia and cerebellum and endarteritis. The one feature which these findings seem to have in common is that they are widespread and not localised to any particular part of the central nervous system. Buchanan *et al.* have therefore suggested that the abnormal movements originate in the cerebral cortex, but only occur when the motor cortex is hyperexcitable, either congenitally, or because of lesions in the circuits which normally modify the activity of the cortex.

INTRACRANIAL HAEMORRHAGE

There are many causes of intracranial haemorrhage, and the relative frequency of those, which are either the main cause of the symptoms and signs or the cause of death, will vary from hospital to hospital and from time to time, especially with regard to the frequency of those due to mechanical trauma.

In 1954 Russell published her findings of the causes of spontaneous intracranial haemorrhage from the post-mortem records of the London Hospital (1912–52). She excluded all varieties in which trauma played a part and all neo-natal haemorrhages. She recorded only cases in which there were significantly large haemorrhages (in the brain stem of 1·5 cm. diameter or more, in the cerebrum and cerebellum 3 cm. or more).

Hypertensive		232
Basal ganglia	151	
Cerebral white matter	21	
Subcortical (cerebrum)	4	
Meninges	6	
Pons and midbrain	32	
Cerebellum	18	
Congenital medial defects of cerebral arteries (92 cases with aneurysm)		96
Blood diseases		36
Acute leukaemia	15	
Thrombopenia	13	
Aplastic anaemia	3	
Other anaemias	3	
Erythrocythaemia	1	
Haemophilia	1	
Mycotic aneurysm		28
Vascular hamartoma		21
Telangiectasis	0	
Multiple cavernous angioma	1	
Arteriovenous angioma	20	
Arteritis (no aneurysm)		13
Pyaemia	10	
Associated purulent leptomeningitis	3	
Neoplasm		9
Arterial degeneration (no cardiovascular hypertrophy)		7
Various		3
Cause not found		16

Comparable figures from the post-mortem records of the National Hospital, Queen Square (1909–56), inclusive are:

Hypertensive		32
Cerebrum	26	
Pons	3	
Cerebellum	2	
Pons and cerebellum	1	
Congenital saccular aneurysms		73
Patients with a single aneurysm	60	
Patients with multiple aneurysms	13	

In the 73 patients there were 88 aneurysms distributed as follows:

Junction of terminal portion of internal carotid and its branches	31	
Junction anterior cerebral and anterior communicating	22	
Middle cerebral at Sylvian point	21	
Basilar artery and its branches	8	
Anterior cerebral at distal points of branching	4	
Junction internal carotid and ophthalmic artery	2	
Blood diseases		1
Mycotic aneurysm		1
Vascular hamartoma		8
Telangiectasis (cerebellar)	1	
Arteriovenous angioma (cerebral 6, cerebellar 1)	7	
Two of these arteriovenous angiomata also had saccular aneurysms, 2 and 4 in number respectively. In one case an aneurysmal rupture was the cause of death. These figures are not included amongst the congenital saccular aneurysms.		
Arteritis (no aneurysm)		0
Haemorrhage into a neoplasm		7
Arterial degeneration (no cardiovascular hypertrophy)		0
Cause not found		4

The London Hospital is a general hospital and the National Hospital, Queen Square, is a neurological hospital, and this probably accounts for the greater frequency of hypertensive cases, blood diseases and mycotic aneurysms in the London Hospital figures.

In the two series there were 3·5 per cent and 3·1 per cent of cases in which the cause of the haemorrhage was not found. Some of these were probably due to a congenital saccular aneurysm or a small, cryptic, venous or arteriovenous malformation such as those described by Crawford and Russell (1956), which was destroyed by the haemorrhage.

The age distribution of the most frequent causes of haemorrhage in the National Hospital series is:

Age period	10–19	20–29	30–39	40–49	50–59	60–69	70–79
Hypertensive		1	2	6	12	9	2
Congenital saccular aneurysms	4	2	14	17	31	3	2
Vascular hamartomata		1	1	2	4		

HAEMATOMYELIA

The expression haematomyelia is usually confined to a large intramedullary haemorrhage, extending over several segments. The haemorrhage is predominantly in the grey matter, which is largely destroyed, but may also spread along the white columns, separating rather than destroying the nerve fibres. The most frequent cause is, probably, bleeding from an angiomatous malformation (Richardson 1938). It has been reported in association with arteriosclerosis, meningovascular syphilis, spinal tumour and syringomyelia.

It is very doubtful whether mechanical trauma ever produces haematomyelia. It is true that, after a severe fracture-dislocation or bullet wound of the spine (Holmes 1915), the naked eye appearances will often be those of a very haemorrhagic pulping of the cord at the level of the injury, together with a thin pencil of bloodstained material which runs upwards and downwards from this site for several segments. Microscopical examination, however, shows that the material is composed principally of disintegrating nervous tissue, which has been produced at the site of the lesion by pulping and haemorrhagic infarction, and has been forced upwards and downwards. It is not haemorrhage and the condition is not haematomyelia.

THE CENTRAL NERVOUS SYSTEM IN HYPERTENSIVE VASCULAR DISEASE

Changes in the vessels

In the presence of arterial hypertension the arteries and arterioles of the brain, like those elsewhere in the body, show hypertrophic and degenerative changes, but in the brain these changes are of a lesser degree of severity (Moritz and Oldt 1937). Baker (1941) found that in benign hypertension, even of long duration, both the small arteries (50–150μ diameter) and the larger arteries showed little change, except in patients over the age of 60, in whom the larger arteries were noticeably affected, with severe intimal and medial changes including fibrosis and eventual degeneration and hyalinisation. In severe and rapid (malignant) hypertension the changes, both hyperplastic and degenerative, are well marked (Rosenberg 1940). The blood vessels of the spinal cord show very little change.

In our experience, in patients who have died from hypertensive haemorrhage, the *arteries* of the circle of Willis and their main branches, including the basal arteries, show hypertrophic and degenerative changes, including muscular hypertrophy and fibrosis of the media, adventitial fibrosis, splitting and reduplication, often eccentric, of the internal elastic lamina, and intimal fibrosis (Fig. 2.52). Sometimes the changes cannot be distinguished from atherosclerosis.

The arterioles show an increase in the thickness of the vessel wall and a reduction in the calibre of the lumen. In the larger arterioles the thickening affects all three coats, with proliferation of the endothelium, thickening or fraying of the internal elastic lamina, hypertrophy of the muscle cells of the media with an increase of the size of their nuclei, and fibrous thickening of the adventitia (hypertensive arteriolosclerosis). Fibrosis and hyaline change may affect the media in some cases (Figs. 2.52, 2.53 and 2.54). In the smaller arterioles there is, in malignant hypertension, often a thickening of the wall of the vessel by a sub-intimal deposit of hyaline acidophilic and fatty material. This may be confined to the intimal region or may involve both intima and media. The appearances are similar to those seen in the renal arterioles. This is probably not a terminal event for, as Pickering *et al.* (1952) found, arteriolar necrosis is present in kidneys and suprarenals removed at operation from patients with malignant hypertension.

The *capillaries* do not usually show any marked histological change, although there may be an increase in reticulin in their walls. In this connection it is interesting to examine the origin of the term 'arteriocapillary fibrosis'. In 1872 Gull and Sutton, writing on 'The pathology of the morbid state commonly called Chronic Bright's disease with contracted kidney' ('Arterio-capillary fibrosis'), describe the changes which they found in fresh and frozen preparations of blood-vessels. They found a 'hyalin-fibroid' formation in the walls of the minute arteries and a 'hyalin-granular' change in the corresponding capillaries. This finding is often referred to, but it should be noted that the cerebral vessels which they examined were the 'minute arteries and larger capillaries of the pia mater'. Nowadays these vessels would be called arteries and arterioles.

Changes in the parenchyma

In Rosenberg's series of 17 patients, who had died with malignant hypertension, multiple infarcts were found in 12 cases. In 4 they were only found microscopically, in 8 both gross and microscopic lesions were present. The regions of ischaemic necrosis were widespread, involving basal ganglia, cerebral cortex, white matter, brain stem and cerebellum. Sometimes adjoining vessels were thrombosed, sometimes not. With such findings we would agree.

The extent and degree of ischaemic necrosis varies from destruction of a small zone of pericapillary tissue to a large infarct. It may take the form of loss of nerve cells within the distribution of a cortical arteriole, or of partial or complete destruction of white matter, as is seen in Binswanger's subcortical encephalopathy. Indirect signs of such lesions having occurred are seen in pericapillary gliosis, and in the enlargement of perivascular spaces secondary to shrinkage of surrounding tissue.

The presence of an ischaemic lesion without a related thrombosed vessel, together with the often transient nature of the clinical symptoms, have been taken as evidence of the occurrence of spasm of arteries or arterioles. This view, vigorously opposed by Pickering (1955), has received support from the experimental work of Byrom (1954).

Byrom has pointed out that, in the human, hypertension is not associated with a more rapid flow of blood through the brain, so that some degree of arterial or arteriolar constriction must occur. This constriction is due to the fact that arteries have intrinsic local tone, largely dependent on intra-arterial pressure. Byrom made rats hypertensive by means of a renal clamp. These rats showed clinical evidence of hypertensive encephalopathy. He observed the cerebral vessels through transparent windows in their skulls and saw arteriolar spasm taking place. By means of *intra vitam* injection of trypan blue he showed that some capillaries were abnormally permeable. Histologically he saw (1) focal cerebral oedema without vascular necrosis, (2) vascular necrosis, (3) haemorrhage.

He considers that hypertensive disease may be dividied into two main grades of severity. In the first the underlying peripheral vasoconstriction is diffuse and so controlled that the distribution of the blood to the tissues remains substantially normal, except where it is locally impeded by secondary degenerative changes in the arterial wall, such as atherosclerosis. In the second, more severe, grade there is, superimposed upon physiological vasoconstriction, a state of focal but widespread pathological spasm. This spasm is a direct local response to the physical strain of excessive intra-arterial tension; a morbid response which can be traced to a simple physiological property of arterial muscle, i.e. its faculty of contracting against a filling tension. It is possible that the arteries are also abnormally sensitive.

The effects of the spasm depend upon its intensity, duration, location and extent. They comprise, in increasing order of severity (1) transient disturbance of function, (2) increased capillary permeability with attendant focal oedema and (3) local necrosis of the arterial wall and/or the tissue supplied. An alternative explanation of arterial necrosis is that blood trapped between two zones of constriction may be squeezed into the vessel wall. Byrom found that the arterial spasm which underlay these various changes could be abolished in the rat by removing its cause, i.e. by lowering the blood pressure.

Although there is much in Byrom's experimental findings which seems directly applicable to man, on the other hand, in considering the occurrence of ischaemic lesions in the brain, especially those without a closely related thrombosed vessel, it is important not to forget either

2.56

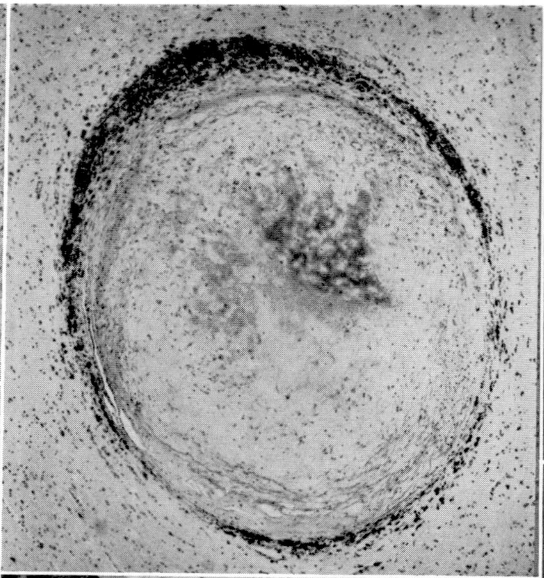

2.53

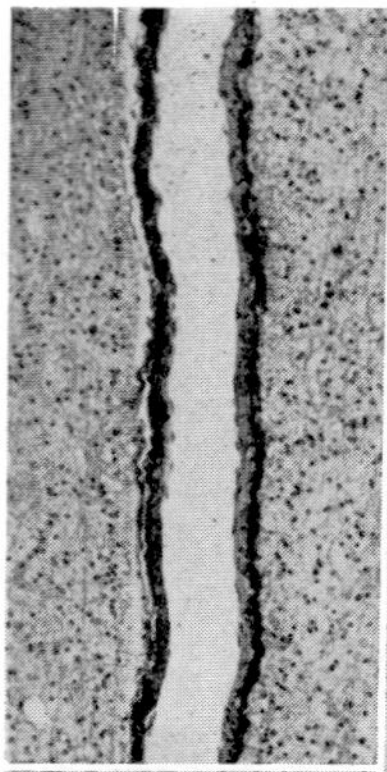

2.54

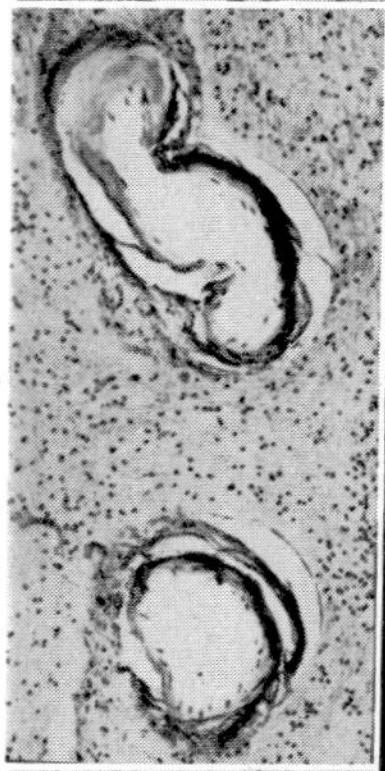

2.55

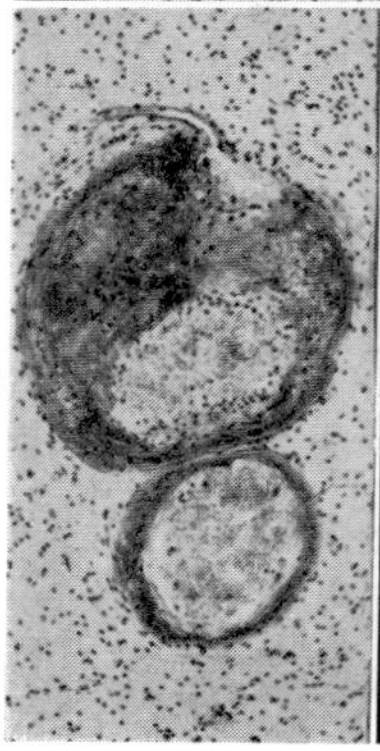

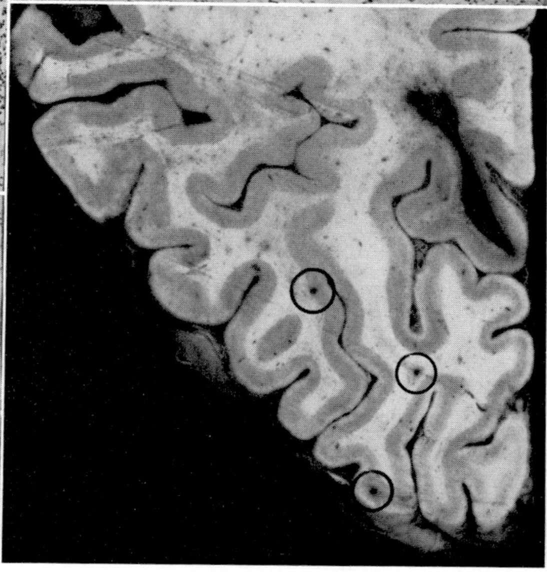

2.57

2.58

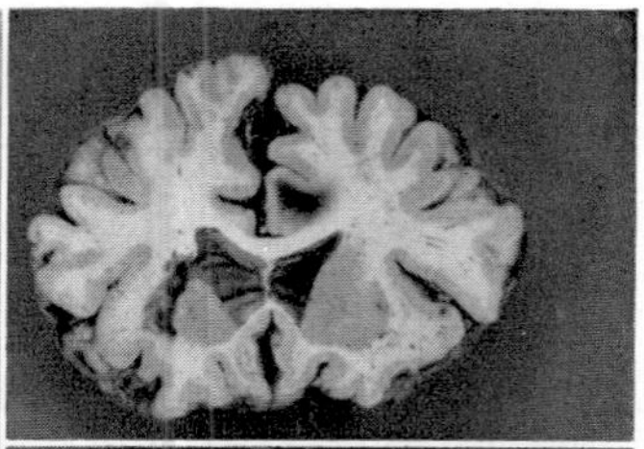

2.59

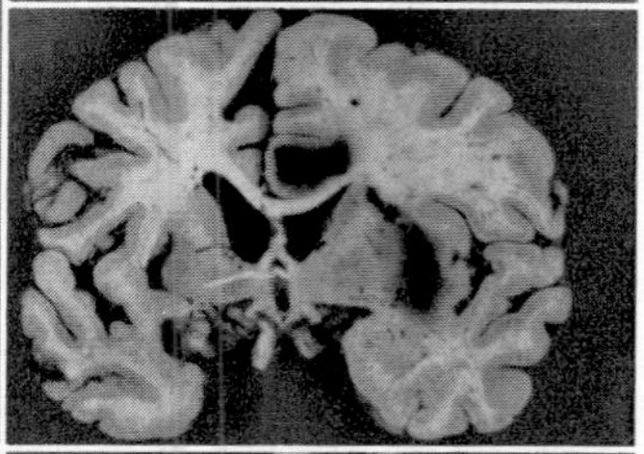

2.60

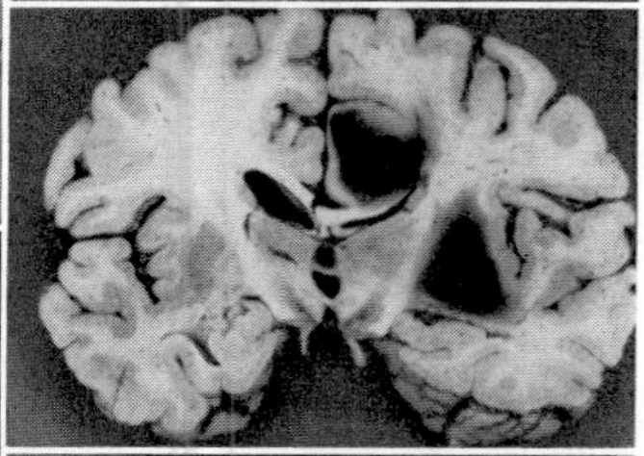

2.61

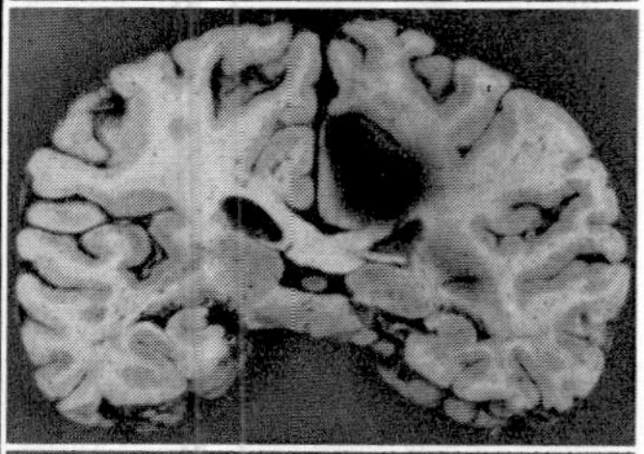

2.62

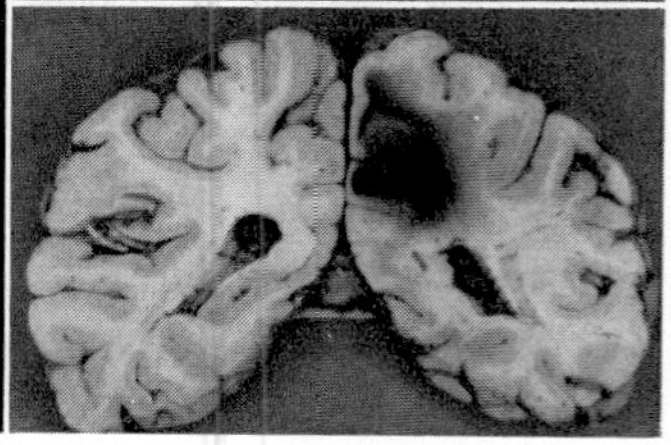

FIGS. 2.53–2.62. *Hypertensive vascular disease.* These pictures illustrate the progressively more serious lesions which may be found in this condition. Figs. 2.53–2.56 are from one brain, Fig. 2.57 from a different case, Figs. 2.58–2.62 from a 3rd case.

FIG. 2.53. Small artery in the superficial cerebral white matter showing muscular hypertrophy. From a man aged 59, B.P. 240/160, heart weight 550 g., died from uraemia. Small frontal and occipital haemorrhages were present. (Celloidin, haematoxylin van Gieson, ×40.)

FIG. 2.54. Another small artery in the superficial white matter showing fibrous degeneration of wall. (×40.)

FIG. 2.55. Small arteries in the superficial white matter showing degeneration of the wall and aneurysmal dilatation. In the lower vessel the wall is necrotic but the lumen contains fluid blood. In the upper vessel the wall is necrotic and dilated but otherwise intact. The lumen is partly occupied by thrombus. A patent capillary is visible in the upper part of the picture. Its lumen is in continuity with the residual lumen of the artery. (×40.)

FIG. 2.56. Microscopic appearance of haemorrhagic lesion in cortex, similar to those in Fig. 2.54. The wall of the original artery is degenerate and there has been haemorrhage into the surrounding tissue. The lumen is completely filled with old thrombus. Around the false aneurysm are phagocytes containing haemosiderin, which appear dark in colour. (×50.)

FIG. 2.57. Horizontal section, occipital region, male, aged 53, B.P. 250/150, left ventricular hypertrophy. Note the miliary aneurysms (circles) in the cortex and white matter. In the upper right-hand side of the picture there is a slit haemorrhage, which probably arose from a lesion similar to that which produces a miliary aneurysm.

FIGS. 2.58–2.62. Same case as Fig. 2.52. Recent haemorrhages (clinically 10 days' duration) are present in the white matter of the cingulate gyrus and the putamen. The cingulate haemorrhage was 9 cm. antero-posteriorly. An old haemorrhagic softening is present in the left corpus striatum.

the state of the main arteries of supply (carotid and vertebral arteries including their cervical portions), which may be atherosclerotic, or the efficiency of the heart.

In malignant (severe) hypertension it is common to find atherosclerosis of the coronary arteries and myocardial insufficiency (Schottstaedt and Sokolow 1953). There may therefore be periods when the heart is unable to force sufficient blood through often organically narrowed arteries and arterioles to keep the nervous tissue healthy; a state of acute cerebral vascular insufficiency arises (Corday *et al.* 1953).

In the brains of persons with severe hypertension there is usually atherosclerosis and hypertensive arteriosclerosis. The degree of this organic obstruction is not uniform throughout the brain and, therefore, with a drop in blood pressure, some parts of the brain will suffer more severely from vascular insufficiency than others. It is possible that this is the cause of the often focal nature of the symptoms and signs.

According to the duration and severity of the general or local vascular insufficiency, which may be mitigated by the opening up of the local collateral circulation, the changes in the nervous tissue may be reversible or irreversible. If reversible there may be transient symptoms and signs, without any local structural lesion which can be found at post-mortem: if irreversible there will be local organic change, but there may not be any thrombosis of the related vessel.

Changes in the cerebrospinal fluid

It is common to find elevation both of the pressure and the protein content of the lumbar fluid. Jefferson (1955) found the mean value of the pressure to be approximately 210 mm. H_2O and the mean value of the protein to be about 66 mg. per 100 ml. The cause of these changes is not known.

Haemorrhage from diseased vessels

This may be divided into at least three forms, in order of magnitude.

(1) Bleeding into vessel walls, perivascular sheaths and closely adjacent parenchyma.

(2) Slit haemorrhages.

(3) Massive haemorrhage, in cerebrum, pons or cerebellum.

(1) *Bleeding into vessel walls, perivascular sheaths and closely adjacent parenchyma.* These are seldom seen in a recent state but are quite often found as old lesions, usually with thrombosis of an arteriole; sometimes as a large group of phagocytes, laden with haemosiderin, around an arteriole with a patent lumen. Such lesions are found in the cerebral cortex, and in the white matter just deep to the cortex. To the naked eye they are often clearly visible, on section of the brain, as dark reddish or brownish-red rounded masses up to about 1 mm. diameter (Fig. 2.57). In the thrombosed lesions the wall of the arteriole is dilated, lacks muscle and shows degeneration of its elastic and fibrous tissue. The degenerate, dilated wall may surround the haemorrhage (Fig. 2.55) or be buried in it, in which case the periphery of the thrombus will be surrounded by phagocytes filled with haemosiderin (Fig. 2.56). Such lesions (Green 1930) are undoubtedly the miliary aneurysms which Charcot and Bouchard (1890) described as being found in every case of massive cerebral haemorrhage, not only within and close to the haemorrhage but also, usually in considerable numbers, in the cortex and subcortex more or less distant from the haemorrhage.

(2) *Slit haemorrhages.* These are quite often present in the brains of hypertensive patients, in the superficial part of the white matter of the cerebral hemispheres. The blood clot is not

rounded but fills a slit-like cavity which runs roughly parallel to the overlying cortex (Fig. 2.57). These slit-like haemorrhages probably arise as a further stage in haemorrhage from vessels as described under (1). Their appearance suggests that the blood, after leaving the vessel, found that the path of least resistance was between the fibres of the white matter in a plane parallel to the cortex. The blood clot in these lesions varies from recent to very old; and the lesions vary in size from very small to those extending for about half the anteroposterior length of the brain (Figs. 2.58–2.62). A somewhat similar type of localised haemorrhage may be found involving the region of the putamen (Figs. 2.59 and 2.60), which is partially or completely replaced by blood clot. In this case the haemorrhage is confined to the lentiform nucleus by the more resistant surrounding bundles of white fibres.

(3) *Massive haemorrhage.* The common sites for massive cerebral haemorrhage of hypertensive origin are (1) the region of the lentiform nucleus, (2) the deep white matter of the cerebellar hemispheres, (3) the pons and midbrain. Courville (1950) gives the relative incidence in his 40,000 autopsies as 938, 124 and 73 respectively.

It is not uncommon, in cases of massive cerebral haemorrhage, to find one or more separate haemorrhages in the midbrain and pons. The brain stem lesion is then secondary to the displacement caused by the cerebral haemorrhage, and is similar to that commonly seen as a terminal event in patients with other kinds of supratentorial space-occupying lesions, e.g. a glioma, abscess, oedema, extradural or acute subdural haemorrhage (see p. 443).

Haemorrhage in the region of the lentiform nucleus has been divided by Courville and Friedman (1942) into a medial ganglionic type, which is usually fatal, and a lateral ganglionic type, which the patient may survive. The medial ganglionic type arises medial to the putamen and usually destroys the hypothalamus and ruptures into the ventricle. Haemorrhages of lateral ganglionic type arise in the putamen, external capsule or claustrum. In some cases the haemorrhage remains relatively localised to the putamen; in other cases it extends posteriorly into the white matter of the occipital lobe.

Massive hypertensive haemorrhage into the cerebellum, or into the pons and midbrain, is almost invariably and rapidly fatal.

Examination of the brain, soon after a massive haemorrhage, reveals clot which is soft and like red currant jelly. When such a clot is removed, the walls of the cavity are ragged. Small vessels can often be found projecting into the cavity and, in these vessels, necrosis of the wall and thrombosis of the lumen are often present. Around the main haemorrhage, numerous petechial haemorrhages are visible in the adjacent grey matter, and in the white matter which is soft, swollen and oedematous. On microscopical examination there is ischaemic necrosis of variable extent in the nervous tissue which forms the wall of the cavity; many of the small vessels which are present have necrotic walls; and the petechial haemorrhages, which are principally of ring and ball type, are around capillaries. These changes at the periphery of a recent haemorrhage appear to have occurred at, or about, the time of the massive haemorrhage. If the patient does not die as a result of the haemorrhage, the blood clot becomes inspissated and turns reddish-brown in colour. Reactionary changes occur in the surrounding tissue, with phagocytosis of haemosiderin and of necrotic cerebral tissue. Astrocytes become swollen, increase in numbers and lay down astrocytic fibres. The amount of nervous tissue which is destroyed is not as much as one might perhaps expect. Massive cerebral haemorrhage has a tendency to track along tissue planes, separating rather than destroying the nervous substance. In this way it differs from a haemorrhagic infarct, due to obstruction of an artery, in which nearly all the tissue within the distribution of the artery undergoes necrosis. This anatomical difference is helpful in deciding whether a lesion, especially an old lesion, was a haemorrhage or a haemorrhagic infarct.

Pathogenesis of hypertensive cerebral haemorrhage

This subject, upon which discussion will probably never cease, has been reviewed by Bouman (1931), Stern (1938) and Globus and Epstein (1952) and considered by Byrom (1954).

The causative abnormality must, presumably, be present in relation to one or more of (1) the circulating blood, (2) the vessel wall, (3) the surrounding parenchyma.

(1) *The circulating blood.* There is no doubt that the arterial and arteriolar blood is at an abnormally high systolic and diastolic pressure. This force will take advantage of any weakness of the vessel wall and find a way out. It should also be remembered that the blood pressure does not remain constantly high, but varies; and may therefore, at times, fall below the level necessary to drive it through organically narrowed arteries and arterioles into the capillary field beyond. In this way there may be periods of ischaemia of the tissue supplied by these vessels and of the walls of the vessels themselves.

(2) *The vessel wall.* Here there may be spasm. At the site of the spasm the vessel wall may become necrotic and weak. Haemorrhage is inevitable if the spasm relaxes and the blood, under high pressure, runs back into a devitalised or necrotic channel.

Structural change in arteries and arterioles is commonly found in the brains of hypertensive patients. In the small arteries there often are changes identical with atherosclerosis, with loss of muscle from the media. Cerebral arteries are weaker than most other arteries in that the amount of medial muscle is slight, there is no external elastic lamina, and but little adventitia. With a damaged internal elastic lamina and little muscle remaining in the media, the artery may be unable to contain the hypertensive blood and haemorrhage may occur, first into the Virchow-Robin space to form a miliary aneurysm (Green 1930) and later into the cerebral tissue. The blood may pass through the wall in the form, at first, of a dissecting aneurysm (Shennan 1915). Alternatively it is possible that the haemorrhage may commence at arteriolar level, for the arteriolar walls are frequently degenerate.

(3) *The surrounding tissue.* As a result of one of the abnormalities already mentioned, or possibly due to a hypothetical circulating toxin, originating from the damaged kidneys, the tissue around a small artery or arteriole degenerates. Foci of perivascular degeneration are undoubtedly a common finding and in cases with atherosclerosis there may be 'état lacunaire' (see p. 111). It is suggested that this entails a lack of normal support for the vessel, which therefore ruptures.

It should be remembered that the same factor or factors may not operate in each case. In a young person, with relatively healthy vessels and rapidly developing severe hypertension, the factor of spasm, if it exists, is likely to be important. In an old person, with long continued hypertension and degenerate vessels, the factor of spasm would be less important.

Changes in the brain in hypertensive encephalopathy

Very rarely, in persons with hypertension due to acute glomerulonephritis, toxaemia of pregnancy or acute lead poisoning, and less often in persons with hypertension due to other causes, there occur attacks of sudden increase of blood pressure, severe headache, impairment of consciousness, convulsions and sometimes focal neurological signs such as hemiplegia, aphasia and blindness. Uraemia is not present. To this clinical entity Oppenheimer and Fishberg (1928) gave the name 'hypertensive encephalopathy'. At post-mortem they found the brain pale, usually almost bloodless. Some brains were oedematous, in others there was no evidence of oedema and they were unusually dry. They did not see any focal lesions, but they do not state whether they examined the brains microscopically.

In patients with long-standing essential hypertension who suffered from attacks of the above nature Adams and Vander Eecken (1953) found the parenchymal and vascular changes, already described in a previous section, which are to be expected in any person with severe hypertension. In addition they found diffuse, but uneven, swelling or oedema of the brain in association with petechial haemorrhages, perivascular exudates and small multiple infarcts in the grey matter.

Clinically, attacks of hypertensive encephalopathy are preceded by an acute rise of blood pressure. Byrom (1954), whose experiments were expressly designed to elucidate the pathogenesis of hypertensive encephalopathy, considers that this sudden additional rise of blood pressure results in focal arterial spasm, with anoxic damage to neurones, and to the capillary walls. The patient may die from the neuronal anoxia before oedema is present to any appreciable amount. Thus the brain at post-mortem may, or may not, appear oedematous and swollen, but will certainly appear pale and bloodless.

Chronic progressive subcortical encephalitis of Binswanger

Described by Binswanger in 1894, this is a very rare type of involvement of the brain in hypertensive vascular disease. Very few cases have been published, the most recent being those of Farnell and Globus (1932) and Davison (1942).

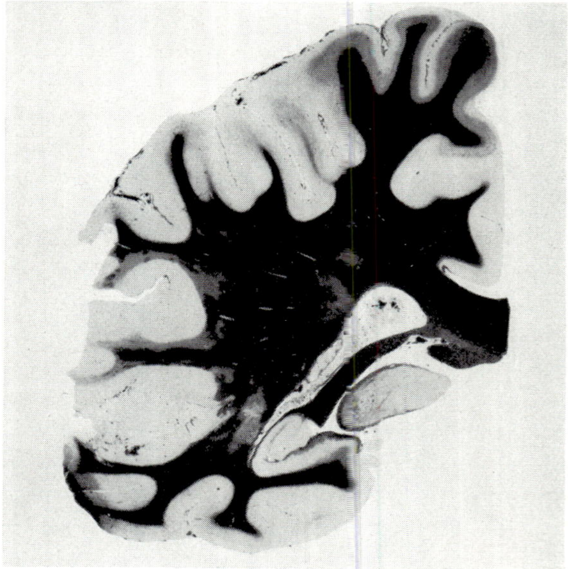

FIG. 2.63. Multiple, often clearly demarcated, foci of myelin destruction in the white matter of a hypertensive patient, of the type seen in Binswanger's subcortical encephalopathy. (Celloidin, Loyez.)

It is found from the age of 50 onwards and affects the cerebrum. The cortex and the subcortical arcuate fibres are intact, or almost intact, but the deep white matter is reduced in amount.

According to Binswanger the disease process is most severe in the occipital and temporal lobes. The condition may be confined to the white matter of one convolution or may affect several convolutions (Fig. 2.63). In severe cases the white matter of whole lobes of the cerebrum is almost completely atrophied, so that there is, in places, very little white matter left. In such cases the temporal and occipital horns of the lateral ventricles will be enormously dilated. In his cases the white matter of the frontal lobes was not significantly affected.

Some of the regions of myelin destruction are sharply delimited, like plaques of disseminated sclerosis; some are less well defined. Where myelin is no longer present there are fat granule cells and proliferated astrocytes and their fibres. The arterioles of the white matter are the site of narrowing, fibrous thickening, and hyaline change, such as is found in hypertension. The arteries of the circle of Willis show atherosclerosis.

ANEURYSM

The word aneurysm means a dilatation of an artery. In relation to the central nervous system we are concerned with:

(1) Congenital saccular aneurysms.
(2) Mycotic aneurysms.
(3) Atherosclerotic fusiform aneurysms.
(4) Spontaneous and post-traumatic arteriovenous aneurysms between the internal carotid artery and the cavernous sinus.
(5) Dissecting aneurysms.

Congenital saccular aneurysms

Frequency. In the large pre-surgical series, discussed by Fearnsides (1916) and corrected by Turnbull (1918), the incidence of congenital intracranial aneurysm was 0·64 per cent (29 persons with 33 aneurysms in 4,547 post-mortem examinations of the head at the London Hospital 1908–13). The extra number of aneurysms is accounted for by 3 persons having, 2, 2 and 3 aneurysms respectively, giving an incidence of multiple aneurysms of 11 per cent. Bigelow (1955) found multiple saccular aneurysms in 16 per cent of his cases. Multiple saccular aneurysms of congenital type are also found upon the cerebral arteries in association with arteriovenous angiomata. In one such case death was due to rupture of an aneurysm (Brihaye and Blackwood 1957).

Age. Although aneurysms have been recorded at the extremes of life, they most commonly cause death during the 5th decade (Carmichael 1950). Of those which give rise to clinical symptoms about half are found after the age of 40 (Meadows 1951). They are not markedly more frequent in either sex (Dandy 1944).

Site. Almost all saccular aneurysms arise at, or very close to, the points of division of arteries (Carmichael 1950). The commonest site is on the middle cerebral artery at its first or second point of branching in the Sylvian fissure (about 30 per cent): the next most common is at the junction of an anterior cerebral and an anterior communicating artery (about 25 per cent): next the junction of the terminal portion of the internal carotid artery and its branches (the middle and anterior cerebral and the posterior communicating) is involved in about 20 per cent of cases. The basilar artery and its branches account for about 12–15 per cent and other arteries (vertebral, posterior cerebral, posterior communicating) for about 12 per cent. Aneurysms are not appreciably more common either on the left or the right side (Dandy 1944).

Naked eye findings. Saccular aneurysms may vary in size from smaller than a pin's head to 30 mm. in diameter, but, as Fearnsides (1916) records, the commonest size is that of a pea.

At post-mortem it is occasionally difficult to find the aneurysm, either because of its small size or because, in rupturing, it has disintegrated.*

Initially the sac lies in the subarachnoid space, but with enlargement and possible leakages the major portion of the sac may be buried in the substance of the brain, or a portion of the sac may protrude through the arachnoid into the subdural space. The blood vessels of the circle of Willis may be generally atheromatous, but sometimes almost the only yellowish thickening

* We recommend an initial careful dissection of the common sites in the unfixed specimen, because after fixation it is more difficult to push away any blood clot which may be present. If this fails to reveal the aneurysm then examine the less common sites; or fix the brain, dissect out the basal vessels and examine all junctional points.

of the vessels is to be seen close to the neck of the aneurysm. The wall of the aneurysm is usually thin and is composed of fibrous tissue. In larger aneurysms the sac is often partly filled with laminated, organised and organising blood clot. Embolism of the arteries distal to the aneurysm, by fragments of the clot which form in it, is very rare or perhaps unknown. Calcification may be present. Brownish pigmentation, fibrous thickening and adhesions of surrounding tissues are signs of old leakage. Occasionally at post-mortem one finds a small aneurysm filled with old pale fibrous tissue: it appears to be healed.

Aneurysms often rupture, usually near the fundus of the sac.

The blood from a ruptured saccular aneurysm may pass:

(1) Into the subarachnoid space (Fig. 2.64).

(2) Into the overlying brain, sometimes forming a false aneurysm, but more often ploughing through the substance of the brain to enter and fill the ventricular system (Figs. 2.65, 2.66 and 2.67). Richardson and Hyland (1941) emphasised the frequency of intracerebral haemorrhage (19 out of their 27 cases of ruptured aneurysm). They noted the two common sites, frontal and temporal, from aneurysms in the region of the anterior communicating artery, or at the carotid bifurcation, or on the middle cerebral artery in the Sylvian fissure.

(3) Much less commonly, into the subdural space.

Distortion, compression and destruction of neighbouring cranial nerves and brain substance may be produced by the sac and by haemorrhage which is not sufficient to cause death. Rupture of an aneurysm is not invariably fatal. In Fearnsides' (1916) series 18 out of 31 cases (58 per cent) died after the first rupture. The other 13 cases gave a history of previous seizures indicating repeated serious bleeding. Of these 1 had five seizures, 1 had four, 6 had three seizures and 5 had two seizures before death.

The mortality and morbidity of cases of ruptured congenital saccular aneurysms, which have not been treated surgically, have been investigated by Hyland (1950) and by Walton (1956). After considering the literature and his own cases of subarachnoid haemorrhage (80 per cent of which he considers to be from aneurysms), Walton's conclusions may be summarised as follows. Of 100 persons who come into hospital with ruptured intracranial aneurysms, 45 will die during the next 8 weeks, 55 will survive this period. Of the 45 who die, 28 will die from the initial haemorrhage (12 within 24 hours, 16 between the 3rd and 14th days); 17 will die from a recurrence of the haemorrhage. Of the 55 who survive the first 8 weeks, 5 will die of a recurrent haemorrhage within the next 6 months, 7 will die for the same reason at a later date (in several cases the follow up was as long as 12 years). Of the remaining 43, one-third will be more or less disabled by residual paralysis, epilepsy, headache or mental symptoms; one-third will suffer from relatively trivial symptoms, and one-third will recover completely.

Microscopical findings. At the neck of the sac the muscle of the media of the artery comes to an abrupt end. At about the same point the internal elastic membrane shows degenerative changes, which appear to be due to the implication of the elastica in an ordinary atheromatous process. The degenerate elastic membrane usually passes only a short distance into the sac, the wall of which is formed of fibrous tissue continuous with the intima and adventitia of the artery. Part of the fibrous wall may be degenerate. In cases where there has been previous leakage, phagocytes filled with haemosiderin, small round celled infiltration and fibrous thickening are present around thesac.

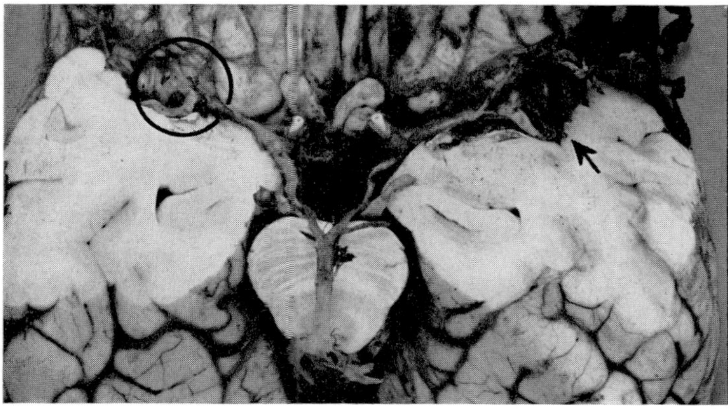

2.64

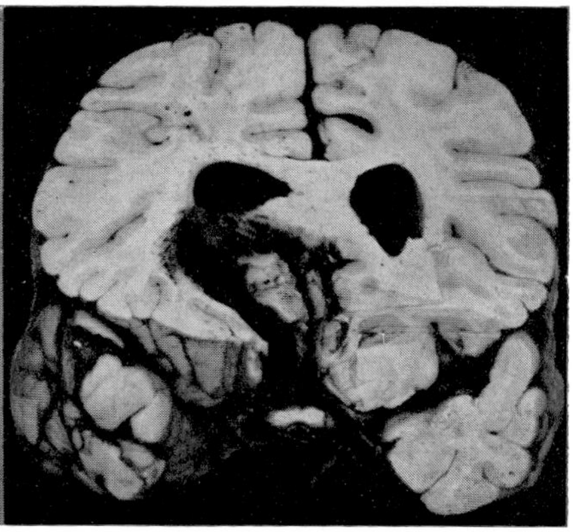

2.65

FIG. 2.64. Ruptured congenital saccular aneurysm of the left middle cerebral artery (arrow). The blood had passed into the subarachnoid space of the insula and of the basal cisterns (from which it was partly removed to display the aneurysm). The aneurysm arose from the point of branching of the artery in the Sylvian fissure. The corresponding point of branching on the right middle cerebral artery is ringed.

FIG. 2.65. Ruptured congenital saccular aneurysm of the right anterior cerebral/anterior communicating artery. The blood has ploughed through the substance of the frontal lobe into the lateral ventricle.

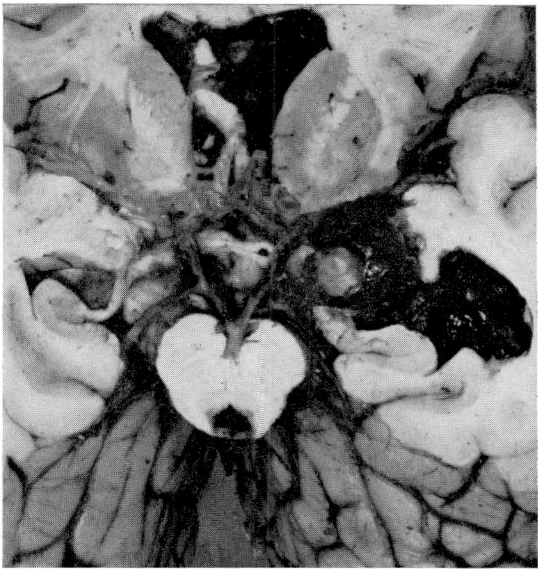

2.66

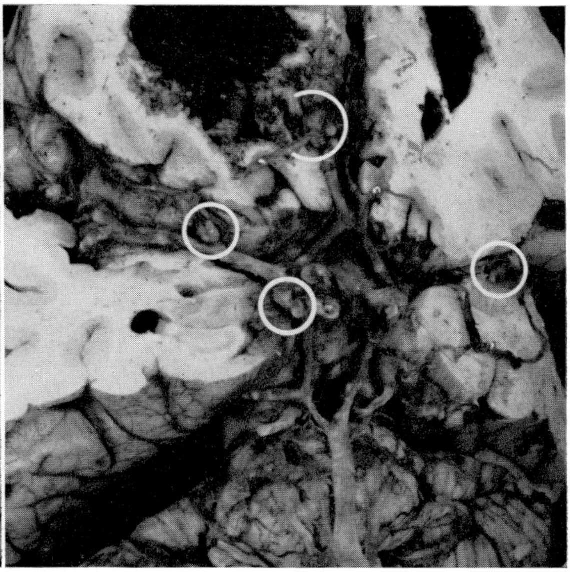

2.67

FIG. 2.66. Ruptured congenital saccular aneurysm of the left internal carotid/posterior communicating artery. The blood has passed laterally through the choroidal fissure into the left lateral ventricle. A lesser amount of blood was present in the right lateral ventricle. The 3rd ventricle, the aqueduct and the 4th ventricle were full of blood.

FIG. 2.67. Base of the brain in a patient with multiple congenital saccular aneurysms (ringed). An aneurysm on the right anterior cerebral artery has bled into the substance of the right frontal lobe and into the lateral ventricle.

Pathogenesis. There is general agreement that the chief aetiological factor in the development of these aneurysms is aplasia or hypoplasia of the muscle coat at the point of branching or junction of the arteries. Such developmental defects are not confined to cerebral arteries but are also present in coronary, mesenteric and pulmonary arteries (Forbus 1930). In the circle of Willis, Glynn (1940) found such defects at 80 per cent of bifurcations, both in cases with cerebral aneurysms and in normal controls. The probable reason for the defect is the way in which the medial coat of an artery and its branches develops. It does not grow in continuity, like the bark of a tree, but develops from separate islands of mesenchyme, which subsequently fuse at the points of junction or branching of permanent vessels or of temporary embryonic vessels which are subsequently absorbed (Padget 1944). If fusion is imperfect then, at these points, the arterial wall is composed only of endothelium, the internal elastic lamina, and a small amount of fibrous tissue: for cerebral arteries have no external elastic lamina and only a rudimentary adventitia.

In the majority of people this thin portion of wall is adequate. In a few people, however, there is evidence that this region is further weakened by degeneration of the elastica. This degeneration is almost invariably associated with appearances indistinguishable from atheroma. Without the support of the elastica, the endothelium and the fibrous tissue yield before the pressure of the blood and an aneurysm is formed (Carmichael 1950).

Other causative factors have from time to time been suggested. Of these hypertension cannot be proved. It may, indeed it must, aggravate the lesion, but, as Fearnsides did not find cardiac hypertrophy in 15 out of his 31 cases, it cannot be considered to be an essential causative factor. Nor should syphilis be considered as other than a most exceptional cause. Turnbull (1918) stated that he had never seen a saccular aneurysm which appeared to be due to syphilis.

Mycotic aneurysm

A mycotic aneurysm forms when the wall of an artery is weakened from within by pyogenic bacteria. The bacteria usually reach the affected portion of the wall in an infected embolus. The commonest source of such emboli are the aortic heart valves in endocarditis, particularly of subacute bacterial type. Less commonly pulmonary suppuration or pyaemia may be the origin. The organisms are usually of low or attenuated virulence; those of high virulence cause leptomeningitis or cerebral abscess. The aneurysms are usually found on the branches of the middle cerebral artery, especially in the lateral fissure (Stengel and Wolferth 1923). Sometimes they are peripherally situated in the distribution of this artery and are multiple.

The embolus becomes adherent to the wall, which shows the usual histological changes of an acute inflammatory process. When the elastica and the media are sufficiently damaged, the wall of the artery shows a localised dilatation, which may progress to rupture and haemorrhage into the subarachnoid space or into the nervous tissue. Mycotic aneurysms are usually small because the process is a relatively rapid one. These aneurysms rarely heal, but with modern anti-biotic therapy this is to be anticipated. Since the aneurysm usually arises from the lodgement of an embolus there will be a varying amount of ischaemic necrosis of nervous tissue in the field of distribution of the artery.

Atherosclerotic fusiform aneurysms of the basilar artery and aneurysms of the intracavernous portion of the internal carotid artery

Fusiform dilatation of the basilar or internal carotid artery is a not uncommon finding in patients with severe atherosclerosis. The elastica and muscularis of the vessel are damaged by the atherosclerotic process and the vessel dilates. The *basilar artery* is often elongated as well as dilated and has a sinuous course. Neighbouring structures are seldom damaged. The dilatation of the *internal carotid artery*, which usually affects both arteries, may be more serious, especially in its intracavernous portion where it is closely related to important structures.

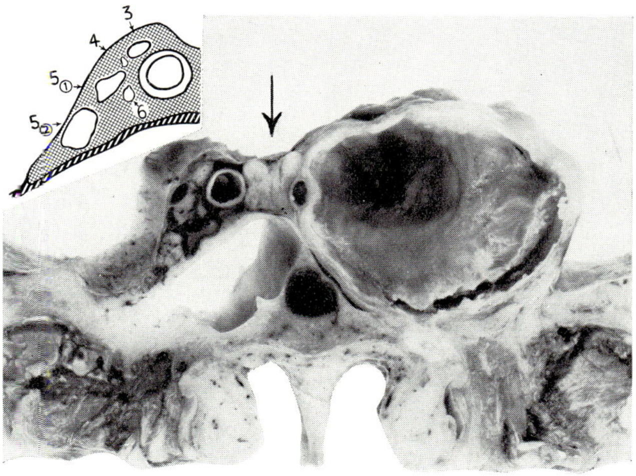

FIG. 2.68. Coronal section of the skull of a patient with an intracavernous saccular aneurysm of the right internal carotid artery. The section passes through the pituitary gland (arrow). On the left of the pituitary can be seen the normal internal carotid artery, the cavernous sinus, and the 3rd, 4th, two divisions of the 5th, and the 6th cranial nerves (see diagram). On the right of the pituitary is the large, partly thrombosed, sac of the aneurysm. The wall of the internal carotid artery is complete at this level, the neck of sac lay further forward. Blood, which had leaked from the aneurysm into the right sphenoidal air sinus, is visible below and medial to the sac of the aneurysm.

Aneurysms in this situation may be either of fusiform shape and associated with atheroma, or of saccular shape (Fig. 2.68), associated with atheroma but presumably developing upon the basis of a congenital saccular aneurysm. Since the ill effects of both types are essentially similar they are considered together. As the aneurysm enlarges it may damage the adjacent 3rd, 4th, 5th and 6th cranial nerves, elevate the dura on the lateral aspect of the cavernous sinus, enlarge the sphenoidal fissure and erode the anterior clinoid process and the lateral portions of the sella turcica (Jefferson 1937 and 1938, Bull and Rischbeith 1957). It may enter the sphenoidal air sinus and bleed into it, producing epistaxis. Thrombosis and calcification occur in these aneurysms: rupture is rare.

Carotid-cavernous sinus aneurysm

As it lies within the cavernous sinus the internal carotid artery is surrounded by venous blood. Any breach in the continuity of the artery will result in an arteriovenous aneurysm. This is usually secondary to mechanical trauma, but less commonly it develops spontaneously, with an unexplained predilection for middle-aged women. Some of these spontaneous cases are secondary to rupture of a congenital saccular aneurysm of the internal carotid artery (Dandy and Follis 1941). Some are secondary to atherosclerotic degeneration of the artery. The consequence of such an arteriovenous communication, here as elsewhere, is a rise in the blood pressure in the venous tributaries of the sinus, with dilatation and tortuosity of the veins and the development of a pulsating exophthalmos. The alteration of the flow of the blood produces a murmur. Secondary enlargement of the heart was not present in Dandy's (1937) 8 cases. Histological descriptions are few, but thrombosis within the aneurysm may occur and is the probable cause of the spontaneous cure which occasionally happens.

Dissecting aneurysms

Dissecting aneurysms of cerebral arteries are rare. Wolman in 1959 found 14 cases in the literature and added 3 of his own. Subsequently a case has been reported by Scott *et al.* (1960). Males were involved only slightly more often than females, ages ranged from birth to 47 years (more frequent in the 4th and 5th decades). The middle cerebral artery was most commonly involved (10 cases), then the basilar artery (5 cases). The plane of dissection has been sub-

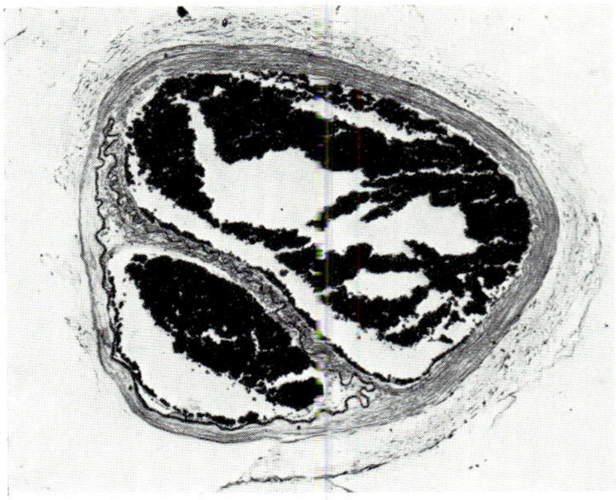

FIG. 2.69. Branch of the right middle cerebral artery, showing blood in the original lumen (with an elastic lamina) and in the false lumen. Verhoeff's elastic stain. (Drs. Norman and Urich's case.)

intimal, splitting the internal elastic lamina and separating it from the media. The cause of the dissection has been ascribed to trauma (3 cases), syphilitic arteritis (2 cases) and to a congenital defect of the media (in Wolman's 3 cases), similar to that considered to be associated with saccular aneurysms. Norman and Urich (1957) were unable to find any indication of the cause, in spite of serial sectioning of the affected vessel, in their case (Fig. 2.69), which was unusual in that death did not occur within a few days of the sudden onset of the illness but about 14 years later.

Neurological complications of the adult type of coarctation of the aorta

In this condition the aorta is narrowed, or occluded, distal to the left subclavian artery, at or just below the aortic insertion of the ductus arteriosus, which is almost always obliterated. The blood pressure in the arteries of the upper part of the body is raised. In the combined figures of Abbott (1928) and Reifenstein *et al.* (1947), which cover 304 cases of the adult type of coarctation, death was due clinically to intracranial haemorrhage in 12 per cent of cases, a diagnosis which was confirmed *post mortem* in 29 of the 36 cases. In 10 cases a ruptured saccular aneurysm of the circle of Willis was found. In the opinion of the authors rupture of an aneurysm, histologically of the type described later as a congenital saccular aneurysm, is the principal cause of intracranial haemorrhage in this condition.

In coarctation the aortic obstruction prevents the arterial blood from reaching the lower

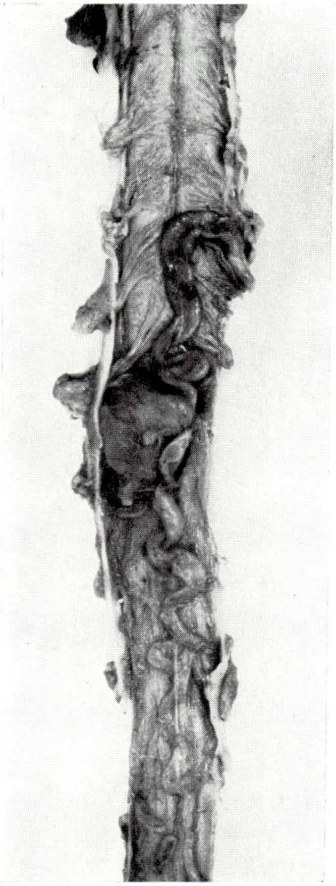

FIG. 2.70. *Coarctation of the aorta.* Ventral aspect of the spinal cord of a girl who, when aged 14, had transient headache and twitching of the legs followed 5 days later by weakness of the right leg. Gradual complete recovery. Aged 16 onset of progressive motor and sensory loss to level of the nipple line. Aged 18 died after negative exploratory laminectomy. Post-mortem, left sided cardiac hypertrophy and coarctation of aorta. The cranial portion of the anterior spinal artery was slightly larger than normal. At C.5, on the left, a dilated and thick walled radicular artery joined the anterior spinal artery. At Th.1 there was a rounded thick walled aneurysmal sac lying partly within and partly anterior to the thin orange-coloured substance of the spinal cord. This sac lay posterolateral to the tortuous dilated anterior spinal artery, with which it communicated through a small aperture in the wall of the artery. It appeared that the aneurysm was a false aneurysm, which had formed as the result of haemorrhage from the tortuous anterior spinal artery. At Th.3 the anterior spinal artery divided into two, one branch passing laterally as an anterior radicular artery on the left side and the other branch continuing onwards for a few more segments until it too joined a radicular artery.

part of the body by the usual route. An anastomotic circulation develops which includes the anterior spinal artery. The blood passes from the heart to the subclavian arteries, via the vertebral arteries into the cranial end of the anterior spinal artery, and via the ascending cervical branches of the inferior thryoid arteries and the branches of the thyreo-cervical trunks into the upper radicular tributaries of the anterior spinal artery. The blood then by-passes the aortic obstruction by flowing down the anterior spinal artery to reach the spinal branches of the aortic intercostals below the obstruction. In such cases the anterior spinal artery becomes enlarged and tortuous, a feature well illustrated by Edwards *et al.* (1948).

This change in the anterior spinal artery does not usually cause any clinical ill effects. Haberer (1903) however found, in a woman of 47 who died 4 months after the sudden onset of a transverse myelitis, that the spinal cord at Th.2 was compressed and necrotic. This he considered to be a compression myelitis secondary to pronounced dilatation and tortuosity of the anterior spinal artery at this level. Greenfield had a case (unpublished) in which there was a saccular false aneurysm of the anterior spinal artery at Th.1 (Fig. 2.70). In each of these cases the anterior spinal artery became markedly dilated and tortuous immediately inferior to the point of entry of an enlarged lower cervical radicular artery, of which indeed the anterior spinal artery appeared to be the continuation.

REFERENCES

Abbie, A. A. (1933) *Brain*, **56**, 233; (1934) *J. Anat.*, Lond., **68**, 433.
Abbott, M. E. (1928) *Amer. Heart J.*, **3**, 574.
Adams, R. D. (1943) *Arch. Neurol. Psychiat.* (Chicago), **49**, 765.
Adams, R. D., Cammermeyer, J. and FitzGerald, P. J. (1948) *J. Neurol. Neurosurg. Psychiat.*, **11**, 27.
Adams, R. D. and Michelson J. J. (1952) *Proc. 1st Internat. Cong. Neuropath.*, Rome, **1**, 347.
Adams, R. D. and Vander Eecken, H. M. (1953) *Annu. Rev. Med.*, **4**, 213.
Allison, R. S. and Morison, J.E. (1941) *J. Neurol. Psychiat.*, **4**, 1.
Antoni, N. (1952) *Proc. 1st Internat. Cong. Neuropath.*, Rome, **3**, 557.
Arkin, A. (1930) *Amer. J. Path.*, **6**, 401.
Atkinson, W. J. (1949) *J. Neurol. Neurosurg. Psychiat.*, **12**, 137.
Bailey, O. T. and Hass, G. M. (1937) *Brain*, **60**, 293.
Baker, A. B. (1937) *Amer. J. Path.*, **13**, 453; (1941) ibid., **17**, 39.
Barnett, H. J. M. and Hyland, H. H. (1953) *Brain*, **76**, 36.
Batson, O. V. (1940) *Ann. Surg.*, **112**, 138.
Beevor, C. E. (1908) *Phil. Tran. Roy. Soc.*, Series B., **200**, 1.
Bertrand, I. (1923) *Les processus de désintégration nerveuse*, Masson et Cie, Paris.
Bertrand, C. (1952) *J. Neuropath. exp. Neurol.*, **11**, 53.
Biemond, A. (1951) *Brain*, **74**, 300.
Bigelow, N. H. (1955) *Arch. Neurol. Psychiat.* (Chicago), **73**, 76.
Binswanger, O. (1894) *Berl. klin. Wschr.*, **31**, 1187.
Blackwood, W. and Dott, N. M. (1952) Personal communication to Society of British Neurological Surgeons and the Association of British Neurologists.
Bolton, B. (1939) *J. Neurol. Psychiat.*, **2**, 137.
Bouman, L. (1931) *Arch. Neurol. Psychiat.* (Chicago), **25**, 255.
Brain, W. R. and Russell, D. S. (1937) *Proc. Roy. Soc. Med.*, **30**, 1024.
Brihaye, J. and Blackwood, W. (1957) *J. Path. Bact.*, **73**, 17.
Bruetsch, W. L. (1942) *Trans. Amer. neurol. Ass.*, **68**, 17; (1949) *Proc. Cong. Neurol. Internat.*, Massol et Cie, Paris, **3**, 297.
Buchanan, D. N., Walker, A. E. and Case, T. J. (1942) *J. Pediat.*, **20**, 555
Bull, J. W. D. and Rischbeith, R. (1957) *Brit. J. Radiol.* (N.S.), in press.
Byrom, F. B. (1954) *Lancet*, **ii**, 201.
Carmichael, E. A., Dix, M. R. and Hallpike, C. S. (1956) *Brit. med. Bull.*, **12**, 146.
Carmichael, R. (1950) *J. Path. Bact.*, **62**, 1.
Charcot, J. M. and Bouchard, C. (1890) *Œuvres complétes de Charcot*, **9**, 3 and 21, Paris.
Chiari, H. (1905) *Verh. dtsch. path. Ges.*, **9**, 326.
Cone, W. and Barrera, S. E. (1931) *Arch. Neurol. Psychiat.* (Chicago), **25**, 523.
Corday, E., Rothenberg, S. F. and Putnam, T. J. (1953) *Arch. Neurol. Psychiat.* (Chicago), **69**, 551.
Costero, I. (1949) *Arch. Neurol. Psychiat.* (Chicago), **62**, 48.
Courville, C. B. (1950) *Pathology of the Central Nervous System*, 3rd edition, Pacific Press Publishing Association, Mountain View, California.
Courville, C. B. and Friedman, A. P. (1942) *Bull. Los Angeles neurol. Soc.*, **7**, 137.
Crawford, J. V. and Russell, D. S. (1956) *J. Neurol. Neurosurg. Psychiat.*, **19**, 1.
Critchley, M. (1930) *Brain*, **53**, 120.
Critchley, M. and Schuster, P. (1933) *Z. ges. Neurol. Psychiat.*, **144**, 681.
Crompton, M. R. (1959) *Brain*, **82**, 377.
Cumings, J. N. (1961) *IVth Internat. Cong. Neuropath. Munich*, **1**, 157.
Dandy, W. E. (1937) *Zbl. Neurochir.*, **2**, 77; (1944) *Intracranial arterial aneurysms*, Comstock Publishing Co., Ithaca, New York.
Dandy, W. E. and Follis, R. H., Jr. (1941) *Amer. J. Ophthal.*, **24**, 365.
Davison, C. (1937) *Arch. Neurol. Psychiat.* (Chicago), **37**, 91; (1942) *J. Neuropath. exp. Neurol.*, **1**, 42; (1944) ibid., **3**, 73.
Davison, C., Goodhart, S. P. and Savitsky, N. (1935) *Arch. Neurol. Psychiat.* (Chicago), **33**, 1143.
Denny-Brown, D. (1951) *Med. Clin. N. Amer.*, **35**, 1457; (1960) *Arch. Neurol. Psychiat.* (Chicago), **2**, 194.
Denny-Brown, D., Horenstein, S. and Fang, H. C. H. (1956) *J. Neuropath. exp. Neurol.*, **15**, 146.

Duguid, J. B. (1948) *J. Path. Bact.*, **60**, 57.
Earle, K. M., Baldwin, M. and Penfield, W. (1953) *Arch. Neurol. Psychiat.* (Chicago), **69**, 27.
Edwards, J. E., Clagett, O. T., Drake, R. L. and Christensen, N. A. (1948) *Proc. Mayo Clin.*, **23**, 333.
Ehlers, H. and Courville, C. B. (1936) *J. Pediat.*, **8**, 600.
Eicke, W. J. (1957) in *Handbuch der speziellen pathologischen Anatomie und Histologie. Lubarsch, O., Henke, F. and Rössle, R.*, Springer, Berlin, **13** *part* 1, *B*, 1536.
Farnell, F. J. and Globus, J. H. (1932) *Arch. Neurol. Psychiat.* (Chicago), **27**, 593.
Fearnsides, E. G. (1916) *Brain*, **39**, 224.
Fisher, C. M., Karnes, W. E. and Kubik, C. S. (1961) *J. Neuropath. exp. Neurol.*, **20**, 323.
Fisher, C. M. (1959) *Neurology*, **9**, 333.
Fisher, M. and Adams, R. D. (1951) *J. Neuropath. exp. Neurol.*, **10**, 92.
Foix, C. and Alajouanine, T. (1926) *Rev. neurol.* (ii), 1.
Foix, C. and Hillemand, P. (1926) *Rev. de Médecine*, **43**, 287.
Foix, C., Hillemand, P. and Schalit, I. (1925) *Rev. neurol.* (i), 160.
Foix, C. and Levy, M. (1927) *Rev. neurol.* (ii), 1.
Foix, C. and Masson, A. (1923) *Pr. méd.*, **31**, 361.
Foley, J. (1955) *Brain*, **78**, 1.
Forbus, W. D. (1930) *Johns Hopk. Hosp. Bull.*, **47**, 239.
Foster, D. B. and Malamud, N. (1941) *Univ. Hosp. Bull. Mich.*, **7**, 102.
Freeman, W. and Jaffe, D. (1941) *Arch. Neurol. Psychiat.* (Chicago), **46**, 115.
Frøvig, A. G. (1946) *Acta psychiat.*, Kbn., Suppl. 39.
Fullerton, H. W. (1955) *Proc. Roy. Soc. Med.*, **48**, 664.
von Glahn, W. C. and Pappenheimer, A. M. (1926) *Amer. J. Path.*, **2**, 235.
Globus, J. H. and Epstein, J. A. (1952) *Proc. 1st Internat. Cong. Neuropath.*, **1**, 289.
Glynn, L. E. (1940) *J. Path. Bact.*, **51**, 213.
Goodhart, S. P. and Davison, C. (1936) *Arch. Neurol. Psychiat.* (Chicago), **35**, 501.
Gowers, W. R. (1893) *Diseases of the Nervous System*, 2nd edition, **2**, 436, Churchill, London.
Green, F. H. K. (1930) *J. Path. Bact.*, **33**, 71.
Greenfield, J. G. (1939) *Brain*, **62**, 129.
Greenfield, J. G., Rickards, A. G. and Manning, G. B. (1955) *J. Path. Bact.*, **69**, 95.
Greenfield, J. G. and Turner, J. W. A. (1939) *Brain*, **62**, 227.
Greenfield, J. G. and Wolfsohn, J. M. (1922) *Lancet* (ii), 603.
Grinker, R. R. and Guy, C. C. (1927) *J. Amer. med. Ass.*, **88**, 1140
Gruber, G. B. (1926) *Zbl. f. Herz. u. Gefasskr.*, **18**, 185.
Guillain, G., Bertrand, I. and Peron, N. (1928) *Rev. neurol.* (ii), 835.
Gull, W. W. and Sutton, H. G. (1872) *Med.-chir. Trans.*, **55**, 273
Haberer, H. (1903) *Z. Heilk.*, **24**, 26.
Hamilton, C. E. and Rothstein, E. (1935) *J. Amer. med. Ass.*, **104**, 2226.
Harrison, C. V. (1948) *J. clin. Path.*, **1**, 197.
Haymaker, W. (1957) in *Handbuch der speziellen pathologischen Anatomie und Histologie. Lubarsch, O., Henke F. and Rössle, R.*, Springer, Berlin, **13**, *part* 1*B*, 1600.
Heptinstall, R. H., Porter, K. A. and Barkley, H. (1954) *J. Path. Bact.*, **67**, 507.
Hiller, F. (1936) in Bumke u. Foerster *Handbuch der Neurologie*, **11**, 328, Springer, Berlin.
Holmes, G. (1915) *Brit. med. J.* (ii), 769.
Holmes, G. (1934) *Jb. Psychiat. Neurol.*, **51**, 39.
Hultquist, G. T. (1942) *Uber Thrombose und Embolie der Arteria Carotid und hierbei Vorkommende Gehirnveranderungen*, Fischer Jena, Stockholm.
Hunt, J. R. (1914) *Amer. J. med. Sci.*, **147**, 704.
Hurst, E. W. (1955) *J. Path. Bact.*, **70**, 167.
Hutchinson, E. C. and Yates, P. O. (1956) *Brain*, **79**, 319; (1957) *Lancet* (i), 2; (1961) *Spec. Rep. Ser. med. Res. Coun., Lond., No.* 300.
Hyland, H. H. (1950) *Arch. Neurol. Psychiat.* (Chicago), **63**, 61.
Jaburek, L. (1936) *Arch. Psychiat. Nervenkr.*, **104**, 518.
Jäger, E. (1932) *Virchows Arch.*, **284**, 526.
Jefferson, A. (1955) *Quart. J. Med.*, **24**, 245.
Jefferson, G. (1937) *Brain*, **60**, 444; (1938) *Brit. J. Surg.*, **26**, 267; (1938) *Arch. Neurol. Psychiat.* (Chicago), **40**, 857.
Johnson, R. T. and Yates, P. O. (1956) *Acta radiol. Stockh.*, **46**, 250.

Jones, E. (1910) *Quart. J. Med.*, **3**, 233.
Kalischer, O. (1914) *Berl. klin. Wschr.*, **51**, 1286.
Kernohan, J. W. (1942) *Trans. Amer. neurol. Ass.*, **68**, 18.
Kernohan, J. W. and Woltman, H. W. (1929) *Arch. Neurol. Psychiat.* (Chicago), **21**, 274.
Kernohan, J. W. and Woltman, H. W. (1938) *Arch. Neurol. Psychiat.*, (Chicago), **39**, 655.
Kiloh, L. G. (1953) *Post grad. med. J.*, **29**, 65 and 119.
Klatzo, I., Piraux, A. and Laskowski, E. J. (1960) *J. Neuropath. exp. Neurol.*, **17**, 548.
Kubik, C. S. and Adams, R. D. (1946) *Brain*, **69**, 73.
Levine, B., Cheskin, L. J. and Applebaum, I. L. (1949) *Arch. intern. Med.*, **84**, 431.
Lhermitte, J. and Barrelet (1934) *Rev. neurol.* (ii), 851.
Lhermitte, J., Fribourg-Blanc, A. and Kyriaco, N. (1931) *Rev. neurol.* (ii), 37.
Lindenberg, R. and Spatz, H. (1939) *Virchows Arch.*, **305**, 531.
Lovshin, L. L. and Kernohan, J. W. (1948) *Arch. intern. Med.*, **82**, 321.
McBrien, D. J., Bradley, R. D. and Ashton, N., (1963) *Lancet*, **1**, 697.
McCormick, H. M. and Neubürger, K. T. (1958) *J. Neuropath. exp. Neurol.*, **17**, 471.
Magee, P. M., Stoner, H. B. and Barnes, J. M. (1957) *J. Path. Bact.*, **73**, 107.
Mair, W. G. P. and Druckman, R. (1953) *Brain*, **76**, 70.
Mair, W. G. P. and Folkerts, J. F. (1953) *Brain*, **76**, 563.
Marcus, H. (1933) *Acta Psychiat. et Neurol.*, **8**, 297.
Martin, J. P. (1941) *Brit. Med. J.* (ii), 537.
Meadows, S. P. (1951) Feiling, A., *Modern Trends in Neurology*, Butterworth, London.
Merritt, H. and Finland, M. (1930) *Brain*, **53**, 290.
Meyer, J. S., Fang, H. C. and Denny-Brown, D. (1954) *Arch. Neurol. Psychiat.* (Chicago), **72**, 296.
Miller, H. G. and Daley, R. (1946) *Quart. J. Med.*, **15**, 255.
Minea, I. (1932) *Bull. Soc. roum. Neurol.*, **13**, 27.
Moore, M. T. and Stern, K. (1938) *Brain*, **61**, 70.
Moritz, A. R. and Oldt, M. R. (1937) *Amer. J. Path.*, **13**, 679.
Moschowitz, E. (1925) *Arch. Int Med.*, **36**, 89.
Neubürger, K. T. (1925) *Z. ges Neurol. Psychiat.*, **95**, 278.
Norman, R. M. and Urich, H. (1957) *J. Path. Bact.*, **73**, 580.
Oppenheimer, B. S. and Fishberg, A. M. (1928) *Arch. intern. Med.*, **41**, 264.
Padget, D. H. (1944) *The circle of Willis, its embryology and anatomy;* in Dandy, W. E., *Intracranial arterial aneurysms*, Comstock Publishing Co., Ithaca.
Pentschew, A. (1933) *Arch. Psychiat. Nervenkr.*, **101**, 80.
Pickering, G. W. (1955) *High Blood Pressure*, J. and A. Churchill, London, p. 257.
Pickering, G. W., Wright, A. D. and Heptinstall, R. H. (1952) *Lancet* (ii), 952.
Plass, E. D. and Matthew, C. W. (1926) *Amer. J. Obstet. Gynec.*, **12**, 346.
Reichardt, M. (1905) *Allg. Z. Psychiat.*, **62**, 787.
Reifenstein, G. H., Levine, S. A. and Gross, R. E. (1947) *Amer. Heart J.*, **33**, 146.
Rich, A. R. and Gregory, J. E. (1943) *Johns Hopk. Hosp. Bull.*, **72**, 65.
Richardson, J. C. (1938) *Brain*, **61**, 17.
Richardson, J. C. and Hyland, H. H. (1941) *Medicine*, Baltimore, **20**, 1.
Rosenberg, E. F. (1940) *Arch. intern. Med.*, **65**, 545.
Russell, C. K. (1931) *Arch. Neurol. Psychiat.* (Chicago), **25**, 1003.
Russell, D. S. (1937) *Proc. Roy. Soc. Med.*, **30**, 1025; (1954) ibid., **47**, 689.
Russell, R. W. R. (1961) *Lancet*, 1422.
von Santha, K. (1932) *Virchows Arch.*, **287**, 405.
Scheinker, M. (1945) *Arch. Neurol. Psychiat.* (Chicago), **53**, 289.
Schottstaedt, M. F. and Sokolow, M. (1953) *Amer. Heart J.*, **45**, 331.
Scott, G. E., Neubürger, K. T. and Denst, J. (1960) *Neurology* (Minneap.), **10**, 22.
Shennan, T. (1915) *Edin. med. J.*, **15**, 245; (1934) *Spec. Rep. Ser. med. Res. Coun.*, Lond. *No.* 193.
Smyth, G. E. (1939) *Brain*, **62**, 41.
Smyth, G. E. and Henderson, W. R. (1938) *J. Neurol. Psychiat.*, **1**, 226.
Spatz, H. (1935) *Dtsch. Z. Nervenheilk.*, **136**, 86.
Spillane, J. D. (1937) *Bull. neurol. Inst. N.Y.*, **6**, 529.
Spiller, W. G. (1909) *J. nerv. ment. Dis.*, **36**, 601.
Stengel, A. and Wolferth, C. C. (1923) *Arch. intern. Med.*, **31**, 527.
Stern, K. (1938) *J. Neurol. Psychiat.*, **1**, 26.

Stewart-Wallace, A. M. (1939) *Brain*, **62**, 426.
Stopford, J. S. B. (1916) *J. Anat. Lond.*, **50**, 131 and 255; (1917) ibid., **51**, 250.
Strauss, H. (1933) *Mschr. Psychiat. Neurol.*, **85**, 1.
Stuart, A. E. and MacGregor-Robertson, G. (1956) *Lancet* (i), 475.
Suh, T. H. and Alexander, L. (1939) *Arch. Neurol. Psychiat.* (Chicago), **41**, 659.
Symmers, E. St. C. (1952) *Brit. med. J.*, **2**, 897; (1956) *Brain*, **79**, 511.
Symonds, C. P. (1952) *Ann. R.C.S. Eng.*, **10**, 347; (1955) *Brit. med. J.* (i), 119; (1956) *Neurology*, **6**, 681.
Taylor, J. E. D. (1952) *Brit. med. J.* (i), 890.
Thompson, G. (1956) *Brain*, **79**, 111.
Tichy, F. (1949) *Arch. Path.*, **48**, 475.
Torack, R. M., Terry, R. D. and Zimmerman, H. M. (1960) *Amer. J. Path.*, **36**, 273; (1959) *ibid.*, **35**, 1135.
Tureen, L. L. (1937) *Res. Publ. Ass. nerv. ment. Dis.*, **18**, 394.
Turnbull, H. M. (1918) *Brain*, **41**, 50.
Vander Eecken, H. M. and Adams, R. D. (1953) *J. Neuropath. exp. Neurol.*, **12**, 132.
Villaret, M. and Cachera, R. (1939) *Pr. med.*, **47**, 267.
Walton, J. N. (1956) *Subarachnoid Haemorrhage*, E. and S. Livingstone Ltd., Edinburgh and London.
Weisman, A. D. (1944) *New Engl. J. Med.*, **231**, 118.
Weisman, A. D. and Adams, R. D. (1944) *Brain*, **67**, 69.
Williams, D. J. (1936) *Brain*, **59**, 175.
Winkelman, N. W. (1942) *Arch. Neurol. Psychiat.* (Chicago), **47**, 57.
Winkelman, N. W. and Eckel, J. L. (1929) *Arch. Neurol. Psychiat.* (Chicago), **21**, 863; (1932) ibid., **28**, 844.
Wolman, L. (1953) *Brain*, **76**, 364.
Wolman, L. (1959) *Brain*, **82**, 276.
Wright, H. P. (1942) *J. Path. Bact.*, **54**, 461.
Zeek, P. M., Smith, C. C. and Weeter, J. C. (1948) *Amer. J. Path.*, **24**, 889.
Zeitlin, H. and Lichtenstein, B. W. (1936) *Arch. Neurol. Psychiat.* (Chicago), **36**, 96.
Zülch, K. J. (1954), *Vth Internat. Neurol. Cong. Lisbon*, **3**, 42.

CHAPTER 3

INFECTIOUS DISEASES OF THE CENTRAL NERVOUS SYSTEM

By J. G. Greenfield

INFECTIONS BY BACTERIA AND FUNGI

Introduction

The central nervous system offers less resistance to infection than any other tissue of the body. As a consequence micro-organisms, such as *fusiformis* and *albicans*, which are commonly regarded as feebly pathogenic, may, when they obtain access to the brain, cause abscesses or meningitis which are often fatal. Other organisms of comparatively mild pathogenicity such as *meningococcus*, *H. brucella abortus* and *cryptococcus neoformans* rarely cause fatal illness unless they invade the nervous system; and among the viruses there are many which produce only mild fever unless they attack the brain or spinal cord, where they may cause severe permanent damage. It is fortunate therefore that the central nervous system is well shielded from infection from without by its bony and dural coverings and that the blood-brain barrier also gives some protection against infection by the blood stream.

In the history of most infectious diseases the search for the causative agent has followed a presumptive diagnosis based largely on the character of the cellular exudate. This remains true for many individual cases in which the clinical diagnosis is uncertain. It is therefore important first to decide, as far as possible, what type or degree of cellular exudate can be accepted as evidence of infection by a living organism. This question has arisen especially in some forms of demyelinating disease and of peripheral neuropathy and in the more acute cases of systemic degeneration, in all of which some degree of cellular infiltration is commonly found especially round the vessels and in the meninges.

It is now recognised that cellular exudation, especially of lymphocytes, can be excited by many chemical stimuli, one of which may be the rapid breakdown of nervous tissue. Spielmeyer (1922) called these reactions *symptomatisch*; the nearest English equivalent is *concomitant*. They are comparable to the reactions seen in acute degenerations and ischaemic necroses in other organs such as the liver, kidney and heart. In doubtful cases the first question is whether the destruction of nervous tissue precedes the cellular exudate or whether both appear at the same time. When this cannot be ascertained an assessment of the relative intensities of exudate and destruction of nervous tissue may give valuable evidence. The type of cell forming the exudate is also important. For example, acute demyelinating processes are often associated with quite thick cuffs of lymphocytes round the vessels in the neighbourhood, but polymorphonuclear leucocytes and plasma cells are usually absent or very scarce. On the other hand mild inflammatory reactions in which plasma cells and their derivatives, Russell and mulberry cells, are prominent, as in some forms of subacute encephalitis, are strong evidence of an infectious aetiology.

Reaction either to infectious or other acutely destructive processes is not confined to leucocytes and other wandering cells. The supporting tissues of the central nervous system also react either by regressive changes or by hyperplasia. Some of the reactions of astrocytes and microglia have already been discussed. Reticulin and collagenous tissue is only present in the meninges and the walls of the vessels, and their reactions are less constant and usually slighter than those of astrocytes, but with the more severe infections and other serious lesions of nervous tissue their reaction may be of major importance. The fact that the only available supply of fibroblastic tissue is in the walls of the vessels delays and may prevent the fibrous tissue encapsulation which plays an important part in the healing of acute inflammatory foci here as elsewhere in the body. In many milder infections, and in demyelinating lesions also, there is some thickening of the walls of small vessels and outgrowth of reticulin or collagenous fibres from them into the surrounding nervous tissue.

Virchow-Robin space

The perivascular or Virchow-Robin space, which surrounds the arteries and veins within the central nervous system down to their finest branches, is a structure peculiar to the central nervous system. It may be considered as an invagination of the subarachnoid space along the vessel walls as they leave this space to enter the nervous tissue. Its inner wall is the adventitia of the vessel walls. Externally it is bounded by a thin layer of collagen or reticulin fibres between which cells may be able to enter and leave the space. When it is empty, as it normally is, its thin outer wall is not easily distinguished from the adventitia of the vessel wall, but when it is filled with lymphocytes or lipid phagocytes, these cells are seen to lie between the adventitia and an enclosing connective tissue layer which stains red with van Gieson's picro-fuchsin and is usually also argyrophilic. Fine trabeculae can be seen under these conditions to join the inner and outer walls of the space in a manner similar to the trabeculae of the subarachnoid space. The Virchow-Robin space is not present around capillaries.

The Virchow-Robin space normally contains occasional lymphocytes and lymphoblasts and numerous mesenchymal or reticulo-endothelial cells lie in its walls. Under many conditions, especially in post-infectious encephalitis, these cells may be seen undergoing mitotic division (Perdrau 1928, Lumsden 1956). It is probable that they also play an active part in the absorption and katabolism of lipids in areas of demyelination or softening. Whether lymphocytes can multiply in the space is less certain. To the writer it seems that the lymphocytic cuffing, which is commonly seen round venules and small arteries in the absence of any cellular infiltration in the surrounding nervous tissue, is most easily explained in this way.

The term *perivascular infiltration* is commonly used in neuropathology to describe these collections of lymphocytes and other cells within the confines of the Virchow-Robin space. In the meninges also cellular infiltrations may be chiefly perivascular, sometimes because they consist of cells which have reached the meninges along the Virchow-Robin spaces. However, in certain forms of encephalitis, especially in that following vaccination, measles and other exanthemata, the cellular increase, although essentially perivascular, is outside the Virchow-Robin space. Extra-adventitial infiltrations such as these usually consist chiefly of microglia and histiocytes, although wandering cells from the blood stream may also take part in them. In some such cases there is also infiltration within the Virchow-Robin space, which is chiefly lymphocytic. A similar combined reaction, inside and outside the Virchow-Robin space, may sometimes be seen in other forms of encephalitis.

The manner in which lymphocytes and lipid phagocytes are confined within the space in pathological conditions and the fact that it may be filled by injecting indian ink or colloidal carbon into the subarachnoid space (Millen and Woollam 1954) make it certain that a potential space, in communication with the subarachnoid space, normally exists around the intracerebral and intramedullary arteries and veins (Weed 1914). It is thought that the current in this space is normally from within outwards so that lymphocytes or other cells which collect around the smaller vascular branches pass along the larger vessels into the subarachnoid space. The Virchow-Robin space appears to be wider round these larger vessels and cuffs of lymphocytes, two, three or more cells thick, may be seen around them in cases where only a single layer of cells surrounds the small venules and arterioles.

The Virchow-Robin spaces may be considered both in constitution and in function as the lymphatic channels of the central nervous system. It seems probable that some protein substances, as well as lymphocytes, plasma cells and lipid phagocytes, may be carried along them to the subarachnoid space since, in its passage over the brain and spinal cord, the cerebrospinal fluid always receives an addition of protein. The γ globulin, which the cerebrospinal fluid often contains in subacute forms of encephalitis, may well be formed within the brain and pass into the cerebrospinal fluid along the Virchow-Robin spaces (Field 1954).

The term *perivascular space* is sometimes also used for a cleavage space between the vessels and the surrounding nervous parenchyma. This space, which is sometimes called the *space of His*, may often be seen in paraffin sections of nervous tissue. Under certain conditions haemorrhages or pools of plasma are seen in the position of this space, separating the vessel walls from the surrounding nervous tissue; but it is very doubtful whether there is any true space here under normal conditions, except perhaps around the larger arteries which enter the base of the brain. As has been seen astrocytes are connected to the walls of the smaller vessels by foot-plate processes and the formation of a space between vessel wall and parenchyma would entail the rupture of these processes. No space in this situation is seen in celloidin sections even when the brain tissue is oedematous (Greenfield 1939) and when present in paraffin sections it is considered by the writer to be a shrinkage artefact. The name *Virchow-Robin space* is therefore used in preference to *perivascular space* to avoid ambiguity.

PYOGENIC INFECTIONS OF THE CENTRAL NERVOUS SYSTEM

Anatomical considerations

The brain and spinal cord are protected from infections from outside by their membranous coverings. The skull also provides an effective shield although emissary veins may carry infection through it to the brain. The dura mater is a valuable barrier against infection and, especially in the spinal cord, may prevent the spread of infection through it for a considerable time. The external layer of arachnoid, possibly largely owing to the layer of endothelial cells which covers its external surface, provides a check to infection passing either from the subdural to the arachnoid space or vice versa, and the pia mater, in much the same manner, acts as a temporary barrier preventing subarachnoid infections from spreading into the brain. Infections in these four situations, *epidural, subdural, subarachnoid* and *intracerebral* or *intramedullary*, are therefore discussed separately, although in many cases they are combined.

Routes of infection

(*a*) Infections of the central nervous system or meninges may come from the blood stream either directly or via the choroid plexus or by first producing a focus of infection in the overlying bone.

(*b*) Infections of the paranasal or aural air sinuses may erode the thin layer of bone which separates them from the dura mater.

(*c*) Fractures of the base of the skull may open a channel via these air sinuses from the outside air to the subarachnoid space, or open cranial wounds may cause a more direct communication by which micro-organisms may gain entrance to the intracranial cavity.

Epidural infections and suppurations

Infections of the intracranial epidural space may produce abscesses which are flattened between the bone and the dura mater, and are usually of small size. They most often result from infection of the para-nasal or aural air sinuses, but may be secondary to osteomyelitis of the cranial bones. When infections erode the bone on the base of the anterior or middle cranial fossae, as in infections of the sphenoidal or ethmoidal air sinuses or the middle ear, they usually spread through the dura mater into the subarachnoid space or the cerebral tissue without producing an epidural abscess. This is probably due to the fact that in the erect posture the brain rests on the base of the skull, displacing cerebrospinal fluid by its greater density. When infections of the frontal or mastoid air sinuses burst through their posterior walls they not infrequently produce a small extradural abscess. These are always associated with inflammation of the dura mater itself and are liable to burst through this into the subdural or subarachnoid space, or to cause septic phlebitis of emissary veins or intradural venous sinuses.

Within the spinal canal epidural infections are usually secondary to osteomyelitis of the laminae or bodies of the vertebrae, and are most often caused by the staphylococcus aureus. The less acute staphylococcal infections in this situation may be more granulomas than abscesses, containing at most only small pockets of pus in inflammatory fibroblastic or fibrous tissue. They are most frequently found in the thoracic region and may extend over several segments of the cord. The focus of osteomyelitis which gave rise to the epidural infection may be small and difficult to find. Sometimes the pus tracks downwards in the epidural space so that the largest collection lies within the lumbar theca, whence it may be drained by lumbar puncture. In many of these cases there is a history of previous infection or of osteomyelitis of other bones. Suppuration of the wound may occur after a granuloma of this kind has been dissected out and must be attributed to the viable organisms still present within it, and not to external infection. Typhoid spine, or infection of the vertebrae with *B. typhosus*, may also produce an epidural abscess or granuloma. The resistance of the dura mater to infection in these cases, as well as in epidural abscesses within the cranium, is demonstrated by the commonly favourable results of surgical procedures which expose the dura mater. In occasional cases there may be a wide spread of infection within the layers of the dura mater. A case of chronic infection in the sacral region spreading in this way to the posterior cranial fossa, and revealing itself first by signs of damage to the lower cranial nerves, was an unusual instance. In this case the dura mater throughout its intraspinal portion was greatly thickened and inflamed and contained numerous small staphylococcal abscesses.

Infections of the pleural cavities or in the subdiaphragmatic and perirenal tissues may extend through the intervertebral foramina into the spinal epidural space. Infection in the reverse direction, from the epidural space to the thoracic or abdominal cavities is rare.

Epidural granulomas due to *tuberculosis* and *syphilis* will be discussed under those headings.

Subdural infections

Infection of the subdural space is most commonly secondary to infections of the paranasal air sinuses. In many such cases the infection seems to spread early to the dural venous sinuses; for example from the frontal sinus to the anterior end of the sagittal sinus, or from the sphenoidal sinus to the circular and petrosal sinuses. From these it may spread to veins entering these sinuses and thence to the subdural space. Subdural abscesses resulting from sphenoidal sinusitis may in this way involve both middle fossae. Infections spreading from the frontal air sinus may reach the subdural space directly, but in some such cases the chief focus of infection appears to be near the coronal suture, suggesting an indirect spread via the sagittal sinus. Infection of the subdural space is also a common result of osteomyelitis of the cranial bones.

All subdural infections are liable to spread widely and to cause phlebitis of veins at some distance from the original focus of infection. Pus is often also collected in pockets of the subdural space which it is difficult to drain, especially alongside the falx or on the upper surface of the tentorium (Schiller, Cairns and Russell 1948). From these pockets it is likely to spread to the subarachnoid space. For these reasons subdural infections have a high mortality. The most common causative organisms here also are *staphylococci* and *streptococci*.

Pathology. The absence of any endothelial lining to the dura mater and the vascular character of its innermost layer makes it the protagonist in the reactions to subdural infection. In the less acute infections it rapidly forms an inflammatory granulation tissue by which the infection may become loculated. As it becomes adherent to the underlying arachnoid the latter becomes involved in the inflammatory tissue and localised abscesses may thus be formed. But these adhesions take some time to form and in the early stages the pus can be wiped off the surface of the arachnoid leaving a smooth glistening surface. In treated cases which recover at this stage the subdural space remains patent, and the dura mater shows few residua except thickening of its inner layer.

Leptomeningitis

The leptomeninges offer comparatively little resistance to infection, although the pia mater contains a vascular bed from which polymorphonuclear leucocytes can migrate freely. In fact the cerebrospinal fluid provides a good culture medium for many organisms. When virulent micro-organisms invade the subarachnoid space they often cause death within a few hours and many kinds of micro-organisms, which have a low pathogenicity for other tissues, may produce serious or even fatal meningitis. Many forms of virus also produce infections of the nervous system which appear to be chiefly meningeal. These are rarely fatal but may cause considerable difficulty in diagnosis.

To some extent the type of micro-organism varies with the route of entry to the meninges. In the pre-antibiotic era meningitis secondary to an infection of the internal ear or the paranasal air sinuses was most often due to streptococci and pneumococci. At the present time micro-organisms with a greater resistance to bacteriostatic agents are probably more common. Infection may also spread from the upper nasal passages via fractures in the cribriform plate of the ethmoid or other part of the floor of the anterior fossa.

Infection by the blood stream from foci in the respiratory tract may cause streptococcal and pneumococcal meningitis and *Haemophilus influenzae* may be similarly conveyed. Meningitis due to this micro-organism has a high mortality in childhood. *Meningococcal meningitis* is also almost always due to blood-borne infection. It follows a stage of septicaemia during which, in severe infections, macular rashes may appear, giving rise to the old name *spotted fever*. It seems probable that the choroid plexus is the site of invasion of the brain in most cases since the diplococci are often most abundant in ventricular fluid. The subacute form of the disease, in which meningeal inflammation is almost confined to the neighbourhood of the cisterna magna, is most easily explained on this theory. It may be assumed that in these cases the meningococcus is of low virulence or the child's resistance high, so that although capable of survival in the ventricles the diplococci are quickly destroyed when they reach the more vascular meninges. Rarer types of infection via the blood-stream are those with *Brucella melitensis* or *abortus*, *B. anthracis*, *Streptothrix actinomyces* and the various fungi, especially *Cryptococcus neoformans* (*Torula histolytica*).

Macroscopic appearances. In a typical case of pyogenic meningitis of a few days' duration the appearance of the brain and spinal cord is quite characteristic. The cisterns at the base of the brain are filled with creamy pus which covers the blood-vessels and appears to stretch the arachnoid membrane which covers them. But there is little if any pus on the surface of this membrane. On the convexity of the hemispheres the pus may be confined to the fissures and their lips, exposing the convolutions. But in some cases these also are covered, sometimes more over one hemisphere than the other. Where exposed the cortex may appear congested, but is often less so than in encephalitis. Pus may be found in the ventricles in flakes mixed with cerebrospinal fluid or lying on the ventricular walls. The choroid plexus may be covered by a more firmly attached layer of pus. The spinal cord is similarly covered by subarachnoid pus especially on its dorsal surface. In more acute cases the quantity of pus is less and the congestion of the meninges greater. Purulent infiltration is often most obvious in the cisterna basalis and over the dorsal surface of the spinal cord. In very acute cases purulent infiltration of the meninges may be much less obvious. The pia-arachnoid covering the base of the brain appears congested and cloudy and there may be fine creamy lines on either side of the cortical veins, over the convexity of the hemispheres. In some such cases the diagnosis of meningitis can only be confirmed by histological examination. On section the brain appears soft, the cortical congestion may be more obvious and the white matter is often oedematous. Small cortical infarcts may be seen in the cerebrum and cerebellum. In cases of longer standing some dilatation of the ventricles with softening of the subependymal tissues may be present. In many cases of *meningococcal meningitis* petechial haemorrhages in the white or grey matter, focal softenings or even small abscesses caused by septic embolism of the smaller vessels may be seen. In infections due to *B. anthracis* the haemorrhagic nature of the exudate and the rapidly fatal course may suggest a spontaneous subarachnoid haemorrhage.

The *histological characters* of purulent meningitis are similar to those of pyogenic inflammation in other body cavities. Large numbers of polymorphonuclear leucocytes, with an admixture of plasma cells, lymphocytes and histiocytes lie between the outer layer of the arachnoid and the pia-mater. The causative bacteria may be seen in or among the pus cells. The meningeal vessels are dilated and there is a varying amount of fibrinous exudate. In some cases the inflammation spreads into the walls of the smaller meningeal vessels causing thrombosis but this is more often seen in tuberculous meningitis. There may be some infiltration along the Virchow-Robin spaces of the cortical veins, and some microglial reaction in the outer cortical layers. Otherwise there is little evidence of inflammatory reaction in the nervous parenchyma. In the walls of the ventricles some stripping of ependymal cells and infiltration of the subependymal veins may be seen. During the later stages mononuclear cells, some of which are phagocytic, appear in greater number. Some of these may be derived from the histiocytes of the meninges, and others from the blood-stream.

In more chronic infections, especially in subacute cases of meningococcal meningitis in which diagnosis is retarded or treatment inadequate, there is proliferation of fibroblasts and eventually of collagen fibres in the meninges. This may lead to loculation of cerebrospinal fluid and so produce well-recognised sequelae. (1) When the meningeal thickening takes place round the basal cisterns it may prevent the free flow of cerebrospinal fluid in an upward and downward direction. Hydrocephalus in such cases may result either because the cerebrospinal fluid cannot escape from the cisterna magna, in which case it is *non-communicating*, or because it is prevented by adhesions and meningeal thickening around the ventral aspect of the pons and midbrain from passing upwards into the middle cranial fossa. This is a common cause of acquired *communicating hydrocephalus* in childhood. (2) Loculation of fluid in pockets of the thickened meninges around the spinal cord may cause paraplegia by pressure. In some epidemics of meningococcal meningitis this sequela has not been uncommon, especially when intrathecal antiserum was the only treatment. In cases treated by antibiotics it is probably rarer, especially when frequent lumbar punctures are performed, but it may still occur. It may also be seen in infections by staphylococci and other pyogenic organisms. Some of the cases of progressive spinal arachnoiditis which occur as sequelae of spinal anaesthesia may be due to infections by micro-organisms of low virulence. In other cases, however, the normal condition of the cerebrospinal fluid during the early period after the anaesthetic excludes bacterial infection. Irritation of the meninges by a chemical contaminant is the most probable cause of this condition (*vide* p. 249). The leptomeninges appear to be very sensitive to chemical irritants and, unless these are quickly eliminated, progressive thickening and adhesions of the pia-arachnoid may cause symptoms of paraplegia or hydrocephalus after an interval of several months.

Encysted loculations of fluid, either in the spinal canal or over the base of the brain, have for long been recognised as a cause of paraplegia, hydrocephalus, vertiginous attacks or symptoms due to pressure on the oculomotor or optic nerves and chiasma. The cause of most cases is unknown. Syphilis used to be blamed for many, but at the present time only a small proportion can be attributed to this cause, and the majority appear to be due to minor meningeal infections. Some seem to be related to trauma. Elkington (1936) in 41 cases of spinal arachnoiditis, obtained a history of spinal injury in 9, of syphilis in 4, of gonorrhaea in 4 and of other systemic infections in 6. In 18 no cause could be ascertained. A rare situation of such encysted collections of cerebrospinal fluid is over the surface of the hemispheres where they cause symptoms of intracranial pressure. The writer has seen two cases of this kind in which a rounded depression, filled with clear fluid and 5–6 cm. in width, was found on the surface of the parietal lobe. This appeared to be the only cause of the symptoms of intracranial pressure which led to death. (See also page 355.)

Cerebral abscess

Aetiology and pathogenesis. Pyogenic micro-organisms may gain access to the tissues of the brain, as to the meninges, either from the blood-stream, from foci of infection in overlying tissues, or from wounds which communicate either directly or indirectly with the outside air. Before antibiotics came into general use the great majority of cerebral abscesses were due to infections of the middle ear and paranasal and aural air sinuses, and this is still a common route of infection. The causative organism varies greatly, and anaerobic strains of streptococci, coliform bacilli, diphtheroids and fusiformis are often present either alone or along with the more virulent streptococci, staphylococci and pneumococci (McFarlan 1943). Infection of the middle ear may spread through the tegmen tympani to cause a temporal abscess, or via the mastoid air sinuses, especially in children in whom the bone is thinner, to produce an abscess in the cerebellar hemisphere. Disease of the frontal, ethmoidal or sphenoidal air sinuses or fractures of the roof of the nasopharynx, especially the cribriform plate of the ethmoid, may cause abscesses in the frontal lobe.

Abscesses arising from blood-borne infection may occur anywhere in the brain but especially at the junction of the grey and white matter. They are commonly but not always multiple. In most cases they are secondary to chronic septic diseases of the respiratory tract such as bronchiectasis, but sometimes the focus of infection is less obvious or more recent (Fig. 3.1). Metastatic staphylococcal cerebral abscesses may occur also after osteomyelitis or other severe staphylococcal infections, or without evidence of previous infection. They are less commonly multiple than those secondary to disease of the respiratory tract.

Abscesses due to gun-shot wounds, most often with lodgement of a small piece of shell casing within the brain, were very common after the First World War; in some such cases the first symptoms of intracranial pressure appeared months or even years after the wound. The use of antibiotics and the more thorough early treatment of wounds greatly reduced the number of such cases in the last war.

Abscesses form much more commonly in the white than the grey matter of the brain. Even when infection has to pass through the cerebral cortex the main bulk of the abscess is deep to this and the channel leading to it through the cortex may be very narrow and difficult to find. The reason for this choice of situation may be that the white matter has a poorer vascular supply than the grey. This not only restricts the migration of phagocytes from the blood-stream but also delays the encapsulation of a focus of infection by fibrous tissue, since in the brain fibroblasts can only be formed from the meninges or the walls of the blood-vessels. The delay in capsule formation and the softening of brain tissue which occurs round an abscess often allow the infection to spread more deeply into the white matter and to produce secondary abscesses, which are connected to the primary abscess either by a narrow channel or by an area of inflamed

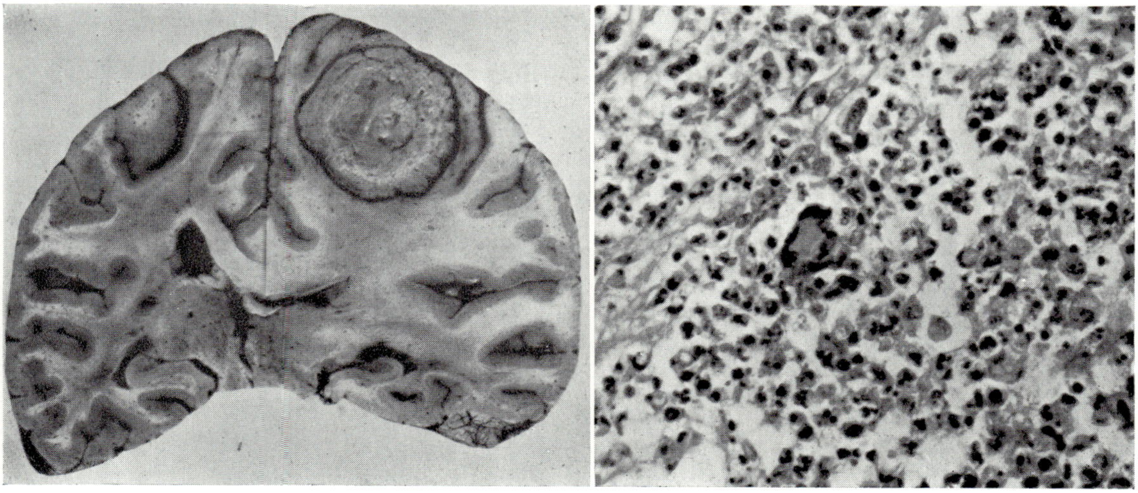

(a) (b)

FIG. 3.1. Actinomycotic abscess of the brain, secondary to lung infection.

(a) Gross appearance on coronal section. (b) Microscopic appearance near margin. Note the giant cell of Langhans type. (By the courtesy of Dr. McAlpine.)

and softened brain tissue. Occasionally a chain of such abscesses may be found. This tendency to spread inwards makes rupture into the ventricles one of the chief dangers in cerebral abscesses.

It is not uncommon to find a firmer capsule around the primary than around the secondary abscesses, or the capsule may be better formed on the superficial than on the deep side of the abscess. Thorotrast, which is sometimes injected into the abscess cavity to make its position and size visible to X-rays, appears also to have a value in encouraging encapsulation. The walls of an abscess treated in this manner often show a zone, several millimetres thick, of concentric layers of collagen fibres between which are innumerable phagocytes filled with thorotrast.

The earliest stage of an abscess is an area of septic encephalitis, that is of softening and congestion of an area of brain tissue, often with numerous petechial haemorrhages. The centre of this area becomes deliquescent and an abscess cavity is thus formed. Its wall is at first poorly defined and may be quite irregular in outline. Gradually a firmer wall appears, sometimes more at one side than the other, and as this grows thicker and more complete the abscess becomes encapsulated. Chronic abscesses, especially those of staphylococcal origin, may be surrounded by a firm concentric capsule of fibrous tissue from 1 to 3 mm. in thickness.

The white matter in the zone surrounding an abscess is usually softened and oedematous so that the capsule may strip from it very easily. Sometimes a firmly encapsulated abscess may appear *post-mortem* as if lying loose in a cavity in the brain tissue. The oedema around an abscess is often very severe and extensive so that, on section of the brain, the white matter is seen to be swollen and often has a yellow or greenish discoloration. The distinction which is sometimes made between brain swelling and oedema, according to whether the tissue feels dry or wet, appears meaningless, since in either case the cause and pathogenesis are the same. As has already been seen there is an excess of fluid between the nerve fibres of the white matter as well as irregular swelling of these fibres and of the cell bodies of the astrocytes. In most cases the bulk of the fluid appears to be interstitial and the term oedema is, therefore, quite appropriate for such cases.

Microscopically the appearances of the wall of a cerebral abscess vary greatly. In the most acute abscesses there is an inner layer of pus, usually with a narrow irregular layer of inflammatory granulation tissue external to it. But in some abscesses and around some part of the wall in many, this layer may be scarcely recognisable. The brain tissue is infiltrated with polymorphonuclear leucocytes and plasma cells near the abscess and with lymphocytes in the more peripheral zones, and there is usually heavy lymphocytic cuffing of the veins both in the neighbourhood and extending some distance from the abscess. The oedema of the white matter appears as a loosening of texture with pools of faintly eosinophilic plasma in some places and swelling of the cell bodies of the astrocytes. Those in the zone nearest to the abscess may have undergone clasmatodendrosis. Along with this there is pallor in the staining of myelin around the abscess.

In more chronic abscesses the layer of granulation tissue is more definite and passes gradually into a collagenous capsule which varies considerably in thickness and density over different parts of the abscess. This has a fairly well defined outer border, but fibroblasts and reticulin fibres may be seen intertwined with neuroglial fibres in the zone outside it. In such cases there is often considerable swelling of the cell bodies of astrocytes, which may assume large spider forms and often have more than one nucleus. Perivascular cuffing with lymphocytes may still be seen in the zone around the abscess in spite of good encapsulation.

The chief differences between abscesses in the brain and those in other parts of the body are thus seen to be due (1) to the paucity of fibrous tissue and the consequent tardiness of fibroblastic activity in the encapsulation of the abscess; and (2) to the very vulnerable nature of the nervous parenchyma. The neuroglial reaction is slow and has little value in the encapsulation of the abscess; in fact the astrocytes are easily destroyed by infection and in the early stages show more degenerative than proliferative change.

Septic embolism

In cases of malignant endocarditis multiple septic emboli may lodge in the small cerebral arteries. These may cause mycotic aneurysms (q.v.) which may enlarge and burst, or multiple small infarcts. It may be difficult to distinguish these from aseptic emboli since neutrophil leucocytes can be seen round both. But septic emboli are more often multiple, they are more heavily infiltrated with neutrophil leucocytes, and streptococci can usually be found in them.

Cerebrospinal fluid

In bacterial infections of the brain or its coverings the constancy and severity of inflammatory changes in the cerebrospinal fluid vary with the site of the infection. When the subarachnoid space is involved evidences of inflammation, in cell count and protein, are always found, as also in many cases of subdural infection. In cases of cerebral or subdural abscess they are more variable and when infection is confined to the cranial epidural space the fluid is usually normal.

Spinal epidural infections, when granulomatous or localised, usually produce the compression syndrome of raised protein with or without xanthochromia (Froin-Nonne syndrome) and some degree of spinal block. More purulent collections may gravitate to the lumbar theca where they may be tapped by lumbar puncture. The pus in such cases is not under pressure and may have to be aspirated: this and its creamy consistency distinguish it from purulent cerebrospinal fluid. Rarely a mixture of epidural pus and normal cerebrospinal fluid is obtained on lumbar puncture. This can be distinguished from the fluid of purulent leptomeningitis by the fact that it contains normal percentages of glucose and chlorides, although pus cells and staphylococci are present in the deposit.

In *purulent arachnoiditis* the most important characteristics of the fluid, apart from the pressure, are (1) its tendency to form a fibrinous or stringy coagulum, (2) the diminution or absence of glucose and (3) the presence of visible bacteria in the deposit. The cell excess may be of any degree and the more purulent fluids contain several thousand cells per cubic millimetre. But in late cases and in some subacute cases the cell count may be comparatively low and may contain a varying proportion of lymphocytes and large mononuclear cells, including plasma cells. The protein rises in proportion to the cell count. Glucose always falls rapidly and often disappears from the fluid. The chlorides also often fall to 650 mg. per 100 ml. or below. The causative organism can usually be seen in films of the centrifugalised deposit either extra- or intracellularly and can be grown on culture. In meningococcal meningitis when diplococci are scanty and, as is usual, intracellular, they are best demonstrated by counter-staining after Gram's method with Pappenheim's methyl green pyronin, which stains the cocci a brilliant red against the green (or purple) of the nucleus.

The differential diagnosis between *diffuse* or *generalised meningitis* and *cerebral abscess* may rest on the examination of the cerebrospinal fluid and the distinction is not always easy. The most typical fluids, in cases of cerebral abscess, are either: (1) a cell count of less than 50 per cu. mm. with 25 per cent or more of neutrophil leucocytes along with a rise in protein to the neighbourhood of 100 mg. per 100 ml., absence of a coagulum and normal glucose and chlorides; (2) a purulent fluid which does not form the stringy coagulum of meningitis, which contains over 30 mg. glucose per 100 ml. and in which no bacteria can be seen in the deposit. Purulent fluids of this kind are not uncommon when the abscess is near the meningeal or ventricular surface and are sometimes responsible for an erroneous diagnosis of generalised meningitis. But all variations between these types of fluid, or more normal fluids, may be found. In some fluids the proportion of neutrophil leucocytes is high when the total cell count is comparatively low, e.g. 50 per cent of 5 cells or 80 per cent of 25 cells, but counts over 100 cells per cu. mm. may be predominantly lymphocytic. Since neutrophil leucocytes may also be found in the fluid from cases of cerebral glioma or embolism, they do not of themselves indicate infection. The protein usually rises rather above the level that might be expected from the cell count, but in some fluids with a cell count of 1,000 per cu. mm. or over it may be only moderately increased. The formation of a fibrin coagulum is rare, whereas it is the rule in generalised meningitis. The chlorides are usually normal but may fall temporarily when the blood chlorides are lowered by vomiting or other cause. The glucose is little reduced and a fall below 25 mg. per 100 ml., or disappearance, is usually evidence of spread of infection to the leptomeninges and generalised meningitis.

The leucocyte count in the blood is almost as fallacious as the temperature in the diagnosis of cerebral abscess since normal counts are found in a large proportion of cases.

NEUROPATHIES CAUSED BY BACTERIAL EXOTOXINS

The soluble exotoxins produced by *Cl. botulinus, tetanus* and *C. diphtheriae* are very powerful poisons of nervous tissue. But they appear to exert this action in quite different ways.

Cl. botulinus, when grown under strictly anaerobic conditions, produces an exotoxin which paralyses first the cranial and later the spinal motor nerves. Botulism follows the ingestion of bottled or canned foodstuffs which have been infected before being sealed. It never results from infection by the living bacillus alone, either via the gastro-intestinal canal or the skin. In mild cases the paralysis passes off in a few days and it is not associated with any structural changes in the nervous tissue. The toxin appears to act at or near the terminal twigs of the motor nerves in such a way as to reduce the potential in the end-plates. It does not appear to interfere directly with the formation of acetylcholine or with the sensitivity of the end-plates to acetylcholine (Thompson and King 1957).

The conditions which are most favourable for the production of *tetanus toxin* in wounds infected by spores are not fully known, but the presence of foreign material, such as rust or earth, splinters of fractured bone or haematomas seems to favour the appearance of symptoms. The toxin appears to reach the nervous system both along nerves (since symptoms often begin in the wounded limb) and via the blood stream, and causes hyperexcitability of spinal and pontobulbar reflexes. Sometimes there is also evidence of motor paralysis. These effects are produced without any known structural alteration in the central or peripheral nervous system, except those associated with local infection in the neighbourhood of the wound, and central chromatolysis in motor neurones exhausted by tetanic spasms. The small haemorrhages in the brain stem or spinal cord which are sometimes present may be attributed to the severity of the muscular spasms.

In cases in which symptoms lasted for more than 5 days Baker (1942) found perivascular zones of demyelination in the grey and white matter of the cerebral hemispheres. In some of the small arteries the walls appeared homogeneous and stained poorly; but vascular changes were less conspicuous than those in the parenchyma, and this he attributed to passage of toxin through the walls of the vessels.

Diphtheritic neuropathy

Paralysis, beginning in the soft palate and affecting the ciliary and vagus nerves as well as those going to the body and limbs, has been recognised as a common sequela of diphtheria for more than a century (Trousseau and Lassègue 1851, Maingault 1854). The discovery of the *C. diphtheriae* by Klebs (1883) and Loeffler (1884) and of the rôle of its exotoxins by Roux and Yersin (1888–90) appeared to establish the pathogenesis of the disease, but the cytochemistry of the action of the neurotoxin is not yet fully understood. The action is a slow one as paralysis may not appear for several weeks after the pharyngeal manifestations of the disease have disappeared. Walshe (1918–19, 1920) and Gaskell and Korb (1946) have reported numerous cases of neuropathy in soldiers in semitropical theatres of war, following cutaneous or wound infections by *C. diphtheriae*. In these cases the characteristic paralysis of accommodation was a very common symptom, but palatal palsy was much rarer than after faucial diphtheria and was often absent. The latent interval between the infection and the onset of paralysis is longer after cutaneous than after faucial diphtheria. In Gaskell and Korb's series of 60 cases it averaged 70·4 days (shortest 23 days, longest 158 days).

Pathology. The histological changes which the diphtheria toxin produces in the nervous system have received comparatively little study in spite of the opportunities offered by the high death-rate of the disease, but general agreement has now been reached between studies of the human disease and the results of experimental work on animals.

In most cases lesions are limited to the peripheral nervous system but all parts of this may be involved from the ciliary nerves to the lumbosacral plexus. They are greatest in the nerve roots, dorsal root ganglia and proximal parts of the cranial and spinal nerves, but may be found also in more peripheral parts of the nerves. They consist essentially of *segmental demyelination* of nerve fibres, that is demyelination involving one or more internodes with preservation of the myelin sheath round the axon proximal and distal to the lesion.

In the cases of Fisher and Adams (1956), in which death occurred from 34 to 80 days after the onset of pharyngitis, myelin degeneration was well established but varied in degree in different cases and different levels of the neuraxis. In the least damaged fibres the sheaths were swollen, vacuolated or fragmented. Others were converted into granular material which stained similarly to myelin but less intensely, and in many fibres the myelin was replaced by phagocytes containing sudanophilic lipid. In severe cases almost all the area in the centre of the ganglia and the neighbouring parts of the nerve roots and spinal nerves showed myelin destruction of this degree. In less severely affected areas small foci of myelin loss, apparently unrelated to vessels, were seen. Minor changes in the axons were also found. Some were swollen and beaded or irregular in calibre but very few were fragmented. Wallerian degeneration in the peripheral parts of the nerves was seen only in 2 cases which survived 52 and 80 days after infection. The roots and intraganglionic parts of the vagus nerve were constantly affected in Fisher and Adams' cases. Owing to the preservation of axons, the cell bodies of the lower motor and sensory neurones showed no axonal reaction or other definite lesion and there was no degeneration in the dorsal columns of the spinal cord.

Of the lesions which may occur in the organs of the body cavity, bronchopneumonia, due to weakness or paralysis of the chest musculature, and interstitial myocarditis are the most common. The heart failure which is a common mode of death in diphtheritic neuropathy may be partly due to this lesion but electrocardiographic studies suggest that it is more often associated with abnormalities of conduction due to lesions of the vagus nerve and cardiac plexus.

Cerebrospinal fluid. The protein-cell dissociation which may be found in acute infective polyneuritis is also common in diphtheritic neuropathy (Queckenstedt 1917). The fluid may be yellowish in colour. In some cases it has formed a heavy coagulum (Greenfield 1921) but this has probably been due to slight blood admixture since pleocytosis is rarely if ever present. The other constituents of the fluid are usually normal.

Experimental. Waksman *et al.* (1957) produced diphtheritic neuritis in rabbits and guinea pigs by injection of underneutralised toxin–antitoxin mixtures. Histologically the disease was a progressive demyelination of the peripheral nervous system without damage to axons or inflammatory cell infiltration—a segmental demyelinative neuropathy. In the guinea pigs the peripheral nerves, in the rabbits the spinal roots and sensory ganglia were involved. Phase and electronmicroscopic studies by Webster *et al.* (1961) upon the sciatic nerves of similarly treated guinea pigs revealed that lesions first appeared and later were most severe in the membrane systems of the Schwann cells, near the nodes of Ranvier, and included the surface membrane, the mexaxon, the myelin sheath and the axon–Schwann cell membrane. There was a striking variation in the severity of the process both within different regions of the same Schwann cell and between adjacent Schwann cells.

TUBERCULOUS INFECTION

Epidural infection

Tuberculous disease of the vertebral bodies or *spinal caries* (Pott's paraplegia) will be considered later (Chapter 13) as a cause of spinal compression. It is very frequently associated with an epidural tuberculous granuloma. In the majority of cases this does not spread more deeply, but in rare cases it may give rise to tuberculous meningitis. In the cranial cavity epidural tuberculosis is very rare except when related to otitis media.

Subdural tuberculous infection

This occurs during the somewhat rare passage of an infection through the dura mater towards the subarachnoid space. Miliary tubercles are also frequently found on the inside of the dural covering of the floor of the cranium in cases of tuberculous meningitis. They may assist in the macroscopical diagnosis of this form of meningitis. More widespread granulomas attached to the inner surface of the dura mater, usually with some spread to the leptomeninges and sometimes to the cerebral cortex, have been described by Boinet (1899) and Chantemesse (1884) under the name *meningite en plaque tuberculeuse.* Pardee and Knox (1927) in reporting a case of this kind used the term *tuberculoma en plaque.* A number of such cases has been described in adults, but none in children. In such cases a history of epilepsy or of symptoms of intracranial pressure may go back for many years. These granulomas form fairly large flattened, sometimes nodular, masses, adherent to the dura externally and in varying degree to the leptomeninges and the cerebral cortex internally. Their outer margin can often be lifted free from the surface of the brain when their central area is more adherent. In some cases their relation to the cerebral sulci suggests a subarachnoid spread. Their size may reach 9 cm. by 6 cm. with a thickness of less than 1 cm. (von Czirer 1914).

Meningeal tuberculosis and tuberculous leptomeningitis

Isolated tuberculomas of varying size may be found in the leptomeninges, and although they often give rise to generalised meningitis, this is not a constant sequela. The name *meningeal tuberculosis* is applicable to such cases. Single tuberculomas on the surface of the brain may originate either in the leptomeninges or in the cerebral cortex and may form rounded or oval masses of the size of a walnut or even of a goose's egg. They compress and destroy the underlying brain tissue and, except for their attachment to the leptomeninges, do not differ from tuberculomas found more deeply within the brain. Multiple isolated meningeal tuberculomas, a few millimetres in diameter, are not very rare as autopsy findings in patients who die of tuberculosis without showing clinical evidence of intracranial disease. They may lie in the fissures of the brain or along the line of the larger cerebral vessels. In most cases they are associated with tuberculomas of similar size within the brain tissue.

Generalised tuberculous meningitis is a very common form of meningitis which was almost always fatal before streptomycin was discovered. It occurs most often in young children, especially between the ages of 6 months and 5 years, but no age is exempt. It is always secondary to disease elsewhere in the body, but in some cases the primary focus may be small and difficult to find, for example a small Ghon's focus in one lung or infection of a cervical or mediastinal lymph node. In children it is most often part of a generalised miliary tuberculosis; in the large series collected by Blacklock and Griffin (1935) 68 per cent of all cases of meningitis were associated with a miliary spread of disease in the organs of the body, and in 81 per cent of all cases of miliary tuberculosis there was also meningitis. In a smaller series with a more varied age incidence, Rich and McCordock (1933) found miliary tuberculosis in 78 per cent. In adults the association with miliary tuberculosis is rather less common. The primary focus is usually in the lung (Blacklock and Griffin, 74 per cent), but cases of abdominal or genito-urinary infection or of tuberculosis apparently limited to lymph nodes or bones and joints may end with meningitis.

Although in the majority of cases of tuberculous meningitis the bacillus is of the human type, a large proportion of cases, especially in children, has been shown to be caused by bovine infection. This proportion differs in different countries and in different parts of the same country. The highest percentages of bovine infection have been found in Scotland (42·9 per cent, Griffith 1934) and in Denmark (40·9 per cent, Jensen 1932). Blacklock and Griffin found a rather lower percentage in Glasgow where the milk was pasteurised, than in the surrounding country (17 and 23 per cent). In their series the highest incidence of bovine infection was in the third year of life and in most cases the primary focus was in the abdomen. Hayes (1954) in the United States records percentages of 15 per cent in children under 5 years of age and 27·5 per cent in a small series of older children.

Various theories of *pathogenesis* have been put forward.

(1) A direct spread to the meninges would appear to be the most obvious cause when their infection is part of a generalised miliary tuberculosis. But Rich and McCordock (1929, 1933) showed that in animals the injection of tubercle bacilli directly into the carotid artery does not cause primary tuberculous meningitis, although it produces miliary tubercle nodules in the brain, meninges and elsewhere in the body. On the other hand an injection of bacilli directly into the subarachnoid space constantly produces generalised meningitis. They therefore postulated that in the majority of cases meningitis was secondary to a small focus in the cortex or leptomeninges, and they found evidence for this theory in 90 per cent of their cases. Their conclusions were supported by Macgregor, Kirkpatrick and Craig (1935), who found superficial foci of older date in 24 out of 27 brains with tuberculous meningitis (Fig. 3.2*b* and *c*). But others have been unable to find foci of this kind in so large a percentage of cases. Beres and Metzler (1938) in 28 cases of tuberculous meningitis found no intracerebral foci in 14 and none in contact with the surface in 3 others. These results are in agreement with the writer's experience. In cases of tuberculous meningitis which have been treated with streptomycin and relapsed or died of hydrocephalus some months later, caseous tuberculous nodules are commonly found among the exudate either over the base of the brain or in the depths of the sulci on the convexity of the hemispheres, but such tuberculomas have probably developed during the course of the clinical disease.

(2) Hektoen (1896) examined the changes in the meningeal vessels in 9 cases of tuberculous meningitis. In all he found invasion of the walls of both arteries and veins by miliary tubercle nodules. In most cases the adventitia and media were more involved than the intima, but in three cases the reverse was true; endarteritis was found in all the vessels in these cases but 'one can examine a large series of sections without finding any changes in elastica, media or adventitia'. These three cases had widespread miliary or subacute tuberculosis of other organs in the body, but no older tubercle nodules in the brain or meninges. Hektoen therefore concluded that the infection had reached the meninges by passing through the walls of small arteries which might be entirely replaced by tuberculous granulation tissue.

(3) A primary focus in the choroid plexus with secondary spread to the walls of the ventricles and subarachnoid space was postulated by Kment (1924) who found tuberculomas in the choroid plexus in 60 per cent of cases. Other workers have found lesions in this site in a smaller proportion of cases (Beres and Metzler 39 per cent). In the writer's experience the choroid plexus

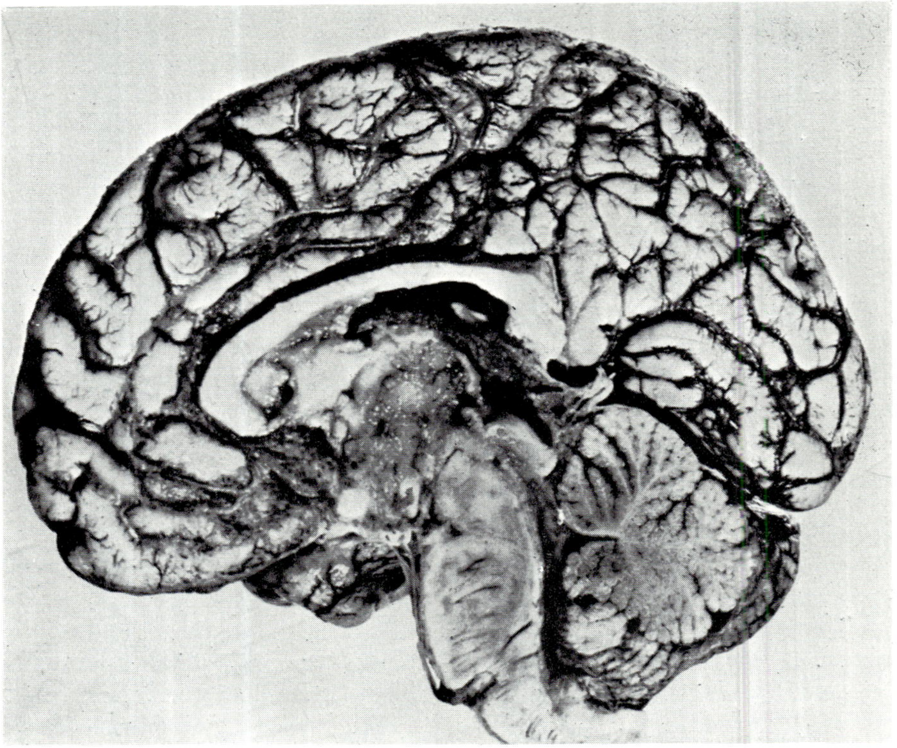

(*a*)

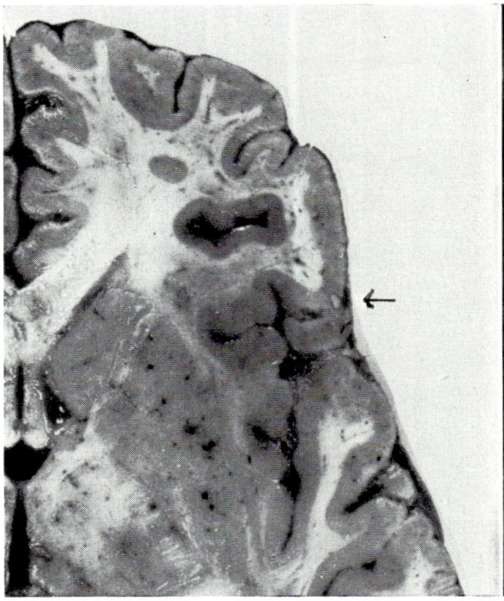

(*b*)

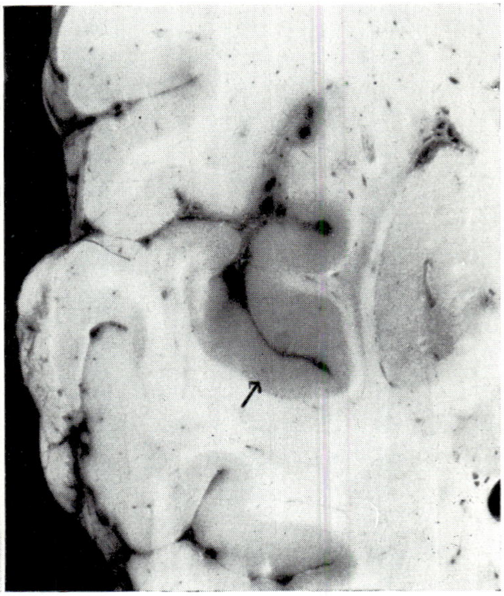

(*c*)

FIG. 3.2. Tuberculous meningitis.

(*a*) View of the mesial surface of the brain. The cisterna basalis is filled with exudate and glistening tubercles are seen on the walls of the dilated 3rd ventricle and septum pellucidum.

(*b*) and (*c*) Rich's foci in tuberculous meningitis. The arrows point to small recent tubercular foci on the surface of the cortex.

is frequently involved but usually with miliary tubercles which might be no older than the disease in the subarachnoid space.

Macroscopical appearance. The appearance of the brain of a case of tuberculous meningitis is usually typical (Fig. 3.2*a*). There is a diffuse greyish opacity of the meninges over the convexity of the hemispheres, and a greyish, gelatinous exudate fills the basal cistern and spreads out from this into the neighbouring parts of the subarachnoid space, covering the front of the pons. The membranes over the cisterna magna are also infiltrated and the dorsal surface of the spinal cord is covered by a gelatinous exudate which is often especially thick in the cervical

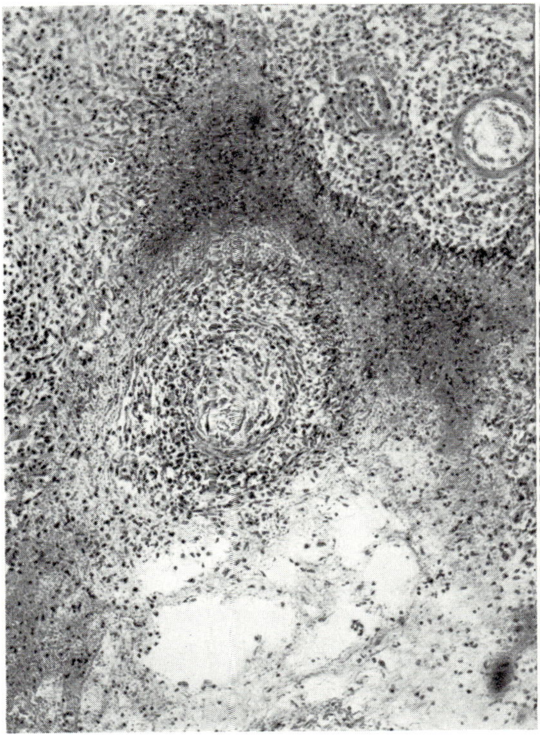

3.3

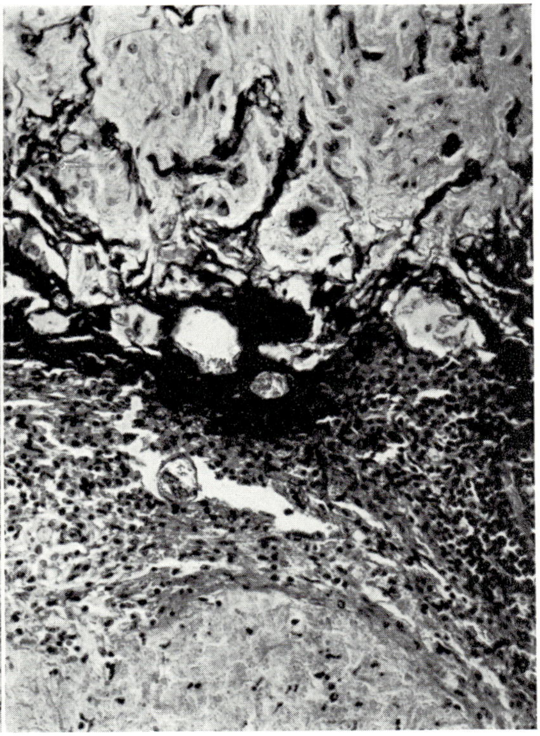

3.4

FIG. 3.3. Tuberculous meningitis, showing an area of caseation and a small inflamed and thrombosed meningeal artery. Note the absence of Langhans giant cells.

FIG. 3.4. Margin of a cerebellar tuberculoma. Zones of lymphocytic infiltration, collagenous fibrous tissue and neuroglial reaction with large irregular glial cells are seen round the caseated central mass (bottom of the photograph).

region. In this exudate individual tubercle nodules may not easily be seen. They are most common in the lips of the Sylvian fissures and near the pre- and post-central veins over the convexity of the hemispheres. They are also common on the inner surface of the dura mater covering the basi-sphenoid, or other part of the floor of the skull, and these may show the nature of the infection in cases in which the exudate looks more purulent. The amount of meningeal infiltration varies with the length of history of meningitis. In rare early cases it may be limited to a small area of the surface of the brain, sparing the base (Macgregor *et al.* 1935). In such cases it usually lies in the neighbourhood of a tuberculoma of the brain or meninges. On section of the brain the tissue is usually soft, especially that surrounding the lateral ventricles which are somewhat dilated.

Microscopically in cases which have lasted for a few weeks the meningeal exudate consists of lymphocytes, plasma cells and large histiocytes lying in a matrix of degenerated and partly caseated fibrin. Giant-celled tubercle nodules may be seen in this exudate, but are often scanty and may be absent. The degree of cellular exudate and of caseation varies from case to case. It is often concentrated around the meningeal vessels. *Myco. tuberculosis* may be abundant or scanty. In the latter case they are most often found in the tubercle nodules.

The meningeal arteries show inflammatory changes in the adventitia and media, and often also in the intima, or secondary proliferation of the intima may occur as in Heubner's arteritis (q.v.) (Fig. 3.3). These inflammatory changes both in arteries and veins may go on to fibrinoid necrosis or complete caseation. The resulting thrombosis leads to infarctions which may be superficial, but often involve the basal ganglia when the perforating vessels are involved. They are most often seen at the base of the brain and the lips of the Sylvian fissures (Smith and Daniel 1947). Elsewhere the outer layers of the cerebral cortex and some of the superficial folia of the cerebellum show microglial reaction, and there is usually some lymphocytic infiltration of the entering veins. Small tubercle nodules are not uncommonly seen in relation to these, but widespread involvement of the cortex is rare.

In streptomycin-treated cases, dying more than 10 weeks after the onset of the illness, the exudate is more fibrous and may be of woody hardness (Daniel 1949, Doniach 1949). It is especially thick round the base of the brain and the cisterna ambiens where it obstructs the circulation of cerebrospinal fluid and thus often leads to hydrocephalus. Lesions in the walls of the vessels, either at the base of the brain or in the Sylvian fissures, may cause anoxic changes or gross infarction, especially in the basal ganglia and hypothalamus; and many small foci of cortical necrosis, or tuberculous granulomata in all stages of activity and healing, may be found, especially in the depths of the sulci.

Cerebrospinal fluid

The importance of early diagnosis of cases of tuberculous meningitis has been greatly increased since the advent of streptomycin therapy. The typical cerebrospinal fluid in tuberculous meningitis is under increased pressure, often over 300 mm. It is clear or very slightly opalescent, and on standing forms a fine cobweb coagulum. The cell count is usually between 50 and 200 cells per cu. mm. and consists chiefly of lymphocytes with plasma cells and other large mononuclear cells; neutrophil leucocytes may also be present in considerable numbers. The total protein is only moderately increased in the early stages, but as the disease progresses it often exceeds 200 mg. per 100 ml. The glucose almost always falls to 20 or 30 mg. or lower but is rarely completely absent. The chlorides fall progressively and often very considerably so that levels below 600 mg. of NaCl are not uncommon. But in the early stages they may be in the region of 700 mg. They are therefore less reliable than the level of glucose. *Myco. tuberculosis* may be found either in the spread out coagulum or in slides made by scraping and drawing up the centrifugalised deposit with a Pasteur pipette (Greenfield and Carmichael 1925). The percentage of cases in which tubercle bacilli can be found varies with the technique and with care may exceed 90 per cent. Guinea-pig injection and culture of the deposit are even more reliable.

Meningeal permeability is greatly increased in tuberculous meningitis, and various tests for this have been devised. Permeability to bromide, as calculated by the ratio of serum/cerebrospinal fluid bromide after intravenous injection or ingestion of the sodium salt, has proved of great value both for diagnosis and in estimating the success of treatment (Taylor, Smith and Hunter 1954). In early tuberculous meningitis these authors found the ratio as low as 1 in half their cases and almost always below 1·3.

The chief diseases which may cause difficulty in differential diagnosis are various forms of meningo-encephalitis due to viruses, including poliomyelitis, cerebral abscess and subacute meningitis due to organisms other than *Myco. tuberculosis* (e.g. cryptococci). Virus meningitis and cerebral abscess are most easily distinguished by the normal level of glucose and usually of chlorides in these conditions, as also by the absence of the typical cobweb coagulum, although this may form in rare cases of poliomyelitis and other virus conditions. The bromide permeabilility in these conditions is only moderately increased, giving serum/cerebrospinal fluid ratios above 1·6. The nature of the cell count and the presence of organisms are the most valuable criteria in distinguishing tuberculous from other forms of ingravescent meningitis. But these very seldom come into question on clinical grounds.

Tuberculomas of the brain and spinal cord

Tuberculous granulomas used to be considered a very common form of intracranial tumour and are still far from rare, especially in areas where tuberculosis is rife. Garland and Armitage (1933) in Leeds found 89 cerebral tuberculomas in 13,000 consecutive autopsy records for the years 1910–31. Of these, 68 ended with tuberculous meningitis. In this series there were 288 other cases of tuberculous meningitis and 153 of other forms of cerebral tumour. Thus cerebral tuberculomas were present in 0·685 per cent of all autopsied cases and formed 33·8 per cent of all forms of intracranial tumour. Such high percentages are probably uncommon in the British Isles. The most common intracranial site for tuberculomas is the cerebellum. In the Leeds series cerebellar tuberculomas were present in 66 cases. They formed solitary masses in 24 of these and in a further 11 cases numerous small tuberculomas were found in the cerebellum and none elsewhere in the brain. The reason for this is not clear, since it cannot altogether be explained by the greater tendency of cerebellar masses to cause hydrocephalus and fatal increase of intracranial pressure. Cerebellar tuberculomas used to be considered as the commonest form of intracranial growth in children. The fact that they are now outnumbered by medulloblastomas and other tumours of the glioma group is probably due to the reduced incidence of tuberculosis in this age group. Supratentorial tuberculomas often cease to enlarge after a time and may become calcified, especially in their outer parts. Cerebellar masses probably less often become quiescent (Stewart 1927). Such masses may be visible on X-ray examination of the skull either as irregular opaque shadows or as rounded or oval shells with a well-defined outer margin. Evans and Courville (1938), in a series of 15,000 autopsies, found 43 cases of intracranial cerebral tuberculoma of which 3 (7 per cent) were calcified. This percentage would no doubt be higher in patients who survive with an intracranial tuberculoma. It is rather more common to find multiple than single intracerebral tuberculomas. They may form rounded or oval masses or may have a more lobular shape from the fusion of several smaller nodules. On section the centre is necrotic but firm and of a cream colour. Evans and Courville state that the centre is never caseous, but this depends on the definition of the word. The capsule, which may be from 1 mm. to 3 mm. in thickness, is grey, gelatinous and rather tough, and a narrow zone of greyish gliotic tissue is present around it; there is much less softening in this zone than in cerebral abscesses. A tuberculoma can often be separated almost cleanly from the brain tissue at operation, but before streptomycin was used this proceeding was almost constantly followed by tuberculous meningitis in cerebellar cases and very frequently also in supratentorial cases.

Tuberculous disease may extend into the spinal cord from the dura mater in cases of Pott's disease. Isolated tuberculomas within the parenchyma of the spinal cord are a rare cause of paraplegia. In this situation they are necessarily of small size. In occasional cases multiple masses within the spinal cord may be associated with multiple intracranial tuberculomas.

Microscopically the capsule of an intracerebral tuberculoma contains varying proportions of collagenous tissue and of giant-celled tubercle nodules. The capsule may vary considerably in thickness round different parts of the mass. Its contents have the usual necrotic appearance of caseous material, and external to it there is a zone of gliosis in which large spider-like astrocytes with thick processes are often found (Fig. 3.4). There is a varying amount of lymphocytic infiltration of the vessel walls in the neighbourhood. In old-standing cases the capsule becomes more collagenous and loses more or less completely its giant-celled nodules and other inflammatory infiltrations. At this stage calcospherites may be present in large numbers, especially in the outer parts of the necrotic centre, and bone may be formed in occasional cases.

SARCOIDOSIS

(*Schaumann's disease*)

Sarcoidosis has been recognised for many years as the most usual cause of the syndrome of uveoparotitis. In these cases the facial nerve is often involved in its course in or near the parotid gland. More recently a considerable number of cases have been reported in which sarcoidosis has affected the meninges, brain or spinal cord. Some of these cases have been associated with the syndrome of uveoparotitis, others with a spread of the disease to lungs, spleen or bones, but in a few there has been no evident disease outside the cranial cavity. As the disease is frequently self-limited, the diagnosis may rest on clinical evidence alone. For example, diabetes insipidus or papilloedema may appear as complications of the uveoparotid syndrome or of other evidence of sarcoidosis. In some such cases the diagnosis rests on a biopsy taken during a craniotomy (Colover 1948, Askanazy 1952), but in a few others full autopsy reports are available (Ross 1955). In the majority of these cases the disease has been localised in one of two situations: (1) the meninges, most often round the base of the brain and in the posterior fossa; (2) the infundibulum and the floor and anterior part of the walls of the third ventricle. The optic nerves and chiasma may also be invaded in these cases. Zollinger (1941) reported a case in which the Virchow-Robin spaces of the vessels in the basal ganglia and pons were distended with granuloma, but there was little invasion of the meninges, and Meyer *et al.* (1953) a similar perivascular invasion of the cerebral and cerebellar cortex with lesions in the overlying meninges. Askanazy (1952) reported a case in which the spinal cord at the upper thoracic level was infiltrated by granulomatous nodules with slighter meningeal lesions. He noted that giant cells may be small and scarce in the nervous tissue and that reticulin is not so abundant as in sarcoid lesions elsewhere in the body. The lesions are always closely related to blood vessels, and even within the brain may be confined in the Virchow-Robin spaces. Granulomas in the floor of the 3rd ventricle may not be recognised as sarcoid lesions unless more typical lesions are found in other organs.

The course of the intracranial disease is usually slow and there may be clinical remissions or arrest of progress, but some cases are fatal within a few weeks. When the disease is limited to the meninges the symptoms are usually those of hydrocephalus or cranial nerve palsies; Jacksonian epilepsy due to meningeal lesions near the vertex of the brain has been reported by Askanazy. When the infundibulum and floor of the 3rd ventricle are invaded there may be diabetes insipidus or other signs of damage to the hypothalamus. Direct invasion of the optic chiasma or nerves may lead to hemianopia or blindness.

LEPROSY

Leprosy has been recognised as an infectious disease since the causal organism, *Mycobacterium leprae*, was discovered by Hansen in 1874. But the failure to grow this organism outside the human body or to transmit the disease to laboratory animals has hindered the study of its pathogenesis. Analogies have, however, been drawn from experiments with rat leprosy due to the very similar *M. leprae murium*. Until the last few years knowledge of the pathology of leprosy has been based on the study of post-mortem material, but this has, more recently, been supplemented by biopsies of early cases and contacts (Khanolkar 1951, 1955). These studies and skin tests with lepromin have shown that infection with leprosy is much more wide-

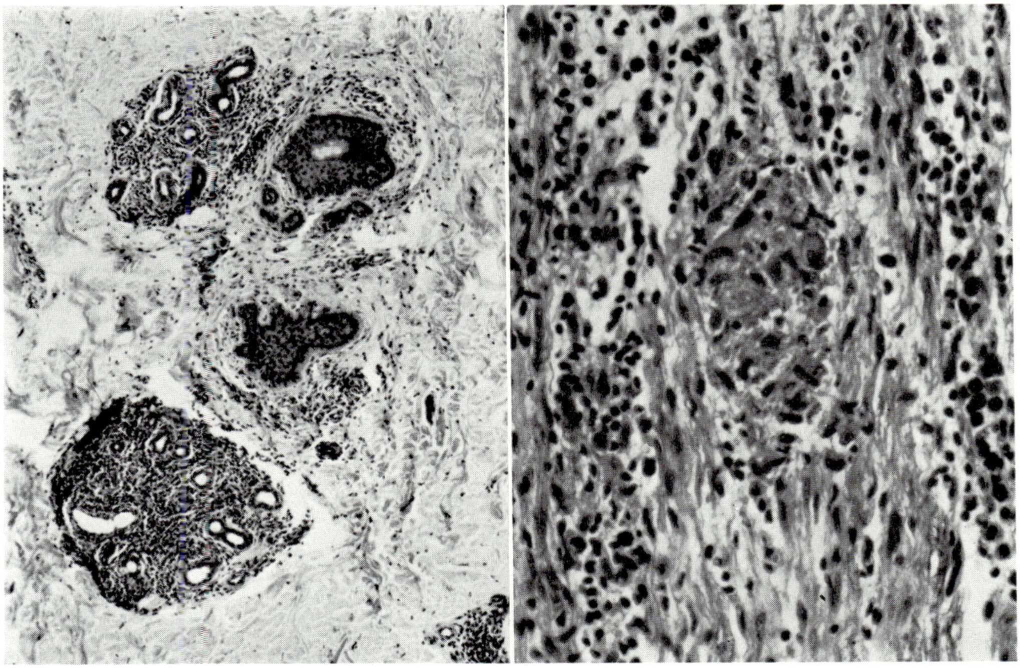

(*a*) (*b*)

FIG. 3.5. Leprosy.

(*a*) Small lepromatous nodules in the sweat glands of the skin. (H. and E. ×70.)
(*b*) Tuberculoid lesion of peripheral nerve showing rounded collections of epithelioid cells and lymphocytic infiltration. (H. and E. ×300.)

spread among contacts than had been supposed, but in many cases remains subclinical. Most lepers have been infected during childhood: the disease is very chronic and is subject to exacerbations and periods of quiescence corresponding to variations in the patient's resistance. In these respects leprosy shows a close resemblance to tuberculosis. Infection takes place through the skin or the mucous membranes of the nose and nasopharynx. Since in cases with ulcerative lesions of the nasal septum, which are not uncommon, the nasal discharge contains large numbers of bacilli, there are abundant opportunities for infection under poor hygienic conditions.

Pathology. The organisms *M. leprae* are slender bacilli about 4μ in length, acid-fast after staining with hot carbol fuchsin but less alcohol-fast than *M. tuberculosis*. They also have less tendency to appear beaded or as long forms. In the tissues they seem to multiply intracellularly and are commonly found in sheaves or bundles in large epithelioid cells (lepra cells). They also may be seen in the tissues massed in rounded or oval spaces up to 100μ in diameter. These collections, which are called 'globi', may result from multiplication of organisms in giant cells which are eventually destroyed or from their collection in lymphatics or tissue spaces (Koppisch 1953).

Two main types of leprosy are recognised, the *lepromatous* or *nodular type* and the *neural, maculo-anaesthetic* or *tuberculoid* type. These are often combined, with preponderance of one or the other type of lesion. Recent work has shown that the initial stages of both types are essentially the same (Khanolkar 1951). As seen in contacts and very early cases in childhood the infection is confined to the sheaths of the small nerves in the dermis where there are foci of infiltration with lymphocytes, histiocytes and a few epithelioid cells. Sparse bacilli may be found in or around the nerve fibres or in the cellular exudate in their neighbourhood. From this earliest stage the disease may progress either to form subcutaneous granulomas (lepromatous form) or to spread up the nerves (neural or maculo-anaesthetic form). In the former case the granulomas begin around the nerves and the sweat and sebaceous glands (Fig. 3.5*a*) but they soon destroy the nerve fibres and for this reason are often described as perivascular. In the early stages of lepromatous lesions cellular exudate is slight but numerous bacilli may be seen both in the axonal space and as clusters in the cytoplasm of Schwann cells. Later they may burst out from these and spread into the surrounding tissues. Lymphocytes, plasma cells and large endothelial cells then appear and, along with fibroblasts, form rounded or trabecular granulomas in the dermis and subcutaneous tissues. Even when these become larger and more solid, they usually spare a thin layer of connective tissue under the epidermis. In chronic lesions the infiltration with small mononuclear cells becomes less and the majority of the cells filling the connective tissue network are lepra cells. These are large oval, mono- or binucleated cells filled with bacilli. Some of the larger cells are vacuolated.

Subcutaneous nodules of this kind are characteristically seen on the face and ears, where they produce the well-known leonine facies, and on the extensor surfaces of the limbs. They also occur under the mucosa of the nose, throat and larynx; those on the nasal septum often ulcerate discharging large numbers of bacilli. Cutaneous ulcers may also occur. The lymph nodes related to infected areas of skin, especially the inguinal nodes, are infiltrated with lepra cells and in post-mortem examinations collections of these cells are commonly found also in the liver, spleen and testes. Diagnosis during life may be made from nasal swabs or scrapings or by puncture or biopsy of swollen inguinal nodes. Biopsy of skin lesions, which are usually anaesthetic, may also be made. In this form of the disease the cutaneous lepromin reaction is usually negative.

In the *neural* or *maculo-anaesthetic* form the infection may be confined to the nerves or may be combined with less florid skin lesions. The posterior auricular, ulnar and peroneal nerves are said to be most often involved, but this may be because these nerves are most easily palpated, and can be felt as thickened, often nodular cords (Ash and Spitz 1945). In this form there are cutaneous areas of hypo- or hyper-pigmentation, but the skin has otherwise a normal texture and appearance. When dissected out the nerves usually show fusiform swellings along their course.

Histologically the peri- and endo-neurial sheaths are infiltrated with lymphocytes and plasma cells and small rounded collections of epithelioid cells, and occasional Langhans giant cells may also be seen (Fig. 3.5*b*). The lesions bear some resemblance to those of tuberculosis and for this reason are called *tuberculoid*. As in tubercle nodules bacilli may be scanty and difficult to find. Caseation is rare but occasionally a local swelling appears on a nerve and undergoes caseation and softening. The nerve fibres are destroyed early in this form of disease. The infection very gradually spreads up the nerves involving some motor as well as sensory fibres and producing fairly large areas of cutaneous anaesthesia and some amyotrophy. It may eventually reach the dorsal root ganglia where bacilli are sometimes seen distending the bodies of the nerve cells. Less often they are found also in the motor neurones of the spinal cord. Whether they reach the nerve cells by passing directly up their axons or less directly via endoneurial tissue spaces is not definitely known. Invasion of other parts of the central nervous system is very rare. As a result of the anaesthesia trophic ulcers may form on the extremities but these do not usually contain bacilli.

In this form of the disease the patient's resistance is relatively high, as is shown both by the paucity of bacilli in the lesions and by the lepromin skin reaction which is usually positive. The decision whether the disease assumes the nodular or the neural form appears, indeed, to depend chiefly on the immunity of the host. When this is low the bacilli, which at first multiply in, or in close relation to, the nerve fibres, burst out from these into the surrounding tissues and are able to multiply in epithelioid cells, producing lepromatous nodules. If the immune reactions are strong the bacilli remain confined to the nerves where they appear to find a specially favourable site for their growth and where they may be protected to some extent from humoral action. In favour of the latter assumption Khanolkar (1951) instances the continued presence of bacilli in the nerves after prolonged and apparently successful sulphone treatment.

INFECTION BY FUNGI

The nervous system may be invaded by various fungi (1) either as part of a general infection, (2) along with involvement of lymph nodes or (3) as apparently the only site of infection. Although most of these organisms have a comparatively low virulence for the tissues of the body invasion of the brain is almost always fatal, since no effective therapy has been discovered. In a few cases surgery has brought about a cure, at least for some years.

The more important fungi which have been known to cause cerebrospinal disease are the yeast-like organisms *Cryptococcus neoformans*, *Coccidioides immitis*, *Histoplasma capsulatum* and *Blastomyces dermatidis*. A few cases of generalised infection with *Candida albicans* have ended fatally with widespread meningitis. Such cases have occurred most often, in recent years, following treatment by aureomycin or chloromycetin. A very few cases of *mucormycosis* of the central nervous system have also been described, some in diabetics. The mould may enter the blood-stream causing multiple thromboses and infarctions or may spread to the meninges from the orbit or nasopharynx.

Cryptococcus neoformans (Sanfelice 1896)

This pathogenic yeast has been given a number of different names of which that given above is the most generally accepted. The name *Cryptococcus hominis* (Vuillemin 1901, Benham 1934) indicates that the organism has been most commonly found as a cause of disease in man, but it was first isolated by Sanfelice in fermenting fruit juices and has since been found in the soil and in lesions in animals. Lodder (1934), after examining 26 strains, classed it as a *torulopsis* but more recent workers retain it among the *cryptococci*. The name *Torula histolytica* (Stoddard and Cutler 1916) was shown by Freeman (1931) to be incorrect as the organism has little tendency to destroy the tissues which it invades. It appears to be the only pathogenic cryptococcus, but several different antigenic strains have been described.

Cryptococcus neoformans is a round or oval body usually varying in diameter from 5μ to 15μ, although it may be as small as 1μ (Cox and Tolhurst 1946). It is surrounded by a thick polysaccharide capsule.

In culture occasional organisms develop short abortive germinal tubes, which have been mistaken for hyphae, but these are rarely seen in tissues or exudates (Moss and McQuown 1953). The organism increases by budding and does not form spores. The capsule consists of a complex mucoid polysaccharide containing xylose, mannose and glycuronic acid (Evans and Theriault 1953). The cryptococcus has little antigenic activity in animals unless the capsules are first removed, and the presence of the capsule may allow the organism to grow in the brain without exciting more than a minimal inflammatory reaction. Cryptococcus neoformans is pathogenic to mice and retains this virulence after prolonged sub-culture.

Although occasional cases in which the disease has been confined to the lungs or lymph nodes have been recognised, cryptococci most commonly cause serious symptoms by invading the central nervous system. The distribution of such cases has been almost world-wide. Several have been reported from England (Rose *et al.* 1958) and various continental countries, and one recently from India, but the great majority of cases have occurred in the more southern parts of the United States and in Australia where Cox and Tolhurst (1946) reported 13 personal cases and found that 8 other cases had been reported in that sub-continent. Mosberg and Arnold (1950) collected records of 172 cases, and many more have been reported since that date, but the disease has now become so well known that many recent cases have gone unrecorded. In the great majority of these cases the brain has been the most important site of infection, but in a few recent cases the disease appears to have been limited to the spinal cord (Lay, Jacas and Oliveras 1951, Carton and Mount 1951). In addition to the intracranial lesions, infections of the lungs, kidneys, lymph nodes or tonsils have been commonly found when looked for in fatal cases. In some cases enlarged lymph nodes removed at biopsy have been mistaken for Hodgkin's disease, but have later proved to contain the fungus. In other cases there seems to have been true Hodgkin's disease as well as cryptococcal infection. It appears probable, in most cases, that the fungus enters the body by the respiratory system, but in some invasion may take place through the skin (Greenfield, Martin and Moore 1938). There is no evidence of transmission from animals and the source of infection is unknown.

The cerebrospinal fluid varies greatly from case to case. In some there is a clear fluid with only a small excess of lymphocytes and protein, whereas in others the fluid is turbid and contains large numbers of lymphocytes; polymorphonuclear leucocytes may also be present. Cryptococci may be found on culture even when the cell count is low. With higher cell counts they are usually to be seen in the centrifugalised deposit or perhaps more easily in the counting chamber. They may be mistaken for lymphocytes in dried films unless the capsules are demonstrated by special techniques. When cryptococci are abundant their mucoid capsules make the fluid viscid. The protein varies greatly and may be normal or may rise to 500 mg. or more per 100 ml. The chlorides are usually reduced and the glucose is reduced or absent.

Pathological appearances. Naked eye examination of the brain shows a diffuse or more localised opacity of the meninges, with flattening of the convolutions and other evidences of increased intracranial pressure. The subarachnoid fluid is turbid, sometimes yellowish and often glairy and may make the surface slippery to the touch. Small tubercle-like granules or nodules, 2 or 3 mm. in diameter, may be seen especially in the interpeduncular space and in the sulci. On section of the brain cortical and subcortical lesions are commonly seen. Freeman classified them as *perivascular* or *embolic*, but it is not always easy to distinguish these two forms. *Perivascular lesions* are seen more often in the grey than the white matter. They appear as distensions of the perivascular spaces with mucoid material. In the cortex innumerable small cysts or flask-shaped cavities opening to the pial surface may be formed in this way. In the basal ganglia and sometimes in the white matter the lesions may follow the vessels for some distance as sleeves of mucoid material with localised cystic formations in places (Fig. 3.6*a*). *Embolic* lesions may appear as simple or multilobulated cysts. They are not uncommon especially in the cerebrum. Stevenson *et al.* (1950) described small single sub-

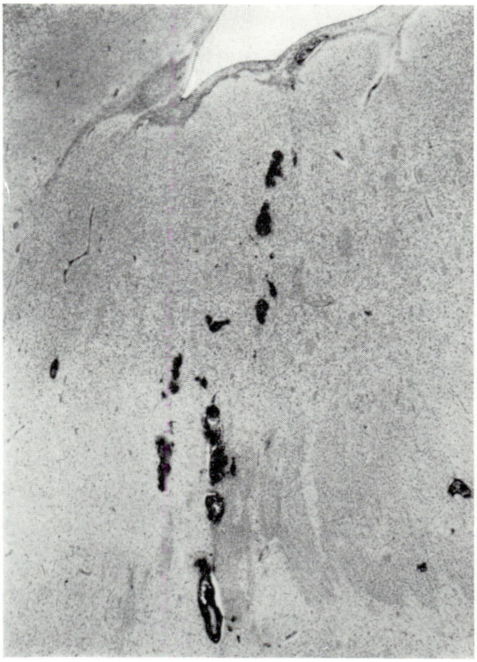

(*a*)

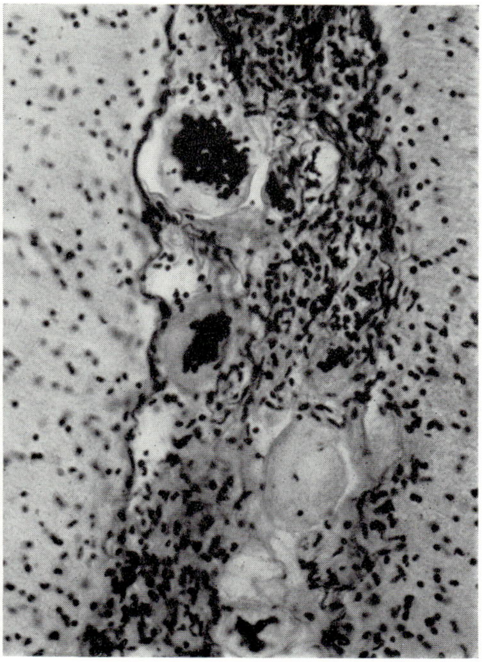

(*b*)

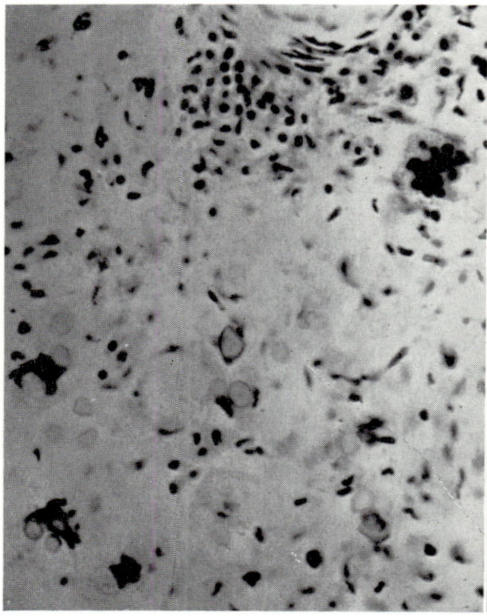

(*c*)

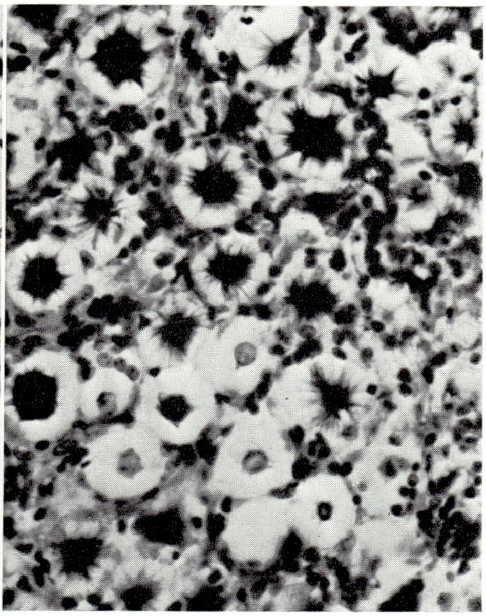

(*d*)

FIG. 3.6. Infection of the brain with *Cryptococcus neoformans*.

(*a*) Low power view showing granulomatous infiltration of the walls of subventricular veins. (Nissl.)

(*b*) Infiltration of the cerebellar meninges with lymphocytes and giant cells. (Haematoxylin van Gieson.)

(*c*) Area of invasion of the brain showing numerous cryptococci, some in giant cells. (Haematoxylin van Gieson.)

(*d*) Masses of cryptococci stained by Toluidin blue without differentiation. The spicules in the capsule are metachromatic mucopolysaccharides.

cortical cysts measuring 1 cm. or less in diameter as chance post-mortem findings in 3 cases, and larger, apparently single, cysts in the cerebellum or spinal cord have been found at operation. The cerebellar lesions are more often purely meningeal and granulomatous, but small cysts may form in the deeper sulci.

Histologically the *meningeal lesions* consist of an irregular granulomatous thickening of the meningeal tissues which are infiltrated by lymphocytes and occasional plasma cells. Multinucleated giant cells are also present in varying numbers (Fig. 3.6*b*). Their nuclei are usually more centrally placed than in typical Langhans cells and cryptococci, often without capsules, can often be seen in them. Capsulated cryptococci are scattered through the meninges either as isolated units or small collections. The solid masses of organisms seen in the intracerebral lesions are more rarely found in the meninges. The *perivascular intracerebral lesions* may be granulomatous like those of the meninges, or the Virchow-Robin spaces may be distended by capsulated cryptococci with less cellular exudate or may show fibrous tissue hyperplasia. Giant cells are sometimes abundant in these lesions. Although often confined to the Virchow-Robin spaces the cryptococci may break out and form solid masses in the surrounding cerebral tissue. The *embolic cysts* and *flask-shaped subcortical cysts* may contain little except masses of encapsulated organisms, which appear to push the surrounding tissues aside rather than to destroy them (Fig. 3.6*d*). Freeman has emphasised the paucity of fat granule cells or neuroglial reaction around these cysts. The cryptococci stain well with basic blue dyes, and when lightly stained show small dark granules near their surface. When more deeply stained the capsules often appear, owing to shrinkage artefacts, as radial spicules which stain metachromatically. They stain by the periodic-acid-Schiff (P.A.S.) method.

In the *lungs* the lesions may be either mucoid or granulomatous (Cox and Tolhurst). Occasionally lesions of broncho-pneumonic type may be seen. Caseation has not been found in human lesions. The *kidneys* also are commonly affected with small granulomatous or abscess-like lesions in cases with generalised cryptococcal infection. Lesions have also been reported in most of the other organs of the body, including the bone marrow. The spleen and lymph nodes are often enlarged and may have the histological appearances of Hodgkin's disease, even when they yield cryptococci on culture or animal inoculation.

Coccidioides immitis (Rixford and Gilchrist 1896)

This is classified by Moss and McQuown (1953) among the *fungi imperfecti* as it has no sexual cycle. It forms arthrospores which may be carried for a considerable distance by the wind, and thus gives rise to a dust-borne disease which infects a large proportion of the population in the semi-arid regions where it is endemic. In addition to the San Joaquin Valley of California, from which most of the serious cases have been reported, it appears to be endemic in parts of Arizona, New Mexico, Central West Texas and the Chaco district of the Argentine and Paraguay. Although it usually causes only a mild transient febrile infection, in a significant number of cases this is followed by a more chronic form of disease with granulomatous lesions in the lungs. Hence the disease may spread to the meninges or brain. It has been estimated that widespread lesions of this kind are 10 times more common among the negro and Mexican populations than among the white races. The organism also causes disease in cattle, sheep, dogs and rodents (Conant 1952, Egeberg 1954).

Within the cranial cavity it causes a granulomatous meningitis or more solid granulomas within the substance of the brain. The spinal cord may be involved either by similar meningeal lesions or by extradural granulomas arising from the bones of the spine (Rand 1930). Histologically the lesions closely resemble those of tuberculosis, but many of the giant cells contain the organisms which appear as large spherical bodies varying from 10μ to 80μ in diameter.

They have a double contour due to a thick highly refractile capsule and often contain a number of endospores. The diagnosis may occasionally be made by growing the organisms from the cerebrospinal fluid, but is more easily made by skin tests or complement fixation tests with the antigen, *coccidioidin*.

Blastomyces dermatidis (Gilchrist and Stokes)

This is a yeast-like fungus which appears in the tissues as rounded or oval bodies about 10–25μ in diameter, surrounded by a refractile capsule. Budding is frequently seen and distinguishes the fungus from coccidioides immitis. Blastomycosis occurs as a rather rare cause of skin lesions in the Northern States of America, especially in the neighbourhood of Chicago and in Caracas, Venezuela. Occasionally it causes systemic lesions especially in the lungs and bones; the brain and spinal cord are more rarely attacked. The brain or its meninges are most often infected by blood spread. This may also happen in the spinal cord, but in most cases paraplegia is due to compression of the spinal cord by an extradural granuloma arising in the vertebrae. A dumb-bell shaped granuloma partly in the spinal canal and partly in the thoracic cavity was described by Craig *et al.* (1940). Le Count (1909) forecast that cerebral lesions 'will undoubtedly be found in a considerable proportion of the systemic infections with blastomyces if they are carefully sought', but 30 years later Martin and Smith (1939) found only 16 cases in the literature.

Pathology. The lesions have considerable resemblance to those of tuberculosis, both macroscopically and microscopically. In the brain they may be confined to the meninges (Wilhelmj 1925) or there may be multiple nodules of varied size in the brain and cerebellum. The meningeal lesions may be diffuse or form a flattened granuloma resembling a *tuberculoma en plaque*, adherent both to the dura and the pia mater. In Gaspar's (1929) case a mass of this kind measured 6·5 cm. in diameter and 2 cm. in thickness. The intracerebral nodules may vary from a few millimetres to 1 cm. or more in diameter. Most of the smaller nodules occur in the cortex or at the junction of cortex and white matter.

Microscopically the granulomas consist of a collection of small nodules, joined by fibroblastic and fibrous tissue. The centres of the more recent nodules contain a collection of neutrophil and eosinophil leucocytes or pus cells, and groups of fungi are usually seen among these. In the larger nodules necrosis of this central core is more evident, but caseation is not seen. This core is surrounded by a zone of macrophages and fibroblasts, and one or more giant cells of Langhans type, often containing isolated fungi, are usually present in this zone. A denser wall of hyalinised connective tissue infiltrated with plasma cells is formed round the nodule. The older lesions consist of one or two giant cells which may contain fungi, lying in a nodule of connective tissue sparsely infiltrated by plasma cells. Gaspar found that the fungus was most easily demonstrated by Levaditi's silver impregnation.

Histoplasma capsulatum

Systemic infections by this fungus are not very uncommon in the Southern and Middle Western States of the U.S.A. and a number of cases have also been reported from Brazil, the Argentine, Panama, Southern Rhodesia and Australia. Occasional case reports have also come from Scandinavia, Germany and Austria. It has appeared in small epidemics in the Middle West States by infection from mines, cellars or towers some of which were full of pigeon droppings (Schwartz and Spitz 1952). Infection in such cases probably takes place by inhalation, as X-ray lesions appear in the lungs within 2 or 3 weeks after infection. Although widespread systemic infection is not rare, very few cases of involvement of the central nervous system have been reported. This may take the form of isolated granulomata in the brain or of more diffuse meningitis. In 23 fatal cases of histoplasmosis occurring in Tennessee, Sprofkin, Shapiro and Lux (1955) found invasion of the brain or its meninges in 6 cases and considered that a more careful examination of the brain in such cases would disclose a still larger percentage of infections.

They describe the exudate over the base of the brain as thick and yellow with occasional discrete greyish white opacities resembling tubercles along the lines of the vessels in the Sylvian fissure. Microscopically it consisted of large mononuclear phagocytes, lymphocytes and a few polymorphonuclear and plasma cells. It tended to form granulomas round the vessels in the meninges and spread along the vessel walls for a short distance into the brain. Neither they nor Schulz (1953) found any giant cells in the meninges. The organisms appeared as lightly staining basophilic structures measuring 2–5μ in diameter, ovoid, pyriform or crescentic, and surrounded by a clear halo. They filled many of the macrophages both free in the exudate and in the adventia of the vessels. They are well demonstrated by the P.A.S. method which stains their inner polysaccharide capsule but not the halo.

Mucormycosis

Infection of the cerebral meninges by the common mucors has been observed in a few cases of diabetes. In most of these a more or less localised meningitis has been caused by spread from an infected paranasal air sinus (Wolf and Cowen 1949) or via the veins from the nasopharynx. In the loose fibrinous exudate containing leucocytes and macrophages, numerous large branching non-septate hyphae are seen. These may spread into the cerebral cortex or by invasion of the walls or lumen of the blood-vessels may cause vascular thrombosis leading to extensive softening of the cerebral tissue (Kurrein 1954).

NEUROSYPHILIS

Syphilis loses nothing of its protean character when it attacks the central nervous system and the variety of lesions which it may produce there is rivalled by no other disease. The incidence of different types of neurosyphilis has changed during the last 40 years and certain forms such as tabes dorsalis and cerebral gummata have become much less common than they were in the early years of the century. This change was contemporary with, and probably due to, the introduction of treatment by arsenical drugs. The effects of penicillin treatment have not yet been fully assessed; but it has certainly made general paralysis and probably other forms of neurosyphilis more curable, so that fewer cases are likely to come to autopsy. But although becoming rarer neurosyphilis has not lost its interest to the neuropathologist, since many of the lesions which it produces are unusual and the pathogenesis of some is far from clear.

Primary and secondary stages

It is generally agreed that the meningeal spaces are invaded by the *Treponema pallidum* during the first two years after infection in a very large percentage of cases. There is much evidence to show that inflammatory changes are present in the cerebrospinal fluid during this stage of the disease in from 30 per cent to 60 per cent of all infected persons. This percentage varies with the adequacy of early treatment and the stage of infection at which it is begun. In some clinics early lumbar puncture is considered inadvisable owing to the supposed risk of encouraging meningeal invasion, and the statistics in these clinics are limited to cases in which lumbar puncture was performed after thorough early treatment. Under these circumstances the percentage of cases with abnormal fluids may fall to 13·9 per cent (Dattner). These figures are taken from days before large doses of penicillin were given in early treatment, and may well have been reduced at the present time. In the majority of cases the increase of cells and protein, which is found in the fluid at early lumbar puncture, disappears rapidly under treatment and does not reappear after this is terminated. It is probable that neurosyphilis is a rare sequel in such cases. In other patients the changes in the cerebrospinal fluid are less easily influenced by treatment, and, according to Ravaut (1934) these patients are candidates for the later forms of neurosyphilis. Moore and Hopkins (1930) and Dattner (1944) consider the type of alteration in the cerebrospinal fluid of more importance. Moore and Hopkins classify abnormal cerebrospinal fluids as (1) those with increased cell count and globulin but no serological changes, (2) cases with cell and protein excess and some other evidence of syphilis, and (3) those in which the Wassermann, Lange and other reactions are similar in character and intensity to those of general paralysis. In their view cases with changes of Type (3) are most likely to develop neurosyphilis, though it may occur in cases with changes of milder types. In their follow-up study they found that of 36 cases with fluids of Type (3) 33 per cent had developed neurosyphilis (7 general paralysis and 3 tabes dorsalis) and doubtful signs were found in a further 39 per cent, whereas of 87 cases with fluids of Types (1) and (2) neurosyphilis had developed in only 8 per cent and a further 27·5 per cent showed doubtful signs. Dattner has collected evidence which shows that neurosyphilis is a more common sequela, and follows infection at a shorter interval, in patients who have received inadequate early treatment than in those who have had none.

This invasion of the meninges during the secondary or latent stage is usually clinically silent. But in a small number of cases meningeal symptoms such as headache and drowsiness or amaurosis, often associated with papilloedema, or cranial nerve palsies or hemiplegia may appear abruptly. In such cases the cerebrospinal fluid shows clear evidence of inflammation, usually containing several hundred cells per cubic millimetre and giving strongly positive globulin and Wassermann reactions (Merritt, Adams and Solomon (1946)). Moore (1929) in a follow-up study of 28 cases with 'neuro-recurrences' of this kind found that they were especially prone to develop some form of neurosyphilis after a comparatively short interval. Fifty per cent of cases, in which he considered that treatment had been inadequate, had developed tabes or meningovascular syphilis and 30 per cent of well-treated cases had general paralysis, tabes or other form of neurosyphilis. In most of these cases signs of the disease had appeared within 5 years of the neuro-recurrence.

In a few cases which have come to post-mortem during the neuro-recurrence a more or less widespread infiltration of the meninges with lymphocytes and sparse plasma cells has been found. Pette (1924), in 3 cases found diffuse meningitis which was greatest over the base of the brain, cerebellum, brain stem and cervical cord and less over the cerebral cortex and lumbar cord. The infiltration, which was chiefly lymphocytic, followed the vessels into the brain stem and spinal cord as thick cuffs, chiefly confined in the Virchow-Robin spaces. In one case the vessels of the corpus striatum and those under the walls of the ventricles were heavily infiltrated. In another there was infiltration and degeneration, going on to necrosis, of the media of some small meningeal vessels along with swelling and concentric proliferation of the intima; numerous treponemas were found in the walls of these vessels (Heubner's arteritis). Swelling of the cell bodies of astrocytes and microglial hyperplasia were seen in the subpial zone of the cerebral cortex, but no deeper lesions. In the spinal cord swollen-bodied astrocytes were more abundant; there were reactionary changes in the nerve cells of the ventral horns and some myelin degeneration around heavily infiltrated vessels in the dorsal and lateral columns. In a case with amaurosis and papilloedema Buzzard and Greenfield (1921) found heavy lymphocytic infiltration of the connective tissue septa and meninges of the optic nerve. In other cases temporary visual impairment with or without papilloedema may be due to hydrocephalus.

Tertiary neurosyphilis

The later forms of neurosyphilis are usually divided into (1) meningovascular and (2) parenchymatous, which includes general paralysis and tabes dorsalis. All types of neurosyphilis have certain features in common such as thickening of meninges and lymphocytic infiltration of these and of the perivascular spaces of small vessels. But in other ways there is a remarkable histological distinction between the meningovascular and parenchymatous types. Thus gummata and the grosser forms of cerebral vascular disease are very rare in cases of parenchymatous neurosyphilis, whereas the typical parenchymatous lesions of the cerebral cortex or posterior columns of the cord are rarely found in cases in which the lesions are chiefly meningovascular. It has been suggested that these differences depend on a difference in the local or general immunity reactions of the patient to the treponema. The lesions in meningovascular cases are essentially the same as those of tertiary syphilis elsewhere in the body and are often combined with such changes, whereas the diffuse exudative and inflammatory process in the cerebral cortex, and the abundance of viable organisms which can usually be found there in general paralysis, link the disease to the mucocutaneous lesions of the secondary stage. But these analogies with the secondary stage do not explain the concentration of the lesions of general paralysis in parts of the brain, such as the pre-frontal cortex and striatum, which are phylogenetically newest. Nor is syphilitic aortitis less commonly found in parenchymatous than in meningovascular cases. It seems clear, however, that in general paralysis there is less tendency than in other forms of late syphilis for the development of those immune reactions which kill off the majority of organisms and hedge in those that remain with dense connective tissue barriers. Dattner found that the absence of allergy, or 'anergy', in cases of general paralysis was of a more general character, since 80 per cent of cases failed to give a skin reaction to tuberculin which was positive in more than 80 per cent of the general population. Other evidence in the same direction is given by the fairly numerous cases in which miliary or larger gummata or ulcerations have appeared in general paralytics after treatment with malaria, which by destroying the treponema may stimulate immunity reactions.

The classification of tabes dorsalis among the parenchymatous forms of neurosyphilis is justified by the concentration of the lesions on the dorsal roots and columns. But although it shares with general paralysis certain characteristics such as absence of gummatous lesions, there are few other resemblances between the pathology of the two diseases. It is true that tabetic degeneration of the dorsal columns may be found in occasional cases of general paralysis, but it is the writer's experience that in most of the cases in which cerebral symptoms appear during the course of tabes, and which are often diagnosed clinically as taboparesis, the cerebral lesions are those of meningovascular syphilis. It is also recognised that primary optic atrophy is commonly associated with tabes dorsalis and sometimes with meningovascular syphilis, but rarely with otherwise uncomplicated general paralysis. It is, however, impossible to classify tabes dorsalis more exactly until its pathogenesis is better understood.

Meningovascular syphilis. As the name implies, meningovascular syphilis attacks the meninges and vessels primarily. The lesions which occur in the brain and spinal cord are as a rule secondary, but certain changes in the subpial zone of the cord and brain stem and in the floor of the fourth ventricle may be an exception to this. Tertiary syphilitic meningitis takes a great variety of forms which are to some extent separable both clinically and pathologically, although all kinds of grouping of lesions and transition forms between those of different kinds are found. In all forms there is widespread, often diffuse, thickening of the pia-arachnoid and infiltration of its meshes with lymphocytes and plasma cells. This is usually concentrated around the meningeal vessels and may follow their branches for a short distance into the brain and spinal cord along the Virchow-Robin spaces. The small meningeal vessels especially show thickening and infiltration of the adventitia and in some there is also intimal proliferation.

In the description which follows the various forms are treated separately, although it is recognised that they are no more than variants in distribution and concentration of the same type of lesion. Clinical symptomatology must also be taken into account in classifying these cases, since they usually come to autopsy owing to a different train of symptoms such as those of intracranial pressure or paraplegia.

Diffuse basal meningitis. The basal meningitis of the secondary stage may be carried over into the tertiary stage with increased fibrosis of the meninges and the formation of small, often miliary, gummata in them. A series of cases of this kind, in which death was due directly or indirectly to hydrocephalus, was reported by Greenfield and Stern (1932). They found the meninges around the fourth ventricle to be so thickened and felted that in most cases the foramina of exit of cerebrospinal fluid from the fourth ventricle were sealed off and the cisterna magna contained little or no fluid. The meningeal thickening was continued over the front of the pons to the cisterna basalis, but was less evident above this level. The basilar artery might

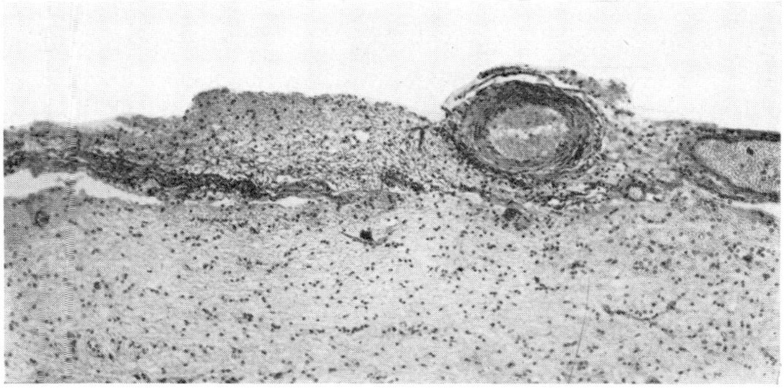

FIG. 3.7. Chronic meningovascular syphilis. Outgrowth of neuroglia through breaks in the pia mater on the ventral surface of the medulla.

be buried in a felt-work of thickened meninges. Firm white or greyish gummatous thickenings in the meninges were also seen, especially in the region of the acoustic nerve and over the front of the pons. On microscopic examination, giant-celled miliary gummata, which were scarcely visible to the naked eye, might be found in the thickened meninges and sometimes also in the superficial parts of the medulla and cerebellum. The floor of the fourth ventricle was covered over, especially towards its lower end, by an outgrowth of neuroglial cells and fibres and often also by a layer of fibroblastic and collagenous tissue, heavily infiltrated with lymphocytes and plasma cells. This formed a diffuse smooth pad which filled the calamus scriptorius, and in some cases covered the greater part of the floor of the ventricle (*vide* Fig. 1.15*b*). On naked-eye examination this did not appear at first sight to be much altered but had lost its glistening appearance. Small ependymal granulations, like those seen in general paralysis, were also seen in the upper and lateral parts of the floor of the ventricle and perivascular infiltration or miliary gummata might be found under the floor of the ventricle. A very characteristic lesion seen in these cases was an outgrowth of neuroglia into the subarachnoid space over the ventral surface of the medulla through irregular breaks in the thickened pia mater. Collagen strands were often intermingled with neuroglial fibres in these outgrowths (Fig. 3.7). This lesion has been described by a few other workers (Martin 1925, Lhermitte 1926). Both it and diffuse neuroglial overgrowth in the floor of the fourth ventricle are very characteristic of tertiary meningeal syphilis, especially when associated with basal meningitis, but they may also be found, especially in chronic cases, when the predominant lesions are in the spinal cord or over the convexity of the brain.

In cases of basal meningitis the meningeal thickening is often continued over the upper cervical segments but is usually less evident over the lower part of the spinal cord. The hydrocephalus may be of the communicating type, but in some cases the foramina of Luschka and Magendie seem to be completely covered by fibrous tissue.

In many such cases symptoms of hydrocephalus are associated with loss of vision due to papilloedema and secondary optic atrophy (Fig. 3.11*a*). The blindness in such cases should be distinguished from the so-called primary optic atrophy of syphilis although the two forms may be combined (Fig. 3.11*b*). Basal meningitis also often causes paralysis of cranial nerves especially the oculo-motor, abducens and acoustic.

Diffuse syphilitic spinal arachnoiditis usually involves principally the leptomeninges. It may reveal its presence by root symptoms and signs or by pressure effects. The nerve roots may be enclosed in small gummata or strangled by local thickening of the meninges. Pockets of cerebrospinal fluid may form in the subarachnoid space and cause local pressure effects on the spinal cord or occlusion of small vessels may cause local softenings. In more chronic cases diffuse degenerative lesions may be found in the spinal cord, which on macroscopic examination appears shrunken and has lost its firm consistency. In transverse sections of such cords there is general pallor of myelin staining along with a narrow zone of more complete destruction of myelinated fibres under the pia mater. This may be most evident in the ventrolateral columns but often surrounds the cord in what has been called a 'syphilitic halo'. Although it involves the fibres of the spinocerebellar tract it is clearly not a systemic degeneration as it passes around both the ventral and dorsal surfaces of the cord and often also along the lips of the ventro-median fissure. Some overgrowth of neuroglial fibres may be seen in this zone but there is seldom the dense sclerosis which might be expected from the amount of myelin loss. This marginal degeneration may be seen throughout the length of the cord as in Martin's case (1925), or may be most extensive in the cervical or thoracic segments. In cases associated with muscular atrophy, which is most often seen in the upper limbs, the corresponding ventral roots appear grey and atrophic and the ventral horns in the affected segments are also shrunken and have lost the majority of their motor neurones. Those that remain may be atrophic or show the peripheral type of chromatolysis. These lesions are often associated with hyaline changes in the walls of the intramedullary vessels. In some cases the vascular lesion may be severe enough to cause local ischaemic softenings in the cord, most often at the thoracic level. The classical picture of syphilitic meningomyelitis is a combination of these meningeal and vascular changes in which either may preponderate.

The pathogenesis of the more diffuse lesions is not clear. Merritt, Adams and Solomon (1946), in an early case of spastic paraplegia without amyotrophy, found heavy infiltration not only of the meninges but also along the vessels in the periphery of the cord. They considered that the syphilitic inflammation of the pia mater directly affected the more superficial parts of the cord. This seems more probable than theories which invoke constriction by thickened meninges or purely ischaemic effects since the meninges are not always greatly thickened and the peculiar peripheral distribution of the degeneration is not seen in vascular occlusions. Although atrophy of the ventral horns and roots is often combined with the characteristic sub-pial degeneration, it cannot be easily explained by the meningitis, which would be expected to damage the dorsal as severely as the ventral roots. In rare cases of *tabetic amyotrophy* the subpial zone of degeneration may be associated with the lesions of tabes dorsalis, but in many cases of syphilitic amyotrophy there is no systemic degeneration of the dorsal roots or columns.

Martin (1925), in whose cases of amyotrophic meningomyelitis changes in sensation were uncommon and when present were slight, suggested that the atrophy of the ventral horns and their neurones might well be ischaemic. The similarity of the atrophy in the ventral horns to that seen in cases of protruding cervical disc gives support to this hypothesis (Mair and Druckman 1953).

Pachymeningitis cervicalis hypertrophica. This name was given by Charcot and Joffroy (1869) to a fairly well-defined form of syphilitic disease of the spinal cord. It is somewhat confusing, as the inflammatory thickening is not confined to the dura mater and in the writer's experience is more evident in the pia arachnoid. In this condition the membranes over the cervical region of the cord form a thick sleeve, in which all three membranes are so united by dense fibrous adhesions that it is impossible to separate them. Its outer layer may be unduly adherent to the posterior common ligament of the vertebrae. Necrotic foci may be found in this gummatous thickening. The cord, to which the membranes are firmly adherent, is usually reduced in size but may be oedematous. The nerve roots passing through the thickened membranes are atrophied and the walls of the blood-vessels share in the fibrous thickening. As a result of vascular stasis and compression the white columns of the spinal cord undergo degeneration, which is usually greatest near the surface, and there is also atrophy of the grey matter and its neurones. This condition is now quite rare but several typical cases have been examined by the writer. It is not clear why in these, as in those of classical literature, the disease was much more evident at the cervical level of the cord than elsewhere. It was usually combined with diffuse letpomeningitis over the lower part of the cord and the base of the brain without involvement of the dura mater at either of these levels.

The symptomatology of pachymeningitis cervicalis hypertrophica was well described by older writers (Gowers 1899, Oppenheim 1911). It is closely related to the pathology, in that symptoms of paraplegia are associated with root pains or paraesthesiae in the upper limbs and with progressive amyotrophy in these or in the shoulders and neck. This may or may not be symmetrical. Areas of anaesthesia or analgesia may be found in the same segmental areas as the muscular wasting. As Gowers pointed out, the loss of skin sensibility differs from that of syringomyelia in affecting all modalities and in being less extensive than the muscular wasting.

Lumbar puncture, in cases of this kind, shows a complete spinal block and the spinal fluid contains a great excess of protein with some excess of cells and strong serological reactions for syphilis. It is probable that the cases on which Froin (1903) based his syndrome of massive coagulation and lymphocytosis in the cerebrospinal fluid had syphilitic lesions of this character.

Large meningeal gummata are now rare. They most often occur either over the convexity of the cerebrum or over the cerebellum, and are usually attached both to the dura mater and to the brain, in which they become embedded. More rarely gummata are confined to the dura mater and skull and produce cerebral symptoms by pressure. Similarly gummata involving the spinal cord usually grow from the leptomeninges and invade the tissue of the cord, but in some cases they are confined to the dura mater or grow from the vertebrae. Gummata of sufficient size to cause pressure symptoms may be associated with other smaller gummatous masses, and a few cases have been described of multiple meningeal gummata of the size of a pea or a bean. Such cases are now very rare, but it is not unusual, in cases of meningeal syphilis, to find small flat gummata resembling dense fibrous thickenings of the leptomeninges; these may be adherent to the dura mater.

Meningeal gummata are usually less sharply circumscribed than tuberculomata and the surrounding meninges are more diffusely thickened. On section they are tough, rubbery and often difficult to cut. The capsule is irregular in thickness and is continuous with fibrous trabeculae which run into or through the gumma. Caseous areas may be seen but do not constitute the greater part of the mass, as they do in tuberculomata. When gummata are embedded in the brain or cerebellum they are surrounded by a zone of oedematous softening which may extend for a considerable distance into the white matter. This may be to some extent ischaemic in origin, and may be determined by involvement of the meningeal veins and arteries in the syphilitic process. *Microscopically* they contain much more collagen than tuberculomas. There is considerable infiltration of the outer layers with lymphocytes and plasma cells; giant cells may also be seen; it is seldom possible to find treponemas. Lymphocytic infiltration of the Virchow-Robin spaces may be found in the surrounding nervous tissue, and there is always a widespread meningeal infiltration which may, however, have a rather focal distribution.

Syphilitic vascular disease

Lesions of the cerebral vessels of varied severity may accompany any form of neurosyphilis, but are most common in meningeal and gummatous forms. In some cases they are the chief

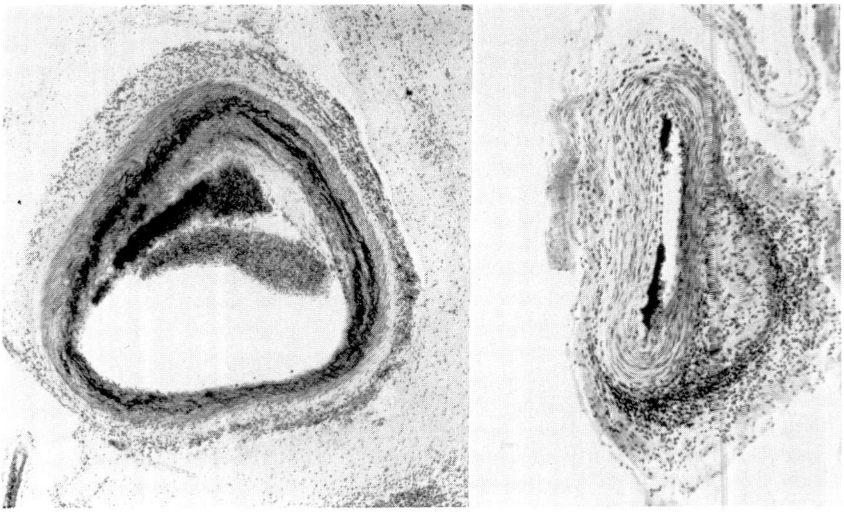

(*a*) (*b*)

FIG. 3.8. Syphilitic arteritis.

(*a*) Heubner's arteritis in a vessel on the surface of the cerebellum. There is infiltration and thickening of the adventitia, thinning of the media, reduplication of the elastica and proliferation of the intima. (Elastin.)

(*b*) A small gumma in the wall of the anterior spinal artery. (Haematoxylin van Gieson.)

cause of cerebral or spinal symptoms. Syphilis was at one time considered to be a common cause of cerebral vascular accidents, since a positive Wassermann reaction was found in a considerable proportion of such cases. In about half of these the cerebrospinal fluid was normal (Greenfield and Carmichael 1925). Syphilitic vascular disease is not now a common cause of cerebral thrombosis, and is a rare cause of cerebral haemorrhage.

The classical lesion of syphilis in the large and medium sized meningeal vessels was described by Heubner in 1874 and is often called *endarteritis obliterans*. It consists of a fibroblastic and eventually collagenous thickening of the intima, which is usually greater on one side of the vessel but may be concentric. This is associated with fibrosis or thinning of the media. The elastica is usually intact. There is an excess of fibrous tissue in the adventitia and lymphocytes and plasma cells infiltrate this coat and often penetrate into the media (Fig. 3.8*a*). In the larger vessels they may be most numerous round the vasa vasorum. Although it is usually called an endarteritis, the writer adheres to the view taken by Buzzard and Greenfield (1921) that the lesion is due in most cases to a primary inflammation of the middle and outer coats, to which the intimal thickening is, for the most part, secondary. The arteritis appears in fact to be due to an extension of the meningeal inflammation to the vessels which lie in the subarachnoid space. It is possible that this inflammation sometimes spreads inwards and directly stimulates the fibroblastic proliferation of the intima and, as in tuberculosis, inflammation of the intima may in some cases be the only early lesion. It follows from this view of the pathogenesis that Heubner's arteritis may result in weakening of the media and aneurysmal dilatation. When such syphilitic aneurysms form they are usually fusiform and are not so liable to rupture and cause haemorrhage as the small berry-like aneurysms which are commonly seen at the points of branching of the larger meningeal vessels. More often the encroachment of the thickened intima on the lumen of the vessel leads to ischaemia or thrombosis.

In the late stages the affected vessels appear firm and creamy white in colour. Although usually more widespread than the lesions of atheroma in the cerebral vessels, syphilitic arteritis rarely affects all the vessels in a uniform manner. In some cases the typical change may be seen only in some of the medium-sized vessels. At this stage lymphocytic infiltration may be scanty and the lesion may be most evident in the media and elastica.

Those with recent experience in syphilis vary greatly in their views as to whether syphilitic arteritis is a common or a rare condition. This may be due largely to differences in the interpretation of vascular lesions in syphilis. Certainly concentric thickening and fibrosis of the media and adventitia, with lymphocytic infiltration in and around the outer coat, is not uncommonly seen in vessels which lie in areas of thickened meninges, and similar thickening, which may go on to hyaline change in the media, is seen in the smaller meningeal vessels. The characteristic intimal thickening is much more rare. This may depend on the acuteness of the initial attack on the vessel walls, since if these are not weakened compensatory thickening of the intima is not so likely to occur. It may well be that the introduction of efficacious chemotherapy, by reducing the severity of the meningitis in the early stages of the disease, has made typical Heubner's arteritis much rarer than it was in the past.

Tabes dorsalis

The lesions in tabes dorsalis are concentrated on the dorsal roots and columns, most often at the lumbosacral and lower thoracic levels. In a typical case there is a moderate or slight, diffuse meningeal thickening which is greater over the dorsal than the ventral surface of the spinal cord. The dorsal roots of the lumbo-sacral enlargement are thin and grey and contrast with the normally thick, white ventral roots. The spinal cord is flattened from before backwards owing to shrinkage of the dorsal columns, which appear grey throughout their width especially in the lower part of the cord. At higher levels the funiculus gracilis may be more severely degenerated than the funiculus cuneatus. The dorsal root ganglia of the lumbar segments may be smaller than normal, but usually they show little change.

In early cases, transverse sections of the lumbar segments of the cord, stained for myelin, show a very characteristic pattern of degeneration. This was described by Charcot and Pierret (1871) and, although called in question by some later writers, has been the most common distribution in the early cases which have been examined by the writer during the last 40 years (Fig. 3.9). Pierret (1871) found the earliest degeneration in a bundle of fibres which passed ventro-medially along the inner border of the dorsal horn, and which he called the *ruban externe*. After Flechsig (1876) had described the zones in the dorsal columns in which myelination occurred at different stages of foetal development, it was realised that the *bandelette of Pierret* corresponded to the outer part of *Flechsig's middle root zone*. Flechsig's view, that the fibres from this zone passed to the cells of Clarke's column, has been neither confirmed nor refuted by more recent work. The association, both in tabes dorsalis and Friedreich's ataxia, of predominantly ataxic symptoms with degeneration commencing in this zone, makes it probable that it carries proprioceptive impressions. In the lumbar segments Flechsig's middle root zone forms a wedge-shaped cap of rather large fibres, lying ventral to the superficial, lenticular, posterior root zone and separated both from the dorsal horns and to a less extent from the dorsal median septum by finer fibres probably of intrinsic origin. When degenerated

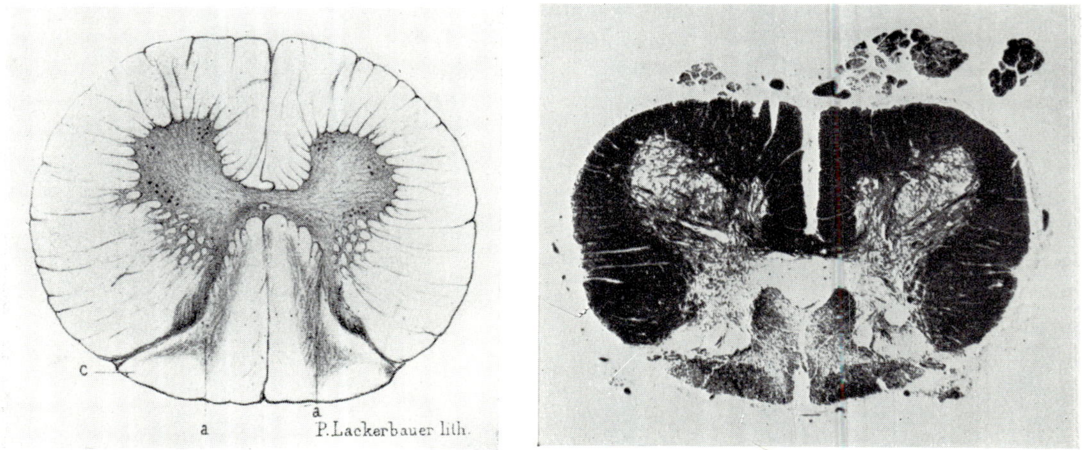

(*a*) (*b*)

FIG. 3.9. Tabes dorsalis.

(*a*) Drawing from Pierret's (1871) article showing sclerosis in *bandelette externe* in a case of cervical tabes (probably picro-carmine). (*b*) Section of lumbar cord in early tabes showing degeneration in the middle root zone. (Myelin.)

in both dorsal columns it forms an area shaped like a butterfly, or like a broad letter 'W'. On passing up the cord the fibres of this system disappear into the dorsal horns and their place is taken by fibres which enter by dorsal roots at higher levels. In the cervical region also degeneration in this system of fibres is often seen in the central part of the funiculus cuneatus in cases in which the upper limbs are involved in the disease (Fig. 3.9*a*).

In some cases degeneration appears as early in the posterior as in the middle root zone. Very rarely it appears to begin in the posterior root zone, but this arrangement is more usual in non-syphilitic, familial cases of trophic ulcers, the *hereditary sensory radicular neuropathy* of Denny-Brown (1951).

In later cases the posterior root zone degenerates and in long-standing cases the whole of the dorsal columns except a narrow *cornucommissural* zone, near the bases of the dorsal horns and the gray commissure, may become cleared of myelinated fibres and filled with a dense feltwork of fibrous neuroglia. On passing up the cord the degeneration becomes greatest in the funiculus gracilis and it may be confined to this tract at the cervical level. In early cases, in which the degeneration in the lumbar segments is almost confined to the middle root zone, the degeneration of the funiculus gracilis at the cervical level may be slight or even absent. In cases of *cervical tabes*, degeneration in the middle root zone of the funiculus cuneatus appears at this level and in occasional cases this funiculus may be severely degenerated.

Degeneration of dorsal roots is found to correspond closely to that in the dorsal columns but in the early stages it is less obvious. It has been frequently observed, in sections stained for myelin, that the dorsal root fibres become less deeply stained on passing through the pia mater. This has been described as the *zone of paling*. It is, however, difficult to be certain whether there is in early tabes a greater disparity than normal between the staining of myelin sheaths external to and internal to the pia mater, or whether the scarcity of large myelinated fibres in this disease makes a normal difference more evident. In later cases or those with severe and rapid onset of symptoms, there may be degeneration of a large proportion of the fibres in the dorsal roots, especially those of larger calibre.

Lesions in the dorsal root ganglia are less definite. They were denied by many of the early workers and do not appear to be at all commensurate with the degeneration in the dorsal roots and columns. But atrophic cells may be found in the lumbar ganglia in severe cases; it is probable that some also have disappeared, but shrinkage of the ganglia makes it difficult to assess the degree of cell loss. Stern (1929) found very little lymphocytic infiltration or other evidence of inflammation in the dorsal root ganglia of her cases.

Lymphocytic and plasma-celled infiltration of the leptomeninges varies greatly in intensity from case to case. Perivascular infiltration within the cord is also common and is not limited to the degenerated tracts. The meningeal vessels in early cases usually show little change except lymphocytic infiltration and some thickening of the adventitia. In cases of longer standing this adventitial thickening, as well as the fibrous thickening of the pia-arachnoid, often become more intense, while the cellular infiltrations may be less, especially in burnt out and well-treated cases. In cases of tabes with cranial nerve palsies, these nerves undergo a similar grey atrophy to that seen in the dorsal roots. The pathological basis of the Argyll-Robertson pupil is not clear, but it probably depends on degeneration of the ciliary ganglion or of its afferent nerves.

Pathogenesis. Various theories of the pathogenesis of tabes dorsalis have been put forward but none has gained general acceptance. The earlier writers considered that the disease began in the spinal cord but did not explain why the dorsal roots also underwent atrophy. Vulpian (1879) seems to have been the first to consider that the lesion in the dorsal roots was primary. Obersteiner and Redlich (1894–5) and Nageotte (1894) considered that both the symptomatology and pathology of tabes could be explained by an inflammatory lesion of the dorsal roots; but their localisation of the lesion differed widely. Obersteiner and Redlich placed the lesion at the site where the root pierces the pia mater. Emphasising the *zone of paling*, which has already been discussed, they considered that syphilitic thickening of the pia mater could strangle the nerve fibres and lead to their degeneration. Their theory did not, however, explain the absence of degeneration in the dorsal columns in meningovascular syphilis. Nageotte held that the main lesion was in what he called the *radicular nerve*, that is in that part of the spinal root which lies between the dorsal root ganglion and the subarachnoid space. In this part of its course the roots are covered by a dural sheath and by an extension into this of mesothelial cells which cover the arachnoid. Nageotte, at this point, found an interstitial radiculitis consisting of an infiltration of lymphocytes and plasma cells and what he considered as embryonic cells, along with fibrosis limited to the posterior root. He considered that the inflammatory changes in this situation varied from time to time and, when severe, damaged a certain number of dorsal root fibres, which were unable to regenerate since most of their course ran in the dorsal columns. If any fibres of the ventral roots were also damaged they were

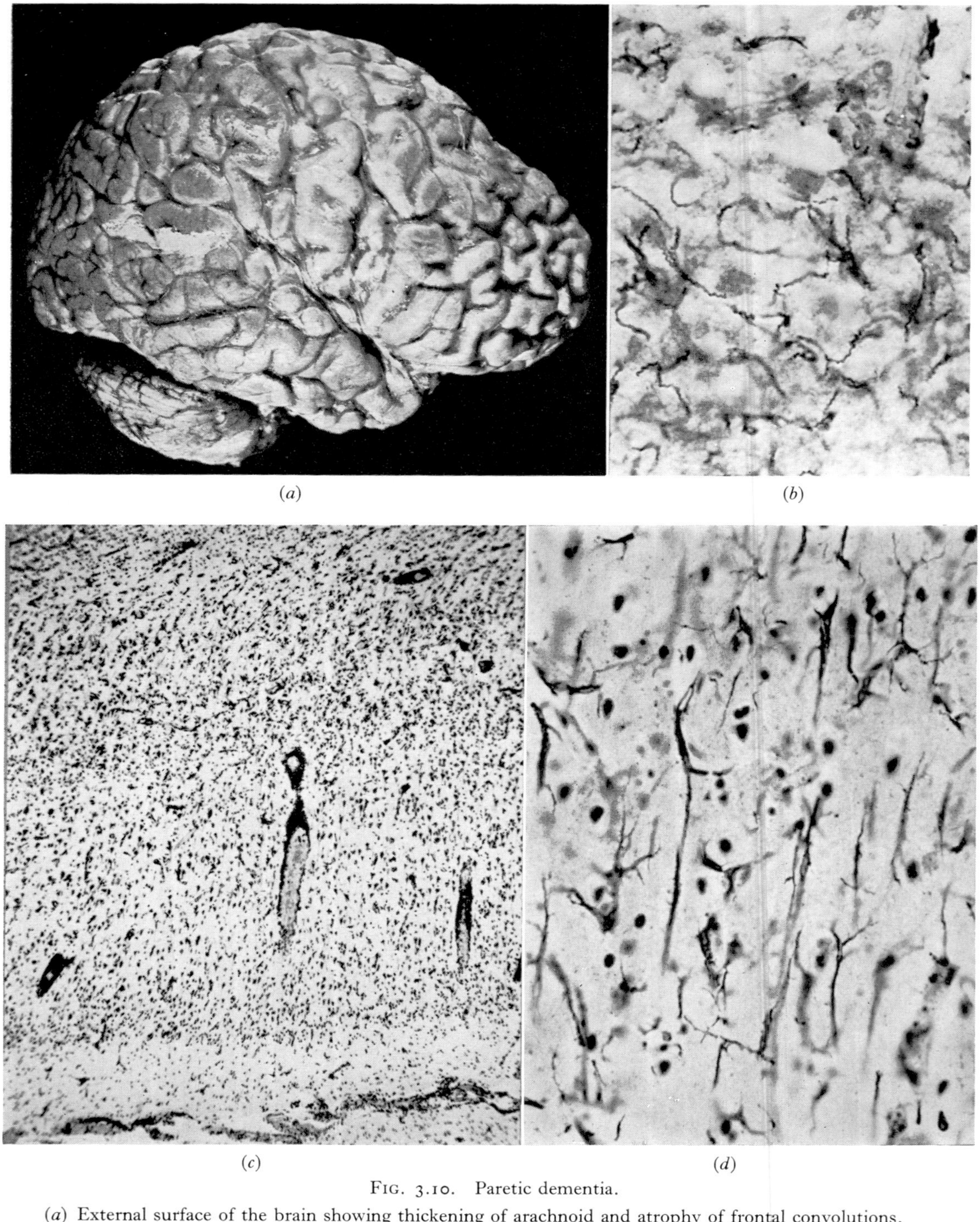

(*a*) (*b*)

(*c*) (*d*)

FIG. 3.10. Paretic dementia.

(*a*) External surface of the brain showing thickening of arachnoid and atrophy of frontal convolutions.
(*b*) Treponemas in cortex. (Jahnel's silver method.)
(*c*) Low power view of the cortex showing loss of definition of the cell layers and perivascular infiltration. (Nissl ×50.)
(*d*) Rod-cell forms of microglia. (Silver carbonate, ×400.)

capable of regeneration, as the degenerated segment was in them peripheral. This theory was later supported by Richter (1921–4) who held that spirochaetes settled down in the *radicular nerve* and there produced a specific type of granulation tissue. This spread into the interstices of the nerve and was later replaced by fibrous tissue which strangled the nerve fibres. The special type of granulation tissue which Richter described was recognised by Hassin (1929) and Stern (1929) as the normal mesothelial covering of the arachnoid. Stern found it to be as abundant, in relation to the radicular nerve, in cases of other spinal diseases as in those of tabes. Richter supported his theory by finding the treponema pallidum in the tissue around the radicular nerve in three out of nine cases of pure tabes and in one out of four cases of tabes associated with spinal syphilis. This finding was confirmed by Jahnel in one case, although Richter himself had been unsuccessful with Jahnel's method. Hassin and Stern confirmed the presence of lymphocytic infiltration, both intradural and extradural, and of dural and slighter interstitial fibrosis in the radicular nerves, but they disagreed with Richter's interpretation and especially with his description of the arachnoidal cap cells as granulation tissue. While therefore it is possible to accept the Nageotte-Richter lesion of the radicular nerve as playing some part in the pathogenesis of tabes dorsalis, the limitation of the disease in almost every case to the dorsal component of the nerve and its special incidence on fibres going to the middle root zone are not easily explained.

Paretic dementia (*General paralysis of the insane*)

Paretic dementia has been a recognised form of insanity for more than 150 years, as it was described by Haslam of Bethlem Hospital (the 'Bedlam' of Shakespearian times) in 1798. The name *general paralysis of the insane* was given to the disease by Calmeil in 1826. Its relation to syphilis was suspected by Esmarch and Jessen (1854) but was not fully confirmed until the introduction of the Wassermann reaction. Noguchi and Moore (1913) by finding treponema in the cortex of general paralytics provided the final proof that the disease was a direct result of syphilitic infection of the brain.

When a patient dies demented after several years of illness the brain presents a very typical appearance. It is shrunken and firmer than normal and is covered with opaque, thickened pia-arachnoid (Fig. 3.10*a*). This thickening partly conceals a convolutional atrophy and, like it, is usually most evident in the frontal lobes and temporal poles, diminishing on passing towards the occipital poles. The pia-arachnoid is unduly adherent to the cortex, and if an attempt is made to strip it small pits and tears are left in the cortical surface. The vessels may be generally thickened, but are not always much altered. There is considerable dilatation of the lateral ventricles and the ependyma, especially of the frontal horns and the 3rd and 4th ventricles, presents a coarsely granular appearance due to the presence of innumerable fine projections on its surface (*vide* Fig. 1.15*a*). These are most evident near the foramen of Monro and in the floor of the 4th ventricle. In old descriptions the dura mater was said to be greatly thickened, containing on section several brownish layers of altered blood. This *pachymeningitis haemorrhagica* appears to have been due to repeated head injuries and is now seldom seen in Great Britain. Abnormal adhesion of the dura mater to the bone has also been described, but this is too common as a post-mortem finding to be significant.

Many cases of general paralysis, however, come to autopsy for various reasons at much earlier stages of the disease. In them the brain at first sight may show little abnormality. There may be slight opacity of the leptomeninges especially over the frontal poles, the base of the brain and the dorsal surface of the spinal cord. On careful examination ependymal granulations will usually be found in the floor of the 4th ventricle and near the foramina of Monro. Otherwise the brain may appear normal. There may be no alteration in the vessels at the base or in the size of the ventricles.

Microscopical examination, at any stage of the disease, shows the lesions to be concentrated on the cerebral cortex, striatum and hypothalamus. In the cerebral cortex the lesions, like the meningeal thickening, are most intense in the pre-frontal cortex, and diminish on passing toward the occipital pole, but they often vary greatly in intensity in different areas. All the cellular elements of the cortex, neurones, neuroglia, microglia, blood-vessels and meninges, are involved in the process. With low magnifications the most obvious change is loss of the cortical architecture so that the different layers cannot easily be distinguished (Fig. 3.10*c*). Examination with higher magnifications shows this to be due to loss of many nerve cells, shrinkage and degeneration of others, and increase in the number of the nuclei of astrocytes and microglial cells. There is also thickening of the walls of the small vessels, many of which contain a single ring of plasma cells in their Virchow-Robin spaces. Heavier cuffs of lymphocytes and plasma cells may be seen round many of the larger cortical venules.

With special stains further details of the lesion can be made out. Many of the nerve cells are sclerotic with hyperchromic nuclei and corkscrew-like apical dendrites. The protoplasmic astrocytes of the deeper cortical layers are not only more numerous, but their processes are thickened and Ranvier-Weigert fibres appear in some of the foot-plate processes. There is also thickening of the subpial layer of fibrous neuroglia, and from this layer neuroglial fibres pass inwards in the outer cortical layers for a varying distance.

The changes in the microglia are even more characteristic. These cells are increased both in number and in size. The bipolar forms which normally are orientated perpendicularly to the surface, have proliferated and become greatly elongated; their nuclei also have increased to twice or more their normal length, and their cytoplasm is often visible, even with basic aniline dyes, for some distance at either pole of the nucleus (Fig. 3.10*a*). To this form of hypertrophic microglial cell Nissl gave the name *rod cell* (Stäbchenzell). Other forms of microglial cell are similarly enlarged and their nuclei tend to assume unusual trilobed or horseshoe forms. This microglial hyperplasia and the infiltration of many of the small cortical vessels with plasma cells and lymphocytes links paretic dementia to other forms of subacute encephalitis such as encephalitis lethargica or sleeping sickness due to Trypanosoma Gambiense. Even more characteristic of paretic dementia is the demonstration, by the Prussian blue or Turnbull's blue method, of unmasked or easily unmasked iron as fine granules in the cytoplasm of many of the microglial cells and in larger irregular masses in the walls of many cortical vessels. This iron-containing material does not stain with haematoxylin as does that which is commonly found in dead cortical nerve cells or in the walls of vessels in the globus pallidus. It may be difficult to demonstrate in the microglia in brains which have remained for some months in formalin, and for this reason Merritt, Adams and Solomon recommend fixation in alcohol. The vascular deposits are less soluble in watery fixatives, and are usually readily demonstrated even in brains which have remained in formalin for years.

The meningeal lesions in general paralysis differ from those of diffuse meningeal syphilis only in the larger proportion of plasma cells which they contain, but this varies from case to case. In some early cases, especially those dying in convulsive attacks, both meninges and cortical vessels may be very heavily infiltrated with cells, the majority of which are lymphocytes, whereas in more chronic or quiescent cases infiltrations may be very scanty in both situations. Heubner's arteritis is found in about a quarter of the cases (Galbraith 1938).

Lesions which are similar in all respects to those in the frontal cortex, but which may be less severe, are usually present in the striatum. No lesions except perivascular infiltration are usually found in the globus pallidus and the line of demarcation in this respect between the two nuclei is often quite striking. It has been suggested that striatal lesions are related to the tremor in the tongue and limbs, but Stern (1932) was unable to trace any correlation between their intensity and the degree of tremor observed during life. Neuronal degeneration, microglial hyperplasia and perivascular infiltration are also frequently present in the thalamus and hypothalamus. In some cases the thalamic lesions are confined to the neurones, and these may be secondary to cortical lesions.

The *Treponema pallidum* has been found in the cortex in a large proportion of cases of paretic dementia (Fig. 3.10*b*). Jahnel (1917, 1922), who studied a large number of brains with a selective silver technique, found that they usually adopted one of three patterns of distribution. (1) In some cases they were diffusely and sometimes rather sparsely scattered. (2) In other cases they occurred in dense local aggregations or swarms which in stained sections might be visible to the naked eye. (3) A perivascular distribution in which the treponemas were found chiefly in and around the cortical blood vessels was much rarer. Very occasionally treponemas have been found within the lumen of vessels but this probably only occurs after death (Jakob 1929). Treponemas have on rare occasions been found in almost every part of the brain but they are most abundant in the frontal cortex and if absent they are unlikely to be found elsewhere.

Ependymal granulations consist of small hummocks of neuroglial fibres containing a few astrocyte nuclei. They either raise the ependymal cells over them or more often break through their line and lie over those that remain. They are usually about 0·5–1 mm. at the base and rise 0·3–0·5 mm. above the level of the ependyma. Except for small-celled infiltration of underlying blood-vessels there is no evidence of inflammation either in or around these granulations and the term *granular ependymitis* which has sometimes been given to the lesion is to that extent a misnomer. In severe cases the median V of the 4th ventricle may be filled with neuroglial overgrowth, but the diffuse neuroglial pad which is common in chronic meningovascular syphilis is rare in paretic dementia. It seems probable that ependymal granulations are formed by the reaction of astrocytes to treponemas which have been deposited on the wall of the ventricle, but Stern (1932) was unable to find any organisms in them in her cases.

The effects of malarial treatment on the lesions of paretic dementia have been studied by a number of workers, all of whom agree that treponemas disappear rapidly after treatment has begun. Stern was able to find a few degenerated forms in the brain of 1 patient who died 16 days after inoculation with malaria, but none in 22 other cases so treated. They may, however, be present in large numbers in the brains of patients who relapse after a course of malarial therapy. Disagreement as to the effects of malarial treatment on the cortical lesions is due, no doubt, to the great variation in the intensity of these lesions before treatment was begun. There appears to be no doubt that there is a gradual or more rapid recession in the number of infiltrating lymphocytes and plasma cells without necessarily any alteration in the relative proportion of these cell types. There may be some shrinkage of the microglial cells but the neuronal and astrocytic changes appear for the most part to be irreversible. There is also a gradual recession in the amount of iron in the microglia and vascular adventitia (Galbraith 1938).

Few observations have been made on the histology of paretic brains after treatment with penicillin. Smith and Morais (1948) examined 2 cases of acquired and 2 of congenital paresis which came to autopsy within a few months after treatment with rather small doses had been begun (2·4 mega in 3 and 4·8 mega in the fourth). In the cases of acquired syphilis the inflammatory changes were comparatively mild, but in the congenital cases there was little reduction in their intensity. Iron was found round the vessels in all cases and in the microglia also in the congenital cases. No spirochaetes could be found in any of these cases.

Norman *et al.* (1959) examined a congenital case in whom the treatment appeared to have been sufficient to arrest the paretic process but not to eradicate the infection completely.

Pathogenesis. Paretic dementia has the histological features of a subacute encephalitis due to infection of the cortex and striatum with the spirochaete pallida. The meningeal and perivascular infiltrations, microglial and astrocytic hyperplasia and proliferation and the degeneration and disappearance of nerve cells are similar to those found in other forms of subacute or chronic encephalitis such as sleeping sickness due to Trypanosoma Gambiense and Dawson's subacute inclusion encephalitis. In the former the iron reaction in the cortex also resembles that seen in paretic brains. The concept of paretic dementia as a syphilitic encephalitis, however, leaves many of its special features unexplained. The local incidence on the frontal lobes and striatum with relative sparing of the occipital lobes and globus pallidus may be compared with that of Alzheimer's and Pick's forms of cortical atrophy, in which the newer areas phylogenetically and those which mature last tend to be specially affected. The damage to nerve cells in the cortex in paretic dementia may be considered as the direct effect of toxins emanating from the spirochaetes or as the result of narrowing of the small cortical vessels by endothelial proliferation (Merritt, Putnam and Campbell 1937). The clearing of the mental confusion which is seen after any treatment which kills the spirochaetes might be explained by either theory. But obvious reduction in the calibre of the cortical vessels is far from being constant and shows little correlation with the mental state.

Another problem concerns the presence of large numbers of spirochaetes in the cerebral cortex at a long interval after the original infection. This may be considered as a prolongation of the secondary stage of the disease in the brain alone. It is possible that any spirochaetes which gain access to the cerebral cortex during the early stages of the disease are protected by the blood-brain barrier from the processes of immunity which normally bring the secondary stage to an end. It has also been suggested (Dattner 1944) that patients with paretic dementia have less tendency to acquire allergic reactions than the general population. Whatever be the explanation it is evident that in paretic dementia there is either failure to produce neutralising or destructive antibodies, or, if these are formed, they fail to reach the spirochaetes. In spite of much investigation this problem still remains unsolved.

Lissauer's dementia paralytica

Lissauer (1901) described a rare form of general paralysis characterised clinically by epileptic or apoplectiform attacks followed by focal signs such as hemiplegia or aphasia. Pathologically, in addition to the usual appearances of general paralysis, there was severe atrophy of convolutions in one or both temporal lobes and the neighbouring parts of the parietal lobe. Merritt and Springlova (1932) studied 8 cases of this kind, two of which were caused by congenital syphilis. In their cases epilepsy was a constant early symptom and hemiplegia, aphasia, apraxia or hemianopia might follow as immediate sequelae, or come on more gradually. In some cases these focal signs were at first temporary but later became permanent. The course of the disease was more prolonged in their cases (7·9 years) than is usual in paretic dementia.

Post-mortem examination showed atrophy which was always greatest in the temporal lobes, but usually involved also the post-central, supra-marginal and angular gyri. In 6 of their 8 cases it was unilateral. The frontal lobes were involved in only 2 cases. The distribution of the atrophy differed from that of Pick's disease in not sparing the first temporal convolution or the cornu Ammonis, in being usually asymmetrical and in rarely involving the medial surface of the frontal pole.

Microscopically there was a pseudolaminar degeneration in the atrophic convolutions affecting chiefly the 2nd and 3rd layers and, where it was most severe, causing a *status spongiosus* of the cortex. Nerve cells with distended cell bodies, in which nucleus and Nissl granules were displaced to the periphery, were found in the 5th and 6th layers. They resembled the cells of

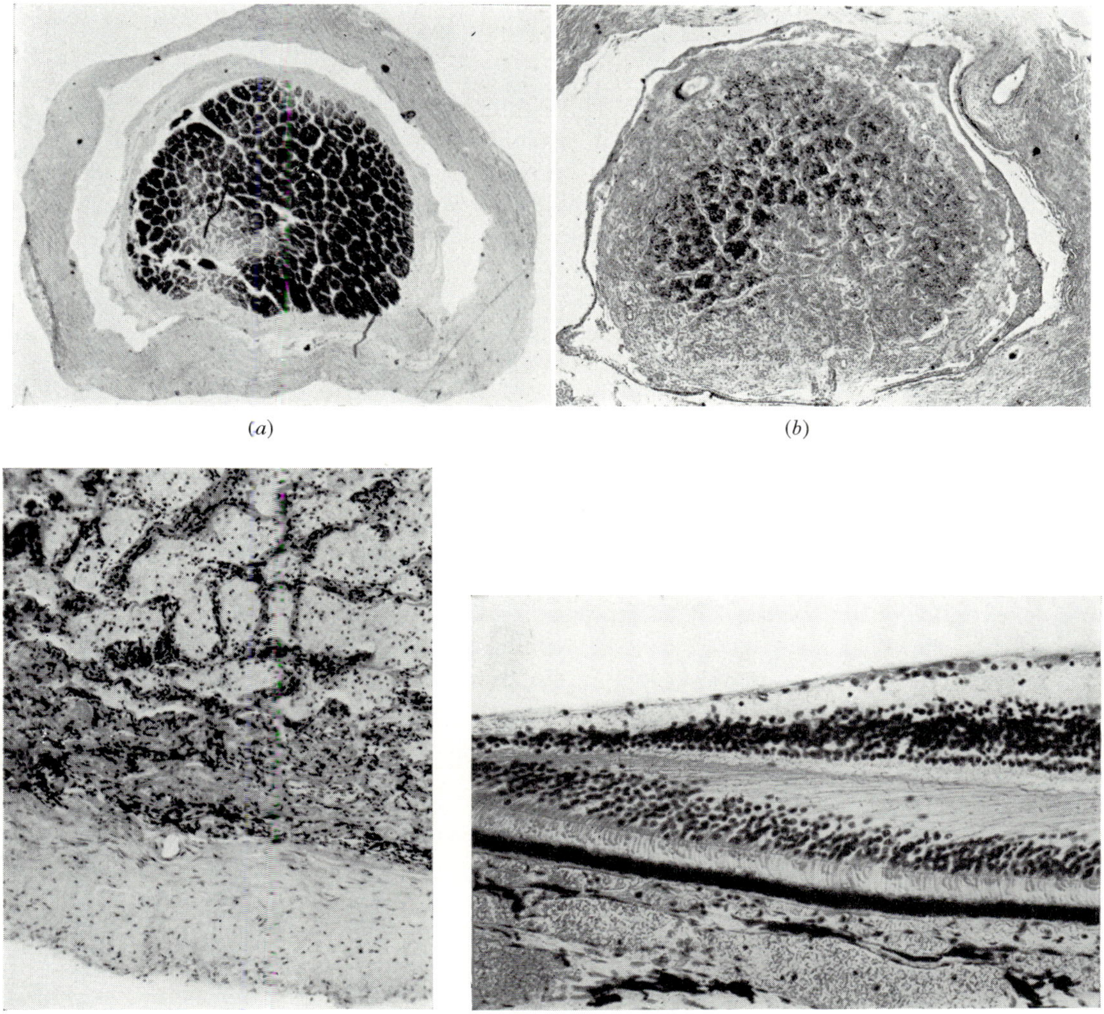

(*a*) (*b*)

(*c*) (*d*)

FIG. 3.11. Optic atrophy in syphilis.

(*a*) Central atrophy of the optic nerve secondary to syphilitic hydrocephalus. The arachnoid is thickened but not adherent to the dural sheath. (Myelin.)

(*b, c* and *d*) Syphilitic optic atrophy. (*b*) Section of the optic nerve showing relative sparing of the more central fibres. (W. P. carmine.) (*c*) Higher power view of the optic nerve showing fusion of dura and arachnoid membranes and lymphocytic infiltration of these and the connective tissue septa. (Haematoxylin van Gieson.) (*d*) Section of retina at the macula in chronic case with almost complete disappearance of nerve cells in the ganglion cell layer, but no other obvious change. (Haematoxylin van Gieson.)

Pick's disease but did not contain argyrophilic inclusions. Other nerve cells had undergone sclerotic changes. There was an increase in numbers and size of the protoplasmic astrocytes, and some formation of neuroglial fibres in the spongy areas. Although the usual exudative changes of general paralysis were present in the less damaged areas of cortex they were slight in the atrophic convolutions. Iron was not seen there, either in the microglia or in the walls of the blood-vessels, nor could treponemas be found. Degeneration of white matter was present under the areas of cortex showing status spongiosus and in small foci elsewhere. The pathogenesis of this lesion is not clear, but it may be related to the lobar or more local atrophies which sometimes follow repeated convulsive attacks.

Syphilitic optic atrophy

Syphilis may produce optic atrophy in several different ways.

(1) *Syphilitic hydrocephalus* and *cerebral gummas* may cause excess of intracranial pressure which leads to papilloedema and secondary optic atrophy. In some cases of hydrocephalus direct pressure on the chiasma and intracranial portions of the optic nerves may cause primary optic atrophy or there may be considerable loss of vision with slight papilloedema (Fig. 3.11*a*).

(2) The condition known as *optico-chiasmatic arachnoiditis* is occasionally due to syphilis. In it the optic chiasma and the intracranial portion of the optic nerves are surrounded by thickened pia-arachnoid. Pockets of fluid, collected in the meshes of this tissue, may compress the nerves or they may be stretched or pressed on by contraction of the fibrous tissue. In either case loss of vision, which is usually bilateral, comes on fairly rapidly, but in some cases there are periods of remission. Bitemporal hemianopia, horizontal field losses or central scotomata are common. The optic discs most often show a combination of papilloedema and optic atrophy.

(3) The classical *primary optic atrophy* of syphilis is often called *tabetic optic atrophy* as it is more often associated with tabes dorsalis than with other forms of neurosyphilis. It is rare in otherwise uncomplicated cases of general paralysis; it may accompany chronic meningo-vascular syphilis, or may be the sole clinical manifestation of neurosyphilis.

Until the end of the nineteenth century syphilitic optic atrophy was considered by most neurologists to be due to primary atrophy of the ganglion cells in the retina, with secondary degeneration of their fibres in the optic nerves. The work of Leri (1904) and Stargardt (1913), however, showed that the primary lesion was a chronic inflammation of the pia mater in the intracranial part of the nerve and the chiasma. They found lymphocytic and plasma-celled exudate concentrated around the vessels in this situation, with fibrous thickening of the meninges and intraneural septa. Leri laid great emphasis on the accompanying endo- and peri-arteritis and considered that the degeneration of the nerve was due to ischaemia. Stargardt found that inflammatory exudate into and around the nerve always preceded degeneration, but he did not think that either was secondary to the other; both, in his view, were directly caused by the treponema. At that time the organism had not been found in or around the nerve, but later Igersheimer (1921) demonstrated treponemas in the sheaths of the optic nerves in a large proportion of cases. Stargardt rarely found evidence of inflammation extending forwards from the optic foramen into the orbit or backwards to the optic tracts and external geniculate bodies.

This work has been fully confirmed by later workers. In long-standing cases there may be considerable fibrous thickening of the pia-arachnoid covering the intra-orbital part of the nerve, with adhesion of these membranes to the dural sheath. But the intraneural septa show little thickening and lymphocytic exudate is slight and usually confined to the neighbourhood of the optic foramen. The exudate is much more evident in the intracranial part of the nerve and may extend into it along the septa or the vessels (Fig. 3.11*c*). Degeneration of nerve fibres, in which the myelin sheaths are usually more severely damaged than the axons, is commonly greatest in the peripheral zone of the nerves, but is often eccentric or irregular; and the whole cross-section of the nerve usually stains poorly for myelin (Fig. 3.11*b*). The degeneration becomes less severe on passing towards the nerve head. It is associated with heavy fibrous gliosis. In the retina there is simple atrophy of many nerve cells, and others show chromatolysis, but even when the degeneration of the nerve appears complete near the chiasma many nerve cells may still be present in the retina (Leri) (Fig. 3.11*d*). There is little gliosis of the layers of nerve cells and fibres, and the outer retinal layers show no changes. In some cases a subpial zone of degeneration extends along the optic tracts (Greenfield and Epstein 1937). The resemblance of this subpial zone of degeneration to that seen in the spinal cord in cases of diffuse meningomyelitis suggests a similar pathogenesis.

Syphilitic optic atrophy often begins in one eye and may be far advanced in this eye before the other is affected. In most cases the progress is slow and vision may not be completely lost for some years. There is evidence that modern treatment may arrest the disease, at least in the earlier stages. The visual fields commonly show peripheral restriction which may be concentric or greater in the temporal fields. Quadrantic loss or hemianopia is less common and central scotomas are seldom if ever found (Paton 1922).

Congenital syphilis

Congenital syphilis may produce lesions in the central nervous system similar to those seen in the acquired disease. Hydrocephalus due to basal meningitis may occur in early infancy. General paralysis, when it occurs, does not usually show itself until towards the end of the first or during the second decade. Tabes is rare. The lesions of general paralysis, when due to congenital syphilis, are often very severe. They differ from those due to the acquired form in being more diffuse and in attacking the cerebellar cortex, often severely. There is considerable loss of Purkinje and granule cells and gross, often irregular, shrinkage of the cortex. A rather dense neuroglial overgrowth is seen throughout the cortex. In the molecular layer it is usually quite irregular, with little of the parallel orientation of fibres which is seen in the cortical glioses of adult life. Binucleated Purkinje cells are often found. They were at one time considered characteristic of congenital syphilis, but it is now recognised that they may occur when the cerebellum is involved at any age or any stage of the disease.

VIRUS DISEASES

Encephalitis or brain fever has been a common clinical diagnosis for several centuries, but knowledge of the aetiology of most forms has only been acquired during the last half-century. Epidemics of encephalitis may have occurred on the continent in 1580 (Schlafkrankheit) and in London in 1673–5 (Sydenham's *febris comatosa*). In the eighteenth century the names *schlafkrankheit*, *schlafsucht* and *febris comatosa* were given to many cases, some associated with influenza, others with malaria and some occurring in small epidemics. Clifton (1724) and Freind (1730) described encephalitis after smallpox and a case of temporary paraplegia following smallpox with a relapse a year later after measles was recorded by Lucas (1790).

Towards the end of the nineteenth century encephalitis was considered to be specially related to influenza. For example, the *nona* epidemics which occurred in Italy in 1890 and 1891 followed an epidemic of influenza. Von Economo (1931) considered that this was probably encephalitis lethargica. Other cases were more haemorrhagic and were called by Oppenheim *acute haemorrhagie encephalitis*. Strumpell (1891) described the pathological appearances in 2 such cases, and the name Strumpell's encephalitis was often used, during the next 25 years, for cases in which hemiplegia or diplegia followed a febrile illness in childhood. Although rabies, which had long been known to be related to the bites of rabid dogs, was shown by Pasteur in 1884 to be due to an invisible virus, a similar cause for other forms of encephalitis does not seem to have been suspected during the nineteenth century. As a rule pathologists tended to attribute them to a bacterial aetiology and *Haemophilus influenza* was often incriminated, especially during epidemics of influenza.

Cases of encephalomyelitis following the infectious diseases of childhood were also reported at the end of the nineteenth and in the early years of the twentieth century. Barlow and Penrose (1886) and Batten (1905) reported cases following measles and Collins and Armour (1912) a fatal case following mumps which, from the illustrations, was clearly of the perivascular, post-infectious type. Batten (1905) reported a series of cases with transient cerebellar symptomatology and (1910) stated that *influenzal meningitis*, by which he probably meant *benign lymphocytic meningitis*, might give rise to symptoms very similar to those of encephalitis. However, until the advent of encephalitis lethargica pathological descriptions of encephalitis were rare and, by modern criteria, unsatisfactory. The histological distinction between the primary and the post-infectious forms was not recognised until the numerous cases which followed vaccination during the years 1922–30 drew special attention to that form.

The demonstration by Landsteiner and Popper (1908–9) and by Flexner and Amos (1914) that poliomyelitis was due to a virus was undoubtedly a milestone in the conception of virus diseases of the nervous system. Clinicians and laboratory workers were thus prepared to recognise the viral origin of *encephalitis lethargica* when this disease appeared in 1917.

Since that time many forms of virus have been found to be pathogenic for the central nervous system of man. Some of these have given rise to serious epidemics or are still endemic in some parts of the world, while others, including some well-known forms of encephalitis in farm animals, have been responsible for isolated cases, sometimes only in those especially exposed to infection such as laboratory workers or veterinarians. Some of the common viruses such as psittacosis, mumps and the Coxsackie virus and the rarer virus of lymphocytic choriomeningitis have so low a virulence for the nervous system that they seldom cause more than transient meningeal symptoms. Attacks by such viruses are clinically grouped under the term *benign lymphocytic meningitis*.

Aetiology and pathogenesis

The nature of viruses and their affinity for nervous tissues. Viruses are generally considered to be the lowest form of life. They are always parasitic on higher living forms, e.g. bacteria or animal or vegetable cells. The viruses which cause encephalitis are of very varied size ranging from the very small virus of poliomyelitis (8–12mμ)* to the large virus of rabies (100–150mμ). The viruses of equine encephalomyelitis and Russian spring-summer (tickborne) encephalomyelitis occupy an intermediate position (15–30mμ).

Caspersson and Hydén have shown that viruses contain nucleoprotein in their structure. In the larger viruses, such as influenza and neurovaccinia, this is in the form of desoxyribosenucleic acid (DNA) whereas in the smaller viruses, such as poliomyelitis, equine encephalomyelitis and louping-ill, it is ribosenucleic acid (RNA). Hydén (1947) considers that viruses grow and reproduce themselves in the nucleus of the cell, in which he finds an excess of DNA in cells infected with rabies, and an excess of RNA, along with an increase in the size of the nucleolus, in cells infected with poliomyelitis and louping-ill. At the same time the nucleoproteins in the cytoplasm of the neurone are depleted resulting in chromatolysis. It is possible that some viruses such as rabies may migrate into the cytoplasm at a later stage and give rise there to intracytoplasmic bodies such as Negri bodies (Marinesco and Stroesco 1931).

Of the many classifications of viruses which have been suggested that of Weston Hurst (1936) is specially useful for those which attack the nervous system. He divided them into:

* Electron microscopy shows it to be rather larger, 25–30mμ (van Rooyen and Rhodes).

(1) *Neurotropic*; those which can parasitise and destroy nerve cells, but have little affinity for other tissue cells. (2) *Pantropic*; those which attack nerve cells directly, but have a much wider range of affinity and may produce obvious lesions elsewhere than in the nervous system. (3) *Viscerotropic*; those viruses which under normal conditions have no tendency to attack the brain. Many of them, however, may cause meningitis, and some can be made more neurotropic by passage from brain to brain in animals.

It must be recognised that no sharp line divides the characteristics of one group of viruses from those of another, and that the neurotropism of viruses varies from one animal species to another and can be altered under laboratory conditions. Rabies is the most characteristic of the stricter neurotropes, but as is well known this virus exists in considerable quantity in the saliva of infected animals and causes inflammatory lesions in the salivary glands. Poliomyelitis which, under laboratory conditions in macacus rhesus monkeys, tends to behave as a fairly strict neurotrope, in the natural infection in man causes enlargement of mesenteric lymph nodes and frequently myocarditis, and can be found in the faeces of patients and carriers. The distinction between a neurotropic and a pantropic virus is, however, well illustrated by contrasting poliomyelitis with the encephalomyocarditis group of viruses. In monkeys these may produce lesions in the spinal cord indistinguishable from poliomyelitis, but are as likely to cause death from myocarditis without lesions in the nervous system. In man they may cause transient meningo-encephalitis, but never permanent paralysis. They may, however, cause death from myocarditis (Koch 1950).

In the *pantropic* group the virus attacks and multiplies in various body tissues and in experimental work can usually be found in the blood at some stage after infection. In the great majority of infected animals the stage of systemic infection is not followed by any evidence of encephalitis. Many of these forms of virus are normally transmitted by the bite of insects. This would only be possible if the virus were present in considerable amount in the blood of the donor; it is extremely rare in poliomyelitis and unknown in rabies. The distinction between the *neurotropic* and *pantropic* groups is only one of degree, but is valid clinically as well as experimentally, in that the proportion of sub-clinical or non-nervous infections is much higher with viruses of pantropic character.

The *viscerotropic* viruses are known chiefly by their effects on organs outside the nervous system, which is rarely attacked. When nervous symptoms occur they are more often due to involvement of the meninges in 'aseptic' or 'benign lymphocytic' meningitis than to damage to the nervous parenchyma. But rare cases of acute encephalitis may be caused by viruses of this kind. For example the common virus of herpes simplex, which is normally parasitic on skin epithelium, but which on inoculation into the eye or the brain of rabbits produces severe encephalitis, may occasionally be the cause of an acute fatal encephalitis also in man or may cause mild transient nervous symptoms (Armstrong 1943, Alm 1951).

Among the many viruses which may cause benign lymphocytic meningitis that of mumps is probably the most common (Hammon 1949). Members of the psittacosis-lymphogranuloma-inguinale group, which are not always classed as viruses, and the Armstrong-Lillie virus of lymphocytic choriomeningitis may cause meningo-encephalitis which is sometimes fatal (Walton 1954). Louping-ill, pseudolymphocytic-choriomeningitis, Coxsackie and the encephalomyocarditis group are other viruses which have caused transient meningeal symptoms.

Viscerotropic viruses may, however, be responsible for acute reactions in the tissues of the brain and spinal cord to which the name *post-infectious* or *para-infectious encephalomyelopathy* is usually given. There is considerable evidence that these are of an allergic character, but the mechanisms of the reaction and the antigen which is responsible for it are so far unknown. Some viruses, for example that of mumps, may cause nervous symptoms by either method.

Epidemiology

Insect-borne epidemics of encephalitis are precipitated or brought to an end by variations in several factors.

(1) *The insect.* In the Saint Louis epidemics of 1933 and 1937 the epidemic was limited to a few weeks in the year from late July to early September. The fact that mosquitoes are most numerous during this period led to the discovery that *Culex tarsalis* and *Culex pipiens* could carry the disease. In addition to mosquitoes, the disease may be carried by ticks which may remain infective for some months, and the disease may spread among birds and mammals in this manner. Eastern and Western equine encephalomyelitis and Japanese B encephalitis have a similar seasonal incidence and may also be carried by mosquitoes. In tick-borne (Spring-summer) encephalitis in Russia the incidence is earlier and corresponds to the season when tick bites occur. Sabin considers that the most important cause of epidemics is the abundance of insect vectors, since many of these have occurred in years when the numbers of mosquitoes has been unusually large.

(2) *The animal reservoir.* These forms of encephalomyelitis are usually transmitted to man from birds or mammals. In the North American forms (Saint Louis and eastern and western equine E.M.) there is evidence that, in addition to horses and mules, both domestic and wild birds form the animal reservoir since anti-bodies have been found both to the Saint Louis and western equine virus in 50 per cent of domestic birds, and also in American robins (50 per cent) and owls (100 per cent). An equally high percentage of horses in an endemic area in the Western States was found to have immune bodies in their serum (Hammon *et al.* 1941). These figures indicate a high incidence of mild infections among susceptible animals. During the brief 1938 outbreak of eastern equine E.M. in New England States the virus was recovered from the brains of pigeons which died in the affected area (Fothergill and Dingle 1938). For Russian spring-summer encephalitis it has been shown that the human disease is endemic only in areas where there are many wild or domestic animals, and recent work suggests that rodents may be of special importance as intermediate hosts. In the small epidemic of Japanese B encephalitis in the Murray Valley of Australia in 1951 the evidence pointed to carriage of the virus to this area by migrating birds. But the part played by an animal reservoir in Japanese B encephalitis has not been so fully investigated as in the North American forms. As is well known an animal reservoir is the only source of human infection in rabies. In most instances the spread is through wolves or canines, but in Trinidad and South America the disease is transmitted to cattle by the bites of bats, and human cases have occurred in the same manner (Hurst and Pawan 1932).

(3) *Immunity in the human population and in the animal reservoir.* Sabin (1949) noted that a very large proportion of the population of certain districts of Korea and China have anti-bodies to Japanese B virus in their serum whereas clinical cases are almost unknown in these areas. This indicates a very wide spread of the disease in sub-clinical form. This is also known to occur in poliomyelitis in which the especial incidence in young children is probably due to the immunity of older children and adults as the results of sub-clinical attacks. A similar spread of immunity occurs among the birds and mammals which form the animal reservoir of a virus, but this is offset by a high birth-rate with the appearance of many young susceptible animals; and variations in the balance between these two factors may cause great variations in the proportions of immune and susceptible animals. Thus in the year following a severe epizootic the number of susceptible animals is likely to be small.

(4) *The phenomena of exaltation and interference in combination of viruses.* In 1932 MacLeod and Gordon investigating louping-ill in Scotland found that another tick-borne virus which caused only a non-lethal fever, was also infecting the flocks. Although this virus had no effect

on the nervous system, sheep infected by both this and the louping-ill virus were much more prone to develop nervous symptoms and die than those infected with louping-ill alone. To this form of interaction between viruses the name *exaltation of virulence* has been given. However, in relation to many viruses it has been found that the presence of one virus interferes with the virulence of infection by a second virus—the *phenomenon of interference*—and this appears to be more common than exaltation of virulence.

Routes of invasion of the central nervous system

The theory that neurotropic viruses travelled to the nervous system by the peripheral nerves goes back to the work of Roux (1888, 1889) in his work on rabies and was strongly supported by Nicolau, Nicolau and Galloway (1929) who found that Borna virus passed out of the central nervous system along the peripheral nerves after intracerebral injection. Fairbrother and Hurst (1930) found evidence that the virus of poliomyelitis commonly passed from one side of the brain to the opposite ventral horn of the lumbar cord, suggesting transmission by nerve tracts within the central nervous system rather than by cerebrospinal fluid. Howe and Bodian (1942) have suggested that the route taken is by the chain of neurones of the extrapyramidal system rather than the more direct corticospinal tract. They showed that monkeys could be regularly infected with poliomyelitis by immersing the cut end of the sciatic nerve in an emulsion of virus; in their experiments the spread of virus up the nerve was at about the rate of 2–4 mm. per hour with a latent period of about 11 hours. Using a strain of equine encephalomyelitis virus, the neurotropism of which had been raised by repeated intracerebral passage, King (1939) found that after intra-ocular injection the virus constantly travelled along the optic pathways, passing by the optic chiasma from the right optic nerve to the left visual cortex (48 hours). This was confirmed by Sabin (1949) in the mouse. But when an unmodified virus is inoculated into the pad of the foot in the guinea-pig, the distribution of lesions in the brain appears to be quite random, suggesting infection by the blood-stream. Sabin (1949) has found evidence that some viruses (e.g. pseudorabies) reach the central nervous system along the sympathetic and para-sympathetic nerves. These experiments and others indicate that the route by which viruses gain access to the central nervous system may be determined by the degree in which they are neurotropic. The more purely neurotropic viruses, such as rabies, may only spread along nerves, whereas a virus with more general tissue affinity may use either the nerves or the blood-stream. Once a virus has reached the nervous parenchyma it appears to be, to a considerable degree, protected from the immune bodies of the blood. Hurst (1936) showed that with the virus of *equine encephaloymelitis* in the monkey, there is a stage after infection during which virus has disappeared from the blood and antibodies make their appearance in increasing quantity. It is at this stage that evidence of encephalitis is likely to appear, and this may increase and lead to death in spite of the presence of large amounts of antibodies in the blood. It is possible that the blood-brain barrier against antibodies may be weakened by the inflammation in the nervous tissues which results from virus action. This mechanism would account for the comparatively short period of activity of the virus in the nervous system in poliomyelitis and some other forms of virus encephalomyelitis.

Histological diagnosis of encephalitis

The reactions of the brain to inflammation are somewhat stereotyped and tend to be similar in all forms of encephalitis. But they vary both in the emphasis on one or another type of reaction and in their distribution through the cerebrospinal axis. The types of reaction found in all forms of encephalitis are:

(*i*) *Cellular infiltration.* In encephalomyelitis, as in other inflammatory processes, the cellular exudate is usually the most obvious histological lesion. In the most acute forms of encephalitis it consists chiefly or largely of neutrophil leucocytes, most of which lie free in the tissues. At a later stage of acute forms and in the less acute forms the exudate consists almost entirely of mononuclear cells, lymphocytes, plasma cells and large mononuclear phagocytes. A single layer of lymphocytes in the Virchow-Robin space of small venules, and thicker cuffs of lymphocytes round the larger vessels are characteristic appearances at this stage. After the first week these cells may be replaced by plasma cells which also can be seen lying sparsely in the tissues. To what extent lymphocytes escape from the vessels and invade the tissues is not easily made out, owing to their resemblance to oligodendroglia and perhaps also to microglia. In certain forms of encephalitis, notably American equine encephalomyelitis, fairly large collections of small hyperchromic nuclei are seen in the tissues apart from vessels and it is probable that some of these cells are lymphocytes.

Morular cells are rare but isolated cells of this kind are found in the more subacute and chronic forms of encephalitis. In sections stained by phosphotungstic acid haematoxylin or other stain for neuroglial fibres (e.g. Holzer) they stand out prominently as purple, mulberry-like masses (*vide* page 218). They are also easily recognised by their intense red staining with Lendrum's phloxin tartrazin stain for virus inclusions.

(*ii*) *Microglial hyperplasia and proliferation* is almost constant but may be restricted in degree and extent. It may be diffuse or focal. Diffuse proliferations are seen in the cortex and brain stem in all polioclastic forms of encephalitis even in the subacute and chronic forms to which reference will be made later. It is sometimes difficult to decide in such cases whether there is an actual excess of microglial cells, but the individual cells are hypertrophied forming rod cells and cells with long curved nuclei similar to those seen in general paralysis. A focal accumulation of microglia or histiocytes round degenerated or dying nerve cells, so-called *neuronophagy*, is typically seen in the ventral horns in poliomyelitis and *glial shrub formations* in the molecular layer of the cerebellar cortex may point to the destruction of Purkinje cells. Glial stars, sometimes related to small vessels, containing ten or more hypertrophied microglial nuclei are also a characteristic of encephalitis. They occur most often in the grey matter but are also seen in the white matter, especially near the cortex. Larger accumulations in which lymphocytes and other mononuclear cells take part are also found in most forms of encephalitis directly due to virus infection, e.g. in the brain stem in poliomyelitis, lethargica, St. Louis and equine encephalomyelitis. They are not usually found in the post-infectious forms. Plasma cells are not common in these accumulations, but may often be seen lying free in the tissues in the more involved areas.

(*iii*) Changes in the *nerve cells* were emphasised by von Economo in his original description and later in his monograph. These are important, though by no means characteristic. They vary from 'slight tigrolysis to swelling and hyalinisation of the cell protoplasm, shifting of the nucleus to the periphery of the cell, pallor and disappearance of the nucleus extending to the formation of ghost cells' (Economo 1931). A very common change is loss of Nissl granules and tendency to eosinophilia of the cytoplasm. Often only a proportion of the nerve cells in any area is involved, especially in the cortex and basal ganglia, but in encephalitis lethargica a very large proportion of the nerve cells in the substantia nigra was frequently destroyed. These cells often seemed to disappear leaving no trace except their melanin pigment which lay free or engulfed in microglial cells. Neuronophagy varies from case to case and from one type of disease to another. Even in poliomyelitis, in which it is very characteristic, one may see in the ventral horns chromatolytic or necrotic neurones with no surrounding phagocytes. In encephalitis lethargica neuronophagy occurred, but was not common. In some of the more recent epidemics and epidemic forms it appears to be more commonly seen.

(*iv*) *Inclusion bodies.* Various forms of inclusion body may be found in neurones, astrocytes and oligodendroglia in virus diseases. Some of those described are now recognised to be non-specific degeneration products, but some are important, especially the Negri bodies of rabies and Type A intranuclear inclusions. The former, which are quite typical of rabies, are fully described along with that disease.

Acidophilic intranuclear inclusions were divided by Cowdry (1934) into Types A and B. Type A inclusions may be amorphous or finely granular; they are spherical and surrounded by a clear halo. The nuclear chromatin is collected in granules under the nuclear membrane, and the nucleolus is also displaced. When fully developed the inclusion may occupy the greater part of the nucleus leaving a clear zone between it and the nuclear membrane, or may entirely fill the nucleus except for a ring of fine chromatin granules. It is generally agreed that this type of inclusion is only found in virus diseases (Pinkerton 1950), but the inclusion itself may contain little or no virus (Francis and Kurtz 1950). It should probably be regarded as a characteristic form of degeneration of the nuclear sap caused by the virus.

Type A inclusions are seen in nerve cells and oligodendroglia in herpes simplex encephalitis and subacute inclusion encephalitis. In both diseases they may be associated with acidophilic cytoplasmic inclusions. These are small and spherical in herpes encephalitis and in the less affected cells in subacute inclusion encephalitis, but in more severely damaged cells in the latter disease they become floccular, crescentic or horseshoe shaped, and eventually the cell body is completely replaced by hyaline material. In cytomegalic inclusion disease Type A inclusions may be found in subependymal astrocytes as well as in the endothelium of small cerebral vessels.

Type B intranuclear inclusions are also spherical but are small and may be multiple. They do not cause displacement of nuclear chromatin or nucleolus. They may become as large as, or slightly larger than, the nucleolus of the large motor cells in which they are found. They were described by Covell (1930) in ventral horn cells in poliomyelitis. In this disease they occur in surviving nerve cells and are best seen after the acute phase of inflammation has passed, or in slightly affected segments of the spinal cord. Although under these conditions and in this situation they are characteristic of poliomyelitis, they resemble very closely the acidophil intranuclear bodies which are normally found in the substantia nigra (*vide* p. 8).

(*v*) *Lesions in the white matter.* Many forms of encephalitis, especially those caused by the more pantropic viruses including the insect-borne forms, produce lesions in the white matter as well as the grey. In some acute forms, such as herpes simplex encephalitis, there is spread of inflammation from the cortex into the underlying white matter, producing softening and necrosis which appears to be independent of vascular lesions. A similar process may result in the cystic spaces seen by Noran and Baker (1943) as a sequel to western equine encephalomyelitis. In subacute inclusion encephalomyelitis (Dawson 1933), as in subacute sclerosing leuco-encephalitis (van Bogaert 1945), which is probably the same disease, the slowly progressive demyelination of the white matter associated with astrocytic gliosis appears to be independent of lesions to cortical nerve cells. The presence of intranuclear inclusions in the oligodendroglia in this form suggests that damage to these cells, on which the nutrition of myelin seems to depend, may play some part in the demyelination.

(*vi*) *Changes in the vessel walls* are by no means a constant feature of encephalitis, but in equine encephalomyelitis they occur so constantly as to be characteristic of the disease. They are described as arteritis of varying intensity, migration of neutrophil leucocytes through the walls of the vessels, necrotic or hyaline changes or fibrin deposition in the walls (Wesselhoeft,

Smith and Branch 1938, Farber, Hill, Connerly and Dingle 1940). Thrombosis is incidental, and some authors describe much vascular disease with little or no thrombosis, but the reverse may occur. Tissue necrosis and ischaemic changes of greater or less degree may complicate or even dominate the picture.

POLIOMYELITIS

(**Poliomyelitis anterior acuta, Heine-Medin disease**)

This common form of encephalomyelitis has been recognised for more than a century. It was described in England by Badham in 1836 and more completely by Heine in 1840 and 1860. Until the end of the nineteenth century it appeared as sporadic cases, but in 1891 Medin reported an epidemic in Sweden and in 1907 Wickman reported another epidemic which had occurred in the same country in 1905, and gave a classical description of the pathology. Since that time there have been many local epidemics in Europe. In the United States, Canada, Australia, New Zealand and South Africa severe epidemics have occurred, and until 1947 the incidence of the disease both in North America and in Australia was considerably higher than in Great Britain. During the 1939–45 war there was a high incidence of poliomyelitis among British, Dominion and American troops in the Near East and epidemics, chiefly among the native population, occurred in Malta and St. Helena. A severe epidemic in South Africa in 1944–5 was attributed to the return of soldiers from the Near East. Great Britain had its first severe epidemic in 1947 and since then has had further epidemics in 1950 and 1955.

Aetiology

Poliomyelitis was first shown to be a virus disease by Landsteiner and Popper (1908–9). Their work was carried further by Flexner and Amos (1914). The virus of poliomyelitis is one of the smallest known, measuring 25–30mμ as seen by electron microscopy. It is regularly present in the nasopharynx of patients for a few days before and after paralysis appears and can be found in their faeces for 1–2 months. It is also present in the faeces of many contacts. During epidemics it has been found in urban sewage and it may survive in polluted cold water for 3 months or more. It is readily destroyed by chlorination of filtered water and by ultraviolet light.

Three serologically distinct types of poliomyelitis virus are recognised. Of these Type I (Brunhilde) is the most common. Type II (Lansing), which is also common, is the least virulent. It has caused no epidemics and only rare fatal infections. Type III (Leon) is also not uncommon in certain areas. Immunity to one type does not protect, in laboratory tests, from infection by another, but second infections in the human rarely cause paralysis. Type II is pathogenic for cotton rats, mice and hamsters as well as for primates; the other types are pathogenic only for primates. Poliomyelitis virus can be grown on tissue cultures containing fresh primate or human (foetal or adult) tissue and can be isolated directly from faeces on to roller tube cultures (Enders 1952). The virus is pathogenic for the cells of the tissue culture which, after about 8 days, degenerate and die; these effects are obvious first in connective tissue and later in epithelial cells.

Epidemiology

The seasonal incidence of poliomyelitis during the later summer months, with a gradual decline in autumn, has been explained in various ways. Flies as faecal feeders and contaminators of food have been blamed for the spread of infection. It has been found that domestic house flies (*Musca domestica*), and especially blow flies (*Phormia regina*), may have virus in their bodies and excreta for several days, and virus has been found in pooled flies about 4 weeks before the appearance of epidemics. Some small epidemics have been attributed to contamination of milk by house flies. On the other hand Gear (1952) has pointed to two outbreaks which occurred in African villages after prolonged spraying with DDT to destroy mosquitoes. As the seasonal incidence of poliomyelitis corresponds with the season for fresh fruit, it has been suggested that the disease may be spread by the contamination of fruit either by pickers or when exposed for sale. These two factors may be related since flies are attracted to fruit. It is, however, generally held that infection is most often spread by carriers, that is subclinical cases, or by direct case to case infection. A few small outbreaks have been traced to water supplies contaminated by sewage. Bathing in polluted streams or in swimming baths has also been blamed for individual cases, but without conclusive evidence.

Poliomyelitis appears to have an almost world-wide distribution, although most epidemics have occurred in temperate climates. The evidence indicates that in more primitive communities infection takes place during infancy chiefly in a sub-clinical form. The absence of epidemics in these communities may therefore be due to general immunity of the population. In these communities the disease is endemic and occurs most often in children under the age of 5 years. On the other hand where sanitary and hygienic controls are stricter, there is less immunity; there is therefore a greater tendency to epidemic spread and a higher age incidence. The natural resistance of different races to the disease must also be taken into account. It has been shown that in Honolulu white races are more prone to the disease than yellow, and both are much more susceptible than Hawaians. Recent outbreaks in St. Helena and among the Eskimos in Northern Canada have the characteristics of spread in a virgin, unsalted community.

Mode of infection

Having gained access to the body by the mouth either by droplet infection or from food or drink, the virus appears to multiply in the intestinal tract. There may be a short period of viraemia as virus has been isolated from the blood at an early stage of infection in the chimpanzee and very occasionally in human cases. Whether it reaches the nervous system along nerves from the intestines or by the blood-stream is not known.

Cerebrospinal fluid

During the initial preparalytic stage, the cerebrospinal fluid is under normal pressure. It contains an excess of cells, usually between 50 and 200 per cu. mm., of which a large proportion, but rarely more than half, are neutrophil leucocytes. The protein is only slightly raised, but occasionally a fine fibrin coagulum may form. Chlorides and glucose remain normal; the gold sol reaction often gives a moderate mid-zone curve. During the progress of the disease the cell count rapidly falls, neutrophil leucocytes disappear early and are rare after the first few days of paralysis. Along with this fall in the cell count the protein rises progressively and may reach levels between 100 and 200 mg. per 100 ml. after the first fortnight. At this stage rarely more than 10 or 20 lymphocytes per cu. mm. are found in the fluid.

Morbid anatomy and histology

Post-mortem examination of a case fatal within the first few days after the appearance of paralysis may show little evidence of disease in the organs of the body cavity. Congestion of the tonsils and swelling of the spleen and abdominal lymph nodes are, however, commonly found. Examination of the heart muscle has shown some degree of interstitial myocarditis in a proportion of cases which varies from 14 per cent (Ludden and Edwards 1949) to 84 per cent (Saphir and Wile 1942). When severe it may be associated with verrucous endocarditis. In the central nervous system the only naked eye abnormality is congestion of the grey horns of the spinal cord and sometimes also of the medulla. This may be associated with petechial haemorrhages or very small areas of softening.

Microscopically the changes vary with the stage of the disease at which the patient dies. In the first few days there is a diffuse infiltration of the ventral horns and the bases of the dorsal horns of the spinal cord with small cells. Most of these appear to be lymphocytes and histiocytes, many probably being of microglial origin; polymorphonuclear leucocytes may also be numerous in the early stages. There is congestion of small vessels, often with some petechial haemorrhages. The infiltration may be so dense as to obscure the changes in nerve cells, but these are always present in degrees varying from slight, diffuse chromatolysis to necrosis with lysis and neuronophagy. In areas where the disease is most severe clusters of histiocytes may

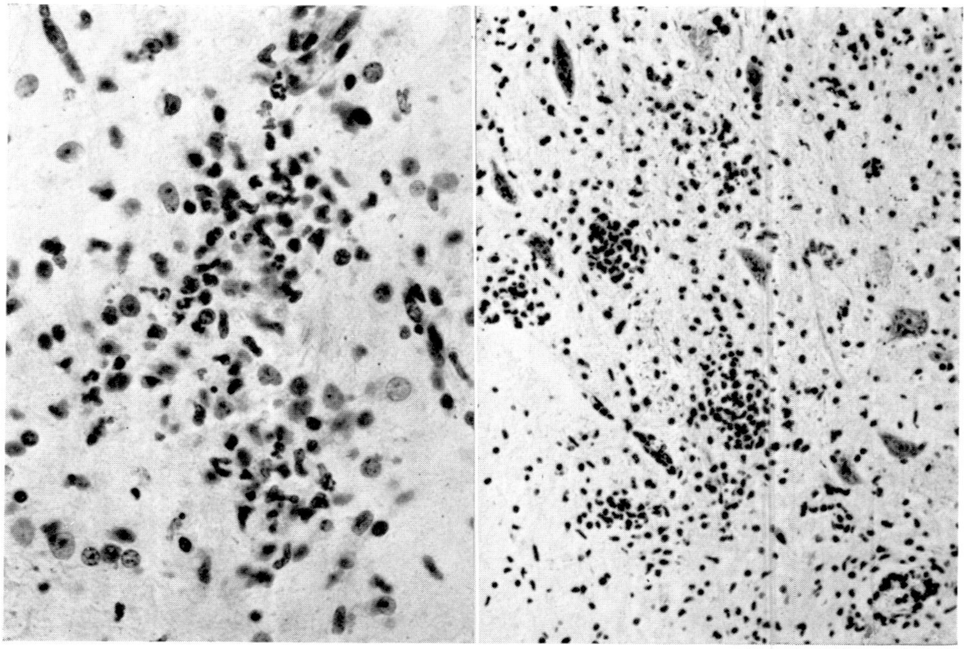

(*a*) (*b*)

FIG. 3.12. Poliomyelitis. Ventral horns of cord in acute stages.

(*a*) Very early lesion with many neurophil leucocytes. (*b*) Stage of histiocytic (microglial) phagocytosis.

cover all the nerve cells in the anterior horns, but in less affected areas some of the neurones are less severely damaged. The characteristic appearance during the early stages is therefore intense diffuse cellular infiltration of the ventral horns, extending a varying distance into the dorsal horns, with clumps of cells engulfing dead neurones. These changes are associated with lymphocytic infiltration of the meninges but this may be slight or patchy (Fig. 3.12).

At a rather later stage, when death occurs after several days of paralysis, the infiltration may be less diffuse and neuronophagy more evident. A number of degenerated nerve cells which are not surrounded by phagocytes may also be seen. The changes in these vary from a moderate degree of central chromatolysis to complete loss of Nissl granules along with degenerative changes in the nucleus. In sections stained with basic blue dyes the more affected neurones appear as ghost cells, but with haematoxylin and eosin the cytoplasm is eosinophilic. Intranuclear eosinophilic inclusion bodies of Type B, which may be found in chromatolytic neurones in the early stages, are now rather larger and more definite in some of the less affected cells in which they may be as large as the nucleolus. At a rather later stage (21 days) their presence in otherwise normal neurones is evidence that these cells were attacked by the virus but have recovered (Bodian 1952). Perivascular infiltration with lymphocytes and a few plasma cells appears during the first few days and increases for a week or more; it may persist for weeks or months.

In cases which come to autopsy after a few weeks or months the most obvious change is loss of anterior horn cells, associated with some perivascular infiltration in the vessels passing from the ventral horns to the surface. There is also loss of myelinated fibres in the ventral horns, often producing large irregularly rounded unstained areas in sections stained for myelin. Small cysts due to loss of nervous tissue are not infrequently found in the ventral horns. Some may be surrounded by haemosiderin, but this is by no means the rule, and most of them seem to result from necrosis of all the nervous tissue in an area rather than from haemorrhages. Bodian (1952) does not consider that they are necessarily due to thrombosis of vessels. Einarson (1952) suggests that the tendency to agglutination of red blood corpuscles (sludge formation) which occurs at the height of the disease may produce temporary plugging of terminal arterioles and so cause areas of necrosis. This may also be a factor in the distribution of the more severe neuronal lesions in the ventral horns (q.v.). At this stage Einarson (1949) and Bodian (1952) found cells showing extreme hyperchromia. These had also been seen by Warburg (1931) in chronic experimental poliomyelitis. Einarson considers that cells in this condition either may go on to atrophy and the formation of cell shadows or may recover, and he thus explains some cases of late return of power in paralysed muscles.

Distribution of lesions

The most severe lesions are usually found in the anterior two-thirds of the grey matter of the spinal cord. In this they vary from one level to another, usually sparing the lower sacral segments relatively or completely. In early fatal cases infiltrative changes of varied intensity are seen also in the formatio reticularis, especially in the medulla but to a less degree also in the pons and sometimes in the midbrain, in the nucleus tecti and sometimes the nucleus dentatus of the cerebellum, in the hypothalamus, thalamus and globus pallidus. They are almost constantly present in the area giganto-pyramidalis of the pre-central gyrus, where some Betz cells may undergo neuronophagy, but are rare elsewhere in the cerebral cortex. In cases of bulbar poliomyelitis dense cellular infiltrations may be seen in relation to most of the nuclei of the motor cranial nerves. In some cases the sensory nuclei are also infiltrated but, whereas there is usually degeneration or neuronophagy of many neurones in the motor nuclei, the nerve cells of the sensory nuclei appear unaffected. Peers (1943) found severe cell loss in Deiter's nucleus and some loss also in the substantia nigra and locus coeruleus, and perivascular infiltration here and in the nucleus ruber. He also found glial shrubs in the molecular layer of the cerebellar vermis.

In convalescent cases the loss of nerve cells in the spinal cord often has a rather characteristic distribution. Although in the most severely damaged segments of the cervical and lumbosacral enlargements every motor neurone may have disappeared, there is in general a tendency for the more lateral and posterior groups to be spared and the greatest cell loss to be found in the more medially placed cell groups (Peers 1943, Elliott 1947). Einarson (1952), who found a similar distribution of lesions in Vitamin E deficiency, considers that it results from a relative hypoxia of the more medially placed cell groups during the height of the disease. He cites the experiments of Krogh (1945), who saw the same distribution of lesions in experimental hypoxia of the lumbar cord and found that the arteries at this level broke up into capillaries in the lateral zone of the ventral horns, whereas the veins arose in the more medial zones. The capillary blood would therefore have lost much of its oxygen by the time it reached the more medially placed nerve cells. This tendency to hypoxia would be increased by the tendency to agglutination of red cells which has already been mentioned. Sharrard (1955) found that the autonomic nerve cells of the intermediolateral tract were specially resistant to destruction. The cells of Clarke's column may be damaged, especially in the 12th thoracic and 1st lumbar segments (Batten 1916, Peers 1943).

Muscles and peripheral nerves

Many changes have been described in the paralysed muscles in poliomyelitis. These include necrosis, loss of striation and hyaline and waxy degeneration of some fibres in the very early stages, and fibrillary splitting and perivascular infiltrations at a rather later stage (Carey *et al.* 1944, Denst and Neubuerger 1950). In the writer's experience, however, there is nothing in the histological appearances of muscles in human cases of poliomyelitis which is inconsistent with the effects of partial or complete denervation. Cellular infiltration is not seen in the first few days and when it appears is limited to perivascular collections of histiocytes and lymphocytes which are commonly found in neurogenic atrophy. This opinion is confirmed by the experimental work of Bowden (1952) who found the lesions in the muscles of monkeys infected with various strains of poliomyelitis virus to differ in no way from those seen after section of ventral roots. There is thus no evidence of a direct attack by this virus on the muscle fibres such as is caused by viruses of the Coxsackie group, and it appears possible that the acute necrotic and degenerative changes in the muscle which have been seen in some cases have been due to simultaneous attack by both viruses (Dalldorf 1952, Rhodes *et al.* 1953). Hypertrophy of some muscle fibres has been described in late cases which have received physical treatment (Denst and Neubuerger 1950) but Bowden was unable to find evidence of this in experimental monkeys.

Batten (1916) noted that the muscular atrophy was followed either by fibrosis or fatty infiltration and that the gastrocnemius muscles were specially likely to show the latter form of change. He found normal muscle spindles in muscles which had otherwise undergone complete atrophy, and relative sparing of muscle spindles has been noted by others.

The changes in the nerves and motor end-plates are less easily assessed. Degeneration of motor end-plates and of the terminal part of the axons occurs at a very early stage, and the nerve fibres whose perikarya have been destroyed undergo Wallerian degeneration. A centripetal degeneration of nerve fibres similar to that described in *simple neuronal atrophy* has also been seen (Carey *et al.* 1944, Bowden 1952). This may be evidence of degeneration which goes on to the death of the motor neurone, or may be associated with temporary neuronal damage from which recovery is possible. If the latter, it may explain some cases of late recovery of muscular power. In experimental poliomyelitis there is evidence that neurites arising from intact nerve fibres may re-innervate paralysed muscle fibres (Bowden 1952, Wohlfart 1955). This phenomenon is recognised as occurring after traumatic lesions of peripheral nerves and may well take place also in human poliomyelitis.

RABIES

Human cases of this once dreaded disease have become rare in Western Europe and practically unknown in the British Isles,* but in Eastern Europe, Siberia, India and some parts

* In 1885 dogs in Great Britain were compulsorily muzzled and since then all dogs brought into the country have been quarantined. The quarantine rules were broken in 1918 when some infected dogs were brought into the country, but fortunately no human cases were caused by them.

of North America, where wolves and wild canine species abound, it is still a serious problem. Some cases in South Africa have been due to bites by meercats or allied species. In South America the paralytic form of the disease has affected cattle and horses since 1908 and was shown by Haupt and Rehaag (1921) to be spread among them by vampire bats. In 1931 it was carried to Trinidad, an island in which, owing to quarantine regulations, rabies was unknown. There it spread, by vampire bats, to cattle and to a number of human cases, which were studied by Hurst and Pawan (1931–2).

Almost all human cases can be traced to the bites of dogs or other rabid animals or to contamination of cuts or abrasions by their saliva. The incubation period varies greatly. It is rarely as little as 2 weeks, more commonly 1–3 months and sometimes, either with or without Pasteur treatment, more than a year. The disease may assume a *restless* type, corresponding to the 'furious' rabies of dogs, or a *paralytic* type. As the old name 'hydrophobia' implies, spasms of the muscles of deglutition on attempting to drink water may be the first or an early symptom.

Aetiology

Rabies is one of the larger viruses. Its size has been estimated by the filtration technique at 100–150mμ (Galloway and Elford 1936) or 150–250mμ (Levaditi *et al.* 1936). The evidence that it reaches the central nervous system along peripheral nerves derives from the observations of Pasteur, Chamberland and Roux (1884), who found virus in the nerves after subcutaneous inoculation. This work was extended by Nicolau, Nicolau and Galloway (1929) who found the peripheral nerves to be infective after intracerebral inoculation of virus. In animals dying of rabies, and in fatal human cases, the virus may be found not only in the central and peripheral nervous systems and in saliva, but occasionally also in many other organs of the body. The milk of infected rabbits and guinea-pigs has been found to contain virus.

Negri and Lyssa bodies. These cytoplasmic inclusions, which are characteristic of rabies, are most numerous in certain areas of the fore-brain which show little or no inflammatory exudate and are rare or absent in areas where other signs of inflammation are severe. Both in the dog and in man they usually abound in the pyramidal layer of the hippocampus, especially towards its posterior end, but they are also common in the cerebral cortex and in Purkinje cells in the cerebellum. They may be scarce in cases of paralytic type. In the dorsal root ganglia and the parts of the central nervous system which bear the chief brunt of the inflammatory disease they are always scarce. They are more abundant and larger in cases with the longest duration of symptoms, in man 4–7 days, and may be difficult to find in patients who succumb during the first 48 hours. Their number appears to bear little relation to the length of the incubation period (Fig. 3.13).

*Negri bodies** are sharply defined, rounded or oval, acidophilic cytoplasmic inclusions which, when suitably stained, show an internal structure. They may lie anywhere in the cytoplasm of the cell body or dendrites and two or more may be seen in one cell. Their size may vary from 1μ to 20μ but usually lies between 5μ and 10μ. The largest bodies are seen in the pyramidal cells of the hippocampus and neighbouring parts of the temporal cortex and in the Purkinje cells of the cerebellum. When present in motor neurones of the spinal cord they may

* Negri (1903), in his description of the cytoplasmic inclusions to which his name is now given, considered that they represented a stage in the life cycle of a protozoal parasite. This view was also held by Levaditi who called them *Glugea Lyssae*, but is not now generally accepted. Marinesco and Stroesco (1931) pointed out the great difference in amount of nuclear chromatin, as seen with the Feulgen technique, between Negri bodies and protozoa such as malarial parasites and coccidia. Covell and Danks (1932), who agreed with this conclusion, were unable to relate them to mitochondria or other normal cell structures.

also be very large. Their form is adapted to their surroundings; for example those in dendritic processes are often oval. The cells in which they lie may show little other abnormality or only minor degrees of chromatolysis. They do not therefore appear to be so incompatible with the continued life of the cell as Type A intranuclear inclusions.

Marinesco and Stroesco (1931) described three types of Negri body. (*a*) Bodies which are homogeneous except for the presence of very small basophil granules. There may be from 2 to 30 granules which lie either centrally or symmetrically arranged towards the periphery of the Negri body. Some bodies of this kind appear to be enclosed in a definite membrane. (*b*) Bodies consisting of an agglomeration of smaller acidophilic bodies ('elementary bodies') each of which, in the larger Negri bodies, may contain a basophil granule. (*c*) Bodies showing an inner core containing only basophil granules and an outer ring of elementary bodies. Marinesco and Stroesco consider that elementary bodies appear first and, by fusion or enlargement and increase in the number of basophil granules, become Negri bodies. They found evidence that elementary bodies arose in the nucleus and passed through the nuclear membrane, thereafter forming Negri bodies.

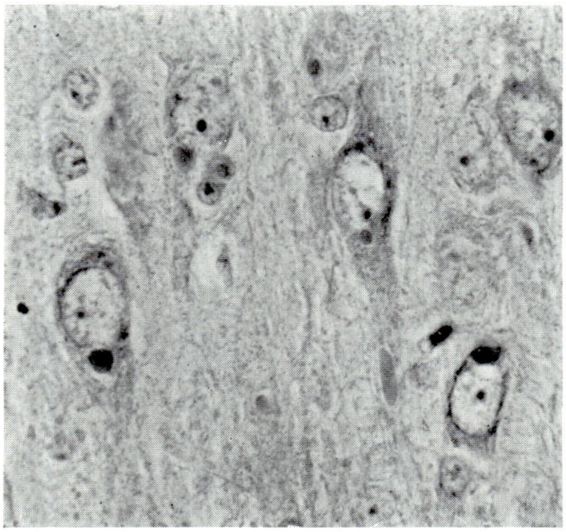

FIG. 3.13. Rabies. Cornu Ammonis in a guinea-pig showing Negri and lyssa bodies.

Negri bodies are only seen after infection by 'street virus'. When the virus becomes 'fixed' by laboratory passage they no longer appear. Wolman and Behar (1952) found that in the earlier stages after infection with street virus in the mouse nerve cells contained basophilic inclusion bodies giving a positive Feulgen reaction (DNA). Later these bodies became embedded in a Feulgen negative matrix which eventually became amorphous and lost its basophilia. Sourander (1956), however, could not demonstrate in the dog either DNA or RNA and concluded that Negri bodies did not contain virus but were a reaction by the protoplasm of the cell to infection with street virus.

The name *Lyssa bodies* was given to simple acidophil, cytoplasmic inclusions with no internal structure. This may be the only recognisable type of inclusion in some cases. But inclusions of this type are not so characteristic of rabies as Negri bodies, as similar acidophilic droplets may be seen in nerve cells in a variety of degenerative conditions which are not related to virus infections.

Morbid anatomy and histology

On naked eye examination the only abnormality may be congestion. Bernsten and Stevenson (1953) describe severe oedema and small subarachnoid haemorrhages in the brain of a 4-year-old child.

Microscopically the distribution of the lesions differs to some extent in the two chief clinical types of the disease. In the *classical type* with restlessness and dysphagia, the chief inflammatory lesions are found in the jugular, Gasserian and dorsal root ganglia, the lower two-thirds of the medulla, locus niger and hypothalamic and tuberal nuclei, usually in that order of severity. Infiltrations may also be seen in the peripheral nerves, spinal cord and cerebral and cerebellar hemispheres. In all the inflamed areas the nerve cells show varying degrees of degeneration and destruction, the slighter degrees of which include chromatolysis which may be central, peripheral or diffuse, or achromatosis and eosinophilia of the cytoplasm with hyperchromasia of the nucleus. In the dorsal root ganglia there is multiplication of capsule cells around many neurones but degeneration of neurones may be present without these. Neuronophagy by polymorphonuclear or microglial cells is common in the jugular ganglion, and may also be seen in other dorsal root ganglia as well as in the spinal cord, medulla and locus niger. In the central nervous system the most severe infiltrative and inflammatory lesions are commonly seen in relation to the sensory and motor nuclei of the 9th, 10th and 12th cranial nerves.

The Babes nodules, which were considered at one time to be characteristic of rabies, are accumulations of microglial cells, either in relation to dead neurones or independent of these. They may be of any size from 10 to 12 cells up to 100 or more. They are now recognised as the neuronophagic or glial nodules which are common in all forms of virus encephalitis.

The classical studies of the nerve cells in rabies by Achucarro (1910) were made on the cornu Ammonis and cerebellum of rabbits infected with *virus fixé*. Negri bodies are not seen under these conditions and the nerve cells show more degenerative changes. Achucarro described increase of granules, both acidophil and basophil, in the nucleus, followed by degeneration of the nucleus and disappearance of the nuclear membrane. Nissl granules disappear early and the cell body shrinks. The neurofibrils at an early stage show local thickenings and with the progress of the disease this becomes more general and intense, filling the whole cell body.

The pathology of the *paralytic form* of rabies was well described by Hurst and Pawan (1932). They had 5 cases in Trinidad, in coloured folk who had been bitten on the feet while asleep by vampire bats. The disease appeared in them about a month after the bite and was fatal in from 5 to 7 days. It began in the foot which had been bitten, usually the left, and gradually spread upwards as a flaccid paraplegia with loss of cutaneous sensibility and of sphincter control. *Post mortem* the spinal cord was congested and its lower half was softened almost to the consistence of butter. There was less congestion of the brain. Meningeal infiltration was slight, and in many places absent, over the cord but perivascular infiltrations, chiefly of lymphocytic type, were abundant. Microglial infiltration in the grey matter was severe, and in some segments was diffusely spread over both ventral and dorsal horns. Focal collections of microglia were also seen in the white columns. Many of the nerve cells were swollen, with severe central chromatolysis; neuronophagy of some cells was seen at all levels and in some of the lower segments of the cord almost every nerve cell had succumbed in this manner. The neurones of the dorsal horns were as severely affected as the motor neurones. In the more severely damaged segments the myelin sheaths in the grey matter had broken up into ovoids or globules.

The lowest levels of the *medulla* showed almost as severe lesions as the spinal cord. Above this in the pons and midbrain the tegmentum was more affected than the ventral half in which only small glial knots were seen. Many of the neurones in the lower brain stem had undergone degeneration in varying degree, but no neuronophagy was seen at these levels. The cerebellum was normal. In the cerebral cortex the lesions were confined to perivascular infiltration and chromatolysis of the larger pyramidal cells. They found no Negri bodies, but were unable to examine the hippocampus. The left sciatic nerves showed lymphocytic infiltration.

In monkeys infected with this strain of virus the changes were very similar. The adrenals were constantly the seat of focal and diffuse round-celled infiltration which was strictly confined to the medulla. Many foci of infiltration were also seen in the salivary glands. Similar inflammatory changes were seen round small ducts of the salivary glands by Bernsten and Stevenson (1953) in their human case.

HERPES ZOSTER

(**Zona**)

Herpes Zoster was shown by von Barensprung (1863) to be associated with a lesion of the dorsal root ganglion corresponding to the level of the skin rash. The pathology of the disease was fully described by Head and Campbell (1900) in a series of 20 post-mortem cases. Since that time the virus nature of the disease has been recognised, and its relation to other viruses, especially those of varicella and herpes simplex, has been explored, with rather equivocal results.

Some workers by injecting the fluid from a zoster vesicle on the scarified cornea of rabbits have got reactions very similar to those caused by herpes simplex but these have not been followed by encephalitis. Other workers have failed to transmit the disease to animals. That zoster has some relationship with varicella has been recognised by epidemiologists for many years, since varicella in children often appears to be caused by contact with a case of zoster. Experimentally the injection of the fluid from a zoster vesicle into the skin of children may produce a local vesicular eruption, or very occasionally has been followed by what appears to be typical varicella. Such experiments, however, have not always been successful. Varicella does not cause lasting immunity to zoster, although second attacks of either disease are very rare, and it has been noted that in the isolated communities of Christmas Island and Tristan da Cunha, where zoster is not infrequent, varicella is unknown. Immunological experiments have been equally equivocal. Some workers have obtained cross complement fixation reactions between varicella fluid and zoster serum and vice versa, but other workers have got negative results from similar experiments. Convalescent zoster serum appears to have no neutralising power on the virus of varicella as tested on the monkey's testis.

Although no certain method of testing for the presence of zoster virus has been devised, it is generally considered that the virus is present in the 'elementary bodies' which may be seen in the fluid of zoster vesicles. These measure about 0·25μ in diameter. By electron microscopy rounded virus-like bodies measuring 145mμ have been found in zoster fluid. Although there do not appear to have been any cases in which the lesions of zoster have been transmitted either to children or to animals from dorsal root ganglia or cerebrospinal fluid, it is presumed that the virus is present in the ganglia as well as in the cutaneous vesicles. If so it probably passes along the nerves from one to the other. Support for this hypothesis is given by the inflammatory changes which are commonly found in the peripheral nerves, but as was shown by Fairbrother and Hurst (1930) in poliomyelitis, the neural transmission of a virus does not always, or even usually, lead to any inflammatory changes in the nerve fibre tracts along which it passes. Opinion is divided as to the direction of this passage as some have postulated that the virus enters through the skin in the area in which the eruption appears. The order of clinical events, pain usually preceding any cutaneous eruption, and the absence, in most cases, of any cut or abrasion of the skin by which the virus could enter, favour the view that the virus first attacks the dorsal root ganglion, gaining access to it either from the blood or from the respiratory or gastro-intestinal tract.

The *cerebrospinal fluid* in cases of herpes zoster constantly shows a moderate or considerable excess of lymphocytes with little increase in protein and no other definite change.

Morbid anatomy and histology

The pathological changes of herpes zoster are usually limited to one dorsal root ganglion or to the sensory ganglion of a cranial nerve, and to the nerve and nerve root close to it. Head and Campbell considered it 'probable that two ganglia are occasionally affected together', but had no instance of this in their series. Others have found slighter changes in one or two dorsal root ganglia above or below that most affected. Head and Campbell also noted that certain of the spinal root ganglia were more often attacked than others. These were the 2nd, 3rd and 4th cervical, the thoracic, from the 2nd downwards, and the 1st lumbar. The ganglia related to the limbs are less often affected. Of the cranial ganglia the Gasserian is most commonly attacked, usually in its internal part which is related to the ophthalmic division. Facial paralysis is a very common complication of cervical, otic or trigeminal herpes, having occurred in 152 of the 267 cases of cephalic zoster collected by Rebattu *et al.* (1933). Ramsay Hunt (1907) postulated that its cause would be found in a lesion of the geniculate ganglion and this was confirmed histologically by Bethlem (1962).

If examined within a few days of the appearance of the rash, the involved ganglion appears congested and swollen and on section is often haemorrhagic, most often in its dorsal part, that is the part farthest from the ventral root. There may also be congestion and swelling of the dorsal root related to this ganglion. *Histologically* the ganglion is in a state of intense inflammation with congestion of vessels and often haemorrhagic necrosis involving a larger or smaller part. The appearances here may resemble those of an infarct and are associated with death of the nerve cells in the area. Surrounding this area there is a zone of infiltration by lymphocytes with a few plasma and polymorphonuclear cells. In this zone the nerve cells show various forms of degeneration of which loss of Nissl granules, with eosinophilia of the cytoplasm, and neuronophagia are the most common. The cellular infiltration also affects the sheath of the ganglion and extends for a short distance peripherally into the nerve. The nerve root and the meninges at its point of entry to the cord also show lymphocytic infiltration. In most cases lesions are also seen within the spinal cord at the level of the affected ganglion. They are usually confined to the side of the lesion (Lhermitte and Nicholas 1924) and consist of excess of microglial cells especially in the dorsal horns and around Clarke's column, but often also extending into the lateral and ventral horns. Some of the nerve cells in the dorsal horn and an occasional cell in the ventral horn may undergo neuronophagy. Central chromatolysis in anterior horn cells is not uncommon. Perivascular infiltration may also be seen within the cord, but is usually slight. A similar involvement of the brain stem often accompanies trigeminal or glossopharyngeal herpes. Although some of these lesions may be explained on the basis of reaction to degenerating fibres of the primary sensory neurone, others are probably the result of a direct attack by the virus on the secondary sensory neurone. This may explain the almost constant failure to relieve post-herpetic neuralgia by cutting dorsal roots.

Involvement of motor nerves is not uncommon, especially of cranial nerves and those of the upper limbs. Denny-Brown *et al.* (1944) found focal infiltrations by lymphocytes along the course of the facial nerve in a case in which paralysis of the facial and hypoglossal nerve on the side of the lesion followed 11 days after zoster in the upper cervical dermatomes; the geniculate ganglion in this case was intact. In cases of thoracic herpes they found infiltration and degeneration of the motor nerve in the neighbourhood of the affected ganglion. Associated with this the motor cells of the cranial nerve nuclei and anterior horns show central chromatolysis. This suggests that the nerves are involved in their course but does not exclude a direct attack by the virus on the motor neurone.

The histology of the cutaneous lesion is known from old studies by Lipschutz (1925) and others, and resembles very closely that of herpes simplex. The epithelial cells in and near the Malpighian layer swell and become ballooned or disintegrate. At the same time fluid collects between the epithelial cells, forming a multiloculated vesicle, and there is invasion of the epithelium and dermis by neutrophil leucocytes. Some of the ballooned cells at the base of the vesicle and occasional connective tissue cells may contain the Type A nuclear inclusions described by Lipschutz, but these are not always present.

ENCEPHALITIS LETHARGICA

A small epidemic of encephalitis with 50 per cent mortality occurred in Vienna in the winter of 1916–17 and was studied by von Economo (1931) and von Wiesner (1917). Thence the disease spread to western Europe and England where 126 cases, 20 per cent of which were fatal, occurred during the first 6 months of 1918. The pathology of these cases was described by Marinesco and McIntosh (1918) and Buzzard and Greenfield (1919). Towards the end of 1918 the disease spread to North America where pathological reports were given by Globus and Strauss (1922) in New York and by Boyd (1921, 1924–5) in Winnipeg. In England the epidemic reached its peak in the year 1924, during which 541 cases were notified in London, 398 in Glasgow and 301 in Sheffield. Thereafter it became less common and very few cases have been known to occur in the British Isles since 1926. Most cases occurred during the winter and early spring months. The disease was rather protean in its clinical manifestations but in a large proportion of cases was characterised by a peculiar somnolent state from which the patient could be wakened easily and completely so as to answer questions rationally, but quickly relapsed into sleep. In mild cases this condition soon passed off but in many cases persisted for many days, and sometimes for weeks or months. In severe cases sleep might deepen to coma leading to death. This lethargic state, from which the disease received its name, was often associated with other symptoms and signs, especially oculomotor palsies, and myoclonus either of the limb or trunk muscles. A mask-like facies was observed in some early cases and this often passed into a more widespread Parkinsonian rigidity, or Parkinsonism might appear after an interval of apparently complete recovery lasting for weeks or months. Another characteristic sequela was 'oculogyric crises' or forced adversive movements of the eyes. Mental regression, often with a marked psychopathic component, was shown by many children who contracted the disease.

Cerebrospinal fluid

The fluid was almost always clear and colourless and without a coagulum. In occasional cases there was evidence of meningeal haemorrhage. The cell count varied greatly; it usually lay between 5 and 20 cells per cu. mm. but might be normal or rise to 100 cells or more. In most epidemics only lymphocytes and mononuclear cells were present, but in the first Vienna epidemic and in the Sheffield epidemic of 1924 neutrophil leucocytes were also commonly found. The protein was usually increased to a moderate degree, with weakly positive globulin reactions, but sometimes appeared low in comparison with the cell count. Increased percentages of glucose were reported by many observers. The chlorides usually remained normal. Lange's gold sol commonly gave mid-zone reactions and sometimes, in subacute cases, strong reactions in the paretic zone.

Von Wiesner (1917) and McIntosh and Turnbull (1920) claimed to have infected monkeys by intracerebral inoculation, but did not pass the disease to other animals. Later workers either failed to infect animals or produced an encephalitis from which the herpes febrilis virus was passaged. The cause of encephalitis lethargica therefore remains undetermined but the disease has the characters of a virus infection and is generally accepted as being of this nature.

Pathological anatomy and histology

In cases dying during the first 2 weeks the cerebral cortex appeared intensely congested and was sometimes described as plum-coloured. On section congestion was evident not only in the grey matter of the cortex and basal ganglia but also in the brain stem, especially under the iter of Sylvius and the floor of the 4th ventricle. Minute haemorrhages round congested vessels were not uncommon. Meningeal haemorrhage was more rare. Microscopically the most obvious lesions in the majority of these cases were perivascular infiltrations either with

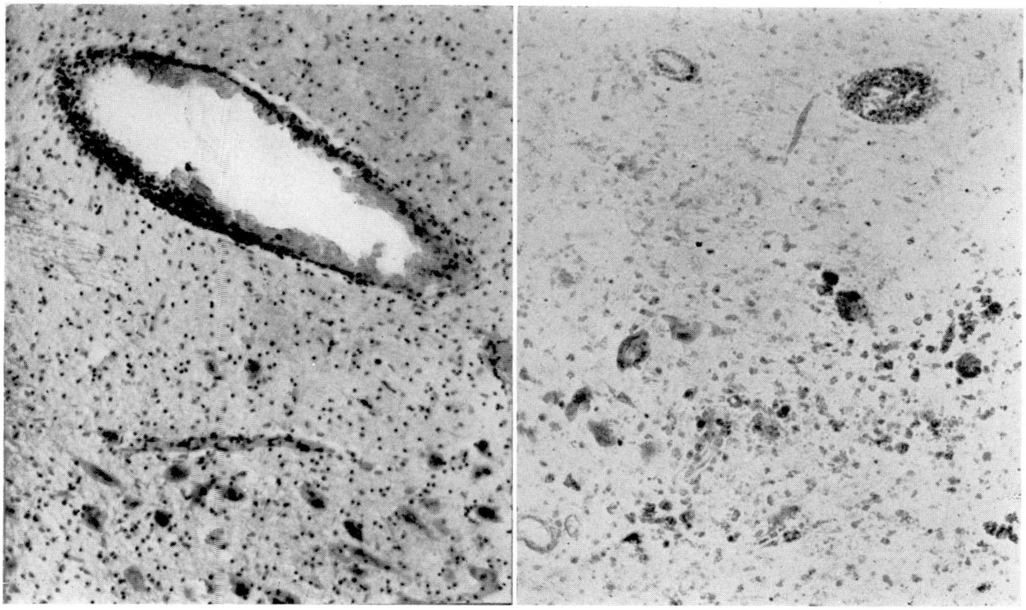

(*a*) (*b*)

FIG. 3.14. Encephalitis lethargica. Substantia nigra.

(*a*) Heavy perivascular infiltration but little loss of nerve cells. (*b*) Severe destruction of pigmented cells leaving granules of melanin pigment in a subacute case. (Nissl.)

lymphocytes or plasma cells (Fig. 3.14*a*). In general, lymphocytes formed thick sleeves round some of the larger veins and single or double rows or incomplete rings round venules. In cases with a history of more than a week many of the smaller vessels were ringed with a single layer of plasma cells. This infiltration of the vessel walls was usually accompanied by a more diffuse increase of small cells in the surrounding cerebral tissue. Some of these cells were haematogenous lymphocytes and plasma cells. Probably many also were derived from microglia, but this cell was not generally recognised during the years when the epidemic was at its height. Cells of these kinds often formed small collections, especially in the midbrain. The intensity of this infiltration of the cerebral tissue was closely related to that of the perivascular infiltrations in the same area. Both forms of infiltration were usually greatest in the midbrain, both in the tegmentum and in the substantia nigra, but it might be present also in the cortex, basal ganglia and lower brain stem and in many cases in the cervical segments of the cord. Meningeal infiltration was always patchy and often appeared to be related to the emergence of infiltrated veins into the subarachnoid space.

Some of the infiltrated venules, and others with no cellular excess in their walls, were surrounded by a circular or crescentic zone of haemorrhage which appeared to have pushed the surrounding tissues away from the vessel wall rather than burst into them. These may have been agonal or may have resulted from post-mortem handling of the brain as the blood corpuscles were always fresh. In cases fatal during the first 3 or 4 days perivascular haemorrhages were often more in evidence than cellular infiltrations, which might be very scarce (Economo 1931).

Lesions of nerve cells were less obvious but were present in most cases. Von Economo used the term *neurophthoria* to describe a degeneration of neurones which often progressed to their disappearance, but was rarely associated with neuronophagy. Marinesco (1918) found diminution in the number of nerve cells in many nuclei in the brain stem, especially in the *locus coeruleus*, where phagocytic cells, filled with melanin granules, gave evidence of cell destruction. He was one of the first to note the special incidence of cellular infiltration and neuronal degeneration on the *substantia nigra* and oculomotor nuclei (Fig. 3.14*b*). In two of his cases the Purkinje cells showed appearances resembling Spielmeyer's homogenising change.

In cases examined after a more protracted illness similar perivascular infiltration, especially with lymphocytes, was commonly found in the midbrain and tegmentum of the pons where there was often great destruction of the melanin-bearing cells of the substantia nigra and locus coeruleus. In a case, fatal on the 23rd day, which the writer examined, most of the cells of the substantia nigra had disappeared and melanin pigment lay free in the tissues or was being absorbed by phagocytic cells. These severe early lesions in the substantia nigra presaged the more complete destruction which was the characteristic finding in cases of post-encephalitic Parkinsonism (Trétiakoff 1921, Lhermitte and Cornil 1921, McAlpine 1923). Cortical lesions were less constant but Buzzard and Greenfield found areas of astrocytic hyperplasia and intense perivascular infiltration in a case with a 6 weeks' history. In another case, in which the illness had lasted for 4 months, they found thrombosis of many small cortical vessels with deposition of calcium salts both in the walls of the vessels and in the thrombus. This condition of the vessels was still more marked in the lenticular nucleus. Many of the vessels showing this change were ringed by lymphocytes. Dürck (1921) in 12 out of 15 fatal cases found calcification, most often in the corpus striatum but also in the nucleus dentatus, hippocampus, cornu Ammonis and thalamus. McAlpine saw similar incrustation in 3 acute and 3 chronic cases of encephalitis. Marinesco and Draganesco (1923) and Lhermitte *et al.* (1924–5) showed that these incrustations contained iron. Weston Hurst (1926) doubted their relation to encephalitis since he found them to be equally common in otherwise normal brains, but later experience with the Japanese B and cytomegalic forms suggests that encephalitis may play an important role in causing vascular incrustations of this kind. In other chronic cases the brains showed scars of the disease chiefly in the hippocampus, corpus striatum, thalamus, hypothalamus and midbrain. These consisted in loss of nerve cells along with neuroglial fibrosis. Lymphocytic cuffing of vessels was not uncommon even in cases surviving for several months, and in many of these cases recent perivascular haemorrhages were found in the walls of the 3rd ventricle.

In cases of *post-encephalitic Parkinsonism* severe diffuse loss of nerve cells in the substantia nigra is a constant finding. In asymmetrical cases this loss may be greater on the side opposite to the greater clinical disability. Some loss of nerve cells and gliosis in the lenticular nucleus and hypothalamus may also be found in these cases, and fibrillary changes resembling those of Alzheimer's disease can usually be seen in some of the pigmented cells of the brain stem (Hallervorden 1935, Greenfield and Bosanquet 1953). A rare sequela is amyotrophy of the limb muscles associated with loss of motor nerve cells in the cervical and lumbar enlargement of the cord and sometimes also with degeneration of the pyramidal tracts (Wimmer and Neal 1928, Greenfield and Matthews 1954). The pathological basis of oculogyric crises is disputed, but in some cases degenerative changes are found in the neurones of the oculomotor nuclei.

SAINT LOUIS ENCEPHALITIS

A severe epidemic involving over 1,000 cases occurred in Saint Louis and the surrounding country during the late summer (August and September) of 1933. A small epidemic which was shown to be due to the same virus occurred in Paris, Illinois, in 1932, and a further smaller epidemic in Saint Louis in 1937. Since then a number of cases have been described in the Middle Western and North Western States of the U.S.A. Hammon and Howitt (1942), in an area in Washington State where an outbreak of encephalitis occurred, found that 72 per cent of patients and 28 per cent of controls had neutralising anti-bodies to the Saint Louis virus. A few horses in this area also had anti-bodies to this virus. The virus, which measures about 20–30mμ, may be transmitted to monkeys, horses, mice and hamsters and may be grown on chick embryos. It appears to infect human cases by the bites of mosquitoes of which *Culex tarsalis* and *Culex pipiens* have been found capable of transmitting the virus. The animal reservoir may be in horses. There is evidence that it is spread in the animal reservoir by ticks which may remain infective for some months, but the seasonal incidence and other epidemiological evidence favours human infection by mosquito bite.

Histologically the lesions varied considerably from case to case, but in all were similar to those of encephalitis lethargica, although they were rather more wide-spread in the brain and brain stem. They are most numerous in the thalamus, substantia nigra and floor of the 4th ventricle (Haymaker 1961). They consist of: (1) *Meningeal infiltration* with mononuclear cells which tends to be focal and greater in the sulci than over the surface of the convolutions. (2) *Perivascular infiltration* chiefly with lymphocytes along with a few plasma cells; this was seen in the cortex, basal ganglia and brain stem, and also in the subcortical white matter and cerebellar peduncles. (3) *Collections of mononuclear cells*, interpreted as glial or histiocytic, irregularly distributed in the grey and white matter; some of these were related to blood vessels, but most appeared to be independent of these. In the basal ganglia and pons they were larger than glial nodules, containing more than 100 closely packed cells. They were also found in the medulla and in both the grey and the white columns of the spinal cord. (4) *Damage to neurones* was most evident in the neighbourhood of, or within, these cellular collections. Weil found severe lesions in the substantia nigra and the anterior horns of the spinal cord. Neuronophagy was, however, rare. Gross softenings were rarely seen. In about 30 per cent of the fatal cases there were renal lesions consisting of petechial haemorrhages and of cloudy swelling and necrosis of the tubular epithelium. Intranuclear inclusions were found in the cells of the convoluted and looped tubules.

*JAPANESE B ENCEPHALITIS**

Severe epidemics of encephalitis have occurred in Japan during the late summer of many years since 1871, but often with an interval of several years during which few cases were seen.

* Japanese B encephalitis was so called by Kaneko and Aoki (1928) when they recognised it as being different from encephalitis lethargica, which had spread to Japan during the pandemic, and which they called encephalitis A. It must not be confused with infection by 'B virus' which is only known as a laboratory infection resulting from the bites or salivary infection of apparently healthy monkeys (Sabin 1949 b). The letter B is often omitted.

An epidemic in Okinawa in 1945 caused a number of fatal cases which were carefully studied by American neuropathologists. Australian X disease, which occurred in 1917–18, 1922, 1925 and 1926 and cases which occurred in the Murray Valley of Australia during the year 1951 appear to have been due to the same virus. According to Rivers and Horsfall (1959) the infection is probably endemic in the Northern Territory and Queensland where the virus is probably maintained by a wild bird–mosquito cycle. During years of excessive rainfall the infection moves South with the migrating birds. The virus has been transmitted to monkeys, horses, sheep, goats and mice, but other laboratory animals appear immune.

Pathology. Naked-eye examination of the brains and spinal cords of acutely fatal cases shows nothing except congestion, but in cases lasting more than a month numerous small, pale, granular or gritty areas are seen on the cut surface throughout the cortex and basal ganglia.

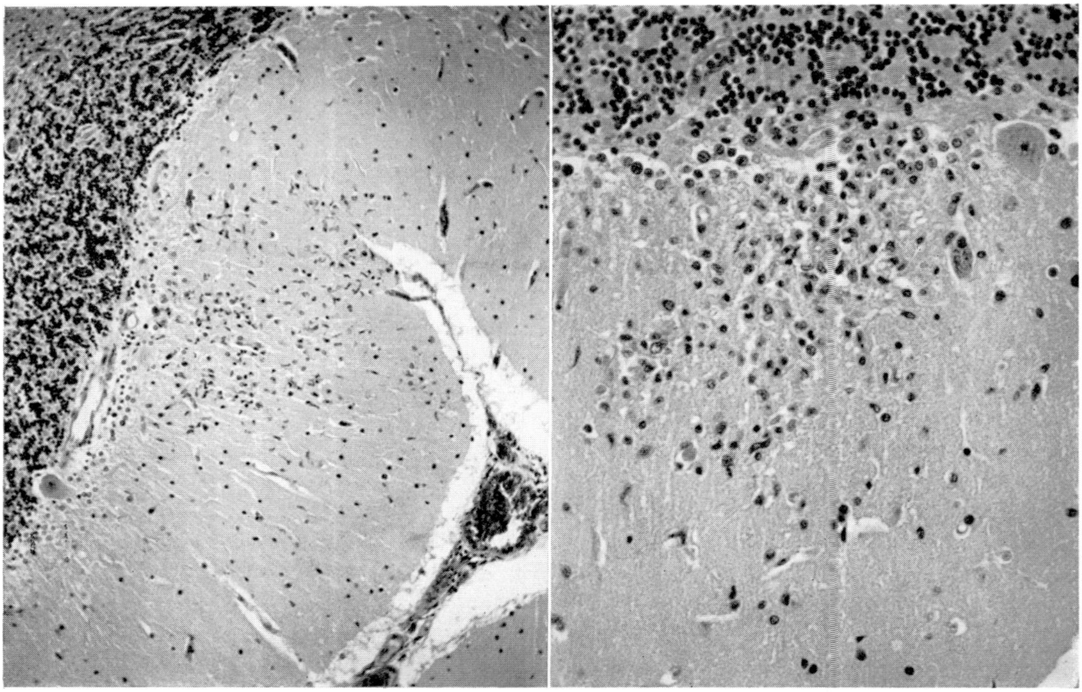

(*a*) (*b*)

FIG. 3 15. Japanese B encephalitis. Shrub formation of microglial cells in the molecular layer of the cortex associated with loss of Purkinje cells. (*a*) ×50, (*b*) ×250. (By the kindness of Dr. Haymaker.)

Areas of softening, some as large as a sparrow's egg, have also been described (Uchiyama 1925). In some still more chronic cases these lesions become so heavily infiltrated with calcium salts that it is impossible to cut the brain with a knife (Zimmerman 1946, 1948). This was noted also in some cases occurring in the Murray Valley of Australia.

Microscopically: (1) meningeal infiltration is usually moderate and concentrated in the sulci. (2) Perivascular infiltration is widespread in the grey matter but mostly restricted to the subcortical zone in the white matter. In early cases it may contain some polymorphonuclear leucocytes. (3) Nodular collections of cells are scattered throughout the cortex, basal ganglia, brain stem and spinal cord. Some, but not all, are related to blood-vessels. They consist chiefly of histiocytic cells which, in older lesions, have the appearance of macrophages (Haymaker and Sabin 1947). In addition to the larger, more solid cell nodules, a more diffuse increase of cells including oligodendroglia and microglia is seen in the basal ganglia and in some nuclei of the brain stem, especially the thalamus, globus pallidus, substantia nigra and nuclei pontis. It is associated with some loss of nerve cells in these nuclei. In the cerebellum nodules are confined to the molecular layer and some loss of Purkinje cells is also found, with glial shrubs in the lines of their dendrites (Fig. 3.15*a* and *b*). In the spinal cord neuronophagy is common especially in the ventral horns, but some is seen also in the dorsal and lateral horns.

In chronic cases Zimmerman found much deposition of calcium in the areas involved. It occurred either as clumps or as long wide bands along the cortical laminae. Foreign body giant cells may be seen among these deposits. In these cases he also found extensive loss of Purkinje cells. Uchiyama also described sclerosis and calcification of the walls of small blood-vessels and deposition of iron-containing material in many vessels in the white matter of the cerebral and cerebellar hemispheres.

EQUINE ENCEPHALOMYELITIS IN MAN

Equine encephalomyelitis, which has been known in North America since 1931, is there due to two serologically distinct types of virus named Eastern and Western. In general the geographical line of separation of these two types is the Appalachian Mountains. In addition to causing very serious epizootics among horses there have been outbreaks in epidemic or endemic form in the population of certain areas. The small epidemic of cases due to the Eastern type of virus which occurred in Massachusetts and Rhode Island in August and September of 1938 drew attention to this disease as a cause of encephalitis in man. Although only 38 cases occurred the death-rate (65 per cent) of this outbreak was alarming. In most cases the disease ran a very acute course, especially in children among whom most of the cases occurred. It was often biphasic with a short remission between the onset of fever and the appearance of neurological signs. In this type of encephalomyelitis the cell count in the cerebrospinal fluid is unusually high, ranging from 250 to 2,000 and including a large proportion of polymorphonuclear leucocytes. Since 1938 only occasional human cases due to the Eastern type of virus have been reported.

The Western type of virus has caused many more cases both in the Western States of the U.S.A. and the prairie provinces of Canada. In 1941 alone 1,700 cases were recorded in Minnesota and North Dakota (Noran and Baker 1945). Most of these have been sporadic and have occurred in persons in contact with horses, but small epidemics such as those in the San Joaquin valley of California in 1937, in Saskatchewan in 1938 and in the Yakima valley of Washington in 1940 have also occurred. Although the death-rate in this type of encephalitis has been lower than in that due to the Eastern type of virus, it has risen to 40 per cent in some epidemics, especially those in which the virus of Western equine encephalomyelitis has been found associated with the virus of Saint Louis encephalitis.

The viruses of Eastern and Western equine encephalomyelitis are small, measuring from 40mμ to 50mμ by electron microscopy. In addition to horses, they are pathogenic for a wide range of mammals and birds including pigs and domestic fowls and pigeons. They are probably transmitted to man in most cases by insect bites, especially by mosquitoes. Both *Aedes* and *Culex* types have been found to harbour the virus under natural conditions and to be able to transmit it by their bite. Ticks and mites may also transmit the virus, and it may be spread in the animal reservoir in this manner.

Morbid anatomy and histology

Eastern type. *Macroscopically* the brain is congested and swollen. The congestion in the brain stem may be so great as to suggest small haemorrhages, but these are rarely found. *Microscopically* inflammatory changes are greatest in the brain stem and basal ganglia but may be widespread in the cerebral cortex and may spread to the cervical cord or even below this. They are both diffuse and focal. In the early stages there is widespread infiltration of meninges and perivascular sheaths with neutrophil leucocytes and occasional lymphocytes and monocytes. Many of the small arteries show acute arteritis with necrosis and fibrin deposition in their walls which are invaded by neutrophil leucocytes. There is also diffuse infiltration of the brain-tissue with neutrophil leucocytes and microglial cells, and where this is most intense many of the nerve cells show degeneration or necrosis. In addition there are discrete or confluent areas of more profound necrosis infiltrated with similar cells (Wesselhoeft, Smith and Branch 1938). Some loss of Purkinje cells and cellular excess in the molecular layer of the cerebellar cortex has been described.

At a later stage the perivascular and meningeal infiltrations are lymphocytic in type; demyelination may be seen in numerous scattered areas of white matter where the inflammatory process has been most severe. Feemster (1938) also described widespread congestion of viscera with numerous small thrombi and severe pulmonary oedema. The Type B intranuclear inclusions described in experimental work with this virus have not been found in human cases.

Western type. In encephalitis due to the Western type of virus the lesions have a similar character and distribution. They are usually less acute; there is less infiltration by neutrophil leucocytes, but more tendency to produce lesions in the white matter. The greatest damage is usually seen in the basal ganglia and the white matter of the cerebral hemispheres where there may be numerous small areas of demyelination or of more severe necrosis of tissues; these are usually perivascular and may form small cysts at a later stage (Weil and Breslich 1942, Noran and Baker 1945). More extensive cystic degeneration of the white matter has been described in patients who have been attacked by the disease during the first year of life (Noran and Baker 1943, 1945). Widespread destruction of Purkinje cells may also be found in children.

RUSSIAN SPRING-SUMMER (TICK-BORNE) ENCEPHALOMYELITIS

Since 1935 a form of encephalomyelitis has been endemic in forest lands of eastern Siberia. The work of various Russian scientists has shown it to be due to a virus, antigenically related to that of louping-ill in sheep, and to be spread by the bite of the tick *Ixodes persulcatus*. More recently cases in more western farm areas of Russia have been found to be due to the same virus, but the tick responsible for the spread of the disease in these regions appears to be *Ixodes ricinus*. This form of disease has spread westwards and many cases have been reported in Slovenia and Styria (Pond and Russ 1955, Verlinde *et al.* 1955). Almost all wild mammals as well as farm animals have been found to be susceptible to the disease, but rodents probably play the chief role in its spread. The virus may remain viable at low temperatures in ticks and may be transmitted to their offspring, and it is considered probable that it is kept alive through the winter in the bodies of ticks. As these only bite in spring and early summer the incidence of the disease is from April to August, most cases occurring during the latter half of May and the first half of June.

Morbid anatomy and histology

The chief incidence of the disease is on the medulla and spinal cord and congestion and petechial haemorrhages are found in these areas.

Microscopically the changes in the medulla and spinal cord are similar to those of poliomyelitis with rather more infiltration of the white matter. Perivascular agglomerations of neuroglial cells and focal infiltrations are described, as well as necrosis of some of the vessel walls. Evidence of inflammation may be present throughout the spinal cord but is usually greatest in the cervical and lower lumbar segments. Numerous microglial shrub formations in the molecular layer of the cerebellum indicate lesions of the Purkinje cells. Inflammatory reactions are also seen in dorsal root ganglia and the Gasserian ganglion.

The weakness and wasting of the muscles of the neck and shoulder-girdle which are common sequelae suggest that the upper cervical segments and the more medially placed cell groups in the cervical enlargement often bear the brunt of the disease.

HERPES SIMPLEX ENCEPHALITIS

As has already been seen herpes simplex virus has also been considered to be the cause of some cases of benign lymphocytic meningitis (Armstrong 1943, Alm 1951). It has also been transmitted to animals from the cerebrospinal fluid of patients with herpes febrilis, as well as from those suffering from other diseases, such as neurosyphilis, on whom its invasion of the central nervous system appears to have produced little if any effect. It was similarly passaged from the brain of cases of encephalitis lethargica, but the lesions of this disease were so dissimilar from those of herpes encephalitis that a common etiology now seems very unlikely. The same problem has arisen in relation to subacute inclusion encephalitis which is regarded by some as a subacute form of herpes encephalitis. However, complement fixation tests with herpes antigen have been negative in the serums of most cases of subacute encephalitis.

In the adult the effects on the nervous system of infection by the virus are seldom more severe than this. In the newborn, however, up to one month old, the effects are severe and are sometimes associated with necrotic lesions of the liver and other viscera. In some of these cases there had been a recent attack of herpes febrilis, and from others the virus of herpes was transmitted to animals. In Wildi's (1951) case a new-born infant was infected with herpes of the skin and conjunctiva from the vulva of the mother and developed encephalitis 5 days after the appearance of the rash.

The virus of herpes simplex measures from 100mμ to 250mμ in diameter. It gives rise to Type A intranuclear inclusions both in the epithelial cells of cutaneous or corneal vesicles and in nerve cells and oligodendroglia in cases of encephalitis. The inclusions are acidophilic, rounded or irregular in shape and often finely granular. They vary in size from 2μ to almost the size of the nucleus in which they lie. Two or more inclusions may be seen in the same nucleus. Unless they fill the nucleus completely they are surrounded by a clear halo and sometimes fine radiating lines can be seen joining the inclusion body to the nuclear membrane. Swan (1943) describes similar fibrillary strands joining two inclusions in one nucleus. The nucleolus is pushed to the side of the nucleus and the chromatin granules become arranged in small clumps under the nuclear membrane. Haymaker (1949) has also described cytoplasmic inclusions in nerve cells. These are rather smaller and rounded and they also are surrounded by a clear halo.

In the cases which have come to post-mortem the encephalitic process has been very severe causing necrosis of areas of the cortex and softening of the subjacent white matter. Haymaker described these areas as 'mushy' and noted that in two cases the cerebral hemispheres had been discarded at autopsy as being too much softened for histological examination. Anatomically such necrotic regions have a characteristic distribution in the grey and white matter of the temporal lobes and the insula.

Microscopically in the most severely affected areas all the nervous tissue is broken down and is being absorbed by macrophages. In areas showing less damage the usual evidences of encephalitis are present, lymphocytes being noticeable. Many cortical nerve cells, both in the neighbourhood of necrotic areas and more diffusely, contain intranuclear inclusions and these are still more abundant in both interfascicular and perineuronal oligodendroglia. Neuronophagy may be a striking feature but has been absent in some cases. In a few cases the vessel walls in areas of necrosis have themselves been necrotic, with fibrinous exudate and polymorphonuclear leucocytes in and around them, but in Haymaker's cases there was no evidence of vascular occlusion in the softened areas. In addition to the cerebral cortex, which has been the area of the most severe damage in all reported cases, inflammatory lesions have been found in the basal ganglia and brain stem, diminishing caudally. The cerebellum has only shown minor lesions.

ACUTE ENCEPHALITIS OF UNCERTAIN ORIGIN
ACUTE NECROTIC ENCEPHALITIS

Greenfield (1950) was perhaps the first to mention cases of acute encephalitis, occurring usually in adults, which are similar clincally and when studied *post mortem* are similar in their basal, temporal distribution and necrotic aspect, to the herpetic encephalitis of the new-born. Histologically the two conditions are similar and similar intranuclear inclusion bodies Type A may or may not be present. The *herpes simplex* virus has not however been recovered from the cases of acute necrotic encephalitis. Twenty-four cases had been published when Brihaye (1958) in his important article from Dr. van Bogaert's laboratory stated that there was no conclusive argument that acute necrotic encephalitis was due to *herpes simplex*. Since then other cases have been published and several are to be found in the Antwerp Symposium on Encephalitides, 1959. Krüeke *et al.* (1952) described the distribution as being in all the temporal gyri, the insula, the posterior part of the orbital gyri and in the cingulate gyri with the most intense and extensive lesions in the temporo-hippocampal and temporo-fusiform gyri and in the insula.

SUBACUTE ENCEPHALITIS OF UNCERTAIN ORIGIN
DAWSON'S INCLUSION BODY ENCEPHALITIS—VAN BOGAERT'S SUBACUTE SCLEROSING LEUCO-ENCEPHALITIS

In 1933 and 1934 Dawson reported two subacute progressive cases of encephalitis in children occurring in Tennessee. They were characterised clinically by involuntary jerking movements of the limbs and mental regression and pathologically by the presence in many cortical neurones of Type A intranuclear inclusions. He failed to transmit the disease to rabbits either by intracerebral, subcutaneous or corneal inoculation of brain tissue, and inoculated mice, guinea-pigs, monkeys, dogs and chickens gave equally negative results. He therefore concluded that the disease was not due to the virus of herpes simplex.

Similar cases were published by Akelaitis and Zeldis (1942) from New York State and by Brain, Greenfield and Russell (1943, 1948) from London. Since that time a number of similar cases in children and adolescents, with a duration of illness varying from 5 weeks to more than a year, has been reported in Great Britain, the United States and Canada.

In 1945 L. van Bogaert, under the title *Subacute sclerosing leucoencephalitis*, reported 3 cases with similar clinical histories, fatal in from 3 to 6 months. He also referred to a case previously reported by himself and de Busscher (1939).

The most unusual feature in the examination of the brains of these cases was the diffuse inflammatory exudate in the white matter in certain areas of the cerebral hemispheres. The fibrous gliosis accompanying this appeared to be out of proportion to the slight demyelination which was present. Subacute inflammatory lesions in the cerebral cortex, thalamus and brain stem were also found. About 50 similar cases have been reported since 1945, many by van Bogaert's pupils, from the continent of Europe. In some of these cases intranuclear inclusions similar to those seen by Dawson were found in cortical nerve cells.

Further experience with subacute progressive cases of this character has made it clear that no dividing line can be drawn either on clinical or pathological grounds between the type of case described by Dawson in which the lesions are limited to the grey matter and Type A inclusions are abundant, and that described by van Bogaert in which inflammatory and sclerotic lesions in the white matter are more evident. While there are great variations in the incidence of the disease on the grey or the white matter, it is a general rule that the more chronic cases show more demyelination and sclerosis of the white matter and that intranuclear inclusions are more easily found in cases which run a short course. This group of cases may therefore be considered as a clinicopathological entity. Although the failure to transmit the disease to laboratory animals makes its aetiology uncertain, Type A intranuclear inclusions such as those found in this disease are generally accepted as evidence of a virus disease (Pinkerton 1950). The characters of the inflammation are also characteristic of virus encephalitis.

In 1939 Pette and Döring described four cases of *nodular panencephalitis* occurring in patients aged 61, 59, 56 and 17 years. Since World War II, in which a considerable part of the histological material was destroyed, the exact position of this encephalitis has been the subject of considerable discussion. The present position is that the encephalitides of Dawson, van Bogaert and Pette Döring are variants of one leucoencephalitis (Pette and Kalm 1953, Petsche *et al.* 1961) or alternatively that the proofs are insufficient to separate these three conditions (Tariska 1961).

Clinical features

This form of encephalitis has several unusual clinical features which may make the diagnosis evident during life. (1) Most of the cases so far reported have been in children or young persons between the ages of 4 and 20 years. (2) There is an ingravescent onset in which psychic changes, such as night terrors or hallucinations, uncontrollable behaviour or mental dullness are often the first symptoms. (3) Either from the beginning or during the middle stages of the disease periodic involuntary movements are present. These may consist of jerking of the face, fingers or limbs, or rapid torsion spasms of the trunk, or of losses of tone causing the patient to stumble or fall. They tend to occur at regular intervals, often once every 5–10 seconds, and the interval may remain the same for many days at a time. (4) A characteristic E.E.G. has been found during the middle stages of the disease in a large proportion of the cases. Its special feature is the periodic succession of high voltage complexes which are usually synchronous in all leads with the involuntary movements. Like these they retain a definite interval which is usually between 5 and 10 seconds. Although their shape and intensity may vary in different leads they usually remain stereotyped in each lead for long periods. They may be present during sleep or when no movements are present. (5) A colloidal gold curve of paretic type has been found in the cerebrospinal fluid in almost every case in which it has been looked for. The cell count is usually low and the fluid otherwise normal. (6) In most cases the disease progresses steadily to a fatal termination in from 6 weeks to 6 months, but the first stage of mental deterioration may be very gradual and prolonged so that the date of onset is uncertain, or the disease may cease to progress during the second stage leaving the patient in much the same condition for months or years.

Morbid anatomy and histology

On naked eye examination the brain may appear normal but often feels unusually firm in its fresh state. Some convolutions may be shrunken and discoloured; more rarely there is local necrosis of the cortex. On section some areas of white matter may appear granular or cheesy; this is most often seen in the occipital lobes in chronic cases (Fig. 3.16*a*). Very occasionally small losses of tissue may be seen either in the white matter or the cortex. The areas of damage to the white matter may resemble to some extent the early stages of Schilder's disease, but the greyish translucent appearance of the later stages of this disease is not seen even in the more chronic cases, and there is no tendency for the subcortical U fibres to be preserved. On the contrary the more damaged areas of white matter are often covered with shrunken sclerotic cortex. But in many cases no abnormality may be seen on section of the brain either in the grey or white matter and it may be difficult for this reason to select for microscopical examination areas which are likely to show the more severe lesions. In general these are most often found in the parieto-occipital and temporal lobes and sometimes also in the precentral gyrus (Osetowska 1961).

Histological examination shows the lesions of a subacute encephalitis. Perivascular infiltrations with lymphocytes and plasma cells and astrocytic and microglial proliferation occur both in the grey and white matter. A slight degree of meningeal infiltration may also be seen in some areas. In the grey matter there is degeneration of many nerve cells which may be chromatolytic or shrunken or may consist only of a hyperchromic nucleus surrounded by some shreds of cytoplasm. A few or many of these may contain Type A acidophilic nuclear inclusions which are usually homogeneous but may be finely granular (Fig. 3.16*c*). Floccular masses of hyaline material may also be seen in their cytoplasm; in the early stages several small oval or rounded bodies may be seen, usually near the cell margin, but sometimes more centrally placed; later these appear to enlarge and fuse into crescentic or horseshoe shaped masses which lie under the cell membrane (Fig. 3.16*d*); in the last stages of degeneration these become more rounded and lie at one side of the nucleus. Both nuclear and cytoplasmic inclusions may be found in the same cell or one type may occur without the other. Cells containing nuclear inclusions always show some alteration of the cell body but this may be no more than slight central chromatolysis. The most typical nuclear inclusions fill the greater part of the nucleus. They are sharply outlined and separated from the nuclear membrane by a clear halo. The radial spikes, which are often seen in herpes simplex connecting the inclusion body to the nuclear membrane, have not been seen in this disease. The nucleolus is pushed to the side of the nucleus but is otherwise normal, and the nuclear chromatin, which may be rather increased in amount, forms small clumps under the nuclear membranes. In the most severely damaged cells, the nucleus is filled with the acidophilic inclusion which compresses the chromatin against the nuclear membrane. At this stage a small irregularly rounded mass of hyaline material at one side of the nucleus may be the only vestige of the cytoplasm.

In the more affected areas of cortex many nerve cells have disappeared; there is an increased number of astrocyte nuclei and some formation of neuroglial fibres may be seen in the deeper cortical layers. Even in less affected areas pairs or quartets of astrocyte nuclei surrounded by thick protoplasmic processes are common. In slightly affected areas the most obvious change

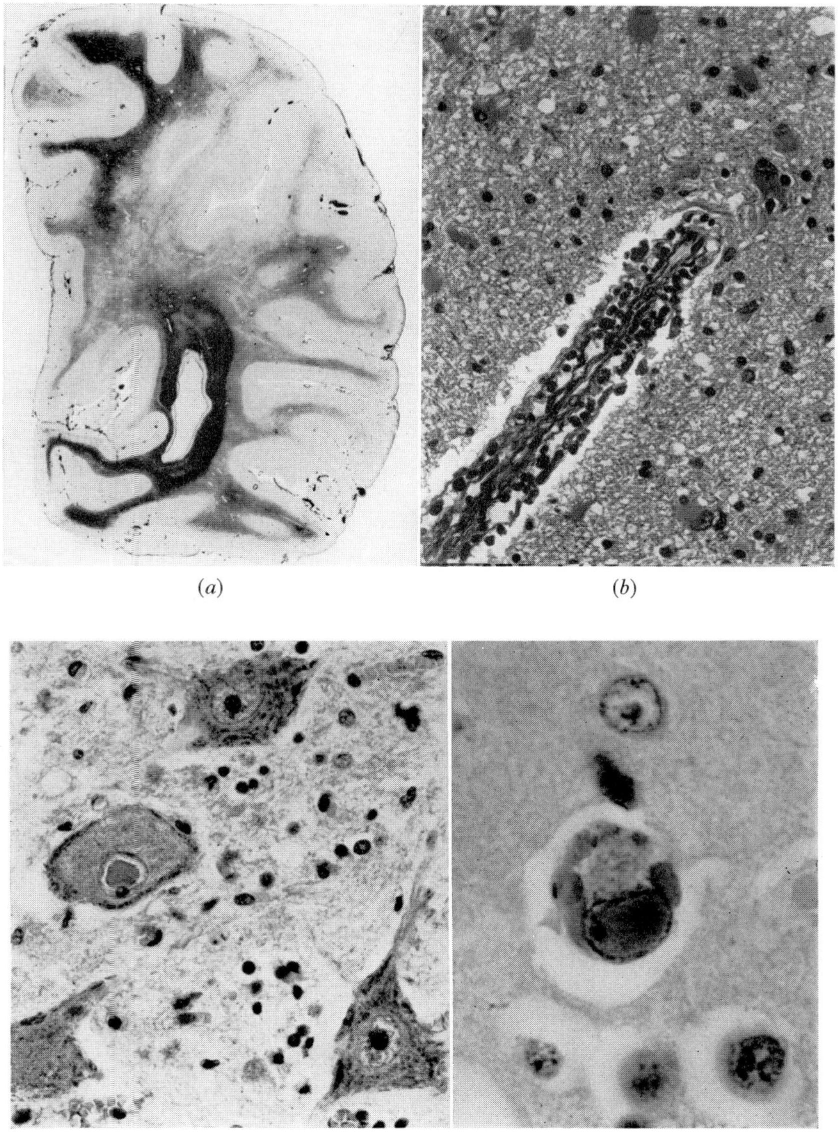

(a) (b)

(c) (d)

FIG. 3.16. Subacute inclusion encephalitis.

(*a*) Section of the occipital lobe in a case of 6 months' duration. (Myelin.)

(*b*) Section of area of white matter in a case of 15 months' duration, showing swollen-bodied astrocytes and perivascular infiltration.

(*c*) Anterior horn cells from 8th cervical segment, one of which shows an intranuclear inclusion and central chromatolysis. (H. and E. ×350.) (Case 2 of Brain, Greenfield and Russell 1948.)

(*d*) Cortical nerve cell with intranuclear and cytoplasmic inclusions; a later stage of degeneration. (Gomori ×1,000.)

is focal increase of microglial nuclei which form small clusters or stars or surround an occasional nerve cell. Even in such slightly damaged areas a few nerve cells containing nuclear inclusions may be found. In some cases a degree of lesion no greater than this, along with sparse perivascular infiltrations, may be found in several widely scattered areas of cortex, with apparently normal cortex elsewhere. Occasional Russell cells or mulberry cells may be found either in the grey or white matter. The more sclerotic areas of cortex show more astrocytic than microglial hyperplasia. Along with this there is great loss of nerve cells especially in the 5th and 6th cortical layers. In such areas nuclear inclusions may be absent or extremely scarce. Malamud, Haymaker and Pinkerton (1950), in a case with a duration of 7 years, found fibrillary degeneration of Alzheimer type in many nerve cells in the cerebral cortex, thalamus and brain stem. Similar changes were seen in the cerebral cortex by Corsellis (1951).

In the affected areas of white matter there is a diffuse or more focal increase of small cells, many of which appear to be early lipid phagocytes. Lymphocytes and plasma cells may also be found free in the tissues as well as in the perivascular infiltrations and some or many oligodendroglial nuclei are filled with acidophilic inclusions. With Sudan IV, cells containing sudanophilic granules may be seen scattered in smaller or larger numbers among apparently normal myelin sheaths. These appearances have more resemblance to Wallerian degeneration in a mixed tract than to the more common demyelinating diseases of the white matter of the hemispheres, and led to the early view that the damage to myelin was secondary to loss of cortical neurones (Brain, Greenfield and Russell 1948). Further experience, however, favours the view taken by van Bogaert that most of the damage to the white matter is independent of cortical lesions. Areas of more complete demyelination with loss of most or all of the myelin sheaths are, however, uncommon (Foley and Williams 1953). This minor degree of demyelination is associated with swelling and some increase in number of astrocytes and with the fibrous gliosis emphasised by van Bogaert (Fig. 3.16*b*). Where the areas are immediately subcortical an early loading of microglial cell processes with sudanophilic granules may also be seen in the overlying cortex. There may be little pallor of myelin staining in areas where sudanophilic degeneration and fibrous gliosis are quite evident, but in many of the more chronic cases fairly large pale areas may be seen. They are most common in the occipital lobes where they usually involve the outer half of the white matter and spare the optic radiations (Fig. 3.16*a*).

Distribution of lesions. In addition to the regions of the isocortex mentioned above the hippocampus is severely involved in some cases but is comparatively normal in others. In the corpus striatum and globus pallidus the lesions are usually slight. In the medial thalamus on the other hand they are often severe. The ventral half of the brain stem is more involved than the dorsal. In most cases microglial proliferation is seen among the nuclei pontis and less constantly in the substantia nigra, nucleus dentatus and inferior olives. Inclusions have on occasion been found in the nerve cells of many nuclei in the brain stem, but most often, and in largest numbers, in the nuclei pontis. In the cerebellar cortex there may be loss of Purkinje cells and microglial shrub formation. Van Buren described typical nuclear inclusions in Purkinje cells. The spinal cord is rarely affected. Brain *et al.* (1948) and van Buren (1954) described inclusions in the nerve cells of the ventral and dorsal horns of the cervical enlargement. Those in the motor cells of the ventral horn are very large, and easily visible with low magnifications. In Brain's case the first symptoms appeared soon after anti-diphtheria inoculations into the arm and, as sometimes happens in poliomyelitis, these may have determined the site of the disease. Degeneration and loss of ventral horn cells and glial stars in the white columns have also been described; Macken and Lhermitte (1950) found sclerosis of the long tracts of the spinal cord.

Radermecker (1949) described lesions in the posterior nerve root ganglia, in the spinal nerve roots and peripheral nerves.

SUBACUTE ENCEPHALITIS OF LATER ADULT LIFE

In 1960 Brierley *et al.* described a subacute encephalitis, mainly affecting the limbic areas (uncus, amygdaloid nucleus, hippocampal region and cingulate gyrus on each side) in patients aged 53, 56 and 58 years who were ill for 3, 7 and 14 months. *Macroscopically*, the cortex of the temporal regions looked abnormal and was not clearly defined from the white matter. *Microscopically*, the leptomeninges showed lymphocytic and plasma-celled infiltration, in the grey matter there was neuronal destruction, glial nodule formation, astrocytic proliferation, perivascular cuffing with lymphocytes and a few plasma cells. Necrosis or inclusion bodies were not seen. The changes spread into the white matter in the most severely affected regions. Virus studies were not carried out.

CYTOMEGALIC INCLUSION DISEASE

This disease, which has been known for many years as a common pathological finding in still-born babies, has come to be recognised as a serious and sometimes fatal febrile illness of infancy or early childhood. It is characterised clinically by petechial or blotchy purpuric rashes, diarrhoea or intestinal haemorrhage and often jaundice, and pathologically by the presence of large granular, acidophilic, intranuclear inclusions and often also small basophilic, cytoplasmic inclusions in swollen epithelial and endothelial cells. These are most often seen in the epithelium of salivary and pancreatic ducts, the convoluted tubules of the kidney, the parenchymal or bile-duct epithelium in the liver and the bronchiolar epithelium and alveolar lining cells in the lungs, but they have also been found in the pituitary, thyroid, parathyroid and adrenal cortex. The disease is not transmissible to laboratory animals but the lesions closely resemble those caused by the salivary gland viruses of various animals, which are transmissible to animals of the same species.

The brains of cases of this kind have not always been thoroughly examined but in a few cases periventricular lesions have been found. The ependyma may appear thickened and rusty coloured and may be coarsely rugose or show finer granulations (Haymaker *et al.* 1954). Some degree of hydrocephalus may be present. Areas of calcification in the periventricular region may be noted on section of the brain. In Kinney's (1942) case there were irregular areas of softening in the basal ganglia and occipital lobe.

Histologically in addition to the deposition of granules containing iron and calcium there is wide-spread subependymal swelling of astrocytes and gliosis which may replace denuded ependyma or cover the ependymal layer in some places. Cytomegalic inclusions may be found in astrocytes and in the endothelium of small vessels. Perivascular infiltration with lymphocytes and plasma cells is usually slight. Although few cases have been reported at the time of writing, this disease may be one cause of hydrocephalus or of the periventricular calcification which is not uncommonly seen radiographically in the brains of epileptic or mentally backward children. Diezel (1954) has produced evidence that micropolygyria may be caused by intra-uterine infection by a virus of this character.

PROGRESSIVE MULTIFOCAL LEUCOENCEPHALOPATHY

This condition was first described by Aström, Mancall and Richardson in 1958. In 1961 Richardson reviewed 10 of his own cases and 12 collected from the literature. The neurological disorder occurred as a relatively short terminal condition in patients, aged 31 to 82 years, who were usually suffering from chronic diseases, viz. Hodgkin's disease (6 cases), chronic lymphatic leukaemia (4), lymphosarcoma (3), chronic myelogenous leukaemia (2), sarcoidosis (2), carcinomatosis (2), miliary tuberculosis (1), coronary heart disease (1) and unknown (old age) (1). They showed symptoms and signs of a diffuse but asymmetrical disorder of the cerebral hemispheres. Hemiparesis, dementia and impairment of vision and speech frequently occurred. The cerebrospinal fluid was often normal.

The pathological lesions, which were multiple, varied considerably in situation, size and stage of development from case to case. They were usually most numerous in the cerebral hemispheres, but the brainstem and cerebellum were often severely affected. The spinal cord, when examined, was not noticeably involved. Within the lesions myelin sheaths were not present and were replaced by phagocytes containing the intensely sudanophilic lipid droplets typical of myelin breakdown. Axis cylinders were relatively spared. Perivascular lymphocytic cuffing was often present. At the periphery of the lesions there was invariably an enlargement of the nuclei of the oligodendroglia, with dense basophilia and loss of nuclear detail. In nearly every case eosinophilic intra-nuclear inclusions were present in these abnormal oligodendroglia. Less constantly many of the astrocytes within the larger lesions were enormously enlarged, with irregular or multiple nuclei. In three cases large nuclei, suggestive of altered granule cells, were present in focal regions in the granular layer of the cerebellum.

Richardson considered that the histological changes in the oligodendroglia and astrocytes were compatible with infection by a virus, which he suggested occurred as a chance complication in patients with an impaired immunological response to infection.

RICKETTSIAL DISEASES

Typhus, scrub typhus (tsutsugamushi) and Rocky Mountain spotted fever

Lesions in the central nervous system are a constant part of the pathology of both European and Oriental (scrub) typhus fevers and are common and may be severe in Rocky Mountain spotted fever. Full descriptions of the pathology of the brain and spinal cord in *European, louse-borne typhus* (*Rickettsia prowazecki*) were given by Spielmeyer (1919) and Wolbach, Todd and Palfrey (1922), in *tick-borne, Rocky Mountain spotted fever* (*Dermacentroxenus Rickettsi*) by Wolbach (1919) and Lillie (1941) and in *mite-borne scrub typhus* (*R. orientalis*) from cases occurring in New Guinea by Weil and Haymaker (1946). In these three diseases the lesions are of the same type with some quantitative differences. They are widely spread throughout the brain, spinal cord and nerve roots but may be more concentrated in the brain stem than elsewhere. The naked-eye appearances of the brain are not very striking. There is usually congestion and maybe some oedema. In scrub typhus Weil and Haymaker describe cloudiness of the pia arachnoid especially towards the vertex of the parietal and occipital lobes both on the convexity and the median surface. Petechial haemorrhages round engorged vessels may be seen especially in the brain stem and corpus callosum.

Microscopically the typical lesions are *typhus nodules* which are present in the brain as well as in the skin and bodily organs. They are small tubercle-like nodules, almost always perivascular in site, and measuring 100–150μ in diameter. They are composed chiefly of histiocytes and microglial cells, and early nodules also contain many neutrophil leucocytes. The earliest changes in their formation occur in the endothelium of capillaries and pre-capillaries and consist in swelling and degeneration often leading to thrombosis. Mononuclear cells, many of which are in mitosis, and neutrophil leucocytes then appear round the vessel. Lymphocytes and plasma cells do not enter into the formation of the nodule but may be seen at its periphery and in perivascular infiltrations. Astrocytes are found in nodules in the later stages and give rise to the neuroglial scar which is the final stage. The nodules do not undergo the necrotic changes commonly seen in tubercles. Rickettsial organisms in pairs or larger numbers may be seen in the endothelial cells included in the nodules, but are less easily found than in skin lesions. Typhus nodules appear to be formed throughout the course of the disease and even after the fever has subsided.

The nodules of *Rocky Mountain spotted fever* differ from those of typhus and scrub typhus chiefly in that they may involve larger vessels in which the muscular fibres of the media may be invaded by the micro-organism. Microscopic infarctions may result from this process, but larger infarctions are not seen (Wolbach 1948). These micro-infarcts are most often found in the white matter of the cerebral hemispheres and in the pyramidal tracts in the brain stem. They are rare before the 12th day but common or constant thereafter (Lillie 1941). The nodular lesions also are usually slight or may be absent during the first 10 days of illness but in the later stages they are constant and may be abundant. Neutrophil leucocytes are less commonly seen in them than in the lesions of European or Oriental typhus.

Typhus nodules are found throughout the central nervous system. In European and Oriental typhus they are more common in the grey than in the white matter, but in Rocky Mountain spotted fever the distribution is more uniform. In the cerebral cortex they are most numerous in the 2nd to the 5th layer. They are also numerous in the basal ganglia and brain stem. Wolbach *et al.* found them especially abundant in the nuclei pontis and inferior olives. In the cerebellum they may be seen in the central nuclei and in the molecular layer; in the latter situation they may be confused with glial shrubs which also are not uncommon. Weil and Haymaker describe similar subependymal nodules which have no apparent relation to vessels. Nodules may also be found in the pars nervosa of the hypophysis but Wolbach *et al.* (1922) found none in the anterior lobe. Degenerative changes are common in the nerve cells which are close to typhus nodules, and may be of any severity from central chromatolysis to neuronophagy. Spielmeyer described the homogenising change in Purkinje cells in typhus fever as occurring independently of typhus nodules. In addition to the characteristic nodular lesions the inflammatory changes common to other forms of encephalitis are also present. Glial stars, rosette formations, or loose-textured collections of cells smaller than typhus nodules are not uncommon in the superficial layers of the cerebral cortex. Perivascular infiltration with lymphocytes and in the later stages also with plasma cells is widespread. The pia arachnoid also is infiltrated with mononuclear cells of various kinds; no increase in the connective tissue of the meninges was seen by Wolbach *et al.* In scrub typhus Weil and Haymaker found the most severe meningeal lesions near the vertex of the parietal and occipital lobes. In the early stages they consisted chiefly of oedema with hypertrophy of trabecular cells. Later there was infiltration by histiocytes and lymphocytes.

Diffuse and perivascular infiltration of *nerve roots* with lymphocytes, plasma cells and histiocytes and degeneration or destruction of the nerve cells of the Gasserian ganglion were described by Wolbach *et al.* Noad and Haymaker (1953) attribute the deafness which may follow scrub typhus to a lesion of this kind in the nerve roots or ganglia of the cochlear nerves. They found damage to myelin, and, less often, to axons in the nerve roots in relation to the denser collections of infiltrating cells.

INFECTIONS BY ANIMAL PARASITES

PROTOZOAL INFECTIONS

Toxoplasmosis

Wolf and Cowen (1937) described a case of granulomatous encephalitis in a 1-month-old baby in which minute nucleated crescentic bodies resembling *Toxoplasma gondii* were found in the lesions. On re-examining a similar case in a 7-week-old infant, which had been reported in 1936 by Richter, parasites of the same kind were found. Since then many cases in new-born infants have been reported from North and South America, Great Britain and the continent of Europe, and from some of these cases the disease has been transmitted to laboratory animals. The parasite may also cause acute encephalitis in older children (Sabin 1941) or pulmonary (Pinkerton and Henderson 1941) or lymph node (Siim 1951, Gard and Magnusson 1951) infections in adults. Siim (1955) divides acquired infections into four clinical types: (1) exanthematous, (2) cerebrospinal, (3) ophthalmic and (4) lymph-node infections. The last appears to be a relatively common and benign form which leaves no sequelae, but babies born of mothers who had this form of infection during pregnancy have suffered from severe cerebrospinal disease (Farquhar and Turner 1949). In babies who survive congenital or neo-natal infection there may be radiological evidence of the disease in the form of small, diffusely scattered or periventricular, calcifications within the brain. These are often associated with epilepsy and mental retardation. They may be accompanied by choroidoretinitis with some degree of optic atrophy, or this may be the only clinical evidence of the disease.

Aetiology. *Toxoplasma gondii* (Gr. *toxon* = a bow) is a crescentic, oval or elongated protozoon consisting of an acidophilic cell body and a polar mass of chromatin. With Wright's or Leishman's stain the cell body stains blue and the polar chromatin red. In some parasites a smaller red staining granule can be seen at the pole opposite to the nucleus. The absence of a kinetoplast distinguishes the parasites from the leishmania stage of trypanosomes. With methylene blue-eosin the cell body stains pink and the chromatin blue. The parasites divide by longitudinal fission which begins in the nucleus. In sections they measure 2–3μ in length by 1·5–2μ in width. Wolf and Cowen give the measurement of the smallest as 0·9μ × 0·7μ and of the largest 3·5μ × 1·8μ. In smears of tissue or of the deposit from the cerebrospinal fluid they appear rather larger. In the tissues they occur either in endothelial cells or free in the tissues. In either situation they may be isolated or in small groups. More rarely pseudocysts containing closely packed parasites or rosettes of parasites, which may arise from the disappearance of the cell membrane enclosing the pseudocyst, are seen. The pseudocysts vary in size from 6μ × 7μ to 15μ × 17μ. The encysted parasites are rather smaller than those that lie free (Fig. 3. 17).

The name *Toxoplasma gondii* is taken from the first mammalian species in which the parasite was found. At first toxoplasmas from different animal species received the name of the species in which they occurred, but according to modern views there is no difference between these various strains. The encephalitozoon cuniculi described and so named by Levaditi, Nicolau and Schoen (1923) may also be a toxoplasma.

Toxoplasma gondii is widely spread in nature among both mammals and birds. It has been found in the urine and faeces of domestic animals and in the milk of laboratory animals. Every mammalian species which has been tested is susceptible but primates appear to be less so than lower animals, and rodents, especially mice, guinea-pigs and rabbits are particularly susceptible. Under natural conditions infection is widespread among rabbits with the result that dogs and cats which feed on rabbits may become infected. In all species the young are more easily infected and more liable to develop cerebral lesions than older animals; for example vaginal infection of pregnant mice may cause a predominantly cerebral infection in their offspring. The same rule applies in human cases. Mothers with only glandular or subclinical infection may give birth to babies with cerebral lesions but all foetuses are not equally susceptible, and one twin may be severely affected when the other shows little evidence of disease.

Pathology. In babies with congenital or neo-natal involvement of the central nervous system, naked eye examination of the brain may show yellowish, depressed and softened cortical areas which vary in size from a few millimetres to 3 cm. in diameter. The pia-arachnoid over these areas is thickened and discoloured. On section of the brain areas of granulomatous inflammation may be seen in all parts of the brain, brain stem and spinal cord. They are often most numerous in the cerebral cortex and basal ganglia and may be confined to these situations. Some are well defined and may have a caseous or cystic centre. Others are more diffuse. A zone of inflammation and necrosis of tissue round the lateral ventricles has been described in some cases. These lesions often feel gritty to the knife when sectioned.

Histological examination may show lesions of three kinds. (1) Large granulomatous areas with a necrotic centre. (2) More diffuse inflammation of the tissues. (3) Miliary granulomas. The last are the most widespread and characteristic. They are often present in the more superficial layers of the cortex where they blend with the thickened and inflamed pia-arachnoid but may be abundant also in the white matter and may be found in the basal ganglia, brain stem, and spinal cord. They are usually about 100μ in diameter. They consist chiefly of large endothelial or epithelioid cells of irregular, oblong or oval shape, along with an admixture of lymphocytes and occasional plasma and other mononuclear cells. Eosinophil leucocytes may also be seen in them. They do not contain giant cells. The large endothelial cells appear to arise from the capillaries and the adventitia of the arterioles which show swelling of their endothelium. The larger granulomas are made up of inflammatory cells of all kinds including neutrophil leucocytes near necrotic areas. The outer zones are invaded by fibroblasts and show capillary dilatation and sprouting. They are surrounded by a zone of oedematous brain tissue in which miliary granulomas may be present. The meninges are diffusely infiltrated and, where they overlie granulomatous areas of cortex, share in this type of inflammation. Parasites may be found in all areas of inflammation. They are chiefly extracellular but many are seen in large endothelial cells (Fig. 3.17). In the larger lesions amorphous deposits of calcium salts are often present, both in necrotic areas and more diffusely; they are rare in the meninges. Many of the nerve cells in the neighbourhood of granulomas are encrusted with calcium or iron salts.

In the *eye* toxoplasmosis may attack the choroid, ciliary body or retina producing small foci of granulomatous inflammation followed by scarring.

Clinical pathology. In infants with severe congenital encephalomyelitis the cerebrospinal fluid is usually xanthochromic and contains a great excess of protein and some increase in cells. In children who survive intra-uterine infection, or who acquire the disease later, the diagnosis may be established by complement fixation tests which should be positive in a dilution of 1 in 8 or more.

Amoebic abscess of the brain

Infection of the brain by *Entamoeba histolytica* causes a rapidly growing abscess and is the most fatal complication of amoebic dysentery. In the great majority of cases it follows abscess of the liver, but sometimes infection spreads to the brain from the lungs. Of the 61 cases collected from the literature by Halpert and Ashley (1944) an abscess was found in the liver in all except 5. When these figures are compared with the prevalence of amoebic dysentery it is clear that abscess in the brain is a very rare complication, but certainly many cases have gone unrecorded. A brain abscess may make its appearance many years after the first attack of amoebic dysentery, in fact it is much more often a late than an early complication of the disease. In many cases the patient does not know that he is a chronic carrier of amoebae, or fails to let his physician know this, so that the cause of the abscess is not recognised until it is too late. This is one of several factors which make amoebic abscess of the brain a very fatal disease.

Amoebic abscesses, in the brain as in the liver, are usually single. They may occur anywhere but are most often found in the cerebral hemispheres. Their contents are reddish-brown or pinkish, creamy fluid, often paler than the characteristic 'strawberry ice cream' contents of liver abscesses. No coagulum forms when this fluid is allowed to stand. It consists of necrotic cells, which are chiefly mononuclear, and unrecognisable débris. Amoebae are not easily recognisable in smears of this material but may be found in wet films. The abscess cavity has ragged and inflamed walls and is surrounded by a wide zone of oedema.

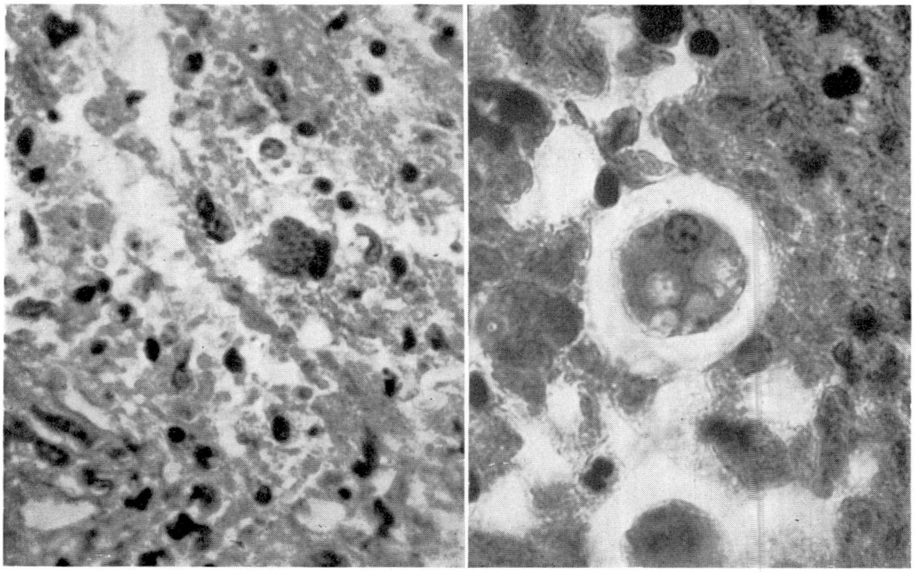

3.17 3.18

FIG. 3.17. Toxoplasmosis. Two large cells filled with toxoplasma parasites (pseudocysts) are seen near the centre of the photograph.

FIG. 3.18. Amoeba histolytica in cerebral abscess.

Microscopically the wall of the cavity is ill-defined and irregular and shows little or no evidence of encapsulation by fibrous tissue. There is an inner zone of necrotic tissue with little nuclear staining and a broad outer zone of vascular congestion, degeneration and necrosis of the nervous tissue and diffuse infiltration by lymphocytes, plasma cells and other mononuclear cells. Neutrophil leucocytes are usually scanty. The astrocytes in the surrounding white matter show the swelling of the cell body characteristic of cerebral oedema. Clasmatodendrosis is seen near the abscess. Amoebae can be recognised by their large size and relatively small, usually eccentric, palely stained nucleus (Fig. 3.18). They are found both in the necrotic tissue and among the infiltrating cells of the abscess wall.

Malaria

Cerebral malaria is almost always due to infection by *Plasmodium falciparum*. The heavily infected red blood cells pack and may block the cerebral capillaries and, in typical cases, this may give the brain tissue, especially the cortex, a greyish colour to the naked eye. In most cases there are also numerous petechial haemorrhages both in the meninges and on the cut surfaces of the brain.

Microscopically granules of brightly anisotropic, dark malarial pigment (related to haematin) lie in lines along every capillary. In addition to ring and ball haemorrhages, small necrotic foci ringed with microglial cells are seen round the blocked capillaries. These resemble the perivascular areas of necrosis seen in fat embolism. In cases that recover from the acute attack they become invaded by microglial cells and form small glial nodules. Small foci of demyelination and rarefaction of the white matter are also commonly found.

Trypanosomiasis

Three forms of trypanosome may attack the human central nervous system, *Trypanosoma gambiense*, *T. rhodesiense* and *T. cruzi* (*Chagas*). The method and results of the attack differ to some extent in the three forms. The African forms produce an initial meningitis which, in the Gambian form, gradually goes on to meningo-encephalitis, the well-known *sleeping-sickness* of the Congo and Uganda. Infection by *T. rhodesiense* is more acute and when untreated usually ends fatally from involvement of the heart before any nervous symptoms appear. When inadequately treated the disease is more subacute and signs of nervous disease may appear for a short time before death.

T. cruzi appears to reach the brain by the blood-stream and produces multiple inflammatory foci in its substance. The heart muscle is also involved in most cases.

Trypanosoma gambiense and rhodesiense

These forms of trypanosome do not appear to have a leishmania stage in their life cycle but in the insect vector develop a crythidial stage in which they multiply. The tsetse fly which is the usual vector of *T. gambiense* is *Glossina palpalis* and that carrying *T. rhodesiense* is *Glossina morsitans*. Both infections are usually transmitted from man to man, but there may be a reservoir in antelopes and domestic animals. Koppisch (1953) divides cases into three clinical types: (1) Those with a chronic course of several years and with changes in the cerebrospinal fluid, but no serious symptoms. (2) Those with severe early symptoms and a course of more than a year, later passing into the stage of *sleeping sickness*. These two forms are commonly caused by *T. gambiense*. (3) Those with an acute or subacute course, fatal in a few months from involvement of the heart and other viscera. Most cases of this kind are caused by *T. rhodesiense*. Changes in the cerebrospinal fluid may be the only evidence during life of infection of the nervous system in these cases, even in those which on post-mortem examination show intracerebral as well as meningeal lesions. In some cases of infection by *T. rhodesiense*, especially those which have received insufficient early treatment, there is a terminal stage of dementia passing into coma (Calwell 1937).

Pathology of African sleeping sickness (*T. gambiense*). On naked eye examination of the brain there is no wasting or convolutional atrophy. In some cases oedema has been observed. The pia-arachnoid is diffusely thickened, or more opaque than normal. Ependymal granulations are not seen. On section of the brain some of the vessels both in the white and grey matter may appear to be surrounded by a grey sleeve, owing to intense infiltration of Virchow-Robin spaces. No haemorrhages or softenings are usually present.

On *histological examination* the most striking abnormality is the perivascular infiltration which is very widespread throughout the central nervous system, but more intense in some areas than in others. In some cases it is greatest in the white matter and it may also be especially severe in the basal ganglia. In a few cases the chief incidence of the disease has been on the spinal cord. Around the smaller vessels the infiltration consists almost entirely of plasma cells, but in the thick cuffs around larger vessels lymphocytes are also found. Large histiocytic phagocytes engulfing plasma cells may be seen in these heavier infiltrations (Bertrand, Bablet and Sicé 1935). Where perivascular infiltration is intense, plasma cells are also found free in the tissues.

Morular cells, which were first described in this disease by Mott (1906), are present in considerable numbers both within and outside the Virchow-Robin spaces in the nervous tissue and in the subarachnoid space. They are more numerous in this disease than in any other condition. They are large spherical or ovoid cells measuring from 12μ to 20μ. The hyperchromic nucleus lies under the cell membrane and the cytoplasm is filled with numerous small globules which measure from 1·5μ to 3μ in diameter, and give the cell the appearance of a mulberry, whence the name. In some all the globules are of the same size; in others they vary considerably.

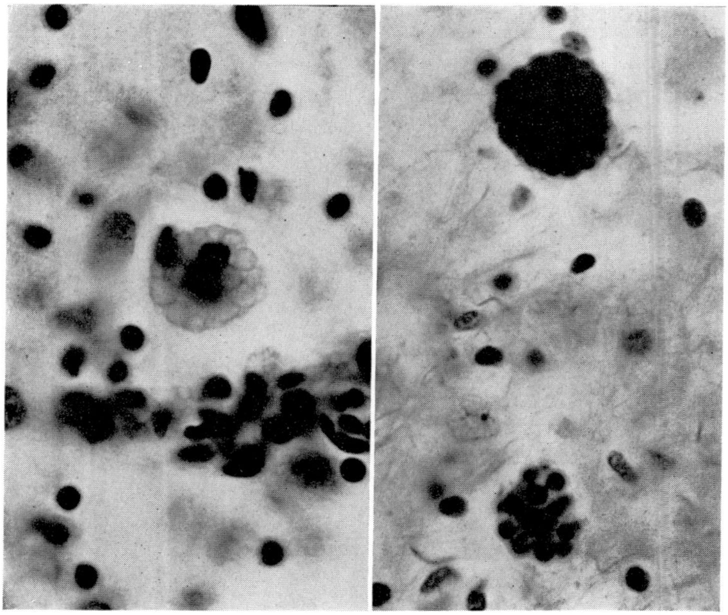

(*a*) (*b*)

FIG. 3.19. Morular cells in subacute encephalitis.
(*a*) Thionin. (*b*) Phosphotungstic acid haematoxylin.

They may appear encapsulated so that the cell has a smooth contour or may, as in a mulberry, form rounded projections on the surface (Fig. 3.19). The globules are acidophilic, staining strongly with acid fuchsin, eosin and phloxin, and also with all stains for neuroglial fibres such as phosphotungstic acid haematoxylin and Holzer's stain. They remain uncoloured by silver impregnations and by fat stains, and are pale blue or unstained in Nissl sections. These cells, which are probably derived from plasma cells, appear to be either the same as Russell bodies or a stage in their formation.

Some hypertrophied microglial cells and rod cells are present in the cortex but are not so numerous as in general paralysis. The astrocytes also are hypertrophied and may be binucleated. There is little loss of cortical neurones; the changes which have been described in nerve cells appear to be chiefly of a terminal character such as Nissl's acute swelling, but a few cells show chronic changes. Some loss of tangential fibres and hyperplasia of neuroglial fibres in the molecular layer of the cortex have also been described but are of minor degree.

Jansen, van Bogaert and Haymaker (1956) found lesions of parenchymatous as well as interstitial character in the cranial and spinal nerve roots and dorsal root ganglia. The interstitial changes consisted of inflammatory exudate and fibrous tissue thickening similar to that found elsewhere in the meninges. In addition there was degeneration of nerve fibres, isolated or in groups and varying in degree from the segmental peri-axial demyelination of Gombault to Wallerian degeneration. This seemed to be primary and independent of the interstitial changes. It appeared likely that both were caused by neurotoxins produced by the disintegration of trypanosomes. The changes in the nerve cells of the ganglia of the dorsal roots and cranial nerves appeared to be secondary to lesions of their axons. In one case a peripheral nerve showed a degree of degeneration of nerve fibres which was quite out of proportion to the degree of inflammatory exudate in and around it.

Clinical pathology. The diagnosis of Gambian trypanosomiasis is best established by finding parasites in the centrifugalised deposit of blood serum or in the juice of enlarged glands. Parasites may be found in the cerebrospinal fluid during the later stages of the disease. Neujean (1950) rarely found trypanosomes in the fluid when the cell count was below 30 per cu. mm. and only in about 10 per cent of cases in which it was between 30 and 100 per cu. mm. With higher cell counts the percentage of positive findings rose sharply and when more than 1,000 cells per cu. mm. were present trypanosomes could always be found. The total protein in the cerebrospinal fluid in trypanosomiasis rises with the cell count and the colloidal benzoin reaction also is usually positive when the cell count has risen above 20 per cu. mm. Hawking (Hawking and Greenfield 1941) found that trypanosomes did not survive *in vitro* at 37° C. in cerebrospinal fluid with a protein level of 100–150 mgm. per 100 ml. for more than 2–4 hours, but remained active for more than 24 hours when the protein level was raised by the addition of serum to 3,500 mg. per 100 ml. The critical percentage of protein appeared to be about 400 mg. per 100 ml. Even in cerebrospinal fluid which naturally contained trypanosomes they died in 1–2 hours at 37° C. From this it would appear that their normal habitat in the subarachnoid space during the early stages of invasion is intracellular rather than free in the fluid.

T. rhodesiense

In two untreated cases of infection by this parasite, in which trypanosomes abounded in the cerebrospinal fluid shortly before death, Hawking and Greenfield (1941) found pericardial and pleural effusions with very little fibrin or adhesions, and severe myocardial infiltration and degeneration. The central nervous system was normal except for mild diffuse meningeal infiltration in both cases and petechial haemorrhages in the occipital lobe in one. There was also slight infiltration of the choroid plexus. The meningeal infiltration consisted chiefly of large histiocytic cells, varying from the size of the large mononuclears of the blood to cells 30–40μ in diameter which were often binucleated or multinucleated. Lymphocytes and plasma cells were relatively scanty. Some of the latter had a vacuolated cytoplasm and resembled morular cells.

Calwell (1937) examined the brains of 17 cases in most of which inadequate treatment had been given in the early stages of the disease. In these the meningeal exudate was usually greatest towards the vertex of the brain. In only one case was it basal. The chief intracerebral lesion was perivascular infiltration which might be found in any part of the central nervous system including the spinal cord. It was common in the medulla and cerebellum, and morular cells were most often seen in those sites, but might also be found in the cortex, meninges, corpus callosum and basal ganglia in descending order of frequency. The choroid plexus was usually infiltrated with plasma cells and fibrinous exudate was sometimes found in it. Calwell found narrow, irregular zones of demyelination around small vessels, most often in medulla, pons, or cortex in 11 of his cases. Trypanosomes were never found in the brain, although they were commonly present in the cerebrospinal fluid during life. In his cases the cell count in the cerebrospinal fluid never exceeded 500 per cu. mm. He noted that with inadequate treatment the Rhodesian type of disease tended to approach the typical picture of *sleeping sickness.*

Chagas' disease

T. cruzi, the cause of South American trypanosomiasis or Chagas' disease, is conveyed by house bugs (usually *Triatoma megista*) which excrete it in their faeces. Mammals, especially the armadillo, are much more commonly infected than man and provide the reservoir of the disease. The human disease, which is relatively rare, usually begins with conjunctivitis and goes on to lymphadenopathy and oedema of the face and limbs. It may undergo spontaneous cure or relapse. When it becomes chronic the heart and nervous system are commonly affected.

The parasite may appear in the blood as a trypanosome, often curved like a letter C, or in cells in leishmania form. The latter form is that usually seen in sections of tissues. Cases in which there is involvement of the nervous system usually end fatally. Post-mortem examination shows congestion and oedema of the brain. Numerous small inflammatory foci, consisting of collections of mononuclear cells of various kinds, are found scattered through the substance of the brain, more in the white matter than the grey. They are commonly seen in the cerebellum, brain stem and spinal cord. They do not appear to be related to vessels. Leishmania may be found in swollen neuroglial cells and large mononuclear cells in these foci. In chronic cases Chagas found old scarred foci as well as recent foci containing leishmania. The *heart* usually shows intense myocarditis, with necrosis and phagocytosis of muscle fibres in some areas. Leishmania may be found in the muscle cells. The skin, spleen, lymph nodes, endocrine glands and voluntary muscle may also contain parasites in leishmania form.

METAZOAL INFECTIONS

Cestodes

Taenia solium (*Cysticercosis*)

The encysted larval stage of the common human tapeworm, *Taenia solium*, is usually passed in the pig; but if ova are ingested by man their shells are dissolved in the stomach and the embryos penetrate the wall of the intestine and are carried to all the organs of the body, including the brain and muscles. In most cases the resulting cysts remain small and in time the larvae die and become calcified. In the brain the cysts may grow for some time but here also they usually remain small, and soon die. In such cases the only symptoms are epileptic attacks, and when these begin in middle life in patients who have lived in India or Central or South America, the possibility of cysticercosis should be considered. Less often cysticerci develop as thin-walled, usually sterile, racemose cysts in the basal cisterns, causing hydrocephalus or cranial nerve palsies. In children, and more rarely in adults, they may develop into larger cysts in the brain, and cause early symptoms of intracranial pressure which may progress to a fatal termination within a few months of the first appearance of symptoms. These three forms or any two of them may be combined.

In the case described by Bickerstaff *et al.* (1952) in which hydrocephalic symptoms were present for 7 years before death, racemose cysts were removed from the cisterna magna at operation, and autopsy revealed numerous small calcified nodules in the brain and a cyst, containing a larva, in the head of the caudate nucleus.

The incidence of human cysticercosis varies greatly in different parts of the world. MacArthur (1933) observed numerous cases of subacute or chronic type in soldiers infected in India. Obrador (1948) in Mexico found that 25 per cent of cases submitted to operation for symptoms of intracranial pressure proved to have cerebral cysticercosis, and large series of surgical cases have also been reported from Chile by Arana and Asenjo (1945) and from Poland by Stepien and Chorobski (1949).*

Clinical pathology Although in chronic cases the cerebrospinal fluid is usually normal, in acute and subacute cases the cell count is raised to between 15–100 cells per cu. mm. and the total protein is also moderately increased. The glucose is often slightly, and may be considerably, reduced. Examination of the deposit often reveals the presence of eosinophil leucocytes, which occasionally form a third of the cells present. The fluid may give colloidal gold curves of meningitic or even paretic type. The complement fixation test is more specific and constant. Obrador (1948), using alcoholic extract of pig cysticerci as antigen, obtained positive results in all his cases, in more than half with a 1:5 dilution of cerebrospinal fluid. Eosinophilia in the blood is less constant and when present is usually low (2–5 per cent, Stepien and Chorobski 1949).

In chronic cases diagnosis often rests on the presence of cysts in the muscles which may be palpable or appear radiographically as small oval, elongated or carrot-shaped opacities. Calcified intracerebral nodules are less easily shown up owing to the density of the skull shadow.

Pathology. External examination of the brain shows in some cases small colourless cysts in the subarachnoid space. When closely grouped they are attached to a central pedicle and resemble a bunch of grapes. They are most often seen in the cisterna magna but may be present in the pontine or basal cisterns or in the Sylvian fissure. The leptomeninges are thickened in their neighbourhood. In other cases small cysts project from the cortex. These may be greyish and glistening with a white mural nodule, or more opaque. On section of the brain numerous cysts measuring about 1 cm. in diameter or smaller spherical nodules may be found. They are most common in the cerebral cortex but a few may be seen in the basal ganglia or white matter and they sometimes project into the cavities of the ventricles. They are rare in the cerebellum. Occasionally cysts lie free in the fourth ventricle and still more rarely in the lateral or third ventricles. The smaller nodules measure 2–4 mm. in diameter and most have a thin greyish corrugated capsule surrounding a paler centre. Some may show no capsule. In chronic cases many of these nodules are calcified and gritty on section. Larger cysts have a tense grey capsule on which, unless they are sterile, there is a mural nodule in which the embryo lies. They contain a little clear fluid.

Microscopically the meningeal racemose cysts and the larger intracerebral cysts have a cyst wall composed of a very thin outer cuticular layer, averaging 3μ in thickness, lined by a wider parenchymatous layer consisting of a meshwork of fine fibrils. This is heavily nucleated immediately under the cuticular layer and more sparsely throughout. The larva in the mural nodule shows a double perioral row of hooklets. Most of the subarachnoid racemose cysts, however, are sterile. Around the intracerebral cysts there is a collagenous capsule derived from the host's tissues. So long as the larva is alive there is little inflammatory reaction and, apart from some gliosis, the neighbouring tissue shows little abnormality. If the parasite has recently died the cyst is surrounded by an inner zone of dead leucocytes, large mononuclear cells and foreign body giant cells, and an outer more vascular zone of granulation tissue forming collagenous fibres. Eosinophil leucocytes may be present in this zone but are rarely numerous (Menon and Veliath 1940). In the smaller nodules a fibrous tissue capsule is separated by a space containing foreign body giant cells from an inner mass of necrotic débris, cholesterol

* These authors recall that Paracelsus in 1650 had noted epilepsy as a symptom of cysticercosis.

clefts and granules of calcium salts surrounding the remains of the parasite. There is no evidence of the cyst wall. The capsule is infiltrated by plasma cells and scanty lymphocytes and large mononuclear cells. Some old nodules consist only of a fibrous tissue scar which in the cortex may be continuous with the fibrous tissue of the meninges. Although calcification usually begins in the remains of the larva, it may start in the capsule. According to MacArthur it is not seen during the first 2 or 3 years after infection.

Cysticercus endarteritis is a characteristic reaction seen in the small intracerebral arteries close to cysts, as well as in the meningeal arteries in the neighbourhood of racemose cysts. The affected vessels show concentric or eccentric fibroblastic or collagenous thickening of the intima or local excrescences sometimes forming bridges across the lumen. The elastica is not reduplicated as in Heubner's arteritis but may be discontinuous in places. There is usually little fibrosis of the media. The adventitia is infiltrated with plasma cells. This form of arteritis differs from that of syphilis in the greater severity of the intimal changes and the slighter lesions in the media. This may be associated to some extent with its greater chronicity.

Echinococcus granularis

Hydatid disease is not uncommon in sheep-rearing countries and very numerous reports have come from Australia, New Zealand, Uruguay and the Argentine (Arana-Iniguez and San Julian 1955). In the British Isles, Wales and Shetland provide the majority of cases. The mature worm lives in the intestine of the dog and ova passed in the dog's faeces infect herbage eaten by sheep in whose liver, lungs or abdominal organs the ova develop into encysted embryos. If dogs are allowed to eat the offal of infected sheep the parasite matures in the dog's intestine and its life cycle is repeated. Human infection arises from the contamination of food by dust containing viable ova or by licking the hands after fondling dogs. The latter method of infection probably accounts for the fact that in the great majority of cases infection is acquired in childhood.

Cases of *primary hydatid cyst of the brain* form about 5 per cent of all cases showing evidence of infestation during childhood, but are much rarer in adults (0·7 per cent, Dew 1934). Of 29 such cases collected by Phillips (1948) from those reported in Australia and New Zealand, only 2 were in adults. This may be explained by the more rapid growth of hydatid cysts in the brain than in the bodily organs or bones. In many cases a cerebral hydatid cyst is associated with a cyst in the liver. The cerebral cysts are usually single, spherical and unilocular, and may be of considerable size. They rarely cause serious symptoms until they reach the size of a hen's egg and they are often very much larger. In Phillips' series 2 had a diameter of 10 cm., 2 contained 600 ml. of fluid and 2 were described as being the size of an orange. Half of these large cysts were successfully removed by operation. Langmaid and Rogers (1940) found 2 cysts side by side, one 8 cm. and the other 6 cm. in diameter. Even larger cysts almost filling a cerebral hemisphere have been described. They are almost always found in the cerebral hemispheres, where they favour the region supplied by the middle cerebral artery, especially the parietal lobe. Owing to their large size they usually lie only a few millimetres below the cortex which is flattened over them and appears bluish. Their outer surface has a characteristic greyish wash-leather appearance. The contents of most cysts are a clear colourless fluid which usually contains small daughter cysts and a granular deposit of scolices. A few cysts are sterile, and some contain turbid or, more rarely, yellowish fluid. If the cyst contents are allowed to infect the brain tissue at operation new cysts are likely to form and may grow rather rapidly. In a case of this kind which came to autopsy 8 months after operation, Phillips found numerous new cysts, some of which were 2·5 cm. in diameter. This gives some indication of the possible rate of growth of hydatid cysts in the brain.

When the scolex is examined under the microscope the head of the embryo, which is usually invaginated, is seen to have a double perioral row of hooklets (Fig. 3.20). The wall of the cyst is 2–3 mm. thick and is readily detached from the surrounding brain tissue: in fact when the cyst is emptied it may free itself spontaneously. It is made up of three layers: (1) The germinal layer which usually has brood capsules attached to its inner surface. (2) A chitinous or cuticular, laminated layer. (3) An adventitial layer of fibrous tissue derived from the tissues of the host. In the brain this layer is usually very thin. The surrounding brain tissue shows little evidence of reaction to the presence of the cyst except fibrous gliosis and lymphocytic infiltration of occasional vessels in the neighbourhood.

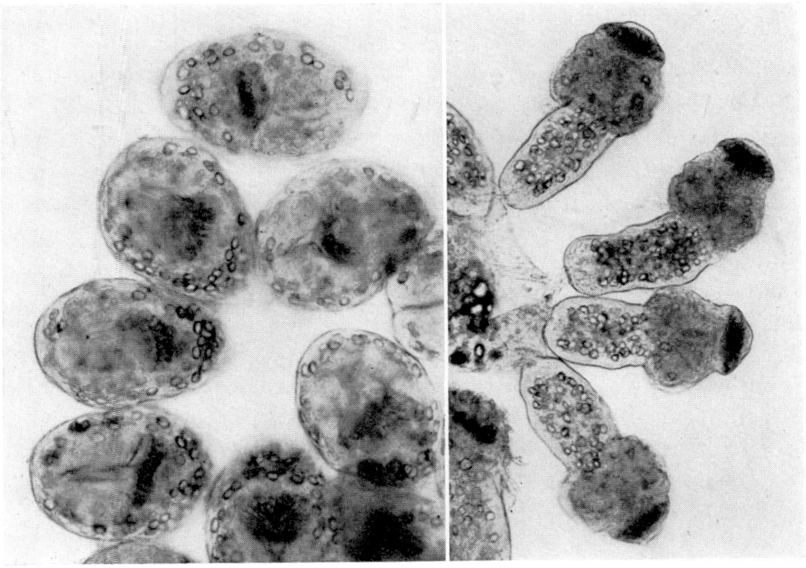

(*a*) (*b*)

FIG. 3.20. Echinococcus granularis.

(*a*) Scolices from the deposit of the fluid from a cerebral hydatid cyst. (*b*) The same after protrusion of the heads.

Secondary hydatid cysts of the brain, which are usually multiple, result from rupture of a hydatid cyst in the heart wall into the cavity of the left ventricle. They are usually met with in adults and are much rarer than primary cerebral cysts.

Hydatid cysts of the vertebrae occur in from 0·3 per cent to 1 per cent of all cases (Woodland 1949). They most often grow in the spongy tissue of the vertebrae, most often in the thoracic or lumbar region and may lead to fracture or subluxation of the spine or, by growing into the spinal canal, may compress the spinal cord. Most of them appear to start in childhood but they grow very slowly and rarely cause symptoms before adult life is reached.

Clinical pathology. In cases of hydatid cysts of the brain without disease elsewhere in the body, the Casoni reaction and complement fixation reactions are usually negative and there is no eosinophilia in the blood. The cerebrospinal fluid also is normal and, except for its increased pressure, gives little help in the diagnosis.

Multiceps multiceps (*Coenurus cerebralis*)

In some sheep-rearing countries, especially South Africa, *Multiceps multiceps* is the common tape-worm of dogs. Its life history is similar to that of *Echinococcus granularis* and it may have an intermediate host in sheep, goats, cattle, horses, gazelles, antelopes and monkeys. In these animals, cysts form in the cerebral ventricles or subarachnoid spaces (*Coenurus cerebralis*). Occasional human cases of this kind have been reported (Becker and Jacobson 1951; Kuper *et al.* 1958).

The cysts, which are unilocular, may be single or multiple, and may vary in size from a few millimetres to 2 or more centimetres. They are most often found in the 4th ventricle or the sub-arachnoid space of the posterior cranial fossa, but may lie in the cisterna basalis where they may compress the optic chiasma. The arachnoid surrounding them is thickened and may form a grape-like collection of vesicles which closely resembles the racemose type of cysticercus. It can, however, be distinguished by the fact that coenurus cysts are always unilocular and often contain several scolices, whereas cysticercus cysts only contain a single embryo.

Microscopical examination of the pedicle will therefore show it to be composed only of connective tissue derived from the arachnoid. The cyst wall is similar to that of a cysticercus, being composed of a thin outer cuticular layer and an inner germinal layer, rich in nuclei. From this scolices project into the lumen of the cyst. The head of these carries a rostellum armed with a double row of hooklets. The cysts may, however, be sterile. In infestations of this type the cerebrospinal fluid is often normal or shows only a slight increase of cells. The complement fixation reaction on the serum with hydatid antigen is usually positive.

Trematodes

Paragonimus westermanii

Owing to its common situation in the lung the ova of this fluke worm are commonly deposited in the brain or meninges, where they become encysted in a fibrous tissue capsule. This later becomes calcified and may thus be visible by X-rays. Kim (1955) in reporting 4 cases with multiple cysts of this kind states that Japanese literature contains reports of about 150 similar cases.

Schistosomiasis

The brain and spinal cord may be the sites of granulomas formed round ova of Schistosoma. These granulomas are most often found in the brain in infestations by *Schistosoma Japonicum*. Of the few cases of spinal cord involvement which have been recorded only one has been due to *S. Japonicum*, the remainder to *S. haematobium* and *S. Mansoni*. The adult worm has not been found in the central nervous system in human infestations. Involvement of the brain in *Japanese schistosomiasis* was recognised as a cause of focal epilepsy by Yamagiwa in 1890, but very few cases were confirmed either by operation or post-mortem examination before 1944. In that year the campaign on Leyte Island in the Philippines resulted in about 1,200 cases of schistosomiasis among American soldiers, among which were 27 cases of cerebral involvement (2·3 per cent). Kane and Most (1948) studied 17 cerebral cases at a hospital where 800 cases of schistosomiasis had been treated (2 per cent). Some who have observed small groups of cases have found cerebral involvement to be more common. Chu (1931) found 2 cases in 39, Egan (1936) 2 cases in 12 and Thomas and Gage (1945) 2 cases in 41. In a disease with which, in some parts of China, a large number of the population are infected (Houghton 1910) even such small proportions of cerebral cases as 2–5 per cent would be impressive, but Houghton did not find many such cases in native Chinese.

In some patients signs of brain involvement occur, along with the typical gastro-intestinal symptoms, from 1 to 2 months after infestation with *S. Japonicum*. In such cases ova are usually abundant in the faeces and the diagnosis is easily made. But when nervous symptoms appear at a longer interval, up to 2 or 4 years after infestation, there may be no evidence of disease elsewhere in the body and ova may be difficult to find in the faeces. The cerebrospinal fluid usually shows an excess of protein with a slight to moderate rise in lymphocyte count. Neither eosinophil leucocytes nor ova have been found in the cerebrospinal fluid.

Kane and Most describe an unusual ophthalmoscopic appearance which may have been evidence of invasion of the choroid or retina by ova. It appeared as 'a billowy white mass which measured 1 by $1\frac{1}{2}$ disk diameters, was triangular and lay in the fork made by branches of the inferior temporal vein, with oedema of the surrounding retina'.

Invasion of the brain by the ova of *S. Japonicum* may be diffuse or focal. When diffuse, miliary granulomas may be found in all parts of the cerebrum. They are most common in the grey matter of the cortex and basal ganglia, but may occur also in the white matter. Bassett and Lowenberg (1949) describe the appearances at operation as 'innumerable, shotty, yellow-orange, glistening, discrete nodules ranging in size from 1 to 2 mm. to a half centimeter in diameter' scattered over the exposed cortical surface which included parietal, temporal and occipital lobes. In other cases a localised, fairly large mass of granuloma, at first sight resembling a glioblastoma multiforme, has been found at operation, or an agglomeration of smaller nodules up to 3 cm. in diameter has been seen on the surface of the brain. Occasionally the dura mater is invaded by granulomas.

On naked-eye examination multiple white nodules of pin-point or pinhead size, or cream-coloured areas resembling minute abscesses, may be seen on the surface of the brain or on section of the excised tissue. This is usually firm and rubbery and when cut may feel gritty from the deposition of calcium salts.

Histological sections show a number of small granulomas containing a smaller or larger number of ova. These are oval measuring 60–90μ in length by 40–60μ in width. Many have a blunt spine midway between the centre and the anterior pole. Paired salivary glands may be seen near the anterior end and a number of germ cell nuclei in the centre and towards the posterior end of the ovum (Fig. 3.21). When they lie singly they may be surrounded by a zone of radially arranged fibroblasts or may be partly enclosed in a multi-nucleated foreign body giant cell. When several lie together there is a central zone of pyknotic and necrotic nuclei and round this a zone of fibroblastic and endothelial cells. A few foreign body giant cells may be present in this zone. External to this there is a wall of varying thickness consisting of collagen fibres infiltrated with inflammatory cells. These vary greatly from case to case. In early lesions the cellular exudate, which consists predominantly of eosinophil leucocytes, is very abundant and there is relatively little collagen. In more chronic lesions the amount of collagen increases and the exudate consists chiefly of lymphocytes and plasma cells with a small number of neutrophil and eosinophil leucocytes. This zone may be very wide, forming the greater part of the granuloma, and giving the mass a firm rubbery texture. It passes externally into a zone of more normal brain tissue in which degenerated or chromatolytic neurones and swollen-bodied astrocytes are seen near the granuloma.

It is clear that the granuloma is formed by the reaction of the tissues to an irritant or toxic substance in the ova. This appears to be present only when they are alive, as, under treatment with antimony, neurological symptoms usually clear up rapidly even when no decompressive craniotomy is performed. The method by which ova reach the brain presents some difficulty. It is unlikely that they come from adult worms lying in their usual situation in superior mesenteric veins, but embolism of ova to the brain might occur if adult worms lay in the pulmonary venules. In this case diffuse dissemination of small lesions would be expected. The larger more focal lesions have usually been found in the occipital, temporal or posterior parietal lobes, and more often on the left side than the right. The condensation of very numerous ova in a localised area of the brain in these cases suggests deposition *in situ* by the female worm lying in a cerebral venous sinus, or large superficial cerebral vein (Greenfield and Pritchard 1937). The usual arrangement at the torcular by which the larger volume of blood passes into the right lateral sinus may account for the preference for the left side.

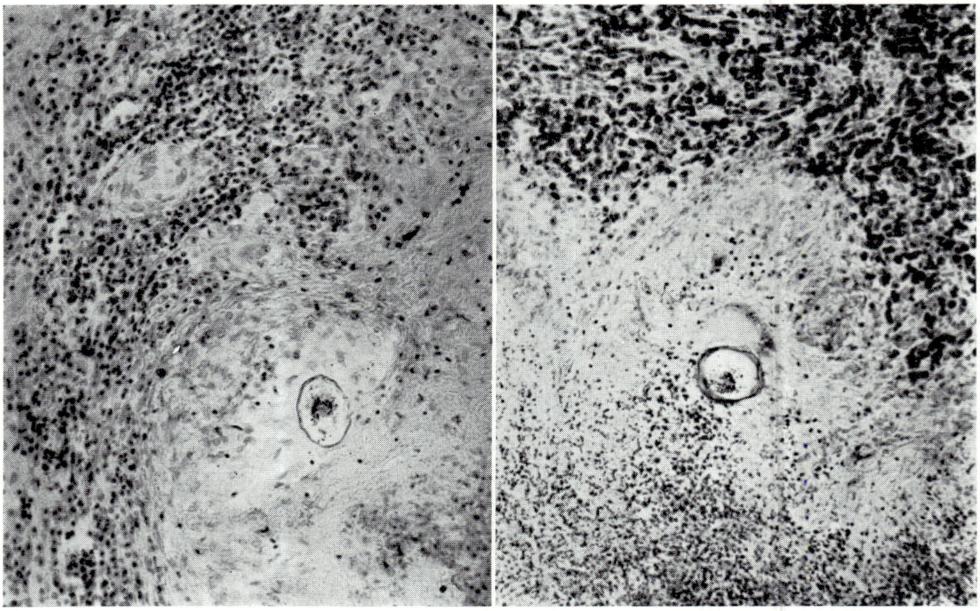

(*a*) (*b*)

FIG. 3.21. *Schistosoma japonicum*. Ova in cerebral granulomas.

In (*b*) a giant cell is partially enveloping the ovum. (*a*) Haematoxylin van Gieson, (*b*) Nissl. (Case of Greenfield and Pritchard 1937.)

Symptomatic involvement of the central nervous system is less common in infestations with either *S. haematobium* or *S. Mansoni* but diffuse deposition of ova may occur without clinical evidence. Gelfand (1950) in Rhodesia by digesting tissue from various parts of the brain and brain stem found ova in 28 out of 50 brains from cases with bilharzial infection. One of these cases died in coma but most were asymptomatic and in none were granulomas macroscopically visible. He also reported a case of myelitis with invasion of the dorsolumbar cord by ova of *S. haematobium*. A few other cases of paraplegia have been reported in which granulomas surrounding ova of *S. haematobium* or *S. Mansoni* have been found. Martinez Niochet and Potenza (1956) collected from the literature 6 such cases which had occurred in Brazil and Venezuela. In most of these the lesions were intramedullary but in 1 (Gama 1953) the conus medullaris and cauda equina were compressed by a meningeal granuloma.

Nematodes

Invasion of the brain by larval forms of round worms is rare by comparison with the frequency of infestation of other bodily organs, but scattered case reports include instances of cerebral invasion by a great variety of nematodes. In many cases they have been chance findings and there has been little evidence that they have contributed in any way to the fatal disease. In other cases symptoms of cerebral disease have been present before or during the final illness or the patient has died in coma. There have also been a number of clinical reports of organic neurological disease which has been attributed, with some evidence, to this cause. In these cases the predominant nervous symptoms may be those of hemiplegia, encephalitis, meningitis or acute psychosis. These symptoms may be transient or there may be recurrent attacks. In some cases with symptoms of encephalitis or meningitis larvae have been found in the cerebrospinal fluid. These cases as well as those of fatal cerebral disease have been most often caused either by larvae of *trichinella* or by one of the forms of *microfilaria*, usually *Loa-loa* or *Wuchereria bancrofti*.

Trichinella spiralis

The rather rare cases of cerebral disease due to invasion by larvae of trichinella have been reviewed by Most and Abeles (1937) who reported a fatal case. They found granulomatous nodules scattered through the brain especially in the white matter and the deeper layers of the cortex. These were of two kinds. Some were composed entirely of microglia and contained no larvae. Others consisted of a more solid collection of mononuclear cells including lymphocytes, histiocytes and plasma cells and often contained larvae. Perivascular lymphocytic infiltrations, which might be quite heavy, were found in the brain and meninges. In addition round and oval cavities filled with amorphous mucinoid material were diffusely distributed in the subcortical white matter and the midbrain. Similar cavities were found by Hassin and Diamond (1926) in the frontal lobes and pons. These authors also noted various degenerative changes in the nerve cells near granulomas. They found numerous trichinella larvae free in the tissues without any cellular reaction round them.

Filariasis

Microfilariae, circulating in the blood, must pass through the cerebral vessels, but they only cause cerebral lesions if they are so numerous as to plug capillaries or if they die and disintegrate in the brain. The latter effect may be produced by therapeutic drugs when the infestation is heavy as in a case reported by van Bogaert *et al.* (1955) from the Congo. In this case the cerebral lesions were severe and widespread. They consisted of small granulomatous nodules not visible to the naked eye, in most of which one or more microfilariae could be found. In addition there were more diffuse inflammatory and vascular lesions. The granulomas were usually perivascular and were made up of microglial cells and lymphocytes with occasional leucocytes. In some there was a tendency to necrosis of the walls of the central vessel and, when microfilariae were numerous, giant cells, probably of histiocytic origin, were formed in them. They were scattered throughout the cerebral and cerebellar hemispheres, including the basal ganglia, but were less abundant in the brain stem. Some folia of the cerebellum showed ischaemic atrophy, and many of the Purkinje cells in the neighbourhood of granulomatous nodules either had disappeared or showed homogenising change. In the cerebral cortex there was a diffuse microgliosis with the formation of rod cells and a more focal increase in astrocyte nuclei. Perivenous lymphocytic infiltrations were found both in the meninges and the brain tissue. In the white matter honeycomb or spongy areas, in which the myelin had undergone lysis, were seen round many blood-vessels. Of the lesions in other organs the most characteristic were in the liver where multiple small necrotic areas surrounded by lymphocytes and containing degenerated microfilariae were found in the portal spaces.

(Revised by W. Blackwood)

REFERENCES

Pyogenic infections of central nervous system

Baker, A. B. (1942) *J. Neuropath.*, **1**, 394.
Elkington, J. St. C. (1936) *Brain*, **59**, 181.
Field, E. O. (1954) *J. Neurol. Psychiat.*, **17**, 228.
Fisher, C. M. and Adams, R. D. (1956) *J. Neuropath.*, **15**, 243.
Gaskell, H. S. and Korb, M. (1946) *Arch. Neurol. Psychiat.* (Chicago), **55**, 539.
Greenfield, J. G. (1921) *J. Neurol. Psychopath.*, **2**, 105; (1939) *Brain*, **62**, 129.
Hurst, E. W. (1955) *J. Path. Bact.*, **70**, 167.
Lumsden, C. E. (1956) *Proc. Roy. Soc. Med.*, **49**, 148.
McFarlan, A. M. (1943) *Brit. Med. J.*, (ii), 643.
Millen, J. W. and Woollam, D. H. M. (1954) *J. Neurol. Psychiat.*, **17**, 286.
Perdrau, J. R. (1928) *J. Path. Bact.*, **31**, 17.
Queckenstedt, H. H. C. (1917) *Dtsch. Z. Nervenheilk.*, **57**, 316.
Schiller, F., Cairns, H. and Russell, D. S. (1948) *J. Neurol. Psychiat.*, **11**, 143.
Thompson, R. H. S. and King, E. J. (1957) *Biochemical disorders in human disease*, Churchill, London.
Trousseau, A. and Lassègue, C. (1851) *L'Union medicale*, **5**, 471.
Waksman, B. H., Adams, R. D. and Mansmann, H. C. (1957) *J. exper. Med.*, **105**, 591.
Walshe, F. M. R. (1918–19) *Quart. J. Med.*, **12**, 14; (1920) *Brain*, **43**, 74.
Webster, H. de F., Spiro, D., Waksman, B. and Adams, R. D. (1961) *J. Neuropath. Exp. Neurol.*, **20**, 5.
Weed, L. H. (1914) *J. Med. Research*, **31**, 21.
Winkelman, N. W. (1952) *Neurology*, **1**, 284.

Tuberculosis

Beres, D. and Metzler, T. (1938) *Amer. J. Path.*, **14**, 59.
Blacklock, J. W. S. and Griffin, W.A. (1935) *J. Path. Bact.*, **40**, 489.
Boinet. (1899) *Gaz. d. Hôp.*, **72**, 390.
Chantemesse. (1884) *Étude sur la méningite tuberculeuse de l'adulte*, Paris.
Daniel, P. M. (1949) *Proc. Roy. Soc. Med.*, **42**, 169.
Doniach, I. (1949) *J. Path. Bact.*, **61**, 253.
Evans, H. S. and Courville, C. B. (1938) *Arch. Surgery*, **36**, 637.
Garland, H. G. and Armitage, G. (1933) *J. Path. Bact.*, **37**, 461.
Greenfield, J. G. and Carmichael, E. A. (1925) *The cerebro-spinal fluid in clinical diagnosis*, Macmillan, London.
Griffith, A. S. (1934) *Lancet* (i), 1382.
Hayes, J. N. (1954) in Tice's *Practice of Medicine*, Prior Co., Hagerstown.
Hektoen, L. (1896) *J. exper. Med.*, **1**, 112.
Jensen, K. A. (1932) *Zbl. Bakt. I. Abt. Orig.*, **125**, 222.
Kment, H. (1924) *Tuberk. Biblioth.*, **14**, 1.
Macgregor, A. R., Kirkpatrick, H. J. R. and Craig, W. S. (1935) *Edin. med. J.*, **42**, 138.
Pardee, I. and Knox, L. C. (1927) *Arch. Neurol. Psychiat.* (Chicago), **17**, 231.
Rich, A. R. and McCordock, H. A. (1929) *Bull. J. Hopkins Hosp.*, **44**, 273; (1933) ibid., **52**, 5.
Smith, H. V. and Daniel, P. M. (1947) *Tubercle*, **28**, 64.
Stewart, M. J. (1927) *J. Path. Bact.*, **30**, 577.
Taylor, L. M., Smith, H. V. and Hunter, G. (1954) *Lancet* (i), 700.
von Czirer, L. (1914) *Centralbl. f. allg. Path. u. Path. Anat.*, **25**, 152.

Sarcoidosis

Aszkanazy, C. L. (1952) *J. Neuropath.*, **11**, 392.
Colover, J. (1948) *Brain*, **71**, 451.
Meyer, J. S., Foley, J. M. and Campagna-Pinto, D. (1953) *Arch. Neurol. Psychiat.* (Chicago), **69**, 587.
Ross, J. A. (1955) *Brit. Med. J.* (ii), 593.
Zollinger, H. V. (1941) *Virchows Archiv.*, **307**, 597.

Leprosy

Ash, J. E. and Spitz, S. (1945) *Pathology of Tropical Diseases*, Saunders, London.
Khanolkar, V. R. (1951) *Indian Council of Medical Research, Special Report series* 19; (1955) *Indian J. Med. Sci.*, **9**, Suppl. 1.
Koppisch, E. (1953) *Pathology* (Anderson), Kimpton, London.

Fungal Infections

Benham, R. W. (1934) *Arch. Dermat. and Syph.*, **30**, 385.
Carton, C. A. and Mount, L. A. (1951) *J. Neurosurg.*, **8**, 143.
Conant, N. F. (1952) in *Bacterial and Mycotic infections of Man*, R. J. Dubos, 2nd Edition, Lippincott.
Cox, L. B. and Tolhurst, J. C. (1946) *Human Torulosis*, Oxford Univ. Press.
Craig, W. McK., Dockerty, M. B. and Harrington, S. W. (1940) *Southern Surg.*, **9**, 759.
Egeberg, R. O. (1954) *Amer. J. med. Sc.*, **227**, 268.
Evans, E. E. and Theriault, R. J. (1953) *J. Bacteriol.*, **65**, 571.
Freeman, W. (1931) *Trans. Amer. Neur. Soc.*, **56**, 203; *J. fur Psychol. u. Neurol.*, **43**, 236.
Gaspar, I. (1929) *Arch. Neurol. Psychiat.* (Chicago), **22**, 475.
Globus, J. H., Garg, K. M. and Bergman, P. S. (1951) *J. Neuropath.*, **10**, 208.
Greenfield, J. G., Martin, J. P. and Moore, M. T. (1938) *Lancet* (ii), 1154.
Kurrein, F. (1954) *J. clin. Path.*, **7**, 141.
Le Count, E. R. (1909) *J. nerv. and ment. Dis.*, **36**, 144.
Ley, A., Jacas, R. and Oliveras, C. (1951) *J. Neurosurg.*, **8**, 327.
Lodder, J. (1934) Die Hefesammlung des 'Centralbureau voor Schimmelcultures', ii Teil. Die Anaskosporogen Hefen. I. Hälfte, Amsterdam.
Martin, D. S. and Smith, D. T. (1939) *Amer. Rev. Tuber.*, **39**, 275.
Mosberg, W. H. and Arnold, J. G. (1950) *Ann. Int. Med.*, **32**, 1153.
Moss, E. S. and McQuown, A. L. (1953) *Atlas of Medical Mycology*, Williams and Wilkins.
Rand, C. W. (1930) *Arch. Neurol. Psychiat.* (Chicago), **23**, 502.
Rose, F. R., Grant, H. C. and Jeanes, A. L. (1958) *Brain*, **81**, 542.
Sanfelice, F. (1896) *Zschr. f. Hygiene u. Infektionskr.*, **21**, 32, 394.
Schulz, D. M. (1953) *J. Amer. med. Ass.*, **151**, 549.
Schwartz, B. and Spitz, L. J. (1952) *Arch. Int. Med.*, **89**, 541.
Sprofkin, B. E., Shapiro, J. L. and Lux, J. J. (1955) *J. Neuropath.*, **14**, 288.
Stevenson, L. D., Vogel, F. S. and Williams, V. (1950) *Arch. Pathol.*, **49**, 321.
Stoddard, V. L. and Cutler, E. C. (1916) *Torula infection in Man*, Monograph No. 6, Rockefeller Inst. med. Res.
Vuillemin, P. (1901) *Rev. gen. de Sc. pures et appli.*, **12**, 732.
Wilhelmj, C. M. (1925) *Amer. J. med. Sc.*, **169**, 712.
Wolf, A. and Cowen, D. (1949) *J. Neuropath.*, **8**, 107.

Neurosyphilis

Achucarro, N. (1910) *Nissl-Alzheimer Arbeiten*, **3**, 143.
Buzzard, E. F. and Greenfield, J. G. (1921) *Pathology of the Nervous System*, Constable, London.
Carmichael, F. A., Kernohan, J. W. and Adson, A. W. (1939) *Arch. Neurol. and Pyschiat.* (Chicago), **42**, 1001.
Charcot, J. M. and Joffroy, A. (1869) *Archiv. de Physiol.*, **2**, 354, 629, 744.
Charcot, J. M. and Pierret, M. (1871) *C.R. Soc. de Biol.*, **23**, 33.
Dattner, B. (1944) *The Management of Neurosyphilis*, Grune and Stratton, N.Y.
Denny-Brown, D. (1951) *J. Neurol. Psychiat.*, **14**, 237.
Flechsig, P. (1876) *Die Leitungsbahnen im Gehirn und Ruckenmark des Menschen*, Leipsic.
Froin, G. (1903) *Gaz. des Hôp.*, p. 1005.
Galbraith, A. J. (1938) *Brit. J. vener. Dis.*, **14**, 197.
Gowers, W. R. (1899) *A Manual of Diseases of the Nervous System*, **1**, 3rd Edition, Churchill, London.
Greenfield, J. G. and Carmichael, E. A. (1925). Macmillan, London.
Greenfield, J. G. and Epstein, S. H. (1937) *Trans. Ophthal. Soc.*, U.K., 1937, **57**, 127.
Greenfield, J. G. and Stern, R. O. (1932) *Brain*, **55**, 367.
Haslam, J. (1798) *Observations on insanity with particular remarks on the disease and an account of the morbid appearance on dissections*, London.

Hassin, G. B. (1929) *Arch. Neurol. Psychiat.*, **21**, 311.
Heubner, O. (1874) *Die Luetische Erkrankung der Hirnarterien*, Vogel, Leipsic.
Igersheimer, J. (1921) *Dtsch. Med. Wochenschr.*, **47**, 738.
Jahnel, F. (1917) *Arch. f. Psychiat.*, **57**, 382 and 847; (1917) *Mschr. f. Psychiat.*, **42**, 58; (1917) *Neurol. Zbl.*, **36**, 402; (1922) *Z. ges. Neurol. Psychiat.*, **76**, 166.
Jakob, A. (1929) *Normale und pathologische Anatomie und Histologie des Grosshirns*, **2**, 794. Deuticke, Wien.
Leri, A. (1904) *Nouv. Icon. Salpêt.*, **17**, 304.
Lhermitte, J. (1926) *Rev. Neurol.* (i), 477.
Lissauer, H. and Storch, E. (1901) *Mschr. Psychiat. Neurol.*, **9**, 401.
Mair, W. G. P. and Druckman, R. (1953) *Brain*, **76**, 448.
Martin, J. P. (1925) Atrophic meningomyelitis, *Brain*, **48**, 153.
Merritt, H. H., Adams, R. D. and Solomon, H. C. (1946) *Neurosyphilis*, Oxford Univ. Press.
Merritt, H. H., Putnam, T. J. and Campbell, A. C. P. (1937) *Arch. Neurol. Psychiat.* (Chicago), **37**, 75.
Merritt, H. H. and Springlova, M. (1932) *Arch. Neurol. Psychiat.* (Chicago), **27**, 987.
Moore, J. E. (1929) *Arch. Neurol. Psychiat.* (Chicago), **21**, 117; (1932) *Medicine*, **11**, 263; (1941) *The Modern Treatment of Syphilis*, C. C Thomas.
Moore, J. E. and Hopkins, H. H. (1930) *J. Amer. med. Ass.*, **95**, 1637.
Moore, J. E. and Woods, A. C. (1940) *Amer. J. Syphilis*, **24**, 59.
Nageotte, J. (1894) *Bull. Soc. Anat. de Paris*, **69**, 808.
Noguchi, H. and Moore, J. E. (1913) *J. exper. Med.*, **17**, 232.
Norman, R. M., Urich, H. and Heaton Ward, W. A. (1959) *B. J. Venereal Dis.*, **35**, 231.
Obersteiner, H. and Redlich, E. (1894–5) Obersteiners *Arbeiten*, **2**, 158; **3**, 192.
Oppenheim, H. (1911) *Textbook of Nervous Diseases*, 5th Edition, Translated A. Bruce, Foulis, Edinburgh.
Paton, L. (1922) *Brit. J. Ophthal.*, **6**, 289.
Pette, H. (1924) *Z. ges. Neurol. Psychiat.*, **92**, 346.
Pierret. (1871) *Arch. de Physiol.*, **4**, 364.
Ravaut, P. (1930) *Monde méd.*, **40**, 566; (1934) *Une nouvelle syphilis nerveuse*, Masson, Paris.
Richter, H. (1921) *Z. ges. Neurol. Psychiat.*, **67**, 1; (1922) *Arch. Psychiat. Nervenkr.*, **67**, 295; (1923–4) ibid., **70**, 529; (1924) ibid., **72**, 318.
Smith, R. H. F. and Morais, V. de. (1948) *J. ment. Science*, **94**, 70.
Spielmeyer, W. (1923) *Z. ges. Neurol. Psychiat.*, **84**, 257; (1924) ibid., **91**, 627.
Stargardt. (1913) *Munch. med. Wschr.*, **60**, 269; (1913) *Arch. Psychiat. Nervenkr.*, **51**, 711.
Stern, R. O. (1929) *Brain*, **52**, 295; (1932) *Brain*, **55**, 145.
Vulpian, A. (1879) *Maladies du Système Nerveux.*

Virus diseases

Achucarro, N. (1910) *Nissl-Alzheimer Arbeiten*, **3**, 143.
Alm, L. A. (1951) Aseptic encephalomyelitis in Gothenburg 1932–1950, *Acta. Med. Scand.*, **140**, Suppl.
Armstrong, C. (1943) *Publ. Hlth. Rep.* (Wash.), **58**, 16.
Barensprung, von. (1862) *Charite-Ann.*, **10**, 123; (1863) ibid., **11**, 99.
Barlow, T. and Penrose. (1886) *Med-chir. Trans.*, **70**, 77.
Batten, F. E. (1905) *Brain*, **28**, 484; (1910) Acute polio-encephalitis in Allbutt and Rolleston's *System of Medicine*, **8**; (1916) *Brain*, **39**, 115.
Bernsten, C. A. and Stevenson, L. D. (1953) *J. Neuropathol.*, **12**, 169.
Bethlem, J. (1962) *Acta. Neuropath.*, **2**, 97.
Bodian, D. (1952) Poliomyelitis, *Proceedings of 2nd Internat. Poliomyelitis Conference*, Lippincott.
Bogaert, L. van. (1945) *J. Neurol. Psychiat.*, **8**, 101.
Bowden, R. E. M. (1952) Poliomyelitis, *Papers and Discussions presented at the 2nd Internat. Polio. Conference*, Lippincott.
Boyd, W. (1921) *Annals of Med.*, **1**, 1; (1924–5) *Quart. J. Med.*, **18**, 153.
Buzzard, E. F. and Greenfield, J. G. (1919) *Brain*, **13**, 305.
Carey, E. J., Massopust, L. C., Zeit, W. and Haushalter, E. (1944) *J. Neuropathol.*, **3**, 121.
Clifton, F. (1724) *Dissertatio inauguralis de distinctis et confluentibus variolis*, Leyden (Lugduni Batavorum).
Collins, J. and Armour, R. G. (1912) *Rev. Neurol. Psychiat.* (Edinburgh), **10**, 361.

Covell, W. P. (1930) *Proc. Soc. exper. Biol. & Med.*, **27**, 927.
Covell, W. P. and Danks, W. B. C. (1932) *Amer. J. Pathol.*, **8**, 557.
Cowdry, E. V. (1934) *Arch. Pathol.*, **18**, 527.
Dalldorf, G. (1952) Poliomyelitis, *Papers and discussions presented at 2nd Internat. Polio. Conference*, Lippincott.
Dawson, J. R. (1933) *Amer. J. Pathol.*, **9**, 7; (1934) *Arch. Neurol. Psychiat.* (Chicago), **31**, 685.
Denny-Brown, D., Adams, R. D. and Fitzgerald, P. J. (1944) *Arch. Neurol. Psychiat.* (Chicago), **51**, 216.
Denst, J. and Neubuerger, K. T. (1950) *Amer. J. Pathol.*, **26**, 863.
Dürck, H. (1921) *Z. ges Neurol. Psychiat.*, **72**, 175.
Economo, C. von. (1931) *Encephalitis lethargica. Its sequelae and treatment*, Oxford Univ. Press.
Einarson, L. (1949) *Acta Orthopaedica Scandinavica*, **19**, 27; (1952) Poliomyelitis, *Proceedings 2nd International Poliomyelitis Conference*, Lippincott.
Elliott, H. C. (1947) *Amer. J. Pathol.*, **23**, 313.
Enders, J. F. (1952) In Poliomyelitis, *Proceedings 2nd Internat. Poliomyelitis Conference*, Lippincott.
Fairbrother, R. W. and Hurst, E. W. (1930) *J. Path. Bact.*, **33**, 17, 1133.
Farber, S., Hill, A., Connerley, M. and Dingle, J. A. (1940) *J. Amer. med. Ass.*, **114**, 1725.
Feemster, R. F. (1938) *Amer. J. public Health*, **28**, 1403.
Flexner, S. and Amos, H. L. (1914) *J. exper. Med.*, **19**, 411; ibid., **20**, 249.
Fothergill, L. D. and Dingle, J. H. (1938) *Science*, **88**, 549.
Francis, T. and Kurtz, H. B. (1950) *Yale J. Biol. & Med.*, **22**, 579.
Freind, J. (1730) *Nine commentaries upon fevers and two epistles concerning the smallpox*, Cox, London.
Galloway, I. A. and Elford, W. J. (1936) *J. Hygiene*, **36**, 533.
Gear, J. H. S. (1952) Poliomyelitis, *Proceedings 2nd Internat. Poliomyelitis Conference*, Lippincott.
Globus, J. and Strauss, I. (1922) *Arch. Neurol. Psychiat.* (Chicago), **8**, 122.
Greenfield, J. G. and Bosanquet, F. D. (1953) *J. Neurol. Psychiat.*, **16**, 213.
Greenfield, J. G. and Matthews, W. B. (1954) *J. Neurol. Psychiat.*, **17**, 50.
Hallervorden, J. (1933) *Klin. Wschr.*, **12**, 692; (1935) *Dtsch. Z. Nervenheilk.*, **136**, 68.
Hammon, W. McD. (1949) The etiology, epidemiology and diagnosis of the virus encephalitides, *Proc. 4th Internat. Neurol. Congress*, **I**, 94.
Hammon, W. M., Gray, J. A., Evans, F. C., Izumi, E. M. and Lundy, H. W. (1941) *Science*, **94**, 305.
Hammon, W. M. and Howitt, B. F. (1942) *Amer. J. Hygiene*, **35**, 163.
Haupt, H. and Rehaag, H. (1921) *Z. Infekt. u. Hyg. d. Haust.*, **22**, 76, 104.
Haymaker, W. (1949) *J. Neuropath.*, **8**, 132; (1961) *Encephalitides. Proceedings of a Symposium at Antwerp*, 1959. Elsevier Pub. Co., p. 38.
Haymaker, W. and Sabin, A. B. (1947) *Arch. Neurol. Psychiat.* (Chicago), **57**, 673.
Head, H. and Campbell, A. W. (1900) *Brain*, **23**, 353.
Heine. (1860) *Spinal Kinderlähmung.*
Howe, H. A. and Bodian, D. (1942) *Neural Mechanisms in Poliomyelitis*, Oxford Univ. Press.
Hunt, Ramsay. (1907) *J. Nerv. ment. Dis.*, **34**, 73.
Hurst, E. E. and Fairbrother, R. (1930) *J. Path. Bact.*, **33**, 17.
Hurst, E. W. (1926) *J. Path. Bact.*, **29**, 65; (1930) ibid., **33**, 1133; (1931) ibid., **34**, 331; (1936) *Brain*, **59**, 1.
Hurst, E. W. and Pawan J. L. (1932) *J. Path. Bact.*, **35**, 301.
Hydén, H. (1947) The nucleoproteins in virus reproduction, *Cold Spring Harbor Symposia Quart. Biol.* **12**, 104.
Kaneko, R. and Aoki, Y. (1928) *Ergebn. inn. Med. Kinderheilk.*, **34**, 342.
King, L. S. (1939 a) *J. Exper. Med.*, **69**, 691; (1939 b) *J. Amer. med. Ass.*, **113**, 1940.
Koch, F. (1950) *Z. Kinderheilk.*, **68**, 328.
Krogh, F. (1945) *Acta physiol. Scand.*, **10**, 271.
Landsteiner, K. and Popper, E. (1908) *Wien. Klin. Wschr.*, **21**, 1830; (1909) *Z. Immunforsch.*, **2**, 377.
Levaditi, C., Paie, C. M. and Krassnoff, D. (1936) *C.R. Soc. Biol. Paris*, **123**, 866.
Lhermitte, J. and Cornil L. (1921) *Rev. Neurol.*, **28**, 185, 587.
Lhermitte, J., Kraus, W. M. and McAlpine, D. (1924–5) *J. Neurol. Psychopath.*, **5**, 195.
Lhermitte, J. and Nicholas. (1924) *Rev. Neurol.*, **31**, 361.
Lipschutz, B. (1925) *Arch. Derm. Syph. Wien*, **149**, 196.
Lucas, J. (1790) *London med. J.*, **11**, 325.
Ludden, T. E. and Edwards, J. E. (1949) *Amer. J. Pathol.*, **25**, 357.
McAlpine, D. (1923) *Brain*, **46**, 255.

McIntosh, J. and Turnbull, H. M. (1920) *Brit. J. exper. Path.*, **1**, 89.
MacLeod, J. and Gordon, W. S. (1932) *J. Comp. Pathol., and Therap.*, **45**, 240.
Magnus, H. von. (1949) *Ugesk. laeger*, **111**, 1451.
Marinesco, G. and Draganesco, St. (1923) *Rev. Neurol.*, **30**, 385.
Marinesco, G. and McIntosh, J. (1918) Reports to the local Government Board, New Series 121, H.M. Stationery Office, London.
Marinesco, G. and Stroesco, G. (1931) *Arch. Roumaines de Pathol. expér. et de Microbiol.*, **4**, 17.
Medin. (1890) *Verhandl. Internat. med. Cong. Berlin*, **2**, 37.
Negri, A. (1903) *Z. Hyg. Infektkr.*, **43**, 507; **44**, 519.
Nicolau, S., Nicolau, O. and Galloway, I. A. (1929). *Ann. de l'Inst. Pasteur* **43**, 1.
Noran, H. H. and Baker, A. B. (1943) *Arch. Neurol. Psychiat.* (Chicago), **49**, 398; (1945) *J. Neuropath. & exper. Neurol.*, **4**, 269.
Pasteur, L., Chamberland and Roux, E. (1884) *C.R. Acad. Sc.*, **98**, 457.
Peers, J. H. (1943) *Amer. J. Pathol.*, **19**, 673.
Pette, H. (1942) *Die akut enzundlichen Erkrankungen des Nervensystems*, Thieme, Leipsic.
Pinkerton, H. (1950) *Amer. J. clin. Pathol.*, **20**, 201.
Pond, W. L. and Russ., S. B. (1955) *Bull. Wld. Hlth. Org.*, **12**, 591.
Rebattu, J., Mounier-Kuhn, P., Dechaume, J., Bonnet, P. and Colrat, A. (1933) *Rev. Oto-neuro-ophthal.* **11**, 333; *Abstr. in Arch. Neurol. Psychiat.* (Chicago), **31**, 1100, 1297.
Rhodes, A. J., Clark, E. M., Knowles, D. S., Shimada, F. T., Ritchie, R. C., Donohue, W. *et al.* (1950) *Canad. J. public Health*, **41**, 183.
Rhodes, A. J., Clark, E. M., Wood, W., Shimada, F. T., Silverthorne, N., McKendry, J. B. J., Duncan, D. and Anglin, C.S. (1953) *Canad. med. Ass. J.*, **68**, 438.
Rivers, T. M. (1948) *Viral and Rickettsial Infections of Man*, Lippincott.
Rivers, T. M. and Horsfall, F. L. (1959) *Viral and Rickettsial Infections of Man*, 3rd edn., Lippincott.
Rooyen, C. E. van and Rhodes, A. J. (1948) *Virus Diseases of Man*, Nelson, Edinburgh.
Roux, E. (1888) *Ann. Inst. Pasteur*, **2**, 18; 1889 **3**, 69.
Sabin, A. B. (1949 a) *Rapports 4me Congrès neurologique International* **I**, 85, Masson, Paris; (1949 b) *J. clin. Invest.*, **28**, 808.
Saphir, O. and Wile, S. A. (1942) *Amer. J. med. Sc.*, **203**, 781.
Sharrard, W. J. W. (1955) *J. Bone Jt. Surg.*, **37**, 540.
Sourander, P. (1956) *J. Path. Bact.*, **72**, 257.
Strümpell, A. (1891) *Dtsche. Archiv. f. klin. Med.*, **47**, 53.
Swan, C. (1943) *Med. J. Australia* (i), 437.
Trétiakoff, C. (1921) *Rev. Neurol.*, **28**, 592.
Uchiyama, T. (1925) *Japan med. World*, **5**, 345.
Verlinde, J. D., van Tongeren, H. A. E., Pattyn, S. R. and Rosenzweig, A. (1955) *Bull. Wld. Hlth. Org.*, **12**, 565.
Walton, K. W. (1954) *J. Path. Bact.*, **68**, 565.
Warburg, B. (1931) *Arch. Neurol. Psychiat.* (Chicago), **25**, 1191.
Weil, A. (1934) *Arch. Neurol. Psychiat.* (Chicago), **31**, 1138.
Weil, A. and Breslich, P. J. (1942) *J. Neuropath. and exper. Neurol.*, **1**, 49.
Wesselhoeft, C., Smith, E. C. and Branch, C. F. (1938) *J. Amer. med. Ass.*, **111**, 1736.
Wickman, I. (1905) *Arbeit. a.d. Path. Instit. Univ. Helsingfors*, **1**, 109, and *Studien uber Poliomyelitis Acuta*, Karger, Berlin; (1907) *Beitrage zur Kentniss der Heine-Medinsche Krankheit.*
Wiesner, R. R. von. (1917) *Wien. klin. Wschr.*, **30**, 933.
Wildi, E. (1951) *Rev. Neurol.*, **84**, 201.
Wimmer, A. and Neel, A. V. (1928) *Acta Psychiat. Kbn.*, **3**, 319.
Wohlfart, G. (1955) *Nordisk. Med.*, **54**, 1075.
Wolf, A., Kabat, E. A. and Bezer, A. E. (1947) *J. Neuropath.*, **6**, 333.
Wolman, M. and Behar, A. (1952) *J. inf. Dis.*, **91**, 69.
Zimmerman, H. M. (1946) *Amer. J. Pathol.*, **22**, 951; (1948) *J. Neuropathol.*, **7**, 106.

Encephalitis of uncertain origin

Akelaitis, A. J. and Zeldis, L. J. (1942) *Arch. Neurol. Psychiat.* (Chicago), **47**, 353.
Aström, K. -E., Mancall, E. L. and Richardson, E. P. Jnr. (1958) *Brain*, **81**, 93.
Bogaert, L. van. (1945) *J. Neurol. Psychiat.*, **8**, 101.

Bogaert, L. van and Busscher, J. de. (1939) *Rev. Neurol.*, **71**, 679.
Brain, W. R., Greenfield, J. G. and Russell, D. S. (1943) *Proc. Roy. Soc. Med.*, **36**, 319; (1948) *Brain*, **71** 365.
Brierley, J. B., Corsellis, J. A. N., Hierons, R. and Nevin, S. (1960), *Brain*, **83**, 357.
Brihaye, J. (1958) *Etude des encephalites herpetiques et des encephalites nécrosantes aiguës*. Editions Acta Med. Belg. Brussels.
Buren, J. M. van (1954) *J. Neuropath.*, **13**, 230.
Corsellis, J. A. N. (1951) *J. Mental Science*, **97**, 570.
Dawson, J. R. (1933) *Amer. J. Pathol.*, **9**, 7; (1934) *Arch. Neurol. Psychiat.* (Chicago), **31**, 685.
Diezel, P. B. (1954) *Virchows Archiv. path. Anat.*, **325**, 109.
Foley, J. and Williams, D. (1953) *Quart. J. Med.*, **22**, 157.
Greenfield, J. G. (1950) *Brain*, **73**, 141.
Haymaker, W., Girdany, B. R., Stephens, J., Lillie, R. D. and Fetterman, G. H. (1954) *J. Neuropath.*, **13**, 562.
Kinney, T. D. (1942) *Amer. J. Path.*, **18**, 799.
Krüeke, W. (1952) *Dtsch. Z. Nervenheilk.*, **169**, 322; (1957) *Nervenarzt.*, **7**, 289.
Macken, J. and Lhermitte, F. (1950) *Bull. Acad. roy. med. Belg.*, 6 Serie, **15**, 205.
Malamud, N., Haymaker, W. and Pinkerton, H. (1950) *Amer. J. Path.*, **26**, 133.
Osetowska, E. (1961) *Encephalitides. Proceedings of a Symposium at Antwerp*, 1959. Elsevier Pub. Co., p. 414.
Petsche, H., Schinko, H. and Seitelberger, F. (1961) *Encephalitides. Proceedings of a Symposium at Antwerp*, 1959. Elsevier Pub. Co., p. 353.
Pette, H. and Döring, G. (1939) *Dtsch. Z. Nervenheilk.*, **149**, 7.
Pette, H. and Kalm, H. (1953) Bergmann-Frey-Schweigk, *Handbuch der Inneren Medizin*, Springer Verlag, Berlin, Vol. 5, Part 3, p. 150.
Pinkerton, H. (1950) *Amer. J. clin. Pathol.*, **20**, 201.
Radermecker, J. (1949) *Revue neur.*, **81**, 1009.
Richardson, E. P. Jnr (1961) *New Engl. J. Med.*, **265**, 815.
Tariska, S. (1961) *Encephalitides. Proceedings of a Symposium at Antwerp*, 1959. Elsevier Pub. Co. p. 541.

Rickettsial infections of the nervous system

Lillie, H. D. (1941) Pathology of Rocky Mountain spotted fever, *Nat. Inst. Health Bulletin*, No. 177.
Noad, K. B. and Haymaker, W. (1953) *Brain*, **76**, 113.
Spielmeyer, W. (1919) *Z. ges. Neurol. Psychiat.*, **47**, 1; (1922) *Histopathologie des Nervensystems*, Springer, Berlin.
Weil, A. and Haymaker, W. (1946) *J. Neuropathol.*, **5**, 271.
Wolbach, S. B. (1919) *J. med. Research*, **41**, 1; (1948) *In Rickettsial Diseases of Man*, Amer. Ass. Advancement of Science, Thomas Adams and Davis.
Wolbach, S. B., Todd, J. L. and Palfrey, F. W. (1922) *The Etiology and Pathology of Typhus*, Harvard Univ. Press.

Infection by animal parasites

Arana-Iniguez, R. and Asenjo, A. (1945) *J. Neurosurg.*, **2**, 181.
Arana-Iniguez, R. and San Julian, J. (1955) *J. Neurosurg.*, **12**, 323.
Bassett, R. C. and Lowenberg, K. (1949) *J. Neuropath.*, **8**, 220.
Becker, B. J. P. and Jacobson, S. (1951) *Lancet* (ii), 198, 1202.
Bertrand, I., Bablet, J. and Sicé, A. (1935) *Ann. Inst. Pasteur*, **54**, 91.
Bickerstaff, E. R., Cloake, P. C. P., Hughes, B. and Smith, W. T. (1952) *Brain*, **75**, 1.
Bogaert, L. van, Dubois, A., Janssens, P. G., Radermecker, J., Tverdy, G. and Wanson, M. (1955) *J. Neurol. Psychiat.*, **18**, 103.
Calwell, H. G. (1937) *Trans. Roy. Soc. trop. Med. Hyg.*, **30**, 611.
Chu, C. F. (1931) *Chinese med. J.*, **52**, 651.
Dew, H. G. (1934) *Surg. Gynec. Obstet.*, **59**, 321.
Egan, C. H. (1936) *J. Roy. Nav. med. Serv.*, **22**, 6.
Farquhar, H. G. and Turner, W. M. L. (1949) *Arch. dis. Childh.*, **24**, 137.

Gama, C. (1953) *J. Intern. Coll. Surg.*, **19**, 665.
Gard, S. and Magnusson, H. J. (1951) *Acta med. Scand.*, **141**, 59.
Gelfand, M. (1950) *Schistosomiasis in S. Central Africa*, Juta, Cape Town.
Greenfield, J. G. and Pritchard, E. A. B. (1937) *Brain*, **60**, 361.
Halpert, B. and Ashley, J. D. (1944) *Arch. Path.*, **38**, 112.
Hassin, G. B. and Diamond, I. B. (1926) *Arch. Neurol. Psychiat.* (Chicago), **15**, 34.
Hawking, F. and Greenfield, J. G. (1941) *Tr. Roy. Soc. trop. Med. & Hyg.*, **35**, 155.
Houghton, H. S. (1910) *J. trop. Med. & Hyg.*, **13**, 185.
Jansen, P., Bogaert, L. van and Haymaker, W. (1956) *J. Neuropath.*, **15**, 269.
Kane, C. A. and Most, H. (1948) *Arch. Neurol. Psychiat.* (Chicago), **59**, 141.
Kim, S. K. (1955) *J. Neurosurg.*, **12**, 89.
Koppisch, E. (1953) *Protozoal and Helminthic Infections* in *Pathology*, edit. by W. A. D. Anderson Kimpton, London.
Kuper, S., Mendelow, H. and Proctor, N. S. F. (1958) *Brain*, **81**, 235.
Langmaid, C. and Rogers, L. (1940) *Brain*, **63**, 184.
Levaditi, C., Nicolau, S. and Schoen, R. (1923) *Compt. rend. Acad. Sc.*, **177**, 985; *Compt. rend. Soc. Biol.*, **89**, 984; (1924) *Ann. Inst. Pasteur*, **38**, 651.
MacArthur, W. P. (1933) *Trans. Roy. Soc. trop. Med. and Hyg.*, **27**, 343.
Martinez-Niochet, A. and Potenza, L. (1956) *Acta Neurol. Latino-Amer.*, **2**, 72.
Menon, T. B. and Veliath, G. D. (1940) *Trans. Roy. Soc. trop. Med. and Hyg.*, **33**, 537.
Most, H. and Abeles, M. M. (1937) *Arch. Neurol. Psychiat.* (Chicago), **37**, 589.
Mott, F. W. (1906) *Reports of Sleeping Sickness Commission*, No. 7, Bale & Danielsson, London; (1907) *Arch. Neurol.* (Lond.), **3**.
Neujean, G. (1950) *Ann. Soc. Belge de Med. trop.*, **30**, 1125.
Obrador, S. (1948) *Arch. Neurol. Psychiat.* (Chicago), **59**, 457.
Phillips, G. (1948) *J. Neurol. Psychiat.*, **11**, 44.
Pinkerton, H. and Henderson, R. G. (1941) *J. Amer. med. Ass.*, **116**, 807.
Richter, R. B. (1936) *Arch. Neurol. Psychiat.* (Chicago), **36**, 1085.
Sabin, A. B. (1941) *J. Amer. med. Ass.*, **116**, 801.
Siim, J. C. (1951) *J. Amer. med Ass.*, **147**, 1641; (1955) *Proc. Roy. Soc. Med.*, **48**, 1067.
Stepien, L. and Chorobski, J. (1949) *Arch. Neurol. Psychiat.* (Chicago), **61**, 499.
Thomas, H. M. and Gage, D. P. (1945) *Bull. U.S. Army med. Dept.*, **4**, 197.
Wolf, A. and Cowen, D. (1937) *Bull. N.Y. Neurol. Inst.*, **6**, 306.
Woodland, L. J. (1949) *Med. J. Austral.* (ii), 904.

CHAPTER 4

INTOXICATIONS

By A. MEYER

The term 'toxic' like the even more general attribute 'degenerative' has been used in the past to designate a *direct* effect upon the neurone and other elements of the nervous parenchyma, as opposed to that operative in inflammatory and vascular disease. Increasing experience and progress in biochemical and histochemical analysis has shown, however, that widely differing processes may be comprehended under these headings. In one important form of poisoning, the toxic action consists in producing anoxia which in turn gives rise to vasodilatation and increased capillary permeability. In poisoning by heavy metals action is likely to be on specific enzyme systems of the cell, mainly those acting on pyruvates. A somewhat similar pathogenic mechanism has been invoked to account for peripheral and central neuropathies in conditions varying from deficiency of B vitamins to diabetes mellitus, carcinomatosis, chronic alcoholism, etc. Again the toxic action of certain viruses is due to their parasitic utilisation of the nucleoprotein of the host cells; different viruses are known to attack different parts of the intracellular mechanisms for protein synthesis.

For such circumscribed metabolic processes, Peters (1936) has coined the term 'biochemical lesion'. Although this term merely indicates that histological lesions are preceded by biochemical dysfunction (a view which has been accepted by most neuropathologists) it has nevertheless attained an almost symbolic significance in drawing biochemistry and histology together. How fruitful a combined chemical and histological approach could be will become apparent in the discussion of various conditions not only in this section, but also in chapters dealing with system degenerations, ageing and the senile and presenile dementias.

Blood-brain barrier

Toxic substances may reach the central nervous system by way of several pathways: through the blood-stream, via the cerebrospinal fluid or along the peripheral nerves and their lymph spaces. Of these, the approach from the blood-stream and the 'barrier' between blood and nervous tissue is by far the most important.

The concept of the blood-brain barrier goes back to observations by Ehrlich (1885) and Lewandowsky (1900) that aniline dyes and sodium ferrocyanide, injected into the blood-stream, stain all tissues of the body except those of the central nervous system. Goldmann (1913) using trypan blue found the tissue of the central nervous system likewise unstained except for the meninges and the choroid plexus. From this latter finding the author concluded that all substances reach the nervous parenchyma by way of the cerebrospinal fluid. This view, firmly advocated by Stern and Gautier (1921), was also held by Mott (1910) and Hauptmann (1925). It was supported by the erroneous assumption, prevalent at the time, that the subarachnoid spaces are continuous with the pericapillary and perineuronal 'lymph' spaces.

A great deal of valuable information has been supplied by experimental work with trypan blue and other acid and basic aniline dyes. It has for example been shown that, while debarred from the rest of the nervous parenchyma, the dye penetrates easily to structures such as the area postrema in the medulla, the region of the tuber cinereum, the neurohypophysis, the pineal gland, the spinal ganglia and peripheral nerves. After heavy intravenous injection of trypan blue the dye is also taken up by microglia in the vicinity of the capillaries. This occurred most markedly in the basal ganglia, thalamus and hypothalamus of rabbits investigated by Wells and Carmichael (1930). Macklin and Macklin (1920) were probably the first to show that the blood-brain barrier was penetrated at the site of injury of the brain (inflicted by stabbing with hot needles). This has been confirmed by Russell (1929), Bakay (1955) and many others, using trypan blue or radioactive tracer substances; anoxia, infarction, epileptic seizures and heavy X-ray irradiation (Clemente and Holst 1954) have been reported to have the same effect.

Since Behnsen's (1926) studies with trypan blue, the barrier is assumed to be more or less undeveloped in the brain of the newborn. 'Kernicterus' is often quoted as an experiment performed by nature in the human brain to show this difference. However, Gröntoft (1954), using trypan blue and radio-active phosphorus, found no significant differences between brains of human and animal foetuses and those in later stages of development. Bakay (1953), who used radio-active phosphorus, arrived at an intermediate conclusion: the blood-brain barrier for P^{32} in the rabbit does function in the foetus, but permeability is greater in the foetus and young than in the adult.

Injection of trypan blue has been much used in order to explore the anatomical site of the barrier. Spatz (1933) located the barrier in the vascular endothelium. He found that after intravenous injection of the acid dye, the walls of the cerebral vessels did not stain—in contrast to what happens in other organs. Spatz' results have recently been confirmed by Gröntoft. Schaltenbrand and Bailey (1928), followed by Tschirgi (1952), on the other hand, believe that the perivascular pia-glial membrane is the more likely site of the blood-brain barrier, while Clemente and Holst believe that the perivascular feet of the astrocytes form the barrier. Yet another structure, the ground substance (Nissl's grey), has been implicated by Hess (1953, 1955), who claimed to have identified it by a positive periodic acid Schiff reaction due to the presence of a neutral mucopolysaccharide. This reaction was negative in the newborn mouse brain but appeared on the 5th day after birth.

Most of the structures implicated in the barrier problem have recently been subjected to renewed microscopic scrutiny. Using the electron microscope, Dempsey and Wislocki (1955) demonstrated that in rats fed $Ag\ NO_3$ in drinking water, silver staining was absent from the central nervous system, except for the area postrema, the tuber cinereum, the neurohypophysis and the pineal gland. In these structures, as in the systemic organs, silver was found in the basement membranes of the capillaries and in connective tissue cells. In those parts of the central nervous system which did not store silver the capillaries were devoid of connective tissue investment. Woollam and Millen (1954, 1955) established that, in the central nervous system, a true perivascular space in communication with subarachnoid spaces, cannot be traced further than the arterioles; capillaries have no such perivascular space. Since the action of silver appears to be in many ways similar to trypan blue, one must assume that absence of trypan blue staining in the central nervous system has the same cause, i.e. lack of a pericapillary space (Peters 1961).

Recent electronmicroscopic investigations (Wickoff and Young 1956, Maynard *et al.* 1957; Hager 1961) have brought greater clarification. There is now fair agreement that the endothelial cells of cerebral and spinal capillaries have a morphology similar to that in other organs. At junctions between adjacent endothelial cells, a terminal bar is found, and there are no fenestrations in this layer. The endothelial layer is outwardly surrounded by a basement membrane which is said to consist of lipids and mucopolysaccharides which give a positive PAS reaction.

Externally, are the endfeet of astrocytes which lie in close apposition to the basal membrane. Although these largely cover the capillary wall—Maynard *et al.* estimate up to 85 per cent of its area—they do not constitute a glial membrane in the original sense of Held, and even less a pial-glial membrane as described by Schaltenbrand and Bailey. The interspaces between astrocytic endfeet are filled with neuropil not yet identified and occasionally by part of a nerve cell body (Hager). As pointed out on page 18, there is little electronmicroscopic evidence for *substantial* amounts of ground substance or intercellular fluid.

Thus, from the morphological point of view, any one, or all three layers of the capillary wall, may well provide the anatomical pathways through which substances carried in the blood may reach the neurones (Peters). There is no indication, however, that any of the layers alone acts as a universal barrier.

Turning now to the more physiological aspects of the problem, there have been many hypotheses regarding the laws governing the passage from blood plasma to intercellular fluid. Friedeman (1942) regarded an easy passage through the barrier as being determined by a positive electrical charge, but recent work has shown that Na, though it has a positive charge, nevertheless penetrates the barrier very slowly. Lipid solubility has been long recognised to be an important factor in certain instances such as chloroform and ethyl alcohol, but this also cannot claim to be a universal factor. Nor can this be said about particle size, though it may well have considerable influence on the passage of protein molecules. In all these researches isotopes have been extensively deployed; the results, however, should be interpreted with considerable care (Brierley 1957).

Present opinion, critically and exhaustively reviewed by Dobbing (1961), tends to deny the implication of any *one* (morphological or physiological) factor to explain all the facts. Once the experiments with trypan blue and similar dyestuffs are explained as resulting from the absence of perivascular spaces around capillaries in the central nervous system, these substances largely lose their significance as indicators of a general barrier function. In the last resort, whether substances enter or are 'excluded' depends on the metabolic requirements, which vary with growth, health and disease, of the neurones themselves and of other cells (MacIlwain 1959).

ANOXIC POISONS AND THE PROBLEMS OF ANOXIA AND SELECTIVE VULNERABILITY

General remarks

Certain poisons exert their toxic action mainly either by preventing oxygen from reaching the nerve cells, or by making oxygen unusable by the inhibition of enzymes, or by removing essential substrates (e.g. glucose) without which no oxidation can take place. Among them are included carbon monoxide, the cyanides and insulin. Since they affect the nervous system in the same way as anoxias of other origin, whether produced by high altitudes or by cardiac or respiratory failure, it will be useful to include them in this section. This will enable us to discuss the problem of anoxia in its totality.

Anoxia has been divided by Barcroft (1925) into stagnant, anaemic and anoxic types, to which the histotoxic type has been added later. This classification is, however, only approximate, the different categories overlapping considerably. From the histological point of view, the most important distinction is between conditions in which only oxygen is absent (anoxic anoxia) and those in which all the substances carried by the blood, including oxygen, are prevented from reaching the tissues (ischaemia, oligaemia). However, this difference is largely offset by the changes of cerebral blood flow which follow oxygen want and which may lead to severe degrees of capillary and venous stagnation and hypotension.

The importance of anoxia (or more correctly hypoxia, as oxygen is reduced and not entirely absent) is brought out by the physiological assessment of oxygen consumption in the brain as compared with other organs. Methods have been introduced which make it possible accurately to determine the arteriovenous gradient and the cerebral blood flow in animals and man. The cerebral metabolic rate can be computed from these two values (Himwich 1951). According to McIlwain (1955), the proportion of oxygen used by the brain is 20–25 per cent of the total breathed; in infants and children up to the age of 4, cerebral respiration accounts for as much as 50 per cent of the oxygen consumed by the whole resting body. Much of this difference is explained, however, by the relatively great weight of the brain in the new-born.

When arterial and cerebral venous blood are analysed, the oxygen saturation is found to fall by 6·7 ml. per 100 ml. of blood while traversing the brain. This fall is greater than that which occurs in most other organs of the body, and equals almost exactly the value of CO_2 increase in venous blood; i.e. the respiratory co-efficient is unity, which points to carbohydrate being the almost exclusive substrate.

During anoxia, labile constituents in the nervous tissue show definite biochemical change. The higher, energy-rich phosphate compounds, such as phosphocreatine and adenosine triphosphate, disappear, while lactic acid and inorganic phosphates increase. There are, however, differences in detail in different types of anoxia to which attention will be drawn.

Anoxia has also been intensively studied from the electrophysiological angle (Brazier 1948, Rohmer *et al.* 1952, Jung 1953 and Meyer and Gastaut 1961). As Jung points out, initial increase in frequency of neuronal discharges is followed by large, slow, delta waves, until finally complete electrical inactivity is apparent. Total O_2 want makes electrical activity disappear in the cerebral cortex after 20 seconds, in medulla and cerebellum after 30–90 seconds.

The vast amount of histological work, both *post mortem* and experimental, has been reviewed by Scholz (1953 a and b, 1957, 1959) and Courville (1953), both of whom have also made outstanding contributions to individual problems. The review by Steegman (1961) is a helpful guide through the hypoxic lesions caused by cardiac and respiratory disease. The varying aspects of this work will be discussed under their respective headings. Only a few general points require to be mentioned here.

The effect of anoxia is a complex one. In the first place, a direct action on the neurone must be assumed; this is followed by capillary and venous dilatation. This latter is initially compensatory and increases the blood flow, but with severe persisting anoxia results in stasis. The changes in the cerebral circulation have been attributed to direct action on the contractile apparatus in the small blood vessels (Ricker 1924, Spielmeyer 1930), which results either in spasm or more often in dilatation and stasis. The view which prevails now is, however, that the dilatation is due to accumulation of CO_2 and, perhaps, even more of lactic acid, which lower the pH in blood and tissue.

The experimental work of Denny-Brown and Meyer and their associates (Denny-Brown and Meyer 1957; Meyer *et al.* 1954, 1958, Denny-Brown 1960, Meyer *et al.* 1961) has done much to clarify the sequence of events. Most of their work was concerned with the cortical effects of the experimental occlusion of larger arteries; they emphasise, however, that the essential events are identical with those occurring in anoxic anoxia. In the cortex, which they could observe through a trephined window, they made simultaneous recordings of the E.E.G., O_2 tension, temperature (cerebral blood flow), pH, CO_2 potential, blood pressure, Na and K movements, etc. During nitrogen inhalation, for example, they noted the fall of O_2 tension before—after a time lag of 5 or more seconds—changes appeared in the E.E.G. A fall of O_2 tension by 30–

50 per cent was followed by decreasing amplitude and slowing of E.E.G. activity. Reduction of O_2 tension by 50–60 per cent resulted in flattening of the E.E.G. When the potential of O_2 was reduced below 8 mm. a flux of Na outward from, and of K into, the extracellular spaces took place. A fall in pH in the ischaemic zone caused capillary dilatation and reduction of vascular resistance. When the fall of blood pressure persisted longer than 2 minutes, microstasis occurred, the capillaries became engorged, endothelial damage (due to anoxia) developed, haemorrhages appeared and the tissue became swollen. Even at this stage, however, reversal may take place on restoration of the blood pressure; if the latter remains low, the process goes on to infarction.

Spasm does not play more than a transient role: this is in agreement with the growing body of opinion that spasm of previously normal cerebral arteries does not occur (Pickering 1951), though it is observed in diseased arteries, for example, in malignant hypertension (Byrom 1954), or after mechanical irritation.

While complete infarctions (anaemic or haemorrhagic) often occur in anoxia, we more often meet with incomplete infarctions where only the neurones become necrotic. For this type of necrosis, Scholz (1953 a and b) has coined the term 'selective neuronal degeneration'.

Much attention has been paid, both in human pathology and in particular in animal experiments, to the duration of anoxia necessary to produce reversible and irreversible damage to nervous tissue. Gildea and Cobb (1930) found neurones of the cerebral cortex to be irreparably damaged after 5 minutes of anoxia, while medullary nerve cells may survive up to 20 or 30 minutes of almost complete cessation of blood supply. Tureen (1936) found that complete stoppage of the blood flow to the spinal cord of cats may, if lasting less than 20 minutes, be followed by recovery. Weinberger *et al.* (1940) reported permanent cerebral damage when the cerebral circulation was interrupted for 3½ minutes; after 7½ minutes the damage was severe and the cats usually died. Meyer and Blume (1934), in experiments with ether, noted permanent damage in cats when the duration of respiratory or cardiac arrest lasted longer than 5 minutes. In a cat, however, no appreciable damage was seen even after an arrest of 10 minutes. Kabat and Schadewald (1941) and Grenell (1946) found damage in the cerebral and cerebellar cortex of dogs who had sustained arrest of 4–6 minutes and made a seemingly full recovery. In a human case of the present writer's experience (1956), severe and widespread lesions occurred after cardiac arrest of only 1 minute. Neubürger (1954), Bourne (1957) and Biemond (1958) have likewise reported damage after arrest or severe hypoxia of about 2 minutes' duration.

There is, thus, both in human and animal cases, wide variation in the endurance of circulatory arrest, and the usual adoption of a limit of safety of 4–5 minutes represents at best only an average figure.

These figures, however, refer to normal body temperature: although during hypothermia the tolerance for O_2 deficiency is considerably increased, cardiac arrest and hypotension resulting in brain damage have been reported to occur (Brierley 1962). In the material of this author the lesions were the same, no matter whether hypothermia had been combined with perfusion or not; they differed from the usual histological picture of anoxic anoxia, occupying chiefly posterior cortical regions and the striatum.

The degeneration of nerve cells during and after anoxia has been carefully studied in human and experimental animal brains by many workers, including Spielmeyer (1922), Gildea and Cobb, Tureen (1936), Grenell and Kabat (1947) and Krogh (1952). Here it suffices to point out that Spielmeyer's ischaemic and homogenising cell degenerations are not the only changes found in anoxic nervous tissue; the remainder, according to Krogh, is made up by nerve cells displaying acute swelling, Nissl's severe change and, more rarely, Nissl's chronic change. Acute swelling and chromatolysis are reversible, while as far as has been ascertained, the other changes are irreversible. The end stage is a hardly stainable cell shadow (ghost cell) which soon disappears completely. Although cells showing ischaemic and homogenising degeneration usually represent only a fraction of degenerating nerve cells, they enjoy, in the writer's experience, a degree of specificity to anoxia and ischaemia greater than any of the other degeneration types. They are, therefore, of considerable diagnostic importance.

Lindenberg (1956) has introduced the distinction between 'morphotropic' and 'morphostatic' necrobiosis: the former develops following sudden exposure to full stagnant anoxia and results, mainly through the accumulation of lactic acid in the tissue, in ischaemic and homogenising nerve cell degeneration; 'morphostatic' necrobiosis is observed when full stagnant anoxia is preceded by a period of critical hypoxia during which the cell metabolites are used up, lactic acid is not appreciably increased and none of the ischaemic cell degenerations occur (though eventually the cells lose their stainability). Although it may be true that ischaemic necrosis is —to a large extent—the consequence of acidosis, it must be noted that in Lindenberg's investigations, death of a person or animal was taken to be the condition comparable to full stagnant anoxia; in human cases agony was regarded as equivalent to preceding hypoxia. This somewhat weakens the author's conclusions, and more stringent experimental conditions seem to be called for. In the present writer's experience, typical pictures of ischaemic or homogenising cell changes do not occur in ordinary autolysis of brain tissue.

Electronmicroscopic contributions to nerve cell changes after hypoxia are still in a preliminary stage. In the Syrian hamster, Scholz and Hager (1959) found the perikaryion of cortical nerve cells swollen and enlarged. The more severely damaged cells exhibited a considerable vacuolic expansion of the endoplasmic reticulum and rarefaction of the ribosome granules. The mitochondria often, though not always, participated in the vacuolisation. Both Altmann (1955) and Büchner (1957) hold a disturbance in the mitochondrial metabolism responsible for this osmotic disequilibrium of the cytoplasmic structures: a view which would be in accordance with the acknowledged role of the mitochondria in oxidative and phosphorilysing enzymatic processes. However, according to Scholz and Hager, the electronmicroscopic evidence in favour of preceding morphological damage to the mitochondria is not yet unequivocal. Little information has yet been obtained on the genesis of ischaemic and homogenising cell degenerations.

Mitochondrial shrinkage (i.e. extreme resting state) has been noted on the electronic screen after barbiturate poisoning (Wilke and Iizuka 1960).

Dead or dying neurones lying in infarcted areas seem to be remarkably resistant to autolysis. Although ribonucleic acid is lost from the cytoplasm, the loss of total protein is relatively small in the cell body; it is more considerable in the dendrites (Dixon 1955).

Carbon monoxide poisoning

Carbon monoxide poisoning is most often due to accidental or suicidal exposure to illuminating gas, but it occurs also from exposure to exhaust gases of internal combustion engines, from incomplete burning of charcoal stoves, and from the development of after-damp in colliery and other explosions. The clinical and pathological sequelae of CO poisoning have attracted attention for a long time. Wilson (1940) quotes pathological observations by Klebs and Pelchen as early as 1888. The review of Sibelius (1906) already contains 200 references. The older workers were mainly interested in the macroscopic lesions in the lenticular nucleus which were conspicuous to the naked eye, and the pathogenesis of this lesion attracted early attention. The discussion of the sequelae of carbon monoxide poisoning entered a new phase in the 1920s following the publication of investigations with modern neurohistological methods (Stewart 1920, Hiller 1924, Grinker 1926, Meyer 1926, 1928 a), Weimann (1930), Hsü and

Ch'Eng (1938), Raskin and Mullaney (1940), Eros and Priestman (1942), Neubürger and Clarke (1945), Roger *et al.* (1952), Dutra (1952), Schwedenberg (1959) among others. Schwedenberg, in a review of 35 cases, which were well documented, found that 24 had a conscious interval, 25 showed pallidal necrosis and 28 had lesions of the white matter which in 3 infants had resulted in its complete dissolution. Examples where the white matter was predominantly affected have been published by Stewart, Grinker, Meyer (1928 a), Hsü and Ch'Eng, Neubürger and Clarke and Schwedenberg.

The toxicity of carbon monoxide consists mainly in its affinity for haemoglobin, an affinity which is several hundred times stronger than that of oxygen. This results in a stable compound, carboxyhaemoglobin, barring the gaseous exchange between blood and tissue. Carbon monoxide has affinity also for the iron of cytochrome oxidase. The importance of this direct effect on cellular respiration for the pathogenesis of lesions following CO poisoning has been re-emphasised by Bänder and Kiese (1955). The inhalation of a 1-per-cent concentration is usually fatal to a resting man in 30–40 minutes and to a working man in 10 minutes. Children, with a higher respiratory rate, die more rapidly than adults. Concentrations of 0·01 per cent produce light headache; of 0·05 per cent severe headache, vertigo and weakness; of 0·01 per cent acceleration of respiration and pulse; and of 0·2 per cent coma (Schumm 1953). However, these figures vary and depend on multiple factors.

In those cases which die from *acute* intoxication in coma or shortly afterwards, all viscera, the blood, the skeletal muscles, etc., display a pink-red colour which is due to the presence of carboxyhaemoglobin. All organs show marked congestion. This is particularly conspicuous in the brain in which marked venous and capillary dilatation is found in both the meninges and in the vessels of the substance of the brain. Haemorrhages are frequent in such early fatal cases, and they may be either petechial, with predilective site in white matter and corpus callosum, or they may be massive in one of the lobes of the brain or in the basal ganglia. According to Weimann, at this stage the globus pallidus may appear anaemic, this anaemia possibly preceding irreparable ischaemic change.

Thrombi have also been described by many observers, but as they are not consistent doubt has been expressed (Hiller 1924 and others) about their primary significance.

The changes after delayed death are of greater pathological interest. It should be noted, however, that only a fraction of cases which undergo coma as a result of acute CO poisoning will later show delayed effects; the overwhelming majority seem to recover completely. In those with permanent sequelae the sequence of events is either that, following prolonged coma, neurological and psychiatric signs indicating permanent tissue damage will manifest themselves on consciousness being regained, or they will appear after an interval of 2–3 weeks during which the patients either appear normal or display only negligible or vague symptoms.

All changes have the appearances and typical localisation of anoxia and/or ischaemia. In cases with short survival of up to approximately 48 hours, macroscopic inspection of the brain usually reveals an increase of weight due to oedema and capillary and venous dilatation, a varying number of petechial haemorrhages and an early necrosis of the globus pallidus (Fig. 4.9).

Occasionally the lesion of the globus pallidus is combined with necrosis of the reticular, iron-rich zone of the substantia nigra. This latter finding was first described by Hiller, but has also been found in other cases of CO poisoning (Meyer 1926) and after cyanide poisoning and respiratory failure in the course of anaesthesia. Cases have been reported, however, in which, despite other severe lesions, the globus pallidus was normal (Meyer 1928 a).

The cerebral cortex, after survival of 1–3 days, may show extensive ischaemic necrosis indicated with Nissl staining by areas of pallor. This may be focal or may take the form of more continuous laminar degeneration of the third and often the second layer, or be confined to the deeper layers and to the superficial white matter. With higher magnification the nerve cells stain badly (ghost cells) and many show the picture typical of ischaemic, homogenising, or Nissl's acute or severe degeneration. Microglial and macroglial proliferation may be seen in their initial stages. Ammon's horn also shows ischaemic necrosis, particularly in area h_1 (Sommer sector) and $h_3 - h_5$ (end-plate). The Purkinje cells in the cerebellum may undergo homogenising change combined with glial shrubs.

In other cases widespread, focally accentuated, degeneration of the cerebral white matter may be more conspicuous than necrosis of the cerebral cortex (Fig. 4.8). Even after a short survival the myelin is less stainable, the myelin sheaths being swollen and fragmented. The axis cylinders also show swelling and fragmentation but to a less degree. The tissue of the white matter has a finely porous appearance, which is independent of the blood-vessels and which is mainly caused by excessive swelling of the oligodendroglia whose nuclei are pyknotic or entirely lost. The macroglia shows both proliferative and regressive changes and there may also be mesodermal proliferation. Jacob (1939), after clinico-pathological analysis of personal and other published cases, has come to the conclusion that this type of degeneration is present predominantly in those cases in which delayed signs of intoxication followed a period of relative normality after the acute intoxication, and that the immediate pathogenesis is oedema due to increased vascular permeability rather than a direct anoxic effect.

In later stages, the early necrotic changes undergo the usual modifications. In Hiller's case, after a survival of 14 days, the lesions in the globus pallidus, reticular zone of the substantia nigra and the deeper layers of the cerebral cortex had progressed to the stage of softening with dissemination of lipid phagocytes, mostly of microglial origin. But more often, this mobile stage of repair does not appear in the cerebral cortex. Only the neurones disappear and are more or less densely replaced by gliosis. Thus the appearances of total, laminar or disseminated focal atrophy develop. In a case with survival of 16 years (Meyer 1926) the cerebral hemispheres, particularly in the frontal and occipital lobes, presented the picture of granular atrophy. In Nissl preparations, the cortex showed irregular focal loss of neurones followed by gliosis and retraction of the surface (Fig. 4.5). A similar case with survival of 15 years has been described by Raskin and Mullaney.

Pathological changes have been reported in many other organs. They include necrosis of heart muscle (Neubürger and Clarke 1945), of skeletal muscle (Loughbridge *et al.* 1958), haemorrhages and centro-lobular fatty degeneration of the liver, haemorrhages in the kidney, etc. In the pathogenesis of skeletal muscle necrosis, posture and pressure play a part cumulative to that of hypoxia; the myoglobinuria resulting from these multiple muscle necroses may result in acute tubular nephrosis.

Observations of CO intoxication in the foetus, following accidental or suicidal poisoning of the mother, are of considerable theoretical interest (Hallervorden (1949), who quotes previous cases by Maresch and Neubürger). In all reported cases the lesions were of striking severity. The damage to the basal ganglia was, if anything, more extensive than in the adult and included the striatum. Microgyria and other signs of arrested development were present. (See Chapter 5.)

Experimental investigations of CO poisoning have been carried out by Photakis (1921), Meyer (1928 b, 1932 b), Ferraro and Morrison (1928), Lewey and Drabkin (1944), van Bogaert *et al.* (1938), Strassmann (1949) and Lund (1956), among others. With the exception of van Bogaert's monkeys they have confirmed the changes described in the human brain, but, through the opportunities they have offered with regard to variation of experimental procedure, species, etc., they have provided additional information of interest to the problem of selective vulnerability.

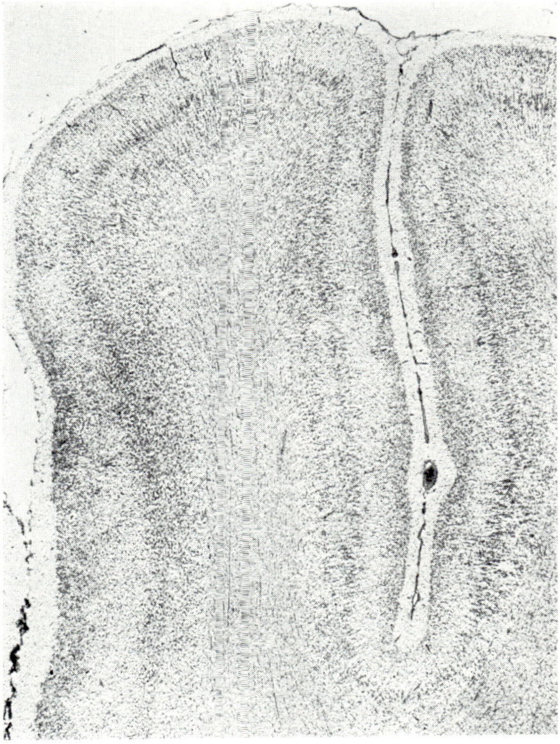

4.1

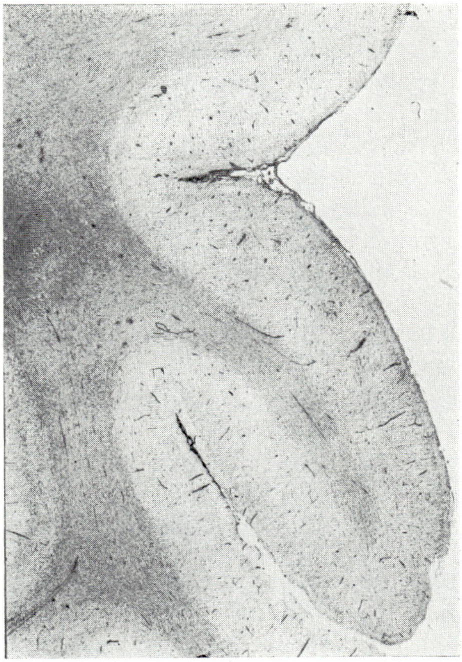

4.2

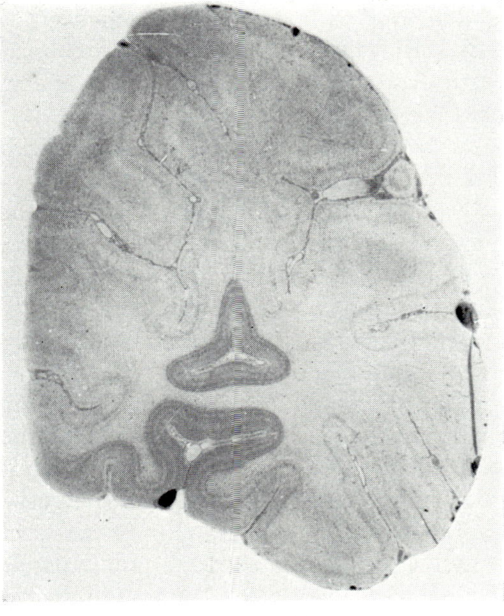

4.3

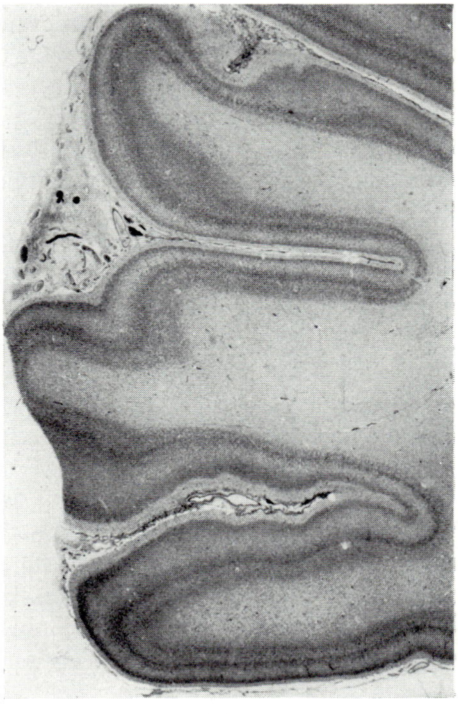

4.4

FIGS. 4.1–4.4. Show acute laminar or total necrosis of cerebral cortex.

FIG. 4.1. Anaesthetic death. (Nissl ×9.)
FIG. 4.2. Hypoglycaemic coma. (Nissl ×6.)
FIG. 4.3. Anaesthetic death, occipital lobe; striate area preserved. (Nissl ×2.)
FIG. 4.4. Death from hanging. (Nissl ×3.)

The *clinical symptomatology* after CO intoxication varies with the extent and localisation of the lesions. The Parkinson syndrome has often been recorded and has been attributed to lesions in the globus pallidus, and, probably, in the reticular zone of the substantia nigra. Choreiform movements may also be connected with lesions of the basal ganglia. Other focal symptomatology includes hemiparesis, aphasias and related symbolic disturbances. In one case, clinically observed by the present writer, alexia was the only residual sign. The widespread damage to the cerebral cortex may give rise to dementia or to amnestic syndromes of the Korsakoff type which occasionally prove to be reversible. Dementia may be so profound as to be confused with the pseudodementia of the Ganser syndrome. When compensation is claimed in such cases the differential diagnosis with hysteria may be difficult (Last and Meyer 1932). The much discussed case of Grünthal and Störring, which showed complete loss of memory, has never been fully accepted as of organic cerebral origin (*vide* Schumm). In several cases (Schumm) the psychosis which followed CO poisoning was of a schizophreniform type and the subsequent discovery of severe anoxic lesions in the brain was a surprise.

Cyanide poisoning

The toxicity of cyanide is generally recognised to be due to its inhibitory action on intracellular oxidative enzymes. Like carbon monoxide it has also an affinity for the iron of cytochrome oxidase. Accidental or suicidal exposure to hydrocyanic (prussic) acid or to sodium or potassium salts of cyanide leads to asphyxia with severe epileptic convulsions which may be a factor contributing to the anoxic lesions in the nervous system.

The cyanides, particularly hydrocyanic acid, have a rapid effect and the result is death in a short time. In such fatal cases of *acute* intoxication pathological changes are few. A pink-red colour of the blood, tissues and skin is frequently seen and there is the characteristic cyanide odour. Cyanide does not combine with haemoglobin, but with its post-mortem derivative methaemoglobin. According to Warburg (1924), like CO, it inhibits cytochrome oxidase by means of its affinity to iron. Although the clinical signs (convulsion, coma) point to an affection of the central nervous system, the pathology in such rapidly fatal cases consists mainly of capillary and venous hyperaemia, and of petechial, subarachnoid and subdural haemorrhages.

Only a few human cases with delayed death have been described, and pathological investigations have not been detailed. Schmorl (1920) saw on macroscopic inspection after 36 hours symmetrical, well-defined areas of softening in the globus pallidus in addition to severe hyperaemia. Edelmann (1921) after 23 hours found general hyperaemia and early softenings in the anterior parts of both striata. Histologically the inner parts of the lenticular nucleus contained haemorrhages and seemed to be more affected than the rest. He also reported signs of inflammation in globus pallidus, cerebral white matter and medulla.

Experimental investigations have amplified the scanty human observations. The first series was carried out in dogs and rabbits (Meyer 1932 a, 1933). Changes similar to those described after CO poisoning were found: ischaemic necrosis of the cerebral cortex, almost ubiquitous in some animals, in others laminar or focal; symmetrical and selective necrosis of the globus pallidus (Fig. 4.10) and reticular zone of the substantia nigra (Fig. 4.20); sector necrosis of Ammon's horn; and necrosis and early softening of the white matter, and in particular of the corpus callosum. In rodents the white matter necrosis predominated, with particular localisation in commissural pathways (corpus callosum and anterior commissure). The myelin was not investigated, because the tissue was fixed for special purposes in 96° alcohol.

In rats given multiple injections of sodium cyanide, Hicks more recently (1950 a) described necrosis in cerebral cortex, corpus striatum, hippocampus, substantia nigra, cerebellum, in addition to the affection of myelinated fibres in the corpus callosum and anterior part of the caudate nucleus. The heart, the organ richest in content of cytochrome oxidase, is not damaged by cyanide whose affinity to the cerebral white matter he explains by its low content of this enzyme. Haymaker *et al.* (1952) also recorded ischaemic changes in cerebral cortex, corpus striatum, substantia nigra and cerebellum.

Emphasis on the white matter and, in particular, on myelin was predominant in the experimental observations of Ferraro (1933, monkeys and cats); Rubino (1935, rabbits); Jervis (1937, cats); Jedlowski (1938, dogs); Hurst (1940, 1942, monkeys); Déchaume and Chambon (1947, dogs), and Lumsden (1950, rats). Lumsden considered this action on the myelinated fibres to be specific for cyanides, with predilection for the corpus callosum, at least in rats: according to him, this effect follows a chain of enzyme reactions which may primarily occur in the mitochondria of oligodendrocytes.

These conflicting findings are nearer to clarification following the study of Levine and Stypulkowski (1959). Experimenting with rats which were given one inhalation of hydrogen cyanide, they succeeded in obtaining and controlling differential levels of intoxication. They found that the lesser degree produced changes in the central white matter, corpus callosum and other commissural systems, while the nerve cells of cerebral and cerebellar cortex, corpus striatum and the pyramidal layer of Ammon's horn were damaged in the deeper level of intoxication. Disorganisation of the oligodendroglia which showed early shrinkage and pyknosis was a striking phenomenon in their material, which confirmed Lumsden's earlier observations. Levine and Stypulkowski regard the effect on cerebral white matter as specific and nonischaemic. Following Hicks and Lumsden they, also, emphasise the pathogenic importance of the low content of cytochrome oxidase in the white matter. It remains to be seen, however, whether this interpretation meets all the complexities of the pathogenesis of cyanide poisoning as well as of CO intoxication in which also inhibition of cytochrome oxidase has been implicated. In particular, it must be proved that the low content of the enzyme in the white matter is *inadequate* to meet metabolic requirements. Hicks himself, on another occasion (1950 b), drew attention to the varying combination of factors which effect the distribution of selective lesions.

These observations on cyanide and—to a lesser degree—on CO poisoning have led to a lively discussion on their relation to human demyelinating diseases (Lumsden 1950, 1957). Although Wolf (1952) denied that conclusive evidence existed in favour of such a relationship, the problem is still under discussion. Cyanide poisoning has been considered also in relation to Marchiava-Bignami disease (*vide* page 264).

Symmetrical and—to all appearances—ischaemic necrosis of globus pallidus and substantia nigra has been described in horses by Cordy (1954) after spontaneous or experimental ingestion of the *yellow star distle*. The condition known as 'chewing disease' leads to Parkinson-like symptoms such as hypertonia of muscle, slow gait and lethargy. The pathogenesis is not known, though the resemblance to the lesions in CO and cyanide poisoning is striking.

Other asphyxiating gases. War gases. Carbon disulphide

Among the older war gases, the pathogenic effects of *phosgene* have been investigated. Phosgene results in irritation and oedema of the walls of the lung alveoli. The changes in the brain are usually haemorrhages of petechial type. Similar changes may be caused by nitrobenzol and other nitric acid compounds, hydrogen sulphide, toluol and benzene. H_2S, like cyanides, seems to have an effect upon respiratory enzymes by the formation of iron-sulphide which results in blackening of the tissue of the brain. Meyer and Blume observed typical ischaemic changes, mainly in the cornu Ammonis and cerebellar cortex, in cats exposed to breathing of CO_2.

The substances available during the Second World War included lewisite and sulphur mustard gases which, in addition to their local vesicant action, were also toxic by absorption. The systemic effects of lewisite are, as is known from experimental work, similar to that of inorganic arsenical poisoning (*vide* page 259).

The so-called 'nerve gases' are known to be more toxic than the formerly used substances. They are organic phosphates and include di-isopropyl fluorophosphonate (D.F.P.), and tetraethylpyrophosphate (T.E.P.P.). Their toxic effect can be explained as an inhibition of cholinesterases. These compounds are used therapeutically in myasthenia gravis and in the management of urinary retention and abdominal distension and their effect upon the clinical symptoms and the electroencephalograms of psychotics has been studied (Rowntree, Nevin and Wilson 1950, Aprison *et al.* 1954). What is known of the *neurohistology* of these toxic compounds will be discussed in the section on trio-ortho-cresyl-phosphate on page 275.

Carbon disulphide is extensively used in the rayon industry and poisoning following exposure to the gas has been reported from time to time. A symptomatology of Parkinsonian syndromes, ataxia, peripheral neuropathies and mental changes has been described (Megro 1930, Alpers 1939, Alpers and Lewey 1940). The pathology in the human and animal brain has been studied by Alpers and Lewey, Ferraro, Jervis and Flicker (1941) and Richter (1945). Alpers and Lewey found widespread acute, subacute and chronic degenerative changes in nerve cells, more severe in animals (dogs) than in man. The Purkinje cells were particularly involved which, probably, accounts for the ataxia which is a prominent clinical feature; but changes in the lenticular nucleus and, in particular, in the globus pallidus were also prominent. The blood-vessels, particularly the arteries of small calibre, showed proliferation of endothelial cells and frequently hyalin changes of the walls, but the pathogenic significance of these changes has not been elucidated. Ferraro *et al.* have also stressed the proliferative changes of the blood-vessels in their experimental studies in cats, of which only one, however, showed softening of the lenticular nucleus, both putamen and the globus pallidus.

In 4 monkeys exposed to repetitive sublethal doses of CS_2 Richter described and illustrated remarkably selective symmetrical necrosis in the globus pallidus and the zona reticularis of the substantia nigra, reminiscent of the lesions which follow carbon monoxide and other anoxic poisoning. The absence of vascular changes in other parts of the central nervous system has led Richter to reject a vascular pathogenesis in favour of direct action on the nervous parenchyma, by anoxia or inhibition of enzymes and co-enzymes. All four of his monkeys presented a clinical syndrome of slowness of movement without paralysis, plastic cogwheel rigidity, flexor postural attitudes and severe action and intention tremor which in Richter's view closely resembled the Parkinsonian syndrome in man.

High altitude and decompression anoxia

The advent of flying in war and peace has directed much work to the effects of high altitude upon the brain, both in fatal cases and in experiments in decompression chambers simulating oxygen tensions at varying altitudes. Pathological changes in human cases have been described by Titrud and Haymaker (1947) and Haymaker and Davison (1950). In the former paper, 2 cases were reported with delayed death after 40 hours and 3 weeks respectively. In the first, conspicuous ischaemic necrosis, usually of a focal kind, was observed in the deep layers of the cortex, the white matter, the striatum, the Sommer sector of Ammon's horn, cerebellar cortex and the anterior horn cells of the cord. The white matter and spinal cord lesions were missing in the second case, which otherwise was similar in the nature and localisation of the changes.

Haymaker and Davison emphasised the importance of factors additional to hypoxia, such as air and fat embolism. They found fat emboli in the lung in 4 of their 5 cases and once in the brain.

There have been a number of *experimental* investigations into the problem by Büchner and Luft (1936), Luft (1937), Altmann and Schubothe (1942), Morrison (1946), Jensen *et al.* (1948) and others. Büchner and his collaborators, in experiments on guinea-pigs, found chromatolysis, vacuolation and ischaemic and homogenising changes in nerve cells beneath the 4th ventricle and, less severe, in Purkinje cells. Altmann and Schubothe, in cats, described severe ischaemic necrosis in the cerebellar cortex, corpus striatum and cerebral cortex. Morrison's experiments were carried out on 25 dogs and monkeys. By varying the intensity and the number of exposures he was able to produce selective lesions confined either to cerebral and cerebellar cortex or to the cerebral white matter and the basal ganglia. White matter lesions occurred with particular frequency when exposure was slight and repeated. Chronic repeated experiments led to exhaustion of the adrenal cortex; diminished glucose production may have been a pathogenic factor.

Anaesthetics and hypnotics

Immediate or delayed death after anaesthesia has been known for a long time. The earlier reports have been reviewed by Bodechtel (1928), Meyer and Blume (1934) and Courville (1939). Beecher and Todd (1954) have recently concluded, from a material of 600,000 anaesthesias, that death associated with anaesthesia occurs in 1 of 1,560 cases. It is not possible to state how frequently, in this series, anoxia was the cause; interestingly the mortality rate rises steeply when a muscle relaxant is used. Maclay (1953) also found this to be so when he reviewed the death rate from convulsion therapy in mental patients (page 564).

Clinico-pathological observations have been recorded, among others, by Bodechtel (1928), Lowenberg *et al.* (1936), Abbott and Courville (1938), Courville (1939), Steegman (1939), Batten and Courville (1940), Winblad (1940), Courville (1941). The anaesthetics most commonly used were nitrous oxide and ether. Steegman used avertin and cyclopropane. The pathological findings were essentially the same with all anaesthetics; in particular, there was no specific clinical or pathological feature that could be solely attributed to N_2O.

More recent case reports include those of Howkins *et al.* (1946), Neubürger (1954), Denst (1953), Courville (1954), A. Meyer (1956) whose 6 human cases have been also included in the paper of Brierley (1961), Bourne (1957), Haberland (1961) and J. E. Meyer (1961). Of these, Bourne's paper is of special interest, because he reports brain lesions in patients who had fainted and suffered hypoxia (of at least 2 minutes' duration), while under anaesthesia in the upright position during dental treatment. Head-up tilt of 20° in combination with the use of hypotensive anaesthesia was suggested also by Brierley and Cooper (1962) to be the cause of cerebral anoxia in a woman who underwent a cosmetic operation.

The sequence of events in almost all published cases is that respiratory and/or cardiac failure develop in the course of the anaesthesia. If this is of sufficient severity to cause permanent damage to the brain the patients either remain comatose and die in the course of a few hours or days or, after regaining consciousness, exhibit permanent clinical sequelae. Batten and Courville (1940) in 10 personal cases, to which they added 11 cases published by previous workers, described states of confusion and stupor progressing to dementia, often associated with spastic signs, rigidity or choreo-athetosis. Milder permanent personality changes have been recorded by Fletcher (1945). Temporary post-anaesthetic restlessness, confusion, convulsions and some permanent mental deterioration may be more common than has so far been acknowledged. Such changes may occur with greater frequency in the higher age groups and may be confused with diagnoses of senile deterioration (Bedford 1955).

Uncomplicated anaesthesia results in a general depression of brain function. Biochemically, this is expressed by the fact that during anaesthesia the values of energy-rich compounds such as phosphocreatine and adenosine triphosphate remain high, and even increase, in the brain tissue, while lactic acid and inorganic phosphates are low: i.e. a behaviour opposite to that seen in anoxia. Cerebral respiration is also moderately depressed, but contrary to previous opinion (Quastel and Wheatley 1932), this inhibition is not now regarded as causing the anaesthetic effect, which is thought to be due to the physical presence of the anaesthetic in the brain and its action on synaptic activity (McIlwain 1955). However if, for reasons not yet fully explained, the depression of cerebral respiration is too great, toxic signs develop, and manifest themselves clinically in respiratory and cardiac disturbances mainly of central origin; they are accompanied by the behaviour of the labile phosphate compounds which is characteristic of anoxia.

The neuropathological sequelae both in type of degeneration and in localisation are clearly those of anoxia. In cases with a few days' survival the cerebral cortex may show confluent or continuous necrosis which may be confined to the 3rd layer (Fig. 4.1), particularly in the depths of sulci, or may involve all layers. In the occipital lobe the visual cortex usually escapes (Fig. 4.3). Many of the nerve cells within the necrotic areas show ischaemic or, more frequently, homogenising degeneration.

Confluent demyelination and glial proliferation in the cerebral white matter, similar to that seen in CO poisoning, may accompany the cortical lesions, or rarely, may even predominate. J. E. Meyer (1961) gives a typical picture of diffuse demyelination and necrosis of the cerebral white matter in a case of acute appendicitis to whom nitrous oxide—ether anaesthesia was administered without complication; the patient, however, remained somnolent and died after about a month from embolism of the lung. The cerebral cortex was normal, but there were lesions in the globus pallidus and cerebellar cortex.

In the cornu Ammonis typical necrosis of the Sommer sector end-plate is usually found (Fig. 4.15). Within the basal ganglia the striatum and the globus pallidus are often affected jointly; their lesion may occasionally combine with a necrosis of the thalamus and the claustrum (Fig. 4.12). The Purkinje cells are usually severely damaged (Fig. 4.17); the majority show homogenising degeneration accompanied by neuronophagia and glial shrubbery (Fig. 4.18).

In a case anaesthetised by nitrous oxide and oxygen, respiratory and cardiac arrest of 1 minute occurred. The patient regained consciousness and *survived for 6 months* in a condition of *profound dementia*. The cerebral cortex was severely damaged in all regions. Many focal lesions extended through almost all layers (Fig. 4.6); in other regions the inner layers of the cortex and the superficial white matter were the site of the lesion. As far as one could ascertain in this much dissected brain the globus pallidus, crowded with lipid phagocytes and proliferating astrocytes, was selectively affected. Part of the amygdaloid nucleus was similarly damaged. Ammon's horn showed glio-mesodermal proliferation in the Sommer sector. Within the cerebellum many lobules, particularly those near the white matter, were atrophic and there was intense gliosis of and around the dentate nucleus (Fig. 4.19).

In one case of anaesthetic death, Neubürger (1954) saw Wernicke-like lesions in the mammillary bodies, in addition to more common changes in other regions. Brierley (1961) observed a similar affection in the case of a 2-year-old child after cardiac arrest of 10–15 minutes. In this latter case there was also unusual cell loss and gliosis in the inferior colliculi with focal softenings in the lateral pontine tegmentum, gracile and cuneate nuclei and in the spinal nucleus of the fifth nerve. Whether such differences in localisation were due to the early age of the patient, remains to be seen. Brierley compares his findings in the brain stem with the somewhat similar localisation in monkeys asphyxiated before birth, reported by Windle *et al.* (Ranck and Windle 1959, Windle 1961). The oxygen requirements of the brain are known to be higher in infancy, although some of the difference may be explained by the relatively large head of the infant (McIlwain 1955). On the other hand, tolerance to anoxia decreases with age (Kabat 1940, De Haan and Field 1959), and the infant animal may metabolise accumulating anaerobic products such as lactic and pyruvic acids, which the adult animal is unable to break down.

Although the physiological action of *barbiturates* has been found to be similar to that of anaesthetics (Quastel 1943, Lucas 1950), gross histological changes of the kind caused by anaesthetics seem to be rare. However, cases in which lesions in cerebral and cerebellar cortex, Ammon's horn, cerebral white matter and the basal ganglia had occurred have been reported by de Groat (1940), Alexander (1942), Jervis and Joyce (1948), Neumann (1951) and Courville (1955), and selective necrosis of the globus pallidus was present in de Groat's and Alexander's cases.

Clinically a wide range of neurological and psychiatric conditions, Parkinsonism, disseminated sclerosis-like pictures have been related to chronic barbiturate poisoning. In some, at least, of these cases the relationship may be coincidental. It is known that certain barbiturates, particularly phenobarbitone, may give rise to allergic reactions, occasionally ending fatally. In constitutionally predisposed persons acute attacks of porphyria may be precipitated by barbiturate medication (page 316).

Spinal anaesthesia and the toxic action of detergents

Sequelae following spinal anaesthesia with local anaesthetics deserve a special section since in most cases both the clinical and the pathological sequelae differ from those following general anaesthesia. Interest has recently been shown both in the United States and in this country as to the nature of these lesions. Several recent papers including one by Greenfield, Rickards and Manning (1955) have given reviews of the literature.

The clinical symptomatology consists mainly of paralyses which in most cases are flaccid, but rarely may be spastic. The commonest signs refer to the cauda equina and these usually occur shortly after the anaesthesia, are often mild and more or less confined to the disturbances of sphincter control. If more severe, they may extend to cranial nerves, especially the 6th, but sometimes also the 7th, 5th or 3rd nerves. In a number of cases paraplegia occurs as a delayed sequel.

Various pathological changes have been reported. One of the earlier observations was made by Spielmeyer (1909) who, both in a human case and after experimental intralumbar injection of novocaine, described degeneration of dorsal and ventral nerve roots, together with marginal degeneration of the spinal cord which was well demonstrated by Marchi's stain. Similar observations have been made by other workers in which other local spinal anaesthetics (pentocaine, percaine, etc.) were used. In addition to this local effect of the anaesthetic, cerebral lesions were occasionally observed which were indirectly due to the involvement of the medullary centres of respiration and circulation. Such clearly anoxic lesions in the brain were observed by Spielmeyer after stovaine anaesthesia and by Bodechtel (quoted from Peters 1951) in a case in which spinal anaesthesia by percaine was combined with rectally applied avertin.

In cases in which severe paraplegia develops as a delayed sequel, subacute or chronic thickening of the pia-arachnoid of varying degrees is often observed at operation or autopsy. Earlier pathological observations of this lesion were made by Weigelt and Michelsen (quoted from Peters); similar more recent observations have been made by workers in the United States (Kennedy *et al.* 1945, 1950). This thickening of the pia-arachnoid was seen also in the 3 cases published by Greenfield *et al.*

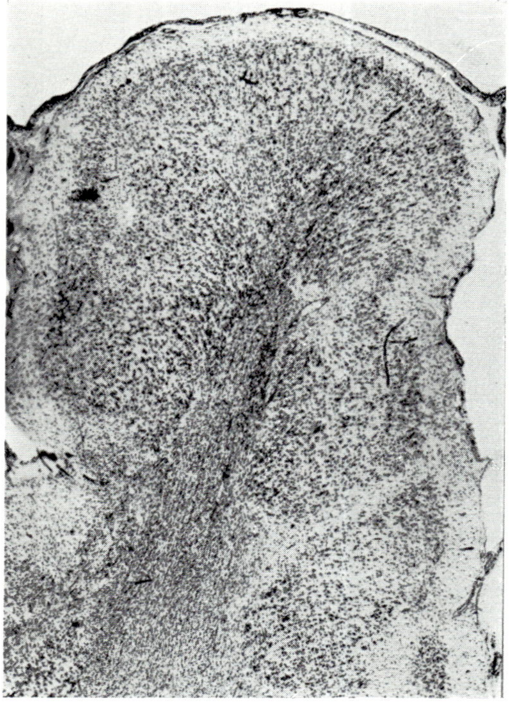

4·5

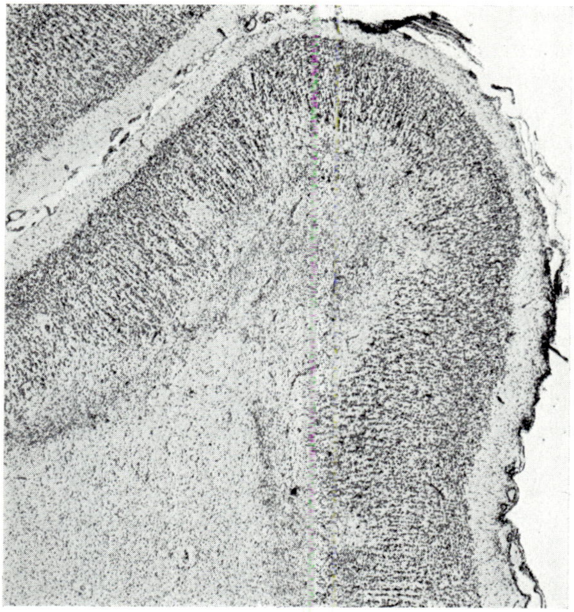

4.6

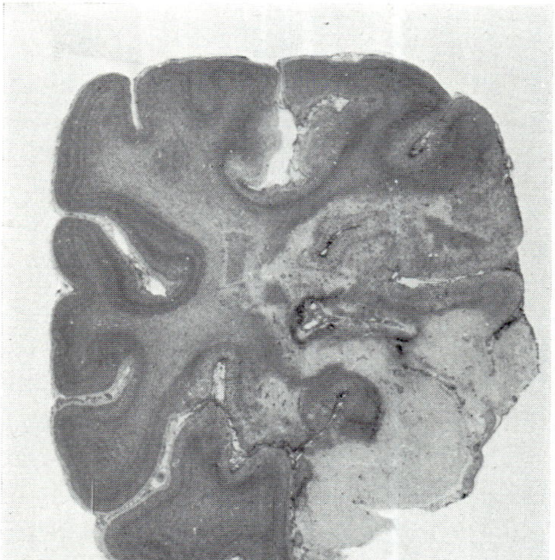

4·7

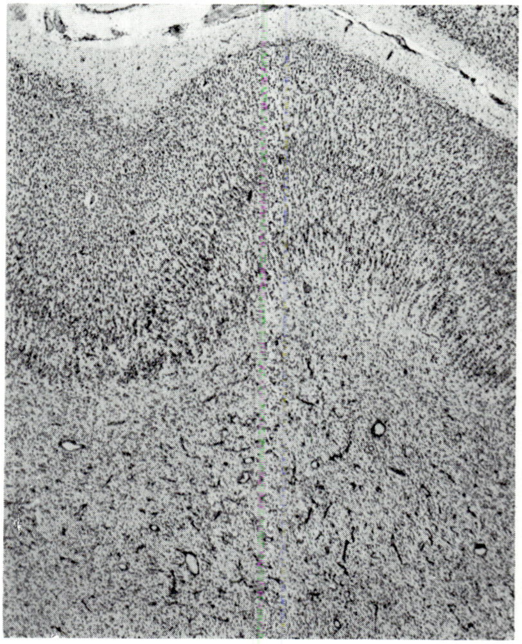

4.8

Fig. 4.5. CO poisoning, 16 years' survival: Focal loss of nerve cells with subsequent gliosis in cerebral cortex and white matter. (Nissl ×20.)

Fig. 4.6. Anaesthetic death, 6 months' survival: Focal loss of nerve cells in all layers of cerebral cortex; gliosis of white matter. (Nissl ×24.)

Fig. 4.7. Hypoglycaemic coma, occipital cortex. Widespread recent laminar necrosis with area of total infarction. (Nissl ×1·5.)

Fig. 4.8. CO poisoning, occipital lobe; recent necrosis of white matter with glial and capillary proliferation. (Nissl ×20.)

The last mentioned authors also describe lesions in the meningeal arteries, consisting of replacement of the degenerated muscular coat by collagen, of stretching, thickening or reduplication of the elastica and of thickening of the intima. They draw attention to more or less comparable findings by Zeckel and Behr (1933), Donat (1937–8), Russell (1937), Macken and Martin (1950), etc. In the case of Russell, in which paralysis developed 1 month after spinal anaesthesia and death occurred after 3½ months, the arterial lesion was a well-defined necrotising (fibrinoid) panarteritis of the perforating branches of the anterior spinal artery, which resulted in extensive softening of the grey matter in the lumbar enlargement.

Greenfield *et al.* considered the lesions to be due either to the spinal anaesthetic itself or, more probably, to some contaminant introduced with it into the spinal fluid. At the time of writing they were unable to decide whether the toxic action was direct or allergic; the latter was suggested by the resemblance of the arterial lesions to those produced in allergic conditions.

With regard to the possibility of contamination, Winkelman *et al.* (1952, 1953) had already suggested the causal importance of *detergents* used for cleaning the syringes with which the injection was made. However, they were not able to advance any positive evidence beyond the fact that a detergent was used in the theatre. This problem has been advanced by the work of Hurst (1955). This author injected various detergents and antiseptics into the cisterna magna of monkeys. Although these were substances of quite dissimilar chemical properties, they all damaged exposed nervous structures such as roots and caused cellular proliferation and fibrosis in the pia-arachnoid, thus obstructing the flow of cerebrospinal fluid; they also caused necrosis of the medial coat of meningeal arteries. The process begins immediately, but there may be no symptoms in the early stages. Arterial necrosis may be caused by one injection, which thus would appear to preclude the assumption of an allergic reaction. Although evidence is still inadequate that any of these or similar substances is implicated in the complications which arise from human spinal anaesthesia, these recent observations are of considerable practical and theoretical interest.

Peters quotes observations of paralysis and sphincter disturbances with degeneration of dorsal and ventral roots, posterior columns and of the marginal zone of the spinal cord following endolumbar injection of a *sulphanilamide preparation.* At the level of the cauda equina the thickened dura was adherent to the pia-arachnoid and the posterior roots were embedded in this fibrous tissue. No inflammation was noticed, but there was evidence of some previous haemorrhage. Sulphanilamide may itself have a toxic action or there may be, again, the concomitant effect of a detergent.

Delayed death from hanging

Delayed death after (usually suicidal) hanging has been of neuropathological interest since Deutsch's (1917) description of symmetrical softening in both lenticular and caudate nuclei with apparent preservation of the thalamus and cerebral cortex. Further cases have been reported by, among others, Bingel and Hampel (1934), Döring (1936), Gamper and Stiefler (1937) and Dublin and Brown (1942). Cerebral cortex and striatum were in all cases severely affected; the globus pallidus was involved in Döring's and Dublin and Brown's cases. In Gamper and Stiefler's case the motor cortex was severely affected. The authors thought that the return of motor function during the interval between hanging and death may have determined the localisation of the lesions in motor centres.

In a personal observation, in a case with death after 3 days in which the patient did not regain consciousness, continuous ischaemic necrosis in the 3rd layer was present in practically all areas of the cerebral cortex, except the visual area (Fig. 4.4). Ammon's horn also showed typical necrosis of the Sommer sector and end-plate. The striatum and globus pallidus

(Fig. 4.11) were intact except for a small area of necrosis in the dorsolateral corner of the putamen. Within the thalamus, the dorsomedial and lateral nuclei were almost totally necrotic, while the intralaminar and midline nuclei were preserved as were all the nuclei of the hypothalamus, and there was a large area of ischaemic necrosis in the ventrolateral part of the amygdaloid complex. The cerebellum showed a moderate degree of homogenising degeneration of the Purkinje cells; the lateral and medial geniculate bodies and the inferior olives were preserved. Ischaemic nerve cell change seems to be more frequent after strangulation than after cardiac arrest and hypoxia.

Hypoglycaemia

Hypoglycaemia may occur during treatment of diabetes, as a result of an islet tumour in the pancreas, in hepatic disease, or in lesions of the brain stem and hypothalamus, and can be artificially brought about as in the treatment of psychoses. An idiopathic variety, giving rise to severe hypoglycaemia in infants, has been added by McQuarrie *et al.* (1949). When sufficiently controlled, insulin coma does not usually result in structural lesions of the central nervous system, but on occasion the coma becomes irreversible and in such cases the brain is found to be severely damaged. A large number of pathological and experimental investigations have been published and these have been reviewed and amplified by Baker (1939), Ferraro and Jervis (1939), Lawrence, Meyer and Nevin (1942), Hoff, Grenell and Fulton (1945) and Courville (1954, 1957).

The findings in the literature show some variation, but there is no doubt that they closely resemble those which occur in other types of anoxia.

Usually the cerebral cortex is extensively involved and presents the picture of either focal or laminar necrosis of the upper layers, or necrosis of all layers. In Fig. 4.2 the normal white matter contrasts strikingly with the pallor of the totally necrotic cortex. Even when all other areas of the cortex are severely damaged the visual cortex is often preserved. The type of degeneration of nerve cells and proliferation of microglia and astrocytes is essentially the same as in other anoxic conditions, but Nissl's severe change and homogenising degeneration markedly predominate over the ischaemic nerve cell change.

Degeneration of the white matter may accompany the cortical lesion, as was reported in one of Richardson and Russell's cases (1952), or occasionally may predominate. A few cases have been reported in which fibroglial proliferation of the white matter was the most prominent lesion (Lawrence, Meyer and Nevin).

The cornu Ammonis is affected in almost every case, presenting the typical necrosis (Fig. 4.16) with variation in its histopathological detail related to the survival period. Grünthal (1947) has published a case, remarkable in that bilateral destruction of Ammon's horn was the only histological lesion, in a patient who was demented through the whole survival period of 6 months.

Of the subcortical centres the striatum bears the brunt of the lesions. This may be almost totally necrotic as it was in case 3 of Lawrence *et al.* (Fig. 4.13). The small nerve cells are more susceptible than the large and after a survival of 14 days most may have disappeared to be replaced by proliferative microglia and astrocytes. The lateral nucleus of the thalamus also displayed ischaemic necrosis. Usually the globus pallidus is found to be intact. Typical necrosis of Purkinje cells has been reported, but in the writer's material it was distinctly less frequent than after, for example, anaesthetic death. The present writer has never in his cases seen indisputable ischaemic necrosis of anterior horn cells, but Williams (1955) has recently reported amyotrophy due to hypoglycaemia.

While the lesions of the cerebral cortex, the striatum and, to a lesser degree, the Purkinje

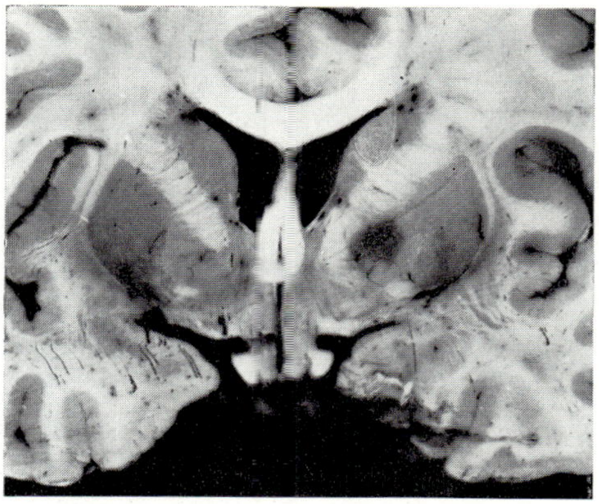

4.9

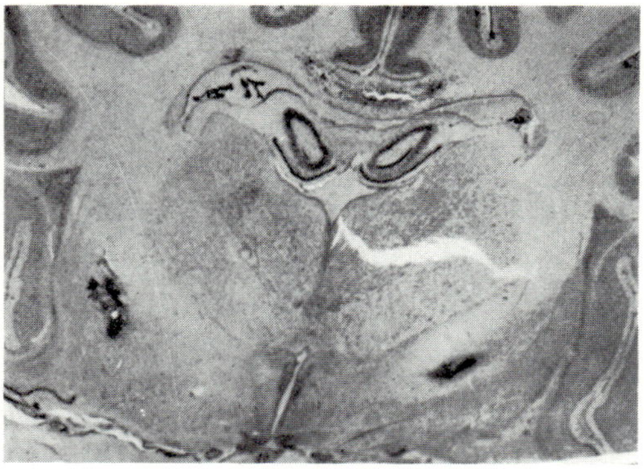

4.10

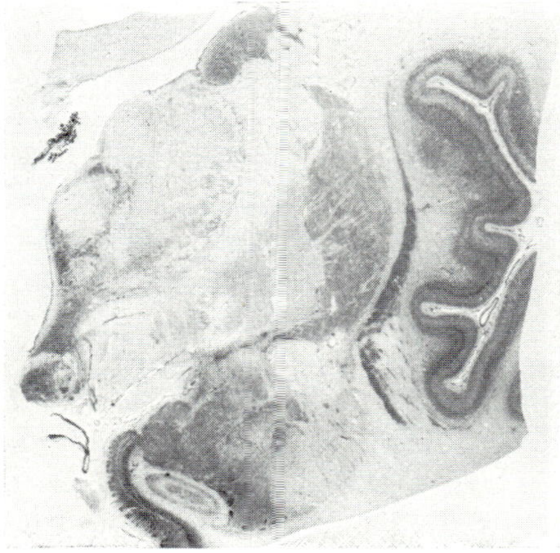

4.11

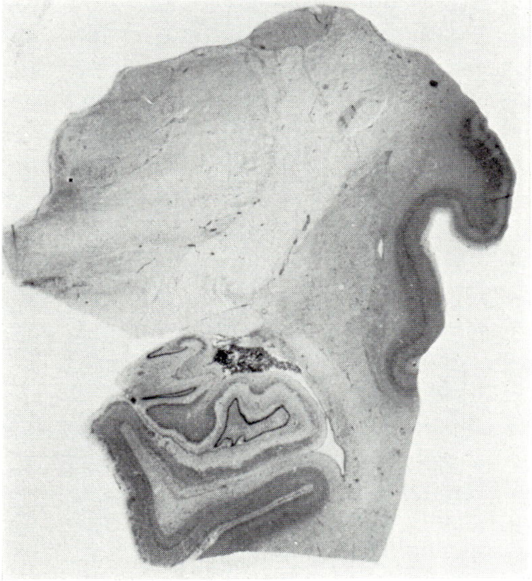

4.12

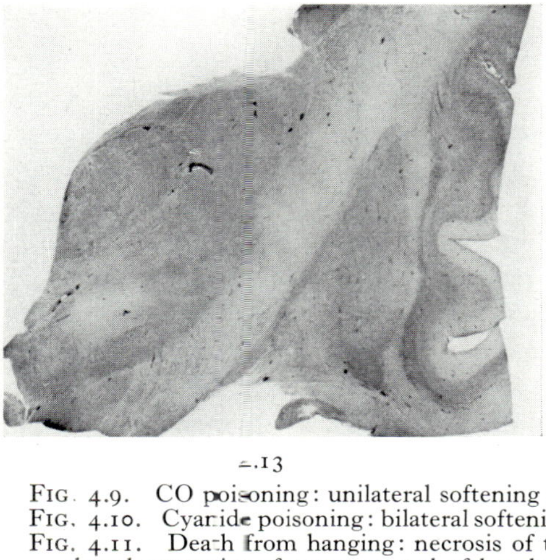

4.13

FIG. 4.9–4.13. Basal ganglia lesions.

FIG. 4.9. CO poisoning: unilateral softening of globus pallidus.
FIG. 4.10. Cyanide poisoning: bilateral softening of globus pallidus and corpus callosum. (Nissl × 2.)
FIG. 4.11. Death from hanging: necrosis of thalamus (except midline and intralaminar nuclei), of dorsal extremity of putamen and of basolateral amygdaloid nucleus; laminar necrosis of insula. (Nissl × 1·5.)
FIG. 4.12. Anaesthetic death: necrosis of corpus striatum, claustrum, thalamus (partial preservation of midline, intralaminar and reticular nuclei). In insula laminar necrosis of 3rd layer; partial necrosis of uncus. (Nissl × 2.)
FIG. 4.13. Hypoglycaemic coma: Necrosis of putamen and lateral nucleus of thalamus; laminar necrosis in insular cortex. (Nissl × 1·6.)

cells in the cerebellum are conspicuous as areas of ischaemic necrosis, it has been stressed by several authors (*vide* Lawrence *et al.*) that almost no nerve cell is entirely normal. From their controlled experiments Winkelman and Moore (1940) concluded that every nerve cell in the central nervous system might be affected. Richardson and Russell reported involvement of some of the hypothalamic nuclei. Large infarctions and haemorrhages have been described, but their incidence in the literature is rare (Lawrence *et al.*). In a personal case a typical laminar necrosis in many parts of the cerebral cortex was associated with extensive infarctions in one hemisphere (Fig. 4.7). The head of the caudate nucleus, the putamen and adjacent areas were also in a state of necrosis, but even in this case, with its unusually severe affection of the striatum, the globus pallidus was better preserved. The appearance of multiple gross infarction in this case renders the possibility of thrombosis (of which there was no macroscopic or histological evidence) unlikely. The case was, however, one of an elderly diabetic with definite atheroma of the basilar arteries, which is likely to have been a contributory factor.

Hypoglycaemia is not an anoxia in the strict sense. Oxygen is available as is indicated by analysis of the arterial and venous oxygen tension, but the arteriovenous gradient is reduced, i.e. oxygen is not used up by the nervous parenchyma because of the absence or considerable reduction of the substrate glucose. For this reason, Lawrence *et al.* have introduced the term of *oxyachrestia* (non-utilisation of oxygen). The similarity between the later stage of hypoglycaemia and anoxia has been emphasised by Gellhorn, Ingraham and Moldavsky (1936), and Himwich. There are also similarities from the biochemical point of view. During hypoglycaemic coma labile cerebral phosphates tend to fall and inorganic phosphate increases, as is the case in hypoxia. Glucose and, to a lesser degree, glycogen are, however, severely reduced, while in hypoxia they show no appreciable change. Lactic acid is unchanged or even decreased in hypoglycaemia while it is increased in anoxic conditions (McIlwain). The compensatory increase of blood flow and vasodilatation is, according to McIlwain, less marked in hypoglycaemia than in anoxia, but this may not apply to the later stages of irreversible coma since, in our experience, post-mortem vasodilation is marked in most cases. In the brains of cats made severely hypoglycaemic, Samson *et al.* (1959) found no appreciable change in the total deoxyribonucleic or pentonucleic acids, whereas glutamic acid, γ-amino-butyric acid and alanine were all reduced.

At present it is not known at what stage and for what reasons a hypoglycaemic coma becomes irreversible. Experience suggested to Lawrence *et al.* that coma of 1–3 hours is usually associated with complete recovery but probably there are, as in other types of anoxia, appreciable individual differences of tolerance. This is also in fair agreement with experimental experience (Schmid 1936, Neumann, Cohn and Katzenelbogen 1942, and Tyler and Ziskind 1940), all of whom found that histological changes were reversible after what was comparable to hypoglycaemic coma induced for therapeutic purposes in man.

Whether irreversibility of coma coincides with the appearance of irreversible histological damage to the nerve cells is not known; it is possible that some biochemical irreversibility precedes the histological degeneration by some time. This would account for a certain incongruity between the clinical signs of deep coma and the severity of the histological changes.

Miscellaneous

Heart disease. Bodechtel (1932) found in 38 cases only 7 without secondary cerebral anomalies. In 13 of his cases the lesions were caused by anoxaemia and presented as areas of pallor and softenings in cerebral cortex, cerebral white matter, Ammon's horn and cerebellum. Lesions of the globus pallidus were not reported by this author, who has amplified his investigations more recently (1953), particularly in a physiological direction. In cases of chronic congenital or acquired heart disease, the emphasis is frequently in the cerebral white matter; increased venous and cerebrospinal pressure is followed by oedema and subsequent gliosis. Scholz (1941, 1953 a and b) has described a combination of degeneration of the globus pallidus, corpus Luysii, reticular zone of the substantia nigra and dentate nucleus as the characteristic syndrome of *pure* oxygen deficiency: it is found in cases of congenital heart disease, asphyxia at birth and in Rhesus factor incompatibility; it has not yet been established, however, whether in all these conditions, hypoxia is the sole or even the most important factor (Haymaker *et al.* 1957–59).

Anaemia caused by severe haemorrhage may be the cause of selective neuronal degeneration in varying regions of the brain, and often includes necrosis of the globus pallidus (Overhof 1933; Scherer 1934; Ulbricht 1948, among others). Baló (1941) found, as a sequel of bleeding peptic ulcers, symmetrical pallidal softening in 5 cases.

Disorders of respiration. Lesions of the globus pallidus have been described by Rotter (1929), following respiratory failure after *head injury.* The importance of anoxia supervening in head injury has also been emphasised by Neubürger (1930), Rand and Courville (1936), Malamud and Haymaker (1946) and Biemond (1958).

With the increase of *poliomyelitis,* attention has focused on the additional part that impairment of respiration may play in the histological picture. Extensive selective neuronal degeneration in the brains of such cases has been described by Steegman and Davis (1950), Alajouanine *et al.* (1952) and Courville and Blossom (1954). It is possible that the ischaemic-like degeneration which Greenfield (1958) occasionally saw in the anterior horns has the same origin.

Status asthmaticus has been known to give rise to severe neurological symptoms: Foley and Paterson (1954), for example, observed cortical blindness and spastic quadriparesis with athetosis as sequelae of an asthmatic attack. Haemorrhagic necrosis of the corpus striatum and of the cerebral cortex was present in a case described by Courville (1956), but the diagnosis was complicated by uraemia and congestive heart failure. In a more convincing case in which symptoms of organic dementia supervened upon a severe attack of asthma, Mattyus (1959) found almost complete destruction of the cerebral cortex, extensive softening of the white matter and bilateral softening of the striatum and globus pallidus. The present writer has seen a typical sclerosis of Ammon's horn in a case (unpublished) which was clinically under the charge of Dr. A. D. Leigh. The patient never had epileptic convulsions.

A superposition of anoxic changes was observed by the present writer in a case (unpublished) of otherwise typical severe post-encephalitic Parkinsonism who suffered from repeated attacks of *laryngeal spasm.* These attacks were described as so severe that there was always danger to life; the patient died suddenly in such an attack while eating an orange. Apart from the typical old post-encephalitic lesions, more recent softening and glio-mesodermal scarring was found in the head of the caudate nucleus, the putamen and the globus pallidus, which had lost its nerve cells and myelin and presented dense gliosis. Ammon's horn and the cerebellum also showed sequelae typical of anoxia.

The problem of selective vulnerability

Although phenomena of regional vulnerability are met in many conditions, those that present themselves in anoxic and vascular disease are particularly striking.

The regions especially affected in human anoxic conditions are the cerebral cortex, striatum, the globus pallidus, thalamus, Ammon's horn and the Purkinje cells of the cerebellum. Particularly vulnerable are the cerebral and cerebellar cortex in the depths of sulci. The 3rd layer of the cerebral cortex is more vulnerable than other layers; necrosis may be confined to this

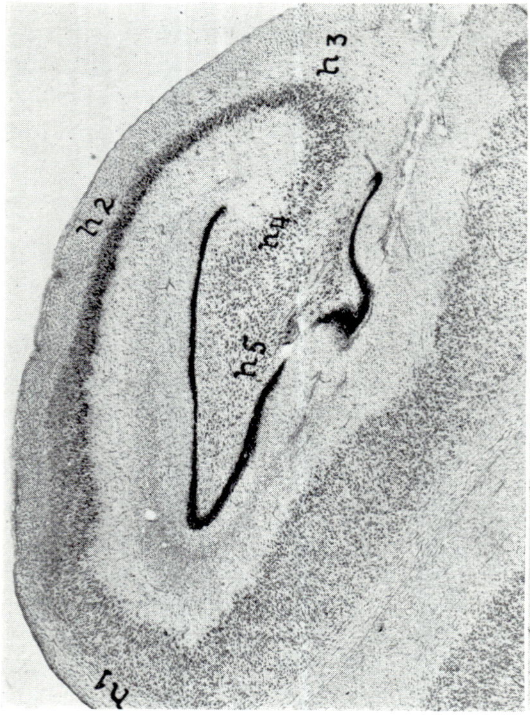

4.14

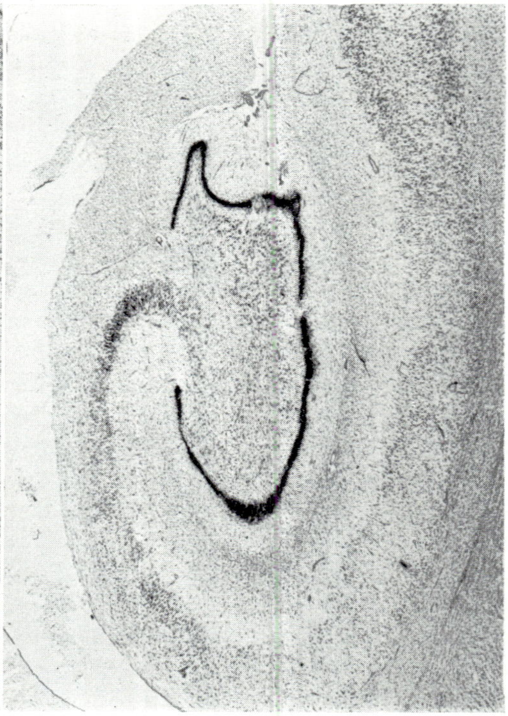

4.15

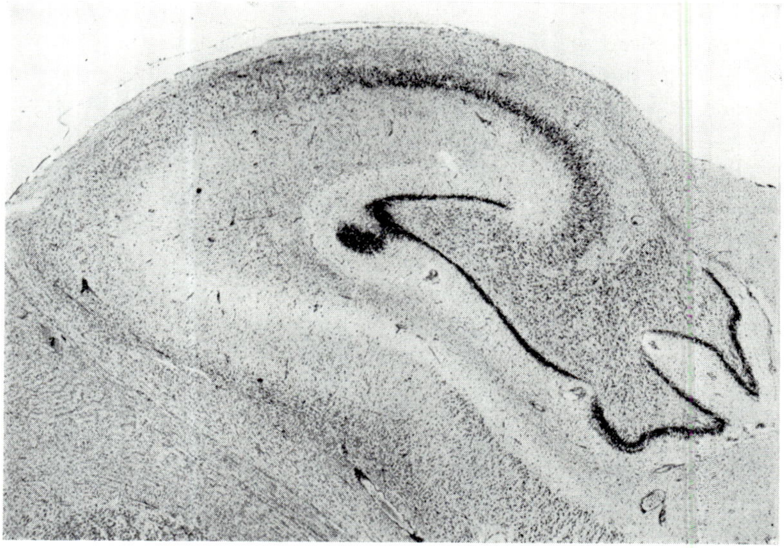

4.16

FIG. 4.14. Normal Ammon's horn, with Rose's fields h_1–h_5 inserted. (Nissl × 10.)
FIG. 4.15. Ammon's horn, anaesthetic death; recent necrosis in Sommer sector (h_1) and partial endplate (h_3–h_5). (Nissl × 12.)
FIG. 4.16. Ammon's horn, hypoglycaemic coma; recent necrosis in h_1 and, less complete, in h_3–h_5 (Nissl × 12.)

layer in a laminar fashion. The occipital area adjacent to the visual cortex is vulnerable while the latter is resistant. Within the cornu Ammonis the Sommer sector (Rose's area h_1) and the end-plate (h_3-h_5) are more susceptible to damage than the rest. In some instances, the cerebral cortex may be intact, the lesion being situated selectively within the white matter. The reticular zone of the substantia nigra, the dentate nucleus, the inferior olives, the corpus Luysii and the amygdaloid nucleus also figure, though less prominently, in the list of selectively vulnerable regions. The hypothalamus, the grey centres of the midbrain, pons, medulla and spinal cord, except for those mentioned above, are as a rule not damaged. The vulnerability of the regions enumerated above should, however, be regarded as *relative*. In many cases of anoxia, for reasons not fully explained, a quite different distribution of lesions may be encountered. When anoxia is very severe, damage may tend to become universal.

In experimental animals, selective findings similar to those encountered in the human brain have been reported after CO poisoning, hypoglycaemia and anaesthetic death. The similarity depends somewhat on the choice of animals; selective necrosis of the globus pallidus, for example, is rare in rodents while it is easily produced in carnivora (Meyer 1936). After sudden arrest of the circulation of the brain Weinberger *et al.* (1940) found that, in order of susceptibility, visual and motor cortex ranked first, followed by Purkinje cells, lateral geniculate body, hypothalamic nuclei, thalamus, globus pallidus and caudate nucleus. Spinal cord and medulla showed great resistance. Grenell (1946) observed a similar gradient, although there were differences in detail. In monkeys asphyxiated shortly before birth, Windle and his associates, as mentioned earlier, described lesions predominantly situated in the brain stem. Some of the discrepancies in these and other experimental investigations are due partly to differences in species and age, and partly to differences in diagnostic criteria. In most human cases, diagnosis of the lesions is based on evidence of *necrosis*, while in the controlled animal experiments, reversible cell degenerations are often taken as evidence of the effect of anoxia.

When the problem of selective vulnerability first arose, two apparently mutually exclusive approaches were given much publicity. The one, promulgated by Spielmeyer (1925) and his school, has become known as the vascular theory of selective vulnerability, while the other, C. and O. Vogt's (1922) concept of pathoclisis, was based on the assumption of general physico-chemical properties of centres or parts of centres. Although such physico-chemical properties were in most instances not known, they were presumed to exist from the characteristics of neuronal architecture.

That the lesions are undoubtedly due to interference with oxygenation must be cited in favour of the vascular theory. Vascular factors seemed therefore likely to explain regional differences of vulnerability. Kolisko (1893), for example, explained necrosis of the lenticular nucleus by the recurrent course of the central branches of the anterior cerebral arteries, consequent on the shift of their origin anteriorwards with the greater development of the frontal region. Alexander (1942) regarded the anterior choroidal artery, which he renamed 'pallido-hippocampo-capsular artery, as particularly vulnerable during disturbances of the circulation of the brain, because it has the longest subarachnoid course and the greatest 'individual length' of any cerebral vessel of similar calibre. But since both in man and in other mammals the greater part of the cornu Ammonis is supplied by the posterior cerebral artery, the anterior choroidal feeding only its anterior part and the amygdaloid complex, Alexander's hypothesis is open to criticism. The lateral geniculate bodies likewise receive a double blood supply, the anterior choroidal being supplemented by the posterior cerebral arteries.

As regards Ammon's horn, Uchimura (1928) believed that the terminal branch which supplies the vulnerable Sommer sector has both a particularly sinuous course and a very fine calibre. Scharrer (1940) stressed the rake-like pattern of the origin of the terminal branches

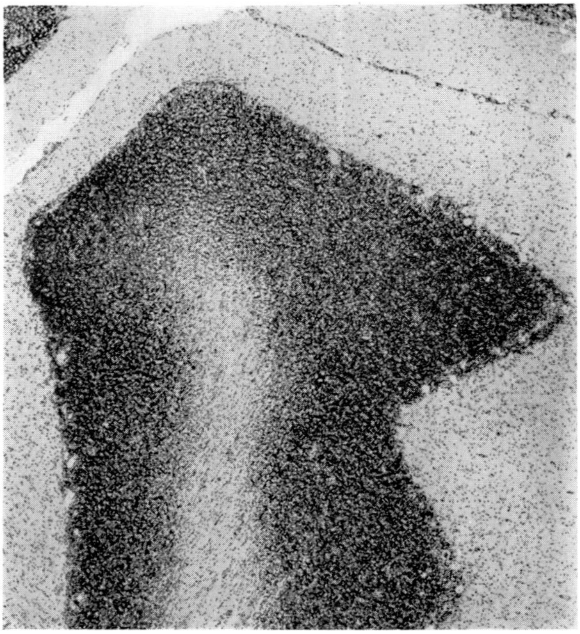

4.17

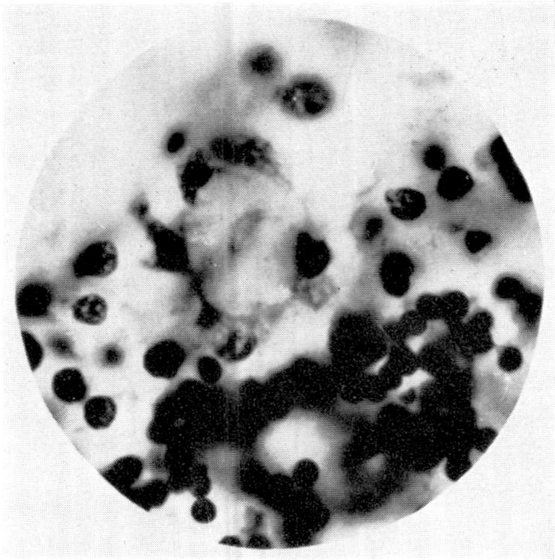

4.18

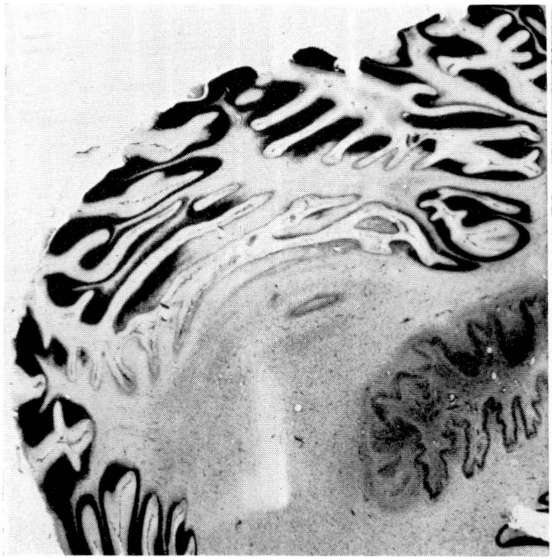

4.19

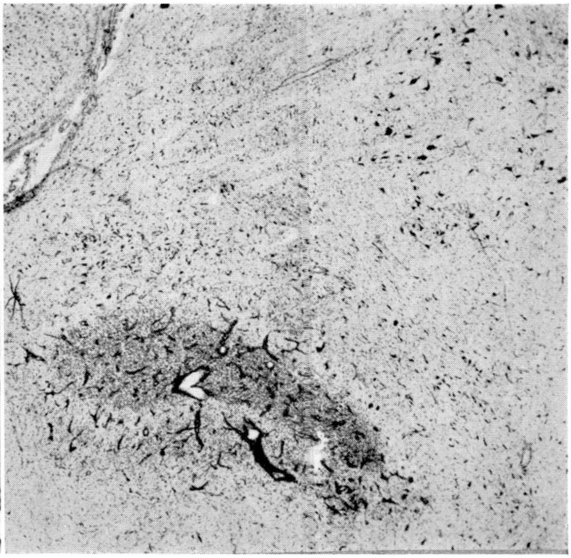

4.20

FIG. 4.17. Anaesthetic death: ischaemic necrosis of most Purkinje cells, microglial 'shrubbery' in molecular layer. (Nissl ×25.)

FIG. 4.18. Anaesthetic death: homogenising degeneration of a Purkinje cell, with neuronophagia. (Nissl ×800.)

FIG. 4.19. Anaesthetic death: survival of 6 months: atrophy of lobules mainly near white matter; gliosis of dentate nucleus. (Nissl ×3.)

FIG. 4.20. Experimental cyanide poisoning: softening of reticular zone of substantia nigra. (Nissl ×20.)

in the opossum and lower mammals. The vertical origin from the main branches of the anterior cerebral, anterior choroidal and posterior cerebral arteries, which in these animals supply the cornu Ammonis, does in conditions of general hypotension expose the area to greater danger.

These explanations on a vascular basis did not, however, satisfy Scholz (1953 a and b) who considers that in no instance of selective vulnerability has an entirely satisfactory explanation so far been forthcoming. Nor, according to him, has the pathoclisis theory on its own been more satisfactory. He has, however, suggested a combination of the vascular and pathoclitic factors which he regards as being not mutually exclusive, but supplementary. Vascular disturbances are usually ubiquitous in the brain, but lead to structural damage only in regions which exhibit an inherent (pathoclitic) susceptibility. However, at present little is known about the metabolic basis of these pathoclitic factors, and it is possible that some may ultimately be related to idiosyncrasies of blood supply and of the probably interrelated O_2 utilisation on the cellular level. This, for example, may apply to the increase of tissue iron and/or to capillary siderosis (pseudocalcium) of many of the vulnerable subcortical centres and of the Sommer sector of Ammon's horn, although the significance of these 'normal' variations is as yet far from clear (Meyer and Blume 1934, Meyer 1936). Reports of increased amounts of ascorbic acid in Ammon's horn and Purkinje cell layer (*vide* Meyer 1936), of zinc (possibly as a component of the enzyme carbonic anhydrase) in areas h_1, h_2 and especially h_3 of Ammon's horn (Maske 1955, Timm 1958) and of 5-hydroxytryptamine in several rhinencephalic centres (Paasonen *et al.* 1957) also require clarification before their significance for selective vulnerability can be ascertained.

Apart from this main development of the problem, there are *additional aspects* which require brief discussion. One concerns the question whether the site of lesions differs after pure anoxia from that following vascular disturbances (ischaemia). The question is of some importance because in ischaemia, in contrast to hypoxia, substances in addition to oxygen are withheld from the nervous tissue. Scholz and his collaborators (Scholz and Schmidt 1952, Orthmayr 1952, Meyer 1953a) have investigated this problem experimentally in cats. Anoxia was produced by temporarily clamping the trachea and, *post mortem*, red blood corpuscles were demonstrated by employing the benzidine stain. The general result of these studies was that in pure anoxias uncomplicated by cardiac arrest, the signs of disturbed circulation in cerebral and cerebellar cortex and in Ammon's horn were not greater than in the subcortical ganglia, while when anoxia was complicated by cardiac arrest, the emphasis of disturbed circulation was on the cerebral and cerebellar cortices. The conclusion drawn by Scholz from these results is that the less the hypoxia is complicated by other factors the greater is the emphasis on those centres such as globus pallidus, corpus Luysii and dentate nucleus whose susceptibility to want of oxygen is, in his view, greatest.

It should be remembered, however, that such differences are only of relative degree. Capillary dilatation is an immediate response to increase of CO_2 tension in the blood. This reaction may vary in degree in different individuals, but stasis is bound to develop when deficient oxygenation of the tissue persists.

The relation between the predominance of *cortical* lesions versus lesions of the *white matter* and the *basal ganglia* has also been the subject of investigations by Hurst (1941, 1942) and his collaborators and by Morrison (1946). Both groups of workers agree that a massive single induction of hypoxia leads to predominantly cortical lesions, while after (single or repeated) mild hypoxia the lesions are confined to white matter and basal ganglia. Although from different premises, this is the same conclusion as that reached by Scholz. The two hypotheses are not irreconcilable because, as mentioned above in the discussion of Scholz' views, the severer the lack of oxygen the more violent will be the vascular reaction, due to the physiological response of capillary dilatation.

It has been known for some time that *boundary* or *watershed zones* between two large arterial systems are more vulnerable than others, because branches supplying these are the most distal. The phenomenon was first demonstrated by Lindenberg and Spatz (1939) in a case of Buerger's disease, but subsequently has been described in a variety of other conditions (Meyer 1953b, Norman *et al.* 1957, and Zülch and Behrend 1961).

Anomalies of the *circle of Willis*, known to be present in 50 per cent of normal brains (Alpers *et al.* 1959; Berry and Alpers 1959), may, during an episode of generalised anoxia or circulatory disturbance, facilitate local infarction, because of pre-existing atresia or absence of some constituent arteries of the circle. The importance of this point has been well illustrated by Meyer and Portnoy (1958), who observed that, after occlusion of the right middle cerebral artery, exposure to hypoglycaemia caused transient additional impairment of function only in the limbs of the opposite side; and by Levine (1960) who, after a similar procedure in rats, found severe hypoxic lesions in grey and white matter almost exclusive to the side of the ligated common carotid artery.

Lindenberg (1955) has accumulated evidence to explain the selectivity of vascular lesions as the sequel to the local pressure which some arterial systems undergo during sudden and considerable *increase* of *intracranial pressure*. Arteries running close to the tentorial edge (such as for example, certain branches of the anterior choroidal, posterior cerebral and superior cerebellar), or arteries which may be pressed against the falx (branches of anterior cerebral) or bone (the stem of the middle cerebral, inferior cerebellar arteries, etc.) are particularly vulnerable. All terminal branches which supply the cerebral or cerebellar cortex in the depths of sulci are similarly at risk. The special vulnerability of Sommer's sector is explained by its proneness to pressure against the tentorium of the long, but not the short branches supplying Ammon's horn.

Lindenberg's important hypothesis falls into line with the herniation theory of Earle, Baldwin and Penfield (1953) in temporal lobe epilepsy (page 558). It has long been recognised that during prolonged hypoxia the volume of the brain increases. Recent observations include those made in man by Richardson *et al.* (1959) and in experimental animals by Denny-Brown *et al.*, Edstrom and Essex (1956) and Spector (1961). It is not known, however, how much of this increase of volume is due to capillary and venous congestion, and how much to fluid escaping from the capillaries into intercellular spaces or into the glial cytoplasm. The term oedema has been somewhat loosely applied to either. However, significant increase of oedematous fluid was observed and measured by Spector.

It is arguable whether compression of arteries is the sole or even the most likely source of tissue necrosis during sudden rise of intracranial pressure. Long before arteries—even those labouring under hypotension—are compressed, one would expect impediment of venous drainage to occur, reinforcing the stasis caused directly by anoxia and hypotension. This point has been effectively demonstrated by Pia (1957), who was concerned, however, with cisternal herniation and its repercussion upon basal veins and the Galenic system rather than with tentorial herniation. One could imagine that raised intracranial pressure and oedema may act as a mechanical irritant on arteries and cause them to constrict temporarily, or that they might produce (mainly in arterioles) just that instability between intraluminal and vessel wall tension which is the condition for Burton's (1954) 'critical closing pressure', resulting in collapse of the vessels (Cavanagh 1962).

It is still an open question whether in most of the hypoxic conditions with which we are dealing here, the increase of pressure is of a degree to result in herniation. Small and Woolf (1957), in a case of severe hypoxic neuronal necrosis, found at operation that the dura was not tense, and the ventricular C.S.F. not under increased pressure. Dissection of the brain, fixed *in situ*, showed no herniation of the hippocampal gyrus at the level of the Ammon's horn. These authors, from experiments of injecting arteries in a number of brains, considered it unlikely that the long branches supplying the vulnerable sector should be regularly occluded by tentorial pressure in contrast to the short branches. It may prove of interest that there seems to be considerable variability in the size of the tentorial opening from brain to brain (Corsellis 1958).

Function of the brain during the interval between the hypoxic episode and death has been thought to influence the distribution of the lesions (Gamper and Stiefler). In a case of delayed death after hanging (page 244) these authors found, among other typical lesions, a striking prominence of necrosis of the motor cortex, which they interpreted as having been caused by violent movements in the interval between hanging and death. Scholz (1953b), in order to give a name to this pathogenic factor, has coined the term *consumptive anoxia*. This factor is obviously of great importance in the anoxia following convulsive activity. At the beginning of certain experimental epilepsies, Jung (1949) found that electrical discharges are particularly high in thalamus, Ammon's horn and the reticular formation of the brain stem. According to this author (Jung 1953) total anoxia results in cessation of electrical activity: in the cerebral cortex within 20 seconds, in medulla and cerebellum only after 30–90 seconds. This longer survival of cerebellar electrical activity is difficult to understand in view of the well-established neuropathological experience of the high vulnerability of Purkinje cells.

Although these variables go far to explain differences in the distribution of lesions in individual cases, many obscurities remain, and the multiplicity of factors involved renders sweeping and dogmatic generalisations difficult (Meyer 1956, Norman 1958). Advance in our knowledge of the anatomy and, in particular, of the physiology of the cerebral circulation and of the chemistry of the centres concerned will eventually contribute to greater understanding of these phenomena.

DRUGS OF ADDICTION

Ethyl alcohol

Acute alcoholic intoxication seldom leads to death, and post-mortem observation is therefore rare. In those cases which have been investigated congestion, oedema and diffuse petechial haemorrhages have been described (Courville and Myers 1954), but with pre-existing cardiovascular degeneration, in particular cerebral arteriosclerosis, renal or hypertensive disease, a toxic dose of alcohol may result in massive haemorrhages or softenings.

According to McIlwain (1955) severe intoxication is accompanied by decreased cerebral blood flow and decreased respiration. The oxidation of ethanol proceeds through acetaldehyde which, normally low, accumulates in the blood following ingestion of alcohol; if acetaldehyde is infused and maintained at a certain level, a nausea akin to alcoholic hangover is experienced, which goes when acetaldehyde is further oxidised. The depressant action of alcohol is, however, due not to these metabolic changes but, as with the other depressant drugs such as anaesthetics and hypnotics, to its physical presence in nervous tissues. Acetaldehyde, like other toxic substances such as the heavy metals (*vide* page 266), combines with lipoic acid which is then no longer available for the oxidation of pyruvates, and this, according to Sinclair (1956), may constitute a possible pathogenic mechanism in some cases of alcoholic polyneuritis.

Chronic alcoholic intoxication

It is possible that continuous repetition of acute intoxication may, over many years, lead to irreversible changes manifest in thickening of the meninges and in a moderate degree of atrophy, which may be general or most marked in the frontal, central and parietal cortex and white matter, and which is accompanied by moderate enlargement of the ventricular system. In such cases the cerebral cortex shows a variety of nerve cell changes (in particular, pigmentary degeneration), and diffuse loss of the supraradiary and tangential myelinated fibres, with or without increase of fibrous glia. These findings, described by earlier workers (Mott 1910 and others), have been largely confirmed and critically discussed by Courville (1955) and his associates, and by Lynch (1960). Astrocytic proliferation with some neuronal degeneration, most marked in the third layer of the frontal cortex, has been described by Morel (1939) in patients who had suffered repeated attacks of delirium tremens followed by memory disturbances, tremor and impairment of speech. A mental syndrome reminiscent of general paresis (alcoholic pseudoparesis) is frequently encountered; delusions, particularly of the auditory type, may accompany the general alcoholic deterioration.

Degeneration may occasionally be more marked in the cerebellar than in the cerebral cortex, as Jakob (1912) first noted. Stender and Lüthy (1931) have described a late form of atrophy of the cerebellar cortex in chronic alcoholics. Lhermitte (1934–35) also emphasised the aetiological importance of chronic alcoholism for cortical cerebellar degeneration; he, with de Ajuriaguerra and Garnier (1938) carried out experiments in rabbits given continuous toxic doses of absinthe; they succeeded, however, in causing chromatolysis of dorsal root nerve cells, Purkinje cells and cortical nerve cells only in such animals in which an additional nutritional deficiency could be implicated. Neubürger (1957) found degeneration of the granular layer as a relatively common lesion in his material of 42 cases of alcoholics.

In all such cases it is often difficult to exclude the effects of indirect or complicating pathogenic factors; cerebral arteriosclerosis or senile involution may play a part in some, whilst in others a concomitant cirrhosis of the liver must be considered as a possible factor. Of the greatest importance is the effect of nutritional deficiencies, whether it results from inadequate or unbalanced food intake or from chronic gastritis or other gastro-intestinal upset; much of the pathology of chronic alcoholism thus becomes a problem of vitamin deficiencies (*vide* chapter 5). The histological changes of pellagra may predominate, particularly the central chromatolysis of nerve cells and, more rarely, the degeneration of dorsal and lateral columns of the spinal cord. In other cases the Wernicke syndrome may be more in evidence, clinically presenting with opthalmoplegia, nystagmus, ataxia and Korsakoff's psychosis. Peripheral neuropathies may accompany either of these syndromes or may occur alone; degeneration of the optic nerves has been reported and in those chronic alcoholics in whom neglect and malnutrition had resulted in deficiency of vitamin B12, subacute combined degeneration of the cord has been described.

Considerable interest was aroused by the description of *degeneration of the corpus callosum* by Marchiafava and Bignami (1903) who included in their paper a case previously published by Carducci (1898). Since then 88 cases have been reported according to the detailed review by Ironside *et al.* (1961). The earlier cases were almost all Italian by birth; more recently cases have been reported from the Americas, France, Switzerland, Spain, Central Europe, etc. The racial and national distribution as well as the main publications have been instructively outlined by Ironside *et al.* Although there is no racial exclusiveness, the high incidence of Latins, and especially Italians, is striking, in contrast to the rarity, for example, among native North Americans and in Great Britain, where—so far—only two cases have been described: the first by McLardy (1951) and the second by Ironside *et al.* Both were Englishmen without traceable Latin or other foreign ancestry. There has been no report of cases from Sweden and Japan.

Almost all reported cases were chronic alcoholics; many were addicted to crude Italian wine and suffered from under-nutrition. There are, however, notable exceptions: McLardy's patient, for example, had neither taste for Italian wine nor, apparently, had he suffered from nutritional deficiency. Ironside's patient, though showing signs of malnutrition, was a heavy drinker of beer and stout At one time the disease seemed to be confined to male persons, but more recently female cases have been discovered.

The main pathology of the condition is a degeneration of the central fibres of the corpus callosum. In the cases of King and Meehan (1936) and Ironside *et al.*, the punched-out lesion had a greater resemblance to ischaemic softening than to any other pathological condition. This lesion in many, though not all, cases is accompanied by degeneration of other symmetrical

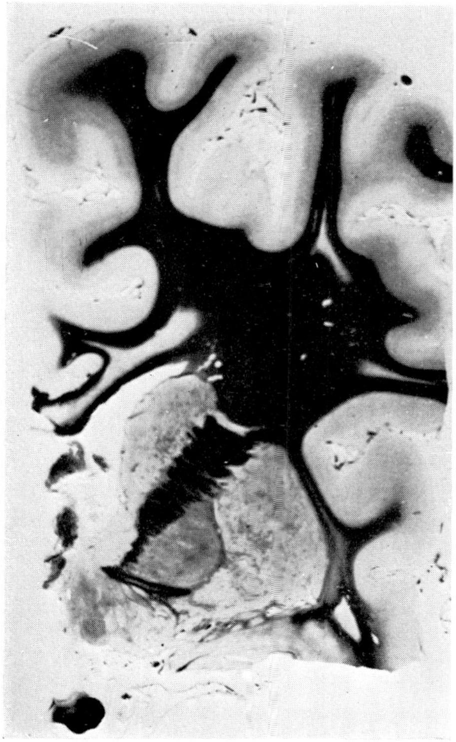

4.21

FIG. 4.21. Marchiafava-Bignami disease (McLardy's case): degeneration of the central fibres in corpus callosum and anterior commissure, and digital white matter. (Heidenhain × 1·5.)

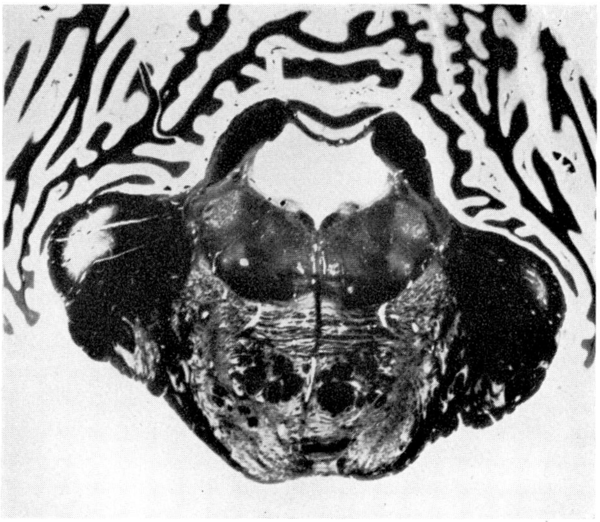

4.22

FIG. 4.22. (McLardy's case): degeneration of middle cerebellar peduncle. (Heidenhain × 2·5.)

pathways such as the anterior commissure and the middle cerebellar peduncles (Figs. 4.21 and 4.22); the centrum ovale and, in particular, the white matter between the centrum ovale and the frontal and parietal gyri may also be involved. Within the lesions demyelination is a consistent feature; the axis cylinders may be affected in some cases, but have been found to be preserved in others. Glial proliferation is not usually marked and myelin breakdown products are often inconspicuous. A striking microscopic feature is the proliferation and fibrosis of blood-vessels within the lesions.

In 2 cases Jéquier and Wildi (1955) observed a combination of the Marchiafava-Bignami findings with the cortical laminar astrocytosis of Morel; among less consistent findings they recorded glial proliferation in the corpus mamillare of one of their cases and slight degeneration of the optic tracts. In the case of Ironside *et al.*, cortical loss of nerve cells with glial reaction was also recorded. McLardy observed demyelination in the most dorsal portion of the optic chiasma. Cirrhosis of the liver is not a constant feature.

The pathogenesis of the condition is at present obscure. The history in many cases of addiction to crude Italian red wine and of malnutrition suggests a nutritional deficiency in the first place, but, as has been indicated, this history does not apply in all cases. Nor is there evidence for the vitamin B_1 deficiency suggested by Lolli (1941) and Bohrod (1942). Intoxication by an ingredient at present unidentified, which may be present specifically in Italian red wine, has been suggested as an alternative; with regard to this hypothesis it may be relevant that lesions of the white matter including the corpus callosum and anterior commissure have been repeatedly described following cyanide, and less often CO poisoning (pages 240–245), particularly in lower mammals. Jéquier and Wildi have considered the possibility that the pathogenesis of the condition may be related to oedema, of which they found histological signs in one of their cases.

This may be the place to mention the *central pontine myelinolysis* described by Adams *et al.* (1959) in 4 patients, 3 of whom had a history of severe chronic alcoholism, and all one of serious malnutrition. The lesion was situated in the centre of the base of the pons and was characterised by demyelination with relative preservation of axis cylinders. Oligodendroglial cells were practically absent. A combination of this lesion with Wernicke's syndrome was present in only one case. The authors, while maintaining reserve about the aetiology of the syndrome, point out the histological resemblance to Marchiafava-Bignami disease. There was no evidence of disseminated sclerosis. Two more cases have been reported by J. H. Adams (1962), who has also amplified previous references.

Methyl alcohol

Methyl alcohol is the most important of the remaining alcohols; its ingestion has given rise to widespread intoxication in periods of prohibition or of war and among poorer populations. One of the earlier clinical reports was given by Wood and Buller (1904), who were able to add almost 200 personal observations in the U.S.A. to the 54 lethal or amaurotic cases which had already been described in the literature. Similar descriptions, although based upon smaller numbers, also appeared at about the beginning of this century, in Russia, Hungary and Germany.

The clinical picture of acute methyl alcohol poisoning has been exhaustively described by Bennett, Cary, Mitchell and Cooper (1953), who observed a mass intoxication in 323 patients at the Graly Memorial Hospital, Atalanta. After a latent period, lasting on an average 24 hours, patients complained of headache, dizziness, anorexia, nausea, weakness and amblyopia progressing to total blindness. The pupils were dilated and reacted sluggishly; sometimes there was hyperaemia of the optic disc with retinal oedema. In all severe cases the outstanding sign was acidosis. The wide individual variability in the length of the latent period is according to Røe (1946) due to the usual, simultaneous or subsequent, ingestion of ethyl alcohol; this prevents or delays the oxidation of the methyl alcohol to formaldehyde and formic acid which is the cause of both the acidosis and of the toxic effect of the alcohol. It is these acids which inhibit oxidative processes in the cells, allegedly by combining with iron in the cytochrome oxydases. Death usually occurs in coma with respiratory paralysis.

In most acute cases autopsy reveals severe congestion and oedema of all organs, including the brain (Pick and Bielschowsky 1912, Jansen 1936, Fink 1943, Orthner 1949). In the brain petechial haemorrhages are widespread, but are most frequent in the neighbourhood of the

3rd ventricle, the aqueduct and beneath the floor of the 4th ventricle. Ischaemic necrosis of all 3 layers of the cerebellar cortex has been reported by Jansen.

Recently Orthner described bilateral necrosis of the putamen which he regards as a selective effect of methyl alcohol poisoning. On naked-eye inspection the centre presents a distinct pallor. Histologically both nerve cells and glia appear to undergo degeneration with little mesodermal reaction, and there may be haemorrhages within the necrotic area.

Degeneration of the ganglion cells in the retina and of the fibres of the optic nerve is a common and characteristic finding. Pick and Bielschowsky have fully described this in human cases and Birch-Hirschfeld (1902) in experimental animals. The choroid vessels were found to be congested and the retina and the optic nerves showed severe oedema. Histologically the ganglion cells in the retina presented a picture of central chromatolysis; the degeneration extended slightly into the inner and outer granular layers. The axis cylinders in the papilla and in the optic nerve were separated by exudate and showed irregular swellings. The changes in the retinal cells and in the optic nerve fibres were regarded as related.

Pick's and Bielschowsky's findings have been confirmed by the majority of subsequent investigators, including Fink, who, on the strength of personal human and experimental observations, concluded that congestion and oedema are the main pathogenetic factors. More detailed histological investigations with modern methods will be required, however, before a final statement on the pathogenesis of the lesions can be made.

Morphine

In large doses, morphine has a depressant action upon respiratory centres in the medulla; acute intoxication may thus lead to respiratory failure with all its attendant anoxic and vascular effects upon the nervous system. In one such case Weimann and von Marenholtz (1928) observed, among other lesions, symmetrical necrosis of the globus pallidus. In other examples of acute poisoning, petechial haemorrhages were the main finding.

In chronic poisoning the lesions in the central nervous system are more difficult to interpret. At concentrations comparable to those causing analgesia, McIlwain considers morphine to have little effect on the metabolism of cerebral tissue; in such doses it is, however, a powerful inhibitor of cholinesterase and this may explain at least part of its side effects. There is no doubt that morphine addiction involves complex mechanisms and these are still being elucidated both from the pharmacological and the endocrinological point of view.

Histological findings in human cases of addiction are few. Penfield and Cone (1926) noted acute swelling of the oligodendroglia. Creutzfeld (1926) and Weimann (1926) saw diffuse fatty degeneration of nerve cells, which, according to the last mentioned author, was most severe in cerebral cortex and Ammon's horn. In other cases of Weimann changes related to disturbance of the circulation predominated, but such disturbances may have been due to complicating factors such as epileptic convulsions or exhausting attacks of excitement. Older observers have described subacute combined degeneration but nutritional deficiency and cachexia may in such cases be an intermediary pathogenic factor.

Experimental histological investigations are few; Weimann (1930), who carried out intoxication in rabbits, guinea-pigs and cats with survival up to 20 days, observed cell changes which were acute in early stages, severe after 8 days and chronic with fatty degeneration after 20 days. Cerebral cortex, corpus striatum and Ammon's horn were especially affected.

Even less is known about the histological effects of *cocaine* intoxication. Like morphine, cocaine also depresses the regulating centres of respiration and circulation in the medulla. In acute poisoning congestion and oedema have been described. After chronic intoxication, fatty degeneration with vacuolar shrinkage of nerve cells have been found both in human and in animal brains.

The changes after chronic *barbiturate* addiction have been described on pages 248 and 316.

INTOXICATION BY HEAVY METALS AND RELATED SUBSTANCES

Metals as a class have, according to Jetter (1953), a diffuse systemic toxicity and are referred to as protoplasmic poisons. The injury caused by them is, however, often most severe at sites of entry and elimination, i.e. to lung and gastrointestinal tract on the one hand and to kidney on the other. The central and peripheral nervous systems also belong to the vulnerable sites of their action. The action of many metals may be as enzyme inhibitors, the primary biochemical lesion being a blocking of metabolic processes by their combination with sulphydril groups of enzyme proteins. This is suggested by the apparent therapeutic effect of 2,3-dimercapto-propanol (BAL, British Antilewisite). Peters (1948) and Thompson (1948) have suggested that their main effect is to inhibit the pyruvate-oxydase system, and is not unlike that which occurs in vitamin B_1 deficiency, although the co-enzyme cocarboxylase does not seem to be directly involved. These complex biochemical relations will be discussed in greater detail in chapter 5.

From the neuropathological point of view, lead, mercury, arsenic, manganese and phosphorus are the most important metallic and related substances which give rise to poisoning.

Arsenic

Arsenic is widely used in industry. Many weed and vermin killers contain it and it was formerly used in paints and also, as liquor arsenicalis, in the treatment of many diseases. Organic arsenicals used against syphilis (arsphenamine) occasionally lead to intoxications and most of the more recent publications dealing with toxic manifestations in the central nervous system come from this source which, with the introduction of penicillin, is now receding in importance.

During the late war arsenical compounds were prepared as war gases. Chlorophenyl-dichlorarsine is the so-called lewisite.

There seem to be no qualitative differences between poisoning by inorganic and organic arsenical preparations. In *acute* intoxications, intense abdominal discomfort, vomiting and diarrhoea and ultimately circulatory collapse dominate the picture. The involvement of the brain manifests itself by headaches, confusion or coma, epileptic convulsions and signs of raised intracranial pressure. Special features of chronic poisoning are cutaneous pigmentation (caused by derivatives of melanin), hyperkeratosis, gastric and other intestinal ulceration and peripheral neuropathies affecting sensory and mixed nerves. Chronic gastrointestinal lesions may give rise to signs of nutritional deficiency and this may well be another source of symptoms resembling vitamin B deficiency (Sexton and Gowdey 1947). Necrosis and eventually a portal type of cirrhosis have been reported in the liver.

The lesions in the central and peripheral nervous systems, which follow arsphenamine intoxication in particular, have been described in a large number of publications, which include those by Globus and Ginsburg (1933), Russell (1937), Scheinker (1944), Krainer *et al.* (1947), Call and Gunn (1949), Peters (1949) and Grzycki and Kobusowna (1951). Diapedetic haemorrhages situated within the corpus callosum, in the deep cerebral white matter near the inferior and posterior horns of the lateral ventricle, in the internal capsule, in the peduncles, and in the peripheral parts of pons and medulla are the main feature in the central nervous system. Foci of perivascular demyelination and necrosis in cerebral cortex and white matter have been described by Russell who suggested they may be due to sensitisation; she emphasised their resemblance to the lesions in post-vaccinial encephalomyelitis and following antirabic treatment. Call and Gunn, Peters, and de Morsier and Feldmann (1951) also consider an allergic pathogenesis for the cerebral lesions.

The amount of arsenic in the brain has been found to be unusually high by Krainer *et al.*, and Call and Gunn. According to Grzycki and Kobusowna, arsenic and its compounds are stored in mesenchymal cells, in the Kupfer cells of the liver, in endothelial cells of the sinuses of the spleen and in the capillary endothelium and microglial cells of the central nervous system.

Arsenical polyneuritis has now become very rare. Clinically it manifests itself in pain, paraesthesias followed by extensor palsy and wasting in forearms or legs, the small muscles of hand and foot being involved first. Histologically myelin and axis cylinders are involved; the distal ends of the fibres degenerate first. Sensory fibres seem to be more affected than those carrying motor impulses. Both in its clinical and histological characters, it resembles alcoholic peripheral neuropathy (Greenfield 1958).

Lead

Inhalation of inorganic lead was, in the past, the cause of many cases of industrial poisoning, for example of tin plumbers during refining and smelting processes, in the manufacture of many lead-containing articles, and very commonly in painters in the process of stripping old paint. This industrial poisoning has now been effectively checked by preventive legislation, so that lead poisoning at present is mainly confined to its domestic occurrence with entrance through the gastro-intestinal tract. Interesting clinical examples of such domestic incidents have recently been published by Gordon and Whitehead (1949), Burrows *et al.* (1951), Millichap *et al.* (1952), Gibb and MacMahon (1955), Marsden and Wilson (1955) and Turner (1955). Millichap *et al.* listed the sources of plumbism in childhood in order of frequency as painted woodwork, nipple shields, toy soldiers, fumes from burning battery casings, drinking water, toilet powder. The earlier Japanese literature (reviewed by Kato 1932) contains numerous reports of lead poisoning present in breast-fed infants, due apparently to the use by the nursing mothers of lead-containing toilet powder.

In *acute* lead poisoning there is a symptomatology of convulsions, delirium and coma, often accompanied by papilloedema and signs of irritation of the meninges; there are also abnormalities in the cerebrospinal fluid manifesting as increase of globulin, cells and sugar.

The well-documented signs of *chronic* lead poisoning consist of epileptiform convulsions associated with varying degrees of dementia, peripheral neuropathy, particularly in motor nerves and muscles, colics, a 'lead line' of the gums and basophilic stippling of the red blood corpuscles. To these may be added signs of impaired cardiovascular and renal function.

Pathology. Chronic intoxication with lead may lead to extensive lesions of the liver and kidney which may give rise to cirrhosis and to chronic interstitial nephropathy. In the liver nuclear acid-fast inclusions, which fill the greater part of the nuclei and stain orange with Masson's trichrome stain, have been found by Wachstein (1949). Similar changes are seen in the convoluted and looped tubules of the kidney. X-ray evidence of skeletal deposits is manifest 3–6 months after the onset of daily absorption of lead. The gastro-intestinal tract shows no gross change; the 'lead line' of the gums is caused by a perivascular deposit of lead sulphide in the submucosal papillae, while basophilic stippling of circulating red blood corpuscles follows the formation of lead phosphate on the surfaces of the red cells.

In the *central nervous system*, oedema seems to be a prominent feature of acute fulminating cases of lead intoxication, particularly severe in the infantile form (Blackman 1937, Alkelaitis 1941, Marsden and Wilson 1955). The cerebral and cerebellar white matter may become necrotic, and the histological picture may simulate that of Schilder's disease (Verhaart 1933, 1934, 1941). Severe oedema in the deep white matter has been experimentally produced and illustrated by Weller and Christensen (1925) in guinea pigs.

The mechanism which leads to subacute and chronic human and experimental lead poisoning has been much under discussion. Direct action on the nerve cell, producing a picture resembling severe cell change has been assumed by Nissl (1892), Lehmann *et al.* (1926), von Meduna (1929) and Ferraro and Hernandez (1932). Spielmeyer (1922) also demonstrated Nissl's severe cell change in a cat poisoned by lead, but, on a different page of his book, he produced a picture of a focus of severe capillary and endothelial proliferation in the deeper layers of the cerebral cortex which Bonfiglio (1910) had observed in dogs. Following Bonfiglio, many authors (Petri 1930; Alkelaitis, Peters 1951, and others) have diverted emphasis to endothelial proliferation and hyalinosis of blood vessels of small calibre in the brain and in most other organs. It is doubtful, however, whether this vascular change can be separated from that caused by renal disease and by hypertension from which many chronic patients suffer. Henderson (1954), in a follow-up study of lead-intoxicated children, found that among 165 who had died, renal or vascular disease was recorded as the cause of death in 108. More recently (van Bogaert 1956, Pentschew 1958), attention has been focused on proliferation of the glia. It is interesting that Mott, as early as 1909, had found a diffuse astrocytic proliferation (investigated with Cajal's method) as the most striking feature throughout grey and white matter in a case of lead poisoning in a coach-painter. It was most marked in the upper layers of the cortex, and out of all proportion to the wasting of neurones. Unfortunately, as Mott himself was aware, the case was complicated by chronic alcoholism, and perhaps by alcoholic pellagra to which the central chromatolysis of anterior horn cells, Betz cells and nerve cells in the motor nuclei of the brain stem should probably be attributed. In the case of van Bogaert, nodular and diffuse proliferation of the glia (mainly astrocytes) was combined with focal or laminar necroses in pons and cerebral cortex respectively. The clinical picture of Parkinsonism was caused by marked gliosis in the substantia nigra, which was not accompanied by loss of nerve cells.

In two cases published by Környey (1931), massive lymphocytic infiltration and microglial proliferation were found to be widespread in the cerebral and cerebellar cortex. The histological picture strikingly resembled dementia paralytica, but the iron reaction in the brain and the Wassermann reaction in blood and cerebro-spinal fluid were negative. The author may have been dealing with one of the now recognised subacute encephalitides occurring in patients who had been exposed to lead intoxication.

De Villaverde (1927) had already noted a certain prevalence of cerebellar lesions following lead intoxication. In several of his infants suspected of lead poisoning, Verhaart (1934) found the cerebellar white matter necrotic, while that of the cerebrum was unaffected. Pentschew (1958) gave a brief description of an acute case with severe oedema of the cerebral cortex and with necrosis of the cerebellar granular layer A case of Biemond and van Crefeld (1939), investigated, however, only clinically, exhibited a distinct cerebellar syndrome.

The *peripheral* neuropathy caused by lead poisoning has been reviewed by Greenfield (1958) whose account will be closely followed here. Although wrist drop, which used to be commonly seen in painters and other workers with lead or lead salts, is probably chiefly due to the direct action of lead on muscle fibres (Reznikoff and Aub 1927), lead may also cause a peripheral neuropathy in which motor nerve fibres are specially affected. The work of Gombault (1880–81) is of special importance as it was the first description of the lesion of the nerve fibre which he called periaxial segmental neuritis (segmental demyelinative neuropathy of Fisher and Adams 1956). He poisoned guinea-pigs with small doses of lead carbonate over a period of several months. Although the animals were not paralysed, their peripheral nerves, when fixed in osmium tetroxide and stained with picrocarmine, showed myelin degeneration in a larger or

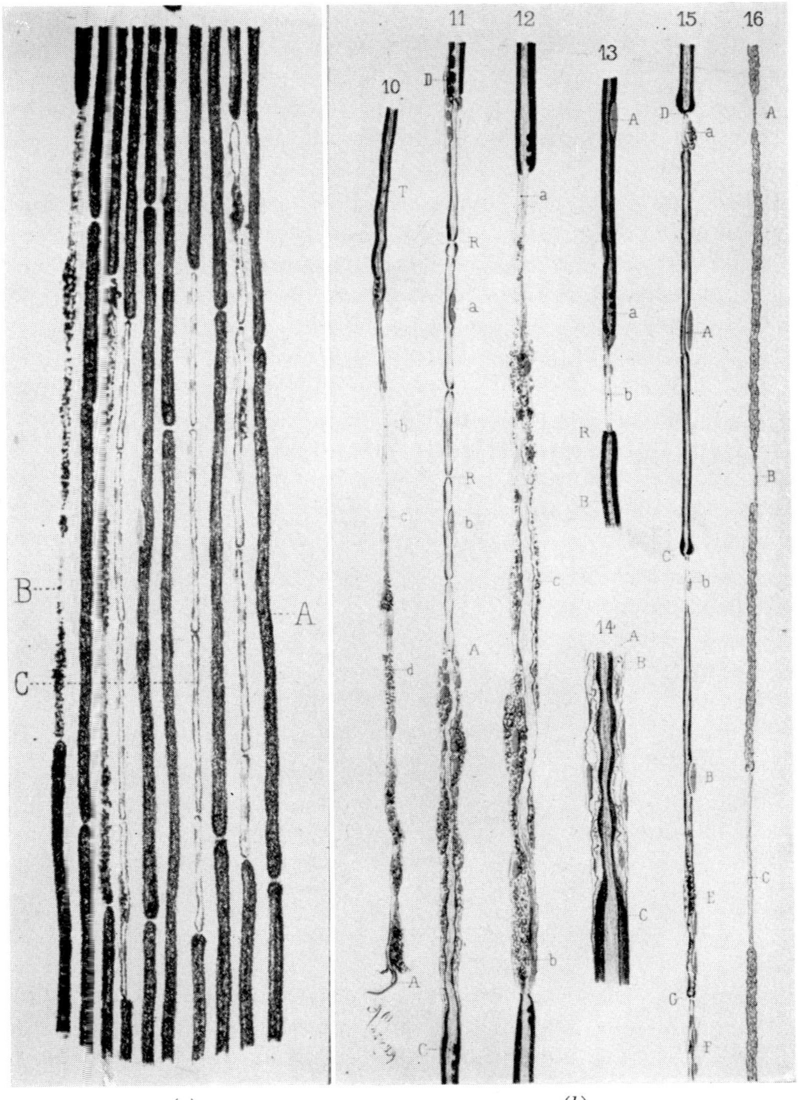

(*a*) (*b*)

FIG. 4.23. Lead neuropathy. Segmental demyelination.

Illustrations from Gombault's article on experimental lead neuropathy. (Osmic acid and picrocarmine.)

smaller proportion of fibres. This was usually limited to a single internodal segment, with normal myelin above and below it (Fig. 4.23). Gombault did not study the axons but concluded, from the absence of Wallerian degeneration, that they were not seriously damaged. Axonal changes were studied by de Villaverde (1926) in guinea-pigs after subcutaneous injections of lead acetate. He found that the distal parts of the nerves showed the most severe lesions, but minor degrees of damage were seen at all levels. In the most affected fibres the axons had disappeared or only oval or irregular argentophilic remains of them were seen. In less affected fibres the axons showed irregular swellings on their course or their neurofibrils were separated by apparently empty spaces. These changes were more common in the larger than in the smaller nerve fibres and could be traced to the motor end-plates many of which showed complete destruction. The reaction of the sheath of Schwann was greater than that seen in Wallerian degeneration.

Organic lead compounds. The most important of these is tetra-ethyl lead or lead benzine. Inhalation of its vapours has been reported to bring about fatal poisoning. Tetra-ethyl lead has its main effect upon the central nervous system and causes delirious states, convulsive seizures and coma. Bini and Bollea (1947), who investigated 2 cases dying after exposure to lead benzine, found severe nerve cell changes particularly in the cerebral and cerebellar cortex. The glia (macroglia and oligodendroglia) showed regressive and progressive change and the endothelial cells contained excess of fat. Focal lesions were found mainly in their first case in the mamillary body and in the grey matter beneath the floor of the 4th ventricle; they were reminiscent of the glio-mesodermal proliferation seen in the Wernicke syndrome. Since the presence of lead in the nervous tissue was not proved histochemically, these authors concluded that the changes were due to the tetra-ethyl radicle whose toxic action appeared to resemble that of acute alcohol and acute ethyl bromide intoxication.

Copper, manganese and mercury

The metal which has recently provoked the greatest interest among clinical neurologists is **copper**, which in hepatolenticular degeneration is deposited in excessive quantities in the liver and basal ganglia (Cumings 1948) and is excreted in the urine. Since occupational poisoning with copper seems to be uncommon, it is likely that these pathological deposits, which accompany lenticular degeneration, are due to faulty metabolism rather than to an intake of toxic amounts of the metal.

The resemblance of the clinical picture of hepatolenticular degeneration to that of **manganese** poisoning has been noted by many observers. Manganese poisoning occurs almost exclusively in workers employed in mining and separating manganese ore. Couper gave the first account of its occurrence in 1837, but it aroused little notice until the beginning of this century, when clinical and clinico-pathological observations began to be published by Embden (1901), von Jaksch (1901), Seelert (1913), Casamajor (1913), Edsall *et. al.* (1919), Charles (1922), Ashizawa (1927), Canavan *et al.* (1934), Jiminez *et al.* (1946), Parnitzke and Peiffer (1954) and others.

The neurological picture has been described as one of a progressive Parkinsonian syndrome with a coarse tremor, often of the intention type, and with attacks of uncontrollable laughter (Edsall *et al.*). Turner reviewing the literature considers that clinically it is more closely related to Wilson's disease than to paralysis agitans. In a case described by the present writer (1930) an extrapyramidal syndrome of rigidity and coarse tremor, which appeared in a man of 46, was accompanied by severe memory and intellectual defect.

Pathological reports of the changes in man have been few. Casamajor found advanced cirrhosis of the liver and chronic interstitial nephritis. In the central nervous system, degeneration of some tracts in the brain stem was noted; changes in the basal ganglia or cerebellum were not recorded.

Ashizawa, in a man aged 33, noticed marked loss of nerve cells in the inner segment of the globus pallidus; the external segment was less affected. Canavan *et al.* found diffuse degeneration of nerve cells in the cerebral cortex, basal ganglia and cerebellum; the changes were most marked in the basal ganglia which were shrunken and showed circumscribed glial scars. Their patient died from cardio-renal disease at the age of 69, 14 years after the onset of the occupational disease; it is not possible, therefore, to exclude lesions arising from the complicating disease. In Stadler's (1936) case, focal softenings and scars were found in the frontal and parietal cortex and disseminated loss of nerve cells in the corpus striatum, particularly in the globus pallidus; lobular sclerosis was present in the cerebellum. Although the cranial blood vessels were normal, Stadler postulated a vascular pathogenesis associated possibly with a functional disturbance of the liver and kidneys. Stadler's case, however, was 56 years old and van Bogaert *et al.* (1945–6), therefore, rightly question the association of the histological changes, of which most were of a vascular nature, with the manganese poisoning.

Experimental investigations into the toxic effect of manganese have been numerous; among these the most important are by Lewy and Tiefenbach (1921), Findlay (1924), Mella (1924), Hurst and Hurst (1928) and van Bogaert *et al.* (1943, 1945–6). Findlay found that a massive dose of manganese chloride is extremely toxic to rabbits, and proved fatal after 22–48 hours. At *post mortem*, the liver showed widespread necrosis. When after smaller doses, the animals survived longer, cirrhosis of the liver developed. Mella caused cirrhosis of the liver in monkeys by intraperitoneal injection of manganese chloride; he found in addition widespread neuronal degeneration and neuroglial proliferation. Clinically the monkeys had displayed rigidity and athetoid movements. Lewy and Tiefenbach found widespread nerve cell degeneration especially marked in the basal ganglia. Hurst and Hurst, while easily producing necrosis of the liver in rabbits and guinea-pigs, failed to observe pathological changes in the central nervous system.

The experimental work of van Bogaert *et al.* has done much to clarify these contradictory experimental results. According to these authors the toxic action of manganese varies with its route of entry. In human intoxication the pathway is invariably by inhalation. Oral, parenteral and intraperitoneal induction require large doses which lead to damage of liver and kidney. The changes in the brain would be secondary and the neurological disturbances, in particular the striatal syndrome, may occur as a functional disturbance which is not necessarily due to an irreversible anatomical lesion. This would explain the transitory nature of some of the clinical neurological and mental signs as well as the inconsistent histological findings in the brains of both humans and animals. Van Bogaert *et al.* succeeded in producing manganese poisoning in a monkey by inhalation of finely sprayed metallic manganese. Since only a small amount of the metal was used in this procedure, no histological changes of the liver, kidney or other viscera, were noted *post mortem* and the main change in the brain was a degeneration of Purkinje cells and a partial disintegration of the granules over a wide area of the cerebellum. The changes were not vascular in origin but resembled the appearance of a system degeneration of the cerebellum and were associated with degenerative changes in the anterior horn cells and the dentate nucleus. The cerebellar changes were absent in a monkey poisoned by parenteral application of a manganese salt. Van Bogaert *et al.* conclude that the central nervous system may be affected without intermediary damage to the liver or kidney.

To Neal (1938) and Brown (1954) we owe a detailed account of the history and the sources of **mercurial** poisoning. Mercurialism, according to Brown, was one of the first recognised industrial diseases. It was known in India in 500 B.C. and was common among gilders of gold, silver and copper in the sixteenth and seventeenth centuries. Prior to this, most cases occurred in those mining mercury. With the introduction of mercury nitrate in the manufacture of fur felt in France in the seventeenth century, most mercurialism occurred in the hatting industry; hence, probably, the expression 'mad as a hatter'. Mercury to-day has many uses in the electrical and chemical industries, in dentistry, in laboratories, in photography, in the production of thermometers and barometers and in the criminal investigations of finger-prints.

Mercuric salts, especially the bichloride, are corrosive poisons which exert a local effect upon the gastro-intestinal tract and a specific toxic action, during excretion, on the epithelium of the proximal convoluted tubules. Although they are of little neurological interest, it should be noted that Noetzel (1955) succeeded in demonstrating in 9 of 14 rats submitted to chronic H_2SO_4 poisoning, degeneration and calcification of the granular layer of the cerebellum which was similar to that produced by Hunter, Bomford and Russell (1940) with organic mercury compounds. In Noetzel's experiments, there was a latent period of 3 months during which the general nutrition of the animals was much reduced. Calcification occurred also in other organs, especially in heart and skeletal muscle.

It has long been known that exposure to metallic mercury or to organic mercury compounds causes a syndrome consisting predominantly of erethysm and tremor. Erethysm is the name given to an obviously organic personality change characterised by fatigue, irritability, emotional instability with varying depressive features, i.e. a change which to some extent resembles the frontal lobe syndrome. It is associated with a tremor, considerably coarser than that occurring in thyrotoxicosis, which affects hands, tongue and legs; the tremor may have an intention quality. The other usual signs of mercurialism such as gingivitis (dark blue line along the gum margins), stomatitis, phthyalism, may combine with the signs described above. The combination of tremor and mental symptoms may give rise to diagnostic difficulties as in a case of Turner, later confirmed as one of chronic mercurialism, in which the initial diagnosis was dementia paralytica. Brown has described a clinical syndrome of amyotrophic lateral sclerosis in a case with a history of chronic mercurialism.

Pathology. Until recently our knowledge of the pathology of mercurial poisoning in the central nervous system was incomplete. Peters (1951) mentions unspecific nerve cell degeneration, softenings, small haemorrhages and perivascular gliosis after chronic intoxication, and in experimental animals degeneration of anterior horn cells. According to this author both direct toxic effect on the neurones and indirect vascular damage have to be considered pathogenically.

Recent clinico-pathological and experimental investigations with organic mercury compounds, particularly with methyl mercury phosphates and nitrates, have thrown more light on the pathology of mercurial poisoning (Hunter, Bomford and Russell 1940, Hunter and Russell 1954). Exposure to methyl mercury salts by inhalation affects the central nervous system predominantly and gives rise to symptoms which include ataxia, dysarthria and visual disturbances. Rats submitted to methyl mercury compounds showed widespread degeneration of the peripheral nerves, posterior columns and the granular layer of the cerebellar cortex, which in one animal contained calcospherites (Hunter, Bomford and Russell). A monkey studied by the same workers showed a diffuse cerebral cortical change with sparing of the cerebellar cortex, but this animal's survival was perhaps too short for the cerebellar change to develop. Hunter, Bomford and Russell also reported on 4 patients suffering from neurological disturbances as a result of industrial exposure to methyl mercury. The predominant clinical features were gross ataxia combined with severe concentric constriction of the visual fields. In 1 case (Hunter and Russell), post-mortem revealed the cortex and subcortical white matter of the area striata in the occipital lobe to be grossly atrophic. Foci of similar but more limited cortical atrophy were found in the left precentral gyrus, the right post-central and the left superior temporal gyrus. These foci affected the depths of the sulci rather than the summits. The cerebellar atrophy in this case is shown in Fig. 4.24. The atrophy is most advanced in the depths of the sulci, the cortex at the surface of the cerebellum being normal apart from a slight loss of granule cells. With higher magnification the main change, both in the human case and in experimental animals, was a selective atrophy of the granular layer with, as a whole, preservation of the Purkinje cells. The dendrites of the latter often display, after silver impregnation, stellate bodies as illustrated in Fig. 4.25. The authors regard this selective lesion of the granular layer as the first example of such a degeneration in man which can be attributed to an exogenous toxin.

Selective lesions of the granular layer have been demonstrated by Upners (1939) after thiophen poisoning in experimental animals. Stellate bodies on the dendrites of the Purkinje cells had previously been seen in amaurotic family idiocy, and in uraemia which developed in a patient suffering from dementia praecox. Hunter and Russell consider that they represent a probably regenerative response of the Purkinje cells to the loss of stimuli normally provided by climbing and basket fibres. Basal ganglia, hypothalamus, brain stem, spinal cord, nerve roots, two posterior spinal ganglia and the portions of sciatic and ulnar nerve available for histological

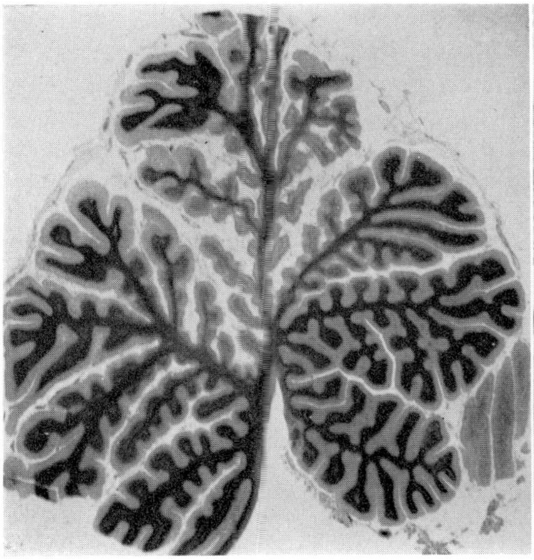

4.24

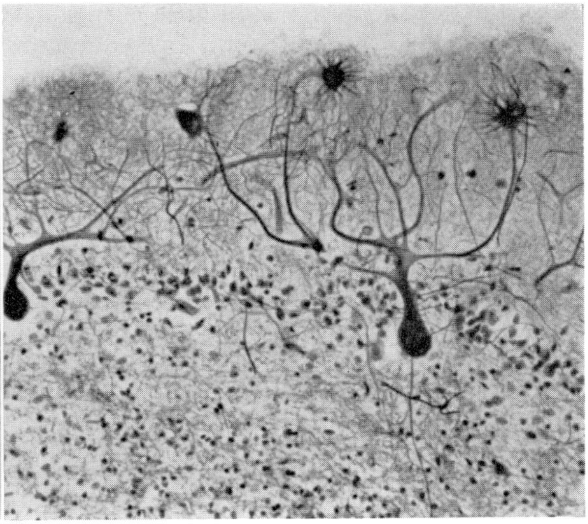

4.25

FIG. 4.24. Section of vermis showing lobular atrophy in declive extending to adjacent lobules. (Loyez' haematoxylin, ×2 (approx.).)
FIG. 4.25. Purkinje cell with stellate bodies. Absence of basket fibres around cell body. (Hortega's double impregnation ×180.)
(Figs. 4.24 and 4.25 are by the kindness of Professor Russell.)

examination were normal. No opinion is advanced by the authors about the pathogenic mechanisms of the lesions. The focal character of the cerebral cortical lesions together with the predilection of lesions for the depth of sulci suggest a vascular (anoxic) factor.

Minamata disease began in 1953 to affect fishermen and their families living around the bay of this name in Japan. Clinical symptomatology and pathology suggested mercurial poisoning as a possible cause (McAlpine and Araki 1958). As a result of intensive research at Kumamoto University, an organic mercury compound effluent from a factory has been isolated from toxic shellfish (Uchida *et al.* 1961). The findings of granular layer atrophy in the cerebellum and of spongiose softenings in visual cortex and other cortical regions closely resemble those in Hunter and Russell's case (Takeuchi *et al.* 1962).

Mercury poisoning has also been suggested as a major etiological factor in *erythroedema polyneuritica* (Pink disease, acrodynia). This condition affects infants in the first 2–3 years, and is characterised by insidious onset, occasionally with raised temperature, and by anorexia, insomnia, loss of weight, and profuse perspiration, particularly of the extremities. Its popular name 'Pink disease' is derived from the red rash (of raw beef colour), and the swelling, coldness and irritation of the hands, feet, cheeks and nose, which is followed by some desquamation. Mental irritability, photophobia and signs of involvement of the peripheral nerves, which is indicated by hypotonia, anaesthesia and loss of tendon reflexes, are consistent signs. The prognosis is universally good with complete recovery; the few fatal cases reported in the literature followed complications such as bronchopneumonia or tuberculosis.

Paterson and Greenfield (1923–4) who examined 2 cases *post mortem* have described polyneuritis affecting the peripheral part of the nerve branches in particular and manifesting itself in considerable degeneration of myelin in the finer nerve bundles. Central chromatolysis of anterior horn cells was widespread and was interpreted as a retrograde reaction to the degeneration of motor nerves. There was some glial proliferation in the spinal grey matter and proliferation of Schwann cells in the ventral roots. Wyllie and Stern (1931), confirming these findings, added central chromatolysis of spinal ganglia and degeneration in the vagal nerve. Kernohan and Kennedy (1928) described in one case central chromatolysis in the Gasserian ganglia and doubtful changes in several nuclei of the brain stem. All investigators found both cerebral and cerebellar cortices to be normal.

With regard to etiology, Paterson and Greenfield favoured infection; in their cases they excluded both dietary deficiency and intoxication by lead, arsenical or other chemical substances. Recent observations have, however, shifted emphasis towards intoxication by mercury in the form of the popular 'teething' powders. Confirming earlier observations by American and Swiss workers Holzel and James (1952) found a higher incidence of mercury excretion in active cases of erythroedema, in striking contrast to the low rate among healthy infants in the same region.

Thallium, tellurium, gold

Thallium is used as rat poison and for depilation. It has an affinity for the nervous system but may act also on the kidneys, heart and blood-vessels. In the clinical symptomatology polyneuritic symptoms predominate. Greving and Gagel (1929) found considerable degeneration of myelin and axis cylinders with corresponding proliferation of Schwann cells in peripheral nerves. According to Scharrer (1933) the posterior columns of the spinal cord are also affected both in the human and experimental animal and there may be degeneration—probably retrograde—of anterior horn cells. Retrobulbar atrophy of the optic nerve is also not uncommon. In addition, various changes have been reported: degeneration in inferior olives and dentate nucleus (Scharrer); slight central chromatolysis in dorsal vagal nucleus (Moeschlin *et al.* 1942); cell changes in hypothalamic nuclei and widespread chromatolysis and vacuolisation of cortical nerve cells, accompanied by slight glial reaction (Bredemann 1954, Prick *et al.* 1949, 1955). Many of the cerebral findings require further scrutiny. It has been suggested that thallium, like other heavy metals, may combine with B vitamins; this may offer a pointer to the pathogenesis of the peripheral neuropathies.

Tellurium is mainly of theoretical interest since it seems possible for it to accumulate in nerve cells without necessarily giving rise to toxic disturbance (Pentschew 1934). In the cat, only the large cells of the red nucleus show structural damage. On macroscopic inspection the grey matter is conspicuous by its blue-grey discoloration, but only by the direct application of a solution of telluric acid to the cerebrospinal fluid do neurological symptoms appear. The storage of tellurium in nerve cells is more consistent than that of other heavy metals.

There is an experimental study by Roberts (1939) of deposits of **gold** in the central nervous system. Following injection of gold salts, the metal was found in nerve and glia cells, particularly in the nuclei of the cranial nerves, the infundibular nuclei, Purkinje cells and anterior horn cells. Courville and Myers (1957) have reported focal subcortical degeneration which they tentatively interpret to be caused by vasospasm following injection of radioactive gold into a pulmonary carcinoma a few weeks earlier.

Phosphorus

Poisoning is not frequent but occurs from sources such as rat poisons, phosphorescent paints and the fumes of phosphorous oxide (Jetter). Wertham (1932) has also recorded a clinico-pathological observation of intoxication in suicide.

Acute poisoning leads rapidly to death by involvement of the central nervous system which is manifest in convulsions, confusional states and coma with terminal respiratory failure. Signs of hepatic failure predominate in subacute poisoning. Peters (1952) has recorded a case in which signs of involvement of the central nervous system occurred as late as 6 years after severe phosphoric burns, but this case was complicated by recurrent abscesses, osteomyelitis and secondary anaemia.

Pathology. Even in rapidly fatal cases extensive fatty degeneration occurs in all viscera including the brain. These changes are particularly striking in the liver, heart and kidneys. In the liver the degeneration begins in the periphery of the lobules. The fatty degeneration of all nerve cells was the outstanding feature in Wertham's case, although death occurred as early as 6 hours after the toxic application. In experimental investigations conducted by Kirschbaum (1924) and Ferraro, Jervis and English (1938), fatty degeneration of nerve cells did not, however, play a major part. The former author found diffuse degenerative changes in cortical nerve cells, with little glial reaction, but which eventually resulted in focal areas of cell loss. Ferraro and his associates describe small perivascular areas of nerve cell loss or of softening, endothelial swelling, haemorrhages and hyperplasia of astrocytes, which they compare with changes occurring in guanidine poisoning. Swelling of the oligodendroglia and, interestingly, of the microglia was a prominent feature.

Phosphorus is a potent protoplasmic poison which leads to depression of cellular oxidations; the sequence of histochemical events is, however, still far from clear.

INTOXICATION BY ORGANIC COMPOUNDS

Tri-ortho-cresyl phosphate *By J. G. Greenfield and A. Meyer.*

This intoxication came to be known mainly during the years of prohibition in the United States, when the substance was consumed as a substitute for alcohol. Adulteration of Jamaica ginger with T.O.C.P. was the cause of nearly 4,000 cases of paralysis in the U.S.A. during the year 1930 before the nature of the poison was discovered by Smith, Elvore and Frazier (1930). About the same time cases were seen in Holland (Ter Braak 1931), as well as on the continent of Europe and in England where T.O.C.P. was sometimes found as an adulterant of 'apiol' or oils used for cooking. In industry it was used for its softening, solvent and extracting properties, and at one time preparations containing cresyl phosphate were included in the treatment of pulmonary tuberculosis.

The paralytic disturbances known as Jamaica ginger paralysis have been also studied by Vonderahe (1931), Smith and Lillie (1931), Sampson (1938, 1942), Staehelin (1942), Aring (1942), Hunter, Perry and Evans (1944), among others. In the American cases foot-drop, followed by more general weakness of the legs and sometimes also of the extensors of the fingers and wrists, came on progressively over a period of about 2 months. In some cases signs of lesions in the spinal cord became obvious as the signs of peripheral neuropathy receded, and late cases often resembled amyotrophic lateral sclerosis with spasticity and peripheral weakness in the legs, deformity of the feet of Friedreich type and wasting of the small muscles of the hands.

In early cases Vonderahe (1931) and Smith and Lillie (1931) found myelin degeneration with slighter changes in the axons in the peripheral nerves. There was no inflammatory exudate. In cases examined in the chronic stages of the disease Aring (1942) found constant degeneration of the pyramidal tracts, greater in the lumbar cord than at higher levels and not evident above the cervical segments. The fasciculus gracilis was also degenerated in some cases and here also the degeneration was greater towards the termination of the tract, that is more in the cervical than in the lower thoracic and lumbar segments. The neurones of the ventral horns were reduced in number and many of the remainder were pyknotic. Similar changes of minor degree were seen in the nuclei of the lower cranial motor nerves. In the peripheral nerves there was loss of some nerve fibres and irregularities on many of the remaining axons. Myelin loss was described as patchy and was associated with considerable endoneurial hyperplasia which might have hindered regeneration.

Cavanagh (1954), in experimental fowls, found the degeneration of myelin in peripheral nerves was not segmental, as had been suggested by earlier workers, but was continuous over the affected fibres in the part examined and resembled the early stages of Wallerian degeneration. It chiefly affected fibres of large calibre and the peripheral parts of nerves contained more degenerating fibres than proximal parts. In the spinal cord degeneration was present in the ventral tracts, in the spino-cerebellar tracts and less intensely in the Goll tracts; it was greatest towards the termination of the tracts. Degeneration of individual fibres was seen also in some tracts of the brain stem. In the cord, as in the peripheral nerves, changes in the axons always accompanied myelin degeneration. Very little chromatolysis was found in the neurones of the ventral horns. The type of degeneration recalled the parenchymatous neuropathy seen in chronic thiamine degeneration (*vide* page 290).

Histological changes similar to those which follow tri-ortho-cresyl-phosphate poisoning have been described as sequelae of other organophosphorus compounds including di-iso-propyl-phosphoro-fluoridate or dyflos and tri-para-ethyl-phenyl phosphate (Fenton 1955; Cavanagh and Holland 1961). It is of interest that this last-mentioned compound, in contrast to the others, has no inhibitory action on cholinesterases. Earl and Thompson (1952) had suggested that the paralysis of T.O.C.P. poisoning may be caused by the inhibitory effect on myelin of pseudo-cholinesterase which is present in Schwann cells and neuroglia. This hypothesis had to be abandoned, however, since it did not explain the degeneration of the axon, and also because other organophosphorus compounds, though capable of the same inhibitory action, produced no paralysis. From a histochemical survey of cholinesterases (both 'true' and 'pseudo') in the spinal cord and brain stem, Cavanagh *et al.* (1961) have recently concluded that there is no simple relation between the sites of lesions in organophosphorus poisoning and the localisation of these enzymes. Nor did these authors find differences in enzyme distribution between those species susceptible and those resistant to organophosphorus poisoning. If, as is still suggested, cholinesterases may play an intermediary role, through their combination with the inhibitor and the subsequent release of the toxic substance (probably a fluoride in the case of dialkyl compounds), there must be other factors, so far unknown, which determine the site of the selective neuronal lesions. This combined histological, histochemical and biochemical approach holds out hope of unravelling some of the complex metabolic factors which determine 'toxic' action on the neurone.

Carbon tetrachloride and related compounds

CCl_4 is used as an industrial solvent. Its toxic effect on the liver and kidneys has long been known, and has been the subject of many clinico-pathological studies. Stevens and Forster (1953) and Cohen (1957) have drawn attention to the early neurological signs of intoxication which consist of headache, vertigo, ataxia, blurred vision, lethargy and coma, and which may appear prior to any manifestation of either hepatic or renal damage. The former, apart from reviewing earlier pathological and experimental investigations, saw perivenous foci of necrosis in the cerebral white matter of one case which were not unlike those occurring in perivenous encephalomyelitis. In another case, emphasis was on the Purkinje cells of the cerebellum which were found to be shrunken, pyknotic and reduced in number, but without glial response. In his 2 cases, Cohen also found venous thrombosis and infarction in the cerebellum with degeneration of Purkinje cells, in addition to perivascular pontine necroses. The pathogenesis of the lesions is still obscure and it must be left to future investigations to decide the relative importance of cerebro-vascular involvement, toxic action on the neurones and the early influence of hepatic and renal dysfunction.

Poisoning by *trichlorethylene* (C_2HCl_3), a chemically related substance, also used as an industrial solvent, seems also to result in a clinical syndrome of optic atrophy, ataxia, spasticity and confusional states (Baker 1958). In experimental dogs, while mild neuronal changes occurred throughout the cerebral cortex, emphasis was on the cerebellar cortex in which many Purkinje cells had disappeared, the remainder showing pyknosis, vacuolation and loss of stainability. The pathogenic difficulties are similar to those with other poisoning by solvents, since kidneys and liver are also damaged. A similar predilection for the Purkinje cells is reported by Baker to occur in benzene and ethyl acetate poisoning.

Aminoquinolines

These substances, including plasmocid (methoxy-diethylamino-propylaminoquinoline), pentaquine, isopentaquine, primaquine and pamaquine—all anti-malarial drugs—have been studied by Schmidt and Schmidt (1948, 1951), Richter (1949) and Löken and Haymaker (1949). These investigations were all experiments on monkeys, except for one fatal human case (Löken and Haymaker) following pamaquine poisoning. Generally it was found that variations of the side chain radicle altered the toxic action; some compounds acted on the heart, others on the haemopoietic system, again others on the central nervous system.

In their earlier publication Schmidt and Schmidt described changes in the spinal cord, the nuclei of the brain stem, diencephalon and extrapyramidal system following acute, subacute and chronic intoxication. With larger doses the histological effect was more widespread than with smaller ones; at half the maximum tolerated doses, plasmocid caused degeneration which was confined to the brain stem nuclei of the proprioceptive pathways, the oculomotor, vestibular and some associated nuclei. In the earlier stages, nerve cell degeneration predominated, in the later astrocytic and fibrous glial and sometimes also microglial proliferation ensued. In their second study, which investigated the effects of pentaquine, isopentaquine, primaquine and pamaquine, the main lesions were in the dorsal motor nucleus of the vagus, supra-optic and paraventricular nuclei and the nucleus of Meynert's commissure; occasionally there was severe injury to the hypoglossal nucleus and mild degeneration of oculomotor nuclei. The Schmidts attribute the severe clinical disturbances of the circulatory system to the lesions of the dorsal vagal nucleus. Richter in macaques identified focal lesions in the thalamus, hypothalamus, red nucleus, substantia nigra, oculomotor and trochlear nuclei, nuclei of the abducens, vestibular and cochlear nerves, in the cuneate nucleus and in the reticular system of the pons and medulla. The lesions consisted of foci of incomplete necrosis, with almost complete loss of nerve cells and microglial proliferation, together with a remarkable proliferation of capillaries and pre-capillaries, which suggested to Denny-Brown a close resemblance to Wernicke's encephalopathy and, consequently, the possibility of an anti-thiamine action.

In Löken and Haymaker's human case there was an area of ischaemic necrosis in the pons, a less severe necrosis in the globus pallidus, and considerable loss of cells with gliosis in the abducens, trochlear and lateral oculomotor nuclei. The authors favour a pathogenesis acting indirectly through anaemia associated with methaemoglobin formation. They do not record lesions in the dorsal vagal nucleus, but Schmidt and Schmidt (1951), who reviewed this case, regard them as likely since the clinical symptomatology was similar to that in their macaques.

Agenised flour

Nitrogen trichloride, known by the name of agene, is used in most wheat-consuming countries to bleach and soften wheat flour. In 1946 Mellanby began a systematic investigation of the possible connection between agene-treated flour and a disease of dogs called 'canine hysteria', which manifests itself by 'running fits'. The problem was taken up in several laboratories, particularly in the United States (Silver 1949, Lewey 1950, and others). Lewey gives a review of these various researches. The action of NCl_3 was found to be toxic to dogs, ferrets and rabbits, but not to guinea pigs, cats, monkeys or man. The electro-encephalogram of dogs suffering from 'canine hysteria' was similar to that of epilepsy in man; symptoms with seizures could be produced in the susceptible animals by feeding or injecting one of the proteins of flour such as gliadin, glutamine, casein, peptide, after treatment with NCl_3.

The toxic agent has now been identified as methionine sulphoximine (Bentley *et al.* 1950). This substance is an antagonist to glutamine as well as to methionine from which it is derived. The changes in the central nervous system of dogs fed on a diet rich in NCl_3 treated flour have been described by Lewey. They consist of necrosis in the deep layers of the cerebral cortex and include the subcortical fibres; the hippocampus shows necrosis identical with that seen in anoxia. The Purkinje cells of the cerebellum, their afferent and efferent pathways, the basket cells and their fibres also show severe degeneration while the nerve cells of the dentate nucleus and the roof nuclei are only mildly affected. The nature and localisation of the changes suggest to Lewey a vascular factor, anoxia or the inhibition of respiratory enzymes as the operative pathogenic factor. A similar pathogenesis was assumed by Hicks and Coy (1958), who on administration of methionine sulfoximine to rats and mice, produced necrosis which was severe in the cerebral cortex (especially the cingular gyrus), corpus striatum and Ammon's horn and less severe in hypothalamus, subthalamic nucleus and thalamus.

Organic tin compounds

While tin in the form of a metal does not seem to be toxic, poisoning by its organic compounds, particularly those containing an alkyl radicle, has been known since the last two decades of the nineteenth century. Interest has recently been renewed because of its importance as a source of poisoning by imperfectly canned foodstuffs. Diethyl tin diiodide has been widely used in France in the oral treatment of boils (quoted from Stoner *et al.* 1955). These authors have undertaken an experimental investigation in rats with di- and tri-ethyl tin compounds. Tri-ethyl tin is the more active compound; its injection causes muscular weakness, tremor and convulsions—symptoms which clearly point to the central nervous system. Naked-eye inspection of the organs reveals little abnormality; tin was not found in the brain nor in any other of the organs. Magee, Stoner and Barnes (1955, 1957) made histological studies of the nervous system of rats and rabbits intoxicated with triethylin compounds. They described in cerebral and spinal white matter and in the optic nerve a remarkable 'interstitial' oedema which, at low magnification, produced a reticular appearance, leaving myelin sheaths and axons intact. When poisoning was interrupted, the animals returned to normal and later—at autopsy—no trace of the oedema or of any lesion could be detected. The pathogenesis remains obscure; no indication of disturbance of the blood-brain barrier could be traced. Gruner (1958, 4 human cases, monkeys and mice) and Cossa *et al.* (1959, 4 human cases) found essentially the same oedematous change, but in addition described more marked ballooning and degeneration of myelin sheaths and axis cylinders, with slight involvement of the cortical grey matter.

Drugs used in psychiatric and neurological treatment

Some of the *tranquillising* drugs of the phenothiazine group are known to produce toxic side effects, expressed especially in extrapyramidal disturbances (usually reversible); all these substances, including reserpine and Rauwolfia, are thought to exert their action upon the hypothalamus and upon autonomic centres in the lower brain stem. A few neuropathological and experimental investigations have been reviewed by Roizin *et al.* (1959) who have also carried out the hitherto most systematic personal investigations on this problem. In their human material (consisting of 3 cases of the literature and of 6 personal cases), they recorded mainly reversible liver changes, and in some cases agranulocytosis. In the central nervous system, diffuse changes such as chromatolysis, increased satellitosis, occasional neuronophagia, and lipid increase were found, perhaps more marked in the basal ganglia and the hypothalamic and mesencephalic regions than elsewhere. In acute experiments on 62 rats, they produced increased sudanophilia of hepatic cells and widespread chromatolysis and increased satellitosis of nerve cells in the brain, again with some emphasis on the basal regions. One chronically-treated monkey, sacrificed after 25 months, showed microglial reaction in the upper cortical layers, and astrocytosis in the cerebral white matter. All chronic monkeys showed a remarkable reduction of testicular size and microscopically, disappearance of spermatozoa with degeneration of spermatogenic cells. In some rats the electron microscope revealed increased osmiophilia and reduction in size of mitochondria. The authors concede that definite conclusions cannot be drawn from the structural changes so far described, including their own findings.

Garland (1957) drew attention to the occurrence of a cerebellar syndrome (dysarthria, nystagmus and ataxia, with or without disturbance of behaviour) in epileptics treated with some of the *hydantoin* drugs (sodium phenytoin, dilantin). Among 31 patients in whom these toxic signs required hospitalisation, overdosage could be incriminated in only 4, while there was obvious individual hypersensitivity in another 3. In a fatal case, Hofmann (1958) found that the Purkinje cells in the cerebellum had practically disappeared, while there was little damage in the cerebral cortex and hippocampus and only mild neuronal changes and some cuffing in striatum and thalamus. The aetiology of the lesions in this case is complicated, as there was a history of symptomatic epilepsy with a background of an undiagnosed infection. The author was aware of this difficulty, but, nevertheless, decided in favour of dilantin poisoning, in view of similar findings experimentally produced in cats by Utterbeck *et al.* (1958).

This is yet another example of predilective toxic action on the cerebellar cortex. It will be remembered that similar predilection has been encountered in chronic alcoholism, and in poisoning by heavy metals and by some organic compounds. It remains to be seen whether a common factor (e.g. vascular, nutritional or hepatic) is involved. Since available evidence is uneven and in many ways incomplete, more systematic experimental exploration is indicated.

REFERENCES

Blood-brain barrier

Bakay, L. (1953) *Arch. Neurol. Psychiat.* (Chicago), **71**, 30; (1955) ibid., **73**, 2.
Behnsen, G. (1926) *Z. Zellforsch.*, **4**, 515.
Brierley, J. B. (1957) *2nd Neurochem. Symp.*, Pergamon Press, London.
Clemente, C. D., and Holst, E. A. (1954) *Arch. Neurol. Psychiat.* (Chicago), **71**, 66.
Dempsey, E. W. and Wislocki, G. B. (1955) *J. biophys. biochem. cytol.*, **1**, 245.
Dobbing, J. (1961) *Physiol. Rev.*, **41**, 130.
Ehrlich, P. (1885) *Das Sauerstoff-Bedürfniss des Organismus*, August Hirschwald, Berlin.
Friedeman, U. (1942) *Physiol. Rev.*, **22**, 125.
Goldmann, E. E. (1913) *Vitalfärbung am Zentralnervensystem*, Georg Reimer, Berlin.
Gröntoft, O. (1954) *Acta path. microbiol. scand.*, suppt. 100.
Hager, H. (1961) *Acta Neuropath.*, **1**, 9.
Hauptmann, A. (1925) *Dtsch. Z. Nervenheilk.*, **89**, 53.
Hess, A. (1953) *J. comp. Neurol.*, **98**, 69; (1955) ibid., **102**, 65; (1958) *J. Anat.*, **92**, 298.
Lewandowsky, M. (1900) *Z. klin. Med.*, **40**, 480.
McIlwain, H. (1959) *Biochemistry and the Central Nervous System*, London (1st edition, 1955).
Macklin, C. C. and Macklin, M. T. (1920) *Arch. Neurol. Psychiat.* (Chicago), **3**, 353.
Maynard, E. A., Schultz, R. and Pease, D. C. (1957) *Amer. J. Anat.*, **100**, 409.
Mott, F. W. (1910) *Lancet* (ii), 1.
Peters, A. (1961) in *Cytology of Nervous Tissue*, Proc. Anat. Soc., p. 20, London.
Peters, R. A. (1936) *Lancet* (i), 1161.
Russell, D. S. (1929) *Amer. J. Path.*, **5**, 451.
Schaltenbrand, G. and Bailey, P. (1928) *J. Psychol. Neurol.*, Lpz., **35**, 199.
Spatz, H. (1933) *Arch. Psychiat. Nervenkr.*, **101**, 267.
Stern, L. and Gautier, R. (1921) *Arch. int. Physiol.*, **17**, 138.
Tschirgi, R. D. (1952) in *The Biology of Mental Health and Disease*, Paul V. Hoeber, New York.
Wells, A. Q. and Carmichael, E. A. (1930) *Brain*, **53**, 1.
Wickoff, R. G. W. and Young, J. Z. (1956) *Proc. Royal Soc.* (*B*), **144**, 440.
Woollam, D. H. M. and Millen, J. W. (1954) *Biol. Rev.*, **29**, 251; (1955) *J. Anat.*, *Lond.*, **89**, 193.

Anoxic poisons

Abbott, C. N. and Courville, C. B. (1938) *Bull. Los. Angeles neurol. Soc.*, **3**, 46.
Alajouanine, T., Bertrand, I., Castaigne, P., Gruner, J. and Pecker, J. (1952) *Rev. neurol.*, **86**, 3.
Alexander, L. (1942) *Proc. Ass. Res. nerv. Dis.*, **21**, 334.
Alpers, B. (1939) *Arch. Neurol. Psychiat.* (Chicago), **42**, 1173.
Alpers, B. J., Berry, R. G. and Paddison, R. M. (1959) *A. M. A. Arch. Neurol. Psychiat.*, **80**, 409.
Alpers, B. and Lewey, F. H. (1940) *Arch. Neurol. Psychiat.* (Chicago), **44**, 725.
Altmann, H. W. (1955) 'Allgemeine Morphologische Pathologie des Cytoplasmas,' in *Handb. d. allg. Pathol.*, edited by Büchner, F., Letterer, E. and Roulet, F., Vol. 2/1, p. 419.
Altmann, H. W. and Schubothe, H. (1942) *Beitr. path. Anat.*, **107**, 3.
Aprison, M. H., Nathan, P. and Himwich, H. E. (1954) *Amer. J. Physiol.*, **177**, 175.
Baker, A. B. (1939) *Amer. J. Psychiat.*, **96**, 109.
Baló, J. V. (1941) quoted from Scholz, Boellaard and Hager.
Bänder, A. and Kiese, M. (1955) *Kli. Wschr.*, **33**, 1, 152.
Barcroft, J. (1925) *The Respiratory Functions of the Blood*, Cambridge University Press.
Batten, C. T. and Courville, C. B. (1940) *Anesthesiology*, **1**, 261.
Bedford, P. D. (1955) *Lancet* (ii), 259.
Beecher, H. K. and Todd, D. P. (1954) *Ann. Surg.*, **140**, 2.
Biemond, A. (1958) *Fol. psychiat. neurol. neurochir.* (*Neerl.*), **61**, 540.
Bingel, A. and Hampel, E. (1934) *Z. ges. Neurol. Psychiat.*, **149**, 640.
Bodechtel, G. (1928) *Z. ges. Neurol. Psychiat.*, **117**, 366; (1932) ibid., **140**, 657; (1953) *Verh. Dtsch. Ges. Kreislaufforsch.*, **19**, 109.

Bourne, J. G. (1957) *Lancet* (ii), 499.

Brazier, M. A. B. (1948) *J. Neurol. Psychiat.*, **11**, 118.

Brierley, J. B. (1961) in *Cerebral Anoxia and the Electroencephalogram*, edited by Gastaut, H. and Meyer, J. S., Springfield, Ill.

Brierley, J. B. (1962) *J. Neurol. Neurosurg. Psychiat.*, **25**, 183.

Brierley, J. B. and Cooper, J. E. (1962) *ibid.*, **25**, 24.

Büchner, F. (1957) Die Pathologie der Zellularen und Geweblichen Oxydationen in *Handb. Allg. Path.* edited by Büchner, F., Letter, E. and Roulet, F., Vol. 4/2, p. 569, Berlin.

Büchner, F. and Luft, U. (1936) *Beitr. path. Anat.*, **96**, 549.

Burton, A. C. (1954) *Physiol. Rev.*, **34**, 619.

Byrom, F. B. (1954) *Lancet* (ii), 201.

Cavanagh, J. B. (1962) personal communication.

Cordy, D. R. (1954) *J. Neuropath.*, **13**, 330.

Corsellis, J. A. N. (1958) *J. Neurol. Neurosurg. Psychiat.*, **21**, 279.

Courville, C. B. (1939) *Untoward Effects of Nitrous Oxide Anaesthesia*, Pacific Press Publishing Association, California; (1941) *Anesthesiology*, **2**, 44; (1953) *Contributions to the Study of Cerebral Anoxia* San Lucas Press, Los Angeles; (1954) *Bull. Los Angel. Neurol. Soc.*, **19**, 135; (1955) *Ibid.*, **20**, 16; (1956) *Ibid.*, **21**, 90; (1957) *A.M.A. Arch. Neurol. Psychiat.*, **78**, 1.

Courville, C. B. and Blossom, R. A. (1954) *Bull. Los Angel. Neurol. Soc.*, **19**, 51.

Déchaume, J. and Chambon, M. (1947) *Arch. Malad. Profess.*, **8**, 119.

de Groat, A. (1940) *Arch. Path. (Lab. Med.)*, **29**, 271.

de Haan, R. L. and Field, J. (1959) *Amer. J. Physiol.*, **197**, 445.

Denny-Brown, D. (1960) *A.M.A. Arch. Neurol.*, **2**, 194.

Denny-Brown, D. and Meyer, J. S. (1957) *Neurology*, **7**, 567.

Denst, J. (1953) *Neurology*, **3**, 239.

Deutsch, H. (1917) *J. Psychiat. Neurol.*, **37**, 237.

Dixon, K. (1955) *Excerpta med., Amst.* Sect. **8**, 772.

Donat, R. (1937–8) *Dtsch. Z. ges. gerichtl. Med.*, **29**, 34.

Döring, G. (1936) *Virchows Arch.*, **296**, 666.

Dublin, W. P. and Brown, R. W. (1942) *Northw. Med.* (Seattle), **41**, 167.

Dutra, F. R. (1952) *Amer. J. Clin. Path.*, **22**, 925.

Earle, K. M., Baldwin, N. and Penfield, W. (1953) *Arch. Neurol. Psychiat.* (Chicago), **69**, 27.

Edelmann, F. (1921) *Dtsch. Z. Nervenheilk.*, **72**, 259.

Edstrom, R. F. S. and Essex, H. E. (1956) *Neurology*, **6**, 118.

Eros, G. and Priestman, G. (1942) *J. Neuropath.*, **1**, 158.

Ferraro, A. (1933) *Psychiat. Quart.*, **7**, 267.

Ferraro, A. and Jervis, G. A. (1939) *Psychiat. Quart.*, **13**, 207.

Ferraro, A., Jervis, G. A. and Flicker, D. J. (1941) *Arch. Path. (Lab. Med.)*, **32**, 723.

Ferraro, A. and Morrison, L. R. (1928) *Psychiat. Quart.*, **2**, 506.

Fletcher, D. E. (1945) *J. nerv. ment. Dis.*, **102**, 392.

Foley, J. and Paterson, J. H. (1954) *Proc. R. Soc. Med.*, **47**, 296.

Gamper, E. and Stiefler, G. (1937) *Arch. Psychiat. Nervenkr.*, **106**, 744.

Gellhorn, E., Ingraham, R. C. and Moldavsky, L. (1936) *J. Neurophysiol.*, **1**, 301.

Gildea, E. F. and Cobb, S. (1930) *Arch. Neurol. Psychiat.* (Chicago), **23**, 876.

Greenfield, J. G. (1958) in *Neuropathology*, Arnold, London.

Greenfield, J. G., Richards, A. G. and Manning, G. B. (1955) *J. Path. Bact.*, **69**, 95.

Grenell, R. G. (1946) *J. Neuropath.*, **5**, 131.

Grenell, R. G. and Kabat, H. (1947) *J. Neuropath.*, **6**, 35.

Grinker, R. R. (1926) *J. nerv. ment. Dis.*, **64**, 18.

Grünthal, E. (1947) *Mschr. Psychiat. Neurol.*, **113**, 1.

Haberland, C. (1961) *Excerpt. Med. Int. Congr. Neurol. series*, **39**, 58.

Hallervorden, J. (1949) *Allg. Z. Psychiat.*, **124**, 289.

Haymaker, W. and Davison, C. (1950) *J. Neuropath.*, **9**, 29.

Haymaker, W., Ginzler, A. M. and Ferguson, R. L. (1952) *Milit. Surg.*, **111**, 231.

Haymaker, W., Margoles, C., Pentschew, A., Jacob, H., Lindenberg, R., Arroyo, L. S., Stochdorph, O., Stowens, D. (1957–9) *Pathology of Kernicterus and Posticteric Encephalopathy* (reprinted from *Am. Ac. of Cerebral Palsy*), Springfield, Ill.

Hicks, S. P. (1950 a) *Arch. Path.*, **49**, 111; (1950 b) *Arch. Path.*, **50**, 545.

Hiller, F. (1924) *Z. ges. Neurol. Psychiat.*, **93**, 594.
Himwich, H. E. (1951) *Brain Metabolism and Cerebral Disorders*, Williams & Wilkins, Baltimore.
Hoff, E. C., Grenell, R. G. and Fulton, J. F. (1945) *Medicine*, Baltimore, **24**, 161.
Howkins, J., McLaughlin, C. R. and Daniel, P. (1946) *Lancet* (i), 488.
Hsü, Y. K. and Ch'eng, Y. L. (1938) *Brain*, **61**, 384.
Hurst, E. W. (1940) *Aust. J. exp. Biol. med. Sci.*, **18**, 201; (1941) *Med. J. Aust.*, **2**, 661; (1942) *Aust. J. exp. Biol. med. Sci.*, **20**, 297; (1955) *J. Path. Bact.*, **70**, 167.
Jacob, H. (1939) *Z. ges. Neurol. Psychiat.*, **167**, 161.
Jedlowski, P. (1938) *Riv. Pat. Nerv.*, **51**, 231.
Jensen, A. V., Becker, R. F. and Windle, W. F. (1948) *Arch. Neurol. Psychiat.* (Chicago), **60**, 221.
Jervis, G. (1937) *Riv. Pat. Nerv.*, **50**, 410.
Jervis, G. A. and Joyce, F. T. (1948) *Arch. Path. (Lab. Med.)*, **45**, 319.
Jung, R. (1949) *Arch. Psychiat. Nervenkr.*, **183**, 206; (1953) *Verh. dtsch. Ges. Kreislaufforsch.*, **19**, 170.
Kabat, H. (1940) *Amer. J. Physiol.*, **130**, 588.
Kabat, H. and Schadewald, M. (1941) *Amer. J. Path.*, **17**, 833.
Kennedy, F., Effron, A. S. and Perry, G. (1950) *Surg. Gynec. Obstet.*, **91**, 385.
Kennedy, F., Somberg, H. M. and Goldberg, B. R. (1945) *J. Amer. med. Ass.*, **129**, 664.
Kolisko, A. (1893) *Wien. klin. Wschr.*, **6**, 191.
Krogh, E. (1952) *1st Int. Congr. Neuropath.*, **1**, 453.
Last, S. L. and Meyer, A. (1932) *Arch. Psychiat. Nervenkr.*, **96**, 73.
Lawrence, R. D., Meyer, A. and Nevin, S. (1942) *Quart. J. Med.*, **35**, 181.
Levine, S. (1960) *Amer. J. Path.*, **36**, 1.
Levine, S. and Stypulkowski, W. (1959) *Arch. Path.*, **67**, 306.
Lewey, F. H. and Drabkin, D. L. (1944) *Amer. J. med. Sci.*, **208**, 502.
Lindenberg, R. (1955) *J. Neuropath.*, **14**, 223; (1956) *Amer. J. Path.*, **32**, 1147.
Lindenberg, R. and Spatz, H. (1939) *Virchows Arch. path. Anat.*, **305**, 531.
Loughridge, L. W., Leader, L. P. and Bowen, D. A. L. (1958) *Lancet* (ii), 349.
Lowenberg, K., Waggoner, R. and Zbinden, T. (1936) *Ann. Surg.*, **104**, 801.
Lucas, B. G. B. (1950) *Proc. R. Soc. Med.*, **43**, 606.
Luft, U. C. (1937) *Beitr. path. Anat.*, **99**, 351.
Lumsden, C. E. (1950) *J. Neurol. Psychiat.*, **13**, 1; (1957) *Proc. 3rd Int. Congr. Neuropath.*, p. 27.
Lund, O. E. (1956) *Arch. Gewerbepathol. Gewerbehygiene*, **15**, 96.
McIlwain, H. (1955) *Biochemistry and the Central Nervous System*, Churchill, London.
Macken, J. and Martin, F. (1950) *Mschr. Psychiat. Neurol.*, **119**, 129.
Maclay, W. S. (1953). *Proc. R. Soc. Med.*, **46**, 13.
McQuarrie, I., Bauer, E. G., Ziegler, M. R. and Wright, W. S. (1949) *Bull. Univ. Minn. Hosp.*, **21**, 35.
Malamud, N. and Haymaker, W. (1946) *Milit. Surg.*, **99**, 397.
Maske, H. (1955) *Naturwissenschaften*, **42**, 424.
Mattyus, A. (1959) *Arch. Psychiat. Z. ges. Neurol.*, **199**, 172.
Megro, F. (1930) *Rev. neurol.*, **49**, 518.
Meyer, A. (1926) *Z. ges. Neurol. Psychiat.*, **100**, 201; (1928 a) ibid., **112**, 172; (1928 b) ibid., **112**, 187; (1932 a) *Nervenarzt*, **5**, 229; (1932 b) *Z. ges. Neurol. Psychiat.*, **139**, 422; (1933) ibid., **143**, 333; (1936) *Proc. R. Soc. Med.*, **29**, 1175; (1956) ibid., **49**, 619.
Meyer, A. and Blume, W. (1934) *Z. ges. Neurol. Psychiat.*, **149**, 678.
Meyer, J. E. (1953 a) *Verh. dtsch. Ges. Kreislaufforsch.*, **19**, 69; (1953 b) *Arch. Psychiat. Z. ges. Neurol.*, **190**, 328; (1958) ibid., **196**, 421; (1961) ibid., **202**, 113.
Meyer, J. S., Fang, H. C. and Denny-Brown, D. (1954) *A.M.A. Arch. Neurol. Psychiat.*, **72**, 296.
Meyer, J. S. and Gastaut, H. (1961) *Cerebral Anoxia and the Electroencephalogram*, Sprinfield, Ill.
Meyer, J. S., Gotoh, F., Tazaki, Y. and Hamaguchi, K. (1961) *Rep. 7th Int. Congr. Neurol.*, p. 427.
Meyer, J. S. and Portnoy, H. D. (1958) *Neurology*, **8**, 601.
Morrison, L. R. (1946) *Arch. Neurol. Psychiat.* (Chicago), **55**, 1.
Neubürger, K. T. (1930) *Handbuch der Geisteskrankheiten*, **11**, Edited by O. Bumke, Julius Springer Berlin.
Neubürger, K. T. (1954) *J. Neuropath.*, **13**, 144.
Neubürger, K. T. and Clarke, E. R. (1945) *Rocky Mountain med. J.*, **42**, 29 (correction 196).
Neumann, M. A. (1951) *J. Neuropath. Clin. Neurol.*, **1**, 145.

Neumann, M. A., Cohn, R. and Katzenelbogen, S. (1942) *Amer. J. Psychiat.*, **98**, 668.
Norman, R. M. (1958) in *Temporal Lobe Epilepsy*, edited by Baldwin, M. and Bailey, P., Springfield, Ill.
Norman, R. M., Urich, H. and McMenemey, W. H. (1957) *Brain*, **80**, 49.
Orthmayr, A. (1952) *Arch. Psychiat. Nervenkr.*, **189**, 126.
Overhof, K. (1933) *Arch. path. Anat.*, **287**, 784.
Paasonen, M. K., MacLean, P. D., Giarman, N. J. (1957) *J. Neurochem.*, **1**, 326.
Peters, G. (1951) *Spezielle Pathologie der Krankheiten des zentralen und peripheren Nervensystems*, Georg Thieme, Stuttgart.
Photakis, B. H. (1921) *Wschr. gerichtl. Med.*, **62**, 42.
Pia, H. W. (1957) *Acta Neurochir. (Vienna) Suppl.*, 4.
Pickering, G. W. (1951) *Lancet* (ii), 845.
Quastel, J. H. (1943) *Trans. Faraday Soc.*, **34**, 12.
Quastel, J. H. and Wheatley, A. H. M. (1932) *Proc. roy. Soc.*, B., **112**, 60.
Ranck, J. B. and Windle, W. F. (1959) *Exp. Neurology*, **1**, 130.
Rand, C. W. and Courville, C. B. (1936) *Arch. Neurol. Psychiat.* (Chicago), **36**, 1277.
Raskin, N. and Mullaney, O. C. (1940) *J. nerv. ment. Dis.*, **92**, 640.
Richardson, J. C., Chambers, R. A. and Heywood, P. M. (1959) *A.M.A. Arch. Neurol.*, **1**, 178.
Richardson, J. E. and Russell, D. S. (1952) *Lancet* (ii), 1054.
Richter, R. B. (1945) *J. Neuropath.*, **4**, 16.
Ricker, G. (1924) *Pathologie als Naturwissenschaft*, Julius Springer, Berlin.
Roger, H., Poursines, Y. and Alliez, J. (1952) *Ann. Méd. Psychol.*, **2**, 144.
Rohmer, F., Gastaut, Y. and Dell, M. B. (1952) *Rev. neurol.*, **87**, 93.
Rotter, R. (1929) *Z. ges. Neurol. Psychiat.*, **119**, 97.
Rowntree, D. W., Nevin, S. and Wilson, A. (1950) *J. Neurol. Psychiat.*, **13**, 47.
Rubino, A. (1935) *Riv. Pat. Nerv.*, **45**, 191.
Russell, D. S. (1937) *J. Path. Bact.*, **45**, 357.
Samson, F. E., Dahl, D. R., Dahl, N. and Himwich, H. E. (1959) *Arch. Neurol. Psychiat.* (Chicago), **81**, 458.
Scharrer, E. (1940) *Arch. Neurol. Psychiat.* (Chicago), **44**, 483.
Scherer, E. (1934) *Z. ges. Neurol. Psychiat.*, **150**, 632.
Schmid, H. (1936) *Schweiz. med. Wschr.*, **17**, 960.
Schmorl, G. (1920) *Münch. med. Wschr.*, **67**, 913.
Scholz, W. (1941) *Z. ges. Neurol. Psychiat.*, **171**, 426; (1953a) *Verh. dtsch. Ges. Kreislaufforsch.*, **19**, 52.
Scholz, W. (1953b) *J. Neuropath.*, **12**, 249; (1957) Die nicht zur Erweichung führenden unvollständigen Gewebsnekrosen in *Handb. Spec. Path. Anat. Histol.*, Vol. XIII, ed. Scholz, W., **1**, B, p. 1284.
Scholz, W., Boellaard, J. W. and Hager, H. (1959) *Toxity Changes in the Central Nervous System*, Tech. Rep. Contr. A F 61 (514–945) U.S.A.F.
Scholz, W. and Hager, H. (1959) in Scholz, Boellaard and Hager.
Scholz, W. and Schmidt, H. (1952) *Arch. Psychiat. Nervenkr.*, **189**, 231.
Schumm, H. (1953) *Fortschr. Neur. Psychiat.*, **21**, 1.
Schwedenberg, T. H. (1959) *J. Neuropath.*, **18**, 597.
Sibelius, C. (1906) *Mschr. Psychiat. Neurol.*, **18**, suppt., p. 39.
Small, J. M. and Woolf, A. L. (1957) *J. Neurol. Neurosurg. Psychiat.*, **20**, 293.
Spector, R. G. (1961) *Brit. J. Exp. Path.*, **42**, 623.
Spielmeyer, W. (1909) *Neurol. Zbl.*, **28**, 69; (1922) *Histopathologie des Nervensystems*, Julius Springer, Berlin; (1925) *Z. ges. Neurol. Psychiat.*, **99**, 756; (1930) *J. ment. Sci.*, **76**, 641.
Steegman, A. T. (1939) *Arch. Neurol. Psychiat.* (Chicago), **41**, 955; (1961) *Rep. 7th Int. Congr. Neurol.*, p. 197.
Steegman, A. T. and Davis, H. V. (1950) *Arch. Neurol. Psychiat.* (Chicago), **63**, 774.
Stewart, R. M. (1920) *J. Neurol. Psychopath.*, **1**, 105.
Strassmann, G. (1949) *Mschr. Psychiat. Neurol.*, **117**, 360.
Timm, F. (1958) *Z. Zellforsch.*, **48**, 548.
Titrud, L. A. and Haymaker, W. (1947) *Arch. Neurol. Psychiat.* (Chicago), **57**, 397.
Tureen, L. L. (1936) *Arch. Neurol. Psychiat.* (Chicago), **35**, 789.
Tyler, D. B. and Ziskind, E. (1940) *Proc. Soc. exp. Biol.*, N.Y., **44**, 622.
Uchimura, Y. (1928) *Z. ges. Neurol. Psychiat.*, **114**, 567.
Ulbricht, J. (1948) *Beitr. Path. Anat.*, **110**, 15.
van Bogaert, L., Dallemagne, M. J. and Wégria, R. (1938) *Arch. int. Méd. exp.* **13**, 335.

Vogt, C. and Vogt, O. (1922) *J. Psychol. Neurol.*, Lpz., **28**.
Warburg, O. (1924) *Biochem. Zschr.*, **152**, 479
Weimann, W. (1930) Intoxicationen, *Handbuch der Geisteskrankheiten*, **11**, Edited by O. Bumke, Julius Springer, Berlin.
Weinberger, L., Gibbon, M. H. and Gibbon, J. H. (1940) *Arch. Neurol. Psychiat.* (Chicago), **43**, 961.
Wilke, G. and Iizuka, R. (1960) *Nervenarzt*, **31**, 519.
Williams, C. J. (1955) *Brit. Med. J.* (i), 707.
Wilson, S. A. K. (1940) *Neurology*, **1**, Butterworth, London.
Winblad, S. (1940) *Dtsch. Z. ges. gerichtl. Med.*, **33**, 73.
Windle, W. F. (1961) *Excerpta Medica. Int. Congr. Ser., No.*, **39**, 81.
Winkelman, N. W. (1952) *Neurology*, **2**, 284.
Winkelman, N. W., Gotten, N. and Scheibert, D. (1953) *Trans. Amer. neurol. Ass.*, **78**, 15.
Winkelman, N. W. and Moore, M. T. (1940) *Arch. Neurol. Psychiat.* (Chicago), **43**, 1108.
Wolf, A. (1952) *1st Int. Congr. Neuropath.*, **1**, 121.
Zeckel, A. and Behr, E. (1933) *Psychiat. neurol. Bl.*, Amst., **37**, 57.
Zülch, K. J. and Behrend, R. C. H. (1961) in *Cerebral Anoxia and the Electroencephalogram*, edited by Meyer, J. S. and Gastaut, H., Springfield, Ill.

Drugs of addiction

Adams, J. H. (1962) *Proc 4th Int. Cong. Neuropath.*, **3**, 303.
Adams, R. D., Victor, M. and Mancall, E. L. (1959) *A.M.A. Arch. Neurol. Psychiat.*, **81**, 154.
Bennett, I. L., Cary, F. H., Mitchell, G. L. and Cooper, M. N. (1953) *Medicine*, Baltimore, **32**, 431.
Birch-Hirschfeld, A. (1902) *v. Graefes Arch. Ophthal.*, **54**, 68.
Bohrod, M. G. (1942) *Arch. Neurol. Psychiat.* (Chicago), **47**, 465.
Carducci, A. (1898) *Riv. di Psicol. Psich. e Neuropat. Fasc. 8–9*, **2**, Rome (quoted from Ironside *et al.*).
Courville, C. B. (1955) *Effects of Alcohol on the Nervous System of Man*, Los Angeles.
Courville, C. B. and Myers, R. O. (1954) *Bull. Los. Angeles neurol. Soc.*, **19**, 66.
Creutzfeld, H. G. (1926) *Z. ges. Neurol. Psychiat.*, **101**, 97.
Fink, W. H. (1943) *Amer. J. Ophthal.*, **26**, 695, 802.
Ironside, R., Bosanquet, F. D. and McMenemey, W. H. (1961) *Brain*, **84**, 212.
Jacob, A. (1912) *Z. ges. Neurol. Psychiat.*, **13**, 132.
Jansen, J. (1936) *Acta path. microbiol. scand.*, suppt., **26**, 146.
Jéquier, M. and Wildi, E. (1955) *Schweiz. Arch. Neurol. Psychiat.*, **75**, 77.
King, L. and Meehan, M. (1936) *Arch. Neurol. Psychiat.* (Chicago), **36**, 547.
Lhermitte, J. (1934/35) *Proc. Roy. Soc. Med.*, **28**, 379.
Lhermitte, J., de Ajuriaguerra, J. and Garnier (1938) *Compt. Rend. Soc. de Biol.*, **128**, 386.
Lolli, G. (1941) *Quart. J. Stud. Alc.*, **2**, 486.
Lynch, M. (1960) *Arch. Path.*, **69**, 342.
McIlwain, H. (1955) *Biochemistry and the Central Nervous System*, Churchill, London.
McLardy, T. (1951) *Proc. R. Soc. Med.*, **44**, 685.
Marchiafava, E. and Bignami, A. (1903) *Riv. Pat. nerv. ment.*, **8**, 544.
Morel, F. (1939) *Rev. neurol.*, **71**, 280.
Mott, F. W. (1910) *Brit. med. J.* (ii), 1403.
Neubürger, K. T. (1957) *Arch. Path.*, **63**, 1.
Orthner, H. (1949) *Zbl. allg. Path. path. Anat.*, **85**, 11.
Penfield, W. and Cone, W. (1926) *Arch. Neurol. Psychiat.* (Chicago), **16**, 131.
Pick, L. and Bielschowsky, M. (1912) *Berl. klin. Wschr.*, **49**, 888.
Røe, O. (1946). *Acta med. scand.*, suppt., 182.
Sinclair, H. M. (1956) *Brit. med. Bull.*, **12**, 18.
Stender, A. and Lüthy, F. (1931) *Dtsch. Z. Nervenheilk.*, **119**, 604.
Weimann, W. (1926) *Z. ges. Neurol. Psychiat.*, **105**, 705; (1930) Intoxicationen, *Handbuch der Geisteskrankheiten*, **11**, Edited by O. Bumke, Julius Springer, Berlin.
Weimann, W. and von Marenholtz. (1928) *Dtsch. Z. ges. gerichtl. Med.*, **12**, 297.
Wood, A. C. and Buller, F. (1904) *J. Amer. med. Ass.*, 972, 1058, 1117, 1213, 1289.

Heavy metals and organic compounds

Alkelaitis, A. J. (1941) *J. nerv. ment. Dis.*, **93**, 313.
Aring, C. D. (1942) *Brain*, **65**, 34.
Ashizawa, R. (1927) *Jap. J. Med. Sci.*, **1**, 173.
Baker, A. B. (1958) *J. Neuropath.*, **17**, 649.
Bentley, H. R., McDermott, E. E. and Whitehead, J. K. (1950) *Nature*, Lond., **165**, 735.
Biemond, A. and van Creveld, G. (1939) *Acta. Paediatr.* (Stockholm), **27**, 51.
Bini, L. and Bollea, G. (1947) *J. Neuropath.*, **6**, 271.
Blackman, jr., S. S. (1937) *Bull. J. Hopk. Hosp.*, **61**, 1.
Bonfiglio, F. (1910) *Histol. histopath. Arb.*, **3**, 359.
Bredemann, W. (1954) *Arch. Psychiat. Z. ges. Neurol.*, **192**, 393.
Brown, I. A. (1954) *Arch. Neurol. Psychiat.* (Chicago), **72**, 674.
Burrows, N. F. E., Rendle-Short, J. and Hanna, D. (1951) *Brit. med. J.* (i), 329.
Call, R. A. and Gunn, D. F. (1949) *Arch. Path. (Lab. Med.)*, **48**, 119.
Canavan, M. M., Cobb, S. and Drinker, C. K. (1934) *Arch. Neurol. Psychiat.* (Chicago), **32**, 512.
Casamajor, L. (1913) *J. Amer. med. Ass.*, **60**, 646.
Cavanagh, J. B. (1954) *J. Neurol. Neurosurg. Psychiat.*, **17**, 163.
Cavanagh, J. B. and Holland, P. (1961) *Brit. J. Pharmacol. Chemotherap.*, **16**, 218.
Cavanagh, J. B., Davies, D. R., Holland, P. and Lancaster, M. (1961) *Brit. J. Pharmacol. Chemotherap.*, **17**, 21.
Charles, J. R. (1922) *J. Neurol. Psychopath.*, **3**, 262.
Cohen, M. (1957) *Neurology*, **7**, 238.
Cossa, P., Duplay, E., Arfel-Capdeville, Lafon, Passouant, Minvielle, and Radermecker, J. (1959) *Acta. Neurol. Psychiat. Belg.*, **59**, 281.
Couper, J. (1837) *J. Chim. Med. Pharm. Toxicol.*, **3**, 233.
Courville, C. and Myers, R. O. (1957) *Neurology*, **7**, 323.
Crescitelli, F. and Gilman, A. (1946) *Amer. J. Physiol.*, **147**, 127.
Cumings, J. N. (1948) *Brain*, **71**, 410.
de Morsier, G. and Feldmann, N. (1951) *Encéphale*, **40**, 97.
de Villaverde, J. M. (1926) *Trav. Lab. Reherch. Biol., Madrid*, **24**, 1, 155, 267; (1927) *ibid.*, **25**, 41.
Earl, C. J. and Thompson, R. H. S. (1952) *British J. Pharmacol.*, **7**, 685.
Edsall, D. L., Wilbur, F. P. and Drinker, C. K. (1919) *J. industr. Hyg.*, **1**, 183.
Embden, H. (1901) *Dtsch. med. Wschr.*, **27**, 795.
Fenton, J. C. B. (1955) *J. Path. Bact.*, **69**, 181.
Ferraro, A. and Hernandez, R. (1932) *Psychiat. Quart.*, **6**, 121.
Ferraro, A., Jervis, G. A. and English, W. H. (1938) *Psychiat. Quart.*, **12**, 294.
Findlay, G. M. (1924) *Brit. J. exp. Path.*, **5**, 92.
Fisher, C. M. and Adams, R. D. (1956) *J. Neuropath.*, **15**, 243.
Garland, H. (1957) *Proc. Roy. Soc. Med.*, **50**, 611.
Gibb, J. W. G. and MacMahon, J. F. (1955) *Brit. med. J.* (i), 320.
Globus, J. H. and Ginsburg, S. W. (1933) *Arch. Neurol. Psychiat.* (Chicago), **30**, 1226.
Gombault, A. (1880–81) *Arch. de Neurol.*, **1**, 11.
Gordon, I. and Whitehead, T. P. (1949) *Lancet* (ii), 647.
Greenfield, J. G. (1958) in *Neuropathology*, Arnold, London.
Greving, R. and Gagel, O. (1929) *Z. ges. Neurol. Psychiat.*, **120**, 805.
Gruner, J. E. (1958) *Rev. Neurol.*, **98**, 109.
Grzycki, S. and Kobusowna, B. (1951) *J. Neuropath.* **10**, 325.
Henderson, D. A. (1954) *Australasian Ann. Med.*, **3**, 219.
Hicks, S. P. and Coy, M. A. (1958) *Arch. Path.*, **65**, 378.
Hofmann, W. W. (1958) *Neurology*, **8**, 210.
Holzel, A. and James, T. (1952) *Lancet* (i), 441.
Hunter, D., Bomford, R. R. and Russell, D. S. (1940) *Quart. J. Med.*, **9**, 193.
Hunter, D., Perry, K. M. A. and Evans, R. B. (1944) *Brit. J. industr. Med.*, **1**, 227.
Hunter, D. and Russell, D. S. (1954) *J. Neurol. Psychiat.*, **17**, 235.
Hurst, E. W. and Hurst, P. E. (1928) *J. Path. Bact.*, **31**, 303.
Jetter, W. W. (1953) in *Pathology*, Edited by W. A. D. Anderson, Henry Kimpton, London.
Jiminez, J. A., Uiberall, C. and Escudero, F. (1946) *Prensa méd. argent.*, **33**, 1684.

Kato, K. (1932) *Amer. J. Dis. Children*, **44**, 569.
Kernohan, J. W. and Kennedy, R. L. J. (1928) *Amer. J. Dis. Child.*, **36**, 341.
Kirschbaum, W. (1924) *Z. ges. Neurol. Psychiat.*, **88**, 487.
Környey, St. (1931) *Dtsch. Z. Nervenheilk.*, **122**, 18.
Krainer, L., Black, D. A. K., McGill, R. J. and Rao, N. V. (1947) *J. Neurol. Psychiat.*, **10**, 171.
Lehmann, K. B., Spatz, H. and Wisbaum-Neubürger, K. T. (1926) *Z. ges. Neurol. Psychiat.*, **103**, 323.
Lewey, F. H. (1950) *J. Neuropath. exp. Neurol.*, **9**, 396.
Lewy, F. H. and Tiefenbach, L. (1921) *Z. ges. Neurol. Psychiat.*, **71**, 303.
Löken, A. C. and Haymaker, W. (1949) *Amer. J. trop. Med.*, **29**, 341.
McAlpine, D. and Araki, S. (1958) *Lancet*, (ii), 629.
Magee, P. N., Stoner, H. B. and Barnes, J. M. (1955) *Excerpta med.*, Amst. (Sect. 8), **8**, 859; (1957) *J. Path. Bact.*, **73**, 107.
Marsden, H. B. and Wilson, V. K. (1955) *Brit. med. J.* (i), 324.
Mella, H. (1924) *Arch. Neurol. Psychiat.* (Chicago), **11**, 405.
Mellanby, E. (1946) *Brit. med. J.* (ii), 885.
Meyer, A. (1930) *Samml. Vergiftungsf.*, **1**, 79.
Millichap, J. G., Llewellin, K. R. and Roxburgh, R. C. (1952) *Lancet* (ii), 360.
Moeschlin, S., Zollinger, H. and Lüthy, F. (1942) *Dtsch. Arch. Klin. Mediz.*, **189**, 181.
Mott, F. W. (1909) *Arch. Neurol. Psychiat.*, London., **4**, 117.
Neal, P. A. (1938) *Amer. J. publ. Hlth.*, **28**, 907.
Nissl, F. (1892) *Z. Psychiat.*, **48**, 1.
Noetzel, H. (1955) *Beitr. Pathol. Anatom.*, **115**, 226.
Parnitzke, K. H. and Peiffer, J. (1954) *Arch. Psychiat. Z. ges. Neurol.*, **192**, 405.
Paterson, D. and Greenfield, J. G. (1923–4) *Quart. J. Med.*, **17**, 6.
Pentschew, A. (1934) *Arch. Psychiat. Nervenkr.*, **101**, 80.
Pentschew, A. (1958) Intoxikationen in *Handl. Spec. Path. Anat. Histol.*, Vol. XIII, ed. Scholz, W. **2** B, p. 1907.
Peters, G. (1949) *Beitr. path. Anat.*, **110**, 371; (1951) *Spezielle Pathologie der Krankheiten des zentralen und peripheren Nervensystems*, Georg Thieme, Stuttgart; (1952) *Dtsch. Z. Nervenheilk.*, **168**, 281.
Peters, R. A. (1948) *Brit. med. Bull.*, **5**, 313.
Petri, E. (1930) Intoxicationen, *Handbuch der speziellen pathologischen Anatomie und Histologie*, **10**. Edited by F. Henke and O. Lubarsch, Julius Springer, Berlin.
Prick, J. J. G., Smitt, W. G. S. and Muller, L. (1949) *Fol. Psychiat. Neurol. Neurochir. Neerl.*, **52**, 95; (1955) *Thallium Poisoning*, Amsterdam.
Reznikoff, P. and Aub, J. C. (1927) *Arch. Neurol. Psychiat.* (Chicago), **17**, 444.
Richter, R. (1949) *J. Neuropath.*, **8**, 155.
Roberts, W. J. (1939) *Arch. Psychiat. Nervenkr.*, **109**, 744.
Roizin, L., True, C. and Knight, M. (1959) *Proc. Ass. Res. Nerv. Ment. Dis.*, **37**, 285.
Russell, D. S. (1937) *J. Path. Bact.*, **45**, 357.
Sampson, B. F. (1938) *Bull. Off. int. Hyg. publ.*, **30**, 2601; (1942) *S. Afr. med. J.*, **16**, 1.
Scharrer, E. (1933) *Z. ges. Neurol. Psychiat.*, **145**, 454.
Scheinker, I. M. (1944) *Arch. Path. (Lab. Med.)*, **37**, 91.
Schmidt, I. H. and Schmidt, L. H. (1948) *J. Neuropath.*, **7**, 368; (1951) ibid., **10**, 231.
Seelert, H. (1913) *Mschr. Psychiat. Neurol.*, **34**, 82.
Sexton, G. B. and Gowdey, C. W. (1947) *Arch. Derm. Syph.*, N.Y., **56**, 634.
Silver, M. L. (1949) *J. Neuropath.*, **8**, 441.
Smith, M. I., Elvore, E. and Frazier, W. H. (1930) *Publ. Hlth. Rep. Wash.*, **45**, 2509.
Smith, M. I. and Lillie, R. D. (1931) *Arch. Neurol. Psychiat.* (Chicago), **26**, 976.
Spielmeyer, W. (1922) *Histopathologie des Nervensystems*, Berlin.
Stadler, H. (1936) *Z. ges. Neurol. Psychiat.*, **154**, 62.
Staehelin, R. (1942) *Schweiz. med. Wschr.*, **72**, 1.
Steiman, S. E. (1939) *Amer. J. Physiol.*, **126**, 261.
Stevens, H. and Forster, F. M. (1953) *Arch. Neurol. Psychiat.* (Chicago), **70**, 635.
Stoner, H. B., Barnes, J. M. and Duff, J. I. (1955) *Brit. J. Pharmacol.*, **10**, 16.
Takeuchi, T., Morikawa, N., Matsumoto, H. and Shiraishi, Y. (1962) *Acta Neuropath.*, **2**, 40.
Ter Braak, J. W. G. (1931) *Ned. Tijdschr. Geneesk.*, **75**, 2329.
Thompson, R. H. S. (1948) *Brit. med. Bull.*, **5**, 319.
Turner, J. W. A. (1955) *Lancet* (i), 661.

Uchida, M., Hirakawa, K. and Inoue, T. (1961) *Kumamoto Medical J.*, **14**, 181.
Upners, T. (1939) *Z. ges Neurol. Psychiat.*, **166**, 623.
Utterbeck, R. A., Oleman, R. and Malek, J. (1958) *J. Neuropath.*, **17**, 516.
van Bogaert, L. (1956) *Mschr. Psychiat. Neurol.*, **131**, 73.
van Bogaert, L. and Dallemagne, M. J. (1943) *J. Neurol. belge*, **43**, 271; (1945–6) *Mschr. Psychiat. Neurol.*, **111**, 60.
Verhaart, W. J. C. (1933) *Z. ges. Neurol. Psychiat.*, **147**, 76; (1934) *Far East Ass. Trop. Med. Trs. 9th Congr.*, **2**, 583 (quoted from Verhaart, 1941).
Verhaart, W. J. C. (1941) *Amer. J. Dis. Child.*, **61**, 1246.
Vonderahe, A. R. (1931) *Arch. Neurol. Psychiat.* (Chicago), **25**, 29.
von Jaksch, R. (1901) *Wien. klin. Wschr.*, **15**, 729.
von Meduna, L. (1929) *Arch. Psychiat. Nervenkr.*, **87**, 571.
Wachstein, M. (1949) *Arch. Path.* (*Lab. Med.*), **48**, 442.
Weller, C. V. and Christensen, A. D. (1925) *Arch. Neurol. Psychiat.* (Chicago), **14**, 97.
Wertham, F. (1932) *Arch. Neurol. Psychiat.* (Chicago), **28**, 320.
Wyllie, W. G. and Stern, R. O. (1931) *Arch. Dis. Childh.*, **6**, 137.

CHAPTER 5

NUTRITIONAL DEFICIENCIES AND DISORDERS

By A. Meyer

Vitamins (like hormones) are organic substances which are needed in minute quantities to maintain the metabolism of the tissues: their absence or lack of absorption causes characteristic diseases. The absence of other substances such as essential amino-acids and essential metallic or non-metallic elements can cause similar effects: these will also be discussed in this chapter in so far as they are of interest to the pathology of the nervous system.

No full historical account can be given here. The interested reader is referred to general accounts such as that of Bicknell and Prescott (1953). Spillane (1947) and Denny-Brown (1947) gave clinical descriptions of their experience of nutritional deficiencies during the recent war and Follis (1948, 1958) has made a comprehensive critical review of the pathological and, in particular, the experimental aspects. Recent work on vitamins as they affect the nervous system has been reviewed by Sinclair (1956) and McIlwain (1955), with emphasis on the experimental and biochemical aspects.

Vitamin deficiencies

Approximately sixteen vitamins have been isolated so far: the majority are now available in synthesised form and include the A, B, C, D, E and K groups. From the neurological and psychiatric point of view the B group is of far greater importance than any other and of this group the main members are thiamine hydrochloride (B_1), nicotinic acid (one of B_2 factors), riboflavin and pantothenic acid (B_2 group), pyridoxine (B_6) and B_{12}(anti-anaemic factor). These will be mainly considered, since the neuropathological significance of others of the B groups such as choline, biotin, inositol and para-amino-benzoic acid is at present little understood.

It must be borne in mind that deficiencies of isolated principles are rare; most deficiencies are multiple or may become so through secondary effects induced by the primary deficiency. Although present in the food, a vitamin may be deficient through lack of absorption, by being destroyed in the gut, or because its full synthesis is prevented by an adverse bacterial flora. This has been demonstrated for thiamine by Najjar and Holt (1943), and for nicotinamide by Ellinger, Coulson and Benesch (1944). It has been estimated that more than 80 per cent of the human requirement of nicotinic acid is synthesised in the intestinal tract by bacterial flora. Variations of storage capacity, rate of excretion and of general requirements which may all be increased or reduced in different metabolic conditions play an important part in the clinical picture of the deficiency. Naturally, deficiency of a vitamin may result in more severe manifestations if, for example, in thiamine deficiency carbohydrates are taken in excess.

Vitamins of the B group particularly play an important role in the metabolism of neurones. Thiamine hydrochloride, in its phosphorylated form, acts as a co-enzyme (cocarboxylase) for reactions which involve the carboxylation of pyruvate; pantothenic acid, which is a part of co-enzyme A, is also essential for the oxidation of pyruvates. Hyperpyruvaemia is, therefore, a characteristic finding in thiamine and pantothenic acid deficiencies and has, in fact, been reported to occur in both beriberi and in the Wernicke syndrome in man (Wortis, Bueding and Jolliffe 1942). According to Sinclair (1961) the oxydation of α-ketoglutaric acid to γ-amino-butyric acid (G.A.B.A.) is prevented in the absence of thiamine; the ensuing depletion of γ-amino-butyric acid in the neurone may be also a factor in the pathogenesis of neuropathies. Nicotinic acid (niacin), as diphospho- and triphospho-pyridine nucleotide, acts as co-enzyme to respiratory enzymes. Riboflavin, a dinucleotide, is a component of a number of dehydrogenase enzymes. Pyridoxine is essential for the metabolism of glutamic acid which is present in considerable amounts in the brain. In most of these reactions other substances are required. For example, in order to decarboxylate pyruvate, thiamine and pantothenic acid must be supported by lipoic acid (6:8-dithio-octanoic acid), which is another co-enzyme. Lipoic acid is formed in the liver and its deficiency may be a sequel of liver disease. According to Sinclair (1956) arsenic, mercury, pyruvate, acetaldehyde or acetoacetate combine readily with lipoic acid which is then no longer available for its reaction with thiamine and pantothenic acid and thus indirectly prevents the carboxylation of pyruvate. If this is, in fact, the behaviour of lipoic acid, the similarity of the neuropathies occurring in arsenical and mercurial poisoning, in chronic alcoholism and diabetes with those seen in vitamin B deficiency would be readily understood, although, in the strict sense, there may be no deficiency of the vitamin. However, this hypothesis has been disappointing, especially from the therapeutic point of view (Sinclair 1961). It may have been an oversimplification to expect that one factor could explain the pathogenesis of all these conditions.

Almost every vitamin has its own antivitamin. Thiaminase, which decomposes thiamine, causes deficiency (Chastek paralysis) in animals fed on raw fish in which this enzyme occurs. Pyrithiamine and oxythiamine are other antagonists of thiamine. Nicotinic acid is 'blocked' by pyridine-3-sulphuric acid (McIlwain 1940) and 3-acetylpyridine (Woolley 1945). Analogues of pyridoxine are deoxypyridoxine and methoxypyridoxine.

In the following account of individual syndromes of deficiencies and nutritional disorders more will have to be said about these important metabolic interlinkages. Here it suffices to underline the complexity of the metabolic background which explains some of the discrepant results experienced by different workers. The present writer is aware that some of the conditions included in this chapter (for example, ergotism and lathyrism) might have found a place in the previous chapter; but they have been retained here because of their relations to nutritional problems.

Thiamine deficiency

The syndromes most closely associated with thiamine deficiency are beriberi and the Wernicke syndrome.

Beriberi occurs mainly in the Far East, and in tropical climates. It has, however, been met in both great wars in other localities, particularly during the periods of famine which occurred in prisoner-of-war camps and in some of the occupied countries in Europe. Acute, subacute and chronic forms are known; furthermore, one has to distinguish between dry and wet beriberi, according to whether oedema is present or absent. Peripheral neuropathies are found more frequently in the chronic forms, where they may occur together with the characteristic heart condition and with oedema. In the infant the condition is usually acute. In such cases, particularly if they are grossly oedematous, the underlying abnormality is likely to be the sequel of a combination of protein deficiency with lack of thiamine (Platt 1958 a). Together with Lu this author (1935) was probably the first to observe marked increase of pyruvic acid and of other bisulfite binding carbonyl compounds in the blood of patients suffering from beriberi.

The heart lesion consists of acute dilatation, particularly on the right side. Oedema starting usually at the ankles spreads upwards in symmetrical fashion. The scrotum may be early involved. Polyneuritis begins distally in the lower extremities, may become widespread and include cranial nerves, the laryngeal nerves, posterior roots and the vegetative nerves.

Retrobulbar neuritis, deafness, the 'burning foot' syndrome, a bulbar myasthenic syndrome and ataxia have all been described in cases of beriberi, but they are now no longer regarded as caused by thiamine deficiency (Denny-Brown 1947, Follis).

Signs of mental disturbance seem to be rare. Platt and Gin (1934) have recorded them in only 4 per cent of cases; when persistent, it is difficult to exclude the Wernicke syndrome.

The pathology of the peripheral neuropathy (reviewed by Greenfield in 1958) was studied in numerous cases by Scheube (1884) and Pekelharing and Winkler (1887, 1893) and little has been added to these classical studies in more recent times. In earlier stages the myelin was mainly affected, but later both myelin and axon were found to be involved. The histological picture was similar to that in Wallerian degeneration, although in the proximal parts of some nerves Gombault's (1880–81) segmental demyelination was seen. Degeneration of myelin was associated with greatly increased numbers of nuclei, chiefly belonging to lipid phagocytes, but Schwann nuclei were also more numerous than normal.

The authors noted that degeneration increased towards the periphery of nerves; it was slight or absent in the large nerve trunks and usually absent in the nerve roots. As Greenfield points out, the primary attack in this parenchymatous type of neuropathy appears to be on the perikaryon, and the nutritive power of the nerve cell may be so impaired that it is no longer able to maintain its long axon which degenerates first in its peripheral part.

Both cutaneous and motor nerves were affected and also the terminal branches of the vagus in the pericardium and heart muscle. The vagus might also be severely involved more proximally, for example in its laryngeal branches; in these and the phrenic nerves the changes were usually earlier than in the nerves of the feet and legs.

With regard to the other pathological manifestations Buzzard and Greenfield's (1921) description still stands; in the wet form anasarca and hydropericardium are present together with congestion of the spleen and with nutmeg liver. In all fatal cases great dilatation of the right side of the heart has been noted. Histologically its muscle shows hydropic swelling of fibres, loss of striation and replacement of necrotic muscle by granulation tissue and fibrosis. Some of the findings recorded as present in the spinal cord are, if not due to other concomitant vitamin deficiency, likely to be secondary to the peripheral neuropathy; for example degeneration of anterior horn cells, of dorsal roots and root ganglia and of posterior spinal tracts.

The brain and its meninges show congestion and oedema. The gross softening, however, within the central nervous system, which has been mentioned in earlier reports (Pekelharing and Winkler 1893, Scheube 1894) is likely to have been due to post-mortem artefact.

The Wernicke syndrome

This syndrome was described by Wernicke in 1881 and was named by him *acute superior haemorrhagic polio-encephalitis*. Although in Wernicke's first case the cause of the syndrome was pyloric stenosis following on sulphuric acid poisoning, the condition was later attributed exclusively to chronic alcoholism by many workers. Neubürger (1936) first drew attention to its wider occurrence in 14 non-alcoholic patients, the majority of whom were suffering from carcinoma of the intestinal tract and especially of the stomach. Campbell and Biggart (1939) and Campbell and Russell (1941) stressed the nutritional aspect as a common etiological link and even suggested deficiency of vitamin B_1. Since then the syndrome has been described in many conditions, such as exhausting infectious disease, chronic gastritis, gastric ulcer and gastric carcinoma, persistent vomiting and especially hyperemesis gravidarum, and pernicious anaemia. The condition following breast milk intoxication observed by several Japanese workers seems identical with that of Wernicke (Tanaka 1934).

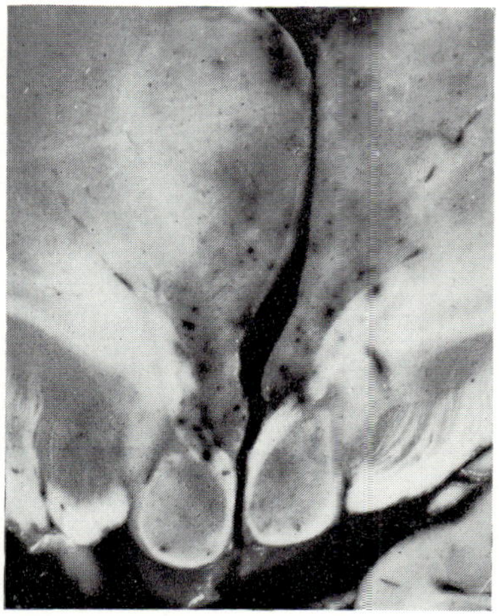

5.1

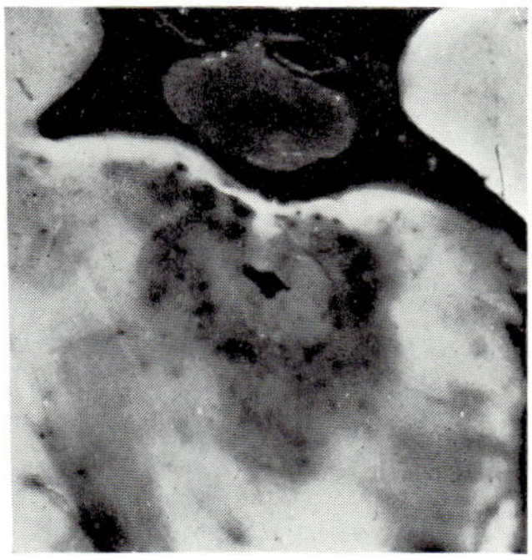

5.2

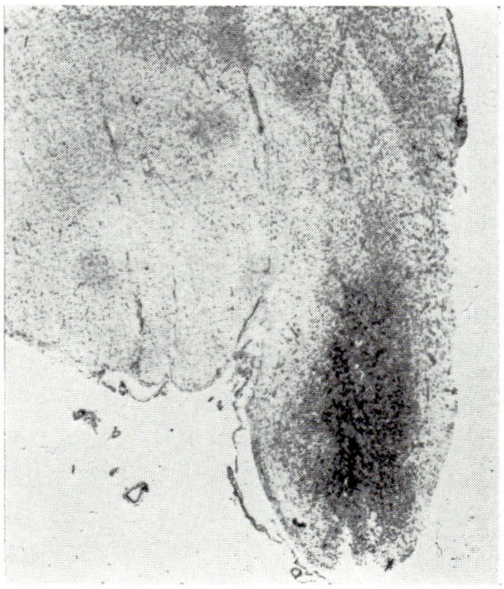

5.3

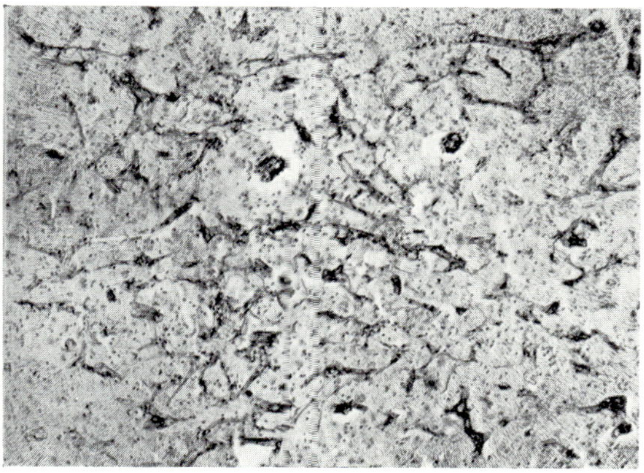

5.4

FIGS. 5.1–5.4. Wernicke syndrome.

FIGS. 5.1 and 5.2. Macroscopic appearance of haemorrhages around 3rd ventricle and aqueduct. (By the courtesy of Dr. J. B. Cavanagh.)
FIG. 5.3. Mamillary body. (Nissl ×7.)
FIG. 5.4. Mamillary body: capillary proliferation. (Holzer ×60.)

The Wernicke syndrome may be acute, subacute or chronic. *Clinically*, it is characterised by disturbances of consciousness and in many cases by ataxia and nystagmus; other less consistent signs are disturbances of the respiration, of vision and peripheral nerves. There is considerable variation of symptomatology from one case to another. In more protracted cases Korsakoff's psychosis is fairly consistently observed.

Pathological descriptions have been given by Wernicke himself, Spatz (1930), Neubürger, Campbell and Biggart and many others. The main lesions are found in the region of the 3rd and 4th ventricles, and of the aqueduct. The mamillary bodies are most consistently involved and, if petechial haemorrhages are present, may be conspicuous on naked-eye view. Other common sites, also occasionally recognisable with the naked eye by their haemorrhages, are the grey matter around the 3rd ventricle and aqueduct (Fig. 5.1 and 5.2), the inferior colliculi and the region of the vestibular and dorsal vagal nuclei. Haemorrhages, however, may be missing or scanty and the lesions can then be demonstrated only histologically. In Nissl preparations the corpora mamillaria stand out by their cellularity (Fig. 5.3), caused by the proliferation and dilatation of capillaries, of which the endothelial and adventitial cells are greatly increased. The proliferating capillaries are well demonstrated by reticulin stains, van Gieson haematoxylin stain and often, as in Fig. 5.4, by Holzer's method. Often there is also considerable proliferation of the macroglia and microglia but the latter is not transformed into lipid phagocytes. The nerve cells show degeneration, occasionally of the ischaemic type, but they have been found to be relatively spared in a number of cases.

The detail of the histological changes is similar when the lesions occur in the other localities mentioned.

Occasionally the emphasis of lesions in the hypothalamus may be not on the mamillary body, but in the anterior part of the centre (Meyer 1944) and may involve the chiasma itself which in the case described showed severe gliosis. Involvement of the optic nerves had also been seen by previous investigators (Campbell and Russell). Calcification of hypothalamic capillaries was present in Meyer's case.

Of other brain stem centres the inferior olives seem to be affected in quite a number of cases: Riggs and Boles (1944) found a lesion in this centre in 11 of 29 cases, while in the series of the present writer it was found in 4 out of 5 cases, and in the absence of appreciable involvement of the cerebellum. The medio-dorsal sector was particularly affected; the histological picture consisted of glio-mesodermal proliferation with homogenising degeneration of the nerve cells.

Earlier investigators have reported spinal cord involvement. Bonhoeffer (1899), for example, found degeneration in the posterior and lateral tracts, but it is likely that here the cause was associated deficiency of other B factors.

The *pathogenesis* of the lesions is still obscure. Most authors regard the vascular changes as primary, resulting in secondary, possibly ischaemic, degeneration of the nerve cells. Scholz (1949) has suggested increased vascular permeability as the primary change, followed by an exudate of high protein content which in its turn stimulates microglia, macroglia and the cells of the blood-vessel wall. The circumscribed occurrence of oedema in this unusual site remains, however, unexplained. A toxic effect of pyruvic acid upon grey matter in the walls and beneath the floor of the 3rd and 4th ventricles and the aqueduct or, alternatively, increased requirements of the vitamin by the affected centres have been suggested as pathogenic possibilities, but, so far, there is no proof for either.

The localisation of the Wernicke syndrome in centres of the hypothalamus and in particular in the corpus mammillare has naturally aroused considerable theoretical interest. The results of experimental investigation indicate that the region of the mamillary body and of the posterior nucleus of the hypothalamus is concerned with the maintenance of consciousness and the waking state. Clouding of consciousness, stupor and coma would then be the natural consequence of their impairment. Gamper (1928) was the first to draw attention to the association of mamillary lesion with Korsakoff's psychosis in the more chronic forms of the Wernicke syndrome, but it should be remembered that this psychosis may be caused also by lesions different in type and localisation. In all their 5 cases of alcoholism Korsakoff, Carmichael and Stern (1931) found widespread nerve cell change in the cerebral cortex (increased lipochrome deposits and central chromatolysis). These changes (as the authors themselves emphasised) appear more closely related to Pellagra than to vitamin B_1 deficiency. Although clinically Korsakoff's psychosis is often preceded by delirium tremens, the pathology of the latter condition has not been clearly established. Widespread nerve cell degeneration of the type common to toxic conditions, and with no special emphasis on the diencephalic region, has been described by many early authors, and more recently by Zahnd (1953). As delirium tremens is a reversible condition, it may be that, during this stage, the pathology is in the nature of a biochemical lesion. Such an explanation might have the support of Huber (1954) who interpreted small recent periventricular haemorrhages and perivascular oedema, found in 9 cases of typical alcoholic delirium, as an initial stage of the Wernicke syndrome.

Other clinical phenomena of the Wernicke syndrome are well explained by the pathology:

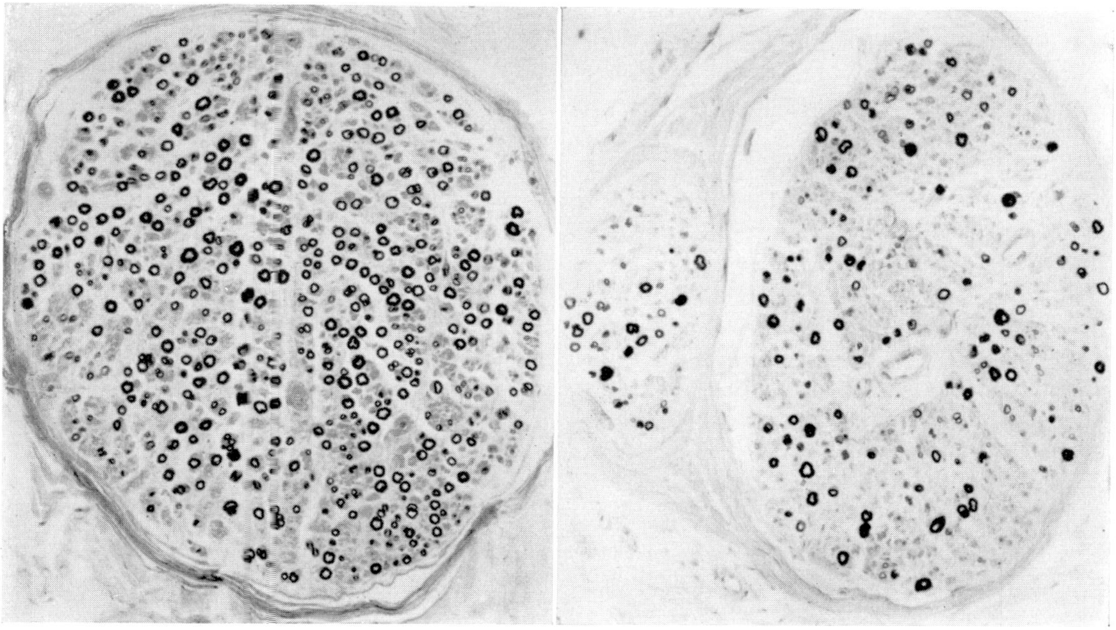

(a) (b)

FIG. 5.5. Alcoholic neuropathy. Sections of fascicles from terminal cutaneous branch of anterior tibial nerve; stained by osmic acid (× 200). (a) Normal nerve. (b) Alcoholic neuropathy.

the disturbance of eye muscles by the peri-aqueductal lesions, ataxia and nystagmus by the affection of the vestibular nuclei, the respiratory disturbance by involvement of the dorsal vagal nucleus and the occasional impairment of vision by involvement of chiasma, optic nerves or by retinal haemorrhages.

Not all cases of the Wernicke syndrome are fatal. Both Neubürger and Campbell and Russell have reported instances of older scars in the characteristic localisation in cases of typical etiology which were found after intercurrent death. One of Campbell and Russell's cases recovered in response to vitamin B_1 therapy. Ule (1959) described an encephalopathy in children which he considered to be qualitatively similar to Wernicke's syndrome, although the lesions affected the lower brain stem and not the mammillary bodies. Neither the history, however, nor the clinical symptomatology, corresponded to that usually found in cases of the Wernicke syndrome. It is possible that the author was dealing with the infantile subacute necrotising encephalopathy, first described by Leigh (1951), and which will be found reviewed on page 407.

Alcoholic peripheral neuropathy. The evidence incriminating lack of some vitamin B factor, especially thiamine, in such cases came first from the response of early cases to parenteral treatment with this vitamin and more recently from the study, in cases of peripheral neuropathy, of the urinary excretion of thiamine or of the blood pyruvate levels, especially after loading doses of glucose (Bueding *et al.* 1942, Joiner *et al.* 1950). The clinical and pathological resemblance of alcoholic neuropathy to beriberi has been stressed by Victor and Adams (1953). According to Greenfield (1958), the neuropathy affects motor and sensory neurones in varying proportions; it is most severe in the distal parts of the nerves, so that the extensors of the feet and toes are most commonly affected, and next to them the extensors of the wrist and fingers. Position sense may be early and severely affected in the ataxic form. This type of sensory loss indicates a greater degeneration of large fibres than of small, and this was confirmed by histograms of the small cutaneous nerve to the toes (Greenfield and Carmichael 1935) (Fig. 5.5). Both they and Aring and Spies (1939) found less evidence of axonal lesions. There was practically no restoration of myelin as long as 11 months after treatment had begun in the cases examined by the latter.

In occasional cases the degeneration of the sensory neurone can be traced into the dorsal columns of the spinal cord, but these may be intact even in severely paralysed cases (Carmichael and Stern 1931). The anterior horn cells, especially in the lower lumbar and upper sacral segments of the spinal cord, often show a varying degree of chromatolysis in severe cases.

Experimental thiamine deficiency. Numerous experimental investigations have been carried out in species ranging from pigeons to primates and, in a limited way, in man. These include the pioneer studies by Eijkman (1897) and Fraser and Stanton (1910), which established the deficiency nature of the lesions. They also include the fundamental investigations in pigeons and rats by Peters and his associates Sinclair and Thompson (1933, 1934), who discovered that, in the absence of thiamine, oxidation of pyruvic acid is prevented.

Hyperpyruvaemia was observed in all species following any appreciable fall of the blood thiamine level. Bradycardia, dilatation of heart and electrocardiographic changes, atrioventricular block and auricular fibrillation were observed in a number of species (Follis *et al.* 1943) and the clinical findings confirmed at post-mortem. Microscopically, the lesions are described as multiple necrosis of heart-muscle fibres. Their pathogenesis is attributed to the known metabolic effects of thiamine deficiency.

In man, in whom only relatively mild degrees of deficiency have been experimentally induced, clinical and electrocardiographic changes in the heart have been recorded (Williams *et al.* 1942).

The evidence for polyneuritis has been criticised by Follis (1948) because in the earlier series of experimental investigations the diet consisted of polished rice, which is deficient in factors other than thiamine. In pigeons, there have, however, been fairly convincing descriptions of neuritis by Bertrand *et al.* (1934), Swank (1940), Swank and Prados (1942), Zimmerman (1943) and Shaw and Phillips (1945). While North and Sinclair (1956) succeeded in producing degeneration in the distal segments of the sciatic and posterior tibial nerves of rats, they emphasised that the tissue was relatively resistant and yielded lesions only after prolonged deficiency. Even then, only 3–5 per cent of the fibres were affected. This may, to some extent, explain the negative results of other experimental investigators. An alternative explanation has been offered by Scriba and Luckner (1949) and Luckner and Scriba (1949), who claimed that a complete experimental equivalent of tropical human beriberi and its triad of heart failure, oedema and peripheral neuropathy could be produced in albino rats, fed on a diet poor in protein as well as in thiamine. Their views are in accordance with those of Platt (1958 a). These authors give, however, no histological detail of the nerve degeneration. North and Sinclair (1957) were unable to produce peripheral nerve degeneration in rats repeatedly submitted to short periods of thiamine (and pantothenic acid) deficiency.

Lesions which more or less resemble those seen in the human Wernicke syndrome have been produced by many experimental workers in animals suffering chronic thiamine deficiency: Prickett (1934) described haemorrhages and (unspecific) nerve cell changes with predilection for vestibular nuclei in rats. Alexander and his collaborators (1938, 1940) produced, in pigeons, haemorrhagic vascular lesions within periventricular grey centres which closely resembled the pseudoencephalitic histopathology of the Wernicke syndrome; these findings have been confirmed in pigeons and dogs by Zimmerman (1939, 1943); in pigeons by Prados and Swank (1942); in mice by Dunn *et al.* (1947), and in rats by Ule and Kammerer (1960). Rinehart *et al.* (1947, 1949) succeeded in obtaining foci of necrosis in the mammillary bodies, corpora quadrigemina, and in the nuclei of the 3rd, 6th, 8th and 10th cranial nerve; in addition, they described similar lesions in unusual sites such as the striatum, globus pallidus, substantia nigra; they failed to produce peripheral nerve degeneration. Alexander (1940) considered the changes of the blood vessels to be primary, attributing antiangionecrotic properties to thiamine. This view is not shared by Prados and Swank, Rinehart and others, who see the vascular proliferation as a reaction to primary neuronal damage—in contrast to the commonly held views on the pathogenesis of the human disease.

Wernicke-like findings in the brain have been reported also in foxes suffering from Chastek paralysis (Alexander *et al.* 1941, Evans *et al.* 1942) and in a similar, spontaneous disease of cats (Jubb *et al.* 1956). In both, a raw fish diet, which contains a thiamine destroying enzyme was implicated. The response to thiamine therapy was marked.

Most recent reviewers including Cruickshank (1952), Sinclair (1956) and Denny-Brown (1958) consider there is suggestive experimental evidence that thiamine deficiency plays a major or at least an initiating part in some essential features of beriberi as well as of the Wernicke syndrome. Follis, who in 1948, had been sceptical about the aetiological role of thiamine, accepts the evidence of the cerebral experimental data, in his 1958 edition, although he remains doubtful about findings in the peripheral nerves of mammals.

According to Sinclair (1956), the sequence of events in so far as they are at present known is as follows: pyruvic acid and apparently also pyruvic aldehyde accumulate; the resulting impairment of metabolism has a particularly noxious effect on those cells which depend entirely on carbohydrate metabolism (nerve cells), use pyruvate extensively (cardiac muscle), or require thiamine (and pantothenic acid) for the synthesis of acetylcholine as many nerve fibres do. Relatively acute and profound deficiency brings about the vascular changes of Wernicke's encephalopathy or the cardiac changes of acute beriberi. In chronic mild deficiency the effect is mainly on the peripheral nerves. The oedema which is a characteristic early symptom of thiamine deficiency appears to be a result of the anorexia induced by the deficiency. It is identical with the oedema which occurs in diets low in calories.

Sinclair's pathogenetic views must, as he admits, be regarded as provisional. They provide only a rough outline of events: they do not explain, for example, why in acute thiamine deficiency, emphasis in some cases is on the heart, in others on the central nervous system; and the selectivity of the lesions, in the human Wernicke syndrome, is not fully explained.

Vitamins of the B_2 group

Pantothenic acid

Deficiency of *pantothenic acid* will be considered first not because it is the most important member of this group, but because it is more closely related to thiamine deficiency than other members. Like thiamine, pantothenic acid is intimately concerned with the oxidation of pyruvate, its absence or 'blocking' likewise resulting in hyperpyruvaemia. As co-enzyme A, it is an important catalyser of the acetylation of acetylcholine. It was for this reason that Follis (1948) and his collaborators thought that many lesions ascribed to thiamine-lack may be caused by deficiency of pantothenate. This, however, has not been confirmed (North and Sinclair 1957).

Pantothenic acid has been proved to be indispensable in a variety of animals. Its absence in rats results in alopecia, greying of the hair and generalised dermatitis; it may also lead to ulceration of the gastro-intestinal tract, particularly of the colon. Haemorrhagic necrosis of the adrenal has been reported in rats, though not in other animals, although a suggestive acute syndrome of sudden prostration, coma, tachycardia and convulsions has been described in dogs deprived of pantothenic acid (Schaefer *et al.* 1942). In monkeys made deficient by McCall *et al.* (1946) ataxia was the main clinical symptom. Follis and Wintrobe (1945) and Swank and Adams (1948) have obtained lesions in the nervous system in swine: they observed degeneration of peripheral nerves, the posterior roots and their ganglia and the posterior columns of the cord. The earliest lesion was central chromatolysis in nerve cells of the posterior root ganglia which was present before degeneration of myelin and axis cylinders could be detected in nerves, dorsal roots or posterior columns. Central chromatolysis was also found in some anterior horn cells; occasionally degeneration was seen in pyramidal tracts.

Pantothenic acid deficiency has not been of appreciable significance in man. It has been suggested (Gopalan 1946, and others) that the 'burning feet' syndrome may be due, at least in part, to pantothenic acid deficiency. Human volunteers in whom deficiency was induced by Bean, Hodges and Daum (1955)—either by a diet devoid of the vitamin or by administration of its antagonist ω-methyl pantothenic acid—showed signs of fatigue and paraesthesias of the 'burning feet' quality which seemed to respond to large doses of the vitamin. The number of subjects was small, however, and Sinclair (1961) considers the aetiology to be undecided.

Nicotinic acid

Pellagra is the condition of outstanding interest in relation to nicotinic acid deficiency; it was known in eighteenth-century Spain and it received its present name (from *pelle* = skin and *agra* = rough) from peasants in Northern Italy. At first intoxication and later bacterial infection were thought to be its causation until, through the clinical studies of Goldberger and Wheeler (1915, 1920), its relation to deficiency was demonstrated both in human patients and in 'black tongue' disease in dogs, which has similar clinical symptomatology.

Clinically pellagra is characterised by lesions of the skin and the mucous membranes, and by neurological and psychiatric disturbances. The skin lesions are characteristic; they begin as erythema and lead on to atrophy. Diarrhoea, glossitis, gastric achylia and anaemia are prominent signs. Changes in the nervous system develop later; polyneuritis, spastic paralysis and ataxia, tremor and rigidity, visual disturbances (particularly retrobulbar neuritis) and deafness have all been described. Mental change may be an early symptom; initially this may be of a 'psychoneurotic' type, which later develops into depressive or excited states, followed in advanced cases by progressive dementia. Epileptic convulsions are not uncommon.

Usually pellagra takes a chronic intermittent course over several years, and morphological lesions of the central nervous system appear only in the later stages.

An acute syndrome has been reported by various authors (Jolliffe *et al.* 1940, Sydenstricker *et al.* 1941, Hardwick 1943, Spillane 1947) and has been named *nicotinic acid deficiency encephalopathy*. The clinical picture consists of clouding of consciousness, cogwheel rigidity and grasping and sucking reflexes. The patients are usually elderly, suffering from organic disease and often living on inadequate diet. Other established signs of B deficiency are frequently present. Patients suffering from this syndrome seem to respond dramatically to nicotinic acid therapy.

A syndrome exhibiting pellagra-like symptoms (light-sensitive dermatitis, cerebellar ataxia and psychotic manifestations has recently been described by Baron *et al.* (1956). Cases described by Hersov (1955), Rodnight and McIlwain (1955), and Hersov and Rodnight (1960), though originally interpreted differently, have been identified as the same condition. It has been given the name 'Hartnup disease' after one of the affected families. Biochemically, it is characterised by a pronounced and persistent amino-aciduria of a special pattern and an abnormally large output of indolic compounds. Baron *et al.* have suggested an enzymatic deficiency in the formation of nicotinic acid from tryptophan. To the writer's knowledge no post-mortem investigations have so far been made.

Pathological studies. Investigations of the nervous system have been carried out by Wilson (1914), Raubitschek (1915), Pentschew (1928), Greenfield and Holmes (1939), Hsü (1942) and Leigh (1952) among many others.

Most workers agree that the change most consistently found in pellagrous brains is central chromatolysis, first described as 'central neuritis' by Meyer (1901). Investigators differ about its distribution. Leigh, in 14 cases, found the highest incidence in Betz cells, followed, in that order, by pontine nuclei (Fig. 5.7), dorsal vagal nuclei, gracile and cuneate nuclei, nucleus ambiguus, descending trigeminal nucleus, oculomotor nuclei, basal ganglia, vestibular nuclei and reticular and arcuate nuclei. Of the six spinal cords available, central chromatolysis of anterior horn cells was seen in four (Fig. 5.6). Hypoglossal and facial nuclei, and the Purkinje cells of the cerebellum, although among the largest neurones, were not affected. Axonal damage is too inconstant in the central nervous system to account for this cell change, which is more likely to be related to a metabolic process associated with the deficiency.

Proliferation of the neuroglia is rare and insignificant. The fibrosis and hyalin change of the blood-vessels emphasised by Hsü was encountered infrequently in Leigh's material; increase of lipofuscin is, according to Hsü, often seen in pellagra, but this likewise was not a prominent feature in Leigh's material.

In addition to central chromatolysis, degeneration of the posterior and lateral tracts of the cord has received much attention. It was the most frequent combination of spinal cord lesions in Wilson's cases. In Wilson's and in Greenfield and Holmes' case, the degeneration was most severe in the fasciculus gracilis, with lesions of lesser severity in the spinocerebellar and crossed and uncrossed pyramidal tracts (Fig. 5.8). Of 13 Chinese soldiers who died from inanition Hsü saw degeneration of the posterior columns in most.

This type of combined degeneration of posterior and lateral tracts differs histologically from the affection of the same fibre systems seen in subacute combined degeneration. The characteristic honeycombed appearance caused by discontinuous degeneration of myelin sheaths in the latter condition is absent in the pellagrous cord which has more of the nature of secondary (Wallerian) degeneration.

Both posterior and anterior roots have been found to be affected in the cases of Greenfield and Holmes as well as of Wilson. Involvement of the peripheral nerves has also been noted by many workers (for example by Wilson, Aring *et al.* 1941, and Greenfield and Carmichael 1935). The last-mentioned authors, counting the fibres in the cutaneous nerves of the toe, found that in pellagrins the highest count was 5,500, whereas in normal nerves the number of fibres per square millimetre lay between 6,500 and 9,000. In severe cases both myelin and axons showed signs of degeneration, while in milder cases only the myelin was affected.

While all these central and peripheral lesions may occur together, experience in the recent

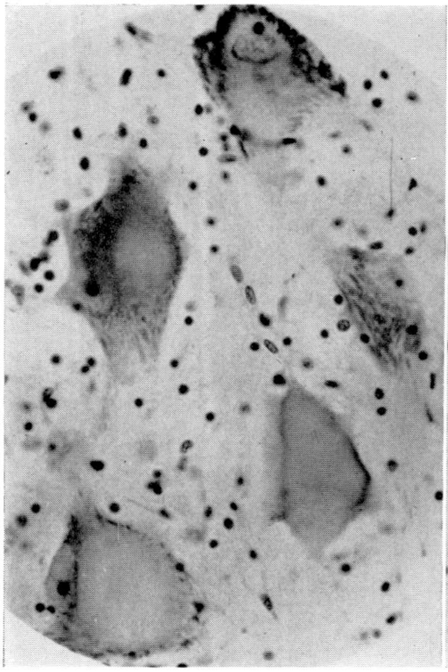

5.6

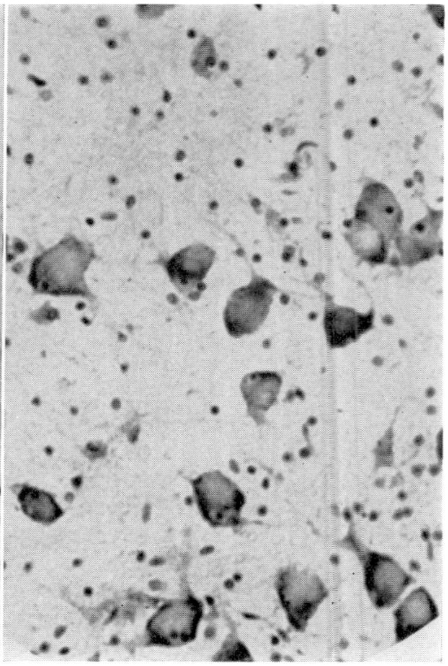

5.7

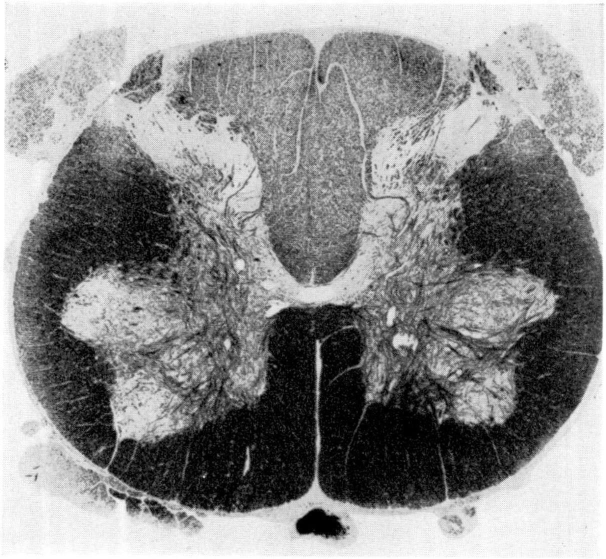

5.8

FIGS. 5.6–5.8. Pellagra.

FIG. 5.6. Central chromatolysis in anterior horn cells. (Nissl ×250.)

FIG. 5.7. Central chromatolysis in pontine cells. (Nissl ×250.) (By the courtesy of Dr. Leigh.)

FIG. 5.8. Lumbar cord in pellagra. Note severe degeneration of the dorsal columns and slighter pallor of the pyramidal tracts. (Myelin.)

war has made it clear that certain component syndromes of pellagra may occur independently. Polyneuritis, for example, is likely to be an admixture rather than an integral part of pellagra and due probably to deficiency of other vitamins, thiamine or other components of the B_2 complex. The combined degeneration of posterior and lateral columns identical with that described in pellagra has been shown to occur as an isolated deficiency syndrome, often combined with retrobulbar neuritis and deafness. Pathological investigations have been carried out only in one case reported by Spillane in which Greenfield observed degeneration in the Sommer sector of the cornu ammonis, central chromatolysis of a few Betz cells and disintegration of Corti's organ. Lesions of Ammon's horn have not been reported to be common in pellagra and related deficiency syndromes. They were, for example, absent in all 14 cases of Leigh's material. In the case under discussion the lesion in Ammon's horn must have been recent since eosinophilic 'ghost' cells were still seen. It is, perhaps, possible that the degeneration of Ammon's horn was due to the terminal condition of the patient who jumped from a water tower and died from multiple injuries 10 days later.

Biochemical and experimental studies. Since Elvehjem *et al.* (1937) showed that nicotinic acid could cure black tongue in dogs, it has been accepted that nicotinic acid deficiency is a major factor in the causation of pellagra. Black tongue is not only clinically similar to human pellagra; Denton (1928), who studied Goldberger's dogs, described lesions of the skin and mucous membranes which were histologically essentially the same as those in human pellagra. Histological changes in the central nervous system were not reported by Denton. Nor did Pentschew (1929) discover histological abnormalities in the nervous system of the macaque which had developed pellagra-like symptoms in the course of poisoning with ergotamine. The degeneration reported by Stern and Findlay (1929) in anterior horn cells in the spinal cord of rats, fed on a diet poor in vitamin B_2, were nonspecific and not comparable with the central chromatolysis of human pellagra. Although Scherer (1944) claimed to have observed central chromatolysis in cranial nuclei and anterior horns of a chimpanzee suffering from hair outfall and paralysis, there is no proof that the underlying condition was a sequel of nicotinic acid deficiency. The results of experiments with analogues of niacin have been equally puzzling. Hicks (1955), using 3-acetyl-pyridine in mice and rats, saw widespread necrosis (eosinophilia of cytoplasm, pyknosis of nuclei) in nerve cells of the spinal and sympathetic ganglia, supra-optic nucleus and the pyramidal layer of Ammon's horn; less frequently in the medial amygdaloid nucleus and in cell groups of the medulla. There had been no convulsions. The lesions could be prevented by antecedent treatment with nicotinamide. Mice kept on a diet devoid of nicotinamide showed no comparable lesions. Coggleshall and MacLean (1958), also experimenting with 3-acetyl-pyridine in mice and rats, obtained lesions confined almost exclusively to Lorente de Nó's areas C3 and C4 of Ammon's horn (though, according to the illustrations, the lesions seem to go beyond the so-called endblade); cell loss in these regions was not, however, accompanied by glial increase. The animals developed an apparent weakness, inspiratory ronchi and urinary incontinence within 6 hours after administration. Of those that survived the acute stage, the majority showed the histological change. The authors discuss the significance of this finding in relation to the particular metabolism of the hippocampus, but like Hicks, they failed to produce lesions comparable to those found in human pellagra. Pinsky and Fraser (1960) gave pregnant mice a single dose of yet another analogue, 6-amino-nicotinamide, and produced weakness within 6–12 hours. Their paper, which does not contain neurohistological investigations, is nevertheless of interest because this temporary inactivation of nicotinamide gave rise to congenital malformations in the off-spring. Experimenting with rats, cats and dogs which were inoculated with 6-amino-nicotinamide, Sternberg and Philips (1958) and Wolf, Cowen and Geller (1959, 1962) described lesions different from those obtained with other antinicotinamides: they were confined mainly to the anterior horns and some nuclei of the medulla, and presented with petechial haemorrhages, chromatolysis, often proceeding to necrosis of nerve cells, and with microglial, endothelial and inflammatory reaction. Wolf *et al.* (1962), reviewing also other recent work, suggest that the difference in localisation and quality of the lesions may be due to action upon different radicles of nicotinamide. This important problem invites further histological and biochemical investigation.

Absence of nicotinic acid from the food is only a partial factor. The greater part of the requirements is met by biosynthesis by the bacterial flora of the intestines, and destruction of these bacteria by certain sulphonamides has been held responsible for pellagrous symptoms. The amino-acid tryptophan seems to be the source from which nicotinic acid is synthesised; the absence of this amino-acid from maize is probably the explanation why an exclusive maize diet often results in pellagra. Moreover, Woolley (1946) has isolated a pellagragenic factor in maize, which may be chemically related to one of the acetyl-pyridins, with anti-nicotinic properties (*vide* McIlwain 1955).

The multiple nature of the deficiency in experimental pellagra has been well demonstrated and to some extent clarified in experiments under varying conditions and in several species by Krehl and collaborators (1945) in dogs and rats and by Wintrobe *et al.* (1945) in swine. A diet poor in nicotinamide but sufficient in thiamine, riboflavin, pantothenic acid and choline, combined with optimal amount of protein has no or few ill effects, but on lessening the protein intake signs of deficiency develop. In such animals chromatolysis in the small nerve cells of the dorsal root ganglia has been reported; but there was no myelin degeneration in peripheral nerves.

From a review of all the experimental and clinico-pathological evidence Follis (1948) concluded that pellagra is the result of a diet poor in protein, reduced in nicotinic acid and probably also containing either toxic or anti-vitamin substances. The classical symptomatology of pellagra is, therefore, not the result of any single deficiency. The neurohistological picture of pure nicotinic acid deficiency is not yet fully known, whether in the human or in the experimental animal.

Riboflavin

Riboflavin was the first constituent of an enzyme system to be isolated (in 1933) and synthesised (in 1935). As riboflavin-phosphate it is part of several 'yellow' flavoprotein enzymes and in combination with adenylic acid functions as co-enzyme in the dehydrogenase group.

In experimental animals of various species the most prominent changes resulting from its lack occur in the skin, eyes and nervous system. The skin lesions, which seem to vary among different species in extent and quality, consist of a dermatitis which brings about atrophy of sebaceous glands and hair follicles. In some species this seems to be most marked in the angle of the mouth and the nasolabial folds. With regard to the eyes Bessey and Wolbach (1939) have drawn attention to abnormal capillary growth in the cornea, which either is due to preceding damage to the epithelium or is a compensatory mechanism to defective cellular oxidative metabolism. Cataracts have been observed in rats and swine.

Myelin degeneration has been described in experimental animals—in peripheral nerves and in the fibre tracts of the spinal cord, and especially in the dorsal column—by Shaw and Phillips (1941) in rats; Street, Cowgill and Zimmerman (1941) in dogs; Lippincot and Morris (1942) in mice and Wintrobe *et al.* (1944) in young pigs. All these lesions have been designated 'equivocal' by Follis—not without justification.

In man the main change, experimentally produced by Sebrell and Butler (1939), is a dermatitis about the mouth resulting in fissure formation (cheilosis) and reddening of the lips. Vascularisation of the cornea, which occasionally results in ulceration, has been reported. It was at one time thought that combined tract degeneration, retrobulbar neuritis and deafness might be due to deficiency of riboflavin, but experimental experience in human volunteers has so far not resulted in any lesion of the peripheral or central nervous system.

Pyridoxine (vitamin B_6)

In 1926 Goldberger and Lillie described a pellagra-like condition in rats fed on a maize diet extracted by alcohol. Later György (1934) and his collaborators excluded nicotinic acid and riboflavin as causative agents and identified another factor, B_6, or lactoflavine as the responsible factor. Pyridoxine seems to be important in protein metabolism.

Pathological lesions have been described in several animal species. They are most prominent in skin, erythropoietic tissue and in the nervous system. The skin lesions consist of pellagra-like symmetrical dermatitis, which, however, is not influenced by sunlight. Anaemia (usually normocytic) develops, the liver may show fatty infiltration and there may be extensive deposits of iron pigment in liver, spleen and bone marrow. Rinehart and Greenberg (1956), amplifying earlier investigations, found intimal proliferation of many arteries, which closely resembled human arteriosclerosis and which developed in monkeys following complete deprivation of pyridoxine for 5–6 months. Blood pressure seems to have been persistently raised. This arterial syndrome was often accompanied by cirrhosis of the liver and by dental caries.

Among the signs of disturbed nervous function epileptiform fits lasting several minutes have been described in rats and pigs (Chick *et al.* 1940, Wintrobe *et al.* 1943). These epileptic phenomena, consisting of grand mal and also of what resembles petit mal attacks, readily respond to therapy. Demyelination of peripheral nerves, dorsal root fibres and of fibres running in the dorsal columns has been described, but early chromatolysis of dorsal root ganglia has not been observed (Folks and Wintrobe, Swank and Adams), although later the cells atrophy and may disappear.

Pyridoxal phosphate is of great importance in the conversion of glutamic acid to γ-aminobutyric acid (gaba) which is now considered to be a principal inhibitor of nerve cell function (Roberts 1961; Tower 1961, *vide* also page 610).

The convulsions of infancy are favourably influenced by pyridoxine (Hunt *et al.* 1954, and others). Deoxypyridoxine, an antagonist of this vitamin, has been reported to bring about in man a peripheral neuropathy which is relieved by pyridoxine (Vilter *et al.* 1953). The cause of the peripheral neuropathy, which may complicate isoniazid therapy, is considered to be that it combines with pyridoxine to form a stable compound which, thus, blocks the latter's function. Pyridoxal phosphate is also required for the conversion of 5-hydroxytryptophan into 5-hydroxytryptamine (serotonin). Deficiency of pyridoxine may thus reduce the level of serotonin in the brain.

Purpura and Gonzalez-Monteagudo (1960) produced in cats a necrosis in the endblade of the hippocampus (areas C_3 and C_4 of Lorente de Nó) which developed within 2 hours after a single injection of methoxypyridoxine. In Nissl preparations the nerve cells appeared shrunken, deeply basophilic and with complete loss of intracellular architecture. In view of the incidence of convulsions, the authors stress that they failed to produce similar changes within so short a time either by hypoxia or by metrazol and strychnine. The animals had been paralysed with succinylcholine chloride. It is of interest that the lesions occurred in the same localisation as those reported above following administration of analogues of nicotinic acid. Confirmation on a systematic basis seems to be called for.

Vitamin B_{12} neuropathy (subacute combined degeneration of the spinal cord). By J. G. GREENFIELD and A. MEYER.

Leichtenstern (1884) reported the association of pernicious anaemia with disease of the spinal cord but he considered that the anaemia came on in the course of tabes dorsalis and did not describe the spinal lesion except as being typical of that disease. Lichtheim (1887) appears to have been the first to recognise that the spinal lesions of pernicious anaemia differed in several respects from those of tabes. They were subacute, as shown both by the short history and by the numerous lipid phagocytes in the damaged tracts of the cord, and they involved both the dorsal columns and numerous areas in the anterolateral columns. They differed also in that there was no thickening of the leptomeninges and only slight atrophy of the dorsal nerve roots in the lumbar region. His pupil Minnich (1892) supplemented these observations by examining the spinal cord of 5 cases of pernicious anaemia with no nervous symptoms, and by finding in them slight degeneration in the dorsal and lateral columns.

The first full clinical and pathological description of the disease was given by Russell, Batten and Collier (1900) who used the name *subacute combined degeneration of the spinal cord.* They were not satisfied with this name but were unable to suggest a better. Other names which have been suggested such as 'funicular myelopathy' and 'posterolateral sclerosis' are pathologically incorrect and have not been generally accepted. The name subacute combined degeneration gives no indication of the constant relation of the spinal lesions to megalocytic anaemia; in fact this was not accepted by Russell, Batten and Collier in some of whose cases there was no obvious anaemia. Nor does it indicate involvement of peripheral nerves and, in some cases, of the brain. For this reason, Richmond and Davidson (1958) have proposed the term Vitamin B_{12} neuropathy and this has been adopted here.

Synthesis of crystalline B_{12} (cyanocobalamin) by Lester-Smith (1948) and Rickes *et al.* (1948) marks the culminating point—hitherto—in the evolution which began with the empirical discovery of treatment of liver for pernicious anaemia by Minot and Murphy (1926–7), the distinction of intrinsic (gastric) and extrinsic factors by (Castle 1929), and the identification and eventual synthesis of folic acid by 1946. Vitamin B_{12} has greatly reduced mortality from subacute combined degeneration by prevention, by cure of early cases and by arrest of the fully-developed disease. Folic acid, however, although it has an effect on megalocytic anaemia, is powerless both in the treatment and in the prevention of the spinal cord syndrome. While B_{12} is now recognised to be Castle's extrinsic factor, the intrinsic factor is still unidentified. The latter is considered by many to be in the nature of a mucoprotein, which serves as a carrier for vitamin B_{12}; this, however, may be, according to Witts (1961), an 'ignis fatuus'. In the human stomach the site of the intrinsic factor is in the wall of the body, whilst in many animals it is found near the pylorus or in the jejunum; this has led to much confusion in experimental research.

The observation by Hurst and Bell (1922) that in cases of subacute combined degeneration achlorhydria was always present, has led to too rigid an identification with Addisonian pernicious anaemia in which there is hereditary atrophy of the gastric mucosa. Richmond and Davison have pointed out, that while Addisonian anaemia is by far the commonest cause of B_{12} neuropathy, one among every seven cases had other aetiologies which included other diseases of the gastric mucosa (such as total or substantial gastrectomy, or gastric carcinoma), malabsorption of vitamin B_{12} as a sequel of organic and functional disorder of the intestine (strictures, fistulae, diverticula, infiltration with tuberculosis or tumour, idiopathic and tropical sprue), and finally following on reduced source of the vitamin in food intake. These authors were able to collect 10 (histologically not verified) cases in the literature which come within these non-Addisonian categories; they were able to add 3 histologically investigated new cases.

Vegetarian diet is poor in vitamin B_{12}. Wokes, Badenoch and Sinclair (1955) and Wokes (1956) interestingly found the serum values of B_{12} significantly low in a group of British vegans which showed also an excess of *p*-hydroxyl-phenyl-pyruvic acid in the blood serum. These abnormalities were most marked during the first 6–10 years of this dietary regime and petered out in later years. Anaemia was slight and no definite signs of neuropathy were recorded. However, Badenoch (1954) has recorded definite clinical signs of B_{12} neuropathy in a 15-year-old boy who was a strict vegetarian and whose symptoms improved dramatically following treatment with the vitamin.

Clinical features. The term *subacute* describes the course of most untreated cases in which nervous symptoms increase fairly rapidly and cause severe disability in a few weeks or months. The course may be more rapid so that the patient becomes unable to stand in 2 or 3 weeks or it may be more gradual and allow the patient to continue at work for a year or more. Russell *et al.* distinguished three stages in the disease. (1) A stage of slight spastic paraplegia with slight ataxia and marked subjective sensations in the lower limbs. These consist of numbness, stiffness or tingling and may precede the onset of motor symptoms by several months. The upper limbs may be similarly affected either at the same time as, or more often after, the lower limbs. Clumsiness in writing is often an early symptom. (2) A stage of severe ataxic paraplegia with marked anaesthesia of the legs and trunk. This stage may come on very rapidly so that a patient who was able to walk on going to bed at night is unable to stand the next morning. This disability is due more to ataxia than to weakness. (3) Their 3rd stage, that of complete paraplegia with absolute anaesthesia leading to death from bed-sores and infection of the urinary tract, is seldom seen in treated patients. The chief danger at the present time is to patients in the first stage, in whom the anaemia is slight and the nature of the early, largely subjective, nervous symptoms is not recognised. While recovery from the first stage is usually remarkably complete under adequate treatment, the transition in untreated patients from the first to the second stage may be so rapid that it cannot be arrested before grave and irremediable damage has been done to the spinal cord.

Heaton *et al.* (1958) found the B_{12} serum level to be lower in 13 patients suffering from tobacco amblyopia than in normal controls. Their patients did not exhibit other neurological abnormalities; amblyopia, however, may be an early symptom of B_{12} deficiency.

A variety of mental changes has been observed. They range from neurasthenia and depression to confusional states, amnesic syndromes and dementia; several workers (Ferraro *et al.* 1945, Mayer-Gross *et al.* 1954) have stressed the frequency of paranoid psychoses. The over-all incidence of mental disorder has been estimated by Woltman (1924) to be 4 per cent of nearly 1,500 cases of pernicious anaemia observed at the Mayo Clinic, but it is not clear whether this figure includes the minor affective aberrations. Epileptic seizures occasionally occur.

Pathology. Russell *et al.* noted that the stress of the disease fell on the mid-thoracic segments of the cord, where a zone of destruction of white matter might be seen all round the cord, affecting not only the long tracts but endogenous and exogenous fibres alike. In severe cases the only intact fibres at this level were those in close relation to the grey horns (Fig. 5.11). On tracing the degeneration upwards it diminished, especially in the ventrolateral columns, until in the upper cervical segments only the dorsal columns, especially the funiculus gracilis, and the spinocerebellar tracts were demyelinated. Degeneration in the pyramidal tract may begin in some cases as high as the medullary pyramids, but these are usually normal. On passing

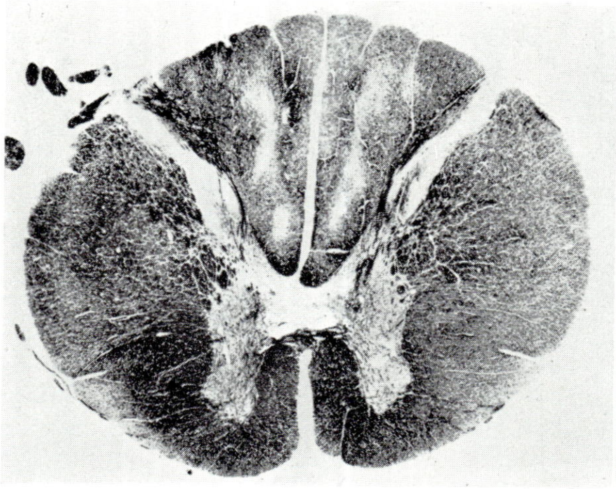

5·9

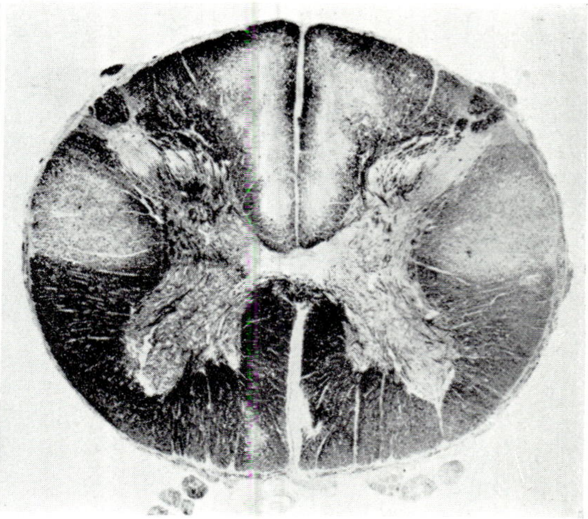

5.10

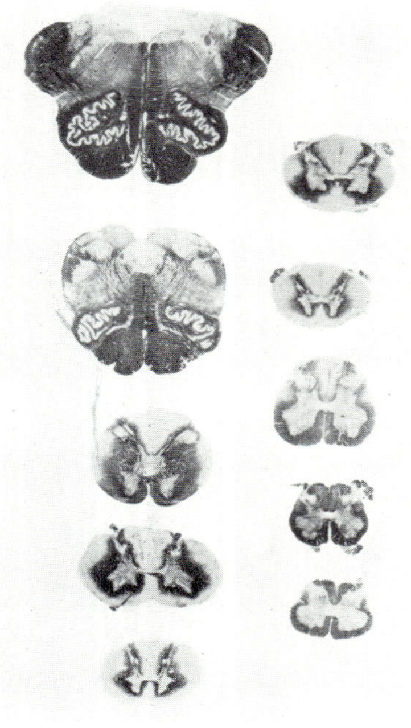

5.11

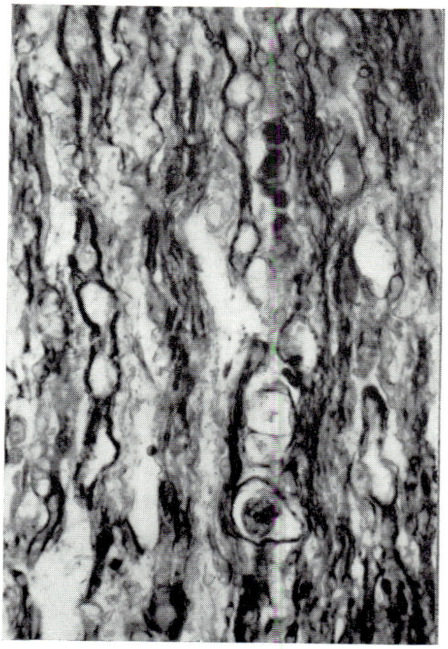

5.12

FIGS. 5.9–5.12. Cord in subacute combined degeneration. (Myelin.)

FIG. 5.9. Early degeneration limited to the dorsal columns.

FIG. 5.10. Fairly early degeneration in dorsal and lateral columns and very early degeneration in one ventral column.

FIG. 5.11. Severe case. Note that there is only Wallerian degeneration in the medulla and the lower lumbar segments.

FIG. 5.12. High-power view of longitudinal section of the dorsal columns in an early case, showing irregular swellings on the myelin sheaths.

downwards also the lesions become more limited until in lower lumbar segments only the pyramidal tracts are degenerated.

The early lesions consist of swelling of myelin sheaths with little change in the axons. The lipid in these swollen sheaths at first retains the characters of myelin, staining darkly with Weigert's chrome-haematoxylin and with iron-haematoxylin lakes, and giving the appearance of 4 bright sectors of a circle under polarised light. At this stage longitudinal sections show a number of fusiform swellings along the course of the myelin sheaths (Fig. 5.12). In some, but by no means all, of these the axons have similar fusiform swellings, but they do not fill the swollen myelin sheaths to the same degree as in traumatic and early ischaemic lesions. The next stage is the breakdown of the myelin sheath into its constituent lipids and the disappearance of the axons. In this way empty spaces form and these tend to fuse together giving the tissue a loose, vacuolated appearance. The myelin breaks down in the same manner as in Wallerian degeneration; numerous lipid phagocytes appear and gradually come to lie within the Virchow-Robin spaces of the small vessels. As a result of the damage to the axons at the levels involved in the primary lesion (usually the lower thoracic segments) there is secondary Wallerian degeneration in the long tracts of the cord, and these may be the only lesions in the cervical and lumbar segments.

The distribution of the lesions is remarkably constant. The earliest lesions usually appear in the centres of both dorsal columns as irregular oval areas separated both from the grey horns and from the surface by intact fibres (Michell Clarke 1904) (Fig. 5.9). In the lateral columns lesions may appear, at the same time or slightly later, in areas on the surface of the cord immediately ventral to the dorsal horns (Fig. 5.10). Thence they spread inwards and forwards and may in severe cases eventually surround the ventrolateral columns. More commonly small and at first separate areas of degeneration appear on the surface of the cord or in the lips of the ventromedian fissure. Neither in the dorsal nor the ventrolateral columns do the early lesions have the distribution of tract degenerations although they may come to involve much of the dorsal columns and the pyramidal and spinocerebellar tracts.

There has been some discussion as to whether in this disease there is demyelination without damage to the axons. In the writers' opinion the pathogenesis is very different from that of demyelinating diseases, but there may be, as has been described, early changes in the myelin without evident lesions of the axon, and if the disease is arrested at this stage it is probable that some loss of myelin will remain. But lesions in the axons follow soon after those of the myelin and lead to typical Wallerian degeneration. In some very early cases, in which the plantar reflexes were of extensor type, Greenfield and O'Flynn (1933) found very slight and early lesions in the lateral columns and it seemed probable that under treatment all signs of involvement of the pyramidal tracts would have disappeared. Therefore the remission and apparently complete cure of the early symptoms by adequate treatment may mean no more than the arrest of the disease at a stage when only a small proportion of the axons in any tract are damaged.

It has also been said that neuroglial scarring only occurs during remissions and especially as a result of treatment. However, Russell *et al.* observed fibrous gliosis in some of their cases, and it has been seen by the writers in untreated cases which had progressed steadily but not very rapidly. The astrocytic reaction seems to depend on the tempo of the disease process. In cases with a short history of rapid increase of symptoms the astrocytes may appear inactive or undergo regressive changes. In less acute cases the cell bodies of the astrocytes swell slightly and their fibres become thicker and more numerous, and in more slowly progressive cases there is often considerable fibrous gliosis in the areas first affected although none may be seen in areas of recent degeneration.

There is little change in the meninges, nerve roots or the grey columns of the cord. The anterior horn cells often contain some excess of lipofuscin but their Nissl granules stain well and there is no displacement of nuclei. In severe cases there may be chromatolysis of the cells of Clarke's column due to the lesions of their axons. Similar changes may be seen in the Betz cells of the precentral gyrus.

More extensive changes in the brain have been reported in a relatively small number of cases by Barrett (1913), Woltman (1918), Adams and Kubik (1944), Ferraro *et al.* (1945) and others. Small, often perivascular ill-defined foci of demyelination within the cerebral white matter are the most characteristic lesions. They may be few in number, detectable only on careful search, or they may be disseminated over wide areas of the corona radiata (Fig. 5.13). The large ascending and descending tracts in internal capsule, cerebral peduncles and pons are, however, relatively spared. The histology of these foci is similar to that of the focal changes in the spinal cord, i.e. fusiform swelling of myelin sheaths and axis cylinders in the most recent foci, followed by destruction of myelin and axons, proliferation of microglia and formation of fat granule cells in foci of longer standing. In some cases astrocytes also proliferate, and this may result in perivascular and diffuse fibrous gliosis of greater severity than is usually observed in the spinal cord.

Apart from these foci of demyelination fibrosis of capillaries and small arterioles, and haemorrhages, may be found. In their cases Ferraro *et al.* described widespread reversible and irreversible (ischaemic) degeneration of cortical nerve cells. Extensive recent ischaemic necrosis of the cortex was found in the case from which Fig. 5.13 has been taken; it probably occurred during collapse and coma shortly before death.

Pernicious anaemia is one of the conditions which have been observed to give rise to the Wernicke syndrome (page 290).

Peripheral nerves. Russell *et al.* found the peripheral nerves normal or only slightly degenerated in most of their cases, but in one more chronic case there was considerable degeneration both in the larger nerves and in the small intramuscular branches. Greenfield and Carmichael (1935), examining the small peripheral cutaneous branch of the anterior tibial nerve, found a constant reduction in the number of myelin sheaths in 4 cases of subacute combined degeneration (Fig. 5.14). In these the average count ranged from 3,000 to 4,400 per sq. mm. whereas in normal subjects of the same age the range was from 5,500 to 9,600 per sq. mm. In 2 of their cases the loss was greatest in fibres with diameters of more than 3μ but in 1 case it was more evenly spread. (In cases of alcoholic peripheral neuropathy examined at the same time a rather greater loss was found, with average numbers of 2,000 to 3,200 per sq. mm. In these the special incidence of the disease on the large fibres was even more marked.)

Clinical pathology. The cerebrospinal fluid usually shows no change except a slight excess of protein. The blood picture varies greatly. Examination of the bone marrow may be valuable in such cases. Estimations of the blood serum show reduction, but rarely complete absence, of B_{12}. Biopsy of the gastric mucosa and measurement of the absorption rate of radioactive B_{12} proved helpful to Badenoch (1954) in separating non-Addisonian cases from those associated with Addison's pernicious anaemia. Only in the latter were the parietal glands in the mucosa atrophic or absent.

Pathogenesis. Although now recognised to be closely related to deficiency of vitamin B_{12} the pathogenesis of subacute combined degeneration is not yet fully explained. That it has little relationship to the degree of anaemia is shown by the appearance of disabling nervous symptoms in patients with only slight anaemia and in those under treatment with folic acid. B_{12} is known to take part in the metabolism of fats, proteins, carbohydrates and nucleic acids. Its absence inhibits the synthesis of RNA and might be expected to have a profound effect on cells such as neurones which have a high RNA content and a rapid protein turnover (Lester-Smith 1956). But an effect on the neurone as a whole or on its axon should produce a predominantly peripheral neuropathy such as is seen with deficiency of B_1 and pantothenic acid. Alexander (1957) observed a lack of myelination in the sciatic nerves of 17-day-old B_{12} deficient chicks, and reversible chromatolysis of nerve cells in the anterior horn and spinal and sympathetic ganglia, together with increase of sudanophilic fat in the peripheral nerves of deficient young rats. This points to a role of B_{12} in the formation and maintenance of myelin and Nissl bodies. Chicks made deficient in B_{12} by Ferguson *et al.* (1955) showed only unspecific lesions (multiple haemorrhages) in the spinal cord and brain. Sinclair (1956) believed that a combination of *p*-hydroxyl-phenyl-pyruvic acid with lipoic acid may produce a substance which is toxic to nerve fibres in the spinal cord; this hypothesis does not however seem to have been sub-

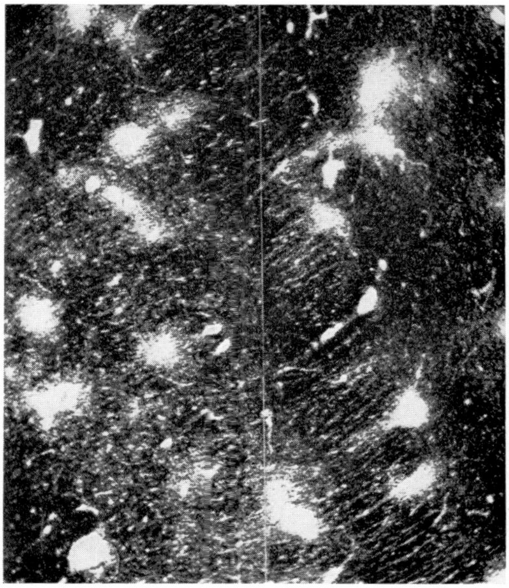

5.13

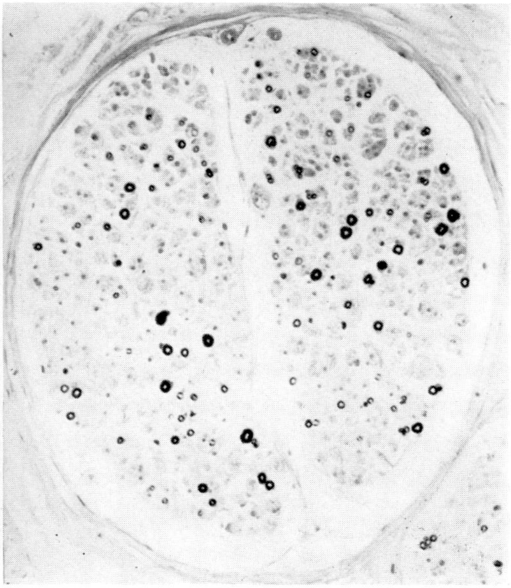

5.14

FIG. 5.13. Subacute combined degeneration. Ill-defined foci of demyelination in the occipital white matter. (Heidenhain's myelin ×20.)

FIG. 5.14. Fascicle of peripheral cutaneous branch of the anterior tibial nerve in subacute combined degeneration. (Osmic acid, ×200.) Compare with Fig. 5.5.a.

stantiated. Thus, all attempts to produce experimentally the specific lesions of B_{12} neuropathy have so far failed.

A spontaneous disease histologically indistinguishable from subacute combined spinal and cerebral degeneration has been observed in monkeys during captivity (cage paralysis). Descriptions of its pathology have been published by (among others) Schroeder (1908), Perdrau (1930), Levaditi *et al.* (1930), Hamerton (1938, 1942) and van Bogaert (1939). Scherer (1944) gave a full report on 20 monkeys exhibiting the disease. The clinical investigations in these reports have been uneven; 3 of Hamerton's monkeys showed achlorhydria which was associated with macrocytic anaemia only in 1 case; otherwise anaemia did not seem to be a prominent feature. Severe diarrhoea often preceded the onset of nervous symptoms. In a few animals in which liver extract was given, the response appeared to be favourable, but whether the condition has any pathogenic or therapeutic relationship to B_{12} is not yet known.

The remaining deficiencies

Biotin. Spontaneous deficiency in man apparently does not occur, but in an experimental group itching, scaling of the skin, anorexia, lassitude and sleeplessness have been described.

No lesions of the nervous system have been described in experimental animals, but muscle fibres in rats have been found to be necrotic and atrophic with a corresponding increase of sarcolemma nuclei. The changes were similar to those seen in alpha-tocopherol deficiency (Follis 1948): biotin deficiency may, therefore, not be the only factor.

Choline. Its metabolism is linked with the sulphur-containing amino-acid methionine. Deficiency of either substance leads to disturbance of phospholipid metabolism and to delay in the transport of fatty acids to fat deposits. Choline is important also for the synthesis of acetylcholine. In experimental animals subjected to its lack, lesions in liver and kidney have been reported. The changes in the liver consist of fatty infiltration with accompanying necrosis of the liver cells, resulting in finely granular cirrhosis (Himsworth and Glynn 1944, Himsworth 1946–7). Pathological changes in the nervous system have not been found, but it may nevertheless be indirectly involved through the affection of liver and kidneys.

Vitamin A, a carotene, is the precursor of the light-sensitive pigment rhodopsin, which is present in the rods of the retina, and deficiency of this vitamin, therefore, leads to nyctalopia. It leads also to keratising metaplasia of the conjunctival and corneal epithelium (xerosis). Degeneration of the cranial and peripheral nerves, grey and white matter of the brain and of the spinal cord has been described by Mellanby (1944) and others, but he, as well as Wolbach and Bessey (1941), have demonstrated that this is due to selective cessation of growth of bone and the subsequent increase of pressure and not to direct action on the nervous tissue. Such lesions are, therefore, confined to growing children and animals and are almost entirely absent in adults. Fluorescence microscopy detects very little of this vitamin in the normal central nervous system (Popper 1941).

Hydrocephalus in young rabbits whose mothers had suffered from vitamin A deficiency is described by Millen *et al.* (1953, 1956). The hydrocephalus is reported as not caused by stenosis of the aqueduct, and its pathogenesis is obscure.

Vitamin D deficiency is of little interest for neuropathology.

In contrast to vitamins A and D, *ascorbic acid* (**vitamin C**) is normally found in appreciable amounts in the cytoplasm of nerve cells, microglia, oligodendroglia, and the epithelial cells of the choroid plexus, although these amounts fall short of that present in the pituitary gland, adrenal cortex and the interstitial cells of the testes. The close relationship of ascorbic acid (demonstrated by a special silver nitrate method as silver granules) to the Golgi apparatus and mitochondria is of considerable histochemical interest (Bourne 1951), particularly in view of the reported increase of oxygen consumption in the presence of ascorbic acid of separated cerebral tissue containing mitochondria (McIlwain 1955). Despite these indications of its influence on the normal functioning of nervous tissue, the pathological findings in deprivation of vitamin C are not particularly noteworthy and are confined to haemorrhages in the central nervous system of patients and animals suffering from scorbutus.

Similar diapedetic haemorrhages in numerous sites have been reported by Ferraro and Roizin (1943) in the brains of fowls and cats deprived of **vitamin K**. Reduction of blood levels of prothrombin follows deficiency of this vitamin. In man, clinical hypoprothrombinaemia with its resultant haemorrhagic manifestations is occasionally seen in patients suffering from obstructive jaundice, diarrhoea, sprue, etc., and in such cases therapy with vitamin K has been successful.

Alpha-tocopherol (vitamin E)

This vitamin was first described by Evans and Bishop (1922) under the name of the reproduction factor. Later, in 1928, Evans and Burr reported muscular paralysis in young offspring of E depleted rats.

Alpha-tocopherol is necessary for the development of the embryo, the integrity of the germinal epithelium in the male and the metabolism of striated muscle. In the absence of the vitamin marked retardation and underdevelopment of the embryo ensues. The spermatozoa show chromatolysis and nuclear changes and striated muscle (including heart muscle) hyalin degeneration and necrosis. Macrophages are filled with acid fast 'ceroid' pigment; the muscular change corresponds to the nutritional muscular dystrophy described in guinea-pigs and rabbits by Goettsch and Pappenheimer (1931). Muscular necrosis in α-tocopherol deficiency has been established as occurring in 19 animal species (Oppenheimer 1956). Acid fast pigment has been described as present in viscera, and by Einarson *et al.* (1938, 1953, 1960) also in nerve cells, glia cells and blood vessel cells of the central nervous system; it can be demonstrated by varying methods which include fluorescence microscopy. Einarson and Ringstead have in addition described degeneration of the posterior roots and of the dorsal spinal tracts—findings which have been confirmed by Luttrell and Mason (1949) and by Malamud, Nelson and Evans (1949). Thus, Einarson's hypothesis that the paralysis is not only myogenic but also neurogenic seems to be confirmed, but the significance of the widespread pigmentary degeneration of cells in the brain and spinal cord of rats suffering from advanced deficiency of the vitamin requires further clarification. In this respect, it is of interest that free cholesterol has been found markedly increased in the muscle and brain of vitamin E deficient rats (Heinrich and Mattill 1943).

Terminal degeneration of mainly afferent axons was the most impressive finding in the grey matter of the spinal cord and the medulla of rats which had been kept by Pentschew *et al.* (1962) on a vitamin E deficient diet for 14½–23 months. The nerve cells were not materially affected, but hypertrophic fibrous astrocytes, some of very large size, were demonstrated with Cajal's method (though not with the Holzer stain). According to the authors the axonal changes are comparable to those found in chronic alcoholism and the Hallervorden-Spatz syndrome.

There is no evidence that vitamin E deficiency occurs in man and there seems to be no connection between such deficiency and the human dystrophic and amyotrophic syndromes, with the exception of infants suffering from diseases such as cystic fibrosis of pancreas or biliary atresia which impede the absorption of food; in these patients the serum level of α-tocopherol (indicated by degree of haemolysis of erythrocytes in H_2O_2) has been found to be persistently low (Nitowsky *et al.* 1956); and Oppenheimer, in such a patient (aged 2 years), claims to have found muscle necrosis.

Protein

Two main conditions are included under this heading: the so-called hunger oedema and Kwashiorkor. These represent, however, only two aspects of a wide range of syndromes.

Hunger oedema has been a prominent feature of many famines. It occurred as a consequence of low calorie diet in Europe during and immediately after the two great wars. Reduction in plasma protein has been considered its main cause, but, according to McCance (1951), this may not be as important a factor as the replacement of fat and of tissue volume by fluid; posture, renal function, salt intake and perhaps hormonal imbalance, all play their part. The central nervous system being the last of the organs to lose weight and tissue volume, there is no specific neuropathology. The central and peripheral neuropathies of vitamin B deficiencies are uncommon.

In contrast, *kwashiorkor*, of which instructive clinico-pathological descriptions have been given by Trowell, Davies and Dean (1954), Follis (1958), Platt (1958 b), and others, is caused by a diet deficient mainly in protein, while adequate or even excessive in starchy foodstuffs. The 'starch dystrophy syndrome' and the 'Mehlnährschaden' of German writers are identical conditions. Kwashiorkor has been reported from poverty stricken areas in Africa, India,

Jamaica and elsewhere. It predominantly affects children between the ages of 6 months and 4 years, but an adult form has also been recognised. Clinically, it is characterised by retardation in growth, muscular wasting, oedema, diarrhoea, a dermatosis resembling pellagra (though not sensitive to sunlight), enlargement of the liver, and a mental apathy and behaviour disturbance which may be profound. If left untreated, the condition is fatal, but even severe manifestations of the syndrome may be restored to normal by adequate diet.

Although investigation of the nervous system has been neglected in the past, it appears that neurological signs are not prominent, although a rhythmic coarse tremor has been reported to occur during the recovery period and to eventually disappear (Kahn 1954, Udani 1960): this also applies to hypotonia and areflexia which have been observed in some cases (Udani). The electroencephalogram may show a cerebral dysrhythmia which occasionally persists after recovery (Udani).

The pathology of kwashiorkor is distinct from that of the marasmus of low calorie diet. According to Davies (1954), subcutaneous fat deposits are not exhausted. The liver shows considerable fatty infiltration, the fat is first deposited in the periphery of the lobule and leads to a fine periportal fibrosis, which is usually halted at an early stage.

The pancreas shows gross atrophy which, according to Davies, may even precede the affection of the liver. Its basic histology is that of an atrophy of the zymogen-secreting cells, which extends to the glands in the small intestine, and to salivary and lacrimal glands. The brain usually shows oedema and congestion. In one case of Udani, cysts and sclerosis were present in the occipital cortex; they were, however, likely to be a coincidental finding. Histological investigation of a case of Kahn which had shown coarse rhythmic tremor during life, revealed nothing but minor histological change which may have been the sequel to a terminal acute gastro-enteritis.

Van Bogaert *et al.* (1962) have reported changes in the muscles of Congolese infants which are considered to be characteristic of kwashiorkor: the muscle fibre itself shows foamy and eosinophilic degeneration and this is accompanied by an intermysial oedema which later results in septal sclerosis. These lesions were not seen in other types of oedema and/or malnutrition.

The salient signs of kwashiorkor have been reproduced in experimental animals, and with particular ease in young pigs, by a 'Gambia diet'. Thus, Platt and his associates were able to study many of the features of this deficiency in strictly controlled conditions. The central nervous system was only slightly (though consistently) affected (Meyer, Stewart and Platt 1961): the histological change consisted of a chromatolysis which was best demonstrated in the somatochrome nerve cells of the anterior horns in the spinal cord and which was accompanied by slight activation of astrocytes and oligodendrocytes. The change has been interpreted as a mainly reversible adaptation to a deficient nutritive supply, rather than as a sign of progressive degeneration and glial replacement. A similar, though more severe, change has been found in the offspring of bitches fed on a low protein diet (Meyer, Pampiglione, Platt and Stewart 1961), although the aetiological problem of this series is still under consideration.

Copper

Deficiency in copper has been established by Bennetts and Beck (1942) as the cause of *enzootic ataxia* or *swayback*—a condition which occurs not only in Australia and England, but has recently also been reported from Greece and Iceland (Spais *et al.* 1961). While in Australia the condition occurs on pastures low in copper, in this country it is found irrespective of the copper content which may even be high. Hypocupraemia is found, however, in both Australian and English ewes. Some conditioning factor may be involved which in England reduces the availability of copper to the animal (*vide* Barlow 1958). The neurological manifestations consist of spastic paralysis, especially of the hind limbs, severe inco-ordination and blindness, occurring in newborn or very young lambs. In the Australian cases severe anaemia was a predominant sign (Bennetts and Chapman 1937). The pathology has been investigated by Innes (1934, 1936, 1939). Demyelination of the white matter is the most consistent feature; its extent ranges from circumscribed symmetrical foci of demyelination to complete destruction of myelin. In the severest cases liquefaction takes place. The cerebral cortex and a thin strip of superficial white matter may line a cavity into which the central white matter has been transformed. Phagocytes filled with fatty breakdown products are present in small numbers, but are not a conspicuous feature because of the rapid course of the disease. Nerve cells in the cortex and elsewhere are little affected and the basal ganglia, the grey centres in the brain stem and the spinal cord are usually spared except for Wallerian degeneration of the descending motor tracts. There is no evidence of myelin aplasia—the demyelination represents destruction of myelin already formed. Gliosis is present to a small degree and there is no evidence of inflammatory exudate.

The spongy transformation of the white matter, extending sometimes to the neighbouring cortex and very rarely affecting the central grey matter is, according to Spais *et al.*, the basis of diagnosis. Lesions in muscles, nerves, anterior horns, spinal tracts and the brain stem—all of which have been described by other workers—are too inconsistent to be included in the typical symptomatology. The condition must be distinguished from aplasia of myelin described in lambs by Markson *et al.* (1959) as 'hypomyelinogenesis congenita' and from the superficially similar demyelination of the 'Border' disease (Hughes and Kershaw 1959), in which hypocupraemia of the ewes is not a feature.

The lesions in swayback are due to oedematous inhibition and subsequent necrosis of the white matter (Spais *et al.*). They cannot be compared, therefore, with the demyelinating diseases in man.

Neuropathies associated with diabetes mellitus, carcinoma and porphyria

(J. G. Greenfield and A. Meyer)

Diabetes mellitus

Neuropathies occur commonly. Their frequency has been estimated by Martin (1953) and Mathews (1955) to be between 30–40 per cent of unselected cases of diabetes; Hirson *et al.* (1953) and Garland and Tavener (1953) found neurological abnormalities among an even higher percentage (50–60 per cent). These cases present predominantly with sensory symptoms such as pain, paraesthesias, sensory loss and areflexia, which are often bilateral. The ankle jerks are lost in most and the knee jerks in about a third of these cases (Martin). Trophic lesions are not uncommon, and may be the first evidence of sensory loss; ataxia and paralysis (foot or wrist drop) are rarer. Pupillary abnormalities, including Argyll-Robertson pupil, have been reported by Martin to occur in 9 per cent of a series of 150 cases with objective evidence of neuropathy.

Symptoms of diabetic neuropathy may occur at any age, but are most common in the fifth and sixth decades of mild chronic cases. In a third of these cases of neuropathy there is also a diabetic retinopathy (Martin). The rate of fetal death and of congenital malformation in the offspring of diabetic mothers is high. In 4 surviving infants Dekaban and Magee (1958) found either severe mental deficiency or cerebral diplegia.

Complete post-mortem examinations of early cases of diabetic neuropathy have been few and most have been concerned with severe forms of the disease to which other factors may have contributed. Fraser and Bruce (1895) found degeneration of myelin extending over many segments, and associated with some varicosity, but with preservation of continuity of the axons.

Woltman and Wilder (1929) examined 3 cases completely and the nerves of limbs amputated for gangrene in 6 other cases. Usually the degeneration of peripheral nerves was diffuse, but in 2 cases it was patchy. They also found consistent thickening of the walls of the small intraneural vessels; others, however, have found no more evidence of arterial degeneration in cases of neuropathy than in other diabetics of the same age. Bosanquet and Henson (1957), in a woman aged 71, who had suffered from severe sensory ataxia, found degeneration in posterior columns, posterior root ganglia, posterior roots and peripheral nerves. It was considered likely that the primary lesion was in the sensory ganglia. Anterior horn cells and anterior roots were virtually intact in their case, although degeneration in some muscles suggested some motor

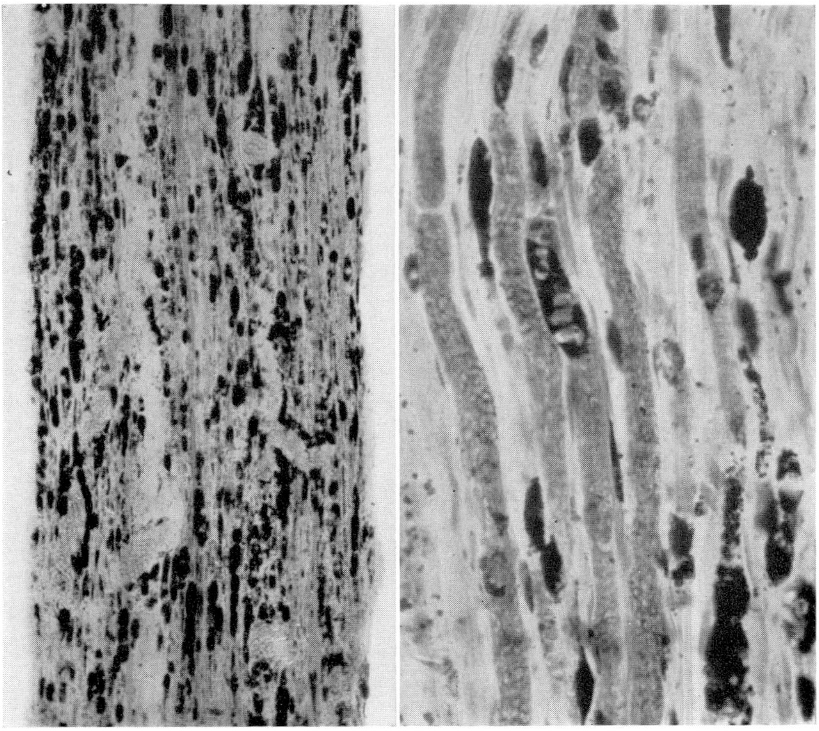

(*a*) (*b*)

FIG. 5.15. Diabetic neuritis.

(*a*) Low and (*b*) high-power views of dorsal nerve root. (Scharlach R. haematin.) The grey cylinders in (*b*) are intact myelin sheaths. (By the kindness of Dr. Bosanquet.)

involvement. There was no vascular disease in the sensory ganglia, although moderate thickening of arterial walls without atheroma occurred elsewhere. Woolf and Malins (1957), in biopsy material, described swelling and fusion of the terminal expansions of the end-plates, with 'soap bubble' formations; they suggested this may be an early indication of 'dying back' from the periphery (Fig. 5.15).

All these lesions may occur in diabetics in whom neither coma nor appreciable acidosis have ever been observed. This in itself renders unlikely Sinclair's (1956) suggestion that lipoic acid may be invalidated by its combining with a ketone body. The failure of vitamin B therapy excludes the possibility of direct deficiency of one of the known members of this group. Sinclair (1961) now suggests a relative deficiency of essential fatty acids as a possible factor in the

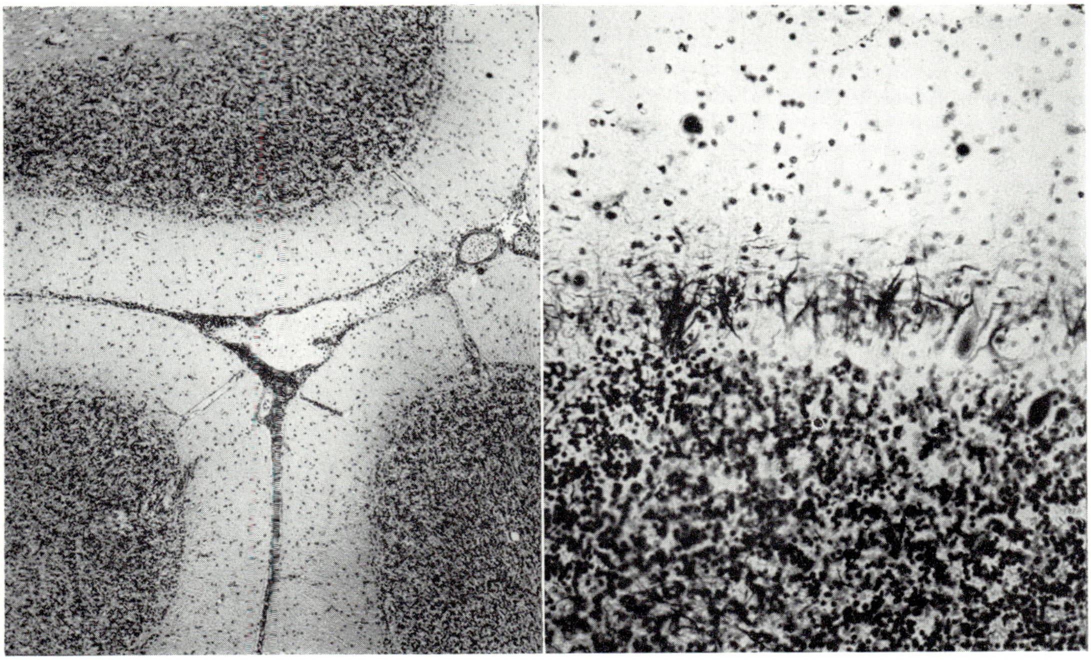

(*a*) (*b*)

FIG. 5.16. Subacute spinocerebellar degeneration. ($3\frac{1}{2}$ months' history. Case 1 of Brain *et al.* 1951.)

(*a*) Cerebellar cortex showing widespread loss of Purkinje cells and lymphocytic exudate in the meninges.

(*b*) Higher-power view showing empty baskets of hypertrophied fibres replacing Purkinje cells. (Bielschowsky's silver impregnation.)

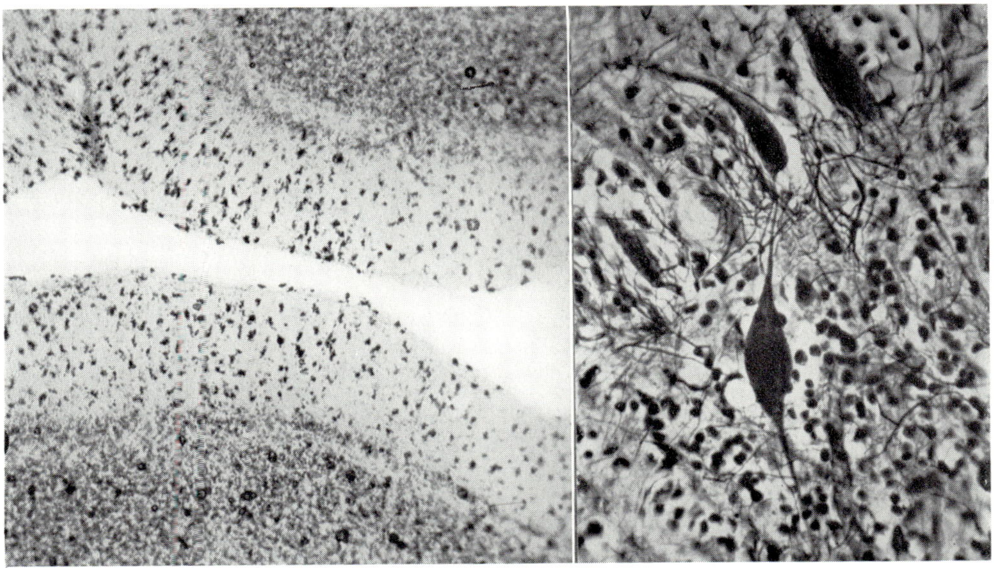

(*a*) (*b*)

Fig. 5.17. Subacute cerebellar degeneration. (6 months' history. Case 2 of Brain, Daniel and Greenfield 1951.)

(*a*) Cortex of cerebellum showing loss of Purkinje cells and phagocytosis of lipid. (Scharlach R. haemalum.)

(*b*) Degenerated Purkinje cell with torpedo-like swelling on its axon.

causation of the neuropathies. In alloxan diabetes of lower animals the E.F.A. requirements are greatly increased because of rapid oxidation of fat. E.F.A. deficiency is also held to cause capillary fragility, and to contribute to the high incidence of atheroma, coronary heart disease and retinopathy in human diabetes.

Carcinoma

Overt vitamin deficiency has been described in the presence of carcinoma: carcinoma of the stomach and the intestines in particular may give rise to the pathological manifestations of the Wernicke syndrome and of pellagra. There are other types of neuropathies whose relationship to specific vitamins is less established. The association of neurological lesions with carcinoma has in fact been known for a long time, but only in recent years has systematic attention been paid to this concurrence which is generally held to be more than a coincidence. The problem and the literature have recently been reviewed by Henson, Russell and Wilkinson (1954),

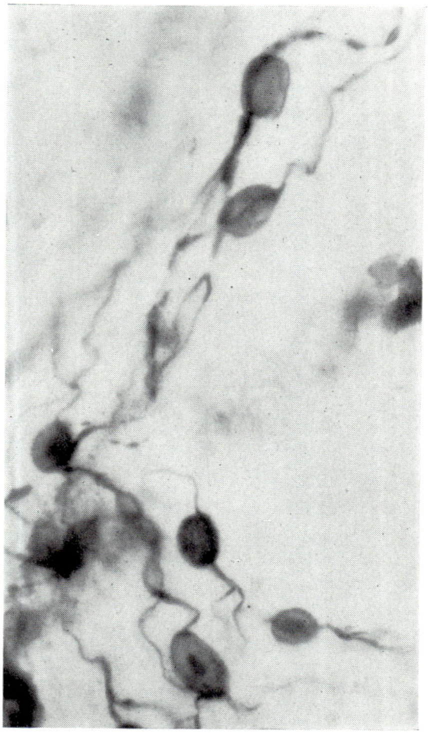

FIG. 5.18. Carcinomatous neuropathy.
Intramuscular nerve twigs showing globular swellings. (From a biopsy. Intravital methylene blue. By the kindness of Dr. A. L. Woolf.)

Heathfield and Williams (1954), Gray, Woolf and Wright (1955) and by Brain and Henson (1958), and each of the reviewers has also contributed new cases.

The last-mentioned authors have made a detailed scrutiny of a material of 42 cases, in 32 of which the site of the carcinoma was in the lung. On the other hand, only a small number (probably below 5 per cent) of sufferers from lung carcinoma develop neurological symptoms. No peripheral neuropathies were encountered by Lennox and Pritchard (1950), nor by Lea (1952), in their large control series in which lung carcinoma was absent. Brain and Henson emphasise the surprisingly small size of the carcinoma in many cases—a fact which has been underlined also by Woolf (1958). Precise classification of the varying types of lesion is difficult, since many levels of the nervous system and also the muscles may be affected in the same patients. To indicate this point Brain and Henson use the term *neuromyopathy*. Nevertheless, it is possible to distinguish several main types:

(1) *Cortical cerebellar degeneration* (Greenfield 1934, Brain *et al.* 1951, 1958). This may occur as a relatively pure form or it may be mixed with other lesions in subcortical centres of the brain (subthalamic nuclei and other brain stem nuclei) and in the spinal cord (degeneration of the spino-cerebellar, pyramidal and posterior tracts, and of the motor cells in the anterior horn). Clinically the picture is one of subacute or even acute cerebellar disorder. Mental changes (initial agitation, confusion, memory defect and eventual dementia) are prominent. Excess of cells and protein and a paretic Lange curve are frequently found, but no organisms were obtained on culture. Histologically, degeneration and disappearance of Purkinje cells is widespread, with moderate loss of granular cells, some damage to basket cells and tangential fibres, and some glial shrub-like proliferation. In some cases only the dentate nucleus or the inferior olives may be affected. The direct spino-cerebellar tracts were among those most frequently affected by degeneration in the cord. Meningeal and perivascular lymphocytic infiltration was so frequent that Brain and Henson speak of an encephalomyelitic form (Figs. 5.16 and 5.17).

(2) *Peripheral neuropathy*. This may occur as a *sensory* neuropathy involving sensory peripheral nerves, dorsal roots, spinal ganglia and the posterior columns of the cord (Denny-Brown 1948); or more rarely as a mixed sensory-motor neuropathy. Again, inflammatory exudate is occasionally present.

(3) *Myopathy*. Myasthenia-like symptoms have been described by Denny-Brown, Henson *et al.* and Heathfield and Williams. Brain and Henson found 8 cases in their material in which these symptoms occurred without any manifestation of myeloneuritic lesions. Post-mortem examination and muscle biopsy have yielded no clues as to the site and nature of the lesion responsible for the myopathy; histological examination of the muscles showed only non-specific abnormalities. Woolf found a remarkable degree of sprouting of the distal extremity of the motor axons in cases of carcinomatous and myelomatous myopathy—not unlike that seen in thyrotoxic myopathy, dystrophic myotonia and myasthenia. Walton and Adams (1958) regarded these patients as suffering from polymyositis which is known to be associated with malignant disease. However, until the histological findings are clearer, the non-committal term carcinomatous myopathy is preferable (Brain and Henson) (Fig. 5.18).

(4) *Mental disorder*. The dementias which accompany the cerebellar neuropathies have already been mentioned. Mental changes of organic type occur also together with other forms of neuropathy or in the absence of neurological signs. They seem, not infrequently, to be early manifestations of carcinoma, particularly of the lung. In the clinical and pathological analysis of several cases, Charatan and Brierley (1956) found no clear-cut histological substrate and had to postulate the effects of toxic or metabolic abnormalities.

The *aetiology* of these 'neuromyopathies' is still obscure. A nutritional or related metabolic disorder caused by the carcinoma has been much under discussion. Denny-Brown (1947, 1948) implicated pantothenic acid because of the close similarity of the dorsal root and posterior column changes to those which are experimentally produced in pigs deprived of this vitamin. He also pointed out the resemblance of the carcinomatous myopathies to the bulbar myasthenia-like syndrome reported in relation to beriberi and pellagra. Other vitamins which have for obvious reasons been considered are α-tocopherol, thiamine and nicotinic acid. However, apart from occasional overt cases of the Wernicke syndrome or of pellagra, no deficiency in these or other vitamins has so far been proved, and extensive therapy with all known vitamins has had no conclusive effect. There may be an indirect deficiency, in so far as the carcinoma is in competition with the demands of normal tissues which may divert substances essential for the metabolism of the neurone. According to Sinclair lipoic acid may be inactivated by keto-acids produced by anaerobic glycolysis of malignant tissue, but therapeutically lipoic acid has proved to be useless. The same author (Sinclair 1961) has made the other suggestion that a partial deficiency in essential fatty acids may contribute to the causation of the neuromyopathies, but no concrete evidence in support of this hypothesis has yet come forth. Brain and Henson rightly point out that if a tumour deprived the body of essential nutritional factors or produced other metabolic or 'toxic' changes, one might expect that such effects would be in direct proportion to the size of the tumour, which is clearly not the case.

The inflammatory changes encountered in some of the neuromyopathic lesions are so marked that the possibility of a *virus infection* cannot be ruled out (Brain and Henson). It may operate in combination with an additional constitutional factor to which only a small proportion of the exposed population is susceptible; or with a process of sensitisation of particular nervous and muscular tissue to some product of the tumour.

Acute porphyria

This condition, to which Vannotti (1954) has devoted a monograph, may be congenital or manifest itself as an acute form in later age periods. The congenital variety is erythroblastic, while the acute porphyrias of later life are usually hepatic in origin. Heredity may be a factor in both forms. Among exogenous factors, alcoholism, ingestion of certain barbiturates, sulphonamides, hepatic adenoma and—as occurred in a recent Turkish epidemic—intoxication by a fungicide have been cited. However, both the classification of the various types and the pathogenic problem are still obscure (Watson 1960). Rimington (1961), who has devoted previous studies to the chemical pathology of the condition, now holds that the biochemical lesion in acute porphyria is an interference with the production of acetylcholine.

In the acute idiopathic form sleeplessness and acute abdominal pain may be the initial symptoms which are followed by polyneuritis or, when severe, by acute ascending paralysis of the Landry type, with confusional states, coma and convulsions.

Erbsloch (1903) examined the spinal cord and peripheral nerves of a case with 10 days' history of weakness. He found no definite changes in the spinal cord or nerve roots, but a varying degree of degeneration of myelin and axons in the more peripheral parts of the nerves.

Since then, many examinations of this form of peripheral neuropathy have been made, the most important recent records in the English language being by Baker and Watson (1945), Denny-Brown and Sciarra (1945) and Gibson and Goldberg (1956). These authors emphasise the irregular, often patchy, distribution of the degeneration in peripheral nerves and its special effect on myelin sheaths, so that often there is no loss of continuity of the axons. Irregular swelling or fragmentation of axons was seen, however, in the more chronic and severe lesions.

Central chromatolysis of motor neurones, corresponding to the duration and severity of the lesion in the peripheral nerves they supplied, was present in all cases.

In Hierons' (1957) case there was degeneration of the fasciculus gracilis and slight degeneration in the lateral columns in the lumbar segments.

In many cases, especially those with cerebral symptoms, lesions which appear to be of an ischaemic character have been found in cerebral and cerebellar cortex, basal ganglia and in the white matter of the hemispheres. Rarely, these consist of small areas of infarction (Hierons); more often of focal cell loss and of ischaemic cell change in the cortex or of pale myelin staining in the white matter.

The pathogenesis of this form of peripheral neuropathy is not clear. The lesions in the brain appear to be anoxic and may well result from constriction of small arterioles, since Baker and Watson and Denny-Brown and Sciarra observed localised spasm in the retinal arteries during attacks of porphyria. These latter authors consider the lesions in the peripheral nerves to have a similar pathogenesis, since in many ways they resemble those produced by experimental ischaemia in nerves (Denny-Brown and Brenner 1944). But, although in many cases the blood pressure is raised during an attack, in others it remains normal. Other authors have suggested an interference with the Krebs cycle of glucose metabolism and Hierons found abnormal pyruvate metabolism in 2 cases. The irregular, patchy or segmental type of lesion in the peripheral nerves is more suggestive of a direct toxic action on the nerve fibres than of a failure in the nutrition of the whole neurone: so far no substance has been definitely incriminated as being toxic to nervous tissue.

Steatorrhoea

This condition is clinically characterised by pale, flatulent and foul-smelling motions. One distinguishes an *idiopathic* form and its infantile equivalent, *coeliac* disease from the tropical form *sprue.* The idiopathic and coeliac cases have to be distinguished from *fibrocystic disease* of the pancreas in the newborn which has a similar symptomatology.

Tropical sprue usually affects white adults living in the tropics.

The aetiology is not yet fully elucidated. The coeliac and idiopathic forms, though they should not be at present regarded as being identical, appear to have a common genetic background, according to Badenoch (1960) who has given a comprehensive review on all aspects of the various conditions giving rise to steatorrhoea. They have also in common frequent anatomical derangements such as blind loops, fistulae and diverticula of the small intestine, in particular, of the jejunum. Since the introduction by Shiner (1956, 1957) of peroral biopsy, clubbing, flattening or villous atrophy of the jejunal or iliac mucosa has been seen in many cases of the coeliac and idiopathic forms, and may even be present in tropical sprue, though in the latter combined with heavy inflammatory change.

Malabsorption may give rise to vitamin deficiency, particularly that of vitamin B_{12}. Badenoch and Bedford (1954) described in two patients the triad of jejunal diverticulosis, steatorrhoea and megaloblastic anaemia.

Neuropathological investigations have been carried out by Martin (1952) and by Smith (1955). Martin described a personality change in 2 cases which developed into progressive dementia. Histologically he found severe nerve cell degeneration in cerebral and cerebellar cortex and in subcortical centres, particularly in the hypothalamus. The material of Smith consists of 20 cases. Peripheral neuropathy, sensory ataxia, cerebellar ataxia, upper motor neurone lesions and mental changes were encountered alone or in varying combinations. In 1 case diffuse loss of Purkinje cells and degeneration of granule cells was combined with demyelination of the posterior and lateral colums of the cord; in a second, there was widespread loss of anterior horn cells, demyelination of lateral and anterior tracts and loss of some Betz cells; in a third case the neuronal degeneration was widespread. The similarity of some of the histological changes to those seen in pellagra was emphasised by the author who (Smith 1962, personal communication) has now collected the material of 9 cases which largely confirm his previous findings.

Lathyrism

This condition was known in ancient times; since the nineteenth century, epidemics have been reported in France, Italy, Algiers and Russia. It is still endemic in India, where it occurs most frequently during famines in the central provinces and in Mysore. A considerable literature has accumulated which has been fully reviewed by Denny-Brown (1947).

Lathyrus sativus, a pea which in times of shortage has been added to bread, has been implicated for most of the outbreaks. However, only a proportion of those who consume bread contaminated by the pea develop signs of disease. Except in times of famine, lathyrus sativa does not seem to have a toxic effect, which suggests that other factors are involved in the production of lathyrism. Shah (1939) has described an epidemic of lathyrism in which lathyrus sativus was absent from food. Lathyrism occurs also in herbiverous animals (horses, pigs, geese, ducks, etc.) which have fed on L. sativus or related peas.

In man, onset of clinical symptoms has been described by Denny-Brown and others as sudden and characterised by pain and paraesthesias of lower extremities, which progress to spastic paraplegia. Loss of sphincter control, impotence and muscular atrophy may follow. Filimonoff (1926) described degeneration of the ventral and lateral pyramidal tracts as the main post-mortem findings in a case dying 35 years after the onset of the disease. Buzzard and Greenfield, in addition to degeneration of the ventral and lateral pyramidal tracts, noted involvement of ascending fibres in the direct cerebellar and dorsal tracts. They emphasised the resemblance of the lesions to those seen in ergotism, but they observed also a honeycombed appearance in marginal parts of the cord.

Experimental investigations (well reviewed by Selye 1957 and German 1960) have become lively since Geiger *et al.* (1933) observed the retardation of growth and abnormalities of bone, cartilage and other mesodermal tissues in rats fed with sweet pea (Lathyrus odoratus). From this paper dates the origin of experimental *osteolathyrism* which subsequently was elaborated by Ponseti *et al.* (1952, 1954); Menzies and Mills (1957), and many others. According to the last-named authors the fundamental change in this disease is the excessive accumulation of intercellular ground substance, chondroitin sulphate, which leads to a general breakdown of collagen fibrils: among the resulting lesions are slipped epiphyses, kyphoscoliosis, degeneration of intervertebral discs, thoracic deformities and a high incidence of dissecting aneurysms of the aorta following the degeneration of elastic fibres. Compression and lesions of the cord by protruding discs or exostoses have been recorded. Osteolathyrism can be also produced experimentally by certain amino-nitriles such as, for example, amino-aceto-nitrile (Selye).

Since these experimental results were obtained in rats which are vulnerable to L. odoratus, but not to L. sativus, they cannot be directly compared with human pathology. The clinical symptomatology of sensory and motor disturbances and the post-mortem finding of a combination of ascending and descending tract degeneration could easily be interpreted as the result of local compression of the cord. On the other hand, there has been evidence of a neurotropic action (Selye's '*neurolathyrism*') of L. odoratus. Several amino-nitriles, in particular β-amino-proprionitrile, have been suggested as the active neurotropic principle of the sweet pea. β-cyano-ethylamine, an analogue of this nitrile, administered to rats by Hartmann *et al.* (1958), caused after 3 weeks hyperactivity, circling movements and intermittent spasms of neck muscles, which were followed by weakness of the hind limbs. Histologically, these authors found chromatolysis and degeneration of ventral roots, which they considered due to direct neurotoxic action, since vertebral deformities were minimal or absent. Although they explicitly excluded central chromatolysis, it should be noted that their figure 3 shows one chromatolytic cell with a definitely eccentric nucleus.

There is hope that these experimental studies will, in due time, throw light on the human forms of lathyrism.

Ergotism

Intoxication by the common 'fungus of rye' has in the past given rise to epidemics, particularly on the Continent. The toxic principles seem to be cornutine and sphacelinic acid: cornutine is responsible for convulsions, while sphacelinic acid by its constrictor action on muscle fibres, particularly those of the vessel wall, results in gangrene.

A consistent finding is degeneration of the long spinal tracts, particularly of the dorsal columns (Buzzard and Greenfield). The change has been likened to tabetic degeneration, but the lesions are less selective and are usually more recent; the arteries show thickening of the media, the smaller arteries are thrombosed.

The pathogenic mechanism is not yet known in detail. The toxic effect may again well be an interference or blocking of enzyme systems in which vitamins are intimately involved (Denny-Brown 1947). Mellanby (1931) has pointed out that the toxic action of ergot is more effective if there is also vitamin A deficiency, and Pentschew (1929) has described the clinical picture of pellagra in a monkey poisoned by ergot. Jervis and Kindwall (1942) also considered that excessive ergotamine administration in migraine may have been one factor in producing a Schilder-like demyelination of the cerebral white matter. A coincidence could not be excluded, however, in this human case.

REFERENCES

Adams, L. D. and Kubik, C. S. (1944) *New Engl. J. Med.*, **231**, 1.
Alexander, L. (1940) *Amer. J. Path.*, **16**, 61.
Alexander, L., Green, K. G., Evans, C. A. and Wolf, L. E. (1941) *Trans. Amer. neurol. Ass.*, **67**, 119.
Alexander, L., Pijoan, M., Myerson, A. and Keene, H. N. (1938) *Trans. Am. Neurol. Assoc.*, **64**, 135.
Alexander, W. F. (1957) *Vit. B12 and Intrinsic Factor*, ed. Heinrich, H. C., p. 372, Stuttgart.
Aring, C. D., Bean, W. B., Roseman, E., Rosenbaum, M. and Spies, T. D. (1941) *Arch. Neurol. Psychiat.* (Chicago), **45**, 772.
Aring, C. D. and Spies, T. D. (1939) *J. Neurol. Psychiat.*, **2**, 335.
Badenoch, J. (1954) *Proc. Roy. Soc. Med.*, **47**, 426; (1960) *Brit. Med. J.*, **2**, 879, 963.
Badenoch, J. and Bedford, P. D. (1954) *Quart. J. Med.*, **23**, 462.
Baker, A. B. and Watson, C. J. (1945) *J. Neuropath.*, **4**, 68.
Barlow, R. M. (1958) *Proc. Roy. Soc. Med.*, **51**, 748.
Baron, D. N., Dent, C. E., Harris, H., Hart, E. W. and Jepson, J. B. (1956) *Lancet* (ii), 421.
Barrett, A. M. (1913) *Amer. J. Insan.*, **69**, 643.
Bean, W. B., Hodges, R. E. and Daum, K. (1955) *J. clin. Invest.*, **34**. part 2, 1073.
Bennetts, H. W. and Beck, A. B. (1942) *Bull. counc. Sci. industr. Rec. Aust.*, **147**, 1.
Bennetts, H. W. and Chapman, F. E. (1937) *Aust. vet. J.*, **13**, 138.
Bertrand, I., Liber, A. F. and Randoin, L. (1934) *Arch. Anat. micr.*, **30**, 297.
Bessey, O. A. and Wolbach, S. B. (1939) *J. exp. Med.*, **69**, 1.
Bicknell, F. and Prescott, F. (1953) *The Vitamins in Medicine*, Heinemann, London.
Bonhoeffer, K. (1899) *Mschr. Neurol. Psychiat.*, **5**, 265, 379.
Bosanquet, F. D. and Henson, R. A. (1957) *Fol. psychiat. neurol. neurochir.* (Neerl.), **60**, 107.
Bourne, G. H. (1951) *Cytology and Cell Physiology*, Clarendon Press, Oxford.
Brain, W. R., Daniel, P. M. and Greenfield, J. G. (1951) *J. Neurol. Psychiat.*, **14**, 59.
Brain, W. R. and Henson, R. A. (1958) *Lancet*, **ii**, 971.
Bueding, E., Wortis, H., Fein, H. D. and Estouronne, D. (1942) *Am. J. Med. Sci.*, **204**, 838.
Buzzard, E. F. and Greenfield, J. G. (1921) *Pathology of the Nervous System*, Constable, London.
Campbell, A. C. P. and Biggart, J. H. (1939) *J. Path. Bact.*, **48**, 245.
Campbell, A. C. P. and Russell, W. R. (1941) *Quart. J. Med.*, **34**, 41.
Carmichael, E. A. and Stern, O. (1931) *Brain*, **54**, 189.
Castle, W. B. (1929) *Amer. J. Med. Sci.*, **178**, 748.
Charatan, F. B. and Brierley, J. B. (1956) *Brit. med. J.* (i), 765.
Chick, H., El Sadr, M. M. and Worden, A. N. (1940) *Biochem. J.*, **34**, 595.

Clarke, J. M. (1904) *Brain*, **27**, 441.
Coggeshall, R. E. and MacLean, P. D. (1958) *Proc. Soc. Exp. Biol. Med.*, **98**, 687.
Cruikshank, E. K. (1952) *Vitamins and Hormones*, **10**, 1.
Davies, J. N. P. (1954) in *Malnutrition in African Mothers, Infants and Young Children* (2nd Inter. African O.C.T.A. Conf.), p. 109, London.
Dekaban, A. S. and Magee, K. R. (1958) *Neurology*, **8**, 193.
Denny-Brown, D. (1947) *Medicine*, Baltimore, **26**, 41; (1948) *J. Neurol. Psychiat.*, **11**, 73; (1958) *Fed. Proc.*, **17** (Suppl. 2, part 2), p. 35.
Denny-Brown, D. and Brenner, C. (1944) *Arch. Neurol. Psychiat.* (Chicago), **51**, 1.
Denny-Brown, D. and Sciarra, D. (1945) *Brain*, **68**, 1.
Denton, J. (1928) *Amer. J. Path.*, **4**, 341.
Dunn, T. B., Morris, H. P. and Dubnik, C. S. (1947) *J. Nat. Cancer. Instit.*, **8**, 139.
Eijkman, C. (1897) *Virchows Arch. path. Anat.*, **148**, 523.
Einarson, L. (1953) *J. Neurol. Psychiat.*, **16**, 98.
Einarson, L. and Ringstead, A. (1938) *Effect of Chronic Vitamin E Deficiency on the Nervous System and the Skeletal Musculature in Adult Rats*, Copenhagen.
Einarson, L. and Telford, I. R. (1960) *Structural Changes in the Nervous System of Monkeys deprived of Vitamin E.*, Aarhus.
Ellinger, P., Coulson, R. A. and Benesch, R. (1944) *Nature*, Lond., **154**, 270.
Elvehjem, C. A., Madden, R. J., Strong, F. M. and Woolley, D. W. (1937) *J. Amer. chem. Soc.*, **59**, 1767.
Erbsloch, W. (1903) *Dtsch. Z Nervenheilk.*, **23**, 197.
Evans, C. A., Carlson, W. E. and Green, R. G. (1942) *Amer. J. Path.*, **18**, 79.
Evans, H. M. and Bishop, K. S. (1922) *Science*, **56**, 650.
Evans, H. M. and Burr, G. O. (1928) *J. biol. Chem.*, **76**, 273.
Ferguson, T. M., Rigdon, R. H. and Couch, J. R. (1955) *Arch. Pathol.*, **60**, 393.
Ferraro, A., Arieti, S. and English, W. H. (1945) *J. Neuropath.*, **4**, 217.
Ferraro, A. and Roizin, L. (1943) *J. Neuropath.*, **2**, 392.
Filimonoff, I. N. (1926) *Z. ges. Neurol. Psychiat.*, **105**, 76.
Follis, R. H., jr. (1948) *The Pathology of Nutritional Disease*, Springfield; (1958) *Deficiency Disease*, Springfield, Ill.
Follis, R. H., Miller, M. H., Wintrobe, M. M. and Stein, H. J. (1943) *Amer. J. Path.*, **19**, 341.
Follis, R. H. and Wintrobe, M. M. (1945) *J. exp. Med.*, **81**, 539.
Fraser, H. and Stanton, A. T. (1910) *Philippine J. Sci.* (Series B), **5**, 55.
Fraser, T. R. and Bruce, A. (1895) *Brit. Med. J.* (i), 1149.
Gamper, E. (1928) *Dtsch. Z. Nervenheilk.*, **102**, 122.
Garland, H. and Taverner, D. (1953) *Brit. med. J.* (i), 1405.
Geiger, B. J., Steenbock, H. and Parsons, H. T. (1933) *J. Nutrit.*, **6**, 427.
German, W. J. (1960) *J. Neurosurg.*, **17**, 657.
Gibson, J. B. and Goldberg, A. (1956) *J. Path. Bact.*, **71**, 495.
Goettsch, M. and Pappenheimer, A. M. (1931) *J. exp. Med.*, **54**, 145.
Goldberger, J. and Lillie, R. D. (1926) *Publ. Hlth. Rep.*, Wash., **41**, 1025.
Goldberger, J. and Wheeler, G. A. (1915) *Publ. Hlth. Rep.*, Wash., **30**, 3336; (1920) *Arch. intern. Med.* **25**, 451.
Gombault, A. (1880–81) *Arch. de Neurol.*, **1**, 11.
Gopalan, C. (1946) *Indian. Med. Gaz.*, **81**, 22.
Gray, K. W., Woolf, A. L. and Wright, E. A. (1955) *Guy's Hosp. Rep.*, **104**, 157.
Greenfield, J. G. (1934) *Brain*, **57**, 161; (1958) in *Neuropathology*, London.
Greenfield, J. G. and Carmichael, E. A. (1935) *Brain*, **58**, 483.
Greenfield, J. G. and Holmes, J. M. (1939) *Brit. med. J.* (i), 815.
Greenfield, J. G. and O'Flynn, E. (1933) *Lancet* (ii), 62.
György, P. (1934) *Nature*, Lond., **133**, 498.
Hamerton, A. E. (1938) *Proc. zool. Soc. Lond.* (series B), **108**, 512; (1942) *Brain*, **65**, 193.
Hardwick, S. W. (1943) *Lancet* (ii), 43; (1950) in *Recent Progress in Psychiatry*, Edited by G. W. T. H. Fleming, Churchill, London.
Hartmann, H. A., Lalich, J. J. and Akert, K. (1958) *J. Neuropath.*, **17**, 298.
Heathfield, K. W. G. and Williams, J. R. B. (1954) *Brain*, **77**, 122.
Heaton, J. M., McCormick, A. J. A. and Freeman, A. G. (1958) *Lancet* (ii), 286.
Hienrich, M. R. and Mattil, H. A. (1943) *Proc. Soc. exp. Biol. Med.*, **52**, 344.

Henson, R. A., Russell, D. S. and Wilkinson, M. (1954) *Brain*, **77**, 81.
Hersov, L. A. (1955) *J. Ment. Sci.*, **101**, 878.
Hersov, L. A. and Rodnight, R. (1960) *J. Neurol. Neurosurg. Psychiat.*, **23**, 40.
Hicks, S. P. (1955) *Amer. J. Path.*, **31**, 189.
Hierons, R. (1957) *Brain*, **80**, 176.
Himsworth, H. P. (1946–7) *Proc. R. Soc. Med.*, **40**, 27.
Himsworth, H. P. and Glynn, L. E. (1944) *Lancet* (i), 457.
Hirson, C., Feinmann, E. L. and Wade, H. J. (1953) *Brit. med. J.*, (i), 1408.
Hsü, Y. K. (1942) *Arch. Neurol. Psychiat.* (Chicago), **48**, 271.
Huber, G. (1954) *Arch. Psychiat. Z. ges. Neurol.*, **192**, 356.
Hughes, L. E. and Kershaw, G. F. (1959) *Vet. Rec.*, **71**, 313.
Hunt, A. D., Stokes, J., McCrory, W. W. and Stroud, H. H. (1954) *Pediatrics*, Springfield, **13**, 140.
Hurst, A. F. and Bell, J. R. (1922) *Brain*, **45**, 266.
Innes, J. R. M. (1934) *Rep. Inst. Anim. Path. Univ. Camb.*, **4**, 227; (1936) *Proc. R. Soc. Med.*, **29**, 406; (1939) *J. Neurol. Psychiat.*, **2**, 323.
Jervis, G. A. and Kindwall, J. A. (1942) *Amer. J. Psychiat.*, **98**, 650.
Joiner, C. L., Thompson, R. H. S. and Watson, D. (1950) *Guy's Hosp. Rep.*, **99**, 62.
Jolliffe, N., Bowman, K. M., Rosenblum, L. A. and Fein, H. D. (1940) *J. Amer. med. Ass.*, **114**, 307.
Jubb, K. V., Saunders, L. Z. and Coates, H. V. (1956) *J. Comp. Pathol. Therapy*, **66**, 217.
Kahn, E. (1954) *Arch. Dis. Childh.*, **29**, 256.
Krehl, W. A., Tepley, L. J., Sarma, P. S. and Elvehjem, C. A. (1945) *Science*, **101**, 489.
Lea, A. J. (1952) *Thorax*, **7**, 305.
Leichtenstern, O. (1884) *Dtsch. med. Wschr.*, **10**, 849.
Leigh, D. (1951) *J. Neurol. Neurosurg. Psychiat.*, **14**, 216; (1952) *J. ment. Sci.*, **98**, 130.
Lennox, B. and Pritchard, S. (1950) *Quart. J. Med.*, **19**, 97.
Lester-Smith, E. (1948) *Nature*, Lond., **161**, 638; (1956) *Brit. med. Bull.*, **12**, 52.
Levaditi, C., Lépine, P. and Schön, R. (1930) *C.R. Soc. Biol.*, Paris, **104**, 986.
Lichtheim. (1887) *Verh. 6th congr. innere. Med.*, p. 84.
Lippincott, S. W. and Morris, H. P. (1942) *J. Nat. Cancer Instit.*, **2**, 601.
Luckner, H. and Scriba, K. (1949) *Dtsch. Arch. Klin. Med.*, **194**, 396.
Luttrell, C. N. and Mason, K. E. (1949) *Ann. N.Y. Acad. Sci.*, **52**, 139.
McCall, K. B., Waisman, H. A., Elvehjem, C. A. and Jones, E. S. (1946) *J. Nutr.*, **31**, 685.
McCance, R. A. (1951) *Med. Res. Counc. Spec. Rep. Ser.*, **275**, 21.
McIlwain, H. (1940) *Brit. J. exp. Path.*, **21**, 136; (1955) *Biochemistry and the Central Nervous System*, Churchill, London.
Malamud, N., Nelson, M. M. and Evans, H. M. (1949) *Ann. N.Y. Acad. Sci.*, **52**, 135.
Markson, L. M., Terlecki, S., Shand, A., Sellers, K. C. and Woods, A. J. (1959) *Vet. Rec.*, **71** (i), 269.
Martin, F. (1952) *Acta neurol. belg.*, **52**, 218.
Martin, M. M. (1953) *Brain*, **76**, 594.
Matthews, J. D. (1955) *Lancet* (i), 474.
Mayer-Gross, W., Slater, E., and Roth, M. (1954) *Clinical Psychiatry*, Cassell, London.
Mellanby, E. (1931) *Brain*, **54**, 247; (1944) *Proc. roy. Soc.* (Series B), **132**, 28.
Menzies, D. W. and Mills, K. W. (1957) *J. Path. Bact.*, **73**, 223.
Meyer, Adolf (1901) *Brain*, **24**, 47.
Meyer, A. (1944) *J. Neurol. Psychiat.*, **7**, 66.
Meyer, A., Pampiglione, G., Platt, B. S. and Stewart, R. J. C. (1961) *Excerpta Medica. Int. Congr. Ser. No.* 39, p. 15.
Meyer, A., Stewart, J. R. C. and Platt, B. S. (1961) *Proc. Nutr. Soc.*, **20**, 18.
Millen, J. W. and Woollam, D. H. M. (1956) *J. Neurol. Neurosurg. Psychiat.*, **19**, 17.
Millen, J. W., Woollam, D. H. M. and Lamming, G. E. (1953) Lancet (ii), 1234.
Minnich, W. (1892) *Z. klin. Med.*, **21**, 25, 264.
Minot, G. R. and Murphy, W. P. (1926) *J. Amer. med. Ass.*, **87**, 470; (1927) ibid., **89**, 759.
Najjar, V. A. and Holt, L. E. (1943) *J. Amer. med. Ass.*, **123**, 683.
Neubürger, K. T. (1936) *Virchows Arch. path. Anat.*, **298**, 68.
Nitowsky, H. M., Gordon, H. H. and Tildon, J. T. (1956) *Bull. John Hopkins Hosp.*, **98**, 361.
North, J. D. and Sinclair, H. M. (1956) *Arch. Pathol.*, **62**, 341; (1957) *J. Nutr.*, **61**, 219.
Oppenheimer, E. H. (1956) *Bull. John Hopkins Hosp.*, **98**, 353.

Pekelharing, C. A. and Winkler, C. (1887) *Dtsch. med. Wschr.*, **13**, 845; (1893) *Beriberi: Researches Concerning its Nature, Cause and the Means of its Arrest*, Pentland, Edinburgh and London.
Pentschew, A. (1928) *Z. ges. Neurol. Psychiat.*, **118**, 17; (1929) *Krankheitsforschung*, **7**, 415.
Pentschew, A. and Schwarz, K. (1962) *Acta Neuropath.*, **1**, 313.
Perdrau, J. R. (1930) *J. Path. Bact.*, **33**, 991.
Peters, R. A. and Sinclair, H. M. (1933) *Biochem. J.*, **27**, 1910.
Peters, R. A. and Thompson, R. H. S. (1934) *Biochem. J.*, **28**, 916.
Pinsky, L. and Fraser, F. C. (1960) *Brit. med. J.* (ii), 195.
Platt, B. S. (1958 a) *Fed. Proc.*, **17** (Suppl. 2, part 2), 8; (1958 b) *Trans. Roy. Soc. Trop. Med. Hyg.*, **52**, 189.
Platt, B S. and Gin, S. Y. (1934) *Trans. Far-East Ass. trop. Med.*, **2**, 407.
Platt, B. S. and Lu, G. D. (1935) quoted from Platt, B. S. (1958 a).
Ponseti, I. V. and Baird, W. A. (1952) *Amer. J. Pathol.*, **28**, 2, 1059.
Ponseti, I. V. and Shepard, R. S. (1954) *J. Bone Jt. Surg.*, **36** (A), 1031.
Popper, H. (1941) *Arch. Path. (Lab. Med.)*, **31**, 776.
Prados, M. and Swank, R. L. (1942) *Arch. Neurol. Psychiat.* (Chicago), **47**, 626.
Prickett, C. O. (1934) *Amer. J. Physiol.*, **107**, 459.
Purpura, D. P. and Gonzalez-Monteagudo, O. (1960) *J. Neuropath.*, **19**, 421.
Raubitschek, H. (1915) *Ergebn. allg. Path. path. Anat.*, **18** (i), 662.
Richmond, J. and Davidson, S. (1958) *Quart. J. Med.*, **27**, 517.
Rickes, E. L., Brink, N. G., Konuisky, F. R., Wood, T. R. and Folkers, K. (1948) *Science*, **107**, 396.
Riggs, H. E. and Boles, R. S. (1944) *Quart. J. Stud. Alc.*, **5**, 361.
Rimington, C. (1961) *Report 7th Int. Congr. Neurol.*, p. 21.
Rinehart, J. F. (1947) *Amer. J. Path.*, **23**, 879.
Rinehart, J. F., Friedman, M. and Greenberg, L. D. (1949) *Arch. Path.*, **48**, 129.
Rinehart, J. F. and Greenberg, L. D. (1956) *Amer. J. Clin. Nutr.*, **4**, 318.
Roberts, E. (1961) In *Chemical Pathology of the Nervous System*, edited by Folch-Pi, J., New York, London.
Rodnight, R. and McIlwain, H. (1955) *J. Ment. Sci.*, **101**, 884.
Russell, J. S. R., Batten, F. E. and Collier, J. (1900) *Brain*, **23**, 39.
Schaefer, A. E., McKibbin, J. M. and Elvehjem, C. A. (1942) *J. biol. Chem.*, **143**, 321.
Scherer, H. J. (1944) *Vergleichende Pathologie des Nervensystems der Säugetiere*. Leipzig.
Scheube, B. (1884) *Virchows Arch. path. Anat.*, **95**, 146.
Scheube, B. (1894) *Die Beriberi Krankheit*, G. Fischer, Jena.
Scholz, W. (1949) *Arch. Psychiat. Nervenkr.*, **181**, 621.
Schroeder, P. (1908) *Arch. Psychiat. Nervenkr.*, **44**, 193.
Scriba, K. and Luckner, H. (1949) *Dtsch. Arch. Klin. Med.*, **196**, 193.
Sebrell, W. H. and Butler, R. E. (1939) *Publ. Hlth. Rep.*, Wash., **54**, 2121.
Selye, H. (1957) *Rev. Canad. Biol.*, **16**, 1.
Shah, S. R. A. (1939) *Indian med. Gaz.*, **74**, 385.
Shaw, J. H. and Phillips, P. H. (1941) *J. Nutr.*, **22**, 345; (1945) *ibid.*, **29**, 113.
Shiner, M. (1956) *Lancet* (i), 85; (1957) *J. Mt. Sinai Hosp.*, **24**, 273.
Sinclair, H. M. (1956) *Brit. med. Bull.*, **12**, 18.
Sinclair, H. M. (1961) In *Chemical Pathology of the Nervous System*, edited by Folch-Pi, J., New York, London.
Smith, W. T. (1955) *Excerpta med.*, Amst. (Section 8), **8**, 860; (1962) personal communication.
Spais, A., Palsson, P. A. and van Bogaert, L. (1961) *Acta. Neuropath.*, **1**, 56.
Spatz, H. (1930) *Handbuch der Psychiatrie*, **11**, Edited by O. Bumke, Julius Springer, Berlin.
Spillane, J. D. (1947) *Nutritional Disorders of the Nervous System*, Livingstone, Edinburgh.
Stern, R. O. and Findlay, G. M. (1929) *J. Path. Bact.*, **32**, 63.
Sternberg, S. S. and Philips, F. S. (1958) *Science*, **127**, 644.
Street, H. R., Cowgill, G. R. and Zimmerman, H. M. (1941) *J. Nutr.*, **22**, 7.
Swank, R. L. (1940) *J. exp. Med.*, **71**, 683.
Swank, R. L. and Adams, R. D. (1948) *J. Neuropath.*, **7**, 274.
Swank, R. L. and Prados, M. (1942) *Arch. Neurol. Psychiat.* (Chicago), **26**, 976.
Sydenstricker, V. P. and Cleckley, H. M. (1941) *Amer. J. Psychiat.*, **98**, 83.
Tanaka, T. (1934) *Amer. J. Dis. Child.*, **47**, 1286.
Tower, D. B. (1961) In *Chemical Pathology of the Nervous System*, edited by Folch-Pi, J., New York, London.

Trowell, H. C., Davies, J. N. P. and Dean, R. F. A. (1954) *Kwashiorkor*, Arnold, London.
Udani, P. M. (1960) *Indian J. Child Hlth.*, **9**, 103.
Ule, G. (1959) *Virchows Arch. path. Anat.*, **332**, 204.
Ule, G. and Kammerer, W. (1960) ibid., **333**, 190.
van Bogaert, L. (1939) *Ann. Inst. Pasteur*, **63**, 315.
van Bogaert, L., Radermecker, M. A., Jansen, P. and Gatera, F. (1962) *Acta. Neuropath.*, **1**, 363.
Vannotti, A. (1954) *Porphyrins, their Biological and Chemical Importance*, Trans. C. Rimington, Hilger & Watts, London.
Victor, M. and Adams, R. D. (1953) *Proc. Ass. Res. Nerv. Ment. Dis.*, **32**, 526.
Vilter, R. W., Mueller, J. F., Glazer, H. S., Jarrold, T., Abraham, J., Thompson, C. and Hawkins, V. R. (1953) *J. Lab. clin. Med.*, **42**, 335.
Walton, J. N. and Adams, R. D. (1958) *Polymyositis*, Edinburgh.
Watson, C. J. (1960) *New Engl. J. Med.*, **263**, 1205.
Wernicke, C. (1881–83) *Lehrbuch der Gehirnkrankheiten, Bd.* 2, Fischer, Kassel and Berlin.
Williams, R. D., Mason, H. L., Smith, B. F. and Wilder, R. M. (1942) *Arch. intern. Med.*, **69**, 721.
Wilson, S. A. K. (1914) *Proc. R. Soc. Med.*, **7**, 31.
Wintrobe, M. M., Buschke, W. H., Follis, R. H. and Humphreys, S. (1944) *Bull. J. Hopk. Hosp.*, **75**, 102.
Wintrobe, M. M., Follis, R. H., Miller, M. H., Stein, H. J., Alcayaga, R., Humphreys, S., Suksta, A. and Cartwright, G. E. (1943) *Bull. Johns Hopk. Hosp.*, **72**, 1.
Wintrobe, M. M., Stein, H. J., Follis, R. H. and Humphreys, S. (1945) *J. Nutr.*, **30**, 395.
Witts, L. J. (1961) *Brit. med. J.*, (ii), 404.
Wokes, F. (1956) *Proc. Nutrit. Soc.*, **15**, 134.
Wokes, F., Badenoch, J. and Sinclair, H. M. (1955) *Amer. J. Clin. Nutr.*, **3**, 375.
Wolbach, S. B. and Bessey, O. A. (1941) *Arch. Path.* (*Lab. Med.*), **32**, 689.
Wolf, A., Cowen, D. and Geller, L. M. (1959) *Trans. Amer. Neurol. Ass.*, **84**, 140; (1962) *Proc. 4th Int. Congr. Neuropath.*, **3**, 447.
Woltman, H. W. (1918) *Arch. intern. Med.*, **21**, 791; (1924) *Amer. J. Psychiat.*, **3**, 435.
Woltman, H. W. and Wilder, R. M. (1929) *Arch. Int. Med.*, **44**, 576.
Woolf, A. L. (1958) *Lancet* (ii), 1121.
Woolf, A. L. and Malins, J. M. (1957) *J. Path. Bact.*, **73**, 316.
Woolley, D. W. (1945) *J. biol. Chem.*, **159**, 753; (1946) ibid., **163**, 773.
Wortis, H., Bueding, E. and Jolliffe, N. (1942) *New Engl. J. Med.*, **226**, 376.
Zahnd, G. (1953) *Mschr. Psychiat. Neurol.*, **125**, 103.
Zimmerman, H. M. (1939–40) *Yale J. Biol. Med.*, **12**, 23; (1943) *Proc. Ass. Res. Nerv. Ment. Dis.*, **22**, 51.

CHAPTER 6

MALFORMATIONS OF THE NERVOUS SYSTEM, BIRTH INJURY AND DISEASES OF EARLY LIFE

By R. M. Norman

I. PRENATAL MALFORMATIONS

Problems of classification

The act of birth marks no particular milestone in the development of the human brain and many years must elapse before approximate structural maturity is achieved. Although the term malformation thus includes in its scope anomalies originating in post-natal life, the latter can usually be more precisely classified on the basis of their aetiology. This is far from being the case in prenatal malformations. Deductions as to pathogenesis drawn in early malformations of the brain are apt to be fallacious, for the immature nervous system does not react to disease in the same way as adult tissue and parts may be absorbed without trace of neuroglial or connective tissue repair. Inflammatory reactions are not seen before the 6th month of foetal life (Eicke 1959). Moreover, it is known from observations on animals that the same anomaly may be produced both by genetic and environmental causes. Considerations such as these lead to the conclusion that in the present state of knowledge malformations of the nervous system are best classified by their morphological features alone.

The findings of experimental teratology

Much light has been thrown on the mechanisms of abnormal development by the study of experimentally induced malformations in animals and a very large literature has grown up around the subject (Gruenwald 1947; Willis 1958). The main exogenous factors leading to congenital malformations have been conveniently listed by Woollam and Millen (1960 a). While these findings are usually not directly applicable to the problems of pathogenesis in man certain important general principles have emerged. It has been shown that each pattern of malformation has for its inception a critical period during which the neuroblasts of the affected region become vulnerable, probably because of their increased metabolic activity at that time. Stockhard (1920), following upon the earlier work of Mall (1908), demonstrated that whatever the effective noxious stimulus to the developing ovum might be, whether oxygen deficiency, mechanical interference or variations in temperature and humidity, it was the stage of development reached at the time of the experiment that was decisive.

More recently deep X-rays have been used with advantage as a damaging agent capable of considerable refinement in respect of the timing and intensity of the lesions inflicted on the developing brain. The systematic studies of Hicks (1952, 1953 a) are particularly instructive. Pregnant rats were subjected to a single dose of ionising radiations on the successive days of their 3 weeks' gestation period and it was found possible to construct a time-table of predictable malformations. The primitive germinal neuro-epithelium was insensitive to the dose of X-rays given, but starting on the 9th day of gestation a similar dose led to severe head deformities with anencephaly. Stenosis of the aqueduct of Sylvius followed radiation on the 11th day and from the 13th to the 18th day various cortical and striatial disturbances and also absence of the corpus callosum were brought about. Minor degrees of damage led to micrencephaly without obvious microscopic loss of nerve cells, while irradiation shortly before birth caused a cerebellar malformation with distortion of the granular layer. The 'stage-specificity' of the changes appeared to be correlated with phases of enhanced metabolic activity of the neuroblasts associated with increased formation of nucleic acids and proteins. During the course of these experiments it was found that the immature brain possessed considerable powers of recovery after injury and damaged areas might apparently be fully restored to normal. This fact accounted for the discrepancies sometimes observed in the expected pattern of the malformations. For example, the eyes alone might be affected, although it was known from other experiments that parts of the cerebrum also must have originally been damaged (Hicks 1954). The late sequelae of irradiation of the brain in rats have been studied by Cowen and Geller (1960) whose paper contains a good survey of the modern literature. Woollam and Millen (1960 b) have shown that the effects of irradiation on the embryo is augmented by thyroxin, insulin and cortisone and diminished by cysteamine, thus suggesting that the sensitivity of the tissues may be dependent on the oxygen saturation.

Experiments using diminished oxygen supply as the teratogenic agent are of special interest since this factor may be concerned in human malformations. Owing to its ability to utilise anaerobic as well as aerobic sources of energy the neuroblast is much more resistant to anoxia and to hypoglycaemia than is the mature nerve cell. Nevertheless, anoxia in chick embryos has been shown to lead to anencephaly, cyclopia and forking of the Sylvian aqueduct, the latter due to the formation of septa by proliferation of the lining neuro-epithelium (Muskett 1953). Ingalls *et al.* (1950) subjected pregnant mice to reduced atmospheric pressures (as at high altitudes) and so produced a gradually increasing degree of anoxia. It was again shown that the more rapidly differentiating structures were the most vulnerable, and that malformations occurred when the oxygen deficiency reached certain critical levels. In later foetal life anoxia may lead to severe and indiscriminate brain damage because of super-added vascular disturbances and anaemic infarction (Hicks 1953 b).

Vitamin deficiencies of various types (panthothenic acid, vitamin E, folic acid) have been shown to cause anencephaly in rats (Giroud 1960). Woollam and Millen (1955) were able to produce hydrocephalus in rabbits with great constancy provided the mother had been deprived of vitamin A for 20 weeks before mating. In this condition no anatomical abnormality of the brain was discovered and the hydrocephalus was considered to be due to hypersecretion of the cerebrospinal fluid. Excess of vitamin A also causes various malformations of the brain in rats (Giroud and Martinet 1954). This effect may be offset by the administration of insulin, or thyroxin B, thus suggesting that the carbohydrate metabolism is disturbed by excess of vitamin A (Woollam and Millen 1960 b). Of the large number of chemical agents that have a teratological effect mention may be made of tumour inhibiting drugs (Murphy 1960). An important recent observation has been the demonstration that actinomycin D is teratogenic to rats and rabbits in extremely small doses, many times less than those recommended for clinical use (Tuchmann-Duplessis and Mercier-Parot 1960).

Selenium poisoning in chick embryos has been investigated by Gruenwald (1958) who found extreme necrosis in certain parts of the brain and spinal cord in addition to malformations and an over-all stunting of growth. Gruenwald draws attention to the presence of necrosis of tissues occurring during normal development and also in certain malformations of genetic origin, and stresses the importance of this disintegration of preformed tissue in the pathogenesis of congenital malformations. This factor may vitiate the deductions often made in human material as to the time of onset of a malformation. There are evidently many variable factors to be taken into account, and it cannot be safely assumed in man that malformation of an organ or part of an organ necessarily implies the action of a noxa at the time of the differentiation of that particular structure (Warkany 1960).

There are thus three main factors to be taken into account in the production of experimentally induced defects: the time of the injury, the nature of the noxa and the extent of the repair. It is important to realise that the ultimate form of the anomaly does not necessarily give any precise indication as to the stage in development at which the abnormal process commenced. A malformation may be the final stage in a gradual retardation of growth and not the consequence of an abrupt cessation of development.

Aetiology

Despite intensive investigations the causation of prenatal malformations in man remains largely undetermined. The problem is complicated by the fact that the same type of structural anomaly may be produced both by genetic and exogenous causes. At first sight it would appear that genetic factors must be of considerable importance, since the commonest malformations of the nervous system (anencephaly, spina bifida and hydrocephalus) often recur in the same form in the same family and the chances of a later sib suffering from one or another of these conditions is greatly enhanced, being roughly 9 times the average expectation (Record and McKeown 1950). The significant aetiological factors in the conditions, however, have been proved to be advancing maternal age or number of pregnancies, so that environmental influences seem to be of decisive moment. Simple Mendelian inheritance has been demonstrated only in a few instances, and, if fresh mutations are responsible for keeping these mainly lethal anomalies in equilibrium, the mutation rate would have to be 'astonishingly high' (Penrose 1949).

Chromosome abnormalities. The new techniques have revealed constant chromosome abnormalities in mongols, the usual anomaly being the trisomic state of chromosome No. 21. In one case, however, a mongol girl had 46 instead of the normal 47 chromosomes (Ford 1960). Trisomy of chromosome 13–15 (D Group) has been found associated with absence of the olfactory bulbs and tracts (arhinencephaly), hypoplasia of one eye and optic nerve, and multiple malformations outside the nervous system (Miller *et al.* 1962). The writer has a similar unpublished case of arhinencephaly in which the chromosome defect has been shown by Dr. Polani to involve chromosome No. 13.

Maternal infections. The demonstration of a relationship between maternal infection during pregnancy and maldevelopment of the offspring has furnished additional evidence of the pathogenetic importance of environmental factors. It is well established that maternal infections other than syphilis may pass the placenta and interfere with development, and Gregg's (1941) original observations on the malign effect of rubella have been amply confirmed. Swan (1949) estimated that no fewer than 93 per cent of the mothers of his 558 collected cases had been infected during the first 4 months of pregnancy. This selected group of patients, however, gives far too high an incidence. The Swedish survey of Lundström (1952) included mothers infected with rubella during the first 4 months of pregnancy and showed that the incidence of still births, neonatal deaths, immaturity and malformations in this group was 17 per cent compared with 6 per cent in the controls. Greenberg *et al.* (1957) put the incidence at 12 per cent. Transmission to the embryo may occur without overt disease in the mother. It is likely that the teratogenic virulence of the virus varies in different epidemics since there are numerous instances of maternal infection in early pregnancy without untoward consequences to the child (Landtman 1948). More recent observations in the effects of maternal rubella and other infections have been summarised by Knobloch and Pasamanick (1962).

In Swan's (1949) large series the commonest abnormalities were microcephaly, cardiac defects, deafness and cataract. Hydrocephalus, absent corpus callosum, mongolism, epilepsy and spastic syndromes were also represented. The deafness is due to defective development of the organ of Corti and is seldom total. The critical stage for the development of the cochlea is about a month later than that for the lens, so that cataract and deafness are not often found in the same individual (Ingalls 1950). Swan however noted that the time of the clinical onset of the maternal infection does not always coincide with the known stage of active differentiation of the affected organ in the offspring and suggested that these discrepancies might be due to variation in the proliferation of the virus or in the resistance of the cells to infection. Very few adequate examinations have been made of the micrencephalic brains following rubella embryopathy. Friedman and Cohen's (1947) case showed absence of the corpus callosum and anomalies of the cerebral cortex. In the two cases described by Mutrux *et al.* (1949) the gyral pattern was normal. The abnormal features were mild hydrocephalus, a small corpus callosum and perivascular and marginal gliosis. Kappers (1959) examined a 6-weeks-old embryo, the mother's infection having taken place a month before miscarriage. The main pathological changes were deep infoldings of the hemispheric neuroepithelium, proliferation and rosette formations in the choroid plexus, endothelial thickening of vessel walls, and a defect in the roof of the rhombencephalon, probably due to necrosis and rupture.

The evidence that other virus diseases are capable of causing malformations is less convincing though on several occasions structural anomalies have been reported following maternal infections occurring in early pregnancy. Cerebral destruction resembling hydranencephaly has been reported in association with infective hepatitis in the mother (Kass 1951). Rubeola, mumps, varicella, infective mononucleosis, poliomyelitis and western equine encephalitis have all been incriminated, though the method of collecting these cases often makes aetiological deductions of doubtful value (Muller 1950). The same doubts arise when the possible teratogenic effect of Asian influenza is considered (Ingalls 1960).

Cytomegalic inclusion body disease (salivary gland virus encephalitis) may also involve the foetal nervous system and lead to hydrocephalus with widespread evidence of inflammation and periventricular calcifications. In Diezel's (1954) case the maternal infection was thought to have occurred in the 4th month of pregnancy, and the infant's brain showed the malformation of micropolygyria in addition to the usual destructive lesions. Several similar cases have now been recorded (Haymaker *et al.* 1954; Crome and France 1959).

Granulomatous meningo-encephalitis is another group of diseases which may attack the developing nervous system, usually in the later stages of foetal life (Wyatt and Tribby 1952). Of these toxoplasmosis (*quod vide*) is the best known. A condition also characterised by hydrocephalus, periventricular calcifications, thickened leptomeninges and eccentric degenerative changes in the smaller blood-vessels has been described as a separate disease by Sabin and Feldman (1948) on the grounds of the negative serological tests ('Sabin's non-toxoplasmic vascular encephalopathy').

Intra-uterine meningitis following staphylococcal infection is another very rare cause of congenital hydrocephalus (Crosby *et al.* 1951). A comprehensive account of the prenatal and perinatal infections of the central nervous system has been given by Wolf and Cowen (1959).

Anoxia. In rare instances the foetus has survived damage due to carbon monoxide poisoning in the mother. Hallervorden (1949) reported the case of a child aged 1 year whose mother had attempted suicide by coal gas inhalation when 5 months' pregnant. The child's brain showed not only softenings of the globus pallidus and putamen but extensive micropolygyria of the cerebral cortex.

Lack of oxygen or other nutritional deficiency has been thought to follow faulty implantation of the ovum and to lead to various malformations. The evidence in favour of this theory is mainly based upon the finding that extra-uterine gestation is associated with a greatly increased incidence of maldevelopments both in embryos (Mall 1908) and in viable babies (Suter and Wichser 1948).

Irradiation. Deep X-ray or radium therapy to the pelvis during the first 4 months of pregnancy has produced many cases of microcephaly (Murphy 1947). Anomalies of the eye (optic atrophy, choroidoretinitis, abnormal retinal pigmentation) are much commoner in these cases than in micrencephaly of genetic origin. Four histologically examined cases in which therapeutic irradiation or radium treatment had been carried out during pregnancy are quoted by Cowen and Geller (1960). Various anomalies of the eyes, cerebral hemispheres and thalamus were present in Johnson's (1938) case. Courville and Edmundson (1958) reported microcephaly with diffuse loss of cortical nerve cells. Cerebellar microgyria with some structural disorientation were the main features of the cases of Miskolczy (1931) and of van Bogaert and Radermecker (1955). It is interesting to note that at autopsy 3 of these brains exhibited meningo-encephalitis. To these cases may be added that of Uiberrack (1942) which showed pachygyria of the cerebral cortex and defective development of the vermis.

Maternal diabetes. Hoet *et al.* (1960) have reviewed the evidence that disturbed carbohydrate metabolism and associated vitamin deficiencies are causal factors in malformations. Arhinencephaly have been reported in the offspring of diabetic mothers (Dekaban and Magee 1958; Dekaban 1959).

Cyclopia

In its most extreme form the cyclopian monster exhibits a centrally placed, diamond shaped orbit containing a single globe showing various degrees of doubling of the intrinsic structures. There are also gross malformations of the mouth and nose, the latter being usually represented by a proboscis placed above the eye. The optic nerves are sometimes absent, one cause for this being that the nerve fibres have been prevented from growing back along the optic stalks because of the primary absence of the choroidal fissures (Gruenwald 1945). Owing to the failure of the anterior telencephalon to divide into two hemispheres a single ventricle without a corpus callosum or septum pellucidum is formed. This 'holosphere' (Yakovlev 1959) is partially roofed by a rudimentary macrogyric cortex in which 9 distinct cytoarchitectonic areas can be distinguished. The hippocampus, fascia dentata and subiculum occupy the entire circumference. The ventricle is closed behind by a thin membrane attached to the thalamus. The basal ganglia form unpaired protruberances in the floor of the holosphere. Except for the absence of cortical projection systems the brain stem and cerebellum are normal. This concentration of primary anomalies in the forebrain region and in the face may be explained as the result of faulty induction by the prechordal mesenchyme. Similarly, the cyclopian eye is not the consequence of a fusion of anlagen, but of faulty induction (Adelmann 1930). The whole subject is well covered by Yakovlev's (1959) account which is based on the examination of 10 specimens.

In the less severe forms of cyclopia the eyes may be separate but microphthalmic, and a flattened nose is present (cebocephaly). The mildest variety is known as *arhinencephaly* and is often associated with hare-lip. As in the cyclops, the olfactory bulbs and tracts are absent and in the great majority of cases there is an unpaired ventricle. The longitudinal cerebral fissure may, however, be present but the hemispheres are connected together in its depths not by a corpus callosum but by a plate of grey matter or by interdigitating gyri. The hippocampal formations have often been described as being unduly small in these brains, but in de Jong's (1927) case they were found to be larger than normal. Hypertrophy of the basal ganglia was a feature of the arhinencephalic brain described by Goldstein and Riese (1925). Stewart's

(1939) specimen was an example of the least severe variety of the condition; hemispheres were fully separated and there was a complete corpus callosum although a distinctly small one. Unilateral absence of the olfactory tract accompanied by similar cerebral anomalies has also been described. Partial separation of the hemispheres with a single ventricular cavity can also occur in the presence of intact olfactory tracts, and general intelligence is not necessarily reduced (Nathan and Smith 1950). An interesting point shown by some cases is that foramina may be present in the cribriform plate despite the absence of the olfactory bulbs—a fact consistent with the development of the olfactory nerves independently of their central connections.

Anencephaly

In this common maldevelopment the brain is either absent or rudimentary ('hemicrania') and there is an associated defect of the cranial vault and scalp. The frontal bones are absent above the supraciliary ridge and the parietal bones and the squamous part of the occipital bone are usually missing. The cervical vertebrae are reduced in number and in rather more than half the cases there is a rachischisis, continuous with the cranial defect, which may reach the lumbar region (Nañagas 1925). In hemicrania the cerebellum and brain stem may be largely spared, but usually the brain is represented by a thin rudiment of highly vascular tissue containing elements of neurones, neuroglia and choroid plexus—the area cerebro-vasculosa. The anterior pituitary may occasionally be identifiable, and its absence or hypoplasia is thought to be correlated with the extremely small adrenals which are a constant feature of the condition. The clinical and pathological features of anencephaly have been well presented by André-Thomas and Ajuriaguerra (1959). There is no doubt that part of the malformation is due to a disintegration of preformed portions of the brain, since in many specimens the eyes are normal though there may be no trace of the optic nerves. The primary defect appears to be defective closure of the anterior end of the neural tube. The process has been followed in rat embryos rendered anencephalic by excess of vitamin A (Giroud 1959). Before the onset of degenerative changes the cellular growth of the various parts of the telencephalon is not greatly disturbed except that development is distorted by the presence of an unclosed neural plate and the cerebral hemispheres are found beneath the everted diencephalon. In *exencephaly* a pendulous cerebral or meningeal hernia covered by normal scalp protrudes from a midline defect in the posterior part of the skull. Much more rarely the whole cranial vault may be absent, as in anencephaly, though the scalp is still present. Vogel and McClenahan (1952) have shown, by the method of injecting fusible metal, that major arteries do not penetrate the areas of cerebral malformation, but are often replaced by a number of slender abnormal branches rising from the internal carotid arteries. In cases in which the cerebellum and brain stem are involved the vertebral system is also disorganised. The authors consider that anomalies of the major arteries occurring between the 3rd and 5th week of foetal life may be an important pathogenic factor in anencephaly. Vogel (1958) has reported anencephaly in one head of a conjoined double twin, again with striking vascular anomalies on that side. Whether these vascular abnormalities are solely responsible for the condition, however, remains doubtful, for Giroud (1960) has observed a normal arrangement of vessels in young anencephalic embryos.

Malformations of the spinal cord

Amyelia, or total absence of the spinal cord, is only found in association with anencephaly. An interesting feature of the condition is the occasionally independent development of many of the spinal ganglia, the posterior roots of which may be seen passing inwards towards the area medullovasculosa as if in search of their non-existent spinal cord—a good example of the principle of 'self-determination' in the formation of the nervous system. The muscles of these monsters are well developed despite the absence of anterior spinal nerve roots.

Much commoner are the various forms of *myelodysplasia* associated with spina bifida. In the most severe of these malformations the neural tube has failed to close (*myeloschisis*). The flattened remnant of the cord which is, in fact, the representative of the neural plate, is covered by a highly vascular mass of connective tissue which may present through the defect in the vertebral column and integument as a raw, red, velvety area. Microscopical examination of such cases usually reveals a large number of coincident developmental errors. The internal structure of the preserved ventral part of the cord may be disorganised at the level of the defect, the anterior cornua being absent or malformed and appearing as islands of nerve cells set in an overgrowth of ependymal and glial tissue. Ectopic nerve cells and fibres together with aberrant ependymal canals may be encountered in the mesodermal tissue with which the dorsal part of the defective spinal cord merges. Spinal root ganglia may also be found occupying abnormal positions in the subarachnoid space. It is generally accepted that the malformation is due to a primary failure of closure of the neural grove, though Gardner (1961) has argued in favour of the old conception of Morgagni that rupture of the closed tube may occur. Patten (1953) studied 3 human embryos with myeloschisis and found a local overgrowth of the unfused lips of the cleft. This principle of excessive growth as a factor in abnormal development is important, as will be seen in the discussion of the Arnold-Chiari deformity.

The other common malformations of the spinal cord which are associated with spina bifida are *meningocele* in which only the meninges herniate subcutaneously, *meningomyelocele* in which the spinal cord as a whole passes into the sac and finally *myelocystocele* in which the central canal is greatly dilated and the thinned-out posterior part of the cord accompanies the meningeal hernia. In the condition of *anterior spina bifida* there is a failure of fusion of the vertebral bodies. Various anomalies may be associated with this, ranging from fistulous connections between intestine and spinal cord, to cysts lined with intestinal tissue within the spinal canal (see Willis 1958 for a full review).

Diastematomyelia. The spinal cord may divide into two halves each of which undergoes subsequent modifications of structure. The extent of the duplication is usually limited to about 10 segments and of the 42 cases reviewed by Herren and Edwards (1940) only 2 occurred at a level higher than the midthoracic. The two cords are often separated from each other by a bony projection or fibrous band arising from the dorsal surface of a vertebral body. This doubling of the cord is often seen adjoining the region affected by myeloschisis. More than half the cases are associated with spina bifida occulta. The cord usually shows an increasing degree of hydromyelia as the point of division is approached from higher levels. This dilatation is succeeded first by a bifurcation of the central canal, then by the appearance of a dorsal cleft reinforced by the downward growth of a connective tissue septum which separates the cord into two halves. Each opposed medial surface of these two divisions of the cord has a fissure containing branches of the anterior spinal artery and probably caused by their inroad during the course of development (Lichtenstein 1940). (Such clefts have often been thought to be the true anterior fissures of a double cord, but this theory would involve the assumption that each 'cord' had rotated through 90°.) Each new half of the cord possesses a posterior and an anterior horn with their roots. In certain instances, the anterior horn becomes secondarily divided into two parts, but the posterior roots remain unpaired. Each half of the divided cord has its own pial investment but the arachnoid and dura may be shared. Very rarely, the two divisions of the cord, instead of lying laterally, are found in a dorso-ventral position (Dominok 1962).

Minor malformations of the spinal cord and status dysraphicus. In spina bifida occulta and also in cases without rachischisis the cord may exhibit a number of *minor malformations*. Although these anomalies do not usually give rise to neurological signs they have been considered of importance by some writers as forming an integral part of the syndrome of status dysraphicus. The conception of this condition as a morbid entity dates from the clinical observations of Fuchs (1909) who distinguished a group of individuals having in common some of the following features: spina bifida, syndactyly, trophic and vasomotor disturbances, sensory disturbances of syringomyelic type, sphincter weakness and skin anomalies such as naevi and hypertrichosis. This syndrome was elaborated by Bremer (1927) who noted the frequency of kyphosis and sternal deformities in the group and who also demonstrated abnormal glial proliferation and small cavities in the region of the dorsal septum in the spinal cords of some of these cases. Bremer stressed the familial concentration of these anomalies and considered that status dysraphicus was inherited as a distinctive constitutional disability. In more recent times this opinion has been supported by Benda (1952) who has described a similar clinico-pathological syndrome ('oligoencephaly') among feeble-minded mental defectives. Among these minor malformations may be mentioned the absence of the posterior septum or the presence of a cleft in this situation, anomalies of the central canal such as patency in adult life, and various distortions and asymmetries of the anterior and posterior horns of grey matter. These findings are important in so far as they indicate the developmental origin of the abnormalities seen elsewhere in the nervous system of these patients, but great care must be taken to exclude the presence of artefacts which may easily be produced by careless removal of the spinal cord (van Gieson 1892).

Syringomyelia and syringobulbia. By J. G. Greenfield

The name *syringomyelia* (syrinx = a tube) is used to describe tubular cavitation of the spinal cord extending over many segments. Cavities which involve only 2 or 3 segments are not

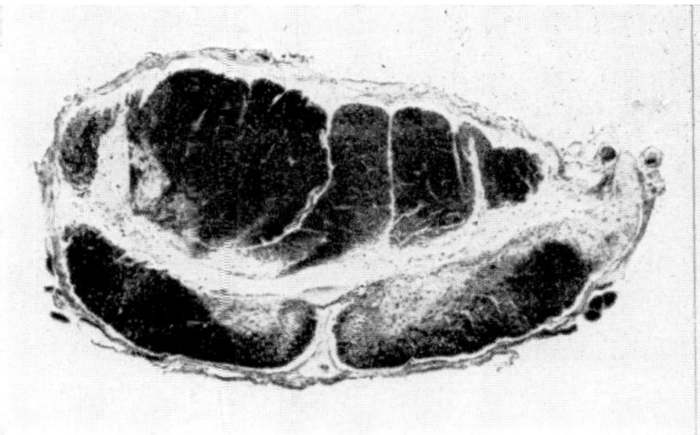

6.1

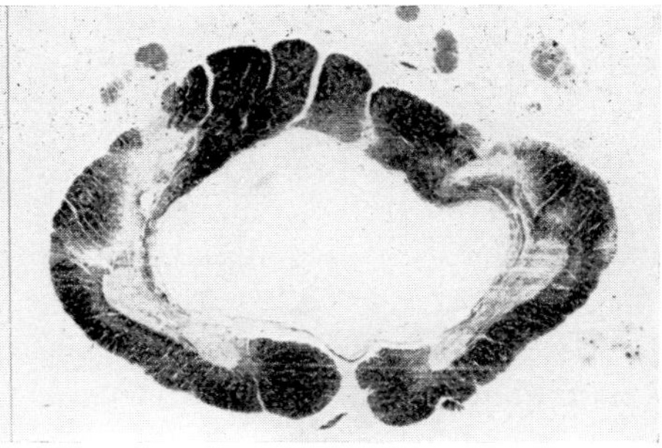

6.2

Fig. 6.1. *Syringomyelia.* Cavity extends into both dorsal horns.
Fig. 6.2. Cavity merges with the central canal.

usually considered syringomyelic, although they may be of essentially similar nature. When the cavitation is merely a distension of the central canal of the cord the name *hydromyelia* or *hydromyelus* is used. The name *syringobulbia* is used for the cavities in the medulla which are often associated with syringomyelia. It is rather less appropriate as these cavities are more often slit-like than tubular. More rarely cavitation extends into the pons and in exceptional cases it may reach the midbrain and internal capsule (Spiller 1906). Clinically the disease usually begins during the 2nd or 3rd decade and is slowly progressive, or the symptoms may increase at first rapidly and then more slowly. They may cease to progress at any time. Unless associated with bulbar symptoms they rarely cause death.

Pathology. When exposed at operation or autopsy the spinal cord appears swollen and tense in the cervical region and may fill the spinal canal. Otherwise it appears normal and there is no thickening of the meninges. The syrinx is filled with clear, slightly yellow serous fluid and when this is allowed to escape the cord becomes flattened, most often in its antero-posterior diameter. On section of the cord the cavity is usually found to be largest in the cervical region but is often absent in the first cervical segment. It extends down through the thoracic segments for a varying distance and usually terminates at the lower thoracic level. The lumbo-sacral enlargement is rarely involved. In typical cases the cavity in the *cervical enlargement* extends transversely across the cord, involving the more dorsal parts of the ventral horns and passing across the midline behind the central canal. It often extends also into the dorsal horns (Fig. 6.1). When very large it occupies most of the cross-section of the cord; the more ventral groups of motor nerve cells lie in front of it but otherwise little grey matter remains, and the lateral and dorsal columns are reduced by compression to a narrow zone of fibres (Fig. 6.2). Extensions in the midline, or more laterally into the dorsal columns, are common and the anterior white commissure is often destroyed either by pressure or by a midline ventral extension of the cavity. A transverse cavity with midline dorsal and ventral extensions, such as is sometimes seen at this level, closely resembles the cruciform shape of the central canal during the stage of foetal development before the alar and basal laminae fuse with one another. That this is more than a chance resemblance is shown by the most usual position of the cavity in the medulla which also lies between the nuclei arising respectively from the alar and the basal laminae. In the *thoracic cord* the cavity very commonly lies in the dorsal horns. It is often unilateral. When bilateral the cavities may be separate or may be joined in the region of the grey commissure and so form a single U-shaped cavity. Serial sections show that cavities which are double at one level usually join into a single cavity at a higher level, and it is usual for the cavity on one side to end at a higher level than the other. More rarely cavities join in the lower thoracic region. Although the grey matter is the common site of cavitation extensions into the dorsal or lateral columns or across the white commissure are not unusual, and the cavity may reach the pial surface at the tips of the dorsal horns at any level.

The walls of the cavity vary greatly in character especially from case to case but also in different parts of the same cavity. In the writer's view these variations depend on the age of the cavity and the degree of tension within it. Where there is a recent extension the wall is irregular and consists of degenerated neuroglial and neural elements. The myelin around it stains poorly, as it does in oedematous white matter, and the appearances suggest tearing of the tissues and transudation of serous fluid into them. When the cavity has been established for a longer time there is neuroglial hyperplasia around it with large fibre-forming astrocytes lying chiefly in a tangential direction. These finally form a dense concentric wall of neuroglial sclerosis which may be 1 or 2 mm. in thickness. It is common to find a thin layer of collagen covering some part of the wall. Thicker strands of collagen, or blood-vessels with hyalinised walls, may be seen passing across the cavity from one wall to another. Where the cavity communicates with the central canal, as it not uncommonly does especially in the cervical region, part of the central wall of the cavity is lined with ependymal cells, but in most places these take no part in the formation of the wall. Where they are present the layer of neuroglial tissue on which they are based is usually thinner than that surrounding the rest of the cavity.

Syringobulbia. Slit-like cavities in the medulla usually lie in one of three positions (Jonesco-Sisesti 1932). (1) The most common is a slit running out in a ventrolateral direction from the floor of the 4th ventricle external to the hypoglossal nucleus. It may communicate with the cavity of the ventricle but sometimes begins ventral to this. It passes outwards and forwards for a variable distance towards the descending root of the trigeminal nerve, usually destroying the fasciculus solitarius and the fibres which pass dorsally from the nucleus ambiguus to join those arising in the dorsal vagal nucleus (Fig. 6.5). A cavity in this position is most commonly limited to the lower half or two-thirds of the medulla where it interrupts the fibres passing from the nuclei gracilis and cuneatus to form the decussation of the median fillet. It may also descend low enough to interrupt many of the decussating pyramidal fibres. At this level it extends

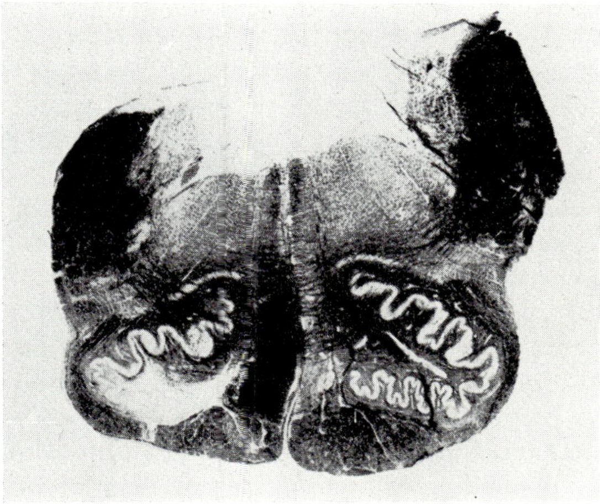

6.3

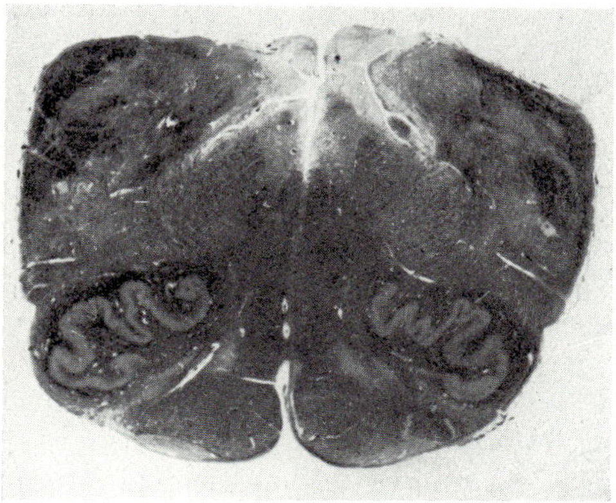

6.4

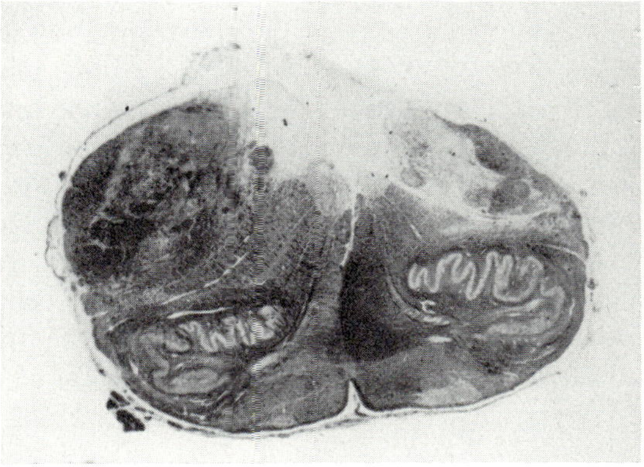

6.5

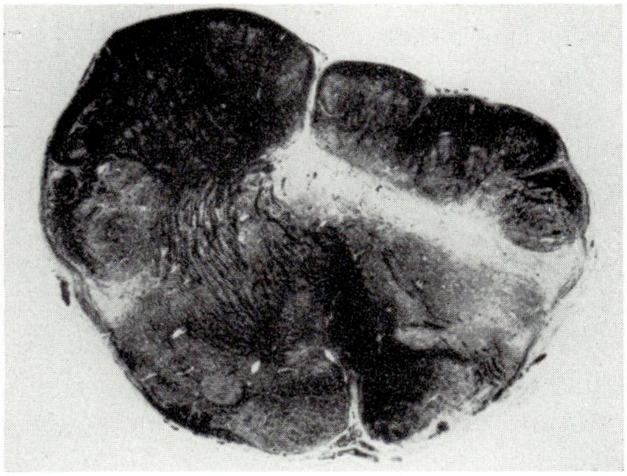

6.6

FIG. 6.3. *Syringobulbia.* Case with ventral slit between olive and pyramid and dorsolateral slit at a lower level which has produced degeneration of the contralateral mesial fillet.
FIG. 6.4. Case with bilateral dorsolateral and dorsomesial slits.
FIG. 6.5. Case with dorsolateral slit producing degeneration of the mesial fillet.
FIG. 6.6. Section at the level of the pyramidal decussation. The lateral extension of the cavity has destroyed the crossed pyramidal fibres.

transversely from the grey matter lateral to the central canal to a position ventral to the substantia gelatinosa and descending root of the trigeminal nerve. Cavities in this position usually have thin walls of neuroglial tissue. Occasionally the slit is replaced by a neuroglial scar which interrupts the fibre systems as completely as a slit or cavity. Such scars are not uncommon at the upper and lower ends of a cavity and may arise from secondary fusion of its walls. These cavities are usually unilateral but may be bilateral and roughly symmetrical (Fig. 6.4). In such a case one cavity extends to a higher or lower level than the other. (2) Almost equally common is an extension of the 4th ventricle along the median raphe for a shorter or longer distance. This is usually lined by ependyma, but occasionally is replaced by a neuroglial scar containing ependymal cells or small ependyma-lined tubules, like those seen in forking of the aqueduct (Fig. 6.4). By interrupting the decussation of fibres passing from the descending vestibular nucleus to the median longitudinal fasciculus these slits may cause nystagmus, but are otherwise asymptomatic. When this median extension is small and is not associated with other cavitation in the medulla it scarcely merits the name of syringobulbia. (3) A rarer position for a cavity is between the pyramid and the inferior olive where it interrupts the emerging fibres of the hypoglossal nerve (Fig. 6.3). These cavities are almost always unilateral; in Spiller's case they were bilateral, although only one was large enough to cause atrophic palsy of the tongue. A cavity in this situation may also damage the ventromedian part of the olive or the dorsal part of the pyramid.

Cavities in the *pons* usually lie in the tegmentum where they may destroy the fibres of the 6th or 7th cranial nerves, or the central tegmental tract. They may pass down dorsal to the olive for a short distance. Extensions of the cavity to a higher level are extremely rare. In Spiller's case the cavity in one pyramid passed up among the corticospinal fibres, destroying also the substantia nigra and ended in the internal capsule and caudate and lenticular nuclei.

Secondary degenerations follow destruction of tracts and fibre systems both in syringomyelia and syringobulbia. The pyramidal tracts may be pressed on by a ventral cavity between the pyramid and medullary olive or a slit at a lower level may interrupt pyramidal fibres during their decussation. In the latter case there is commonly some retrograde degeneration of the pyramidal fibres in the medulla. Or a large cavity in the cervical region may destroy much of the pyramidal tract by compression. The *spinocerebellar tracts* may degenerate owing to destruction of their cells of origin in the grey matter of the cord or of the fibres leaving these. The fibres passing in the *dorsal columns* may be compressed or destroyed by extensions of the cavity in the cord. In cases of syringobulbia the fibres relayed to the thalamus from the nuclei gracilis and cuneatus are commonly destroyed as they pass towards the decussation of the medial fillet so that there is more or less complete absence of the median fillet on the side opposite to the lesion (Figs. 6.3 and 6.5); retrograde degeneration occurs in the nerve cells of the nuclei gracilis et cuneatus. Fibres passing to the spinothalamic tracts are very commonly involved either at or near their cells of origin in the dorsal horns or as they cross the midline in the central commissure. The dorsolateral cavities in the medulla commonly interrupted some of the fibres passing inwards from the descending trigeminal nucleus to the fillet. The destruction of the motor fibres arising in the nucleus ambiguus and hypoglossal nuclei and of the tractus solitarius has already been mentioned.

The *symptomatology* of syringomyelia is closely related to the destruction of nerve cells and fibres. Wasting of the muscles of the hands and fore-arms is related to lesions of the postero-lateral cell groups in the ventral horns of the cervical cord. Dissociated anaesthesia results from damage to spinothalamic fibres and autonomic symptoms to destruction of the cells of the intermedio-lateral tract in the upper thoracic segments. Anaesthesia to all forms of sensibility is usually attributable to a combination of a spinothalamic lesion either with a lesion in the dorsal columns or more often with a cavity in the medulla which interrupts the decussating fibres going to the medial fillet. Loss of appreciation of position and vibration may also result from a lesion of this system of fibres. The position of the medullary cavities explains the paralyses of the lower cranial nerves and the facial and corneal analgesia. Rarely extensions into the pons may cause paralysis of one abducens nerve or of conjugate deviation to one side, or by destruction of the central tegmental tract may lead to the syndrome of palato-laryngeal nystagmus. Nystagmus on lateral deviation of the eyes, which is very common in cases with dorsolateral slits, is most easily explained by the destruction of fibres which pass from the descending vestibular nucleus to the medial longitudinal fasciculus.

Hydromyelia and secondary syringomyelia

The name *hydromyelia* or *hydromyelus* is given to congenital dilatations of the central canal of the cord. They are not uncommonly found in routine post-mortem examinations and they occur in a large proportion of cases of meningomyelocele and of cases of the Arnold-Chiari malformation in older patients. They vary greatly in size and extent, from narrow slits confined to a few cervical segments, to fairly large tubular cavities running through most of the length of the spinal cord. The smaller cavities are either transverse slits or are triangular on cross-section with their base lying transversely in the grey commissure and their apex in

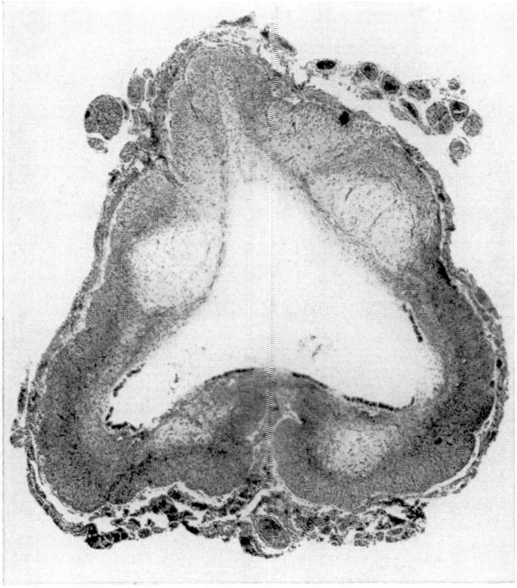

6.7

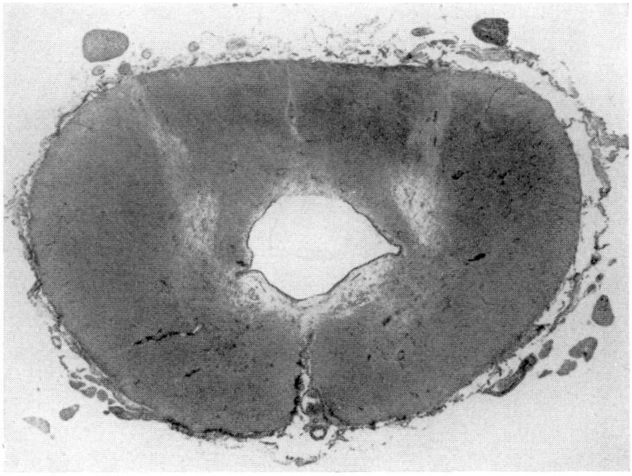

6.8

FIG. 6.7. *Hydromyelia* in a case of Arnold-Chiari malformation in a new-born child with early gliosis replacing lines of ependyma in the dorsal extension.
FIG. 6.8. Hydromyelia in a man of 25 who died of poliomyelitis. Both hydromyelia and Chiari's Type 1 deformity were clinically silent.

relation to the dorsomedian septum (Figs. 6.7 and 6.8). Anteroposterior slits are less common. Larger cavities are sometimes cruciform recalling the shape of the foetal canal. The wall is lined by ependymal cells but this covering is often incomplete especially in the corners of the cavity. Where ependyma is absent it is replaced by thickening of the subependymal neuroglia which may project as granulations into the lumen of the cavity. In some cases, especially when hydromyelia is associated with the Arnold-Chiari malformation in the adult, only the ventral wall of the cavity may be covered by ependyma and the remainder by a thick firm layer of neuroglial fibres. Or a syringomyelic cavity may have formed at one side of a hydromyelia. Such cases form a link between hydromyelia and syringomyelia, and are apt to be assigned to one or the other category according to whether or not the cavitation has produced the classical symptoms of syringomyelia during life.

Secondary syringomyelia may be associated with trauma, chronic arachnoiditis or tumour, or may result from the absorption of the blood in a haematomyelia. The cavities resulting from trauma or haematomyelia usually lie either in the base of the dorsal horns or in the more ventral part of the dorsal columns. Although in most cases traumatic cavities are associated with severe transverse lesions of the cord, from which they run upwards and downwards for a few segments (Holmes 1915), they may also be found in cases with no severe local damage. Cavities associated with chronic arachnoiditis, of syphilitic, bacterial or other origin, are usually limited to a few segments. They are probably due to vascular factors, such as ischaemia associated with venous stasis.

The cavitation associated with spinal tumours presents a more difficult problem. In some cases there is only a small cavity which extends for 1 or 2 segments above and below the tumour. Such cavities may arise as a result of transudation from the tumour. In other cases the cavities may be very extensive and may involve most of the spinal cord above and below the tumour. Such cavities are most often associated either with tumours of ependymal character or with haemangioblastomas. In the former case it is possible that the cavitation was a true syringomyelia and preceded the growth of the tumour. In 2 cases examined at the National Hospital, Queen Square, an ependymal tumour at the midthoracic level was associated with cavitation which extended from the 2nd cervical segment to the conus terminalis. This had all the characters of a syringomyelic cavity but had not caused any anaesthesia or other symptoms above the level of the tumour. The cavitation associated with haemangioblastomas of the spinal cord may, like the cerebellar cysts, be caused by transudation from the tumour acting over many years. Such cavities also are often very extensive. Brain *et al.* (1943) reported a case with a tumour at the 9th thoracic level, and cavitation extending from the medulla to the conus terminalis, and in the case of Craig *et al.* (1941) the cavity was almost equally extensive. It would appear that cavities associated with tumours extend into the lumbosacral enlargement more often than those of simple syringomyelia. The venous congestion which is often found below the level of a spinal tumour may be a contributory factor to this lumbosacral extension.

The association of syringomyelia with cerebral tumours on which Langhans (1881) based his theory of pathogenesis has been found in the writer's experience in less than 0·1 per cent of autopsies on cases of cerebral tumour. This is probably a chance association since asymptomatic cavitation of the cervical cord is not very rare.

Aetiology and pathogenesis. Although anatomical considerations indicate that syringomyelia has a developmental basis it is rarely familial. The so-called 'hereditary lumbosacral syringomyelia' has been shown to be an affection of the dorsal root ganglia and primary sensory neurones (Denny-Brown 1951). The inclusion of syringomyelia in the large group covered by the name *craniorachischisis* appears justified on anatomical grounds but this brings us little nearer to an understanding of its cause. It is often associated with evidence of skeletal maldevelopment such as dolichocephaly, platybasia and spina bifida. Kyphoscoliosis and asymmetry in size of the breasts are not uncommon but are probably related causally to the lesion in the spinal cord.

The evidence for a developmental basis rests chiefly on the constancy of the position of the cavities in the medulla. In the spinal cord also it is not unusual to find dilatation of the central canal, almost amounting to hydromyelia, below a typical syringomyelic cavity (Taylor *et al.* 1922). It is also possible in some cases to trace the development of a syringomyelic cavity from hydromyelia, for example in cases of the Arnold-Chiari malformation in the adult. But this is only true for a minority of cases.

Several different factors may be combined in the pathogenesis of cavitation in syringomyelia. (1) Instability in the lines of junction of the alar and basal laminae with each other. (2) The constant movements of flexion and torsion to which the cervical cord and lower medulla are exposed. (3) The tendency for cysts within nervous tissue to undergo alterations of tension and so to enlarge.

(1) As has been seen the cavitation, both in the spinal cord and especially in the medulla, tends to occur along lines of fusion which take place comparatively late in foetal life. The ventral cavity in the medulla may thus be related to the migration of the olivary cells from the rhomboid lip across the median raphe to their final position behind the pyramids. Many of the older writers have described the cells in the walls of a syringomyelic cavity as of embryonal character (Gowers and Taylor 1899). There is little evidence of this in the cases examined by the writer. Ependymal cells are often seen in the tissue in front of the cavity; in those that result from a hydromyelia they may also be found under its lateral walls; but these cells do not differ from those seen in the gray commissure in normal cords. The theory that cavitation takes place by the breakdown of abnormal neuroglial tissue does not appear to rest on any firm histological basis since in neither the medulla nor the spinal cord does the character of the neuroglia round a cavity differ in any respect from that which may be found in other pathological conditions.

(2) The reason why syringomyelic cavities tend to begin in the cervical region of the cord, and attain their greatest size there, may well be related to the great mobility of the cervical spine. Bending of the neck in all directions and torsion when the head is turned (Schaltenbrand 1951) must impose stresses and strains on the cervical cord to which it is less subject at lower levels, and which may well cause small tears of the tissues in the centre of the cord. Movements of the head on the atlanto-occipital joint must affect the lower medulla in a similar way.

(3) Once cavitation in the spinal cord has begun it may be enlarged by transudation of fluid into it under pressure. This expansion is more likely to occur in the grey matter than in the firmer columns of white matter and owing to the restricting investment of pia mater must take place chiefly upwards and downwards. It is favoured by anything which increases venous congestion in the body cavity, such as muscular effort, since there are no valves on the veins draining the spinal cord, but it may also depend to some extent on the electrolyte content of the blood. In this relation the fact that a syringomyelic cavity usually ceases at the 2nd cervical level and has no communications with the 4th ventricle may be of considerable importance.

Arnold-Chiari malformation

This name is given to a congenital malformation of the lower brain stem and lower part of the cerebellum which is very constantly present in cases of meningomyelocele and, in its milder forms, may also be found in older children and adults with or without other disease of the spine or spinal cord. As there has been some uncertainty as to how the Arnold-Chiari malformation should be defined, especially in cases in the later age groups, it is essential to give, in summary, the original descriptions.

Chiari (1891) described three types of cerebellar malformation which he had found in cases of apparently congenital hydrocephalus. In Type I the medulla was displaced downwards into the spinal canal and was covered on its dorsolateral surface by peg-like processes arising from the amygdalae and lower part of the cerebellar hemispheres. These prolongations might be asymmetrical or unilateral and might reach only to the atlas, but in many cases they passed to the lower border of the axis, so that their lower end was opposite the origin of the 3rd cervical nerve roots. Their tissue might be sclerosed or softened. As an example of this type he cited the case of a girl of 17 in whom the malformation had caused no symptoms during life. There was some widening of the lateral and 3rd ventricles but no great enlargement of the head (circumference 51 cm.).

In Type II along with a similar malformation of the lower parts of the cerebellum there was an elongation of the 4th ventricle which also extended into the spinal canal. A typical case of this kind in a 6-month-old baby with fairly severe hydrocephalus (head circumference 43 cm.) was reported. In this case there were heterotopic nodules of grey matter, the size of beans, in the walls of the lateral ventricles. The cerebellum was small and the tentorium less vaulted than normal. The pons was elongated; its lower quarter lay below the level of the foramen magnum and was flattened from before backwards. The medulla lay entirely in the spinal canal and reached to the lower border of the axis. The lower cranial nerves were thus considerably elongated. Where the medulla joined the spinal cord there was a swelling the size of a bean which covered the upper 9 mm. of the spinal cord and reached to the 5th cervical pair of nerve roots and the disc between the 4th and 5th cervical vertebrae. This swelling contained a pouch-like prolongation of the 4th ventricle. It was covered on its dorsal and lateral surfaces by flattened protrusions of cerebellar tissue arising from the amygdalae and the lower part of the vermis. The cervical portion of the cord was abnormally short (24 mm.) and its roots were crowded together. The upper pairs of posterior roots appeared between the spinal cord and the overlying mass arising from the lower medulla. The thoracic cord contained a cylindrical cavity filled with clear serum. At the lower thoracic level the cord split into two halves and passed into a meningomyelocele at the junction of the thoracic and lumbar cord. Below the 5th lumbar segment the two halves rejoined to form a cylindrical band which ended opposite the first sacral vertebra.

The details of the meningomyelocele and the hydromyelia vary from case to case but Chiari's description of the deformity of the cerebellum and lower brain stem may be applied with little alteration to the condition as it has since been found in almost every fatal case of meningomyelocele.

Chiari's Type III was represented by a single case of cervical spina bifida in which there was herniation of the cerebellum through the bony defect. This unusual case may be grouped among the occipital meningoencephaloceles.

In a later report Chiari (1895) gave fuller details of his other cases of Types I and II. In only 1 of his 14 cases of Type I was a meningomyelocele present. Seven of these were in children under the age of 10 years and 6 in adults. The case of the 17-year-old girl, already described, was the only one in the second decade of life. In 3 cases there was some dilatation of the central canal of the spinal cord. Type II was found in 7 cases in all of which there was also a lumbar meningomyelocele or spina bifida. The malformation, as he described it, was always associated with hydrocephalus of congenital type and never with hydrocephalus coming on at a later age, but he recognised that the more common cerebellar pressure coning might occur in cases of the latter type.

Meanwhile Arnold (1894) had drawn attention to the malformation in reporting a case of meningomyelocele, without hydrocephalus. But his description, although detailed, is less complete than the earlier description by Chiari.

Schwalbe and Gredig (1907) gave the name *Arnold-Chiari malformation* to Type II which they found to be always associated with meningomyelocele, and this condition was introduced to English readers by Russell and Donald (1935) who reported 10 similar cases. McConnell and Parker (1938) reported 5 cases of Chiari's Type I in older children and young adults in none of whom was there any X-ray evidence of spina bifida, and Aring (1938) described a similar case from the laboratory of the National Hospital. Since then many cases of both types have been described. In many adult cases of Type I no spina bifida has been present and in the majority of these the diagnosis has been made at operation. These cases of Type I are of special importance as the severe and often incapacitating symptoms which may be produced by the malformation can, in most cases, be relieved by operation.

It is clear from this summary that the early literature gives no justification for distinguishing the cerebellar malformation as *Arnold's deformity* and the medullary malformation as *Chiari's*

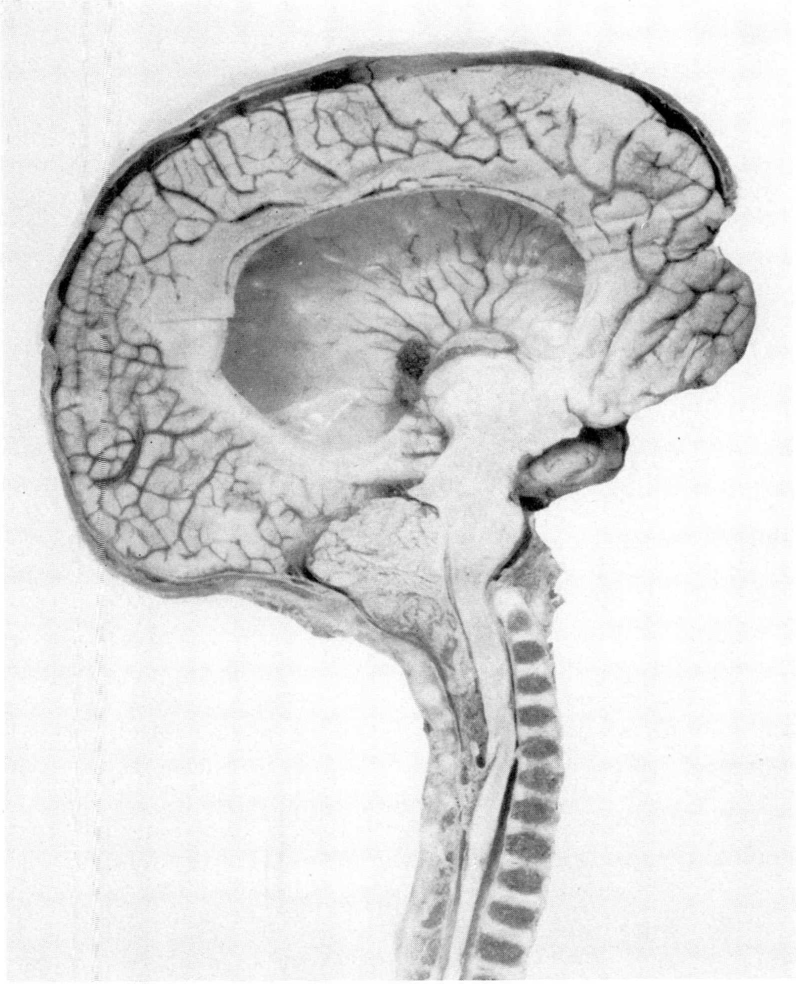

FIG. 6.9. *Arnold-Chiari malformation* and hydrocephalus in 7-week-old infant. (By courtesy of Prof. Moncrieff and the photographic department, Mr. D. Martin, Hospital for Sick Children.)

deformity (List 1941, Lichtenstein 1942). Indeed if Arnold's name had not been included by Schwalbe and Gredig it might well be omitted since Chiari's earlier description was more complete. It is also unfortunate that the latter authors confined their attention to infantile cases associated with meningomyelocele. The milder cases which are found in older children and adults should, in fact, be called *Chiari's Type I malformation*, as has indeed been the practice in recent German literature.

Naked-eye appearances (Fig. 6.9). A few points may be added to Chiari's description. In both grades of the malformation the lower part of the pons and the upper medulla are thinned as well as elongated, so that the upper medulla may have a smaller area in cross-section than its lower end. The finger-like processes of cerebellar tissue are bound to the back and sides of the medulla and spinal cord by arachnoidal adhesions which may be quite firm. These are not found in the more common cerebellar pressure cones. The enlarged lower end of the medulla usually ends abruptly in a depression, below which the cervical cord is of normal size. In severe cases the herniated lower end of the dorsal half of the medulla, containing the 4th ventricle, overlies the upper cervical segments so that on transverse section it may be quite separate from the cord. It is, however, formed entirely from the dorsal half of the medulla. It seems therefore that the elongation and downward displacement of the lower pons and medulla is greater in its dorsal than in its ventral part. At the same time histological examination of these parts of the brain stem shows no evidence of gross displacement of nuclei or fibre systems except occasionally in the inferior olive. There is no cisterna magna as the herniated tissue fills the foramen magnum which is often more funnel-shaped than normal. Daniel and Strich (1958) have reviewed the pathological findings in 26 cases of the Chiari Type II deformity and several points emerge which are not generally appreciated. The tentorium cerebelli is attached close to the margins of a large foramen magnum and has an unusually wide incisura. The cerebellar 'tail' derived from the vermis is often placed terminally within the 4th ventricle and is completely covered by ependyma. The tectal plate in the region of the quadrigeminal bodies is shaped like a beak directed downwards and backwards. At the site of the gracile and cuneate tubercles the spinal cord is bent back upon itself in a Z-shaped kink. The basilar artery lies in a deep groove in the pons and may be covered by medially placed tonsils. The nerve roots of the cervical cord run upwards or horizontally to their foramina of exit; in the upper thoracic region they gradually take a more downward direction and usually appear normal in the middle and lower thoracic segments. The lower cranial nerves are elongated by the downward displacement of their level of origin from the lower pons and the medulla. An asymmetry of the malformation, such as was found by Chiari especially in older children and adults, may result in the lower cranial nerves being more stretched on one side than the other with a correspondingly unilateral symptomatology, as in the case of Penfield and Coburn (1938). In this case, in which an upper thoracic meningomyelocele had been repaired in early childhood, the whole cerebellum was displaced downwards leaving a space filled with cerebrospinal fluid between its upper surface and the tentorium. This has not been found in other cases but the intracranial portion of the cerebellum is often smaller than normal or has shown degenerative changes such as torpedoes on the axons of the Purkinje cells (Aring 1938). Sandbank (1955) found heterotopic areas of grey matter both in the walls of the lateral ventricles and in the cerebellar white matter between the nucleus dentatus and the cortex. Cameron (1957) has found congenital stenosis or forking of the aqueduct in several cases.

Since the report by Russell and Donald (1935) Chiari's Type II had been recognised in Great Britain and the United States as a common or almost constant accompaniment of meningomyelocele. But there has been some uncertainty as to the status of Type I. Some would relate it constantly to spina bifida if not at the lumbar, at least at the sacral level, whereas to others it is only a severe grade of cerebellar pressure coning. The writer's opinion, based on a post-mortem examination of 9 adult cases of this type, is not in agreement with either view. The ages of these cases varied from 20 to 59. Four were cases of syringomyelia with symptoms characteristic of that disease; in 4 cases the symptomatology was closely related to the malformation and in 1 case, in which death was due to poliomyelitis, there were no previous symptoms. In this last case and in 1 other there was hydromyelia. In none was spina bifida found on removal of the spinal cord. This experience, although much less than Chiari's, agrees with his both in the absence of spina bifida and in distinguishing the malformation from cerebellar pressure cones. This distinction is based on (*a*) the form of the cerebellar prolongations which are peg-shaped or finger-like and often appear to be independent of any general downward displacement of the cerebellum. (*b*) Their fibrovascular adhesion to the back and sides of the medulla. (*c*) The elongation of the lower brain stem especially in its dorsal half so that the 4th ventricle is narrower and longer than normal. (*d*) The symptomatology, which usually includes paresis or paralysis of some of the lower cranial nerves, often especially on one side, along with ataxia, clumsiness of the hands and nystagmus.

Aetiology and Pathogenesis. Three chief theories of pathogenesis are current.

(1) The downward displacement of the medulla and cerebellar tonsils is thought to be due to traction resulting from fixation of the lower end of the spinal cord to the walls of a meningomyelocele. As the spine grows faster than the spinal cord the tip of the conus normally rises in the spinal canal during infancy and childhood until, when growth is completed, it lies at the level of the second lumbar vertebra. Fixation of the cord at an early stage of intrauterine life would thus exert a general traction on the spinal cord which might be transmitted to the brain stem (Lichtenstein 1942). This theory oversimplifies the problem. It does not explain why the elongation is greater in the dorsal than the ventral half of the brain stem, nor why the lower end of the 4th ventricle is displaced downwards so as often to overlap the upper cervical segments. Chiari's observation that the cervical portion of the cord was shortened and its nerve roots unduly crowded together is equally difficult to explain on this theory. Its extension to explain cases of Type I malformation with sacral spina bifida appears to have little justification since the sacral nerve roots and filum terminale are normally anchored at this level.

(2) The malformation may be simply the result of hydrocephalus and increased intracranial pressure acting from a fairly early stage of foetal life (Gardner and Goodall 1950; Gardner 1959). These authors also relate the associated hydromyelia to increase of cerebrospinal pressure transmitted to the central canal of the spinal cord. They do not account for the absence of the malformation in most cases of congenital hydrocephalus, nor for its common association with lumbar meningomyelocele, since the neural groove closes before the choroid plexus becomes active.

(3) List (1941) and Russell (1949) consider that the malformation is part of a developmental dysplasia originating at about the 3rd week of embryonic life, that is at about the time of closure of the neural groove. The frequent association of the malformation with congenital anomalies in the bony structures in the neighbourhood of the foramen magnum, such as assimilation of the atlas, basilar impression, platybasia or fusion of the cervical vertebrae (Klippel-Feil deformity, List 1941) are easily explained on this theory. Microgyria and craniolacunia (Ingraham and Scott 1943) and heterotopias of grey matter are malformations which arise later in foetal life.

Barry *et al.* (1957) have put forward a theory of pathogenesis based on the examination of foetuses with myeloschisis, in which, from the age of 10 weeks (90 mm. c.r. length) onwards, there was herniation of the cerebellum and medulla into the cervical canal. They consider that the primary abnormality is an overgrowth of the central nervous system in relation to its craniovertebral encasement, beginning at the 4th week of development. At the lumbosacral level this prevents the vertebral arches from joining in the midline. At the cranial level the large brain displaces the tentorium downwards and causes herniation of the medulla and lower parts of the cerebellum into the cervical canal. At this level the condition becomes stabilised by the adhesion of the meninges both to the herniated neural tissue and to the arches of the vertebrae, so that when, during later development, the intracranial pressure recedes the brain stem is pulled on, elongated and deformed. They found that the traction effects of anchorage of the cord at the lumbosacral level were dissipated within 4 segments, and consider that the hydrocephalus is a sequel to, rather than the cause of, the protrusion of the medulla and cerebellum into the cervical canal. Daniel and Strich (1958) also believe the deformity is due to abnormal growth of the cerebellum and brain stem in early foetal life and they suggest that a failure in the formation of the pontine flexure may be an important factor.

Russell and Donald (1935) also consider that the hydrocephalus, with which the malformation is often associated, is due to downward displacement of the 4th ventricle so that its foramina for the exit of cerebrospinal fluid open into the spinal canal. As the cerebellar protrusions plug the foramen magnum, the cerebrospinal fluid is unable to reach the intracranial subarachnoid space and to be absorbed from there, but must be absorbed from the spinal canal. Lichtenstein (1942) confirmed that the fluid from the spinal canal did not reach the intracranial cisternae and sulci but considered that the narrowing of the iter of Sylvius, associated with the elongation of the brain stem, played a more important part in causing hydrocephalus. In older patients with Chiari's Type I deformity, hydrocephalus, which is rarely severe, may be caused by the close apposition of cerebellar tissue to the back and sides of the medulla.

Aqueductal malformations leading to hydrocephalus. By R. M. Norman

Obstructive hydrocephalus is commonly caused by narrowing or closure of the Sylvian aqueduct and four main types of this anomaly have been described by Russell (1949).

(1) *Stenosis* of the aqueduct may be said to be present when narrowing occurs without abnormal gliosis in the surrounding tissue (Fig. 6.10). The normal aqueduct varies considerably in cross-section at different levels. Two constrictions regularly occur, the first beneath the middle of the superior corpora quadrigemina, the second at the level of the intercollicular sulcus. Between these two narrowings the aqueduct shows a well-marked dilatation or ampulla. Woollam and Millen's (1953) measurements indicate that considerable differences in cross-section also occur between individual specimens at the same situation in the aqueduct; thus at the commencement of the ampulla the average cross-section in 10 cases was 0·9 sq. mm. but the individual variation ranged from as little as 0·2 sq. mm. up to 1·8 sq. mm. In order to establish that stenosis is the cause of hydrocephalus it is therefore necessary to employ control sections made at different levels. According to Alvord (1961) the development of hydrocephalus is determined not only by a reduction in size of the aqueductal lumen but also by the length of the aqueduct, the viscosity of the C.S.F., and differences in pressure between the third and fourth ventricles.

There is a rare hereditary variety of this condition. In the family described by Bickers and Adams (1949), congenital hydrocephalus was confined to 7 males in two generations and a simple aqueductal stenosis was proved at autopsy in one of the sibs. In a similar case examined by the writer the pedigree also indicated inheritance by a sex-linked Mendelian recessive factor (Edwards *et al.* 1961).

(2) *Forking of the aqueduct* is present when two main channels of greatly reduced dimensions are found one behind the other in the midsagittal plane of the brain stem and separated by normal intervening tissue. The dorsal channel shows considerable branching and adjacent groups of ependymal cells may also form short tubules, while the ventral passage is usually a narrow slit. Serial sections show that each main channel may communicate with the other or may enter the ventricle independently or end blindly, but there is usually an aqueductal lumen of some sort to be seen, however functionally inadequate it may be. There may be associated maldevelopment of neighbouring structures, such as fusion of the corpora quadrigemina or of the oculomotor nuclei, and spina bifida is commonly present (Cameron 1957).

The term 'atresia' is inappropriate for this condition (Russell 1949). In brains without hydrocephalus a secondary channel may occasionally be present for a short distance ventral to an aqueduct of normal appearance, but since the cross-section of the latter is not reduced there is no obstruction to the circulation of the cerebrospinal fluid.

(3) *Septum formation.* The caudal end of the aqueduct may be occluded or partially obstructed by a thin neuroglial membrane. Certain of these cases are associated with granular ependymitis of the ventricular system suggestive of an infection during foetal life.

(4) *Gliosis of the aqueduct.* In this condition a narrowing of the aqueduct or its subdivision into two or more smaller channels is found in conjunction with a well-marked proliferation of

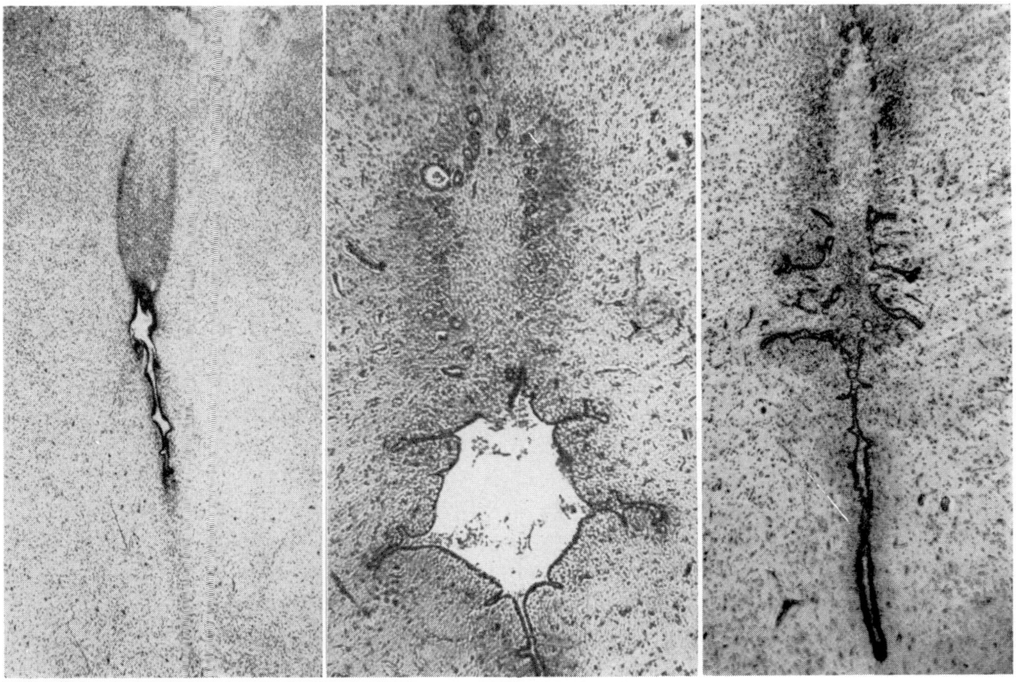

6.10 6.11 (*a*) 6.11 (*b*)

FIG. 6.10. *Stenosis of the Sylvian aqueduct* in still-born hydrocephalic infant. Note the nucleus dorsalis which is a conspicuous feature in early life.

FIG. 6.11 (*a* and *b*). Gliosis of the aqueduct. In its dorsal part the outline of the aqueduct is indicated only by ependymal cells. The ventral part becomes a narrow, ependyma-lined slit.

fibrillary glia. This surrounding zone of gliosis evidently marks out the area of the pre-existing aqueduct, since its peripheral edge is outlined by disorderly groups of ependymal cells (Fig. 6.11). The narrowed lumen itself has no ependymal lining. This gliotic stenosis may be present at only one part of the aqueduct, in which event the anterior part of the channel shows dilatation. Unlike cases of forking the glial type of obstruction is not associated with other maldevelopments of the brain stem or elsewhere.

The pathogenesis of the gliosis is obscure. The condition appears to differ from the primary type of gliosis, with polypoid granulations projecting into the aqueduct, which has occasionally been reported in von Recklinghausen's disease. Russell (1949) has pointed out that whereas the ependyma is highly vulnerable and has little regenerative power, the subependymal glia is readily stimulated to proliferation. Bacterial toxins are thus conceivable pathogenetic agents. Granular ependymitis in the ventricular system below the level of the obstruction would be in favour of an infection. Gliosis of the aqueduct is usually associated clinically with an insidious onset of signs of raised intracranial pressure in early life, but it may also occur in adults. The resulting hydrocephalus thus belongs in the majority of instances to the class of post-natal malformations.

Dandy-Walker syndrome

In this condition the cerebellar hemispheres are widely separated caudally by an enlarged 4th ventricle, the roof of which is represented by a thin, bulging membrane lined by ependyma and composed of neuroglia, connective tissue and blood vessels. This membrane arises from the brain stem in the same way as a normal roof, but laterally it is attached in a curved line to the dorsomedial aspects of the lateral lobes, though the whole cavity is lined by ependyma. The cerebellar vermis may occasionally be absent, but more usually its posterior part is small and abnormally developed. The fastigium is flattened and part of the poorly developed nodulus is incorporated in the adjoining roofing membrane. The choroid plexus may be rudimentary and placed caudally in the ventricle. The finding in many well-examined cases that the foramen of Majendie is not present and that one or both the lateral foramina have also failed to develop has given rise to the theory that the congenital internal hydrocephalus that is often associated with this malformation of the 4th ventricle is causally related to atresia of the foramina (Gibson 1955). This view has been strongly opposed by Brodal and Hauglie-Hanssen (1959) who maintain that the malformation of the posterior vermis and 4th ventricle must have originated at a time prior to the development of the foramina of Majendie and Luschka. A similar type of malformation occurs as an inherited condition in mice. Affected embryos show an abnormal development of the roof of the 4th ventricle at an early stage, before the choroid plexus and the foramina are formed. In man it is apparent that the malformation is not necessarily associated with congenital hydrocephalus, and signs of raised intracranial pressure may first appear in childhood or adult life. Nor are the foramina necessarily closed in the cases of congenital hydrocephalus. It is likely that in such cases there is a narrow margin of safety with respect to the circulation of the cerebrospinal fluid because of the pre-existing malformation.

The condition must be distinguished from cystic conditions of the roof of the 4th ventricle. Gardner *et al.* (1957) have described arachnoid cysts lying above the foramen of Majendie and arising from a splitting of the membrane. In the adult case reported by Kramer (1954) arachnoidal cysts incorporating malformed paraflocculi had occluded the lateral foramina and had caused hydrocephalus.

As a corollary to the enlargement of the posterior fossa the backward growth of the cerebral hemispheres and the associated shift of the venous sinuses may be impeded. Hence arises the pathognomonic clinical picture of dolicocephaly with mainly occipital expansion (Benda 1954) and the X-ray appearance of the lateral sinus and torcula in an abnormally elevated position in the parietal bone (Taggart and Walker 1942).

While this malformation often leads to severe generalised internal hydrocephalus, it does not necessarily do so, and on the average these patients live longer than those with the infantile form of the Arnold-Chiari deformity. Taggart and Walker (1942) suggested that the cerebrospinal fluid might permeate through the thin membranous roof or be absorbed by its vessels, thus maintaining an equilibrium. There is also the possibility that one or all the foramina may open after a delay, in which event there would be no progressive hydrocephalus and the 4th ventricle would not be so severely distended.

Cerebral atrophy due to hydrocephalus

Characteristic changes take place in the wall of the hemispheres when a rise in intraventricular pressure causes an expansion of the brain within the yielding calvaria of the infant skull. Whereas pressure from without, as by the accumulation of fluid in subdural hygroma, causes compression but little atrophy of the brain, unless vessels are occluded, in infantile hydrocephalus the stretch put upon the distended cerebral wall causes rapid thinning of the white substance. The enlargement of the ventricles is not a uniform process and depends not only upon the site of the block in the circulation of the cerebrospinal fluid but also on the duration of the hydrocephalus. In subarachnoid block, for example, the lateral ventricles are the first to enlarge, followed later by the 3rd ventricle, the aqueduct and 4th ventricle. The corpus callosum is elevated and thinned and the septum pellucidum fenestrated or destroyed. Extreme thinning of the floor of the 3rd ventricle is common and is associated with erosion of the clinoid processes, and damage to the hypothalamus may lead to infantilism or to precocious puberty. The atrophy of the periventricular white matter is due to ischaemia following the compression of capillaries by the rising intraventricular pressure (De 1950). The grey matter of the cortex is remarkably resistant, perhaps because of its rich blood supply, and Penfield and Elvidge (1932) have pointed out that since the axons of the unaffected cortical neurones must be preserved the brunt of the atrophy has fallen upon their collaterals. Microscopically, the most obvious changes are first seen in the neuroglia. There is a reduction in the numbers of oligodendroglial and astrocytic cells and the processes of the latter tend to become elongated and wavy. Compound granular corpuscles are found in small numbers in the atrophied white matter and may lie in a linear band some distance from the ependymal surface, thus giving the impression that 'all the myelinated fibres at a certain depth had been simultaneously destroyed' (Penfield and Elvidge 1932). With the continued increase in the hydrocephalus the cerebral atrophy becomes severe and eventually the wall of the hemisphere is reduced in places to a thin membrane. It is always the vertex which is most atrophied since it lacks the buttressing support of the basal ganglia. For this reason the axons of the motor neurones originating in the paracentral and upper parts of the precentral gyrus undergo a greater stretching than do those supplying the upper extremities, so that paraplegia is common in severe hydrocephalus while the arms retain a useful degree of function (Yakovlev 1947).

Rupture of the ventricular wall may lead to the formation of smooth-walled, cystic cavities in the white matter. These diverticula may open into the subarachnoid space and lead to relief of symptoms. Tandon and Harkmark (1959) have described a case in which rupture of the suprapineal recess into the superior cistern had led to a temporary improvement in a patient with a tumour of the brain stem. Spontaneous rupture of the lamina terminalis has also been reported.

During compression the superficial blood-vessels show a compensatory increase which may give a false impression of congenital microgyria (Penfield and Elvidge 1932). True polygyria, however, may be present in congenital hydrocephalic brains and may perhaps be regarded as the expression of a compensatory hyperplasia of the parenchyma itself since the weights of these brains when drained of their fluid often exceed the normal (Potter 1953).

Malformation of the corpus callosum

The telencephalon possesses three commissures, the hippocampal, the anterior and the callosal, which all develop in close proximity to the lamina terminalis. The fibres of the corpus callosum first make their appearance in the 3rd month when they begin to cross the midline in the upper part of the lamina and in the neighbouring fused parts of the medial pallial walls. A thickening of the lamina terminalis has already been produced by a fusion of two plates which act as a bridge facilitating the passage of the interhemispheric fibres. Subsequent expansion of the corpus callosum takes place mainly in a backward direction, so that by the 5th month of foetal life a miniature replica of the adult structure has been formed.

If callosal fibres fail to cross the midline the convolutional pattern of the medial wall of the hemisphere develops in an abnormal manner. The septum pellucidum is necessarily absent, the cingulate gyrus is imperfectly formed or is displaced below the surface and in its place a number of radially placed convolutions are present (Fig. 6.12). This arrangement has been compared by Kirschbaum (1947) to the drawing-in of gyri around a prenatal porencephalic

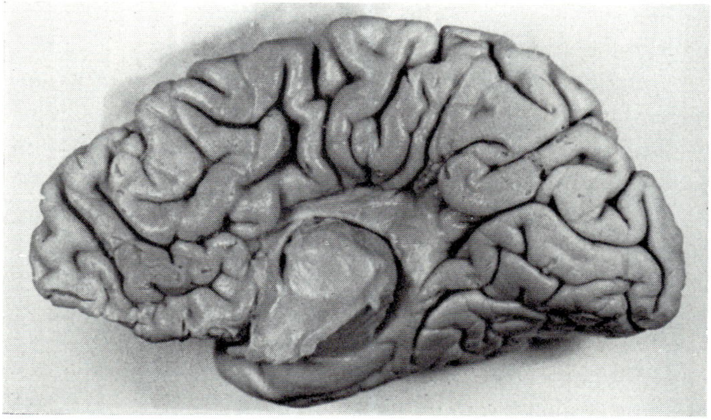

6.12

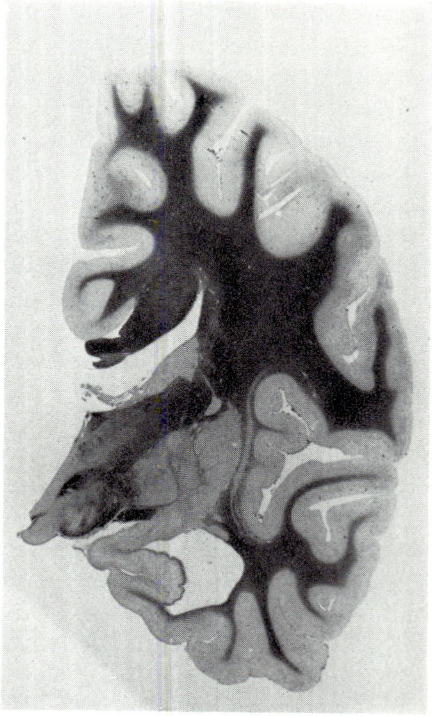

6.13

FIG. 6.12. *Absent corpus callosum.* Note the absence of the posterior part of the cingulate sulcus and the radiate arrangement of the sulci.

FIG. 6.13. Coronal section of a hemisphere showing the longitudinal callosal bundle.

defect. Another abnormal feature often present is the separation of the calcarine from the parieto-occipital fissure. The two halves of the body of the fornix are also separated throughout their course and in some cases the anterior commissure is larger than normal.

When the hemisphere is sectioned in the coronal plane the anterior horns of the lateral ventricles are short and slit-like. In many cases a prominent rounded bundle of myelinated fibres is seen lying above and in contact with each half of the body of the fornix (Fig. 6.13). This is the callosal bundle of Probst (1900) which takes its origin from the white matter of the frontal pole, passes through the inner part of the roof of the lateral ventricle lying internal to the body of the fornix, and merges with the white matter enclosing the posterior horn, reaching its largest diameter at about the level of the optic chiasma. The consensus of opinion is that this aberrant bundle is formed by uncrossed fibres of the corpus callosum. De Lange (1925) showed that, in a brain in which only the anterior half of the corpus callosum was present, an uncrossed bundle of fibres was continuous on either side posteriorly with the crossed part of the corpus callosum and divided into forceps major and minor as in the normal brain to enclose the posterior horn of the lateral ventricle. The fibres of the callosal bundle, in hemispheres in which the corpus callosum was completely missing, behaved in the same way. Moreover, in this case (as in one of Kirschbaum's), the fronto-occipital tract appeared as a distinct structure, thus disposing of an earlier theory that this tract might be the callosal bundle. It is not easy, however, to rule out the possibility that the longitudinal bundle is a normal uncrossed component of the corpus callosum which has undergone hypertrophy and has become unmasked by the failure of the crossed fibres to develop. Some support is given to this theory by Becker's (1952) demonstration that a bundle of fibres, running in an anteroposterior direction and in close proximity to the corpus callosum, makes its appearance in new-born puppies after complete destruction of one hemisphere.

The longitudinal bundle is not an invariable finding in acallosal brains and in cases in which it is absent there are apt to be multiple coincidental malformations of brain or viscera and spina bifida is common. The interhemispheric defect may be partially filled by a lipoma, a meningioma or cysts derived from the 3rd ventricle (paraphysial cyst) or from the arachnoid membrane. Large heterotopias of nerve cells lying deep in the central white matter and lining part of the walls of the lateral ventricles were present in one of Kirschbaum's (1947) cases and were thought to have prevented the development of the longitudinal bundle.

Hypoplasia of the corpus callosum is not uncommon among mental defectives. As in the case of complete absence of the commissure, the cause of the mental retardation must be sought elsewhere in the nervous system, since it is well established that callosal maldevelopment is not incompatible with a normal mentality. In the brain examined by de Lange (1925) an exceptionally thick granular layer was found in all areas of the cerebral cortex, including the precentral gyrus. The internal granular layer of the calcarine cortex did not show its normal subdivision into three laminae—a feature which should be visible in the 7 months' foetus. An unduly small brain is a commonly associated anomaly in mentally retarded patients.

Aetiology. Heredity has not been shown to play a part in the causation of this condition in man, though in the mouse absence of the corpus callosum and the presence of a longitudinal callosal bundle may be inherited as a Mendelian recessive (King 1936). Absence of the corpus callosum has been found in association with micropolygyria or heterotopias lying within the territory of an anterior cerebral artery and the suggestion has been made that these anomalies may have been due to a developmental defect in vascularisation (de Morsier and Mozer 1935; de Morsier 1951, 1952). This view has been opposed by Marburg (1949) on the grounds that the anterior and middle cerebral arteries have not fully differentiated at the time the corpus callosum begins to develop and that, if a vascular process is to be postulated as the cause of callosal suppression, there should be much more widespread interference in the growth of the hemispheres than is in fact found.

Malformations of the septum pellucidum

In brains with absent corpus callosum or with arhinencephaly the septum is necessarily missing, while in severe hydrocephalus it is destroyed or fenestrated. In brains having a corpus callosum Gross and Hoff (1959) describe various anomalies of the septum which are often associated with prenatal porencephaly or heterotopic formations in the region of the insula and claustrum. These range from complete absence to hypoplasia. In one type of malformation the lateral ventricles are defective in their frontal horns and the corpus callosum partially fused with the caudate nuclei. The two laminae of the septum pellucidum are widely divergent and closely applied to the surfaces of the caudate nuclei, thus forming the boundaries of a single ventricular cavity. These maldevelopments are often associated with atrophy of the optic nerves and tracts (de Morsier 1956) which is attributed by Gross and Hoff to stretching of the nerves during the abnormal development of the brain, rather than to a primary dysplasia.

Micrencephaly

The arbitrary brain weight of 900 g. is usually accepted as the upper limit for micrencephaly in the adult. In the majority of instances the departure from normal standards is obvious enough and a brain weight even as low as 25 g. has been recorded in an infant who survived

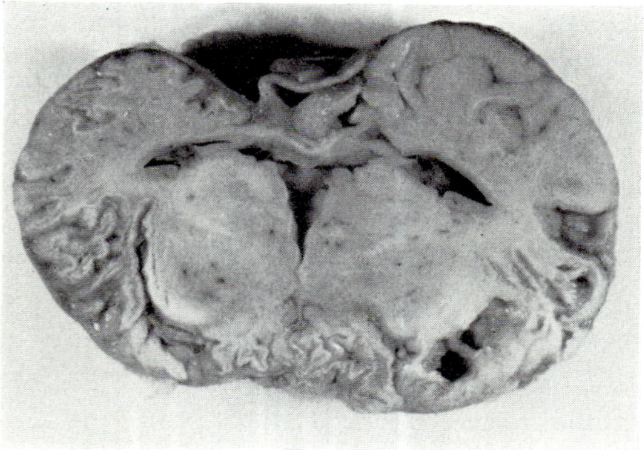

FIG. 6.14. *Widespread ulegyria* following post-meningitic vascular disease, probably prenatal in origin. From a 6-month-old infant. Brain weight 243 g.

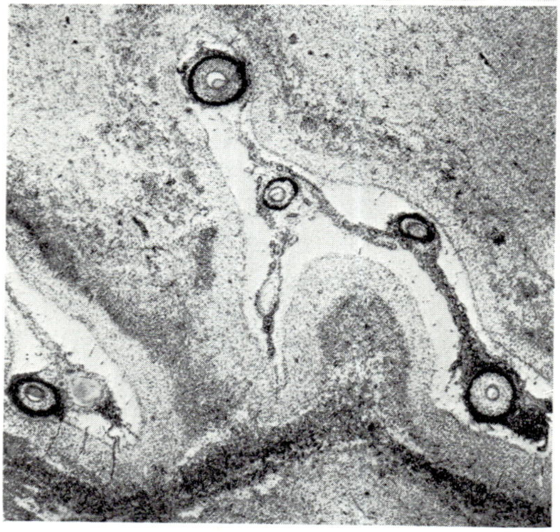

FIG. 6.15. An area of ulegyria. The meningeal arteries show calcification of the elastica and intimal fibrosis.

4 months (von Monakow 1926). The rudimentary cerebral cortex of this tiny brain possessed a recognisable area gigantopyramidalis and there were hypertrophied and uncrossed pyramidal tracts (Yakovlev and Wadsworth 1946; Minkowski 1955).

Destructive processes starting before birth usually lead to obviously malformed brains of small dimensions, as in porencephaly. Unless there is an associated hydrocephalus little or no postnatal growth of the head occurs since the sutures tend to ossify prematurely. Widespread ulegyria follows arteritis of meningeal vessels (Figs. 6.14 and 6.15), but since the signs of meningitis in early infancy are easily overlooked it is often difficult to establish with certainty that the onset of an infection was prenatal, except in well-known conditions such as toxoplasmosis or syphilis (Laurance 1959).

Familial microcephaly. This type of small-headedness has long been recognised as a distinctive clinical entity and may be inherited as a Mendelian recessive. The small cranium with its receding forehead and superabundant, furrowed scalp contrasts strikingly with the more normal dimensions of the face with its prominent nose and large ears. The naked-eye appearance of the cerebrum is also highly characteristic. The brain, including the cerebellum which is often disproportionately large, usually weighs from 500 to 600 g. The convolutional pattern is greatly simplified and somewhat resembles that of the higher anthropoid apes (Conolly 1950), the gyri being relatively broad for the size of the brain (Fig. 6.16). The cortical nerve cells are usually well developed but there are numerous minor anomalies of architectonics including abnormal variations in the depth of individual layers—often in the direction of a marked reduction but sometimes tending towards undue thickness.

Nerve cells irregularly orientated or disproportionately large for the layer in which they are

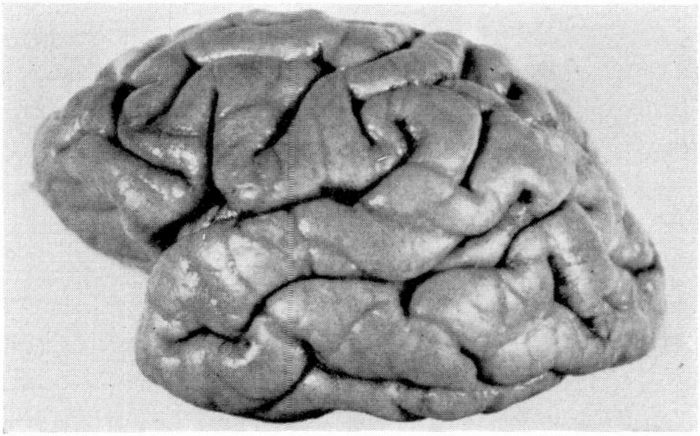

FIG. 6.16. *Familial microcephaly.* Note the simple convolutional pattern with relatively broad gyri.

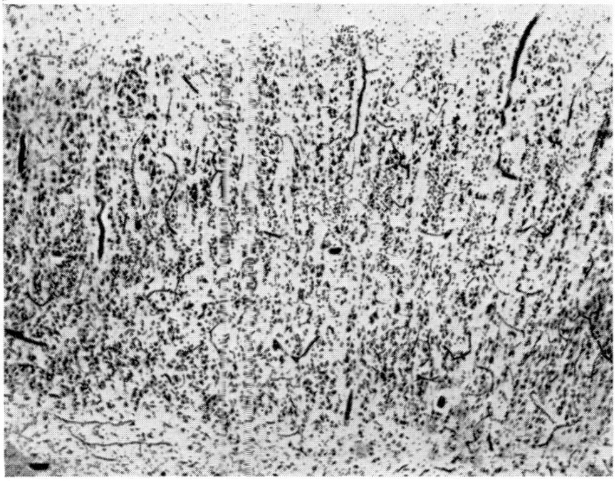

FIG. 6.17. The cerebral cortex shows typical columnar grouping of the nerve cells.

found may also be present and heterotopic aggregations, some of considerable size, are commonly seen in the subcortical white matter. By far the most striking histological abnormality, though one not peculiar to this form of micrencephaly, is the frequent grouping of the cortical nerve cells in columnar blocks separated from one another by acellular strips (Fig. 6.17). The latter are occupied by radially disposed bundles of myelinated fibres. Sometimes only the superficial nerve cells exhibit this clustering together and then an appearance is given which is reminiscent of the glomerular formations seen normally in the hippocampal gyrus. Myelination of the central white matter, basal ganglia and long fibre tracts is normal and the corpus callosum often appears unduly massive for such small hemispheres. The caudate nucleus also may be disproportionately large, even for a normal brain—an example of what von Monakow has termed 'hypergenesis'.

Micrencephaly with cerebral calcification. Jervis (1954 b) collected from the literature five examples of this condition and added two of his own. The brain is symmetrically reduced in size and weighs about half the normal. There is no obvious convolutional shrinkage but the lateral ventricles are somewhat enlarged. The most striking feature is the presence of very coarse and confluent mineral deposits which are sufficiently massive to be recognised macroscopically and visualised during life in X-rays of the skull. The putamen, globus pallidus, dentate nucleus and the deeper cortical layers are mainly affected by this change.

Smaller amounts of this substance, which is mainly calcium carbonate with an admixture of iron salts, are widespread throughout the brain, occurring free in the tissues or as droplets in the walls of vessels. After decalcification a strongly P.A.S. positive matrix is left behind. The loss of nerve cells sometimes seen in the cerebral cortex, thalamus and cornu Ammonis may well be a post-epileptic phenomenon. A conspicuous, patchy demyelination is found in the central white matter and the tegmentum of the midbrain, accompanied by a variable degree of fibrillary gliosis. The usual products of myelin breakdown are not in evidence. In Hallervorden's (1950) 2nd case signs of an inflammatory process were present in the form of meningeal thickening and infiltrations, subintimal fibrosis of vessels, granular ependymitis and microglial rod-cells in the cortex. A sibling of this patient had also suffered from micrencephaly with calcification.

Jervis calls attention to the close relationship of this condition to Fahr's 'non-arteriosclerotic cerebral calcification'. In one of his cases Jervis was able to exclude a general disturbance in calcium metabolism, as in the hypoparathyroidism which may be a feature of Fahr's disease. He inclines to the view that both the calcifications and the patchy demyelination are due to circulatory disturbances and alterations in vascular permeability occurring in the course of an encephalitis of unknown origin, but the familial character of some of these cases is difficult to reconcile with this hypothesis. Calcification of approximately the same distribution are found in a number of inflammatory and degenerative diseases (Erbsloh and Bochnik 1958) and it is evident that the aetiological factors concerned are multiple.

The writer has examined the brains of two siblings suffering from microcephaly, cerebral calcification, dwarfism, nerve deafness and retinitis pigmentosa, the clinical features of which were described by Neill and Dingwall (1950). Massive pericapillary calcifications were present in the putamina, thalami and in the cerebellar white matter superficial to the dentate nuclei. In the larger vessels the calcification was mainly in the adventitial coat. The deposits in the cerebral cortex were found mainly in the depths of the sulci in the arterial boundary zone regions, and the granular layer of the calcarine cortex was also involved. Cerebellar atrophy was present and calcified Purkinje cells were a conspicuous feature. There was patchy demyelination of the centrum ovale and brain stem but this was not related to the calcifications nor was it perivascular (Figs. 6.18–23). The ventricles were denuded of ependyma, there was dense subependymal gliosis, and the choroid plexuses were atrophic. The latter findings suggested a specific degenerative process. A similar distribution of cortical calcifications has been noted in an adult case of Fahr's disease and supports the view that a vascular pathoclitic factor, possibly a peculiarity of capillary permeability, is concerned in the calcifying process (Norman and Urich 1960).

Megalencephaly

Excessive brain weights of the order 1,600–2,850 g. have been recorded in individuals of normal or exceptional intelligence as well as in epileptics and mental defectives (A. Jakob 1927).

6.18 6.19

.20 6.21

.22 6.23

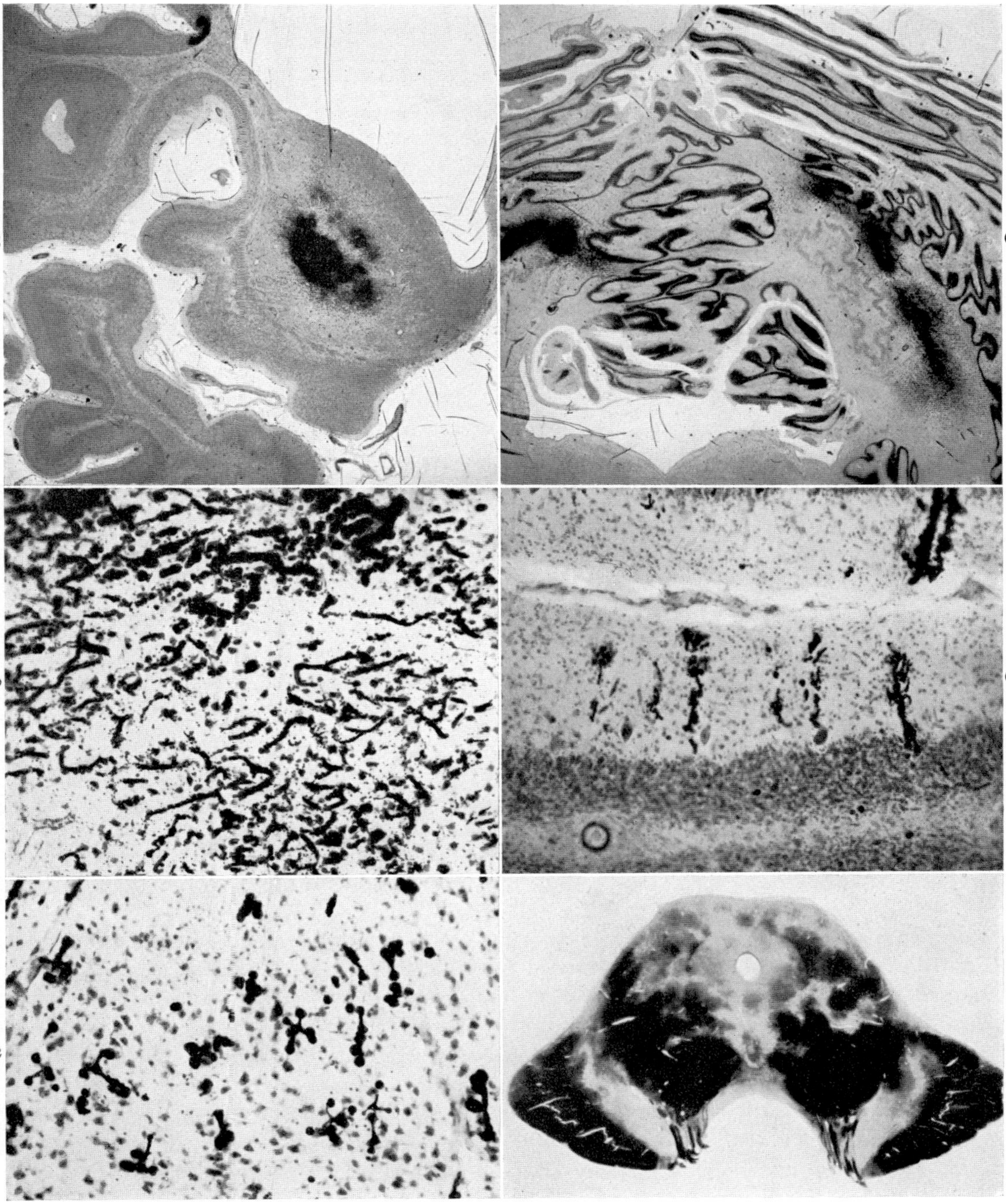

FIGS. 6.18–6.23. *Familial microcephaly with cerebral calcification.*

FIG. 6.18. Calcified capillaries forming dense aggregations in the putamen and caudate nucleus. Note the calcification in the base of the second frontal gyrus. (Carbol azure.)

FIG. 6.19. Cerebellum showing calcifications in white matter dorso-lateral to dentate nuclei. (Carbol azure.)

FIG. 6.20. Typical pericapillary calcifications. (Carbol azure.)

FIG. 6.21. Calcified dendrites of Purkinje cells. (Carbol azure.)

FIG. 6.22. Calcified microglial cells in cerebral grey matter. (Carbol azure.)

FIG. 6.23. Midbrain showing patchy demyelination of the tegmentum. (Kultschitsky-Pal.)

The term 'megalencephaly' has, however, a pathological connotation and should be reserved for heavy brains having additional structural anomalies, and of these three main varieties may be distinguished.

(1) First, megalencephaly may be associated with a diffuse overgrowth of the protoplasmic macroglia (Volland 1910, Schminke 1920, Hallervorden 1926, Weil 1933). As in tuberous sclerosis, a malignant transformation of the astrocytes may sometimes occur. Thus in Weil's case (that of a 7-year-old child with a brain weight of 1,856 g.) the brain stem and cerebellum contained a glioblastoma. In these examples of neuroglial overgrowth the nerve cells often show abnormalities of an unspecific sort, such as irregularities of stratification, the presence of isolated cells or groups of cells of disproportionately large size (as in pachygyria) or heterotopias in the subcortical white matter. A disproportionate enlargement of the spinal cord due to blastomatous glial overgrowth has also been reported in megalencephaly of this type (Kastein 1940, Ferraro and Barrera 1935).

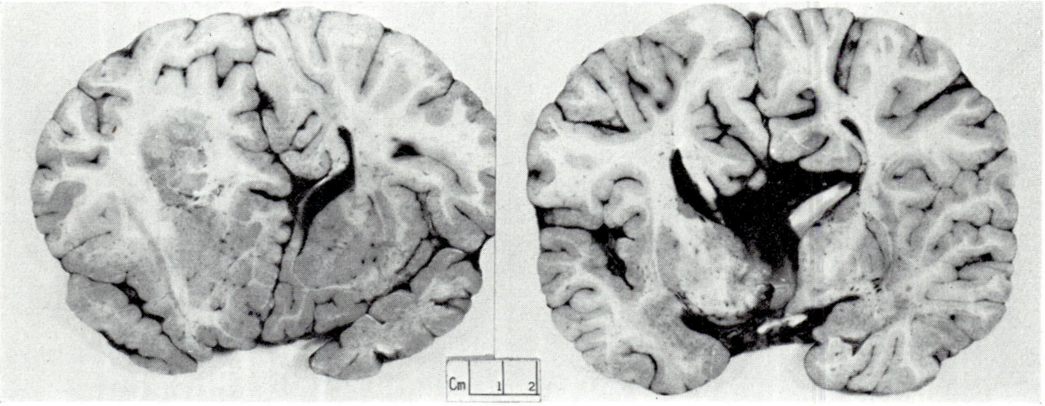

6.24 6.25

FIG. 6.24. *Megalencephaly* with mutiple cerebral anomalies. Note the large hetertopias in the white matter of the left lobe and the longitudinal callosal bundle on the right side.
FIG. 6.25. A more posterior level showing absence of the corpus callosum, abnormal gyral pattern and polygyria in right temporal lobe.
From a child of 3 years with total brain weight of 1,554 g. (cerebellum 186 g.).

(2) In a second type of abnormally large brain the generalised increase in size is not associated with any neuroglial preponderance. In Wilson's (1934) case both grey and white matter were uniformly massive, but in the example recorded by Peter and Schlüter (1927) the corpus callosum and centrum semi-ovale did not participate in the general enlargement. In the latter case the depth of cerebral cortex was notably increased without there being obvious anomalies in cyto-architectonics. In another case (Peter 1928) the cerebellum was disproportionately enlarged and the Purkinje cells showed various irregularities of alignment and size.

(3) In a third and heterogeneous group of cases, megalencephaly is an incidental feature of some other malformation or degenerative condition. Tuberose sclerosis may be associated with a heavy brain (Borremanns *et al.* 1933) and syringomyelia has also been reported (Benda 1952). In one of the writer's cases, that of a child of 3 years with a brain weight of 1,554 g., there were multiple congenital malformations (abnormal gyration of the cerebral cortex, massive heterotopias in one frontal lobe with partial atresia of the lateral ventricle, longitudinal callosal bundles, and an absent olfactory tract on the side of the heterotopic formations) (Figs. 6.24 and 6.25). Excessive brain weights have frequently been reported in the

infantile form of amaurotic family idiocy (Aronson *et al.* 1955). In these cases there is always a great excess of fibrillary neuroglia in the cerebral white matter, often with status spongiosus and widespread absence of myelin. In view of these findings it is not surprising that megalencephaly has also been reported in late infantile metachromatic leucodystrophy and also in 'spongy degeneration of the white matter'.

Porencephaly

The term 'porencephaly' was originally introduced by Heschl (1859) to designate a congenital defect extending from the surface of the cerebral hemisphere into the subjacent ventricle. During the passage of years the name has lost any precise meaning it may have once possessed and it is now commonly used for any excavation or cystic cavity occurring in the brain of a young individual. It is an advantage to separate from such a heterogeneous group the cerebral softenings associated with birth injury or postnatal vascular lesions. There then remains a by no means uniform class of case properly labelled 'prenatal porencephaly'—the qualification 'prenatal' being applicable to porencephaly associated with unequivocal signs of prenatal malformation elsewhere in the brain (Fig. 6.26). The prenatal porencephalies so defined may be usefully subdivided into two groups: those showing evidence of old destructive processes and those which are distortions of growth with no concomitant pathological findings such as glial scarring or calcifications.

The studies of Yakovlev and Wadsworth (1946) have thrown light on the morphogenesis of the latter sort of porencephaly. These authors have drawn attention to a special type of maldevelopment which is characterised by symmetrically placed clefts in the cerebral cortex, a condition named by them 'schizencephaly'. These clefts, which involve the whole depth of the cerebral wall, lie in the line of primary fissures and their walls may be fused together forming a 'pia-ependymal seam', the line of junction of the molecular layers being marked by a streak of myelinated fibres and by elements derived both from the pia mater and the ependymal layer. The heaped-up grey matter of these approximated walls is unduly thick and is unlaminated. Dense aggregations of poorly differentiated cells are arranged in nests and large neurones with heavy chromatin and sometimes with two nuclei may be present. In the depths of the line of fusion these nerve cell layers may become coterminous with heterotopic collections of ependymal matrix cells or they may even extend into the subjacent caudate nucleus. There is no sign that a destructive process has been at work and there is no hydrocephalus, although the occipital horns of the lateral ventricles often show the relative dilatation of 'colpocephaly'. Yakovlev and Wadsworth consider that these clefts arise at points of localised agenesis in the cerebral wall before the end of the 2nd month, at a time prior to the closure of the roof of the prosencephalon and before the 3 layers of His have differentiated.

An entirely different appearance is given to the brain when this type of maldevelopment is complicated by hydrocephalus. Provided the cerebral wall in the region of the clefts is not protected by the buttressing effect of the basal ganglia an expansion may take place, the lips of the clefts open out, and large bilateral gaps bridged over by a thin roofing membrane appear on the surface of the hemispheres. Thus at first sight an impression is given of gross cortical destruction, whereas in fact the brain wall has yielded to pressure at weak spots caused by limited areas of defective growth. Owing to the primary malformation having occurred so early in development retrograde atrophy of the thalamus is not present. Parts of the original clefts with their pia-ependymal seams may be found in the tissue lying at the margins of the defects and provide important evidence in support of this theory of the pathogenesis of the porencephaly.

6.26

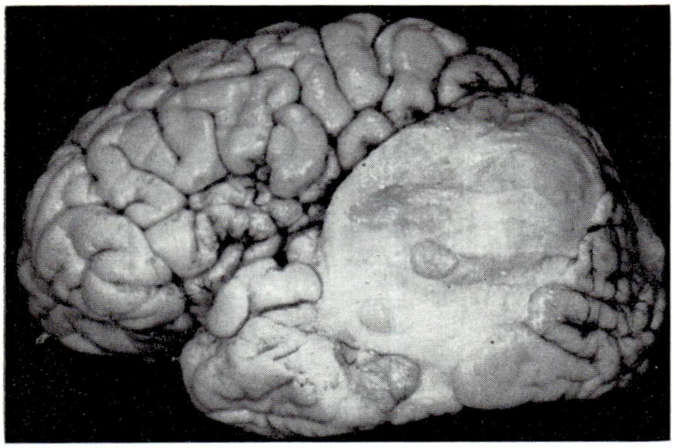

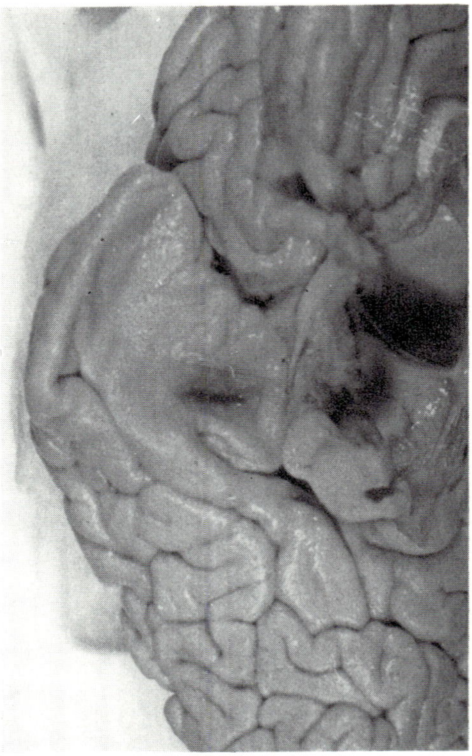

6.27

6.28

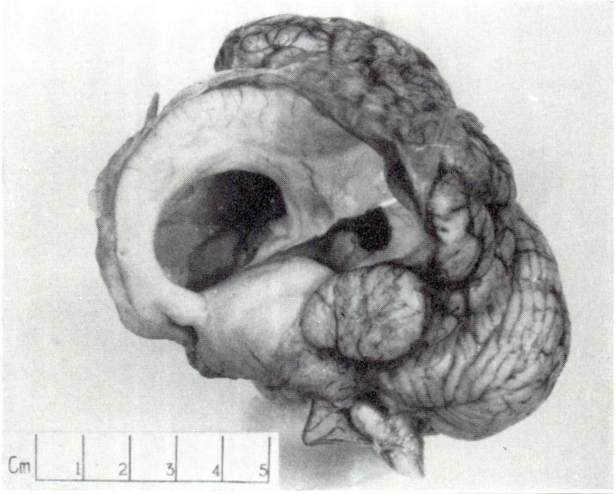

FIG. 6.26. *Prenatal porencephaly*. Note the islands of nervous tissue in the membranous wall of the expanded ventricle. There is a patch of micropolygyria in the upper bank of the Sylvian fissure. The condition was bilateral.

FIG. 6.27. Smooth depression in the undersurface of the temporal lobe caused by an arachnoidal cyst (which has been stripped off). The surrounding gyri are of normal pattern. A similar condition was present in the left temporal lobe.

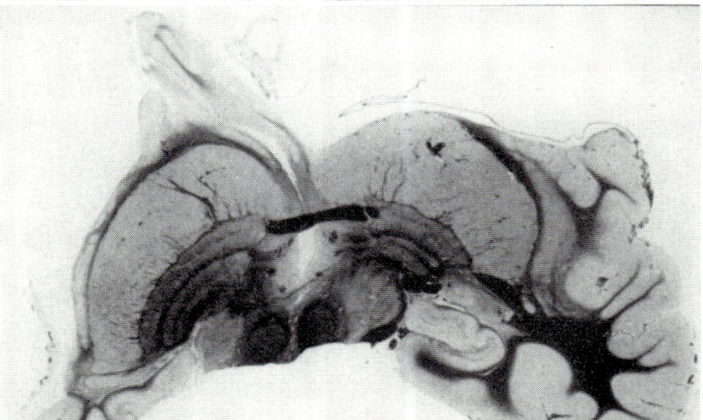

6.29

FIG. 6.28. Bilateral and approximately symmetrical porencephaly of the frontoparietal areas. The cavities were roofed in by a thin membrane (as in hydranencephaly) which has been removed on the left side; much of the remaining cortex showed micropolygyria. Note the large basal ganglia forming the floor of the unpaired ventricle.

FIG. 6.29. Coronal section through the hypertrophied corpora striata which are abnormally rotated inwards. Part of the thin roofing membrane is seen attached to the preserved cortex on either side. (Heidenhain's myelin).

In some specimens these large symmetrical defects in the cerebral wall occupy most of the frontal and parietal lobes. The contour of the brain is, however, preserved by a centrally placed arch of tissue which forms the superior attachment of the membranous covering of the ventricles and resembles in appearance the handle of a basket (Fig. 6.28). This remnant of grey matter was considered by Yakovlev and Wadsworth to represent the hypertrophied induseum griseum or hippocampal rudiment, but, in brains in which the pathological process has originated at a somewhat later date, the tissue is evidently derived from residual isocortex. In the brain examined in detail by Norman *et al.* (1958) the preserved 'handle' of the basket-shaped brain contained grey matter derived from the cingulate gyrus. The putamina and caudate nuclei may be hypertrophied and are seen as prominent elevations in the floor of the single ventricular cavity (Fig. 6.29). In Yakovlev and Wadsworth's specimen (case 3) the thalamic projection fibres took an aberrant course, the majority entering the pyriform cortex while those from the medial nucleus ended in the caudate nucleus. In the writer's case the thalamic projection fibres all entered the striatum.

It is evident that the argument in favour of this type of malformation arising in embryonic life as the result of 'agenesis', and not at a later stage perhaps from a vascular lesion, largely depends upon the interpretation given to the pia-ependymal seam. This type of cleft formation is not always to be found in bilateral porencephaly of prenatal origin, as, for instance, in the typical 'basket-brain' described by Cohn and Neumann (1946). Wedge-shaped defects in the roofs of the posterior horns of the ventricles were present in the writer's case, but these were filled by neuroglial fibres, not by dysplastic grey matter, and there were signs of an old necrotising process elsewhere in the brain. In such cases the thin layer of tissue lying beneath the meninges and covering the cerebral defects resembles that found in hydranencephaly (q.v.) and may be interpreted as the atrophied and gliosed outer layer of a cortex which has undergone pathological change, possibly due to vascular lesions. No doubt the process of hydrocephalic stretching postulated by Yakovlev and Wadsworth applies equally to these encephaloclastic porencephalies, though they probably originate at a somewhat later date. It is certainly true that signs of old destructive lesions may sometimes be found at the margins of these pori where partially eroded tissue and much calcified débris may be present. The prenatal origin of the process, however, is shown by the radial arrangement of the marginal gyri and, more decisively, by micropolygyria. In the majority of instances it seems more reasonable to ascribe both the porus and the microgyria to the action of a single pathological process, occurring about the 3rd–5th foetal month, than to suppose that later softening has occurred in an area of cortical malformation (Schob 1930).

The varieties of porencephaly so far described arise from a focal disturbance of growth in the developing wall of the hemisphere and it is axiomatic that neighbouring or related structures exhibit malformation. This rule does not seem necessarily to apply when cerebral growth is inhibited by slow pressure from without, and deep indentations of the brain can be caused by the presence of arachnoid cysts without the presence of associated cortical maldevelopment in the neighbouring tissue. Starkman *et al.* (1958) have brought forward evidence that these intra-arachnoid collections of fluid may arise as congenital malformations of the leptomeninges. In a case of the writers both temporal poles were deformed by smooth-walled, roughly circular depressions, the floors of which became progressively thinned and atrophic as the centre was approached. There was no communication with the inferior horn of the lateral ventricle but on one side the ependyma was exposed over a small area (Fig. 6.27). These cavities were filled by cysts formed by a splitting of the arachnoid membrane, the outer layer of which formed the roof of the crater and preserved the normal contour of the temporal lobe. The surrounding cortex was normally convoluted and showed no malformation.

Hydranencephaly

In this condition a prenatal destructive process has reduced the greater part of the cerebral hemispheres to membranous sacs. The lateral ventricles are enormously dilated but the infant's head is not enlarged at birth, though it may increase rapidly in size shortly afterwards. The affected areas are mainly those supplied by the internal carotid arteries, while those receiving blood from the vertebral system tend to be spared. The latter include the basal portions of the temporal and occipital lobes, the hippocampi and amygdaloid nuclei, brain stem and cerebellum. More rarely lesions also involve the midbrain, cerebellum, or are unilaterally distributed. The wall of the membranous sac is composed only of two layers, the leptomeninges and a thin shell of gliosed tissue representing the remnants of the cortex, mainly its molecular layer. Blood pigment may be present in the meninges covering the sac-like hemispheres (Lange-Cosack 1944). There is no ependymal lining but the ventricular surface is smooth and covered by a narrow layer of condensed glial fibrils (the 'membrana gliae limitans'). These appearances distinguish hydranencephaly from congenital hydrocephalus, in which condition the atrophy mainly affects the white matter, and also from the bladder-like porencephalic brains due to extensive softening of the centrum semi-ovale. In this latter type of porencephaly the cortex may be largely reduced to a thin membrane but the ependymal wall of the ventricle is preserved and forms the inner boundary of the excavated hemisphere. The cortical destruction is never so uniform or so symmetrical as in hydranencephaly. There are, however, transitions between hydranencephaly and other encephalomalacias of early life (Norman *et al.* 1958) and in some cases there is anatomical evidence of an obstruction to the flow of C.S.F., thus linking the condition to foetal hydrocephalus. The classification of such cases presents difficulties (Crome and Sylvester 1958).

Angiographic studies in hydranencephaly have given variable results. In the case described by Thelander *et al.* (1953) the vascular pattern was normal in both the arterial and venous phase. In that of Poser *et al.* (1955) the anterior cerebral arteries appeared rudimentary and the posterior cerebrals pursued an anomalous distal course.

Pathogenesis. The distribution of the lesions in hydranencephaly suggests that some obstruction to the blood flow in the territories supplied by the internal carotid arteries has occurred in foetal life, though how this has been brought about is unknown. Pressure on the foetal neck by the cord or by amniotic bands, or even direct trauma, or infection, in an attempt to procure abortion have been suggested (Lange-Cosack 1944), but do not carry conviction. Another suggestion is that the internal carotid arteries may be compressed against the sphenoid bones as a consequence of swelling of the foetal brain due to anoxia (Walsh and Lindenberg 1961). Thrombosis of the branches of the internal carotid arteries must also be considered as a possibility for Becker (1949 b) was able to produce softenings equivalent to hydranencephaly by injecting paraffin in olive oil into the carotid arteries of new-born puppies. The experiments of Vogel and McClenahan (1952) are also relevant. These workers occluded major cerebral arteries in 6-day-old chicks by electrocauterisation. Marked retardation in cortical development occurred and the forebrain in survivors often remained as a thin-walled cyst.

Pachygyria (*Lissencephaly, Agyria*)

This variety of cerebral malformation has two essential features: a reduction in the number of secondary gyri and an increased depth of the grey matter underlying the smooth part of the cortex. In extreme instances the only indentation visible over the convexity and external aspect of the brain is a Sylvian fissure the course of which is shorter and more obliquely placed than normal (Fig. 6.30.) Operculation is defective and the insula exposed. It is more usual to find the primary fissures and a few sulci present to a limited extent. Thus in Greenfield and Wolfsohn's (1935) specimen the calcarine and parieto-occipital fissures and the Rolandic, olfactory and orbital sulci were represented by shallow grooves. The brain as a whole is usually small and underweight ('microcephalia vera') but the lateral ventricles are relatively large, a relationship also present in the foetus and not due in the majority of cases to obstructive hydrocephalus. The term 'colpocephaly' has been applied to this condition by Yakovlev and Wadsworth (1946).

The hemispheric walls underlying the smooth parts of the cerebral cortex are composed of four main layers: (1) externally a molecular layer of normal proportions; (2) a layer of nerve cells which represents the true cortex and which may be shallower and more densely packed than is normal; (3) a much deeper and diffuse layer of grey matter in which the neurones tend to be arranged in broad columns separated by plume-like bundles of myelinated fibres which radiate from the deepest layer; (4) the 4th layer is a thin rind of white matter adjacent to the ventricle (Figs. 6.31, 6.32 and 6.33). A conspicuous feature of the 2nd or cortical layer may be the presence of large cells with coarse tigroid bodies resembling giant cells of Betz, scattered irregularly throughout the layer or sometimes arranged in a superficial row (Fig. 6.35). In those parts of the brain where the primary fissures or sulci have been formed the lamination of the cortex may be normal. The thin layer of central white matter and the fibres passing upwards from it towards the surface are well myelinated and often show dense fibrillary gliosis. Heterotopic islands of nerve cells of considerable size may also be present in the centrum semi-ovale (Fig. 6.36) and may bulge into the ventricular cavity giving a mamillated appearance to the ependymal surface (Fig. 6.39).

Lissencephaly ('smooth brain') and pachygyria may affect the central areas of the cortex in a symmetrical fashion as in the case of Fitzgerald (1940), in which absence of the pyramidal tracts was associated with spastic cerebral diplegia. Pachygyria is not uncommonly confined to one hemisphere and is then associated with a spastic hemiplegia. When only a small area of the cortical surface is involved, so that one or two broad gyri (macrogyria) are present, the condition has a superficial resemblance to tuberose sclerosis (Fig. 6.34) owing to the dense gliosis usually found in the affected cortex and also to the presence of large abnormal neurones in these areas. However, the bloated multinucleated neuroglial cells, bizarre giant cells and other features of Bourneville's disease are never seen.

The cerebellar cortex may also exhibit localised patches of agyria but in this case the disordered architecture ('cerebellar microgyria', q.v.) has no relation to any normal stage of development. As in the cerebrum, heterotopic islands of nerve cells are sometimes seen in the cerebellar white matter (Fig. 6.37).

The agyric cerebral cortex is a singularly clear-cut instance of a malformation explicable in terms of retardation of normal development, the structural pattern of the hemispheric wall having much in common with the foetal hemisphere at the 3rd and 4th month. At this stage the neuroblasts are passing outwards from the germinal centres of the matrix towards their ultimate destination in the mantle layer. The zone of their passage, the intermediate zone of His, will eventually be filled by the myelinated fibres of the centrum semi-ovale. In pachygyria, however, a considerable proportion of the neuroblasts never reach the mantle layer and are left behind as a diffuse heterotopia which undergoes subsequent expansion by virtue of the continued maturation and growth of its constituent elements. The more superficial sheet of nerve cells, which, with its molecular layer ('marginal veil'), forms the true cortex, is more compactly arranged and may form shallow infoldings, though never showing normal lamination.

Evidence of retarded development may also be present in other parts of the brain. In several cases the inferior olives have been found broken up into heterotopic groups of cells

6.30

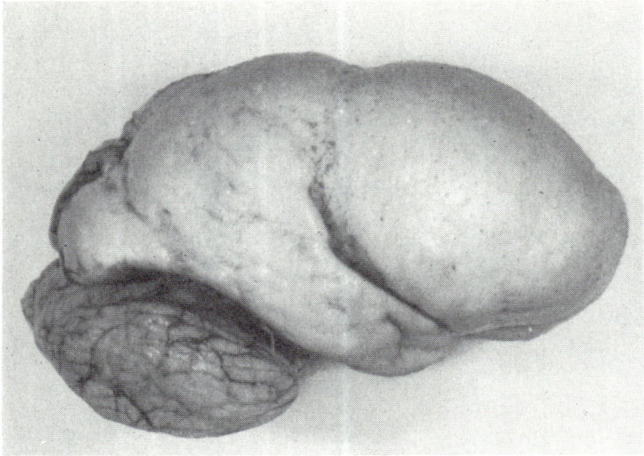

6.31

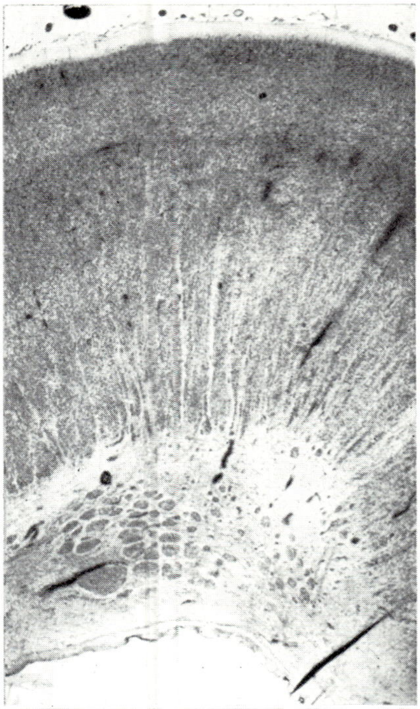

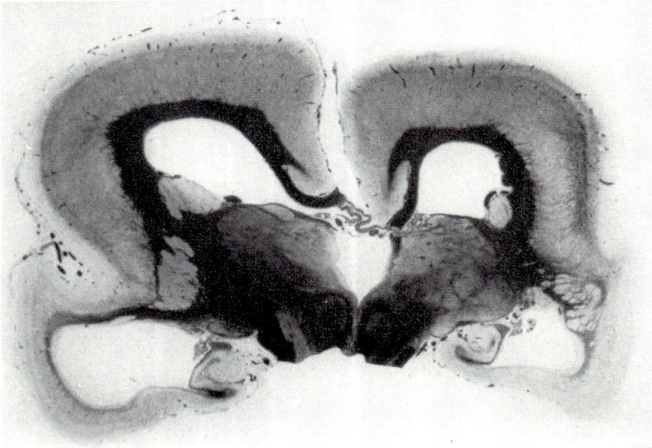

6.32

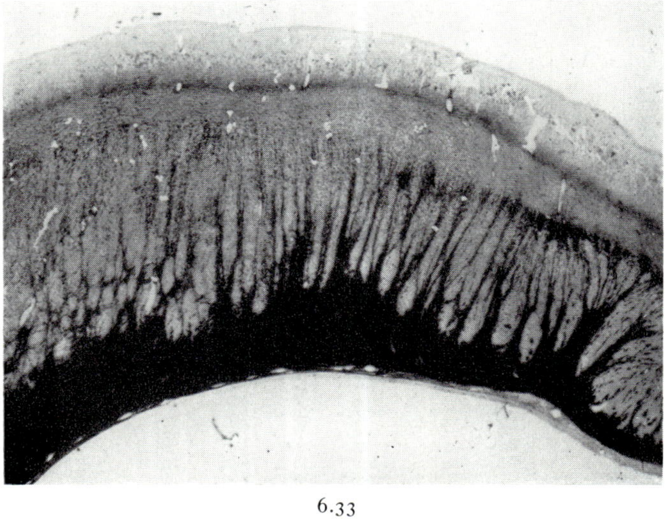

6.33

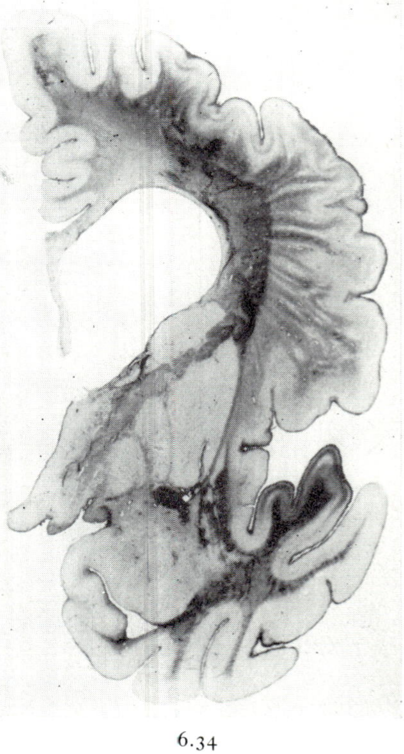

6.34

FIG. 6.30. *Agyria and Pachygyria.* External appearance of brain.

FIG. 6.31. Section through the wall of the hemisphere shown in Fig 6.24 to show the great depth of grey matter. Note the numerous heterotopias in the narrow white matter. (Carbol azure.)

FIG. 6.32. Coronal section of the brain in Fig. 6.24 to show the relative proportions of grey and white matter, and the well-developed thalami and cornua Ammonis. (Heidenhain's myelin.)

FIG. 6.33. Section through the hemispheric wall showing the plume-like radial fibres traversing the deeper layer of the grey matter. (Kultschitsky-Pal method.)

FIG. 6.34. *Pachygyria.* Upper bank of Sylvian fissure shows increased depth of grey matter and a few shallow sulci. There is generalised fibrous gliosis of white matter which was not associated with poverty of myelin. (Holzer).

6.35

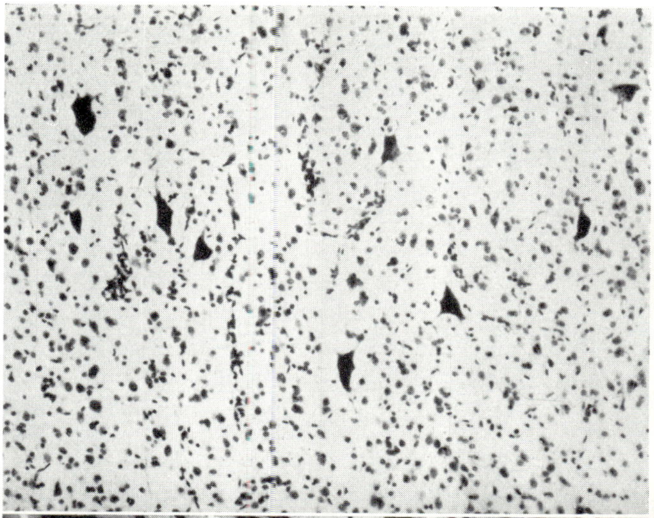

6.36

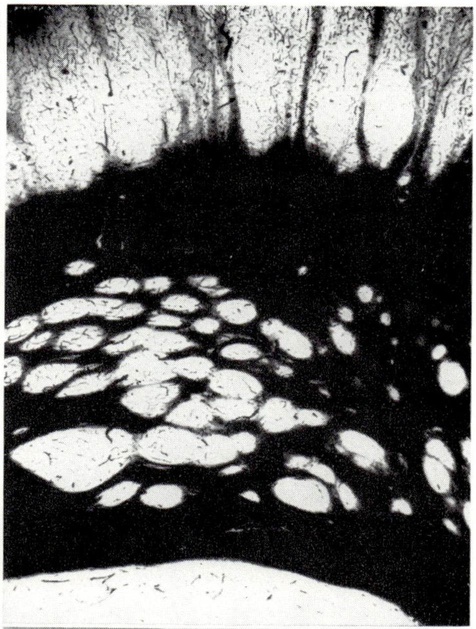

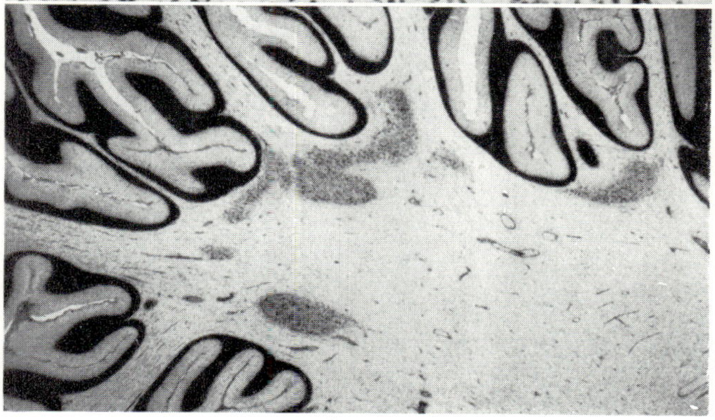

6.37

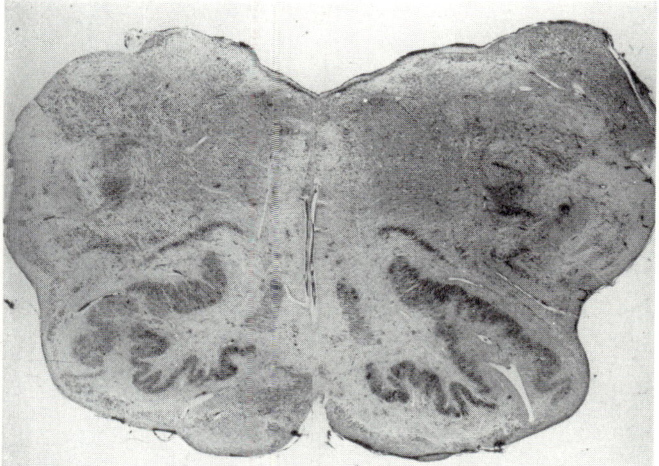

6.38

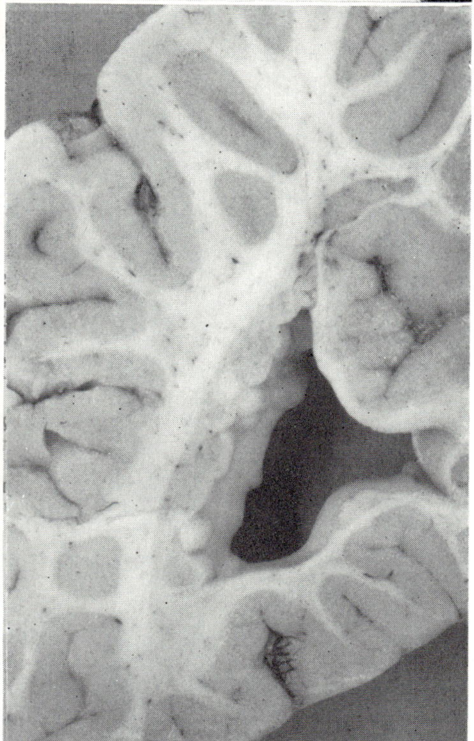

6.39

FIG. 6.35. *Agyria and Pachygyria.* Large, abnormal neurones in the pachygyric 'cortex'. (Carbol azure.)
FIG. 6.36 Heterotopic islands of nerve cells in central white matter of agyric brain. (Heidenhain's myelin.)
FIG. 6.37. Heterotopic islands of nerve cells in the cerebellar white matter in a case of cerebral pachygyria. (Carbol azure.)
FIG. 6.38. Malformation of the inferior olives in a case of agyria. The dorsal cell band has lagged behind in its migration from the rhombic lip and has not been properly incorporated into the nucleus. (Carbol azure.)
FIG. 6.39. Another form of heterotopia—islands of nerve cells lie deep to the central white matter, having remained in the position of the original matrix layer. Note the characteristic bossed appearance of the ventricular wall.

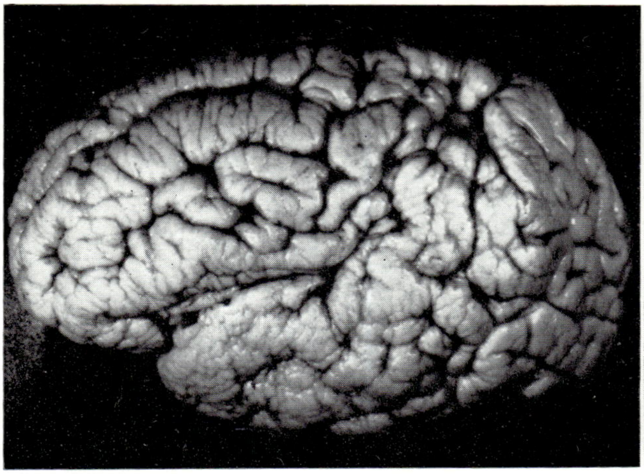

6.40

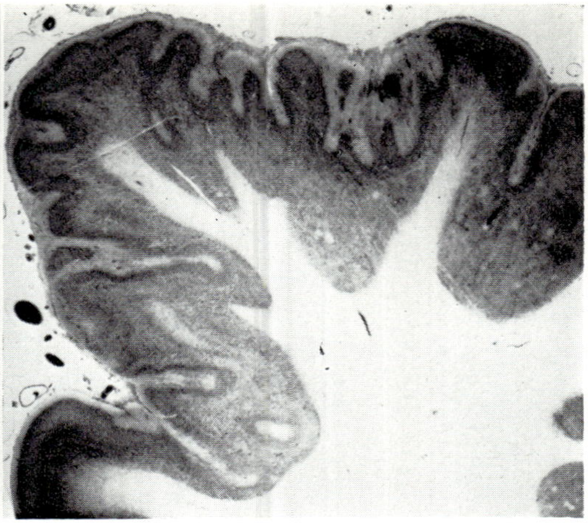

6.41

6.42

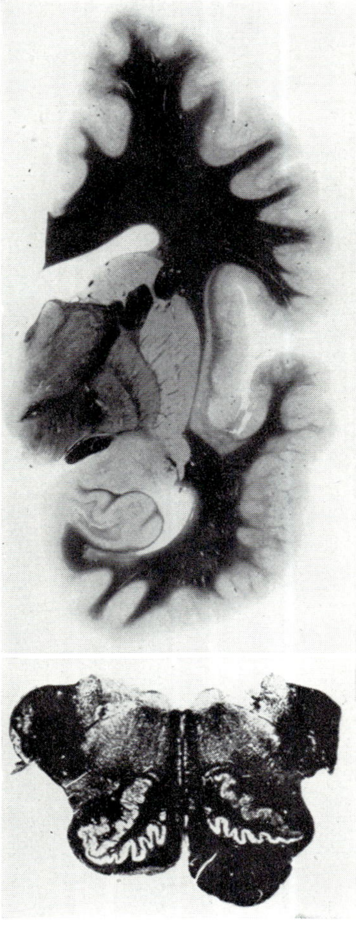

6.43

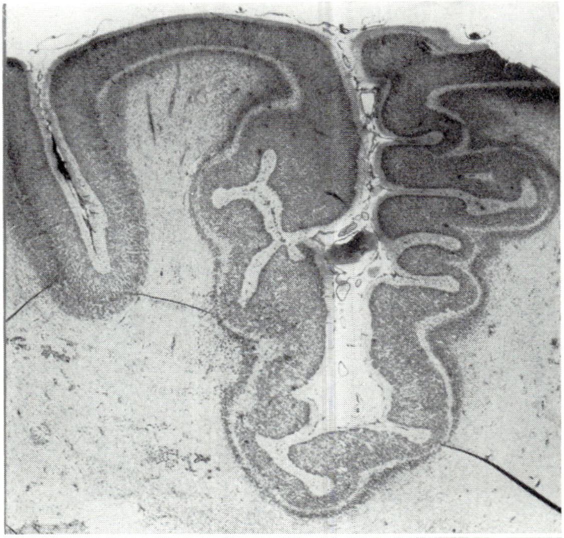

6.44

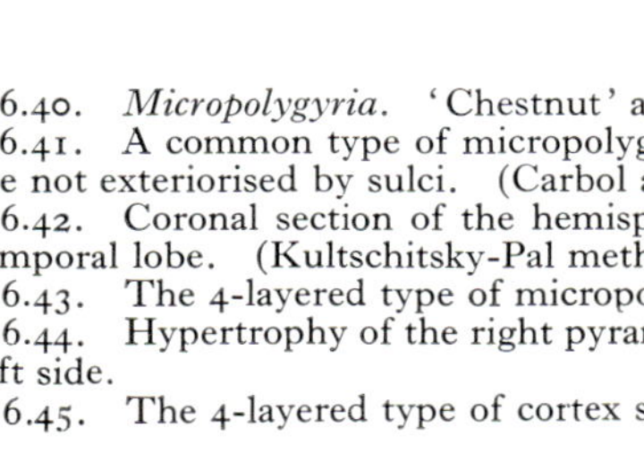

6.45

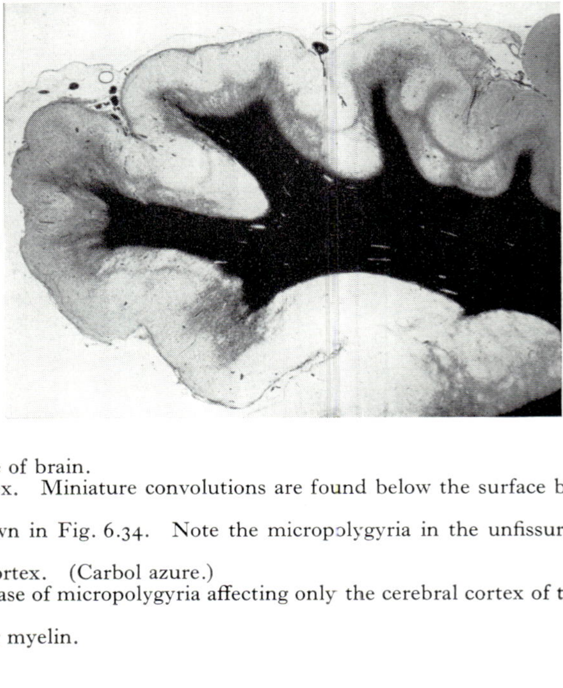

FIG. 6.40. *Micropolygyria.* 'Chestnut' appearance of brain.
FIG. 6.41. A common type of micropolygyric cortex. Miniature convolutions are found below the surface but are not exteriorised by sulci. (Carbol azure.)
FIG. 6.42. Coronal section of the hemisphere shown in Fig. 6.34. Note the micropolygyria in the unfissured temporal lobe. (Kultschitsky-Pal method.)
FIG. 6.43. The 4-layered type of micropolygyric cortex. (Carbol azure.)
FIG. 6.44. Hypertrophy of the right pyramid in a case of micropolygyria affecting only the cerebral cortex of the left side.
FIG. 6.45. The 4-layered type of cortex stained for myelin.

lying in the restiform bodies and thus marking the path taken by the neuroblasts in their migration from the rhombic lip during the 2nd month (Bruschweiler 1927, 1928, Greenfield and Wolfsohn 1935, de Lange 1939, Druckman *et al.* 1959). Less severe malformation of the olives was seen in Walker's (1942) case in which the normal convolutions of the nucleus had been largely replaced by clumps of cells. A somewhat similar minor maldevelopment occurred in one of the writer's cases, the dorsal cell band of each olive being poorly convoluted and distinctly separated from the ventral portion (Fig. 6.38).

Micropolygyria

The old-established name of microgyria is often loosely applied to any type of abnormally small convolution, irrespective of whether this is the consequence of prenatal malformation or of a destructive process occurring at birth or in infancy. An excessive formation of secondary sulci may complicate the otherwise normal convolutional pattern of the brain and the small convolutions so formed, which may suitably be termed 'polygyria', do not necessarily exhibit gliosis or shrinkage. There is, however, another and a more important prenatal cortical anomaly now to be described which is known in the German literature as 'microgyrie' and which may conveniently be referred to as 'micropolygyria' (Schob 1930) in order to avoid ambiguity.

The external aspect of this micropolygyric cortex (Fig. 6.40) does not usually give the impression of convolutional richness but rather of broad and irregular gyri the surfaces of which are wrinkled like a chestnut kernel or finely bossed like morocco leather. It is only after section of the brain that the propriety of the name becomes apparent, for then one sees a wealth of small plications formed by bands of nerve cells lying deep to the surface (Fig. 6.41). These miniature convolutions are submerged because their molecular layers remain fused together and intervening sulci are not formed. Their 'crowns', however, project slightly above the general level of the brain surface, thus giving rise to the characteristic bossed appearance previously mentioned. The extent of the malformation varies considerably from brain to brain. It may be present only as a small patch, usually in the neighbourhood of the Sylvian fissure, or it may extend over much of the lateral cortical surface. The cingulate gyrus, calcarine cortex and hippocampus are spared. In some micropolygyric brains the Sylvian fissure takes an almost vertical course with gyri lying parallel to it on either side like the pleats of an accordion—the so-called 'carnivor' type of convolutional pattern. When the central convolutions are involved the pyramidal tracts are absent or severely stunted and the clinical state of spastic diplegia is produced. Micropolygyria affecting only one hemisphere (Fig. 6.42) is not uncommon and leads to a hemiplegia clinically indistinguishable from that following destructive lesions at birth. The pyramidal tract of the normal side may be hypertrophied and displace the inferior olive dorsally (Fig. 6.44). This phenomenon, which is also sometimes found in the sound pyramidal tract in cases of hemiplegia occurring at birth or in early postnatal life, is due to a relative increase in the number of fibres of large calibre at the expense of the fine fibres. The total number of axons in the hypertrophied pyramid does not exceed the normal (Verhaart 1950). As in the agyric brain, the lateral ventricles are often larger than normal and the central white matter hypoplastic ('colpocephaly'). In some instances the thin hemispheric wall is not strong enough to resist even the normal pressure of the cerebrospinal fluid and a mild degree of hydrocephalus with enlargement of the head occurs.

The appearance of the nerve cell layers in micropolygyria usually varies in different parts of the cortex. The commonest pattern is a wavy, festoon-like arrangement of the nerve cell ribbon with non-separation of the molecular layers. These submerged 'gyri' may be relatively large with central cores of white matter pointing towards the surface like the fingers of a glove.

Sometimes a more complex 'glandular' formation is seen in which tubular columns of cells ramify in tortuous plications. Yet another well-differentiated pattern shows a multifoliate structure somewhat resembling the structure of the normal cerebellar cortex though without the separation of the folia by sulci. It is not unusual to find sheets of nerve cells and their fused molecular layers heaped up one upon another so that the total depth of grey matter is greatly increased, and some of these deeper gyri may, in cross-section, be mistaken for heterotopias. Only in a minority of cases, however, is micropolygyria associated with massive heterotopic collections of nerve cells in the periventricular white matter.

On microscopical examination there is usually no indication of differentiated lamination in the malformed areas, and a normal granular layer is never found. The nerve cells may be of immature type having a poorly developed cytoplasm compared with the size of the nucleus. There is no attempt at the formation of radial bundles and tangles of myelinated fibres may be present in sufficient density to suggest état marbré. The molecular layers commonly show abnormally dense strands of myelinated fibres running parallel to the surface. As in agyria, marked fibrillary gliosis of the whole white matter of the brain without any corresponding demyelination is a feature of some, but by no means all, micropolygyric brains.

Another pattern of abnormal cortex may be found in these brains, the four-layered type of micropolygyria; this deserves a rather more detailed description, because of the light it may throw upon the formal pathogenesis of the malformation. In this variant the grey matter consists of a molecular layer and 2 layers of nerve cells, separated from each other by an acellular strip containing myelinated fibres, which constitutes the 3rd layer (Figs. 6.43 and 6.45). Bielschowsky (1924 a) considered that only the outer 2 layers constituted the true cortex of the micropolygyric brain, the 3rd layer being the analogue of the normal subsulcine or U fibres, while the rather vaguely demarcated 4th layer of nerve cells was heterotopic, representing as it were the stragglers of the main body of migrating neuroblasts which had arrived too late to be incorporated into the cortex proper. There is thus a marked resemblance between this variety of microgyric formation and the pachygyric cortex. In the latter, however, the heterotopic layer is much deeper and occupies most of the cerebral wall, thus indicating an earlier onset of the process of retardation in the neuroblast migration. Another link between the two conditions is that the same type of cerebellar malformation may be present in both. This so-called 'cerebellar microgyria' (q.v.) is characterised by the absence of a normal folial pattern; instead, the granular cells, molecular layers and Purkinje cells form a complex and anarchical arrangement beneath patches of smooth cerebellar cortex.

The four-layered type of cortex may not be present in brains showing widespread micropolygyria and a mere slowing of neuronal migration cannot by itself explain the extremely varied and complex formations that are encountered (Crome 1952). One is thus forced back to the more general and vaguer conception of a disturbance in the relationship of factors governing the harmonious synthesis of the parts of a developing organ (Diezel 1954). Micropolygyria has been reported in cases in which foetal anoxia and foetal infection were certainly the responsible agents. Hallervorden (1949) has reported the malformation in a child 1 year of age, whose mother had attempted suicide by coal gas inhalation when 5 months' pregnant. In addition to micropolygyria the infant's brain showed softening of the globus pallidus and putamen. Cytomegalic inclusion body disease is commonly associated with micropolygyria (Crome and France 1959). Interference with the blood supply of the developing cortex had evidently occurred in this latter case and this factor may well be of importance in others. In this connection it has been shown by de Morsier (1952) that the localisation of various prenatal anomalies, including micropolygyria and heterotopias, may be strictly confined to the territories of main cerebral arteries. The frequency of minor vascular malformations in the micropolygyric cortex has also been stressed by Bertrand and Gruner (1595). The meningeal network of vessels is very abnormal and instead of perforating branches of the usual size numerous small vessels of varying dimensions penetrate the cortex obliquely. Vessels reaching the 3rd layer of myelinated fibres tend to run along in the course of these fibres and supply the festoons of nerve cells from below while the deepest cortical layer is supplied from the white matter. The anterior surface of the pons may show deep indentations from vessels pursuing an abnormal course, and the nuclei pontis are occasionally divided into lobules surrounded by myelinated fibres following the ramifications of these vessels. Similar vascular anomalies accompany the disordered cortical architecture of the cerebellum. These findings give some support to the original theory of pathogenesis put forward by Bielschowsky (1917–18 a). From this point of view, micropolygyria is essentially the outcome of an attempt to compensate for an initial disturbance of growth caused by abnormal vascularisation of the cortical grey matter. A minor malformation of the cerebral cortex which may be found in micropolygyric or in otherwise normal brains is the condition of 'brain warts'. These are elevated nodular collections of fusiform and stellate neurones, usually in the superficial part of the crowns of gyri in the frontal lobes. There is often a central artery running up from the deeper layers and the myelinated fibres of the gyral core fan out to enclose the base of the nodule (Grcevic and Robert 1960).

Cerebellar malformations

Agenesis. It is doubtful whether complete absence of the cerebellum occurs, since careful examination usually reveals a small nodule of recognisable cerebellar tissue (Stewart 1956). In a case of this sort examined by the writer the posterior columns throughout the spinal cord were separated by an ependyma-lined cleft, and uncrossed pyramidal tracts were seen as prominant bundles in the anterior columns. The latter malformation has been studied in detail by Verhaart and Kramer (1952). Absence of one hemisphere is much less rare (Figs. 6.46 and 6.47) and is associated with anomalies of the contralateral inferior olive (Fig. 6.48), which may take the form of atrophy rather than maldevelopment, as in Lichtenstein's (1943) case in which the foliated outline of the degenerated nucleus was clearly visible.

Hypoplasia. The small cerebellum frequently seen in mongols is an example of hypoplasia. A mild unilateral stunting in cerebellar growth is often found in brains showing malformation or long-standing destruction of large areas of the cerebral hemisphere of the opposite side. This condition is much commoner than crossed cerebellar atrophy (q.v.).

Palaeocerebellar aplasia. Partial or complete aplasia of the vermis is due to the failure of the two alar plates of the rhombencephalon to unite in the formation of the corpus cerebelli. The two halves of the cerebellum are separated by a midline cleft and the hemispheres and their peduncles are reduced in size. Various associated nuclear atrophies have been described, including those of the inferior olives, and of cuneate and arcuate nuclei (Lyssenkow 1931). In the condition described by Martin (1949, 1950) in which the neocerebellum as well as the rostral part of the vermis and the flocculi were severely underdeveloped, the dentate nuclei were represented by islands of nerve cells and the lateral vestibular nuclei were atrophied. In partial aplasia of the vermis it is usually the portion lying behind the fissura prima that is involved, the nodulus and uvula being absent and not merely stunted in development as usually occurs in cases of atresia of the foramina of the 4th ventricle.

Ponto-neocerebellar hypoplasia. Brun (1917, 1918 a, 1918 b) described under this title a cerebellum with hypoplastic, flattened, lateral lobes and well-developed vermis and flocculi (Figs. 6.49, 6.50 and 6.51). In the cerebellar hemispheres the mossy and climbing fibres are largely absent. The ventral part of the pons is unduly small and its transverse fibres and the nuclei pontis markedly reduced in numbers (Fig. 6.52). The dentate nuclei are composed of isolated clumps of cells, a malformation also present in the cases of Brouwer (1924) and Biemond (1955). Biemond suggested that this malformation of the dentate nucleus may be the primary event, the other cerebellar changes being of a secondary character.

In this condition the small volume of the neocerebellum must be attributed to hypoplasia. The minor losses of Purkinje cells and patchy thinning of the granular layer in Biemond's case

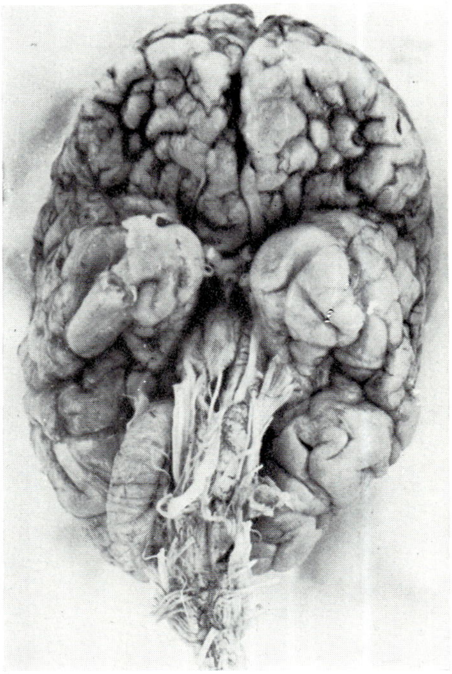

6.46

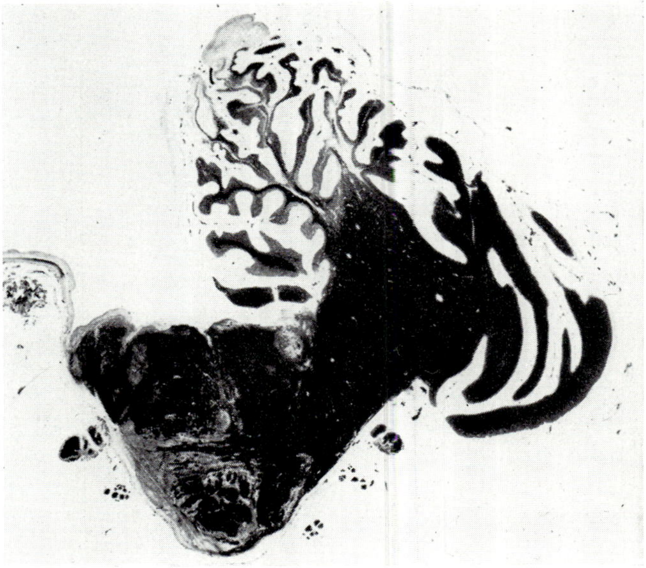

6.47

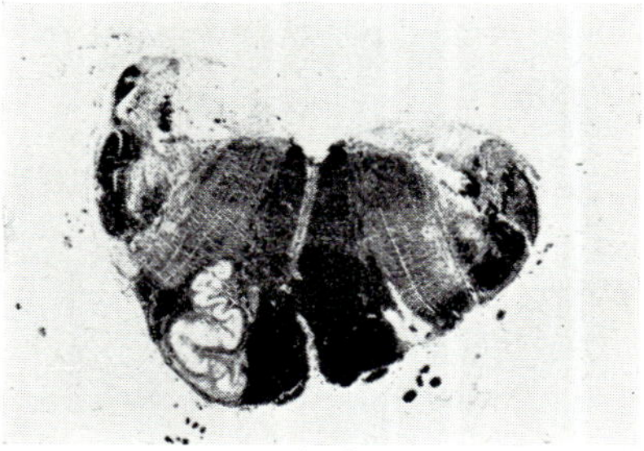

6.48

FIGS. 6.46 and 6.47. *Cerebellar agenesis*: only a rudimentary right hemisphere is present. From a case of the Klippel-Feil deformity.

FIG. 6.48. Malformation of the inferior olives from the same case as in Fig. 6.46. Note the small size of the olive contralateral to the cerebellar defect.

would not account for the great reduction in the size of the hemispheres. However, in other parts of the nervous system signs of a degenerative process may sometimes be found. Thus in an example of ponto-neocerebellar hypoplasia occurring in an infant of 3 months, the writer found both dentate nuclei almost completely degenerated and gliosed, except for the most dorsal convolutions (i.e. the part connected with the vermis) where groups of cells had survived. The original crenated outline of the nerve cell bands was, however, clearly distinguishable. This lesion was evidently related to the atrophy of the nucleus ventralis lateralis of each thalamus.

A severe loss of nerve cells was also found in the inferior olives, particularly in the dorsal convolutions, and this was also accompanied by marked fibrillary gliosis. The ventral pons was about half as thick as in the newborn and showed a great numerical reduction in its transverse fibres and in the nerve cells in the nuclei pontis. The remaining cells were often of small size suggesting a retardation in development, but a heavy gliosis of the region was nevertheless seen. On the other hand, the small lateral lobes of the cerebellum showed no evidence of degeneration. In the brain stem certain nuclei with cerebellar connections were either absent or very poorly developed, their sites showing no traces of a destructive process (Norman and Urich 1958). Gross and Kaltenback (1959) have also noted the combination of malformation and system degenerations in their case.

Ponto-neocerebellar hypoplasia has been found associated with cerebral pachygyria in one instance (Kramer 1956).

Cerebellar microgyria. In this condition the normal foliated lobules fail to develop over a variable extent of cortex, which thus presents a smooth and unconvoluted surface. Microscopical examination reveals a complicated pattern of interlacing strands or islands of granular cells interspersed with relatively acellular strips representing the molecular layer (Fig. 6.53). These areas contain numerous displaced Purkinje cells which have few arborisations and appear as retort-shaped forms when impregnated by silver (Fig. 6.54). They tend to orientate themselves in the normal way at the junction of the aberrant molecular and granular layers and their cytons are often enclosed by normal basket fibres. Tangential fibres are seldom seen in these ectopic molecular layers, but numerous unmyelinated fibres are found passing in different directions. Since this malformation is generally associated with cerebral micropolygyria it has been called 'microgyria' of the cerebellum; but the name 'cerebellar agyria' would seem to be more appropriate, since little or no suggestion is conveyed of minature folia or of microgyric formations and this type of cerebellar anomaly may also be present in brains showing agyria (pachygyria) of the cerebral hemispheres (Walker 1942, Warner 1953). A cerebellar malformation of this type was found in the unique case described by van Bogaert and Radermecker (1955). The mother had been treated by radium for carcinoma of the cervix during the fifth month of pregnancy.

Congenital cerebellar atrophy

A distinction between cerebellofugal and cerebellopetal types of atrophy was first made by Bielschowsky (1920) who noted that in certain cases of amaurotic family idiocy the brunt of the destructive process had fallen upon the afferent elements, so that the granule cells, mossy fibres and climbing fibres had largely disappeared, whereas the cells of Purkinje were preserved. This distribution of lesions is thus the converse of what is found in the cerebello-olivary degenerations of later life in which the Purkinje cell layer is invariably the most severely affected part of the cortex.

Although this contrast is not an absolute one and 'pure' types are by no means the rule, this classification according to the predominant locality of the lesions is a useful one and is applicable to the two types of congenital cerebellar atrophy now to be described.

Congenital cerebellar atrophy of granular layer type. The cerebellum is much diminished in size and shows shrinkage and sclerosis of the folia (Fig. 6.55). In some cases the vermis is much less affected (Ule 1952). Microscopically it is seen that the granule and Golgi cells are absent or very scanty over the greater part of the cortex and the mossy fibres have also disappeared (Fig. 6.56). The Purkinje cells, on the other hand, are numerous and very conspicuous partly because of the small size of the shrunken folia and also because the majority of the cells are scattered throughout the molecular layer (Fig. 6.56). These ectopic neurones are

6.49

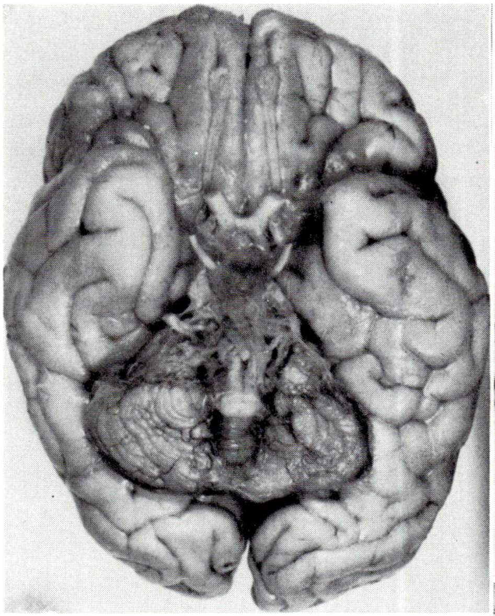

6.50

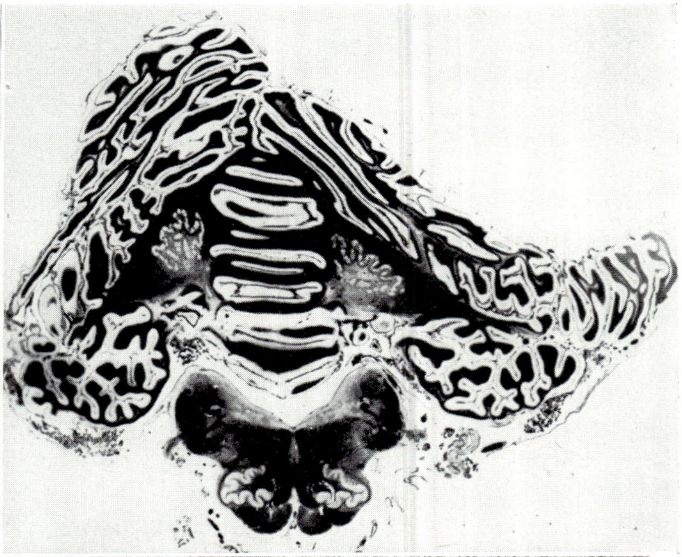

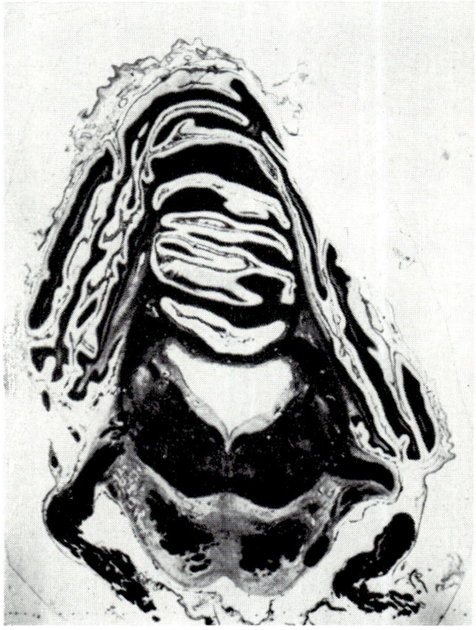

6.51

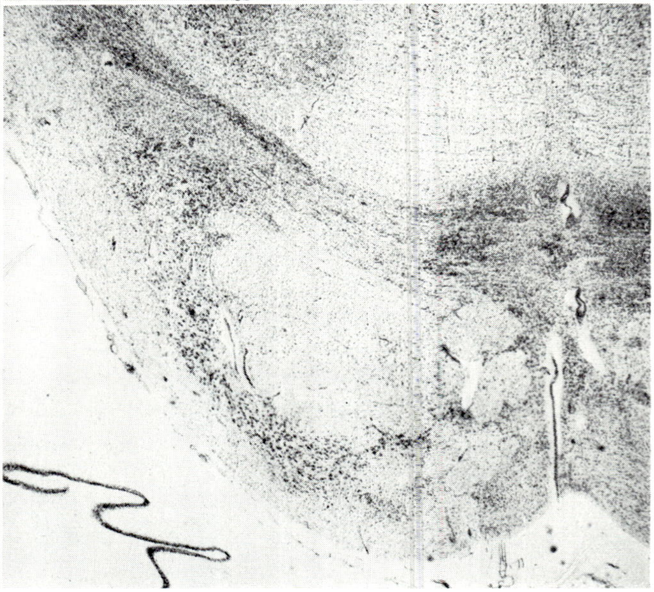

6.52

FIG. 6.49. *Pontoneocerebellar hypoplasia*. The cerebellum is small and flattened—'like a pressed fig'.
FIG. 6.50. Note the relatively large vermis and flocculi compared with the lateral lobes.
FIG. 6.51. Showing the poorly developed pes pontis and lateral lobes of cerebellum.
FIG. 6.52. The nuclei pontis are very poorly represented.

of anomalous shape, resembling retorts or spindles, and are devoid of basket or climbing fibres. The tangential fibres of the molecular layer are generally preserved but their descending branches, instead of forming distinct pericellular baskets, tend to be arranged in a thin, uniformly spaced, curtain which passes downwards to end in the denuded granular layer. As in other types of cerebellar disease the dendrites of the Purkinje cells often exhibit terminal club-shaped expansions which bear short filamentous processes (Fig. 6.57). It is, however, a characteristic feature of this condition that the radial branches of these 'asteroid bodies' often form a peculiarly dense brushwork (Fig. 6.58). When such a formation is attached to a dendritic stalk its origin is obvious, but similar asteroid bodies are often seen in isolation in the molecular layer, their fine radial fibres arranged around a central nuclear structure the peripheral portion of which is denser than the central. These dendritic swellings are not so coarse as the cactus-like formations in amaurotic idiocy and they do not contain lipid. They are best explained as a reaction to pathological change on the part of the damaged but surviving Purkinje cell and they exemplify what Bouman (1934) has called 'hyper-differentiation', to which category also belong the numerous axonal 'torpedoes' which are commonly seen in this and other cerebellar disorders. It is noteworthy that no case of granular atrophy has been accompanied by retrograde atrophy of the inferior olives, so that it seems improbable that the olivocerebellar tracts contribute to the mossy fibres of the granular layer.

A heavy fibrillary gliosis is seen in the molecular layer but gliosis is mild in the territory of

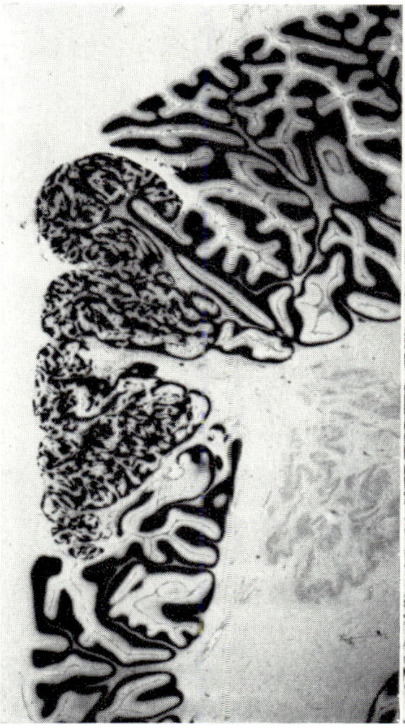

6.53

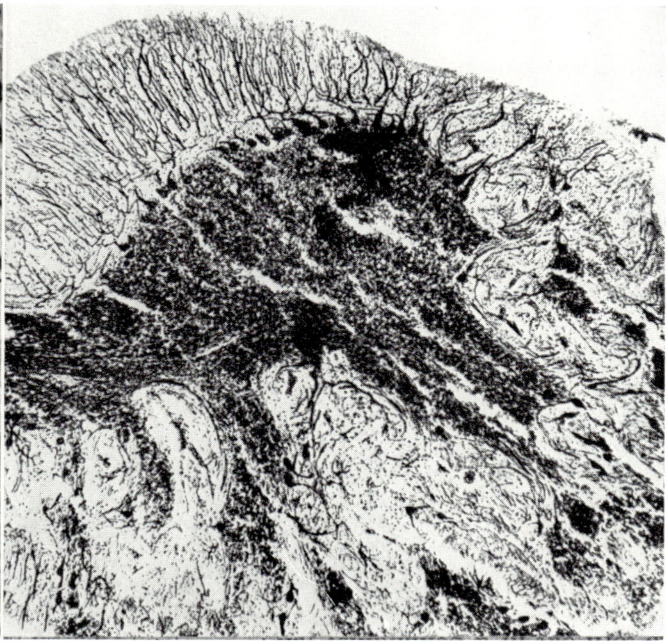

6.54

FIG. 6.53. *Cerebellar microgyria*—the granular layer is disorganised.

FIG. 6.54. Showing transition between normal and malformed cerebellar cortices. Cajal's silver nitrate pyridine method for the cerebellum.

the missing granules (Fig. 6.59). This neuroglial fibrosis is in part derived from the Bergmann astrocytes but the usual radial arrangement of the fibrils is replaced by a wilder, anisomorphic type of gliosis. It is unlikely that traction by gliosis is responsible for the grossly abnormal position of so many of the Purkinje cells, although it must be remembered that dislocation of previously normally aligned Purkinje cells into the molecular layer is a well-known phenomenon in diseases of the cerebellum (Schob 1921). A more probable explanation of the ectopic position of the cells is that, owing to the degeneration of the granular layer at a stage prior to the final organisation of the cerebellar cortex, the migrating Purkinje cells have themselves been implicated in the pathological process. This view is supported by the observation that in folia

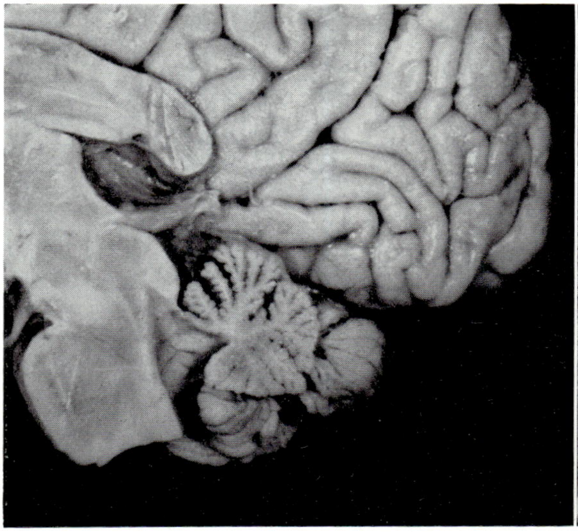
6.55

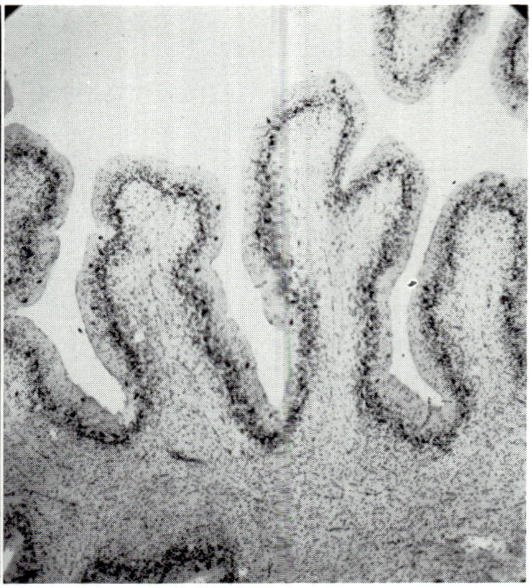
6.56

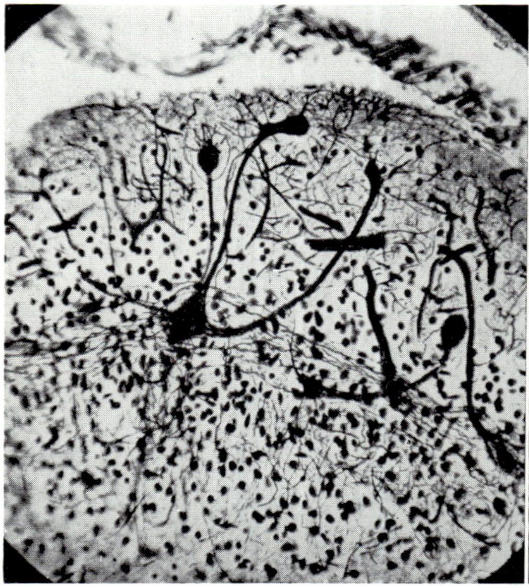
6.57

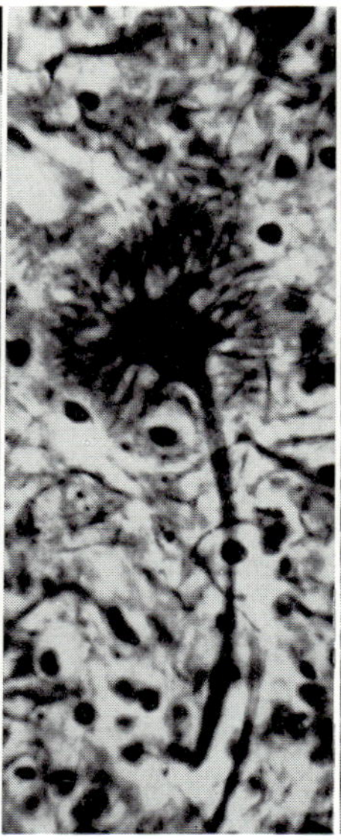
6.58

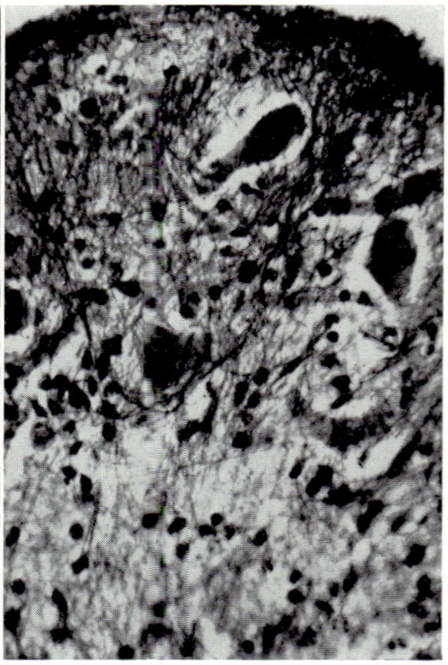
6.59

FIG. 6.55. *Congenital cerebellar atrophy* (granular layer type) showing small size of cerebellum and shrinkage of dorsal vermis.
FIG. 6.56. Atrophy of the granular layer and preservation of the Purkinje cells many of which are present in the molecular layer. (Cresyl violet.)
FIG. 6.57. Cactus-like expansions of the dendrites of the Purkinje cells. Note the tangential fibres lying low in the molecular layer. (Cajal's silver nitrate pyridine method for the cerebellum.)
FIG. 6.58. Dendritic expansion with fine terminal brushwork of fibres. (Bielschowsky.)
FIG. 6.59. The fibrillary gliosis is mainly in the molecular layer. Heterotopic Purkinje cells are seen. (Holzer.)

where the Purkinje cells are in normal alignment there is always a well-formed granular layer.

The aetiology of this primary form of granular atrophy is unknown, though in the writer's cases (Norman 1940) there was the likelihood of familial incidence. The condition is invariably associated with severe mental defect, though no characteristic pathological changes have been demonstrated in the cerebrum. From the clinical point of view there may be little evidence of ataxia, a feature shared by other cerebellar disorders of early life.

Congenital cerebellar atrophy with loss of Purkinje cells. One is on far less certain ground in placing this variety of cerebellar disease in the prenatal class and only rarely can the decision be taken with reasonable confidence. This hesitation arises from the well-known vulnerability of the Purkinje cell to the vascular disturbances associated with epilepsy which may lead to widespread destruction of these cells. Certainly, if lesions appropriate to epilepsy or birth injury are found elsewhere in the brain, the prenatal character of the cerebellar atrophy becomes improbable. There are, however, a few recorded cases in which cerebellar degeneration has evidently occurred very early in life and has led to a small cerebellum and widespread loss of Purkinje cells, especially in the hemispheres. In Scherer's (1933) case of a 2-year-old idiot the granular layer had also suffered slightly. Jervis (1950 c) described a familial case in which the granular layer showed widespread and severe rarefaction, but the substantial involvement of the Purkinje cells and the regular alignment of the survivors seems to put this case in a different category from that of primary granular layer degeneration.

A corollary to the degeneration of Purkinje cells is the presence of empty basket fibres. Axonal torpedoes and swollen dendritic 'antlers' may also be seen among the survivors. When the loss of Purkinje cells is considerable the dentate nucleus always shows characteristic changes in the form of a loss of myelinated fibres and an exceptionally heavy gliosis in the amiculum or 'fleece'. Secondary glial proliferation in the olives is found in long-standing cases but the amount of retrograde cell loss is very variable.

Cerebro-cerebellar atrophy

Lesions of one cerebral hemisphere sometimes lead to a degeneration of Purkinje and granular cells in the cerebellar hemisphere of the opposite side. With few exceptions, the cerebral lesions in the recorded cases have been extensive, have originated in early life and have taken several years to produce their effects. The cerebellar atrophy commonly involves the semilunar and quadrangular lobes and is usually distributed in a patchy way. The vermis and flocculus are rarely affected. There are two suggested pathways by which the chain of degeneration may reach the cerebellum from the cerebral cortex. The first, or prograde way, is along the corticopontine tracts, the ipsilateral nucleus pontis and the opposite middle peduncle to the granular layer of the cerebellum and thence to the Purkinje cells. The second, or retrograde way, is from the precentral cortex (areas 4 and 6) to the ventrolateral nucleus of the thalamus, thence via the superior cerebellar peduncle to the opposite dentate nucleus and so to the Purkinje cells and lastly to the granules. When the cerebral lesions are widespread it is not unusual to find both the thalamus and the cerebral peduncle degenerated, in which case it is only by determining whether the nucleus pontis or the dentate nucleus is the more affected, that a conclusion can be reached as to which path may have been taken by the degenerative process. The most comprehensive account of the subject is that given by Verhaart and van Wieringen-Rauws (1950). From their review of 38 reported cases these authors conclude that cerebro-cerebellar atrophy is unpredictable, and even under apparently favourable conditions the barrier of the pontine or dentate nucleus may not be penetrated. There is, moreover, no sharp topographical relation between the cerebral and cerebellar lesions and the occurrence or extent of the latter may depend upon some innate tendency towards degeneration on the part of the cerebellum itself.

The tuberose sclerosis complex (Bourneville's disease)

The first recorded instance of patchy sclerosis of the cerebral cortex was given by von Recklinghausen (1862), whose case also showed multiple myomata in the heart. The name tuberose sclerosis was first applied to these cortical changes by Bourneville who described 10 cases in a series of papers published during the years 1880–1900. Although Bourneville had noted that facial and renal anomalies might be present it was not until H. Vogt's paper of 1908 that the clinico-pathological syndrome was adequately delineated. Since the term 'tuberose sclerosis' applies only to one feature of a protean disorder it is more precise to designate the condition 'the tuberose sclerose complex' as suggested by Moulton (1942), unless the eponymous title of 'Bourneville's disease' is preferred. The term 'epiloia' was introduced by Sherlock (1911) to indicate the commonly encountered triad of adenoma sebaceum, epilepsy and mental deficiency.

In the fully developed disease an extraordinary diversity of lesions may be encountered, brain, skin, kidneys, heart, bones and lungs being involved in characteristic ways. Many of these anomalies belong to the category of 'hamartoma', that is to say, they are congenital malformations with a potentiality for growth which does not exceed that of the normal tissue in which they are situated.

Central nervous system. The brain may be of normal weight but some reduction is common in low-grade mental defectives. Frank micrencephaly, as in one of Bielschowsky's (1923–4 b) cases, is exceptional; so also is the very heavy brain recorded by Borremans *et al.* (1933). The convolutional pattern is usually within normal limits, although minor disturbances may be caused by the presence of the pathognomonic sclerotic patches or *tubera* in the gyri. When the leptomeninges are removed these tubera are easily distinguished by their pallor and stony-hard consistency which contrast with the appearance and feel of the neighbouring convolutions. There are two main varieties of tuber which have been named after Pelizzi (1901) who first described their points of difference. His first type is characterised by a hardening, blanching and widening of a gyrus, the crown of which is flattened and smooth (Fig. 6.62). The other variety is a rounded, flattened nodule, the surface of which is roughened and dimpled and which is sometimes slightly elevated above the level of the neighbouring gyri from which it is superficially demarcated by a surrounding sulcus (Fig. 6.60). On microscopical examination, the sclerosed areas show an enormous increase in the number of astrocytic nuclei, the nerve cells being usually scanty or their lamination grossly disturbed. The histological picture is often dominated by groups of very large cells of bizarre shape, many of which exceed the size of giant Betz cells (Fig. 6.61). Their outlines are vague in Nissl preparations but a minority may suggest nerve cells by their pyramidal or spindle shape and the coarse tigroid bodies they contain. A much better demonstration of their morphology is obtained by metallic impregnation methods. The commonest form of abnormal cell in tuberose sclerosis is a large oval plump cell, rather like a swollen-bodied astrocyte, which often contains two or three peripherally placed nuclei with prominent nucleoli (Fig. 6.63). These cells do not possess processes. Many of the giant cells have a more obvious relationship either to neurones or to astrocytes. The neuronal derivatives may be shown by Bielschowsky's method to contain neurofibrils (Fig. 6.65), while the large glial types often stain well with Hortega's silver carbonate or Cajal's gold sublimate (Fig. 6.66 and 6.67). These giant cells are most numerous in the tubera, especially near the central umbilication. They are uncommon in the molecular layer and more frequent in the outer zone of the grey matter than in the deeper layers. Isolated examples may be found in any part of the cortex or subcortical white matter and in the latter situation substantial groups are often seen around blood-vessels. In rare instances the majority of the large cells are to be found in the central cores of white matter where they show up as conspicuous heterotopias. Many of the large cells contain conspicuous vacuoles (Fig. 6.64) which have been shown to contain glycogen (Helmke 1937).

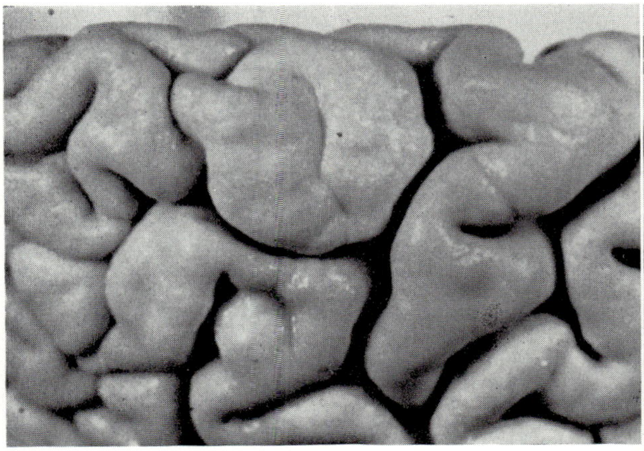
6.60

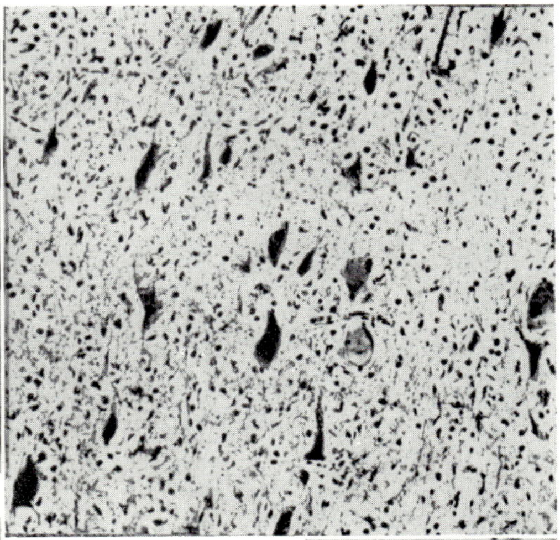
6.61

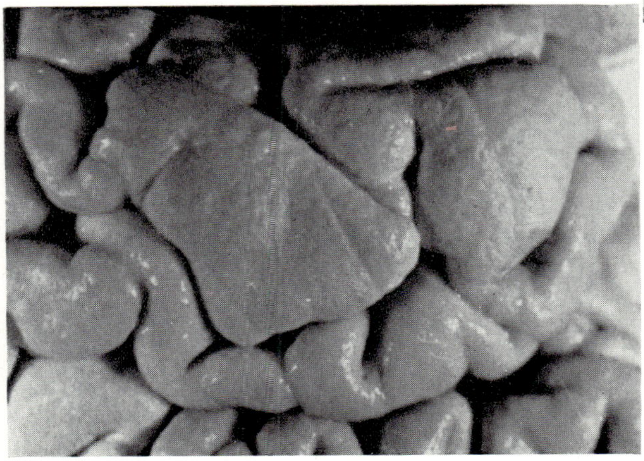
6.62

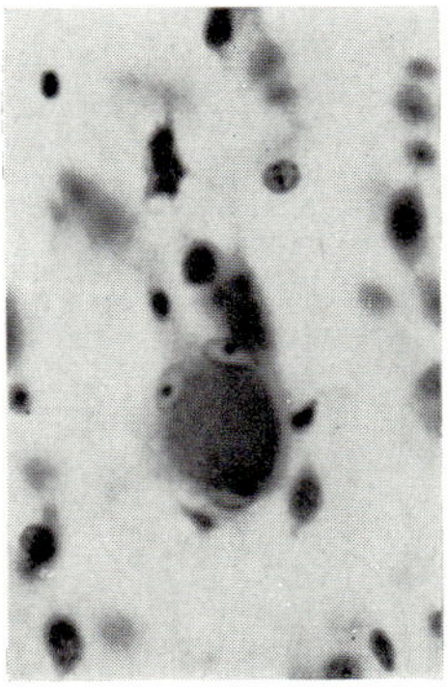
6.63

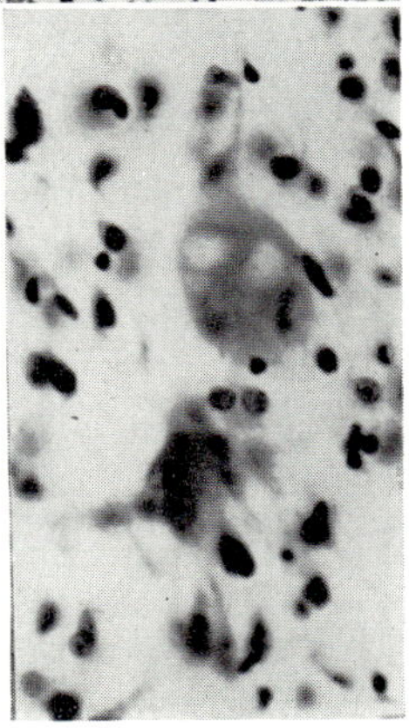
6.64

FIG. 6.60. *Tuberose sclerosis*—a cortical tuber (Pelizzi type 2).
FIG. 6.61. A group of giant cells in an area of tuberose sclerosis. (Hortega's silver carbonate method for astrocytes.)
FIG. 6.62. A cortical tuber (Pelizzi type 1).
FIG. 6.63. Multinucleated large glial cell of anomalous type. (Carbol azure.)
FIG. 6.64. Anomalous cell showing vacuolation. (Carbol azure.)

As might be expected from their very firm texture the tubers exhibit a great proliferation of fibrillary astrocytes. The Holzer stain reveals dense fibrillary gliosis in the outer part of the molecular layer, particularly in the region of the central depression of the tuber where sheaves of coarse fibres form interlacing and brush-like patterns (Fig. 6.68). In comparison, the outer part of the grey matter is usually less gliosed, but a dense overgrowth of fibrils is usual in the deeper layers and in the adjoining white matter. Bundles of glial fibres connect these two zones of gliosis, passing through the less affected cortex in radial fashion. The central part of the cortex in such sclerosed gyri may occasionally show rarefaction of the tissues with status spongiosus. Glial anomalies are not, however, confined to the tubera. A well-marked fibrillary gliosis may be present throughout the white matter of the brain; and in non-tuberose parts selective staining readily reveals atypical astrocytes.

Myelination is disturbed in the sclerotic convolutions, the cortex containing irregular tangles of fibres and the central cores and subcortical white matter showing patchy areas of rarefaction

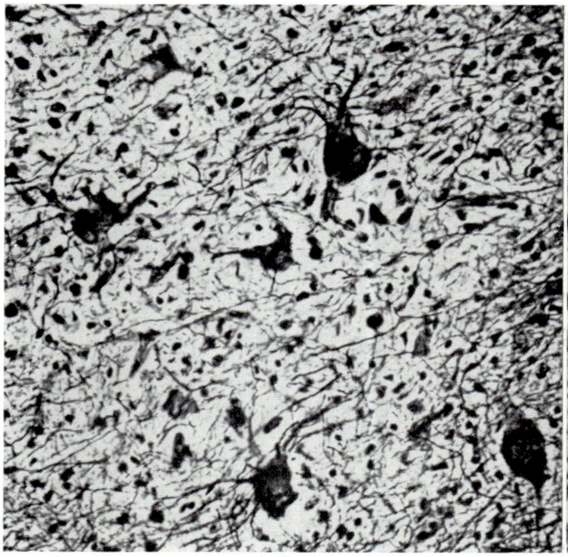

6.65

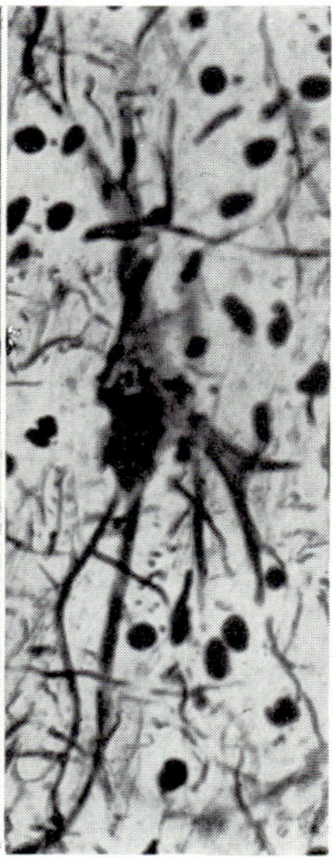

6.66

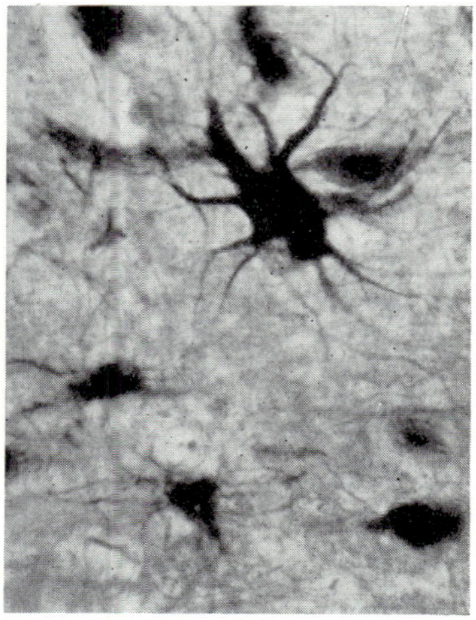

6.67

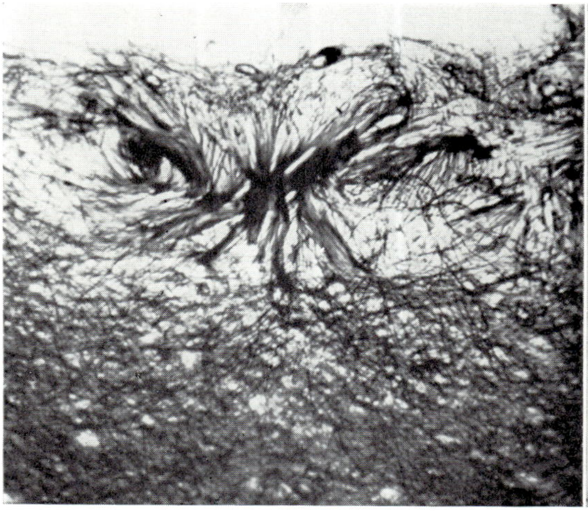

6.68

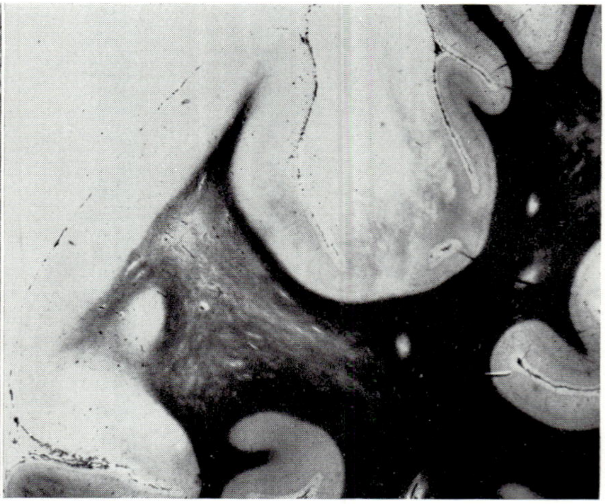

6.69

FIG. 6.65. A group of large abnormal cells of neuronal type in an area of tuberose sclerosis. (Bielschowsky.)
FIG. 6.66. Giant cell of astrocytic type. (Hortega's method for astrocytes.)
FIG. 6.67. Giant astrocyte. (Cajal's gold sublimate method.)
FIG. 6.68. *Tuberose sclerosis.* Sheaf-like bundles of neuroglial fibres in superficial part of a cortical tuber. (Holzer.)
FIG. 6.69. Myelin poverty in an area of neuroglial sclerosis. The flat margin of the central core of white matter lies beneath a cortical tuber and is a characteristic feature of myelin preparations. (Heidenhain's myelin.)

(Fig. 6.69). More sharply defined, circular areas devoid of myelin are caused by the presence of small fibrocellular tumours to be described later.

This account of the cellular abnormalities met with in the cerebral cortex applies in the main to other parts of the central nervous system. The cerebellar manifestations have been fully reviewed by van Bogaert *et al.* (1958). Tubers occur infrequently but heterotopic clusters of giant cells are not uncommon in the white matter. Monster cells in the layer of Purkinje cells are rare (Fig. 6.70). It is not unusual to find widespread loss of Purkinje cells and well-marked lobular atrophy, these changes being attributable to epilepsy. Giant cells and patchy glial overgrowth also occur in the basal ganglia and less frequently in the brain stem and spinal cord.

An important pathological feature of this disease is the presence of multiple small tumour-like nodules of a fibrocellular character. Their site of predilection is the sulcus terminalis from which they project into the lateral ventricle like the 'gutterings of a candle'. They are partially embedded in the substance of the thalamus or caudate nucleus and vary in size from a few millimetres to a centimetre or more in diameter (6.71). They are also commonly seen beneath the ependyma of the lateral ventricles. In the cerebral cortex nodules of similar type are usually found in the subcortical white matter just below the floor of a sulcus and they are also occasionally present in the cerebellum or brain stem. Whatever may be their situation these tumours show little variation in their structure and are composed of aggregations of large round or oval cells, intermingled with leashes or whorls of fibrillary glial tissue (Fig. 6.72). The nuclei of these large cells are often multiple, and elongated or irregularly lobulated forms lie at the periphery of the cell and may even entirely ring its margin. These cells may be seen to contribute long fleshy processes to the fibrous stroma of the tumour, the central parts of which often contain numerous blood-vessels with greatly thickened walls. Fibrillary astrocytes, many of which are hyperplastic, also take part in the tumour and may predominate in the smaller subependymal nodules. Conspicuous iron-calcium deposits, either in the form of concentric spherules or larger confluent masses, are also a characteristic feature of these tumours and the neighbouring blood-vessels may also show extensive calcification. Rings of collagen or reticulin may often be demonstrated around the concretions. When this calcification is sufficiently massive to show in X-ray photographs the position of the nodules in relation to the lateral ventricles may be of diagnostic importance during life. It is also obvious that if much increase takes place in the size of a nodule situated near the foramen of Monro or the opening of the aqueduct of Sylvius the flow of cerebrospinal fluid may become obstructed. Not only may a slow enlargement take place during postnatal life but a malignant transformation of these tumours into astrocytomas or glioblastomas may occur. Diffuse infiltrative tumours of the hemisphere are a well-recognised complication of tuberose sclerosis. In the example recorded by Kufs (1949) the left cerebral hemisphere was generally enlarged and contained in the white matter a massive spongioblastoma. An interesting feature of this case was that only in the hemisphere containing the tumour were there signs of tuberose sclerosis. In a smaller number of cases the tumour has contained numerous abnormal nerve cells in addition to glial derivates of a more or less primitive type. Globus (1938), in particular, has drawn attention to 'spongioneuroblastomas' of this sort in tuberose sclerosis. In Jervis's (1954 a) case the anomalous neurones were thought to be derived from normal elements which had undergone metaplasia.

Closely allied to these subependymal tumours are the retinal phakomata described by van der Hoeve (1921). Both the large nodular type which usually lies at the edge of the nerve head, and the smaller multiple, flattened forms that are present elsewhere in the fundus, have basically the same type of structure and primarily involve the nerve fibre layer of the retina. They are composed in varying proportions of glial fibres and vaguely outlined large cells with fleshy

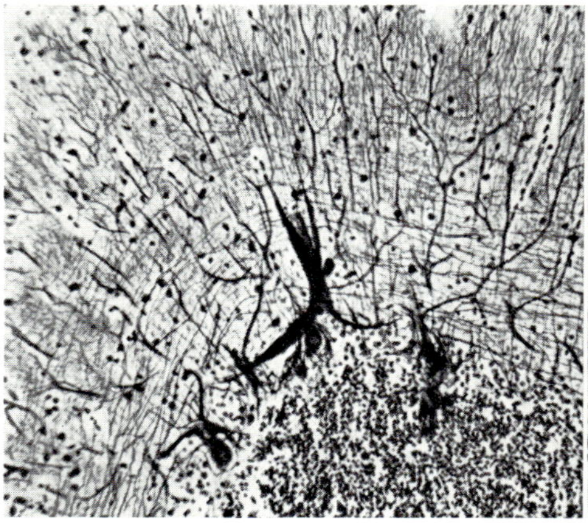

6.70

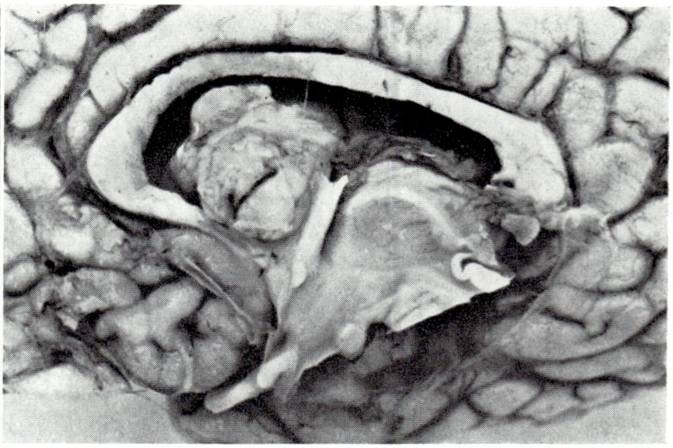

6.71

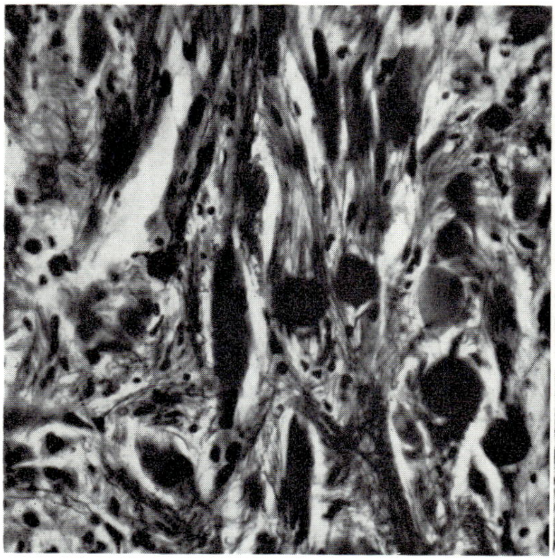

6.72

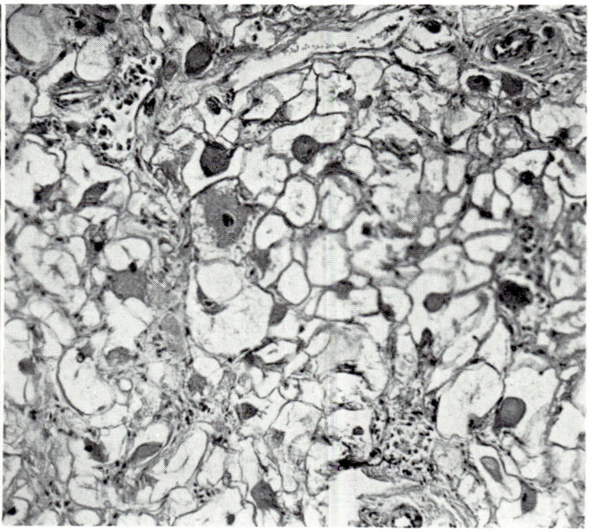

6.73

FIG. 6.70. A large abnormal Purkinje cell from a case of tuberose sclerosis. (Cajal's silver nitrate method for the cerebellum.)

FIG. 6.71. A ventricular tumour of large size arising from the caudate nucleus. The usual glial nodules seen in this region in tuberose sclerosis are considerably smaller.

FIG. 6.72 A common type of ventricular tumour in tuberose sclerosis. Large oval cells are seen enmeshed in a neuroglial stroma. (Hortega's method for astrocytes.)

FIG. 6.73. Typical microscopic appearance of one of the multiple rhabdomyomatous nodules found in the tuberose sclerosis complex. (H. and E.)

cytoplasm which are probably abnormal forms of retinal neuroglia. Neuroglial fibrils are often present in whorls, recalling the appearance of the cerebral tumours, and calcifications or even ossification occurs at their centres. The larger tumours may be partially cystic and an associated angiomatous condition of the choroid has often been noted. The continued growth of these nodules may disorganise the eye, but it is not certain that true malignancy occurs. In Hall's (1946) case a small tumour mass was also found in the lens but, as the author pointed out, this was probably heterotopic and not metastatic in origin.

Visceral anomalies

Heart. Batchelor and Mann (1945) reviewed 63 recorded instances of rhabdomyoma and found that tuberose sclerosis was an associated feature in half the cases, though this is probably a conservative estimate. Rhabdomyomata may have three different distributions in the heart muscle: as a solitary tumour, usually at the apex of the left ventricle, as multiple small nodules and, exceptionally, as a diffuse involvement of the myocardium as in Schminke's (1922) case. Multiple rhabdomyomata are by far the commonest finding. They present as small, rounded, pale areas, rarely exceeding a centimetre in diameter, projecting from, or flush with, the surface of the ventricular, papillary or auricular muscles. Microscopically, the tumours are composed of a loose network of interlacing fibrils many of which possess the striations of skeletal muscle. These fibres may be seen to radiate from large rounded bodies with a granular, eosinophilic cytoplasm resembling the foetal heart muscle cells of Purkinje (Fig. 6.73). These elements, set against the spongy background of the tumour, suggested the appearance of spiders in their webs to Cesaris-Demel (1895) and have since his day been known as 'spider-cells'. They represent primitive striated muscle cells which have become grossly vacuolated by intracellular accumulations of glycogen. In later life these 'congenital nodular glycogen tumours', as Batchelor and Mann prefer to call them, undergo regressive changes, their mass decreasing in size and being finally largely replaced by connective tissue or fat (Steinbiss 1923) in which isolated cells of Purkinje type may still be found.

Apart from rhabdomyoma, cardiac anomalies are of rare occurrence in the tuberose sclerosis complex. Occasional stenosis of the great vessels has been reported (Rehder 1914, Schuster 1914, Critchley and Earl 1932), and in 1 case a large congenital diverticulum, lined by thick fibro-elastic tissue resembling that of the aorta, was found in the left ventricle (Norman and Taylor 1940). A feature of interest in this case was the presence of rhabdomyoma cells in the tissue adjoining the malformation.

Kidneys. Tumours are more commonly found in the kidneys in this condition that in any other organ, their frequency being estimated by Critchley and Earl (1932) as 80 per cent. Whitish or yellow nodules, generally measuring less than 2 cm. in diameter, are seen projecting from the surface or wholly embedded in the renal cortex. Cysts may also be present and in one of Inglis's (1950) cases glomeruli were demonstrated projecting into the walls of some of the smaller ones. Microscopically the solid parts of the tumour are composed of leashes of spindle-shaped cells, often with elongated nuclei the sides of which are parallel and the ends blunt. An admixture with smaller, rounded cells may often be seen and bands of hyaline material may be found passing through the tumour. There is a very variable content of fat cells and blood-vessels. The elongated tumour cells of the kidney have been generally considered to be of mesenchymal origin but Inglis (1950) has suggested that this type of tissue, as also the somewhat similar spindle-shaped cells of the lung nodules and other visceral tumours, are derived from the neurolemma.

Lungs. Pulmonary tuberose sclerosis is a rarity, only 13 cases having been recorded up to the time of J. Dawson's article of 1954. Unlike most of the visceral manifestations of tuberose sclerosis the pulmonary variety leads to serious illness in adult life. The condition is commoner in women and often presents clinically as a pneumothorax. The outer surfaces of the lungs are covered by small subpleural cysts and much of the pulmonary tissue is replaced by cystic spaces embedded in matrix composed in varying proportions of fibrous tissue, smooth muscle fibres and blood-vessels. Compactly arranged nodules containing large muscle fibres are also a common feature.

Other organs, including the thyroid, liver, suprarenal, duodenum and ovary, have been reported to contain hamartomas of a fibrocellular character.

Skin anomalies. J. Dawson (1954) has drawn attention to an early description of the highly characteristic feature of adenoma sebaceum which was given by Addison and Gull (1851) in the following words: 'a peculiar eruption extending across the nose and slightly affecting both cheeks. It consisted of shining tubercles varying in size to that of ordinary acne. They were of lightish colour with superficial capillary veins meandering over them giving them a faint rose tinge.' These pale nodules are usually known as the Balzer type of adenoma sebaceum while the more vascular red type is named after Pringle. Microscopically the nodules consist of an overgrowth of the sebaceous glands, connective tissue and small blood-vessels. Adenoma sebaceum is rarely present at birth and may not appear until puberty. An admixture of fibrous and angiomatous tissue also characterises the subungual fibromata of the fingers and toes, a condition considered by many to be equal in importance to adenoma sebaceum in the clinical diagnosis of the tuberose sclerosis complex.

Bones. There are not many recorded instances of bony anomalies associated with tuberose sclerosis, probably because few patients have been thoroughly examined radiologically. The calvaria may show a mottled appearance which is due to areas of increased density of both the inner table and the diploic trabeculae (Dickerson 1955). In Hall's (1946) case there was also hyperostosis of the petrous bones. Perhaps the commonest X-ray finding is the presence of small areas of rarefaction in the metacarpal and metatarsal bones. These lesions closely resemble those found in neurofibromatosis, but their relationship to any local neural abnormality is improbable since the rarefactions are due to a fibrous dysplasia of the bone (Dickerson 1955). Up to the present only 1 case of tuberose sclerosis has shown the peculiar condition of 'rheostosis' which is characterised by an irregular hyperostosis running down the shaft of a bone in one limb. The anomaly is regarded by Weber (1939) as the bony analogue of linear naevi.

Pathogenesis. The disease is inherited as a dominant and the mutation rate is high (Gunther and Penrose 1935). The earlier writers, notably H. Vogt (1908) and Alzheimer (1904), regarded tuberose sclerosis as essentially the product of defective histogenesis and this view has been endorsed in more recent times by Schob (1930) and Globus (1932). The element of malformation is perhaps most obvious in the heterotopic collections of cells frequently seen in the subcortical white matter, though these are never so conspicuous a feature as in the grosser maldevelopments of micro- or pachygyria. The peculiar character of the giant cells, however, strongly suggests an earlier origin of the abnormalities than the time of the migration of neuroblasts, and it is considered probable that the disease exemplifies a primary defect of differentiation on the part of the primordial neuro-epithelium (Globus 1932). Thus the sclerosis characteristic of the disorder is regarded as a primary anomaly of the neuroglia and it is perhaps surprising that genuine neoplasia is not more common when this background of disturbed balance of cellular growth is taken into account.

Much has been made of the so-called blastomatous features of tuberose sclerosis. Bielschowsky attempted to explain the multiple cerebral abnormalities of the condition as direct consequences of spongioblastic overgrowth. This theory, however, does not account satisfactorily for the large nerve cells which may be so conspicuous a feature of the disease. It is improbable that these are an expression of compensatory hypertrophy conditioned by the local glial overgrowth since nerve cells of giant size are to be found in areas where the gliosis is relatively insignificant. The pathological findings outside the nervous system also provide substantial evidence in favour of the purely dysontogenetic nature of the disorder. In the heart the large muscle cells of the rhabdomyomata, while retaining an imprint of their embryonic prototype, possess none of the proliferative tendencies so often associated with cells of 'primitive' morphology. Rehder (1914) believed that these myoblasts are aberrant derivatives of primordial cells capable of forming both the specialised Purkinje fibres and the ordinary cells of the myocardium, a theory that at once suggests the analogous formation of giant cells in the brain from the indifferent cells of the matrix.

Bielschowsky (1914 a) emphasised the resemblances between the lesions of neurofibromatosis and tuberose sclerosis and proposed to classify the latter condition as the central form of von Recklinghausen's disease. However instructive such histological comparisons may be, the fact should not be lost sight of that tuberose sclerosis and von Recklinghausen's disease are genetically distinct conditions and any pathological affinities that they may possess are due to the influence of unrelated dominant genes upon the same embryonic layers (Borberg 1951). The same proviso applies to other conditions in which isolated features reminiscent of tuberose sclerosis may be found. Thus large abnormal neurones may be seen in certain cases of pachygyria in which there may also be a dense overgrowth of neuroglia. Giant cells of neuronal type and a deranged cortical architecture have also been recorded in the brain of a case of Albright's disease (Jervis and Schein 1951).

Encephalofacial angiomatosis (Sturge-Weber Disease)

This neurocutaneous syndrome is characterised clinically in its complete form by naevus flammeus of the face, buphthalmos, hemiparesis of the contralateral limbs, epilepsy, mental defect and radiological evidence of intracranial calcifications. The latter sign is very rare below the age of two years. The clinical and pathological delineation of this disease has taken many years and many names have been attached to it in the course of time, but if an eponymous title is to be preferred the name of Sturge certainly deserves commemoration. Sturge was not only responsible in 1879 for the first clinical account of the essential features, but he also correctly deduced that an underlying naevoid condition of the brain was probably present in his patient. It was not, however, until nearly 20 years later that Kalischer (1897, 1901) recorded the first post-mortem examination and revealed the prophesied cerebral vascular anomaly. This patient was only 18 months old and the limited pathological examination showed no calcifications. Dürck (1910) was the first to note the cerebral calcification and Weber (1922) described their typical gyriform radiographic contours, though according to Krabbe (1934) priority for their demonstration should be given to Wissing of Copenhagen. Krabbe (1934) himself made the important point that these calcifications occurred in the cortex and not in the meningeal vessels.

Somewhat similar curvilinear shadows of calcification are occasionally encountered in other conditions such as oligodendroglioma, brains injured by irradiation, lead encephalopathy (Lichtenstein 1954), Fahr's disease or in the cases of progressive facial hemiatrophy reported by Merritt *et al.* (1937). The wide extent and uniform pattern of the phenomenon as seen in Sturge's disease is however virtually a pathognomonic picture.

It is advisable to limit the definition of Sturge's syndrome to cases showing at least two of the major signs, that is to say, facial naevus combined with either intracranial angioma or with angioma of the choroid of the eye (Louis-Bar 1944). This criterion rules out many superficially allied conditions such as spinal cord angiomas with cutaneous naevi of metameric distribution (Cobb 1915), cutaneous naevi associated with cerebellar symptoms (Louis-Bar 1941), and the familial non-calcifying meningeal angiomas of Divry and van Bogaert (1946). The inclusion of these and the other vaguely related naevoid states within the nosographic limits of the disease would be unjustified. The localisation of the facial naevus is extremely important in the definition of the disease and only those cases in which it involves the supra-ocular region should be admitted. A complete record of the literature has failed to show a single case in which cerebral angiomatosis or gyriform calcification is present in association with a facial naevus limited to other areas of the face (Alexander and Norman 1960).

Neuropathological findings. The essential intracerebral anomaly is an excessive vascularity of the pia mater and in the majority of cases the occipital or parieto-occipital region of the brain is alone affected, the dura and skull being much more rarely involved. The majority of the meningeal vessels are of small venous type and lie in tortuous folds several layers deep in the subarachnoid space, giving a dark purple colour to the leptomeninges. The meningeal arteries frequently show conspicuous calcification of the subintimal layer (Fig 6.76). This is an early manifestation and was present in a 3-month-old child examined by the writer. Groups of vessels with thick muscular coats but no elastic laminae may also be present among the superficial veins. Abnormal vessels rarely penetrate the cortex but an occasional abnormal convoluted vessel may be seen (Craig 1949) (Fig. 6.77). Beneath these hypervascularised meninges it is usual to find that extensive strips of the outer part of the cortex contain massive deposits of a crystalline material which imparts a gritty sensation on cutting with the knife. Microscopically, the molecular layer and outer part of the pyramidal cell layers are seen to be largely replaced by concretions having the staining reaction of an iron-calcium mixture and varying in size from small spherules to enormous confluent masses of irregular outline (Fig. 6.74). In areas where these calcifications are less dense one can see the early stages of the process in the form of granular incrustations of the walls of the smaller blood vessels.

Not only the outer cortical layers are affected, but calcification may also pick out selectively the deeper laminae (Fig. 6.75). Scattered calcospherites and calcified capillaries are also common in the central cores of the affected gyri and in the subcortical white matter. Calcification of the larger veins may be present here. These changes in the white matter occur early in the disease, before there is any concentration of calcifications in the superficial layers of the cortex.

In some cases there is evidence of ischaemic cortical damage in addition to the destruction of tissue from the confluent growth of the calcifications. Laminar cortical necrosis with intense fibrosis of vessels and powdery calcium deposits of dystrophic type may be a prominent feature, particularly in the calcarine region (Fig. 6.78). After decalcification an amorphous substance which stains positively with P.A.S. remains behind. This represents the original perivascular colloidal matrix upon which the mineral salts have been deposited in successive layers (Mallory 1896).

Wohlwill and Yakovlev (1957) have described enlargement of the Gasserian ganglion in this condition. There was marked proliferation of the capsule cells and ectopic ganglion cells were present in the root. In one case a cavernous angioma was seen between the dural sheath and the nerve roots. The same authors have found angiomatous malformations in the lung, ovary and intestine in Sturge-Weber disease.

Chemical analysis of the brain shows that the mineral deposits are mainly composed of calcium phosphate and carbonate and that there is no excess of iron (Wachsmuth and Löwenthal 1950, Tingey 1955). The Prussian blue reaction given by the concretions is probably due to absorption of the available iron normally present in the tissues. Prolonged formalin fixation substantially increases the amount of iron found chemically.

Pathogenesis. There is some evidence that the Sturge-Weber disease is caused by partial chromosomal trisomy, but that in the majority of cases a translocated extra segment may not be demonstrable microscopically (Patau *et al.* 1961). Certainly, there has been no reported familial instance of the true syndrome.

The combination of skin and pial angiomata is explicable in a general way as a malformation of the embryo's primitive vascular plexus which precedes the formation of separate vessels for the supply of integument, skull and meninges. In the early stages of development the small telencephalic vesicle and the eye are closely approximated and the integument of the embryo's forehead might well share that part of the vascular plexus which supplies the occipital portions

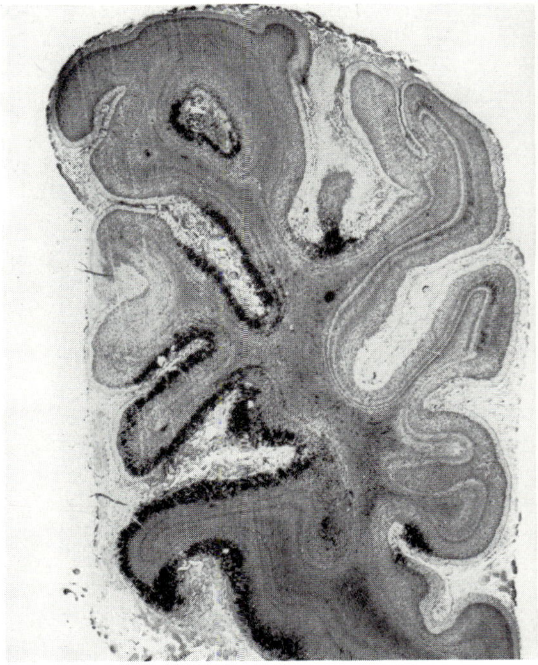

6.74

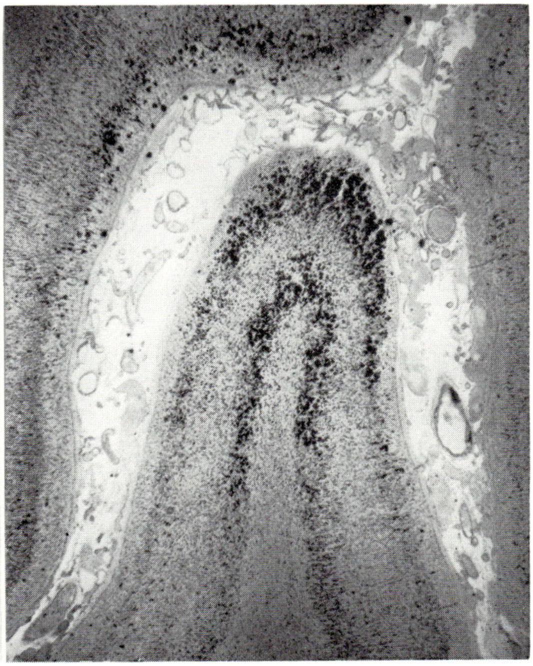

6.75

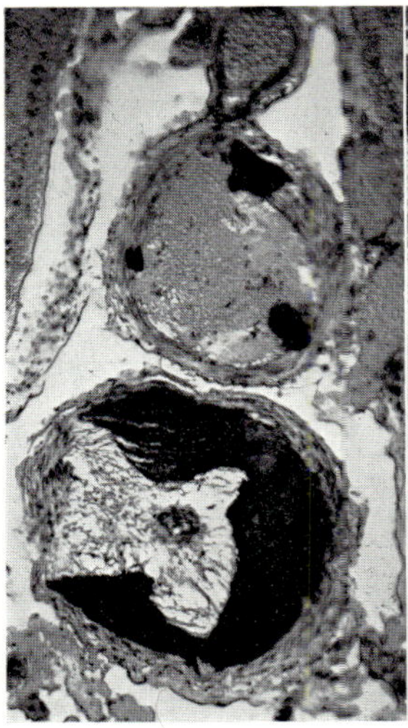

6.76

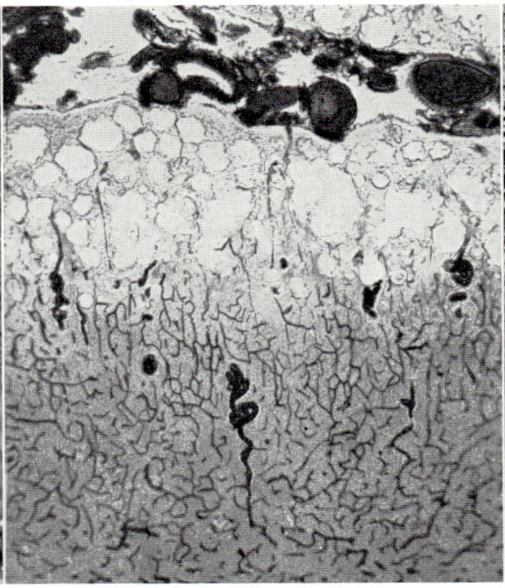

6.77

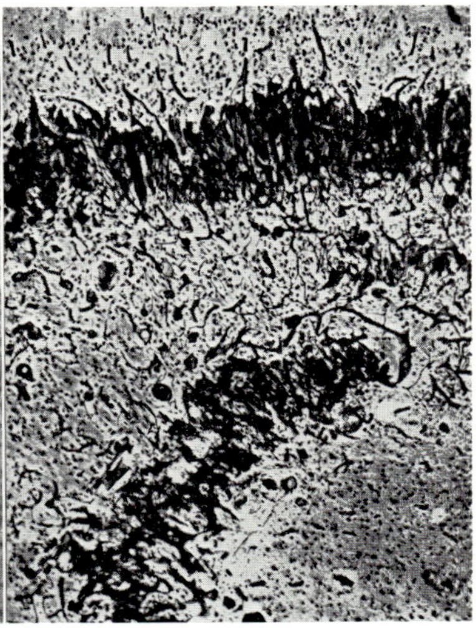

6.78

FIG. 6.74. *Sturge-Weber's disease.* Low-power view of section through occipital pole showing the venous angioma and dense calcifications mainly in the outer layers of the cortex. (Carbol azure.)

FIG. 6.75. The calcifications also affect the deeper cortical laminae. (Carbol azure.)

FIG. 6.76. Calcified meningeal arteries. (Carbol azure.)

FIG. 6.77. Abnormal convoluted blood-vessels in the non-calcified layers of cerebral cortex. (Masson's trichrome.)

FIG. 6.78. Adventitial fibrosis occasionally found in areas of laminar calcification. The calcium deposits are peculiarly dense and powdery in these areas. (Gomori's reticulin.)

of the brain. The later anatomical separation of these two vascular territories occurs as the result of the subsequent growth backwards of the hemisphere. The embryological development of the blood vessels in relation to this syndrome has been well discussed by Thieffry *et al.* (1961). The rarity of dural and diploic hypervascularity remains an enigma. Kautsky (1949) developed the thesis that the vascular anomaly is primarily neurogenic in origin, but against the traditional view that the distribution of the facial naevus corresponds to one or more divisions of the trigeminal nerve several objections may be raised. Alexander in his monograph has pointed out how frequently these territories are transgressed and how often the naevus fails to reach the mid-line. Moreover, in some patients the philtrum is spared, the boundary of the naevus conforming to the defect of hare lip, and it seems probable that the distribution is determined in part by the layout of the fissures in the developing face (Alexander and Norman 1960).

The pathogenesis of the intracortical calcifications is also in doubt. As in all types of calcification the mineral deposits are laid down in a strongly P.A.S. + ve polysaccharide matrix and it is generally held that some abnormality of permeability of the vessels is induced by the circulatory abnormalities conditioned by the meningeal angiomatosis. A case can be made for the importance of an angiomatous malformation formed by vessels of narrow calibre, since gyriform calcification is not found in association with the larger sized penetrating venous angiomas. Yet the angiomatosis in Divry and van Bogaert's (1946) case was not associated with calcification. One is forced to conclude that the rarity of overt malformation in the cortical vessels does not preclude some functional anomaly that may be a factor in the calcifying process. The building-up of crystalline hydroxyl-apatite in the larger concretions is probably a function of mesenchymal tissue (Bochnik 1953).

Mongolism

The external appearance of the mongol brain is much more diagnostic of the condition than are the microscopical findings. The weight of the fully-grown brain seldom exceeds 1,200 g. and is usually nearer the 1,000-g. level. The brain is abnormally rounded and short with a steeply rising, almost vertical occipital contour. The convolutional pattern usually shows no gross departure from normality, but there may be asymmetries on the two sides and the insula is often exposed on account of the poor development of the 3rd frontal gyrus. Compared with the brain of a normal adult there is a poverty of secondary sulci, but the ape-like simplification of genetic micrencephaly is never found. Very characteristic of the mongol brain, though not peculiar to it, is narrowness of the superior temporal gyrus (Fig. 6.79). This anomaly is often bilateral and is present in about half the cases. Conspicuous smallness of the cerebellum and brain stem in comparison with the cerebrum as a whole is also a common feature.

Benda (1947) believes that most of these abnormalities of shape have been impressed on the developing brain by the retarded growth of the mongol skull and has pointed out that the crowns of gyri may be flattened, that the sagittally arranged sulci may show S-shaped distortion and that fibrous union may bind contiguous parts of convolutions together.

Many microscopical anomalies have been described in mongolism but they are all shared by other forms of severe oligophrenia. Davidoff (1928) reported patchy cerebral calcifications and a poverty of nerve cells in the 3rd cortical layer of his cases (Fig. 6.80). In the writer's experience this finding is not very common, but irregularities of grouping certainly occur so that relatively acellular areas adjoin those which display an increased density due to the presence of clusters of small nerve cells. Systematic cell counts in random sections indicate that the nerve cells are, in fact, often increased on the average per unit area. This seeming paradox may be related to the small size of the brain as a whole since, as a general rule, the more underdeveloped the state of the brain the closer together are the cortical neurones. Benda (1947), however, believes that an active destruction of the nerve cells associated with anoxia and oedema takes place in mongols dying in infancy. The same author lays stress upon the poor myelination of the grey and white matter and has demonstrated striking poverty of myelin in the subsulcine or U fibres of the cortex. Meyer and Jones (1939) were the first to demonstrate a conspicuous fibrillary gliosis of the central white matter in many, but by no means all, mongols. There was often no corresponding pallor in myelin preparations, although patchy areas of demyelination were sometimes seen, as they were in Davidoff's cases. Benda has reported

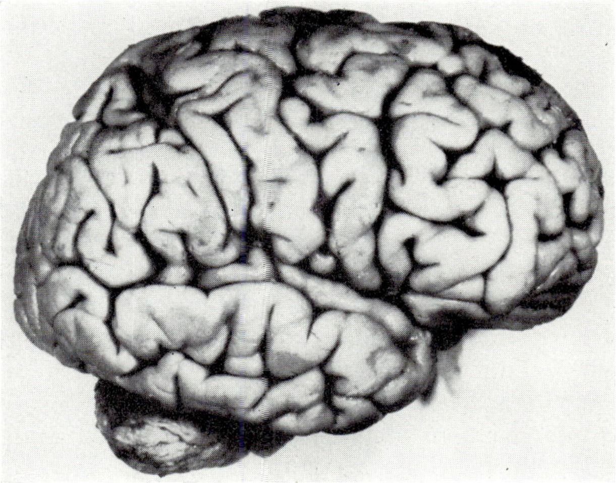

6.79

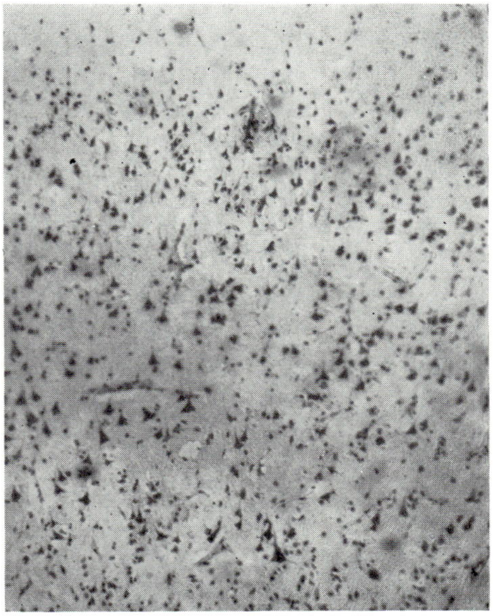

6.80

FIG. 6.79. *Mongolism.* Brain showing small cerebellum, flattened occipital contour and poorly developed superior temporal gyrus.
FIG. 6.80. Angular gyrus of a mongol showing diffuse loss of nerve cells in the 3rd layer. (Cresyl violet.)

frequent minor malformations in the spinal cords of mongols and draws attention to a finding which he considers peculiar to the condition, namely the fusion of the columns of Clark so that the nerve cells occupy a strip of grey matter lying behind the central canal. Except for undoubted signs of retarded or mildly perverted development, the mongol brain thus shows few pathological changes which cannot be explained on the basis of intercurrent disease. Whether such fortuitous lesions are in some way related to abnormal constitutional factors, such as general circulatory asthenia or endocrine anomalies, cannot be precisely determined at the present time. Certainly the frequent association of congenital heart disease is an important factor. Arterial and venous thromboses are well-known complications of Fallot's tetralogy, as are embolism and cerebral abscess due to detachment of vegetations from congenitally malformed or infected valves.

Middle-aged mongols often show clinical signs of premature senility and this may be reflected in the brain by the presence of senile plaques and Alzheimer's neurofibrillary change (Jervis 1948).

Congenital facial palsy and ophthalmoplegia

The clinical syndrome of congenital facial diplegia, often associated with ophthalmoplegia, multiple defects of muscles and skeletal deformity, has been fully reviewed by Henderson (1939). There have been few detailed and unequivocal pathological reports, but in the case of Spatz and Ullrich (1931) aplasia of the abducens nuclei, hypoplasia of the facial nuclei and development anomalies of the oculomotor and trochlear nuclei were clearly demonstrated. When congenital unilateral facial paralysis is present in the absence of ophthalmoplegia the most likely cause is damage to the facial nerve at birth. The pathological findings in Raing and Fowler's (1903) case can well be explained on this basis, as Stewart (1930) pointed out, since the Marchi stain revealed degeneration of the facial nerves throughout their course. Richter (1960), however, in an infant with unilateral facial palsy and congenital musculo-skeletal anomalies who died at the age of one month, found only a few nerve cells in one facial nucleus and no sign of a degenerative process in the scanty intramedullary portion of the nerve. He considered the lesion due to developmental hypoplasia of the nucleus and not to secondary causes.

II. CEREBRAL BIRTH INJURY

In the following sections the term 'birth injury' will be used in a broad sense to cover all types of lesion occurring during parturition. Some writers prefer to draw a sharp distinction between mechanical trauma and cerebral anoxia, including in the latter category a variety of ischaemic lesions. This apparently logical classification tends to obscure the complex interplay of the pathogenetic factors often involved. For example, it might seem that compression of arterial trunks or branches owing to distortion of the brain during head presentation might properly be classed as the result of mechanical trauma, yet such a process may certainly be facilitated by neonatal shock, itself an expression of severe anoxia.

Experience has shown that certain patterns of lesions recur in cases of presumed birth injury and it is upon the basis of such findings that deductions as to pathogenesis may be attempted.

Subdural haemorrhage. If the foetal skull is subjected to severe anteroposterior compression, and particularly when the direction of this force is asymmetrical, the falx cerebri is stretched and in turn may pull upon one leaf of the tentorium cerebelli with sufficient tension to cause its rupture (Chase 1930). Tears in the free margin of the tentorium may involve veins draining into the Galenic system and blood from this source usually collects in an infratentorial situation. With more serious lacerations, rupture of the straight or transverse sinuses may occur with tearing of the great vein of Galen. These injuries are apt to take place during precipitate or breech deliveries. Tearing of the superior cerebral veins at their entrance into the sagittal sinus may follow excessive overriding of the parietal bones and is the commonest cause of chronic subdural haematomata (Guthkelch 1953). Rupture or thrombosis of the sinus itself has been a sequel of the overlapping of the parietal by the occipital bone (Craig 1938).

Chronic subdural haematoma. Blood from a torn superior cerebral vein usually collects over the convexity of the hemisphere, lying above the level of the Sylvian fissure and sometimes extending from the frontal to the occipital poles. The haemorrhage may be bilateral. After clotting has taken place organisation leads to the formation of a thick outer layer adherent to the dura and composed of fibrous tissue containing numerous large sinusoidal vessels. The arachnoidal surface of the haematoma becomes covered with a thin membrane composed of flattened connective tissue cells (Inglis 1946). Further haemorrhages may occur from the sinusoidal vessels of the dural membrane and a progressive expansion of the original lesion is brought about in this way or by osmosis (see Chapter 6). In long-standing cases calcification or ossification of the inner connective tissue layer may take place. Severe damage to the brain results not only from pressure upon the underlying tissues but also from compression of arteries against the edge of the tentorium owing to displacement of the cranial contents (Lindenberg 1955). The enlargement of the head, seen in infants with large subdural effusions, may in part be due to a hydrocephalus of communicating type which follows obstruction of the subarachnoid space beneath the haematoma (Elvidge and Jackson 1949).

Subarachnoid haemorrhage. After severe leptomeningeal haemorrhage the surface of the brain is covered by a thin, easily detached, jelly-like layer of blood-stained meninges. In Craig's (1938) series of cases the parieto-occipital lobes were commonly affected and early softenings, oedema and microscopic haemorrhages were seen in the outer layers of the grey matter. These bleedings are generally regarded as asphyxial in origin and are very common in still-born infants.

Intraventricular haemorrhage. Fatal intraventricular bleeding is almost exclusively found in premature infants and usually originates from one of the anterior terminal veins or, less often, from the choroidal veins. It is usually asphyxial in origin and may occur as a prenatal, natal or postnatal phenomenon.

Intracerebral haemorrhage

Large extravasations into the substance of the brain are unusual, but multiple petechial haemorrhages associated with congestion and oedema are not uncommon, and it is likely that these less lethal types of lesion may lead to neurological sequelae in survivors. Schwartz (1924, 1927) has described in detail the distribution of these haemorrhages and their subsequent evolution. He regards them as of venous origin, those in the cortex being related to the tributaries of the superior longitudinal sinus, while the more centrally placed haemorrhages occur in the drainage area of the great vein of Galen. Bilateral bleedings into the periventricular white matter of the frontoparietal and occipital regions are seen in the distribution of the anterior and posterior terminal veins and of the vena lateralis ventriculi. In the basal ganglia the most characteristic lesion is partial destruction of the head of the caudate nucleus and this may be accompanied by intraventricular haemorrhage. The thalamus also is often involved (Wald 1930), the putamen and globus pallidus rarely, though punctate bleedings are sometimes seen in the external segment of the latter. Dekaban (1962) has described bilateral haemorrhagic infarction of the occipital lobes which he suggested was the result of compression of the posterior cerebral arteries.

The evolution of the haemorrhagic lesions. Schwartz (1924, 1927) studied a large material derived not only from cases of immediately fatal birth injury but also from individuals who survived for periods of days, weeks, months and years. It was apparent that the small haemorrhages so often regarded by other investigators as the consequence of terminal asphyxia were only a minor indication of much more extensive damage which later led to widespread cavitation or neuroglial scarring. These progressive changes were most easily followed in the cerebral white matter in the drainage areas of the terminal veins. By the end of 24 hours the original haemorrhages were seen to be interspersed with yellowish-grey areas radiating from the region of the lateral ventricle towards the cortical grey matter. Liquefaction of the central zone then occurred, and by the 4th day the texture of the peripheral tissues became loosened and fat-granule cells appeared. The stage of organisation began at about the 8th day when the astrocytes at the margins of the cavity began to proliferate. After weeks or months, according to the size of the areas involved, fibrillary gliosis was well established and contained in its meshworks numerous groups of fat-granule cells (the stage of 'presclerosis'). Finally (the stage of sclerosis) the area was converted into a loose neuroglial scar.

When the tissues were more mature or the vascular disturbances less intense the general structure of the ground substance was preserved, and instead of liquefaction and cavity formation the process was one of destruction of axis cylinders and replacement by fibrillary neuroglia. The early stages were marked by the appearance of large numbers of lipid phagocytes, the so-called 'encephalitis' of Virchow. This is a pathological phenomenon associated with tissue breakdown and readily distinguishable from the normal increase in neuroglial cells which is always found in regions undergoing myelination (Roback and Scherer 1934).

In the cerebral or cerebellar cortex wedge-shaped areas of necrosis may appear under the pial haemorrhages. Schwartz also described processes of dissolution and rarefaction in the gyri, leading either to hollow convolutions bounded superficially by the preserved molecular layer, or to gyral shrinkage and patchy destruction of nerve cells ('Sclerotic microgyria').

Periventricular lesions in the new born are not necessarily haemorrhagic. Banker (1960) describes as a frequent finding in premature infants the presence of coagulation necrosis, giving the macroscopic appearance of waxy or white streaks. In a later paper Banker and Larroche (1962) point out that these lesions tend to lie in the arterial boundary zones of the white matter, and it would seem that venous stasis may not be the only factor involved in their production.

Late neuropathological sequelae of birth injury

The following varieties of long-standing lesion may be found singly or in combination with one another in the brains of patients suffering from cerebral palsy attributable to birth injury.

Cortex. Ulegyria (atrophic sclerosis; mantle sclerosis; sclerotic microgyria). In this condition the general convolutional pattern of the cortex is preserved but individual gyri or groups of gyri show varying degrees of shrinkage and sclerosis (Fig. 6.81). The most characteristic feature is the localised destruction of the lower parts of the walls of the convolution with relative sparing of its crown. The bulbous neurone-bearing crown and upper portion of the affected gyrus may be supported only by a narrow fibrous stalk from which all neural elements have disappeared ('mushroom' gyrus). Thus from the surface the uncut brain may have a deceptive appearance of normality since the greater part of the damage is hidden. In its minimal form this type of lesion expresses itself merely as a thinning of the grey matter in the depths of the sulcus, and may easily be overlooked in myelin preparations, though the associated gliosis, which shows up as sharply defined, semi-lunar scars, is obvious enough in sections stained by Holzer's method (Figs. 6.86 and 6.87). The transition between the severely damaged and less affected regions tends to be abrupt so that clear-cut complementary myelin and neuroglial pictures are the rule. The middle zone of the less affected cortical grey matter often shows a thin streak of laminar atrophy (Figs. 6.90 and 6.91), the margins of which contain abnormally dense aggregations of myelinated fibres. This phenomenon is termed 'hypermyelination' and collections of myelinated fibres in the form of plaques, networks, or whorls, are a common feature of ulegyria (Figs. 6.82 and 6.83). The white matter subjacent to the affected gyri usually shows considerable gliosis associated with a thinning of myelinated fibres or small cystic spaces. Lesions of the medullary core of the convolution vary from a thin linear strip of sclerosis, marking an area devoid of myelin, to gross cavitation. The most advanced stage of dissolution is seen in the 'hollow gyrus' the outline of which is maintained largely by the remaining molecular layer.

A condition resembling the 'granular atrophy' of the adult cortex may sometimes be present, both the walls of convolutions and their crowns presenting multiple small bosses due to the separation of islands of nerve cells by fibrillary neuroglia. More commonly, the cortex shows narrow vertically disposed areas of clearing which correspond to the course of cortical branches of meningeal arteries. Sometimes one half of a gyrus is destroyed and occasionally the whole convolution is represented as a thin leaf-like structure composed mainly of neuroglial fibres. The meninges covering sclerotic microgyria of this sort show fibrous thickening but are rarely adherent to the cortex. In these areas of ulegyria the small meningeal arteries often show calcification of the elastica and thin eccentric plaques of subintimal fibrosis (J. E. Meyer 1949). These changes are more frequently seen in the depths of the sulci. In the atrophic grey matter it is usual to find considerable proliferation of the adventitial coats of the blood-vessels, but connective tissue plays little or no part in the attempted repair of the encephalomalacia.

There are certain commonly recurring patterns in the distribution of these lesions. In the first place, ulegyria may be present in boundary zones between main arterial territories (J. F. Meyer 1953, Norman *et al.* 1957). It is a characteristic feature of these lesions that both hemispheres may be involved in roughly symmetrical fashion. Thus the 2nd frontal gyri may be selectively involved, the lesions arching round the frontal pole and affecting a narrow strip of the orbital surface (Fig. 6.99). Boundary zone lesions of the parietal lobe reveal themselves most clearly as areas of atrophic sclerosis running in an anteroposterior direction through the upper part of the lobe and separated from the great longitudinal fissure for the greater part of their extent by a strip of preserved cortex. The middle temporal gyrus, lying between the main territories of the middle and posterior cerebral arteries, though theoretically at risk, has not yet been found affected in cases of birth injury.

Secondly, ulegyria may be limited to the fields of individual arterial branches. The territories supplied by the calcarine and posterior temporal branches of the posterior cerebral artery are often bilaterally involved (Norman and Urich 1962). The lips of the calcarine fissures are distorted by worm-like corrugations which on section are seen to be clusters of miniature gyri arising from an atrophied parent stalk (Figs. 6.84, 6.88 and 6.89). The remnants of the visual cortex often show a characteristic hypermyelination of the stria of Gennari (Fig. 6.85). Lesions referable to the middle cerebral artery may be extensive, in which event there is usually a large cystic softening in the Sylvian region which is fringed by ulegyria (Fig. 6.95); occasionally the areas affected are those supplied by the parietal branches in their more distal distribution (Norman 1961). The post-central gyrus seems to be particularly vulnerable but the pre-central gyrus often escapes damage or shows atrophy only in the depths of its posterior wall (Figs. 6.86 and 6.87).

When ulegyria is widespread there is always a well-marked fibrillary gliosis of the whole of the centrum semi-ovale and an associated dilatation of the lateral ventricles. In such cases there is usually a slight general shrinkage of convolutions that are not obviously atrophied, except in so far as their central cores are rather narrow and gliosed. The number of subsidiary sulci is often increased in these areas and the impression of polygyria is given (Brouwer 1949). The whole of the corpus callosum is usually very thin but is nevertheless apparently well myelinated.

Cerebellar ulegyria (Fig. 6.100) is much less common than its cerebral counterpart. The territory of the superior cerebellar artery is usually involved, with or without its branch to the dentate nucleus (Norman and Urich 1962). As in the cerebral convolutions, the more deeply situated folia bear the brunt of the destructive process and boundary zone lesions may be present. Unlike the lobular atrophy of epilepsy cystic softening may be present and there may be widespread ferrugination of Purkinje cells.

6.81

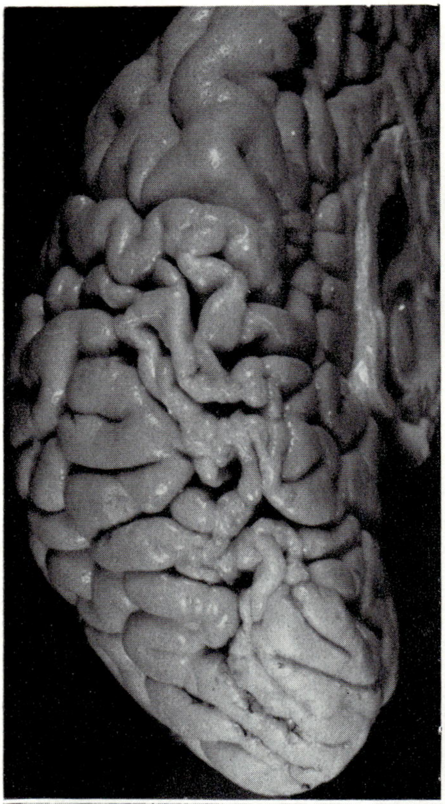

6.82

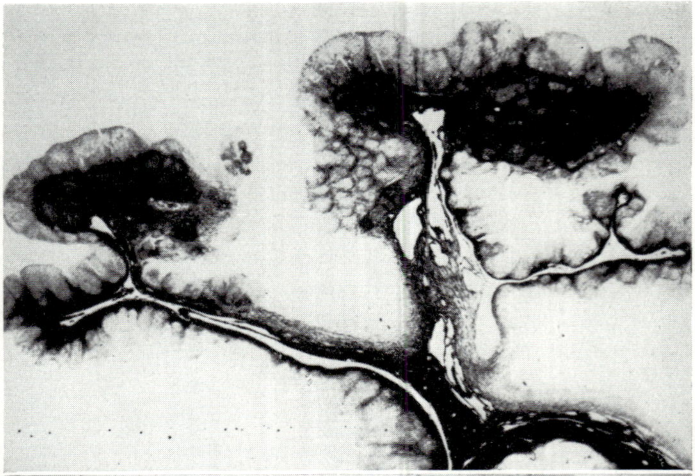

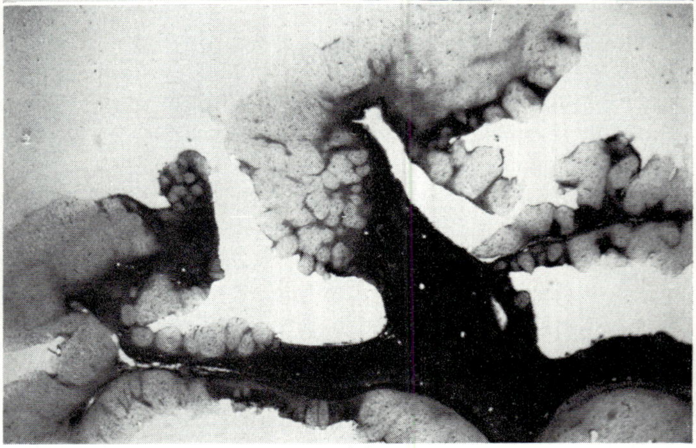

6.83

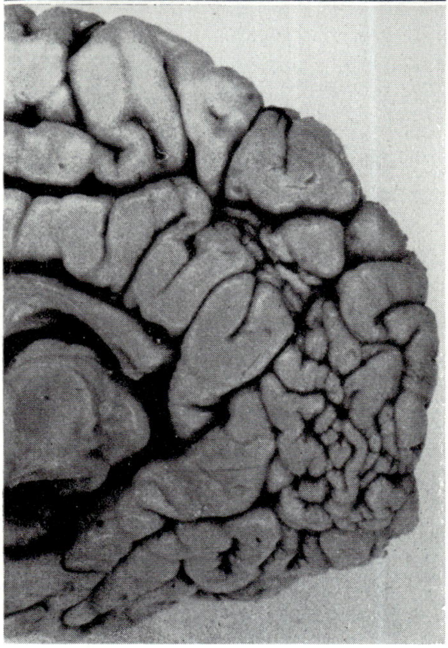

6.84

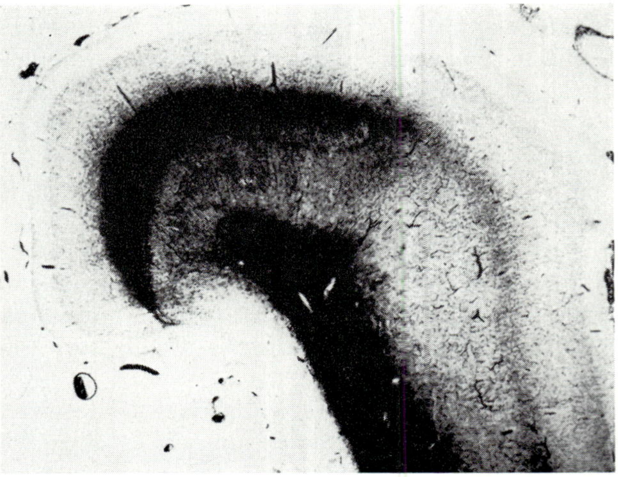

6.85

FIG. 6.81. *Birth injury*. Typical ulegyria of the superior parietal lobule.

FIGS. 6.82 and 6.83. Hypermyelinated ulegyria. Note the linear streaks of necrosis in the central cores of the gryi. (Corresponding Kultschitsky-Pal and Holzer preparations.)

FIG. 6.84. Ulegyria of the calcarine cortex spreading a short distance along the lips of the cingulate sulcus.

FIG. 6.85. Hypermyelination of the stria of Gennari in an area adjoining partial destruction of the calcarine cortex. (Heidenhain's myelin)

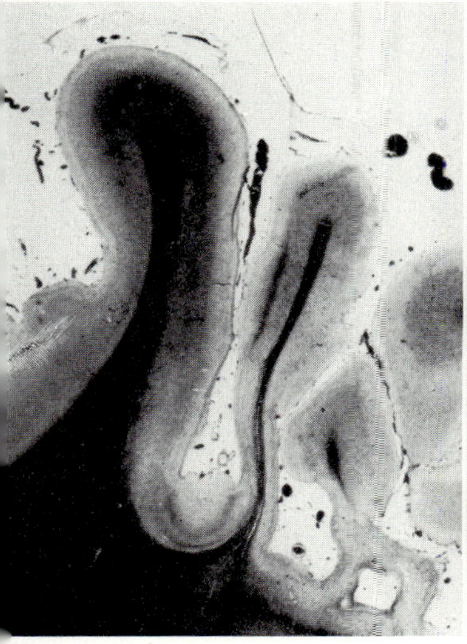

6.86

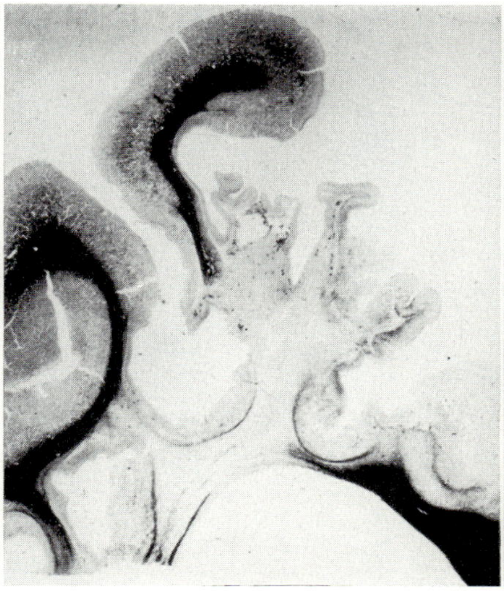

6.88

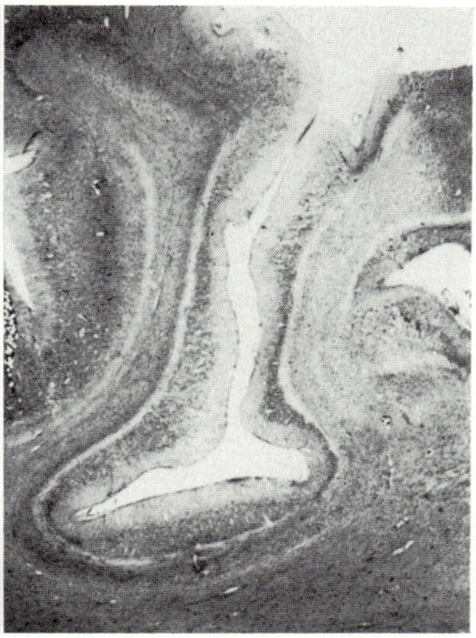

6.90

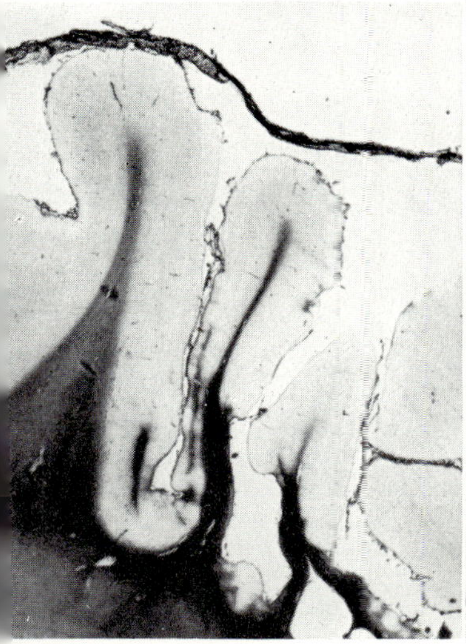

6.87

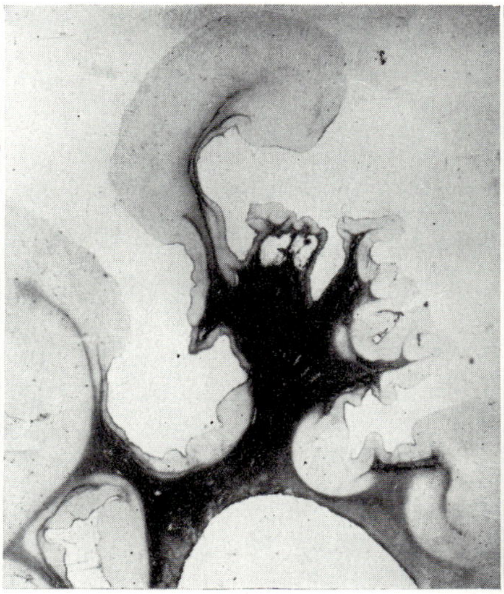

6.89

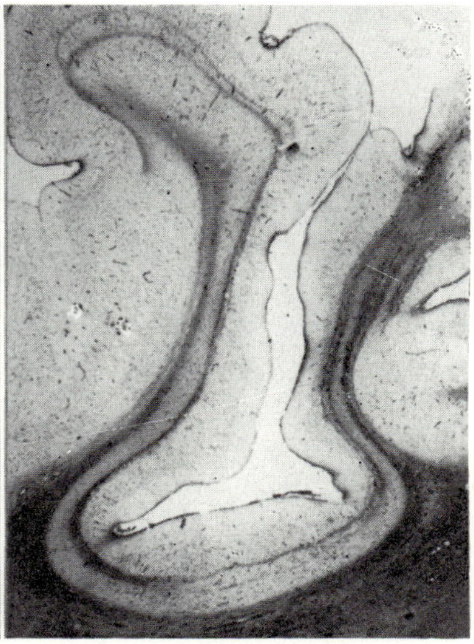

6.91

FIGS. 6.86 and 6.87. *Birth injury.* Corresponding myelin and neuroglial preparations to show typical distribution of ulegyria in the central region. The precentral gyrus (on the left) is relatively intact. (Heidenhain and Holzer.)

FIGS. 6.88 and 6.89. Cluster of small sclerotic microgyric formations (from the ulegyric area illustrated in Fig. 6.84). (Kultschitsky-Pal and Holzer.)

FIGS. 6.90 and 6.91. Laminar loss of nerve cells and gliosis in the deeper part of the gyral walls and floor of a sulcus. (Carbol azure and Holzer.)

Sclerosis and cavitation of the centrum semiovale

A characteristic central lesion of birth trauma, almost its hall-mark, is a rarefaction or cavitation of the tissues adjoining the lateral angle of the lateral ventricle on one or, more often, on both sides (Fig. 6.92). When there are not obvious cystic spaces in this paraventricular region, a discoloration or puckering may be visible in the fresh specimen, while staining for myelin or for neuroglial fibres always reveals a much wider area of destruction than would have been

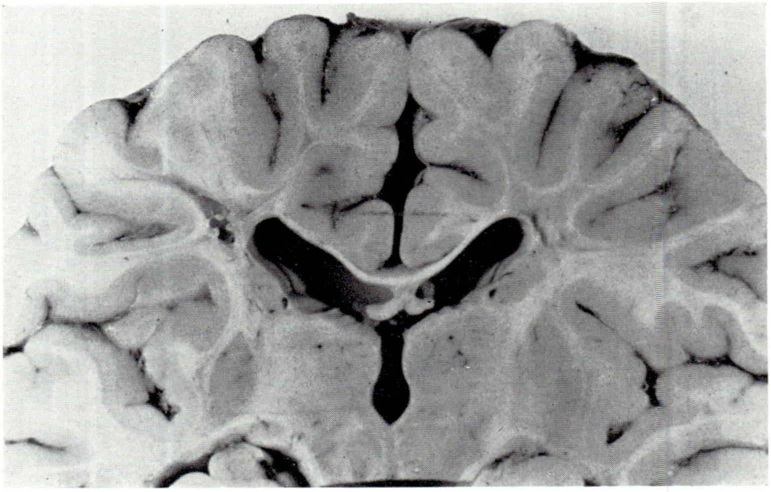

6.92

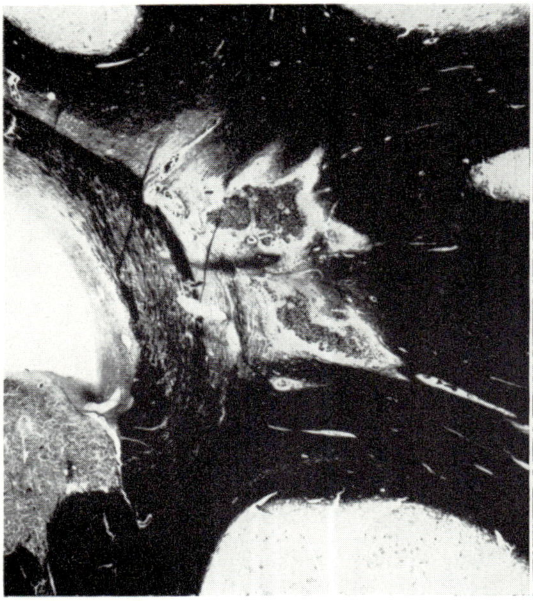

6.93

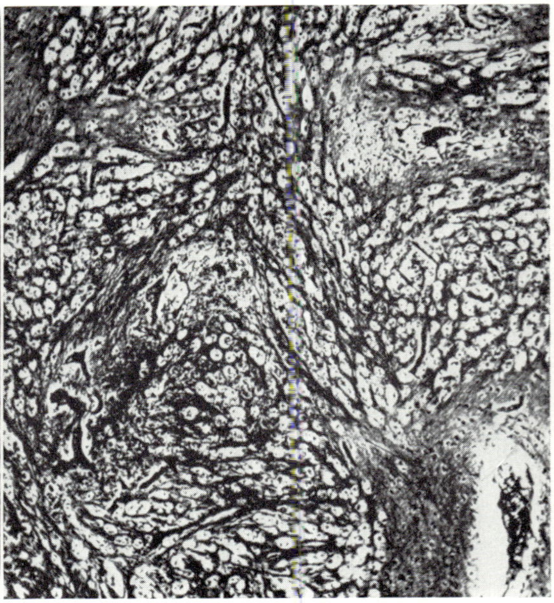

6.94

FIG. 6.92. *Birth injury*. Coronal section of the brain showing paraventricular softenings, more marked on the left. The ventricles are dilated. (From a spastic idiot aged 4½ years, who showed bilateral état marbré of the medial thalamic nuclei.)

FIG. 6.93. Paraventricular softening in an 8-month-old idiot. Large aggregations of fat granule cells are still present.

FIG. 6.94. Microscopic appearances of area of softening shown in previous figure. Fat granule cells are enmeshed in strands of fibrillary neuroglia. (Schwartz's stage of 'presclerosis'.) (Hortega's method for astrocytes.)

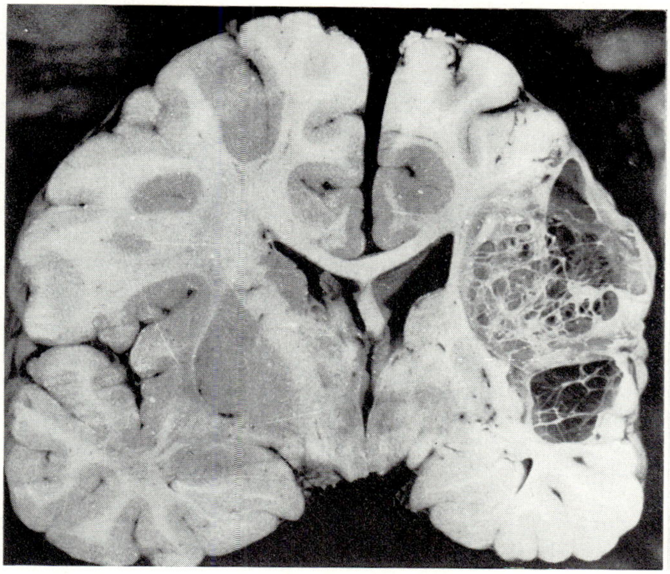

6.95

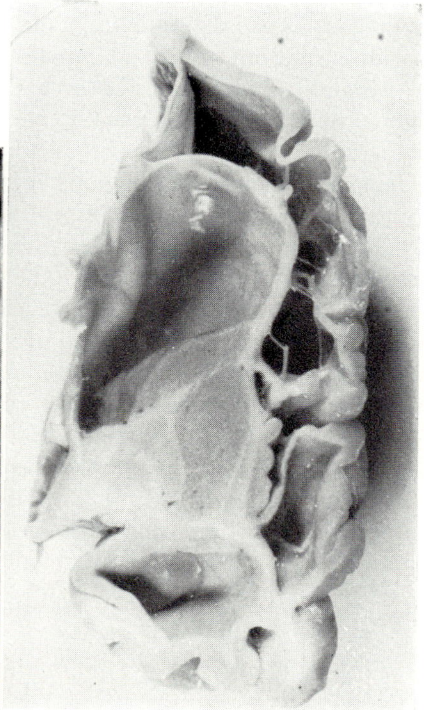

6.96

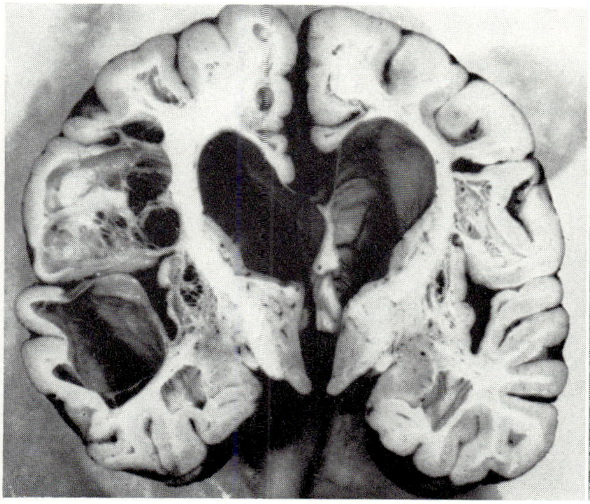

6.97

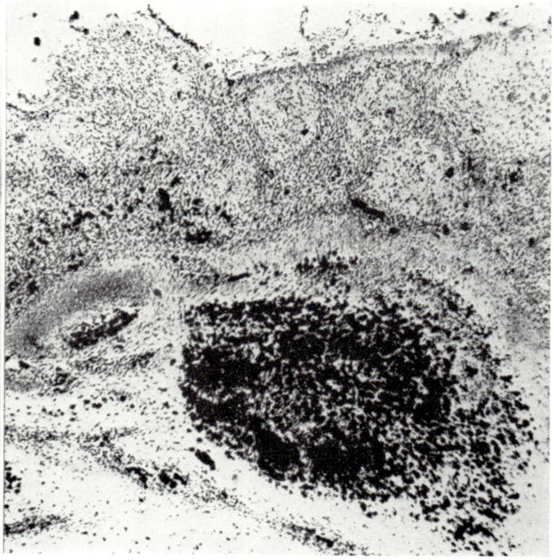

6.98

FIG. 6.95. *Birth injury.* Unilateral softening of middle cerebral arterial distribution. État marbré was present in the putamen and caudate nucleus of the affected side.

FIG. 6.96. Extensive cavitation of the central white matter ('central porencephaly'). The condition was bilateral. (8-month-old idiot. Twin birth: other twin dead in utero for several days.)

FIG. 6.97. Cystic encephalomalacia of subcortical white matter. Note the bilateral softening of the putamina.

FIG. 6.98. Accumulations of fat granule cells in subcortical white matter (same brain as in Fig. 6.96). (Scharlach R. and haematoxylin.)

anticipated from naked-eye inspection alone (Fig. 6.93). Even 8 months after birth large aggregations of fat granule cells may remain enmeshed in the loose glial scar (Fig. 6.94). This lesion is referred to in the French literature as 'sclérose cérébrale centro-lobaire' (Marie *et al.* 1959) and has sometimes been confused with that of a true demyelinating disease. A layer of intact myelinated fibres usually intervenes between the paraventricular softening and the ependyma but, occasionally, a diverticulum is seen which communicates directly with the ventricle. The site of the original opening may show tags of remaining ependyma which distinguish this condition from other varieties of unilateral hydrocephalus.

In contrast to this more localised paraventricular softening of the white matter a condition known as 'cystic degeneration' (Benda 1945) may be present. In such cases the greater part of the centrum semi-ovale is replaced by a series of trabeculated cavities (Figs. 6.96, 6.97 and 6.98) and the cortex itself may be converted into a thin rind by the erosion of the medullary cores of the gyri and the obliteration of the sulcal pattern. Extensive though this destruction is, these 'bladder-like' central porencephalies (Schwartz) of birth injury are found in brains showing a much greater amount of preserved or partially preserved cortex than is seen in prenatal hydranencephaly and there is often a tendency for the parieto-occipital areas to be predominantly affected. In a few cases with a history of birth injury there are changes in the superficial veins and arteries suggestive of old thrombosis (Crome 1958).

Basal ganglia

Corpus striatum. The survivors of haemorrhage from the anterior terminal vein may show severe atrophy of the caudate nucleus, amounting to its almost complete disappearance at some

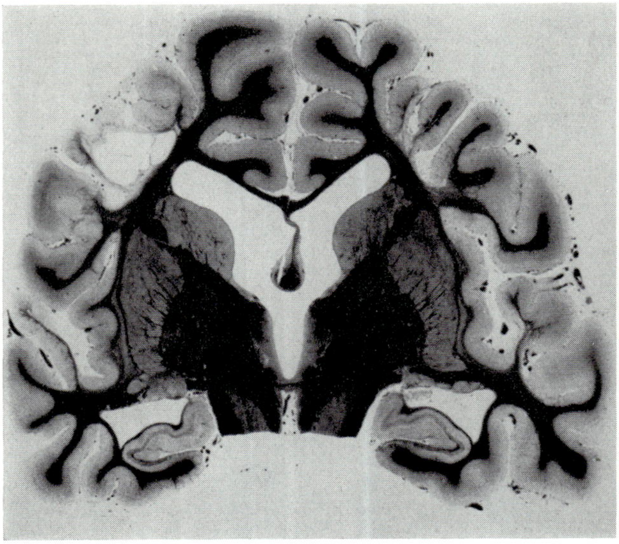

6.99

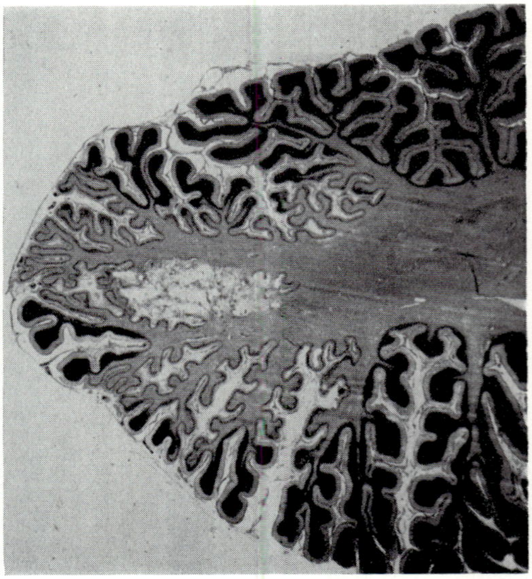

6.100

FIG. 6.99. *Birth injury.* Boundary zone lesions of both second frontal convolutions. (Heidenhain's myelin.)
FIG. 6.100. Boundary zone lesion of the semilunar lobules. (Carbol azure.)

levels. More commonly, the residual damage is confined to the subependymal zone of the caudate nucleus where small cystic softenings may be seen (Schwartz 1949). In a few of these cases transventricular adhesions of fibrillary neuroglia may be found passing to the corpus callosum or septum pellucidum (Norman and McMenemey 1955). Cavitation of the putamina has also been described (Pfeiffer 1939) (Fig. 6.97).

État marbré (*status marmoratus*). This condition is frequently caused by birth injury, though not exclusively so, and is of considerable importance because of its association with the athetoid form of cerebral palsy. État marbré may be said to be present when myelinated nerve fibres are found in aggregations considerably in excess of what is normal for that particular region of the nervous system. In their typical form, as seen in the corpus striatum, these fibres are arranged in coarse networks or bundles which in myelin preparations resemble the veining of marble (Fig. 6.101). There is a tendency for these anomalous myelinated fibres to be more numerous around the large blood-vessels and in one of the writer's cases dense rings of closely packed fibres surrounded some of the vessels of the medial thalamic nucleus and showed little or no spread to the intervening tissue (6.105). The normal myelinated fibre bundles of the putamen or caudate nucleus are not affected. The abnormal networks, together with the intervening and surrounding tissue, usually show a fibrillary gliosis of moderate degree (Fig. 6.102). As in the cerebral cortex, hypermyelination is not seen within an area of severe sclerosis though it may be present at the margins. The nerve cells of the affected part are usually conspicuously reduced in numbers, but the large neurones of the putamen and caudate nucleus appear to be less vulnerable and may be preserved in an otherwise devastated field. On the other hand, a few cases are on record in which gliosis and neuronal loss were not demonstrated (Alexander 1942, Carpenter 1955). In brains of apparently normal persons an increased density of myelinated fibres may often be seen in the most dorsal part of the putamen, but this is unaccompanied by gliosis or nerve cell loss, and cannot be regarded as pathological.

In many instances the marbling of the striatum is accompanied by lesions in other parts of the brain. The favoured sites of nerve cell loss are the ventro-lateral part of the caudate nucleus, the dorsal and anterior part of the putamen, the thalamus, particularly its lateral nucleus, the external segment of the globus pallidus, the amygdaloid nucleus, the uncus and the h_2 segment of Ammon's horn, the inferior wall of the hippocampal gyrus, the cerebellar vermis and the walls of the Rolandic sulcus. These changes are usually bilateral. A characteristic depression due to sclerotic atrophy is often seen in the paracentral lobules. The middle and posterior parts of the putamen are more severely affected than the anterior, the gliosis being denser and unaccompanied by marbling (Norman 1963).

État marbré is to be distinguished from état fibreux (C. and O. Vogt 1920), though these states may merge into each other in the birth injured brain (Norman 1947). In état fibreux (status fibrosus) a diffuse loss of nerve cells with gliosis causes shrinkage of the tissues and a crowding together of the remaining myelinated fibres, so that the impression is given of an abnormally rich myelination of the area. The head of the caudate nucleus is markedly flattened and shows a superficial condensation of the myelinated fibres running along its inner and ventricular portion. In the putamen the usual site of the fibre increase is in the outer part of the nucleus adjoining the external capsule. This condition is usually attributable to post-epileptic encephalopathy.

Thalamic birth injury. Extensive retrograde atrophy of the thalamus is always found when widespread cortical or subcortical damage is present. Severe neuronal devastation, however, often occurs independently of cortical lesions. État marbré may be found in association with striatal marbling or as an isolated phenomenon, most commonly seen in the dorsomedial nucleus (Fig. 6.104). In interpreting these changes it must be borne in mind that there is normally a considerable variation in the myelin content of the dorsomedial nucleus (Fig. 6.103) (Alexander 1942), so that an associated loss of nerve cells should be demonstrated before the condition is regarded as pathological. It has been suggested that involvement of the thalami may be a

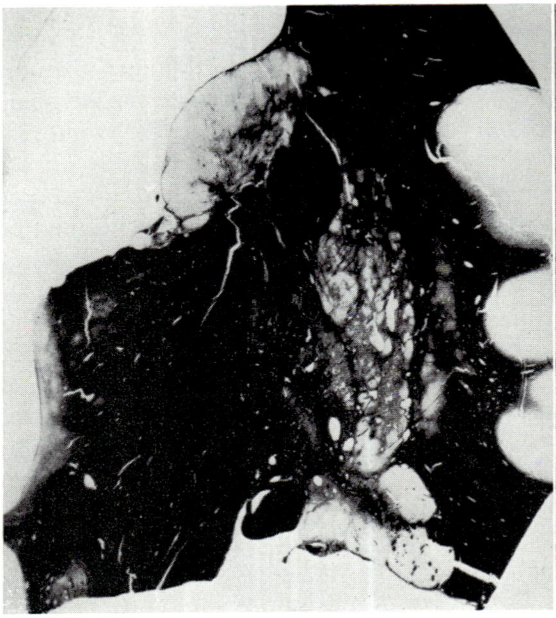

6.101

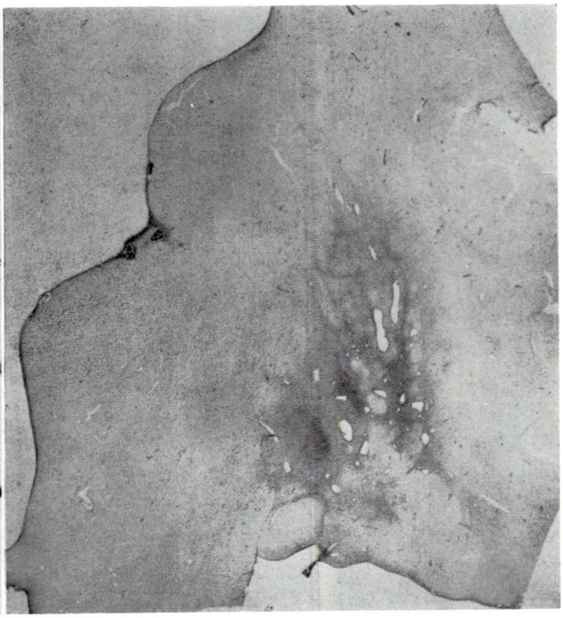

6.102

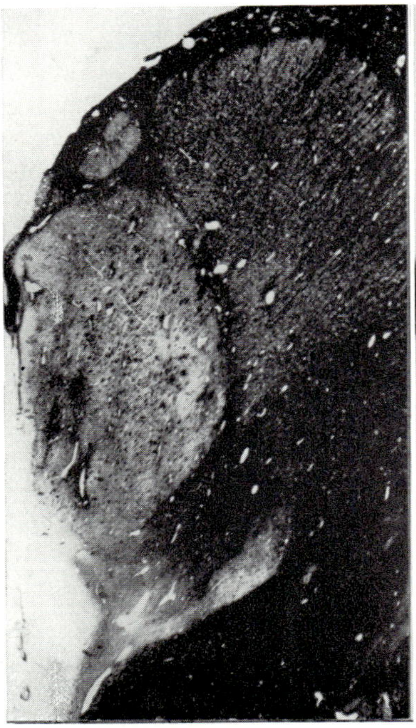

6.103

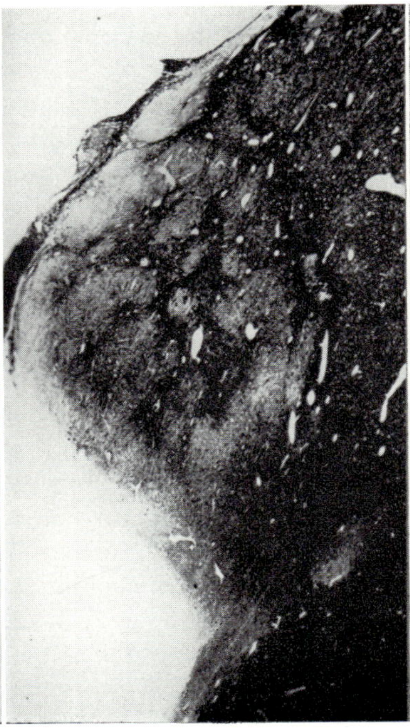

6.104

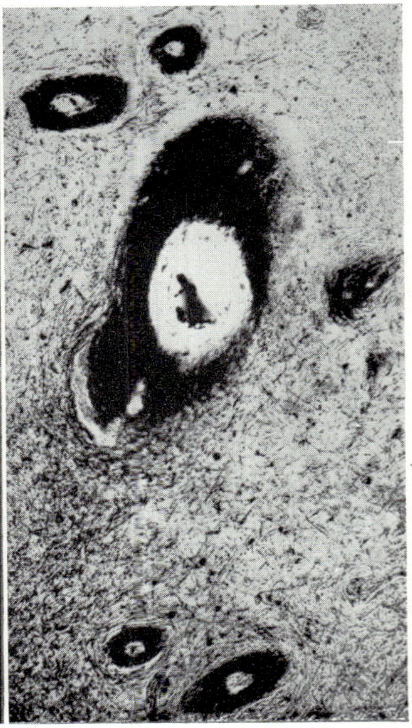

6.105

FIG. 6.101. *État marbré* of caudate nucleus and putamen. Note the slight pallor of the outer segment of the globus pallidus. (Kultschitsky-Pal.)
FIG. 6.102. Corresponding section to Figs 6.101. Gliosis of putamen and globus pallidus. (Holzer.)
FIG. 6.103. Normal myelination of the dorsomedial nucleus of the thalamus. (Kultschitsky-Pal.)
FIG. 6.104. État marbré of the dorsomedial nucleus of the thalamus (same brain as in Fig. 6.92). (Kultschitsky-Pal stain.)
FIG. 6.105. Perivascular hypermyelination in dorsomedial nucleus of thalamus—an unusual form of état marbré.

factor of importance in the severe mental deficiency which is found in certain cases of athetosis (Norman 1947, Malamud 1950). Bilateral or unilateral damage to the thalamus, sometimes in the form of small cystic softenings may be reasonably attributed to compression of the branches of the posterior cerebral arteries, particularly when they are associated with lesions in neigh-

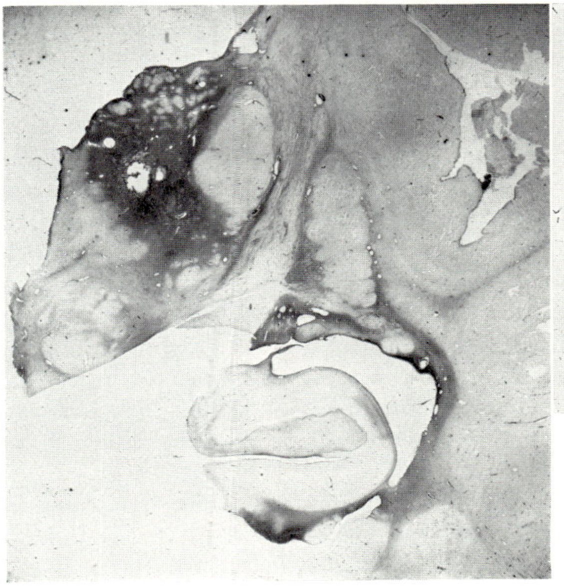

6.106

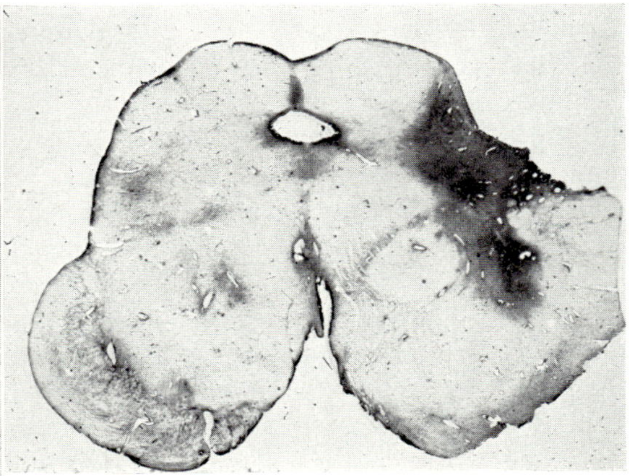

6.107

FIG. 6.106. The thalamus shows dense gliosis. Note the scar in the ventral wall of the hippocampal gyrus (due to pressure by the edge of the tentorium), and the milder gliosis in the Sommer sector and end plate of Ammon's horn. (Holzer.)

FIG. 6.107. Same brain as Fig. 6.106. Glial scar in lateral part of midbrain probably due to local compression. (Holzer.)

bouring parts of the brain, such as the geniculate bodies, Ammon's horn or midbrain (Walsh and Lindenberg 1961; Norman and Urich 1962 (Case 3)) (Figs. 6.106 and 6.107).

Pathogenesis of cerebral birth injury

Although conflicting opinions exist as to the importance or otherwise of birth injury as a cause of cerebral palsy, few would deny that there is ample opportunity for damage to the brain to occur during parturition. Several theories of pathogenesis have been put forward since the time of Little (1862), who suggested that 'capillary apoplexies' following asphyxia might be responsible for spastic birth palsies. The more important of these theories will be reviewed and their applicability to the lesions already described will be indicated. It is obvious that these pathogenetic mechanisms are not mutually exclusive.

Mechanical trauma. The effects of tearing of dural septa and veins during excessive moulding of the foetal head have already been mentioned. It is a debatable point whether less severe stress may also lead to significant lesions. A rise in the vertical diameter of the skull causes upward displacement of the apex of the tentorium, so that kinking of the great vein of Galen is likely to occur at its point of confluence with the less mobile straight sinus (Holland 1920, 1922). Le Gros Clark (1940) has drawn attention to the presence of a vascular structure resembling an arachnoid granulation, which may be found above and behind the pineal gland

and which, under circumstances just described, might facilitate obstruction of the vein of Galen. It is a plausible hypothesis that this mechanism, by causing severe congestion in the drainage area of the internal cerebral veins, may play a part in the production of bilateral lesions of the basal ganglia and central white matter. Whether this venous engorgement is brought about by the mechanism just described, or by asphyxial congestion, or by pressure differences as postulated by Schwartz (q.v.), it is undoubtedly true that in some fatal cases of birth injury the great vein of Galen has shown extraordinary dilatation (Turnham and Rössler 1942, Schwartz 1961).

Asphyxia. The intraventricular or subependymal haemorrhages arising from the anterior terminal veins in premature infants are commonly associated with severe asphyxia and it seems established that venous congestion from this cause may lead to the ultimate bursting of the vessel (Gröntoft 1954). Blood-vessels in premature infants are fragile structures, as Ylppö (1919) showed in his classical paper, and the anatomical situation of the anterior terminal vein favours rupture since it lies beneath the ependyma and embedded in the growth centres of the matrix which have not as yet disappeared. According to Gruenwald (1951) the walls of the veins lying in this undifferentiated tissue are thinner than those in the normal white matter. It is unnecessary to postulate mechanical trauma as a factor in this type of haemorrhage since coincident tearing of the tentorium is rarely found in premature infants and similar terminal vein bleedings occur both in foetuses dead in utero and in infants succumbing to asphyxial attacks in postnatal life.

Asphyxial anoxaemia is thought by some writers to be of great pathogenetic significance in cerebral palsy (Wyllie 1951, Courville 1953). In infants asphyxiated at birth, but who have survived for 2 or 3 days, widespread 'areas of paling' may be found especially in the striatum, globus pallidus, thalamus, nucleus subthalamicus, Ammon's horn and the amygdaloid nucleus. Homogenising change in the Purkinje cells is also common. In such cases the cerebral cortex may escape except for paling and ischaemic nerve cell change in the central gyri. It is probable that extensive lesions of this sort are highly lethal but that the survivors will show the pattern of lesions associated with état marbré of the basal ganglia. In longstanding cases it is often difficult on histological grounds to distinguish between these anoxic lesions occurring at birth with those of a later, post-epileptic encephalopathy since most of the sites of predilection are common to both conditions (Weller and Norman 1955, Norman 1958).

The calcification of the elastica and the eccentric subintimal fibrosis often seen in the wall of small meningeal arteries in areas of ulegyria are probably due to local anoxia (J. E. Meyer 1949).

Prenatal anoxaemia must also be taken into account since oxygen reserves are low in late foetal life. The hazards of even a normal birth may thus be aggravated and it is reasonable to suppose that what otherwise might have been reversible changes in the neurones may be converted into irreparable damage by the added stresses of labour. Interference with placental function probably accounts for some of the cases of cerebral palsy which follow Caesarian section performed for placenta praevia (Clifford 1941). Schwartz noted as a rare finding that the pathological changes present in the central white matter of some of his neonatal cases were so advanced as to make it certain that the commencement of the process had ante-dated birth, and in a recently examined case the writer has seen extensive cystic degeneration of the brain in an infant who survived birth by only 24 hours. In two instances extensive cystic softening of the central white matter of the brain has been reported in infants of low birth weight whose mothers had suffered from severe anaemia in pregnancy. In both cases the treatment of the anaemia had caused serious reactions in the mother shortly before the onset of labour (Norman 1952, Sharpe and Hall 1953). The relationship between foetal anoxia and lesions of the centrum semi-ovale and basal ganglia is most clearly demonstrated in infants who have survived the mother's attempted suicide by coal gas inhalation during late pregnancy (Maresh 1929, Neubürger 1935).

Venous Lesions: Schwartz's theory of venous stasis. Schwartz's (1924, 1927, 1961) studies on an unrivalled material convinced him that the great majority of cerebral birth injuries originated from venous lesions. In his view intense congestion of the venous sinuses and their tributaries could be brought about by blood being drawn into the presenting head after rupture of the membranes. It is generally admitted that the differential between intrauterine and atmospheric pressures is responsible for caput succedaneum or cephalhaematoma, but the novelty of Schwartz's theory was to ascribe intracerebral lesions to the same mechanism. From this standpoint birth injuries to the convexity of the cerebral cortex are to be related to circulatory stasis, thrombosis or haemorrhage in the drainage system of the superior longitudinal sinus, while lesions of the basal ganglia and centrum semi-ovale depend upon similar disturbances in the territory of the great vein of Galen.

This theory of the pathogenesis of cerebral birth injury was elaborated by Schwartz with great thoroughness and has exerted considerable influence. Bilateral ulegyria, spreading out from the margins of the great longitudinal fissure and involving the medial surface of the hemisphere as well as the upper part of the convexity, certainly suggests an antecedent sinus thrombosis and a number of cases are on record in which this pattern of lesions has been associated with obliteration of part of the superior longitudinal sinus (Norman 1936, Benda 1952). But it does not follow that lesions of a venous distribution are necessarily brought about by the mechanism postulated by Schwartz. Even with the Galenic lesions, which were so well described by Schwartz, the alternative mechanism of production described by Holland (q.v.) may carry greater conviction (Haller *et al.* 1956).

Compression of vessels in the depths of the sulci, whether by mechanical distortion of the brain substance or by the effect of oedema, is a likely explanation of the special vulnerability of the gyral wall so characteristic of ulegyria. The long narrow streaks of necrosis passing down the medullary cores of atrophic gyri into the central white matter (Fig. 6.82) are evidently related to the distribution of veins.

Cerebral oedema associated with venous engorgement is also a probable factor in the production of diffuse gliosis or confluent cavitation in the centrum semi-ovale. This problem of tissue anoxia due to venous stasis has been well discussed by Wolf and Cowen (1956), who have drawn attention to the occurrence of softenings in the cerebral white matter in infants suffering from cyanotic heart disease. Lindenberg (1963) believes that when white matter softenings occur in arterial boundary zones the two factors of venous congestion and systemic hypotension are involved, both being related to heart failure.

Arterial lesions. Granular atrophy of the cortex occurring in boundary zones between main arterial territories was first described by Lindenberg and Spatz (1939) in the brains of elderly individuals suffering from a form of obliterative endarteritis. Lesions of a similar distribution, for example, those affecting the 2nd frontal gyri, have since been reported in conditions associated with severe fall in systemic blood pressure (Zülch 1954, Mettler *et al.* 1954). The finding of boundary zone lesions in cases of birth injury (Meyer 1953), thus suggests that neonatal shock (asphyxia pallida) has occurred. The mode of production of these lesions is not fully understood but an explanation has been put forward based upon an analogy with an irrigation system supplying a series of fields with water. If there is a drop in the head of pressure it will be the last field which will suffer first (Zülch 1955). An important factor may be the presence of meningeal anastomotic channels between the major arterial territories, which may perhaps facilitate the short-circuiting of part of the peripheral vascular bed (Becker 1949 a).

Lesions situated in the territory of individual arterial branches are brought about by a different mechanism. It is well known that in conditions of raised intracranial pressure displacement of the brain substance can stretch or compress arteries against the edge of the tentorium or the side of the foramen magnum, and it is thought that the same mechanism may be operative in head presentations associated with considerable cranial deformity. It has been suggested that during birth the uncus herniates into the incisura tentorii, causing compression of the anterior choroidal artery, and this may lead to ischaemia of the uncus and amygdaloid nucleus (Earle *et al.* 1953). Cerebral displacement may also cause temporary occlusion of branches of the posterior cerebral artery supplying the cornu Ammonis and adjacent parts of the temporal lobe, the thalamus (interpeduncular branches) or the calcarine cortex (Lindenberg 1955, Walsh and Lindenberg 1961). Lindenberg has brought forward evidence indicating that in states of raised intracranial pressure, such as may be brought about by oedema of the brain or by a subdural haematoma, branches of the middle cerebral artery may be compressed, the sites of predilection being at the limen insulae and at the posterior end of the Sylvian fissure.

It is an important consideration that lesions attributable to arterial compression have been found in brains also showing typical boundary zone lesions, since a low systemic blood pressure would clearly favour compression of the vessel wall (Norman *et al.* 1957). Indeed, without the intervention of this factor of reduced blood pressure, it might be difficult to conceive the soft brain tissue exerting sufficient force to occlude the lumen of an artery.

It is often difficult to assess the relative importance of these two closely associated factors. No doubt if ischaemic lesions lie in the territory of a vessel which can be kinked or compressed against a rigid structure like the tentorium it is unnecessary to stress the possible additional element of shock, but the situation is very different when compression by brain tissue alone is postulated. This applies to the bilateral patches of ulegyria often found in the upper part of the parietal lobes in cases of birth injury and these may well represent 'last field' lesions aggravated by local pressure. The remarkable symmetry of these lesions, and also of those of the calcarine cortex frequently associated with them, suggests the intervention of another pathogenetic factor besides compression, namely, a fall in systemic blood pressure below a critical level (Norman and Urich 1962). This theory of pathogenesis is greatly strengthened by analogous findings in cases of vascular disease in the adult. Hutchinson and Yates (1956, 1957) have shown that, in persons whose vertebral arteries in their cervical course are stenosed by atheroma, symmetrical infarction of the cerebellum and calcarine cortex may be precipitated by extraneous factors leading to a sudden fall in systemic blood pressure. Another factor operative at birth may be a local impediment to the flow of arterial blood in the vertebral arteries following intramural haematomata. Yates (1959) has recently demonstrated this lesion in a large number of infants dying in the perinatal period.

Pathogenesis of état marbré. The dense overgrowth of axis cylinders present in areas of marbling was first thought to be a prenatal malformation by C. and O. Vogt (1920). More recently Alexander (1942) put forward the theory that état marbré of the corpus striatum was due to the aberrant ramification of the fibres of the frontopontine tracts. The writer has seen a few cases in which very coarse myelinated bundles have broken up the lateral thalamic nuclei into islands of nerve cells and in which there has been a great reduction in the size of the thalamus, striatum and globus pallidus on each side. Such findings suggest that in rare instances a prenatal disturbance of development may interfere with the normal growth of the thalamic projection fibres. The great majority of writers on the subject have followed Scholz (1924), who first suggested that the fibre overgrowth was the consequence of a regenerative activity on the part of injured nerve cells. It is an incontestable fact that marbling of the cerebral cortex is very common at the margins of vascular lesions due to birth injury; and in the adult similar formations may be seen as the sequel of carbon monoxide poisoning or in granular atrophy of the cortex associated with arterial hypertension. Widespread état marbré of the corpus striatum or thalamus, on the other hand, has no counterpart in the vascular lesions of adult life.

The great majority of cases of état marbré of the basal ganglia appear to follow birth injury, a few follow meningitis or a feverish illness in infancy (Malamud 1950) or are the sequels of nuclear jaundice or epilepsy. The relationship of état marbré of the corpus striatum and thalamus to birth injury has been amply demonstrated pathologically by cases in which these lesions have been found in association with typical birth injuries of the cerebral cortex or centrum semiovale (Benda 1945, Norman 1947, Sylvester 1960). In such cases the marbling of the basal ganglia is often asymmetrical and may be attributed to focal vascular lesions. The more usual symmetrical pattern of lesions described in the previous section is also evidently associated in many cases with a history of abnormal birth and neonatal distress, but the pathogenetic factor or factors responsible for this singularly stereotyped distribution are still obscure. Venous stasis in the Galenic system has been suggested as a likely factor, following Schwartz's early work (Norman 1947, Benda 1952, Schwartz 1961, Malamud 1962). Anoxia is strongly suggested by the involvement of so many areas known to be vulnerable in other conditions of clearer pathogenesis. Some of the lesions in the hippocampus, particularly those in the resistent sector h_2 and in the inferior wall of the hippocampal gyrus may be dictated by vascular compression due to anoxic brain swelling (Norman 1963). The often selective involvement of the cerebellar vermis and central gyri of the cerebral cortex are more difficult to explain, but have their counterparts in one or two of Windle's (1963) asphyxiated monkeys. The fact that symmetrical état marbré is usually a feature of full term infants may be of importance in this connection, since it is possible that by this time certain neurones are more dependent upon aerobic metabolism, especially the central gyri of the cerebral cortex which myelinate early. There is also reason to believe that an inherited factor may be operative in those few cases of striatal marbling in which another relative has suffered from athetosis. Up to the present, post-mortem examinations on both the athetoid members of the family have only been carried out in two instances. Koch (1949) recorded two identical twin idiots with double athetosis. One had striatal marbling and slight pallidal demyelination, the other only pallidal changes and no état marbré, though in this last case the neuropathological investigation was by no means extensive. Van Bogaert (1950) has described the only example of état marbré verified in a brother and sister, both of whom showed thalamostriate marbling and cerebellar atrophy of lamellar type. Both patients were severe epileptics, a fact of possible pathogenetic significance. Van Bogaert explained the familial character of the disease on the basis of an inherited vascular anomaly which predisposed the individual to lesions of the type under discussion. He also pointed out that coincidental vascular lesions of a similar sort may occur in system degenerations and cited the example of état marbré appearing in the setting of familial myoclonus epilepsy (van Bogaert 1929).

III. POSTNATAL DISEASES

Nuclear Jaundice (Kernicterus)

Yellow staining of circumscribed parts of the basal ganglia, brain stem and cerebellum had been noted by Orth (1875) in certain cases of neonatal jaundice, but the first detailed pathological account of the condition was given by Schmorl (1903) who introduced the descriptive name of 'kernicterus'. The following structures are most commonly picked out by the yellow or orange pigmentation: the nucleus subthalamicus, cornu Ammonis, globus pallidus, dentate nucleus, inferior olives, the cranial nerve nuclei in the floor of the 4th ventricle, the cerebellar vermis and the flocculus. The putamen, thalamus and grey matter of the spinal cord are less often affected and staining of the caudate nucleus is rare. The cerebral cortex and central white matter may show patchy yellow areas and if there is any coincidental focus of softening in the centrum semi-ovale the edges of that area are deeply jaundiced (Dublin 1949). The comprehensive study by Haymaker *et al.* (1961) should be consulted for further details, particularly for changes in the brain stem nuclei.

Microscopic appearances. In frozen sections, or celloidin sections cleared without the use of xylol, benzene or chloroform, the icteric areas are seen to contain golden yellow granules which not only encrust the nerve cells and the commencement of their processes but also diffusely colour the interstitial tissue. It is important to note that nuclear masses which are heavily pigmented to the naked eye may show no discernible nerve cell damage on microscopic examination (Claireaux 1950) (Fig. 6.113). This applies particularly to the dentate nuclei and inferior olives. Even in the first few days striking changes are to be seen in the most vulnerable areas, namely, the subthalamic nucleus, Ammon's horn and the globus pallidus. When the subthalamic nucleus is examined under the low power the impression may be given that

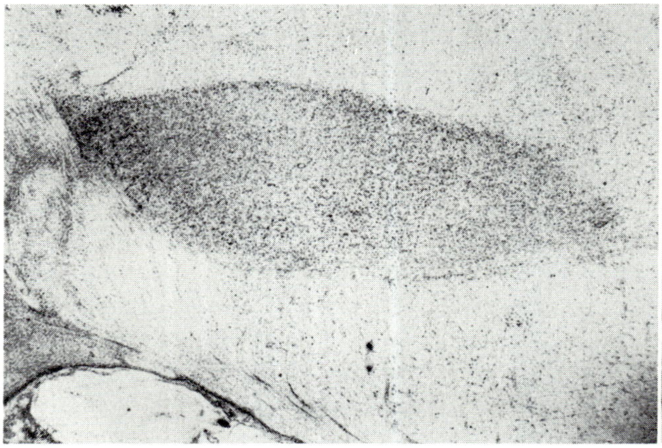

6.108

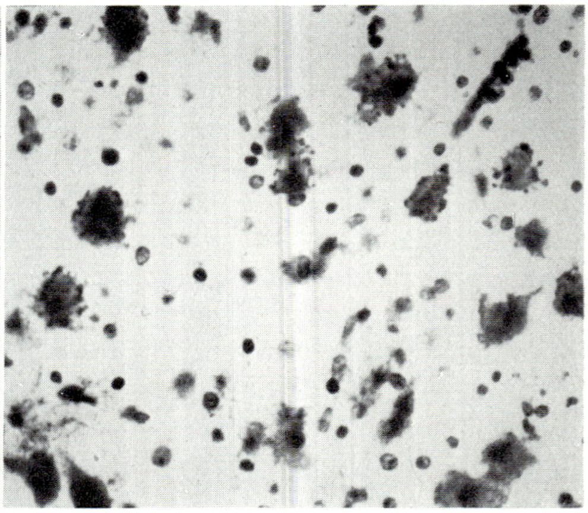

6.109

FIG. 6.108. *Nuclear jaundice of prematurity.* Rt. nucleus subthalamicus showing early degeneration of nerve cells. Death on 9th day. (Carbol azure.)

FIG. 6.109. Nuclear jaundice. Rh. incompatibility. Degeneration of nerve cells in nucleus subthalamicus with incrustation of the Golgi networks. Death on 2nd day. (Carbol azure.)

almost every nerve cell has disappeared (Fig. 6.108) but with higher magnification the individual neurones are revealed as shrunken structures (Figs. 6.109 and 6.111) with their cytoplasm staining yellow or, if the pigment has been removed by the processing of the section, staining a uniform pale blue in Nissl preparations or a pink colour with eosin. The nucleus is usually pale and crenated and contains only a fine speckling of chromation while the nucleolus has lost its basophilic properties. The capillaries of the area are unduly prominent and the astrocytic nuclei appear rather more numerous than usual, perhaps because of tissue shrinkage. Not uncommonly the inner half of the subthalamic nucleus is well preserved, while the outer shows the severe changes just described. In the cornu Ammonis the pyramidal nerve cells exhibit a greater variety of pathological change. The commonest finding is chromatolysis and considerable swelling of the cyton with enlargement, pallor and eccentricity of the nucleus. Necrotic, yellow staining cells are frequently seen here also, while some may show the appearances of homogenising or ischaemic nerve cell change, often with incrustation of the Golgi network. Neuronal damage is usually only present in certain sectors of the pyramidal cell band. It is common in Sommer's sector or in the end folium, but frequently the so-called resistant sector may be symmetrically implicated. This element of regional or 'topistic' (Vogt 1942) vulnerability is sometimes exhibited by the globus pallidus where shrinkage and chromatolysis or the ischaemic change of neurones may be localised in either the outer or inner segment.

In cases which recover and later show symptoms such as athetosis or chorea, the neuronal necrosis expresses itself in clear cut, often symmetrical areas of nerve cell loss, dense gliosis and poverty of myelination (Figs. 6.110 and 6.112). These chronic changes involve the areas already mentioned as being pigmented in the acute form of the disease (Fitzgerald *et al.* 1939) and in almost all survivors the bilateral pallido-Luysial and hippocampal atrophies are striking lesions. The deafness commonly present in these children has been attributed to degeneration of the cochlear nucleus (Gerrard 1952) but the nuclei were not abnormal in two deaf patients

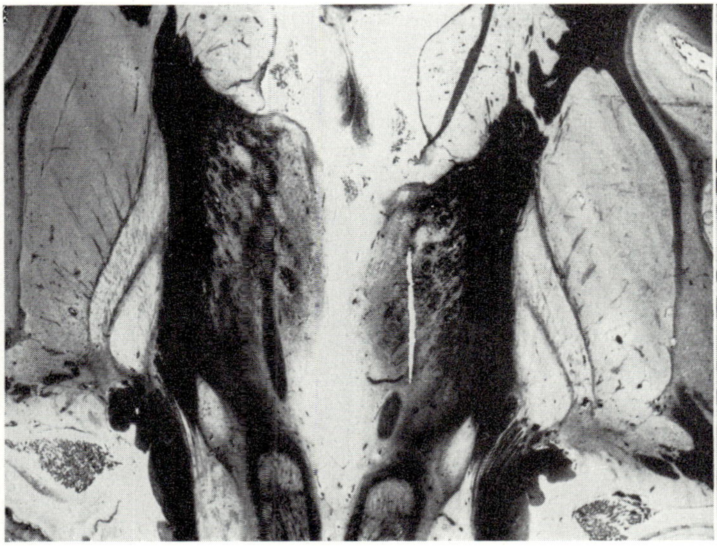

6.110

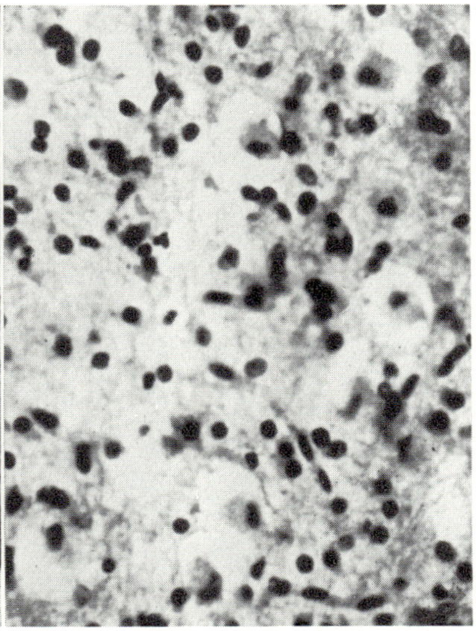

6.111

FIG. 6.110. Late sequelae of nuclear jaundice showing myelin poverty of each globus pallidus and nucleus subthalamicus. Death at 13 months. (Heidenhain.)

FIG. 6.111. Nuclear jaundice of prematurity. Degeneration of nerve cells in nucleus subthalamicus. Death on 6th day. (Carbol azure.)

studied pathologically by Haymaker *et al.* (1961). Investigations on the inner ear are lacking. In a few of the chronic cases the neuronal destruction has been exceptionally widespread. Deschamps and van Bogaert (1948) described disappearance of anterior horn cells and demyelination of the posterior columns of the spinal cord. In another case van Bogaert (1951) found, in addition to pallido-Luysial atrophy, lesions in the thalamus, red nucleus, substantia nigra and corpora quadrigemina. The oculomotor, vestibular and dorsal vagal nuclei were also affected, as well as the nucleus of Roller. The cerebral cortex, apart from the hippocampus, has rarely been found to be damaged, but conspicuous areas of nerve cell loss were noted by Crome (1955) in 2 cases. Severe necrotising lesions reminiscent of birth injury were described by Jervis (1950 b) in a case of B factor sensitisation. He observed cavitation of the subcortical white matter, severe cortical and pallidal damage and also *état marbré* of the putamen.

Pathogenesis. A full account of the possible biochemical factors responsible for nuclear jaundice will be found in the reviews of Haymaker *et al.* (1961) and of Blanc and Johnson (1959). The former is of particular interest because of its critical examination of the commonly held view that the necrosis of nerve cells in this condition is primarily due to the toxic action of unconjugated bilirubin on vulnerable grisea. Haymaker and his colleagues advance the hypothesis that the cells are dead or severely damaged before they absorb bilirubin and suggest that this is due to a deficiency of an unknown liver factor responsible for the supply of energy to, or its utilisation by, the central nervous system (the 'antihypoxidin' factor of Pentschew (1949)). There is, however, no difference of opinion about the cause of the jaundice. High levels of unconjugated bilirubin occur because of the low activity of glycuronyl transferase in the immature liver, and may be aggravated by any factor causing haemolysis, or by the administration of sulphonomides which compete for the binding sites of bilirubin on the plasma albumen. Deficiency in the glycuronyl transferase mechanism is inherited as a Mendelian recessive in the Crigler-Najjar (1952) type of familial non-haemolytic jaundice and in the Gunn strain of rats, the latter being a valuable experimental model for the study of the condition. Jervis (1959) has described the neuropathological findings in an adult patient with persistently high levels of bilirubin who had suffered from rigidity, dystonia, deafness and mental deficiency dating from

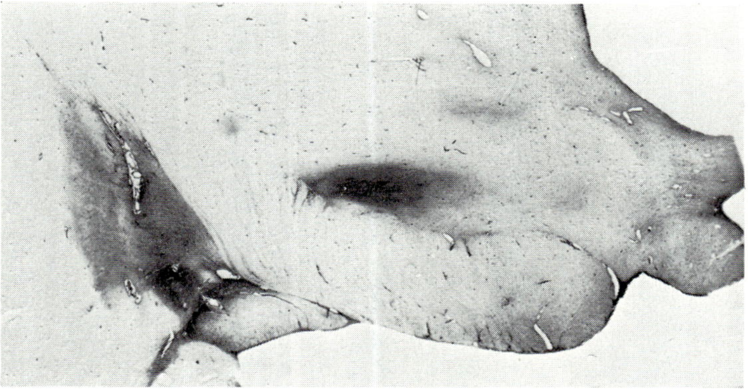

6.112

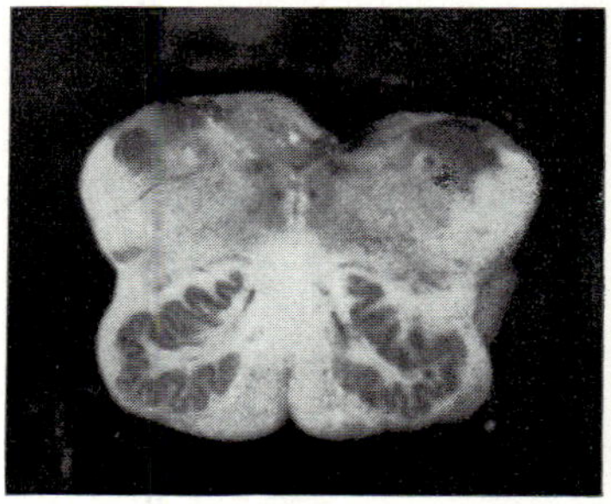

6.113

FIG. 6.112. Late sequelae of nuclear jaundice. Gliosis of globus pallidus and nucleus subthalamicus. Death at 15 months. (Holzer.)

FIG. 6.113. Icteric staining of the vestibular nuclei and inferior olives. The latter showed no appreciable damage on microscopic examination. Fresh specimen.

early infancy. The lesions were similar in distribution to the sequelae of nuclear jaundice of other aetiologies, except that the cerebellar cortex was more severely atrophied. He regarded the condition as due to histotoxic anoxia following the action of bilirubin on vulnerable grisea.

In vitro experiments have shown that bilirubin interferes with oxidation, but in living tissues it is not known what circumstances are necessary to permit the substance to leave the capillaries and enter the cell. Although the explanation usually offered is that the blood-brain barrier is more permeable in neonatal life there may, in fact, be an unexplained delay in the onset of neurological signs despite long periods of hyperbilirubinaemia, as in the patient with familial jaundice described by Rosenthal *et al.* (1956). It is also well known that infants may not develop nuclear jaundice in spite of bilirubin levels well above the danger mark of 20 mg. per cent. However this may be, the recent successful production of experimental nuclear jaundice in kittens by Rozdilsky and Olszewski (1961) is an important link in the chain of evidence pointing to the primary toxicity of bilirubin, and it seems unnecessary to postulate an additional liver defect or an anoxic process to account for the neuronal changes in this condition.

Acute encephalopathies of vascular origin occurring in early life

The majority of cases belonging to this category conform clinically to the classical picture outlined by James Taylor (1905) in the following words: 'a child, hitherto healthy, suddenly becomes ill without any apparent cause, between the ages of 1 month and 6 years. The early symptoms are severe and consist of convulsions, fever, often vomiting and always coma. The limbs remain flaccid for some days, after which the flaccidity begins to lessen and the limbs become spastic'. It was to explain this mysterious form of infantile encephalopathy that Strümpell (1884) introduced his theory of a primary polio-encephalitis, but the intervening years have brought very little clinical evidence and no pathological confirmation of a relationship between anterior poliomyelitis and cerebral palsy of this type (Rothman 1931, Stewart 1948). No doubt this group of encephalopathies contains many examples of vascular thrombosis precipitated by sepsis or dehydration and there is the additional and highly important factor of the severe epilepsy which so often ushers in the illness and which in many cases appears to be responsible for much of the cerebral damage.

Sinus thrombosis. There is clinical evidence that partial thrombosis of the superior longitudinal sinus may lead to infantile hemiplegia (Mitchell 1952) or quadriplegia (Schlesinger and Welch 1952). The middle fifth of the sinus is the site of predilection for thrombosis and it is necessary for the clot to extend into the superior cerebral veins for a sufficient distance to obstruct the collateral circulation before haemorrhagic infarction of the cortex occurs (Bailey and Hass 1937). The veins open into the inferior angle of the lumen of the sinus and mural thrombosis in this situation will not interfere with the Paccionian bodies which are mainly present in the upper angles of the cavity (Martin 1941). The anatomical variations in the arrangement of the superior longitudinal, lateral and straight sinuses are of considerable importance in understanding the clinical and pathological sequelae of the spread of thrombosis, particularly in cases of middle ear disease (Woodhall 1939).

There have been few adequate studies of the late neuropathological sequelae of infantile sinus thrombosis. One difficulty is that the sinus may completely recanalise and leave no residual sign of thrombosis. Another confusing point is the possibility that sinus thrombosis may have occurred in an infant whose brain has already been damaged from another cause, for example by birth injury. In cases of cerebral palsy supposedly due to sinus thrombosis the gyral shrinkage and atrophy, with or without subcortical cystic degeneration, should occupy the region primarily affected by haemorrhage and oedema in the acute cases, that is, the upper part of the convexity, including the medial surface. The intensity of the cerebral destruction should also shade off as the fissure of Sylvius is approached, unless thrombosis has spread to the Sylvian veins via the vein of Trolard. This type of distribution was found by the writer in a case of sinus thrombosis which had presumably occurred at birth or shortly afterwards (Norman 1936) and in an anatomically proven case of longitudinal sinus thrombosis which had led to unilateral cerebral atrophy (Dekaban and Norman 1958). In other cases, in which sinus thrombosis was inferred but not proved, there was marked demyelination and gliosis of the dorsal parts of the central white matter of the hemisphere in addition to the cortical ulegyria (Woolf 1955).

Arterial lesions. Thrombosis of the middle cerebral artery is the commonest arterial lesion in acute infantile hemiplegia. Careful examination of the vessels has not often been carried out in these cases but plaques of subintimal fibrosis associated with splitting of the internal elastic lamina have been noted in the middle cerebral trunk or in its branches by Bertrand and Bargeton (1955) in several hemispherectomy specimens. Mair (1952) has also reported similar findings. Opinion differs as to whether these changes should be regarded as the result of

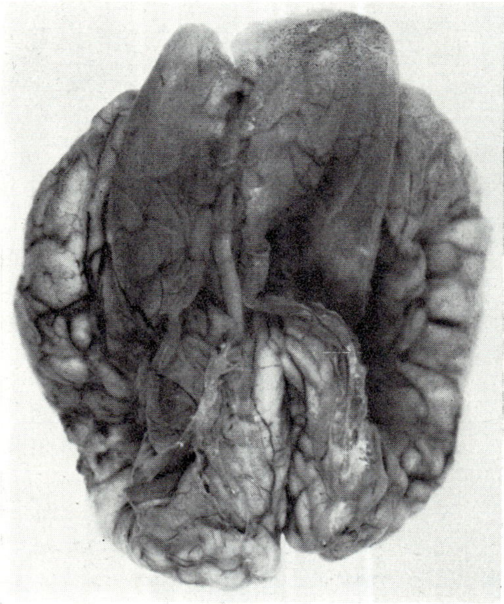

6.114

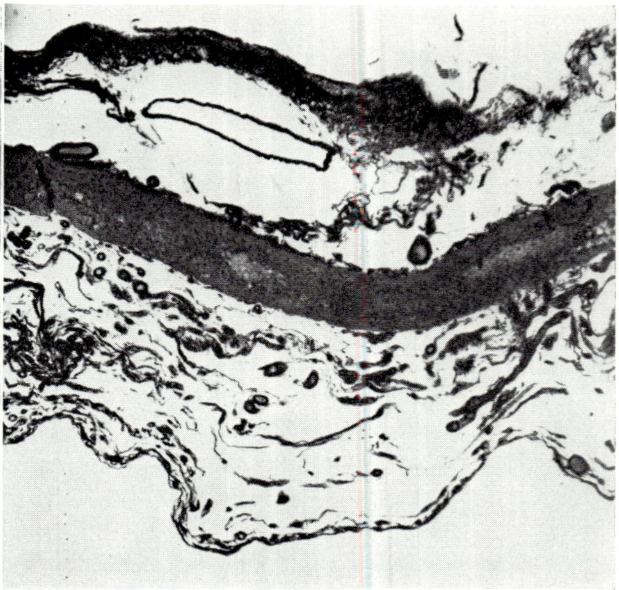

6.115

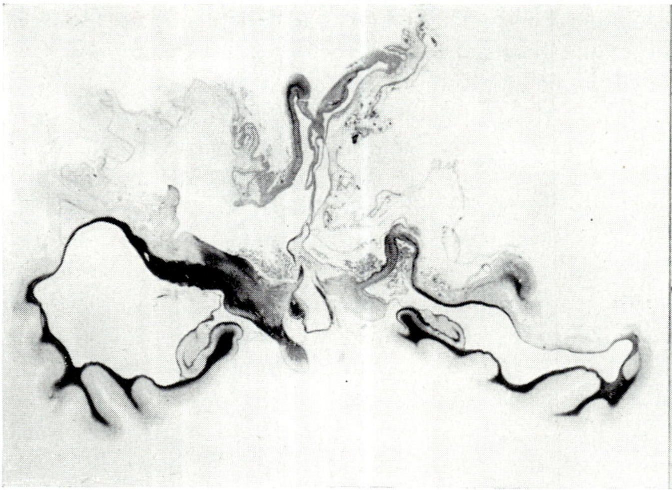

6.116

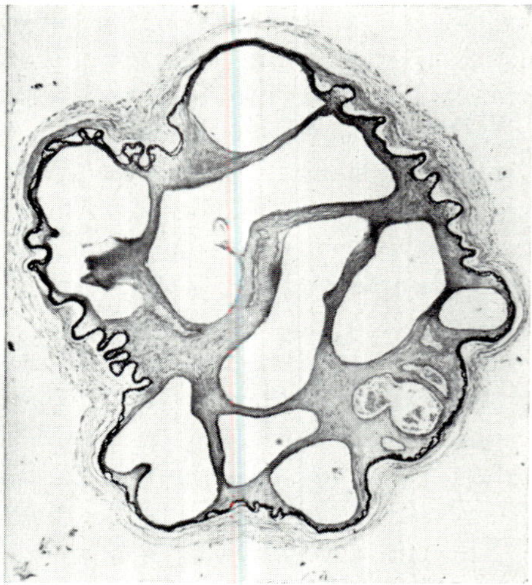

6.117

FIG. 6.114. *Porencephaly*. Superior surface of brain showing bladder-like remnants of frontal and parietal lobes. Case of arrested pneumococcal meningitis with thrombosis of anterior and middle cerebral arteries of both sides. Death at 12 years. (11 years after the original illness.)

FIG. 6.115. Structure of the membranous wall of the hemisphere. From without inwards (1) leptomeninges, (2) gliotic band of residual cortex, (3) meshwork of connective tissue and blood-vessels derived from white matter and separated from the ventricle by (4) a thin layer of fibrous tissue, the 'pia accessoria'. (Masson's trichrome.)

FIG. 6.116. Coronal section of the brain showing preservation of areas supplied by the posterior cerebral arteries. (Heidenhain's myelin.)

FIG. 6.117. Middle cerebral artery in the subarachnoid space at base of brain (Fig. 6.114) showing recanalisation. (H. and E.)

organisation of thrombus, as seems probable, or as endarteritis following a previous infection. Certainly thrombosis of meningeal and larger arteries commonly follows arteritis in tuberculous or other forms of meningitis. In a case of healed pneumococcal meningitis of many years standing Smith *et al.* (1957) found evidence of recanalisation of the anterior and middle cerebral arteries at the base of the brain (Fig. 6.117). Almost complete destruction of the hemispheres had occurred in the areas supplied by these 4 vessels (Fig. 6.114 and 6.116). The bladder-like wall of the atrophied hemisphere consisted of 4 layers, the leptomeninges, the narrow gliotic cortical ribbon and a loose meshwork of connective tissue and blood-vessels separated from the ventricle by a very thin layer of fibrous tissue, the 'membrana pia accessoria' (Fig. 6.115). The latter 2 layers are not found in prenatal hydranencephaly and may be absent in parts of the cyst walls overlying old softenings in cases of birth injury.

Infantile atheroma is a possible rare cause of hemiplegia and the case reported by Ford and Schaffer (1927) may perhaps belong to this category. Dissecting aneurysm of the middle cerebral artery (see page 133) is another rare cause of infantile hemiplegia (Norman and Urich 1957).

Embolism from congenital heart disease or thrombosis associated with polycythaemia are not uncommon complications of mongolism. Prenatal embolism of the internal carotid artery of obscure origin has been reported by Clark and Linell (1954). Carmichael has suggested that a clot detached from the severed umbilical vein might under certain circumstances enter the arterial side of the circulation through the as yet unclosed foramen ovale. Neonatal paradoxical embolism of this sort would be favoured by states of asphyxia leading to a rise in pressure in the right auricle. This hypothesis could explain some of the mysterious cases of unilateral middle cerebral softenings, apparently present from birth, which are often vaguely ascribed to birth injury for want of a more plausible theory of pathogenesis.

Post-epileptic encephalopathy

The realisation that status epilepticus or a series of major fits may severely damage the immature brain has shed considerable light upon the origin of several infantile encephalopathies the pathogenesis of which was formerly obscure. At the same time, this knowledge may add to the difficulty of interpreting lesions which are found in cerebral diseases complicated by epilepsy since the confusing element of a double pathology is introduced. It is particularly in the investigation of illnesses apparently starting after fits in infancy that this difficulty presents itself. Many birth-injured children are epileptic and the possibility that some of the brain damage may have been superimposed upon the original anoxic or ischaemic lesions sustained during birth has to be taken into account. Similarly, an acute infantile hemiplegia may be ushered in by fits associated with prenatal cerebral malformations and this sequence of events is not uncommon in tuberose sclerosis and Sturge-Weber disease. As Scholz (1951) has emphasised, there is nothing specific about those post-epileptic manifestations, but the overall distribution of the lesions in a given case is suggestive of an epileptic pathogenesis. These cases of post-epileptic brain damage present a recurrent pattern of lesions. To the well-known changes in the hippocampus and cerebellum may be added extensive laminar atrophy of the cortex, widespread thalamic lesions, and often partial destruction of the corpus striatum, dentate nucleus and inferior olive. The relative immunity of the globus pallidus and the calcarine cortex is an interesting reminder that the sites of predilection for the brain damage caused by fits are not always identical with those produced by compression of arteries. The cortical lesions are often predominant in one hemisphere and lead to hemiatrophy and hemiplegia. In such cases the clinical picture may be one of progressive aggravation of the paresis, the march of which seems correlated with the successive seizures. From the neuropathological standpoint the progressive character of the destructive process may be inferred by the finding of recent neuronal lesions side by side with those of older date. The neuropathology of epilepsy is described in detail in another chapter, but brief mention may be made here of certain aspects of the subject which are highly relevant to any consideration of cerebral palsy of postnatal onset.

Cerebral hemiatrophy (*Progressive lobar sclerosis of Schob*)

In these cases the birth history and neonatal development are usually normal and the first sign of trouble is a severe fit or series of fits, usually experienced in early life, after which a persistent weakness of one side of the body is observed. The fits recur and, in apparent association with them, mental defect and hemiplegia or quadriplegia become established. At postmortem it is usual to find one hemisphere somewhat smaller than the other and its convolutions shrunken, especially in the temporal lobe where gyral atrophy may be pronounced (Figs. 6.118 and 6.119). Microscopically there are extensive pseudolaminar losses of nerve cells over large

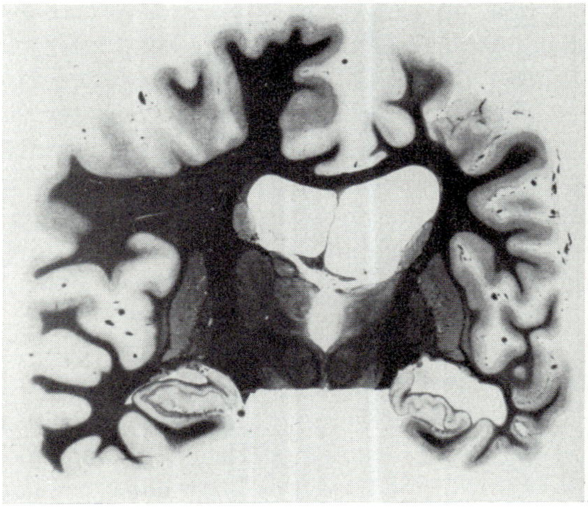

6.118

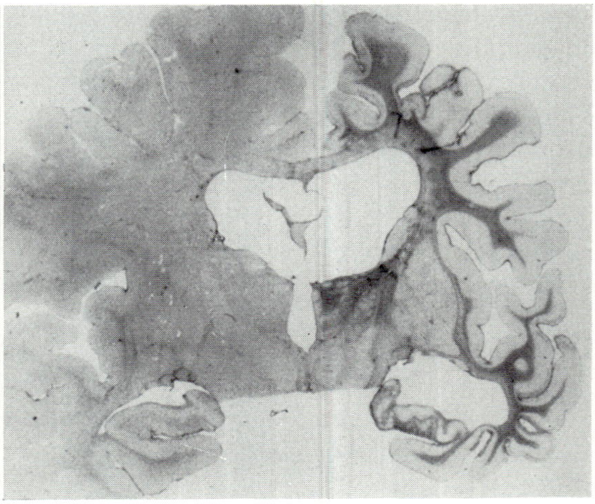

6.119

FIG. 6.118 and 6.119. *Post-epileptic encephalopathy.* Myelin and Holzer preparations of a brain showing post-epileptic hemiatrophy.

areas of the cerebral cortex, and these are not always confined to the macroscopically smaller hemisphere. The outer cortical layers are often diffusely affected so that the large pyramidal cells of the 3rd layer form the most superficial part of the grey matter. Here and there, especially in the middle and inferior temporal gyri, the cortical cell losses may be more severe and almost the whole grey matter may be denuded. Even so, the sharply outlined areas of neuroglial scarring and severe myelin loss, which are so characteristic of the ulegyria of birth injury, are never seen.

When the precentral gyrus is involved by laminar atrophy the deeper layers are usually well preserved and the pyramidal tract remains intact despite the contralateral spastic hemiparesis (Fig. 6.120). The condition of 'intracortical hemiplegia' (Speilmeyer 1906) or 'hemiplegia with intact pyramidal tracts' (Bielschowsky 1916) has been attributed to the widespread laminal cell losses in the cortex, on account of which the cells of origin of the pyramidal tract no longer receive their normal afferent impulses. Penfield (1954) states that dexterous, voluntary movements are still possible after excision of the gyri surrounding the precentral gyrus. The 'patterned flow of impulses' received by the motor cortex cannot, therefore, be transcortical in origin as has often been assumed, but must depend upon the integrity of the thalamic connections.

In severely demented patients the cerebral cortex of both hemispheres may show laminar atrophy but even in these cases one hemisphere is usually the more affected and is macroscopically smaller.

Changes characteristic of epilepsy are almost invariably present in the cornu Ammonis, uncus and amygdaloid nucleus of the atrophied side and often also in the hippocampus of the less affected hemisphere. The cerebellum frequently shows a lobular atrophy mainly affecting the deeper folia. État fibreux of the caudate nucleus is not uncommon. État marbré of the putamen may occur but seldom to the extent found after birth injury. The changes in the thalamus vary from small losses of nerve cells to massive atrophy. Since the centromedian nucleus is conspicuously exempt from pathological change unless the putamen has also been damaged, this thalamic atrophy appears to be largely retrograde from the cortex, an explanation first put forward by Bielschowsky (1916) and supported by Meyer *et al.* (1955) in their case of severe cerebral damage following status epilepticus.

Hemiatrophy with status spongiosus. In the type of cerebral atrophy just described the pathological findings are consistent with a process of selective destruction of nerve cells occurring mainly in certain vulnerable regions of the nervous system. A much smaller number of cases is on record in which the lesions of the affected hemisphere are far more extensive and severe (Fig. 6.121). The leptomeninges are thickened and adherent to the underlying cortex, which is reduced to an outer rind of densely gliosed tissue of varying depth and an inner zone of loose neuroglial fibrils merging imperceptibly into the equally spongy, gliosed demyelinated centrum semi-ovale (Fig. 6.123). The cingulate gyrus and the calcarine area are the least affected parts of the cortex. The lateral ventricle of the atrophied side and the 3rd ventricle are dilated and the thalamus shrunken. Cases belonging to this group have been described by Siegmund (1923), Hallervorden (1939), Clark and Russell (1940) and Norman (1956). In Hallervorden's case the less affected hemisphere showed a small area of gyral status spongiosus, but with this exception the unilaterality of the cortical degeneration has been a remarkable feature. There has also been a clinical association with an initial bout of severe fits and these cases have shown the typical post-epileptic pattern of lesions outside the cerebral cortex. In the writer's case the preservation of part of the visuosensory cortex was striking (Fig. 6.122).

The pathogenesis of this extraordinary condition remains obscure, despite the obvious association with epilepsy. In the writer's case the internal carotid artery on the same side as the hemiatrophy showed a large plaque of subintimal fibrosis with splitting of the internal elastic membrane beneath it. These changes suggested an old mural thrombus and were only present at the level of the carotid syphon. While the cerebral findings were evidently not those of infarction, it is possible that the initial status epilepticus in this case might have been precipitated by embolism or severe arterial spasm. Hallervorden's (1939) theory of the effect of cerebral oedema due to serous transudation is a plausible explanation for the widespread spongy degeneration of the tissues. The same author attributed the common laminar lesions of the grey matter to oedema spreading along the more loosely constituted cortical layers. An abnormal permeability of the vessel walls could be induced by an infective process, but there is little to suggest encephalitis in the clinical histories of these cases nor does the involvement of only one hemisphere favour such a conception.

Alpers' disease (poliodystrophia cerebri progressiva)

In a small group of cases closely allied both clinically and pathologically to the previously described post-epileptic encephalopathies, the claim has sometimes been made that the cerebral destruction is due to a primary degeneration of the grey matter. The illness usually starts in early life with convulsions. A progressive neurological condition characterised by spasticity, myoclonus and dementia ensues; this is often terminated by status epilepticus. Histological examination reveals extensive pseudo-laminar destruction of nerve cells in the cerebral cortex,

6.120

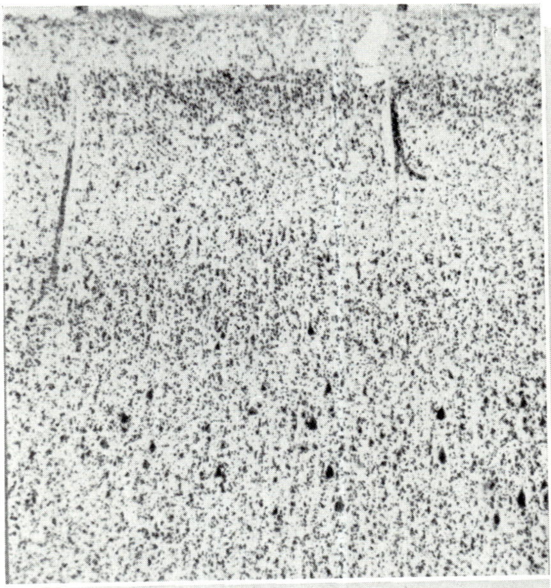

6.121

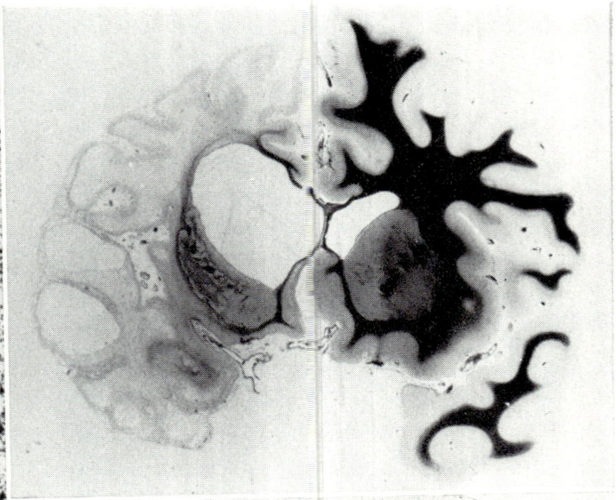

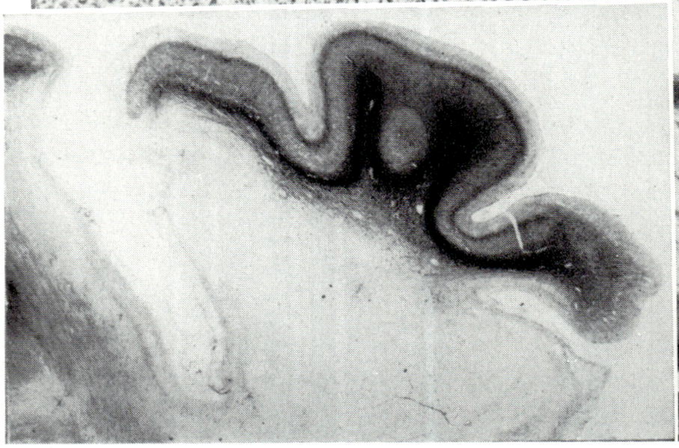

6.122

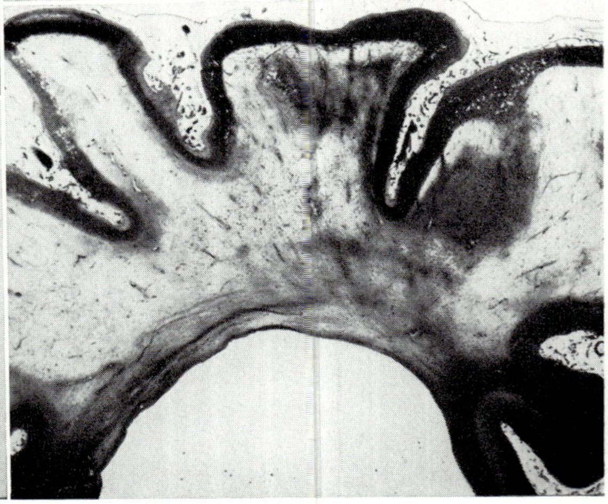

6.123

FIG. 6.121. Typical laminar atrophy of the outer layers of the motor cortex in epilepsy. (Carbol azure.)

FIG. 6.122. Hemiatrophy with status spongiosus. Note the shrinkage of left caudate nucleus and myelinised scar in putamen. (Heidenhain's myelin.)

FIG. 6.123. Same case as in Fig. 6.112 showing preservation of part of the visuosensory cortex. (Kultschitsky-Pal.)

FIG. 6.124. Part of the atrophied wall of the hemisphere showing dense gliosis of the superficial cortical layers and spongy state of the central white substance. (P.T.A.H.)

usually most severe and accompanied by status spongiosus in the 3rd and often the 5th layer. There is an increased activity of the microglial cells the processes of which contain neutral fat.

Degenerative changes are common in the striatum, thalamus and cerebellum, while in a few cases lesions in the globus pallidus, subthalamic nucleus and substantia nigra have been noted. One cerebral hemisphere may be particularly affected, as in the original case of Alpers (1931) whose name is often attached to this clinico-pathological syndrome.

In 3 cases, those of Alpers (1931), Christensen and Krabbe (1949) and Kramer (1953), minor developmental abnormalities in the form of 'immature' ganglion cells in the cerebral cortex were considered to be of pathological significance. Kramer also reported conspicuous groups of nerve cells in the white matter and underdevelopment of the cerebellar vermis and flocculi.

The disease may appear in a setting of apparent familial incidence, as in the brother and sister described by Ford *et al.* (1951), in both of whom the neuropathological examination revealed the characteristic lesions. In the family described by Kramer (1953), however, only one sib showed the typical changes of progressive degeneration of the cortical grey matter, the other affected member being an idiot from birth with multiple cystic softenings in the brain. In a recent paper Alpers (1960) has admitted seven other cases into this category, those of Freedom (1927); Christensen and Krabbe (1949); Ford *et al.* (1951: 3 cases); Kramer (1953); and Jervis (1957). Closely similar changes in the grey matter, but accompanied by demyelination in the centrum ovale or cerebellum have been reported by De Jong and Bebin (1956); Löken and Hörsdall (1961) and Liu and Sylvester (1960).

While it is likely that this group of encephalopathies contains examples of true degenerative disease, the frequent history of severe fits and the distribution of the changes makes it difficult to discount the anoxic effects of convulsions. On the other hand the widespread status spongiosus of the cortex, the involvement in some cases of the substantia nigra and pallidum, and particularly the case of Christensen and Krabbe (1949) in which no fits had been observed, indicate that epilepsy is not necessarily of pathogenetic significance.

Infantile subacute necrotising encephalomyelopathy

In 1951 Leigh reported the case of a male infant aged 7 months, dying within a period of 6 weeks from a neurological illness characterised by somnolence, optic atrophy, deafness and spasticity of the limbs. Examination of the brain showed bilateral areas of brownish discoloration in the tegmentum of the midbrain and pons and in the central grey matter of the medulla. The thalamus, substantia nigra, inferior olives and the posterior columns of the spinal cord were similarly affected. Microscopically these areas showed a conspicuously increased number of capillaries and precapillaries. The nerve cells showed a variety of degenerative changes ranging from swelling and central chromatolysis to shrinkage and neuronophagia, but the frequent presence of interspersed normal neurones was a remarkable feature. The microglia was extremely active and numerous fat granule cells were present at the periphery of the lesion. The astrocytes were also increased but the interstitial tissues were loosened and spongy rather than firmly gliosed. Considerable demyelination was seen in the affected areas and in the optic nerves.

Feigin and Wolf (1954) described three closely similar cases, adding the findings of involvement of the dentate nuclei where small cavities were present, degeneration of the nucleus subthalamicus, and occasional haemorrhages from the dilated and tortuous capillaries. In one of Richter's 3 cases extensive focal necrosis had occurred in the caudate nucleus and putamen and there was patchy spongy degeneration of the cortex and white matter in the cerebral hemispheres and cerebellum. Reye (1960) has described 4 further examples of this distinctive pathological entity in young children. He confirmed the spread of the disease to the basal ganglia and the occasionally severe cerebellar involvement, and also reported degeneration of the posterior columns of the spinal cord. In 3 cases there was also demyelination of the posterior roots and of the peripheral nerves.

The aetiology of this condition is not known. Although the tegmental changes are reminiscent of Wernicke's encephalopathy, no case has yet shown involvement of the mammillary bodies, nor is there any clinical evidence of dietary deficiency being a factor.

Infantile progressive spinal muscular atrophy of Werdnig and Hoffmann

Few diseases have been more adequately described by the original authors than this infantile and often familial form of neurogenic muscular atrophy. The pathological findings of Werdnig (1891) and Hoffmann (1893) have been repeatedly confirmed by later workers, so much so that Greenfield and Stern (1927) regarded the classical features of the condition as stereotyped. Yet the remarkable fact emerges from a consideration of the literature that repeated efforts have been made to detach cases from this singularly homogeneous group and to force them into the category of amyotonia congenita (Oppenheim's (1900) 'myatonie congénitale'). The benign course of the motor disability in Oppenheim's cases is in strong contrast to the progressive character and usually rapidly lethal outcome of Werdnig-Hoffmann's disease. Amyotonia congenita is, in fact, merely a descriptive title, clinically expedient, which covers a number of probably separate entities having in common the feature of hypotonia which becomes less disabling with advancing years. The infantile myopathy associated with the names of Batten (1903) and Aldren Turner (1940) and the family reported by Shy and Magee (1956) are the only members of this group which have up to the present been clearly defined. It is important to note that spinal muscular atrophy often starts in foetal life, as Beevor first showed in 1902. This early onset was not a feature of the original cases of Werdnig and Hoffmann, but the presence of congenital neurological abnormalities is evidently of no value in distinguishing the condition from Oppenheim's syndrome.

Pathology

Muscles. The characteristic feature in the skeletal and tongue muscles is the presence of groups of small fibres, the majority measuring less than 5μ in diameter. These patchy areas are easily picked out by the abnormal crowding together of the sarcolemmal nuclei and chains of these nuclei indicate the site of completely atrophied fibres. The majority of partially atrophied fibres retain their transverse striation and except in long-standing cases there is little evidence of fibrosis or fat replacement. The juxtaposition of these atrophied and normal muscle bundles is usually sufficiently clear-cut to indicate the neurogenic origin of the atrophy, but in some muscles comparatively normal and shrunken fibres may be seen in the same bundle. An important distinction from the findings in infantile myogenic atrophy is the almost invariable normality of the diaphragm (de Lange 1937). Large muscle fibres exceeding 50μ in diameter may be present in certain cases, but are unusual. In estimating whether fibres are hypertrophied the fact must be borne in mind that during the first year of life the width of skeletal muscle fibres very rarely exceeds 20μ (Brandt 1950).

Nerve endings. As in other forms of anterior horn cell disease the neurone dies back from the periphery. Studies by Coers and Woolf (1959), using the intra-vital methylene blue method, have shown that the intramuscular nerve bundles may appear normal or contain mainly large sensory 1a fibres. Distally the nerve fibres develop characteristic lozenge-shaped beads and form a plexiform tangle, the filaments of which end in diminutive terminal expansions. Collateral sprouting, a sign of reinervation, is commonly seen.

Peripheral nerves. The most obvious abnormality in Greenfield and Stern's (1927) cases was an unduly high proportion of very small myelinated fibres. Severe demyelination or evidence of recent myelin breakdown has occasionally been reported.

Spinal cord. The anterior nerve roots are abnormally thin and show a marked poverty of myelinated fibres, though evidence of recent degeneration is often lacking. Their intramedullary course is accompanied by fibrillary gliosis.

In the majority of cases a conspicuous loss of anterior horn cells is easily demonstrable at all levels of the cord and may amount in some segments to 90 per cent (Conel 1940). The spaces left by the degenerated cells are clearly outlined in myelin preparations as the 'empty cell-beds' described in Werdnig's first case. A mild fibrillary gliosis may be present in the affected grey matter. This widespread distribution of lesions is not always found in patients dying early in the course of the disease. Thus in de Lange's (1937) case, in which death took place at 20 days, degeneration of the anterior horn cells was found only in the cervical and thoracic regions. Some of the remaining anterior horn cells have often been described as hypoplastic, though in view of the fact that small cells are common in infants this observation is difficult to substantiate. Many are undoubtedly poor in Nissl substance and others stain darkly and have tortuous processes, but according to Conel (1938) the latter change is of doubtful pathological significance. Unequivocal evidence of concurrent nerve cell degeneration is usually to be found in the form of swelling and chromatolysis of some of the remaining anterior horn cells resembling axonal reaction (Fig. 6.124). In the later stages the cell is represented by a uniformly staining globular mass or 'ghost cell'; or typical figures of neuronophagia by microglial cells may be seen (Fig. 6.125). The swollen nerve cells have a characteristic appearance in Bielschowsky preparations. The intracellular neurofibrils have disappeared and the centre of the cell is occupied by a dark-staining argyrophil mass, sometimes of annular structure, the nucleus of the cell having disappeared or having been displaced to the margin (Figs. 6.126 and 127). This form of active nerve cell degeneration is typical of the younger cases of Werdnig-Hoffmann's disease but may be absent in the rarer cases belonging to older age groups. It was not found, for instance, in the 13-year-old patient described by Greenfield and Stern (1927).

Clarke's column may be involved in the degenerative process but a careful search of a large number of sections is usually necessary to demonstrate this (Conel 1940). On the other hand, routine examination of posterior root ganglia may reveal one or two obviously chromatolytic cells per section (Fig. 6.128). In the atypical case described by Ajuriaguerra *et al.* (1950) the lesions of the ganglia were very severe and accompanied by demyelination of the posterior roots and posterior columns.

The myelination of the spinal cord has in the majority of cases been regarded as normal. Pallor of the pyramidal tracts, varying considerably at different levels of the cord, was noted by Werdnig (1891) and by Hoffmann (1893) who were unconvinced that these lesions represented tract degenerations. Similar changes were also present in the posterior columns of one of Werdnig's cases. These findings have been confirmed in a number of instances by later authors who have also reported pallor of the spinocerebellar tracts. Radermeker (1951), who has summarised the literature on the subject, rejects the notion that these lesions are artefacts on the ground that in his cases the myelin defect was accompanied by a dense and localised gliosis, but this coincidence appears to be exceptional. In the writer's cases an abnormal gliosis could often be demonstrated in regions of the cord which were apparently well myelinated.

Brain stem. The hypoglossal nucleus is usually severely affected and in Conel's (1940) case had lost 50 per cent of its cells. Swollen, chromatolytic nerve cells are often present. Pathological cells of a similar type are also to be found here and there in the nucleus ambiguus, facial, abducens, trochlear and oculomotor nuclei. Lesions of the motor nucleus of the trigeminal nerve are rarer but were noted by Werdnig and others. Occasional swollen cells and figures of neuronophagia have also been seen in the nucleus supraspinalis, formatio reticularis, and the lateral vestibular nucleus.

Suprasegmental lesions have been especially emphasised by Radermaker (1951, 1953) who has described pathological changes in the substantia nigra, the nucleus subthalamicus, thalamus, dentate nuclei and cerebellar cortex. Thalamic lesions have also been described by Gruner and Bargeton (1952) and were conspicuous features of the writer's cases (Fig. 6.129). In one of the latter there were also developmental and degenerative changes in the cerebellum and a pallido-Luysial atrophy (Norman 1961 a).

Cerebral cortex. There are a few reports in the literature of small, underdeveloped Betz cells or even of absent Betz cells in the motor cortex (Burdick *et al.* 1945) but as Brandt (1950)

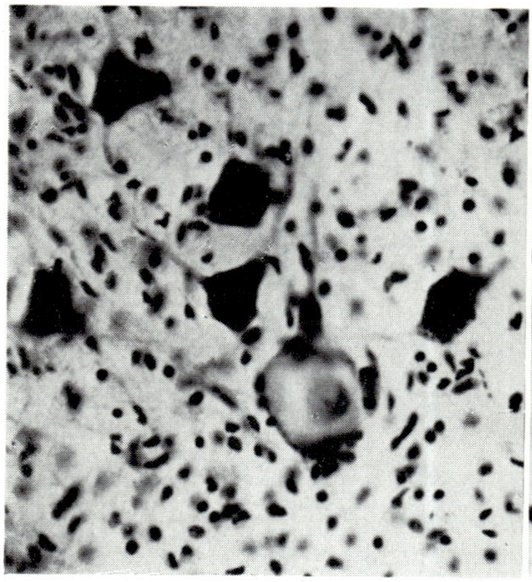

6.124

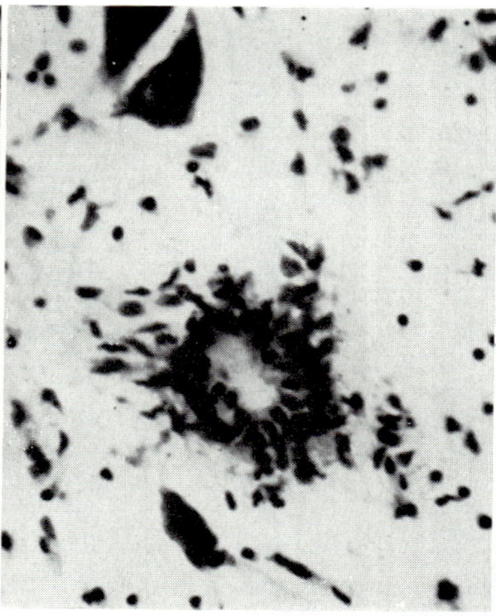

6.125

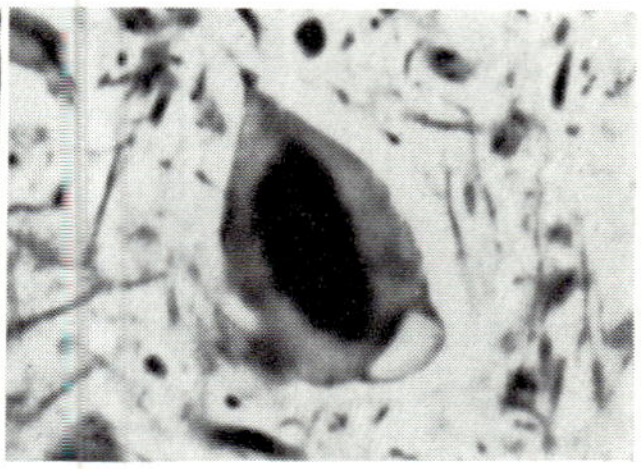

6.126

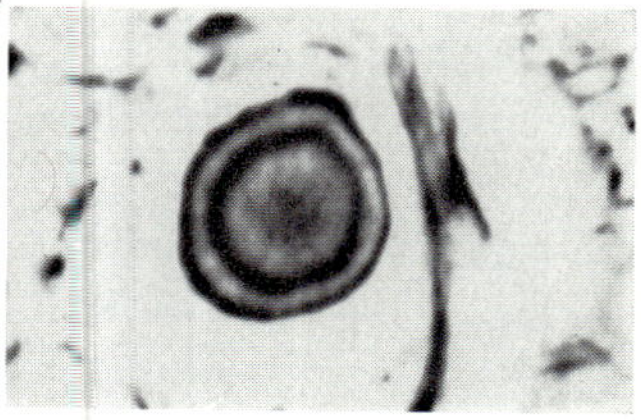

6.127

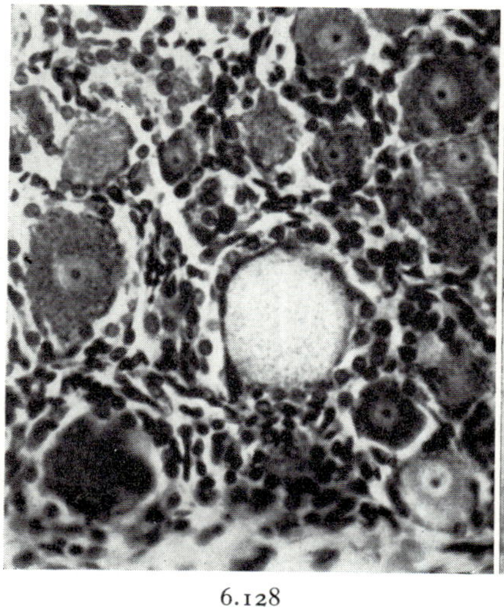

6.128

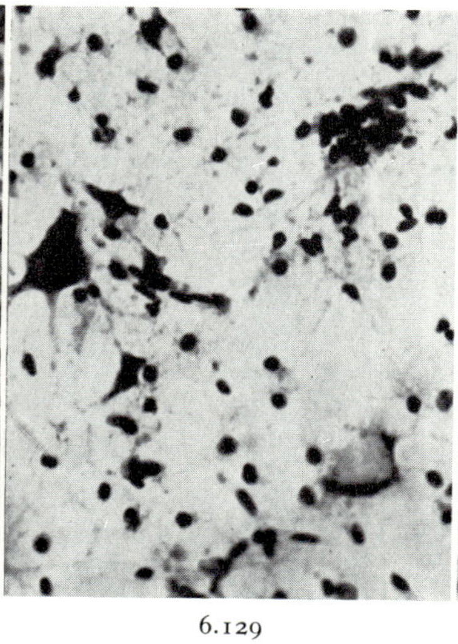

6.129

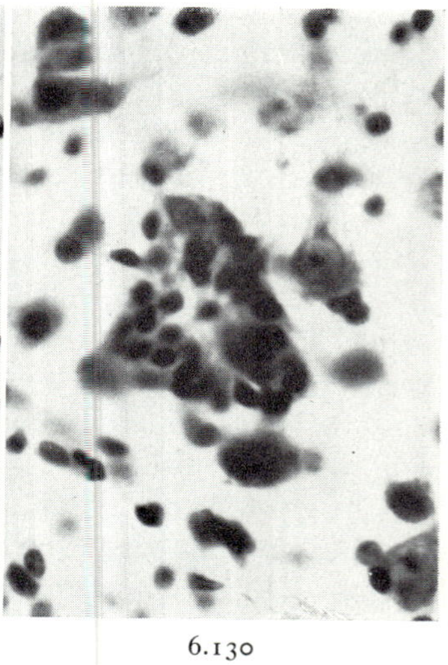

6.130

FIG. 6.124. *Werdnig-Hoffmann's disease.* Anterior horn cell showing typical chromatolytic swelling (Carbol azure.)

FIG. 6.125. Neuronophagia of an anterior horn cell. (Carbol azure.)

FIGS. 6.126 and 6.127. Two nerve cells from the hypoglossal nucleus showing degenerative changes. (Bielschowsky.)

FIG. 6.128. Posterior root ganglion showing one chromatolytic cell. (Carbol azure.)

FIG. 6.129. Thalamus. One degenerate nerve cell and a figure of neuronophagia are shown. (Carbol azure.)

FIG. 6.130. Neuronophagia of a large pyramidal cell in the 5th layer of the precentral gyrus. (Carbol azure.)

has pointed out, the great variability in the appearance of these cells in infants makes it advisable to accept such findings with reserve. Far more convincing is the observation of Conel (1938) who found 4 obviously pathological giant pyramidal cells in the motor cortex after an extensive search. In 2 cases of Werdnig-Hoffmann disease the writer also found evidence of nerve cell degeneration in the 5th layer of the precentral gyrus (Fig. 6.130).

Arthrogryphosis multiplex congenita

This syndrome of congenital deformity and rigidity of the extremities has variable pathological features. In some cases only the muscles are affected, in others there have been marked abnormalities in the spinal cord and motor roots. The anterior horn cells may be grossly depleted, but signs of progressive neuronal degeneration are absent. Bargeton *et al.* (1961) have recently reviewed the literature and have added a new pathological variant which is characterised by plaques of collagen in the anterior spinal roots. The mechanism of the contractures occurring in this syndrome is not understood (Adams *et al.* 1953).

Progressive cerebellar degeneration in childhood

The commonest type of cerebellar degeneration in children is that associated with symmetrical telangiectasia of the bulbar conjunctiva and parts of the skin, a syndrome often called ataxia-telangiectasia' or named after Louis-Bar (1941) who first described the condition,

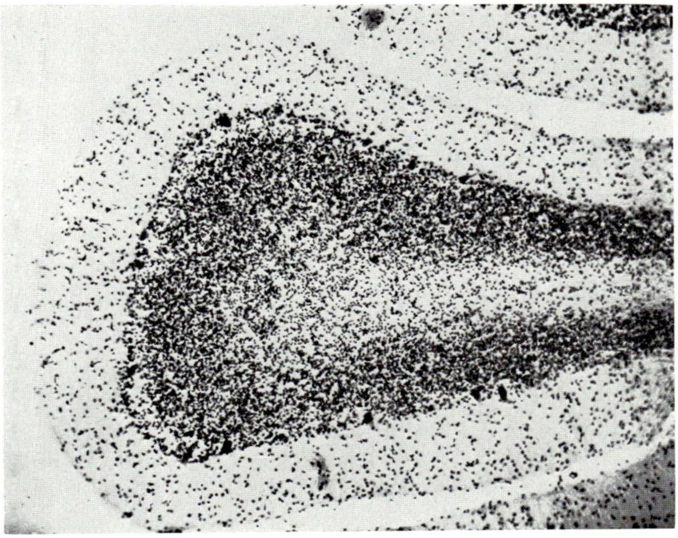

FIG. 6.131. *Ataxia-telangiectasia.* The cerebellum shows severe loss of Purkinje cells and diffuse rarefaction of the granular cell layer (25μ section). (Carbol azure.)

clinically. Korein *et al.* (1961) have summarised the clinical findings in 23 cases, and over 50 have been recognised up to the present time (Sedgwick and Boder 1960). The few neuropathological reports available have shown the expected cerebellar atrophy and little else. There is a reduction in the numbers of Purkinje cells and a diffuse thinning of the granular layer (Fig. 6.131). The vermis was especially affected in the familial cases of Biemond and van Bolhuis (1959). Centerwall and Miller (1958) reported minor additional lesions in the frontal cortex and substantia nigra and noted the presence of abnormally large veins in the cerebral and cerebellar meninges. The latter finding was not present in Biemond's cases or in an example of the syndrome examined by the writer. The cerebellar degeneration is not, therefore, to be regarded as conditioned by a vascular anomaly. Although some of these patients develop athetosis, no pathological basis for the hyperkinesia has yet been demonstrated in the basal ganglia.

As in the adult, system degenerations involving the cerebellum may arise in childhood, though they are much rarer. Malamud and Cohen (1958) have described a syndrome characterised by cerebellar ataxia, later masked by extrapyramidal rigidity, which was inherited as a sex-linked recessive. In addition to diffuse loss of Purkinje cells, degenerative changes were present in the dentate nucleus, thalamus and pallido-Luysial system.

The Hallervorden-Spatz Syndrome. By A. Meyer

The names of Hallervorden and Spatz have been given to a rare condition to which they first drew attention in 1922. Approximately 30 pathologically verified cases of this syndrome have been described to date; it is however difficult to give an exact figure, since the position of some cases in the group is still uncertain. In this total are included a few cases described before 1922 and identified retrospectively: a case of Fischer (1911), the macroscopically investigated case of Rothmann (1915) and the case, Oscar M., of the Vogts (1920).

Reviews of the condition include those of Kalinowsky (1936), Peters (1951) and a comprehensive one by Eicke (1957).

Clinically the condition is characterised by progressive rigidity, first in the lower and later in the upper extremities; an equino-varus deformity of the foot has been recorded as the first presenting sign in several cases. Rigidity is often preceded or accompanied by choreic or athetoid movements, more rarely by torsion dystonia. Both rigidity and involuntary movements may extend to the muscles of the face, tongue and palate, resulting in difficulties in articulation and swallowing. Progressive mental deterioration is a frequent, though not constant, manifestation. Epileptic convulsions have been reported only in the cases of the Vogts (1920), Meyer and Earl (1936), Vincent and van Bogaert (1936) and Fünfgeld (1929–30). In almost all cases the onset was in the first or second decade, and death occurred usually before the thirtieth year of life. Later onset has been recorded, however, by Onari (1925), Hallervorden (1930) and Eicke.

In several reports the condition was found to be *familial*, with incidence frequent in other siblings, though almost never in the ancestors or wider family. Hallervorden and Spatz encountered a clinically identical condition in five of nine siblings; three more children had died early from unknown causes. Onset in the cases they described was between 7 and 9 years, with death occurring at the ages of 16 to 27. Of these one brain was fully investigated, whilst sections from a second brain revealed identical pathology. Familial cases with post-mortem findings have also been reported by Winkelman (1932), Kalinowsky (1927), Urechia *et al.* (1950) and Messing (quoted from Eicke). Eicke includes also the familial cases briefly reported by Fischer (1933), but these were complicated and Fischer himself considered them to be examples of a new syndrome.

Pathology. On macroscopic inspection of the brain the rust-brown discoloration of the globus pallidus and the reticular zone of the substantia nigra is in most cases a striking finding. This discoloration is caused by a very considerable increase of the normal pigment in these centres. In its natural state the pigment has a yellowish-brown colour and, with thionin or cresyl violet, stains in numerous shades of yellow, green and blue. It may be intracellular, in nerve cells, hyperplastic astrocytes, and microglial cells, or may lie free in the tissue, usually as large granules surrounding the blood-vessels. Part of it gives a strong iron reaction. This colourful picture is in almost all cases enhanced by the presence of strongly siderophilic incrustations of the medium-sized blood-vessels and capillaries and of free-lying mulberry concretions (the pseudo-calcium of the German schools).

Apart from the consistent pigmentary increase the other changes within the pallido-reticular zone are more variable. Severe degeneration and loss of nerve cells has been reported in some cases; in others, particularly in familial cases, this may be slight or negligible. Demyelination, particularly of the fine fibres, is usually present, but was absent in some cases. Proliferation of astrocytes and glial fibrosis is found in most cases, though to a variable degree.

The finding of large oval discs staining faintly with thionin and lying between the extracellular pigment granules has aroused some discussion: they are now regarded, as was originally suggested by Hallervorden and Spatz, as being derived from swollen axons. Their occurrence may be widespread beyond the pallido-reticular zone. A histochemical analysis reveals them as consisting of mucoprotoids, according to Seitelberger and Gross (1957) and Gross *et al.* (1957), who suggest the term 'neuro-axonal mucoprotoid dystrophy' for the condition. Neither the axonal changes nor the pigment deposits alone are regarded by these authors as specific signs; in combination, however, they consider them to have considerable diagnostic value.*

Eicke described a remarkable increase of capillaries in the reticular zone in one of his cases: although the resemblance to Wernicke's encephalopathy was striking, the corpora mammillaria and other predilective sites of the latter syndrome were not affected.

In many cases histological changes in other parts of the brain and in the spinal cord have been reported, but again they vary greatly in intensity and were slight in some of the familial cases. Hallervorden and Spatz described loss of nerve cells in the cerebral cortex and the Purkinje cell layer of the cerebellum; this finding has been confirmed in other cases. Jervis (1952) found pigment, histochemically indistinguishable from that of the pallido-reticular zone, in the cortex of a case in which the Hallervorden-Spatz syndrome was associated with amaurotic family idiocy. The striatum was found to be involved by Kalinowsky and Onari. The corpus Luysii showed considerable demyelination and gliosis in the cases of the Vogts, and in that of Meyer and Earl who also reported gliosis in the dentate nucleus and inferior olives. Retinitis pigmentosa accounted for visual disturbances in the cases of Winkelman, Kalinowsky and Helfand (1935). Degeneration of the pyramidal tract was seen in 5, and of the posterior tracts of the spinal cord in 2 cases.

Diagnosis and nosology. Although the clinical observation of progressive rigidity with or without involuntary movements and mental deterioration, commencing towards the middle or end of the first decade, may suggest the Hallervorden-Spatz syndrome, a reasonably certain diagnosis can only be made *post mortem.*

Differential diagnosis from the clinically similar progressive juvenile striato-pallidal (Hunt 1917), pallidal and pallido-Luysial (van Bogaert 1946) syndromes is pathologically straightforward. In these conditions the pigment is not appreciably increased, nor is the reticular zone affected.

The separation of the Hallervorden-Spatz syndrome from *état dysmyélinique* of the Vogts presents greater difficulties. In fact, earlier investigators (Hallervorden and Spatz, Hallervorden, Meyer and Earl) more or less identified the two conditions. It is now increasingly realised, however, that état dysmyélinique is ill-defined and contains, in addition to possible cases of the Hallervorden-Spatz syndrome, conditions caused by anoxia and injury at birth, by Rhesus factor incompatibility and by other infantile diseases. In such cases the lesions appear soon after birth, are not markedly progressive, and are usually severe and widespread. In contrast, in what is now conceived to be the Hallervorden-Spatz syndrome, onset is usually

* See also the recent comprehensive review of this subject by Cowen, D. and Olmstead, E. V. (1963). *J Neuropath.*, **22**, 175.

towards the second half of the first decade, is preceded by normal development, and progression is marked. The important lesions are more or less confined to the pallidum and the reticular zone; when lesions occur elsewhere they are, on the whole, variable or slight. Within the pallido-reticular zone, emphasis is on the striking increase of pigment rather than on neuronal degeneration. The condition thus approximates to a system disease (though in the form of a localised storage of iron-containing pigment rather than of degeneration), to which Helfand has given the name of 'status pigmentosus'. Most of the familial cases and some of the solitary ones (particularly those of Helfand, Vincent and van Bogaert, and 2 cases of Eicke) would correspond to this description.

This more restricted definition of the syndrome renders the position of some of the remaining solitary cases dubious. It is probably no coincidence that in seven of these—almost half of their total—onset was at or soon after birth (Eicke). Their claim to inclusion in the syndrome should therefore be submitted to further scrutiny. Meyer and Earl's case may serve as an example: owing to poor history, no definite statement could be made as to whether the case was solitary or familial nor whether there had been progression. It is likely, however, that onset had been soon after birth. Post-mortem, selective involvement of globus pallidus and zona reticularis was striking; nerve cell loss, demyelination and gliosis were severe, however, whilst pigmentary increase was only moderate. Moreover additional lesions were described in the corpus Luysii, dentate nucleus and inferior olives, a combination which recalled, as the authors themselves pointed out, the pathology of kernicterus.

Increase of pigment in globus pallidus and substantia nigra reticularis has been reported, however, in other conditions, ranging from central neurofibromatosis (Gamper 1929), myopathies (Hallervorden), dementia praecox (Fünfgeld) and epidemic encephalitis (van Bogaert 1939–40) to rheumatic encephalopathy (Benda 1949) and amaurotic family idiocy (Jervis). Each investigator insists that the increase was definitely outside the physiological range. In at least 1 case of Benda's material, and in Jervis's case, the amount of pigment was of the same magnitude as that described in Hallervorden and Spatz' original publication. Hallervorden suggested that in such circumstances the pigment increase is usually not associated with neuronal or glial changes, but these latter changes may be slight also in some cases of otherwise indisputable Hallervorden-Spatz syndrome. The question therefore arises whether status pigmentosus may be precipitated by other, particularly by inflammatory, conditions (Benda), or whether there may be a coincidence of two independent conditions, as suggested by Jervis. A relationship to lipid storage diseases seems to have obtained some, though yet unconfirmed support from the histochemical observations of Zeman and Scarpelli (1958), who in two cases of Hallervorden-Spatz disease found widespread ganglioside and sphingomyelin deposits in nerve cells and ependymal cells. The neurones in the corpus striatum, in the 5th and 6th layers of the cerebral cortex and in the reticular substance were ballooned and their nuclei eccentric.

Aetiology. The nosological difficulties are aggravated by our almost total ignorance of the origin and of the significance of the normal, as well as of the pathological, pigment. Eicke suggested that perhaps a deficiency of an enzyme might be responsible, but was unable to adduce concrete evidence. Helfand noticed in his case, in addition to the status pigmentosus, abnormalities in the formation of melanin pigment in the substantia nigra and locus coeruleus, and consequently suggested a more fundamental disturbance in pigment metabolism; his findings, however, have not been generally confirmed. Pentschew *et al.* (1962) commented on the resemblance of the axon swellings to those which they had observed in experimental vitamin E deficiency. Metabolic investigations will help to clarify the aetiological problem, but, so far, they are only in their infancy.

IV. THE NEURONAL STORAGE DISEASES

The products of abnormal lipid or carbohydrate metabolism may accumulate within the nerve cells causing a distention of the cyton and peripheral displacement of the nucleus and neurofibrils. In Niemann-Pick's disease this process of storage is shared by neurones, reticulo-endothelial system and the parenchyma of liver, spleen and other organs. In Gaucher's disease, in which the reticulo-endothelial cells of liver and spleen are constantly affected, the nervous system may be involved in both the infantile and juvenile forms. In the amaurotic family idiocies, on the other hand, the metabolic disorder is usually localised in the nervous system, only a minority of cases showing visceral involvement. In the metachromatic type of leucodystrophy the nerve cells participate to some extent in the storage of sulphatide, but, since the predominant changes are found in the white matter, this condition is described in the chapter on demyelinating diseases.

Another condition commonly classed as a lipidosis is gargoylism. In this disease lipid metabolism appears to be deranged in the nerve cells but not in the parenchyma of the liver or other affected visceral organs where there is a massive deposition of polysaccharides. Finally, in the rare cardiomuscular form of glycogen disease the nerve cells participate in the carbohydrate storage.

In recent years the focus of interest in the lipidoses has moved away from histological features towards the more fundamental problem of the underlying biochemical abnormalities (Cumings 1960). The task of classification based on chemical or histochemical criteria is, however, by no means an easy one since the lipids are usually present in the form of mixtures and there is variation in their proportions not only from organ to organ but from family to family.

The amaurotic family idiocies

The first member of this group of closely related diseases to be identified was the infantile form, the characteristic ophthalmological picture of which was described by Tay in 1881. The clinical and neuropathological features were described later by Sachs (1887). The familiar character of the condition became apparant when the sister of Sachs' original patient developed the same disease and it was then that the name 'amaurotic family idiocy' was introduced (Sachs 1896). With the passage of time there has come into use a classification of different clinical types of amaurotic idiocy dependent upon the age of onset of the disease. Thus in addition to the classical infantile form of Tay-Sachs there are now descriptions of congenital, late infantile, juvenile, early adult and late adult variants. With certain exceptions to be noted in the older cases the clinical features of progressive mental deterioration with blindness, epilepsy, myoclonus and spasticity or hyperkinesis are shared by the whole group. All the variants are inherited as simple Mendelian recessives, though occasional dominant transmission has been reported in the juvenile and adult forms (van Bogaert 1953). Broadly speaking, the earlier the onset the more florid is the cerebral lipidosis and the more rapid the fatal outcome. In the older age groups, on the other hand, there is a tendency for certain parts of the brain to be preferentially selected by the disease process and in the adult variety the line between lipidosis and system degeneration may be very finely drawn.

At first sight it would appear that the introduction of so many transitional forms had converted what at one time seemed to be a number of separate clinico-pathological entities into a continuous series. In point of fact, a sufficient number of cases are on record to enable a clear-cut distinction to be made between the two most common variants of amaurotic family idiocy, namely, the infantile and the juvenile or, as they are preferably called, Tay-Sachs disease and Batten's disease. A decisive clinical point of difference lies in the contrasting ophthalmological features of the two conditions, the cherry-red spot and large white halo of Tay-Sachs disease never having been found in the same sibship as the macular and retinal pigmentary degeneration of the Batten type (Wyburn-Mason 1943, Danis *et al.* 1957).

Tay-Sachs disease

Macroscopically the brain usually shows generalised atrophy with thickened leptomeninges, excess of fluid in the subarachnoid space, gaping sulci and shrunken convolutions of a rubbery consistency. The optic nerves are unduly thin and the cerebellum may show a marked reduction in size owing to obvious sclerotic atrophy. In several instances the brain has been exceptionally large and heavy with weights of the order of 1,450 g. (Holmes 1911), 1,530 g. (Savini-Castano 1913), 1,690 g. (Bielschowsky 1920–1), 1,980 g. (Jervis 1940) and 2,300 g. (Steegmann and Karnosh 1936). There may be minor abnormalities of gyral pattern but micropolygyria has only been reported on one occasion (Ostertag 1925). Microscopically the leptomeninges show mild fibrosis and contain small numbers of lipid-laden macrophages. The architectonics of the cerebral cortex may be disorganised in places because of severe loss of nerve cells, but in general the normal stratification is preserved. It is usual to find every nerve cell body in the cerebral cortex greatly enlarged and with a round, ovoid or pyriform contour, the nucleus being displaced to the periphery, most frequently towards the apical dendrite. The Nissl bodies have disappeared except in some of the larger nerve cells, such as the giant cells of Betz, in which they may be confined to a small area usually at the apex of the cell (Fig. 6.132).

In frozen sections untreated with lipid solvents the cell bodies are seen to be filled with a finely granular or more diffusely distributed material having the following staining reactions: colourless or a feeble pink or yellow with Scharlach R., dark grey with the Kultschitsky-Pal method (maximal after 4 days mordanting according to Weston Hurst 1925) (Fig. 6.134), bright pink with the P.A.S. stain and a rosy red with Cajal's gold sublimate (Globus 1942). There is no blackening with osmic acid and the material is not doubly refractile. These staining reactions are influenced by changes in the composition of the lipid mixtures stored within the cells, so that regional differences are common and there is considerable variation from family to family. The material is usually readily soluble in cold acid alcohol, ether or chloroform, though in some instances a small amount of insoluble lipid may remain in the cells.

When the granular material has been dissolved many of the larger cells are seen to contain a fine reticulum which stains blue with basic dyes. With Bielschowsky's stain it is evident that the neurofibrils have been displaced to the periphery, where they form a condensed ring continuous with the axon and dendrites. Ovoid expansions of the apical dendrites are also a feature of the pyramidal nerve cells in amaurotic idiocy (Fig. 6.133). They may be very common in some cases, rare in others. These expansions are usually larger than the body of the parent cell and contain a much greater amount of the same type of lipid. In addition to this phenomenon of neuronal storage, which in Tay-Sachs disease is virtually ubiquitous throughout the nervous system, the cerebral cortex often shows in places a reduction in the number of nerve cells. This change is somewhat masked by the great swelling of the remaining neurones but in the more patchy areas of destruction, lipid phagocytosis and gliosis are easily recognised and certain cortical layers, most commonly the fourth, may be selectively affected (M. Vogt 1929). Status spongiosus affecting in particular the deeper layers is also not uncommon. One may assume that in these areas the nerve cells show a special vulnerability to the generalised metabolic disturbance. Bird (1948) considers that in amaurotic idiocy the distended cells may finally burst and their débris become absorbed. Degenerative changes of another sort may be seen in the cortical nerve cells of patients in whom life has been prolonged

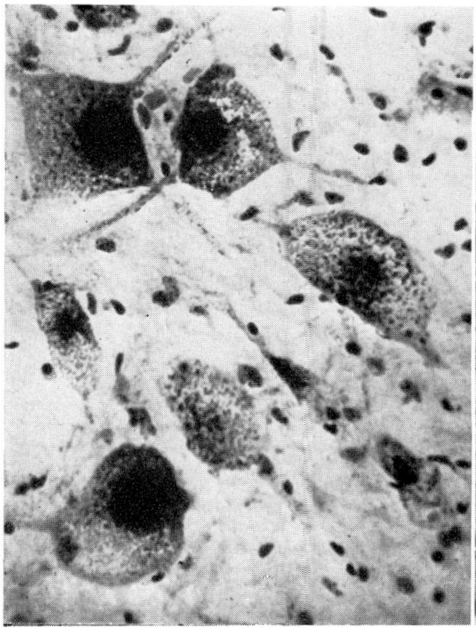

6.132

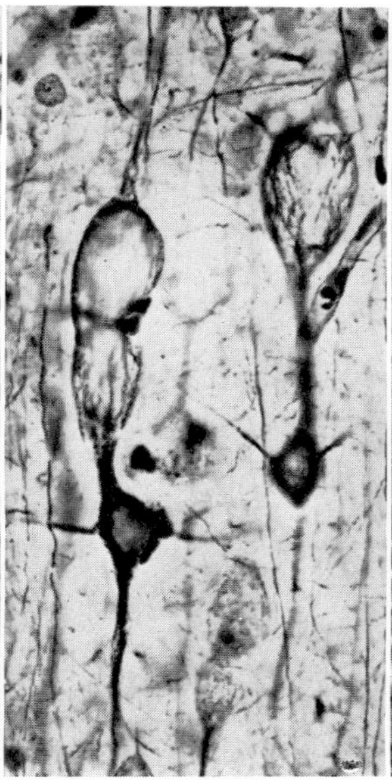

6.133

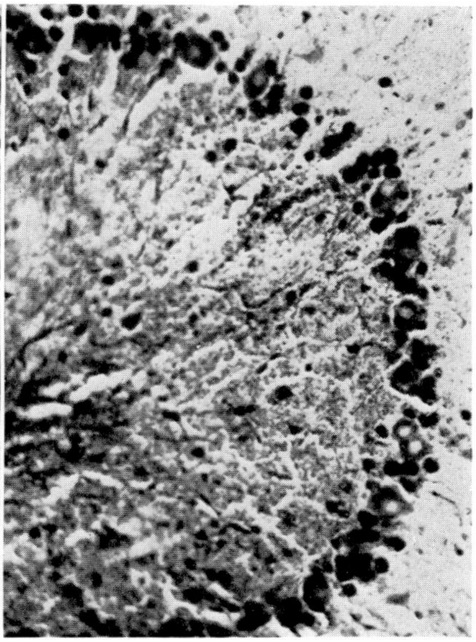

6.134

6.136

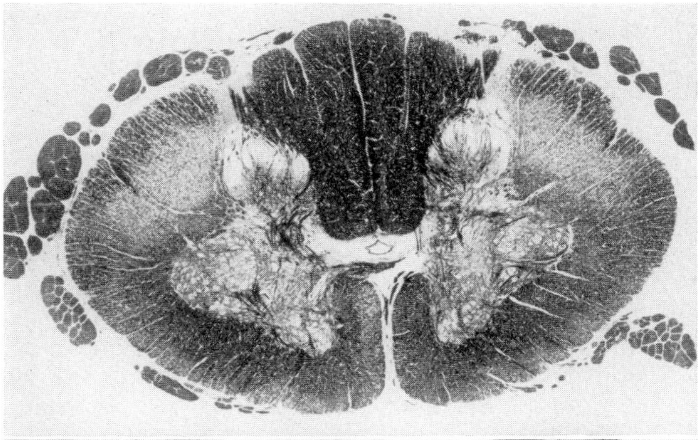

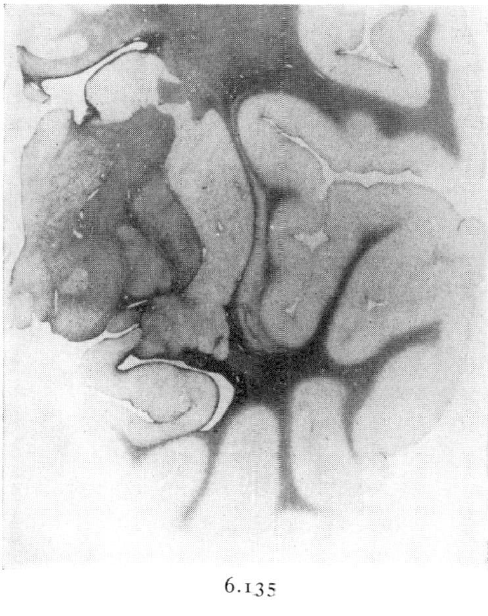

6.135

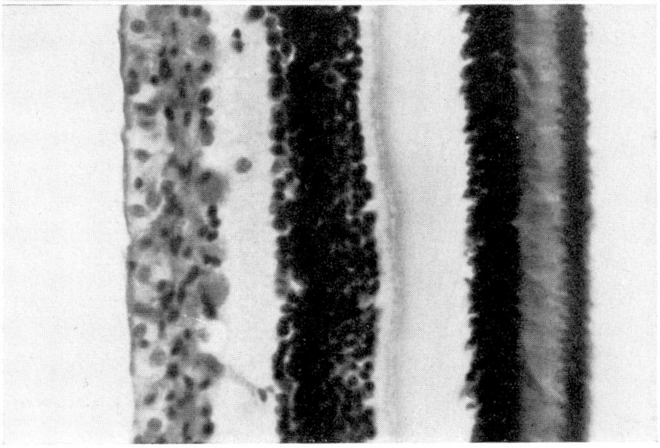

6.137

FIG. 6.132. *Cerebral lipidosis.* Anterior horn cells showing the swelling typical of Tay-Sachs or Niemann-Pick's disease. (Carbol azure.)

FIG. 6.133. Distension of apical dendrites in Tay-Sachs disease. (Bielschowsky.)

FIG. 6.134. Cerebellum in Niemann-Pick's disease showing staining of the lipid in the Purkinje cells and microglial phagocytes with haematoxylin. (Kultschitsky-Pal stain on frozen section.)

FIG. 6.135. Gliosis of white matter in Niemann-Pick's or Tay-Sachs disease.

FIG. 6.136. Pyramidal tract degeneration in a case of Tay-Sachs disease.

FIG. 6.137. Tay-Sachs disease. Retina near the fovea showing degeneration and lipidosis of the ganglion cells. The remaining cells and some large phagocytes stain pink with the P.A.S. stain (grey in photograph). (P.A.S. and haematoxylin.)

beyond the normal span for Tay-Sachs disease. Only a comparatively small number of the large inflated cells are present in the cerebral cortex of such cases. Instead there is a marked reduction in the nerve cell content, most of the survivors being represented by small rounded cells with one or sometimes two shrunken and pyknotic nuclei. They are filled with the same poorly sudanophil lipid as are the neurones elsewhere in the brain, but their content is denser or more coarsely granular and stains more deeply in Nissl preparations. These shrunken cells with degenerated nuclei apparently represent the later stages of a more chronic degenerative process. Somewhat similar nerve cell changes were described by Jervis (1952 a) in a case of Tay-Sachs disease which had survived to the age of 11 years. Striking accumulations of an iron-containing pigment similar to that found in the Hallervorden-Spatz disease was present in the globus pallidus, the red zone of the substantia nigra, the thalamus and to a less extent in the dentate nuclei, hypothalamus and cerebral cortex. In the latter site the microgliocytes were hyperplastic and contained phagocytosed pigment.

Electronmicroscopical studies by Terry have shown that the intra-neuronal lipid granules in Tay-Sachs disease are multilaminated structures differing sharply in their morphology from the lipid aggregates in the juvenile form (Terry *et al.* 1962). Chemical analysis of concentrates of the granules obtained by differentiated centrifugalisation showed a 30–40 per cent content of ganglioside (Samuels *et al.* 1962).

Increase in *neuroglial fibres* in the cortical grey matter is, generally speaking, not a marked feature except where severe neuronal destruction has taken place. Usually only a moderate gliosis of the molecular layer spreads into the superficial cortical layers for a short distance. Microglial proliferation, on the other hand, may be conspicuous especially in the more degenerated areas and fat-granule cells containing neutral fat with or without a doubly-refractile component of cholesterol esters are scattered throughout the grey matter, and are often particularly common in the molecular layer and outer zone of the cortex, while large aggregations are seen round some of the blood-vessels. Some of these microglial phagocytes contain the same poorly staining lipid as is found in the nerve cells, so that it would appear that a breakdown of the lipid into simpler forms is carried out within these cells. Scanty neutral fat globules are also present on the surface of the cell bodies of the astrocytes.

Profound disturbances of *myelination* occur in many cases. The fibre systems of the cerebral cortex are always severely impoverished and the remaining sheaths show marked beading. Pallor of myelin staining is present especially in those parts of the centrum semiovale which myelinate late, and the pyramidal tracts and corticopontine and pontocerebellar fibre systems may show a system-like degeneration (Fig. 6.136). The cerebral white matter shows considerable fibrous gliosis (Fig. 6.135). In another group widespread status spongiosus is present throughout the white matter of the hemispheres and in these cases the brain weight is usually greatly increased. These are the examples previously mentioned of megalencephaly in Tay-Sachs disease. There is evidence that this disintegration of the white matter may be associated with the chronicity of the disease process, since it has been found in patients suffering from Tay-Sachs disease whose lives have been exceptionally prolonged by modern methods of medical treatment (Aronson *et al.* 1955). It is unlikely, however, that this massive destruction of the white matter is due entirely to antecedent degeneration of nerve cells, since there are chemical changes which form a link with the leucodystrophies (Bérard-Badier *et al.* 1958; Thieffrey *et al.* 1960).

The *cerebellum* shares in the generalised neuronal storage of lipid, the cell bodies of the Purkinje cells being swollen and their dendrites frequently showing antler-like expansions also filled with lipid (Fig. 6.134). In cases with naked-eye shrinkage of the cerebellum there is usually marked destruction of both the Purkinje cell and granular layers with accompanying severe fibrous gliosis. This glial overgrowth is most clearly seen in the molecular layer where the thickened and proliferated fibrils of the Bergmann cells form a dense palisade.

Elsewhere in the nervous system the same distension of nerve cells with lipid is always present. The *thalamus* is often severely affected, with great cell loss and gliosis mainly in the nuclei concerned with the cortical projection systems. In the larger nerve cells of the *brain stem* and *spinal cord* (Fig. 6.132) the lipid infiltration is often less massive than elsewhere and some of the Nissl substance may be preserved. The pathological findings in the retina are of special interest in view of the clinical importance of the eye changes in distinguishing the Tay-Sachs and Batten types of amaurotic idiocy. The ganglion cells are swollen with lipid, this change being most marked near the fovea (Fig. 6.137). At the margins of the fovea the ganglion cells show a considerable reduction in number and are intermingled with large phagocytic cells of a greater diameter than the nerve cells themselves (Greenfield 1951). The inner and outer nuclear layers, on the other hand, are normal. These findings are consistent with the explanation given for the occurrence of the cherry-red spot in amaurotic idiocy, namely, that this appearance is due to the normal colour of the fovea being accentuated by the surrounding whitish flare. This whitish ring, which is the abnormal feature of the macular region, is probably due to the increased opacity of the tissues consequent upon the lipid infiltration of the ganglion cells. The thinning of the nerve cell layer in the margin of the fovea may also make the red of the choriocapillary layer more evident. When the ganglion cells have degenerated entirely, as may happen in long-standing cases, the cherry-red spot is no longer seen.

Chemistry. In a series of papers dating from 1939 and summarised in his 1955 article, Klenk demonstrated that in Tay-Sachs disease the grey matter contains a notable excess of gangliosides. These complex substances are sphingolipids closely related to sphingomyelin and cerebroside and contain galactose, glucose chondrosamine and neuraminic acid groups, the latter component giving the sensitive colour reaction by which ganglioside is estimated by Klenk's method. Ganglioside is also significantly increased in the white matter in this condition, but its site of storage is not known.

The relationship of Tay-Sachs disease to Niemann-Pick's disease. Bielschowsky (1928) examined the central nervous system in Pick's original case and found that the changes in the nerve cells were identical with those of Tay-Sachs disease. The main difference in the cerebral pathology is that in Niemann-Pick's disease storage of lipid also occurs in the endothelium of blood-vessels, in arachnoid cells and in macrophages present in the connective tissue stroma of the choroid plexus. Bielschowsky's view that both conditions are variants of one nosological entity was strongly contested over many years by Schaffer (1930), who maintained that there were distinguishing histological features, particularly in the cerebellum. This claim received support from the comparison made between the two conditions by Norman *et al.* (1959 a). Not only did the nerve cells in their Niemann-Pick's brain stain very feebly or not at all with P.A.S., but the microglial phagocytes were much more intensely haematoxyphilic (Fig. 6.125). The chemical differences are more decisive. Ganglioside in Niemann-Pick's disease never reaches the high level of infantile amaurotic idiocy. In the infantile form of Niemann-Pick's disease there is a substantial storage of sphingomyelin and cholesterol in the brain, the liver and spleen. Only in the older children suffering from this disease may this absolute increase of sphingomyelin or phospholipid be lacking (Crocker and Farber 1958). Finally, the visceral changes in the two diseases are entirely different. The writer's example of Tay-Sachs' disease with visceral involvement closely resembled Turban's (1944) case and showed in frozen sections empty foam cells and vacuoles devoid of lipid in the parenchymatous cells in the liver, spleen and other organs. Chemical analysis showed a marked increase in hexosamine, suggesting a storage of polysaccharides. In Niemann-Pick's disease, on the other hand, the histiocytes and parenchyma were filled with haematoxyphil lipid.

The Batten type of amaurotic family idiocy

Batten (1903) gave the first clinical description of a juvenile form of amaurotic idiocy affecting a brother and sister, the symptoms starting at the age of 5 years and 6 years respectively. This variant differs from Tay-Sachs disease in its later onset, in the slower progress of the dementia, with death at about 18 years, and in the ophthalmological findings. The latter consist in pigmentary peppering of the macula with a later spread of the pigmentary degeneration to involve the whole retina. Optic atrophy may, however, occur without pigmentary changes. The disease has no predilection for the Jewish race. The neuropathological features were first described by H. Vogt (1905) and Spielmeyer (1905). In 1914 b Bielschowsky reported an additional 'late infantile variant' of amaurotic idiocy but subsequent experience has indicated that this intermediate form belongs either to the Tay-Sachs' or to the Batten group (Tingey *et al.* 1958).

Histological features. The neuronal swelling and lipidosis in the juvenile form is virtually ubiquitous but the degree of distension of individual nerve cells is seldom so marked as in Tay-Sachs disease. This is particularly so in the cerebral cortex where the nerve cells are often more pyriform in contour and may contain recognisable Nissl bodies in that part of the cyton which is free from lipid (Fig. 6.138). Since the disease at its inception affects relatively mature neurones it is usual to find much better staining of neurofibrils and dendrites than is the case in Tay-Sachs disease (Fig. 6.140). Pyramidal cells showing expansion of the apical dendrite are uncommon and severe neuronal loss or nerve cells with shrunken and pyknotic nuclei are seldom seen except in the subacute or late infantile variant. Several authors have drawn attention to the striking vacuolation of many of the thalamic nerve cells in which unusually coarse lipid granules are present (Lemieux 1954).

The intraneuronal lipid differs in several particulars from that present in Tay-Sachs disease, since it stains a bright orange with Scharlach R., does not blacken with the Kultschitsky-Pal method and is usually almost insoluble in ordinary lipid solvents. Thus frozen sections immersed in chloroform-methanol mixture for a week at 60°C may retain abundant Scharlach or P.A.S. staining material in the nerve cells.

Myelin. Myelination is not seriously affected in the juvenile cases, though a slow atrophy without accumulation of breakdown products leads to some thinning of cortical and subcortical fibres.

Fibrillary gliosis is usual in the white matter of the brain and spinal cord only in some of the subacute, younger cases. Most of the juvenile cases show an increase in the numbers of fibrous astrocytes in the deeper cortical layers, and these cells usually contain a substantial amount of the insoluble lipid. In the Swedish cases this participation of the macroglia in the lipid storage was remarkably selective in its distribution, involving mainly the neostriatum and the cerebral and cerebellar cortices (Sjövall and Ericson 1933).

Microglia. There are usually no phagocytic cells containing neutral fat in the cortical grey matter, but a few cases have shown numerous rod cells and hypertrophied branched forms containing flecks of lipid in their processes (Jervis 1941). (Fig. 6.114).

Selective vulnerability of certain centres is a feature of some of the older cases and the lipidosis may apparently occur in some parts of the brain before others. Extrapyramidal syndromes may thus be associated with specially severe changes in the substantia nigra or corpus striatum (Meyer 1931, Schob 1930).

The cerebellum is often severely degenerated and gliosed (Fig. 6.142) and may show a more

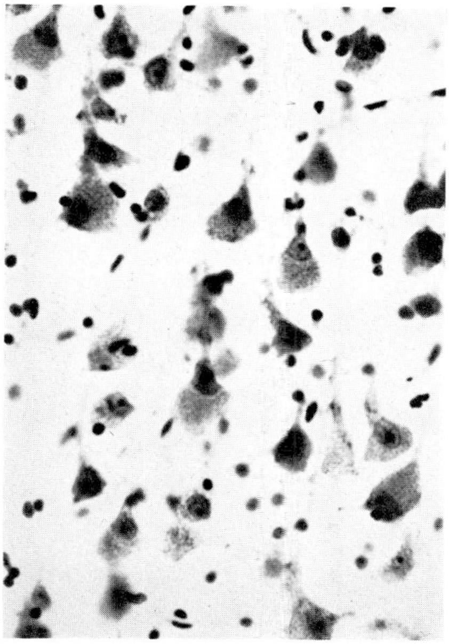

6.138

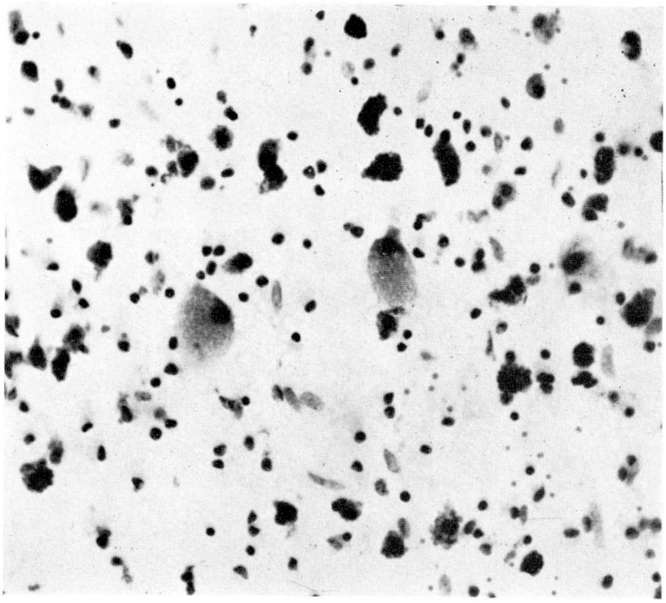

6.139

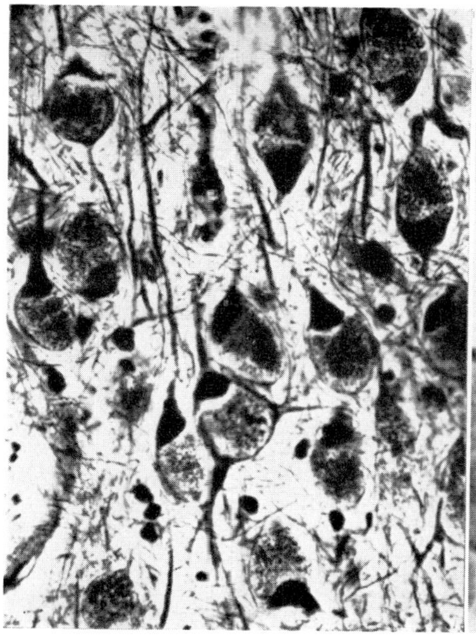

6.140

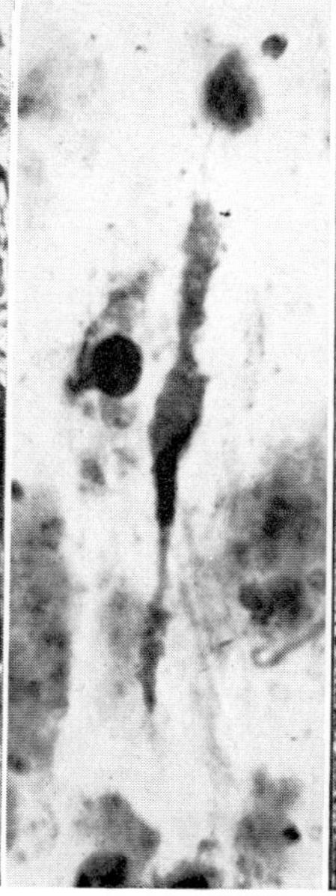

6.141

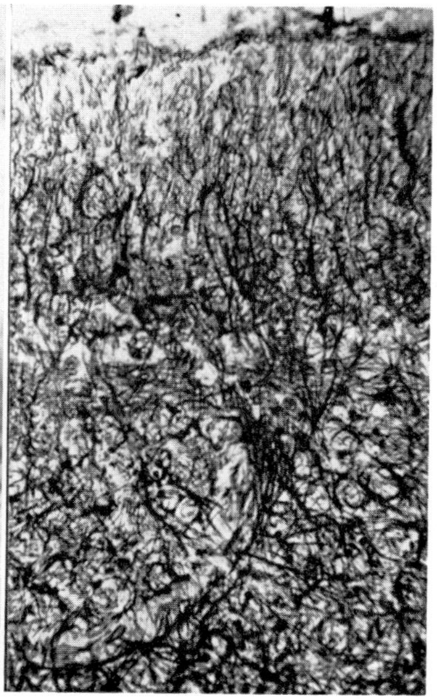

6.142

FIG. 6.138. *Batten type of amaurotic family idiocy.* Nerve cells of the 3rd cortical layer showing the swelling of lipidosis. (Carbol azure.)

FIG. 6.139. Subacute type of Batten's disease. Cerebral cortex. Two swollen nerve cells remain in a field containing shrunken lipid-laden nerve cells and microglial phagocytes. (Carbol azure.)

FIG. 6.140. Pyramidal nerve cells of the cornu Ammonis showing displaced neurofibrils and distension with lipid granules. (Bielschowsky.)

FIG. 6.141. Lipid-laden microglial rod cell from the cerebral cortex in Batten's disease. (Hortega's method for microglia.)

FIG. 6.142. Gliosis in the cerebellar cortex. (Holzer.)

or less selective loss of the granular cells together with the basket and tangential fibres (Fig. 6.143). The Purkinje cells always contain lipid (Fig. 6.144) and their dendrites frequently exhibit massive expansions shaped like antlers or cacti which also store the same material (Figs. 6.145 and 6.146). Large fusiform swellings on the axons of the Purkinje cells ('torpedoes') are also common (Fig. 6.148).

The *retinal lesions* differ from those found in Tay-Sachs disease. The outer nuclear layer, together with the rods and cones degenerate and disappear. This change seems to start at the

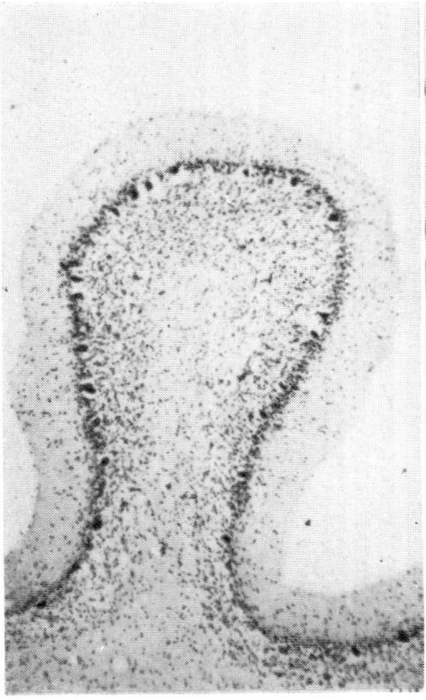

6.143

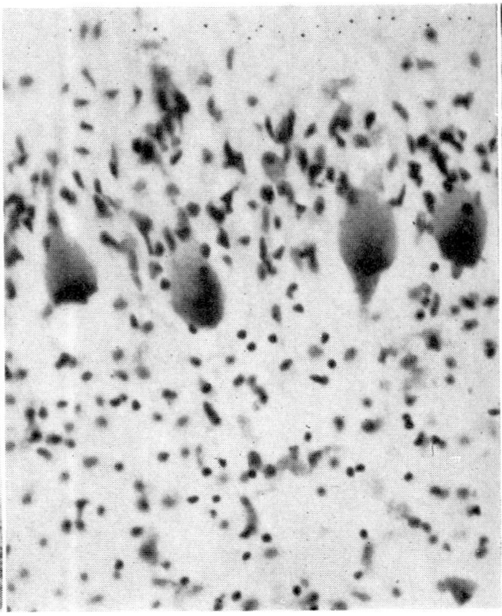

6.144

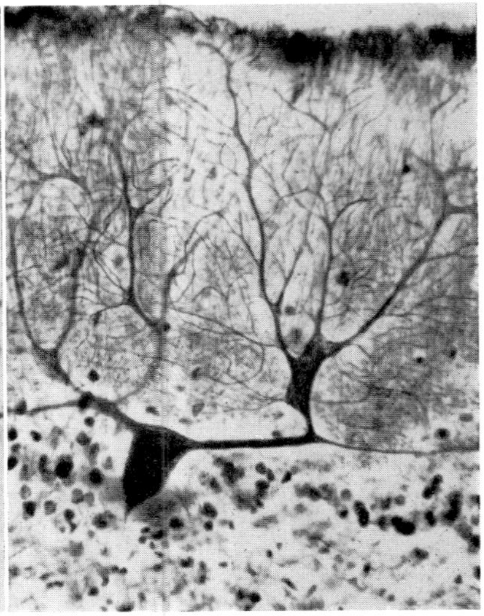

6.145

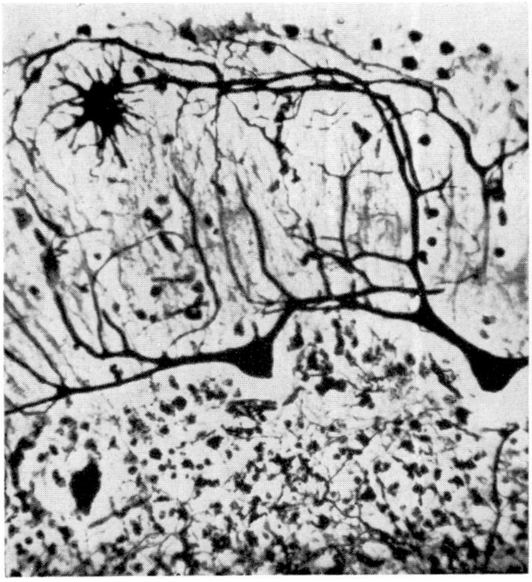

6.146

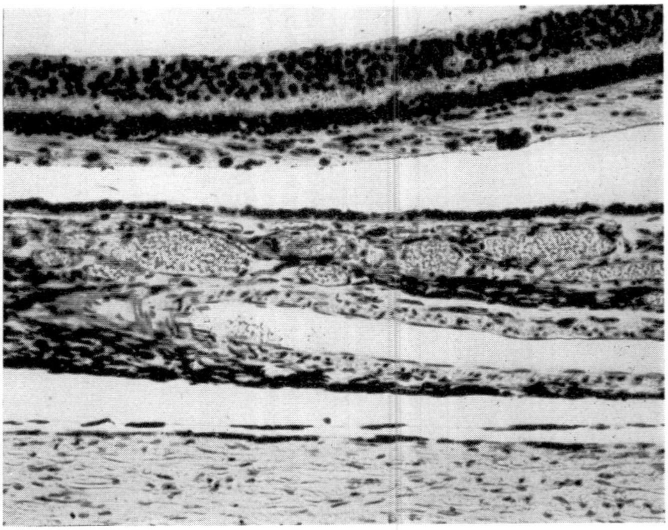

6.147

FIG. 6.143. *Batten's disease*. Atrophy of the granular layer of the cerebellum. (Carbol azure.)
FIG. 6.144. Swollen Purkinje cells and absence of granular layer.
FIG. 6.145 and 6.146. Two forms of dendritic expansions in Purkinje cells. (Cajal's silver nitrate pyridine method.)
FIG. 6.147. Retina. Preservation of the ganglion cell and inner nuclear layer. Degeneration of the outer nuclear layer and of the rods and cones. Migration of pigment from the choroid. (H. and E.)

fovea and spreads later to the more peripheral parts of the retina, the affected layers being replaced by neuroglial tissue in which migrated pigment is a conspicuous feature. The ganglion cells are usually preserved though there is some lipid storage in them as elsewhere in the nervous sytem (Greenfield and Holmes 1925) (Fig. 6.147).

Visceral lipidosis was first described in the juvenile form of amaurotic idiocy by Schob (1930) in a case showing enlargement of the spleen and lymph nodes. In 21 of the Swedish cases Sjövall (1934) also demonstrated small collections of reticulo-endothelial macrophages containing material similar to that present in the nerve cells.

Chemistry. Klenk (1953) found no marked excess of ganglioside on the chemical analysis of the grey matter in 6 juvenile cases. An unfixed brain analysed in the writer's laboratory also showed no increase over normal either in lipid hexosamine or in neuraminic acid. Histochemical methods by Diezel (1954), however, have suggested that the nerve cells store a ganglioside containing neuraminic acid. Seitelberger *et al.* (1957) have reached the same conclusion in both the juvenile and late infantile forms. The relative insolubility of the P.A.S. staining material in the neurones of the Batten type may be due to the ganglioside being bound to protein.

Other forms of amaurotic family idiocy

The adult-type of Kufs. The tendency already noted in the juvenile cases for certain centres to be affected more than others becomes accentuated in the rarer adult form of the disease

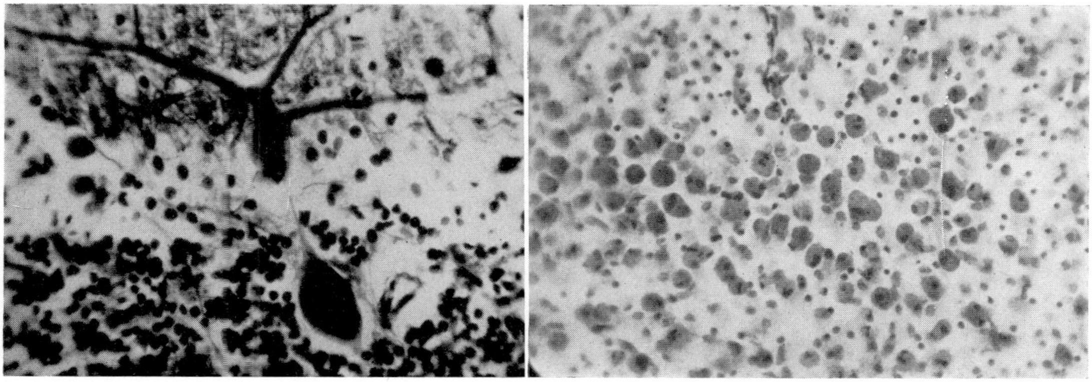

6.148 6.149

FIG. 6.148. Axonal 'torpedo' in a Purkinje cell from a case of Batten's disease with intact cerebellar granular layer. (Bielschowsky.)
FIG. 6.149. *Congenital amaurotic idiocy.* Swollen cortical nerve cells. (Cresyl violet.)

which Kufs described in 1925 and in 1931. The lipidosis is seldom so widespread and the condition may be difficult to distinguish from a presenile pigmentary atrophy or the consequences of terminal cachexia. Vision is often unimpaired and myoclonic epilepsy may be a prominent feature. In an affected family reported by van Bogaert and Borremans (1937) mental deterioration was noted in one sib at the age of 15 years and this was followed by a neurological illness of predominantly cerebellar symptomatology. This patient died at the age of 62. The degree of lipidosis in the nerve cells was so slight as to make the diagnosis of amaurotic idiocy doubtful, but the subsequent neuropathological examination of another sib confirmed that this disease was in fact present (van Bogaert 1952). In this 2nd case the neuronal swelling was much more obvious and the areas chiefly affected were the corpus striatum, hypothalamus, subthalamic nucleus, dentate nucleus and cerebellar cortex. Only a minority of cells in the cerebral cortex showed lipidosis and these were most frequently seen in the 3rd and 4th layers. The intracellular material stained a yellowish colour with Scharlach R. and was mixed with fine granules having the properties of neutral fat. The disease may present clinically as a progressive cerebellar ataxia and in one such case there was a terminal psychosis characterised by ideas of grandeur (Derwort and Noetzel 1959). The papers of Mattyus (1962) and of Zeman and Hoffman (1962) should be consulted for histochemical details. The pathological and genetic relationships existing between the adult and juvenile forms of amaurotic idiocy have been fully explored by the latter authors. It seems likely that only those adult cases without optic atrophy represent a distinct genetic entity. This clinical type is the subject of a recent paper by van Bogaert (1962).

A useful review of the 19 adult cases so far recorded will be found in the paper of Fine *et al.* (1960). These authors point out that the cerebellar degeneration may be of the granular layer type and that in rare instances there are signs of progressive muscular atrophy due to anterior horn cell degeneration and lipidosis.

In Hallervorden's (1938) adult case there had been pre-existing mental defect. In addition to scattered neuronal lipidosis, most evident in the basal ganglia and substantia nigra, Alzheimer's neurofibrillary change was found in the cornu Ammonis, hypothalamus, thalamus and corpus striatum. Pigmentary changes of the Hallervorden-Spatz type was a feature of Moschel's (1954) adult case.

Retina. In an adult case with no visual impairment Greenfield (1951) found coarse P.A.S. positive granules in the ganglion cells, the change being particularly marked near the fovea where some large phagocytes were intermingled with the nerve cells.

Visceral lipidosis. In Kuf's 1st case (1925) lipid storage was seen in the Kupffer cells of the liver.

Chemical analysis. Two adult cases reported by Cumings (1960) showed no significant increase in ganglioside. In two of the writer's unpublished cases a similar negative finding was recorded. The brains were from a brother and sister, without amaurosis, and the material in one instance had been analysed before fixation.

Congenital amaurotic family idiocy

Up to the present this variety of lipidosis has been described only in one non-Jewish family in which closely similar neuropathological findings were present in three sibs (Norman and Wood 1941, Brown *et al.* 1954, unpublished case). The infants lived only for a few days or weeks and the onset of the lipidosis had clearly been prenatal. The brains are extremely small in this variant, weighing in two instances only 87 g. and 65 g., and they show retarded convolutional development especially in the frontal lobes. There is a very large external hydrocephalus and no obvious microcephaly but the skulls are abnormally shaped. In the cerebral cortex the great majority of the surviving nerve cells are spherical (Fig. 6.149) and of smaller size than those in Tay-Sachs disease, only the giant cells of Betz retaining an approximately pyramidal shape. The nuclei are often shrunken, crenated and pyknotic and there may be two in a cell. The better developed nerve cells in the basal ganglia and brain stem show swelling of a degree comparable to what is seen in infantile amaurotic idiocy and all are filled with an insoluble material staining yellowish red with Scharlach R. and a bright pink with P.A.S. There is a marked astrocytic gliosis throughout the whole brain. No neutral fat is present in the cortical grey matter, but extracellular droplets are common in the centrum semi-ovale where very widespread crystalline deposits of cholesterol esters encrust the bodies of the astrocytes and are also present in macrophages. Myelination is absent above the level of the midbrain and severely retarded in the brainstem and spinal cord. There is severe atrophy of the cerebellum involving both the Purkinje and granular cells. In the retina of the unpublished case the ganglion cells had degenerated and large macrophage cells containing P.A.S. positive material were scattered throughout the remaining layers which in many places showed considerable disorganisation. Small groups of lipid-containing macrophages were present in the spleen, liver and lymph nodes.

Chemical analysis in one case showed a slight excess of ganglioside in the cortex and great excess of cholesterol in the white matter. These cases thus differ in their pathological features from Tay-Sachs disease, while from the clinical point of view the congenital character of the illness, the tiny brain, the shadow of which is visible in X-rays of the skull, and the absence of the cherry red spot in a fundus showing optic atrophy and almost complete absence of retinal vessels, are distinguishing points from other lipidoses of early infantile onset.

Gargoylism

First described by Hunter (1917) and then in greater detail by Hurler (1919), this syndrome consists of mental deficiency, hepatosplenomegaly, corneal clouding and dwarfism. The skull is large, even when there is no complicating hydrocephalus, while the widely set eyes, strongly marked eyebrows and depressed bridge of the nose give to the face the grotesque quality which first suggested the name of gargoylism to Ellis and his co-workers (1936). The condition is usually inherited as a simple Mendelian recessive, but a rarer sex-linked form has been described in which there are no corneal opacities (Millman and Whittick 1952). *Formes frustes* are not uncommon (Jervis 1950 a) but the nervous system seldom escapes involvement and the consequent mental deficiency is usually severe and occasionally progressive.

Central nervous system. The leptomeninges may contain lipid deposits and macrophage cells and are often considerably fibrosed (Fig. 6.154), in Magee's (1950) case reaching the extraordinary thickness of 1 cm. The mild internal hydrocephalus found in cases showing this meningeal thickening is probably due to partial occlusion of the subarachnoid space by fibrosis (Russell 1949). The nerve cells show swelling of the cyton closely resembling that seen in the juvenile form of amaurotic idiocy. The stored material stains orange with Scharlach R., greyish black with sudan black and is strongly positive to P.A.S. and Feyrter's thionin. It is not doubly refractile. After treatment with the more powerful lipid solvents, the P.A.S. staining material is removed, but an insoluble Scharlach staining residue remains behind (Bishton *et al.* 1956).

The distension of the nerve cells of the cerebral cortex is always conspicuous and large pyriform cells are the rule (Fig. 6.150 and 6.151). These changes are not always ubiquitous and cells of normal appearance in Nissl preparations may be found in most areas. Elsewhere in the brain there is considerable regional variation in the degree of neuronal lipidosis. The cells of the nuclei pontis may be very slightly affected while those of the thalamus show severe distension. There is often a striking contrast between the large and small neurones of the putamen and caudate nucleus, the former being much more swollen. Patchy areas of nerve cell loss and gliosis are infrequent and, except where there has been recent destruction of nerve cells, there is little evidence of microglial activity. The whole of the white matter may show a mild fibrillary gliosis though there is little or no defect of myelination. A peculiar feature of gargoylism is the presence in the centrum semi-ovale and medullary cores of the gyri of greatly enlarged perivascular spaces (Fig. 6.151). These are filled with a reticulum of collagen fibrils derived from the adventitial coat of the vessels, the perivascular astrocytes contributing relatively few fibres. Small groups of fat-granule cells may be present and in Naidoo's (1953) case, where the changes were particularly marked, the marginal tissues showed heavy gliosis and

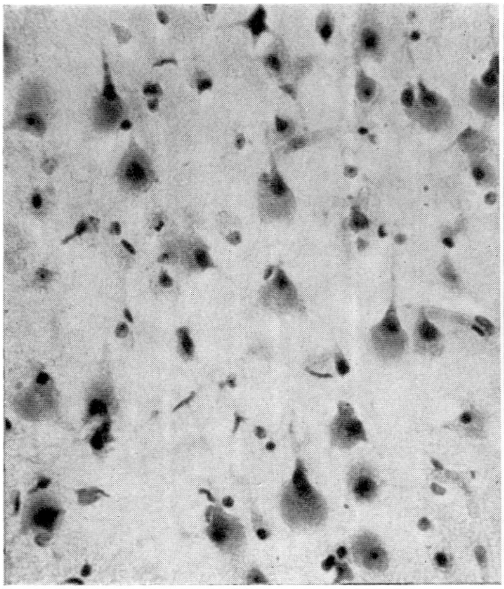

6.150

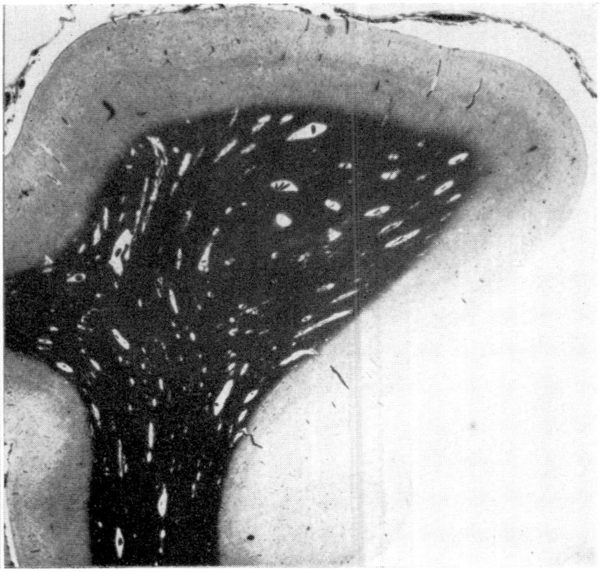

6.151

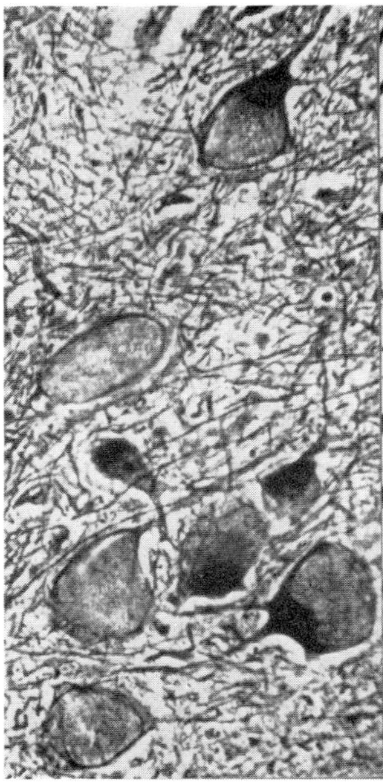

6.152

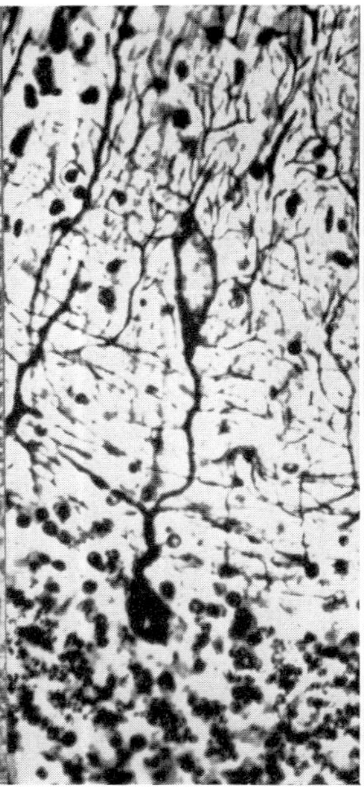

6.153

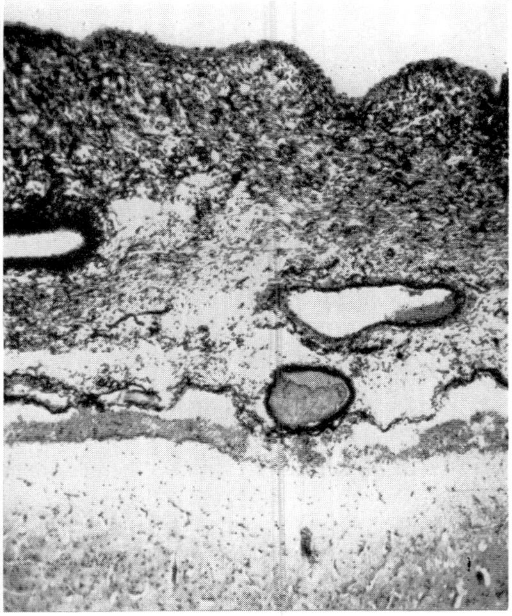

6.154

FIG. 6.150. *Gargoylism.* Swollen nerve cells from the 3rd layer of the cerebral cortex. (Carbol azure.)
FIG. 6.151. Perivascular lacunæ in the central white core of a gyrus. (Heidenhain's myelin.)
FIG. 6.152. Nerve cells of the hypoglossal nucleus showing distension and peripheral displacement of neurofibrils. (Bielschowsky.)
FIG. 6.153. Cactus-like expansion of a Purkinje cell dendrite. (Cajal's silver nitrate pyridine method.)
FIG. 6.154. Fibrosis of the leptomeninges. (Masson's trichrome.)

some demyelination, as though from pressure atrophy. Very large perivascular cavities have also been found bilaterally in the thalamus and striatum (Norman *et al.* 1959 b).

In the cerebellum the Purkinje cells exhibit moderate lipidosis and large oval dendritic swellings containing lipid have occasionally been described (Jervis 1950 a, Bishton *et al.* 1956) (Fig. 6.153) but severe cerebellar atrophy as in amaurotic idiocy has not yet been reported.

Visceral storage. The parenchymal liver cells contain large vacuoles which usually appear empty in formalin and even in alcohol-fixed material. Jervis's (1950 a) demonstration of a lipid substance in the liver resembling that of the nerve cells is exceptional. Using fresh frozen sections of liver Dawson (1954) found an intracellular material which stained both as a lipid and by the P.A.S. method. Liver biopsy has shown that the stored material is not glycogen (Henderson *et al.* 1952). In the spleen the cells lining the sinusoids are similarly affected. The heart is usually enlarged, the muscle cells showing vacuolation and the mitral valve often being thickened and fibrosed. The coronary arteries frequently show severe eccentric narrowing due to subintimal fibrosis and here, also, vacuolation is seen in the connective tissue cells. The pathological findings in the bones vary from case to case. Sometimes no microscopical abnormality is present despite the clinical dwarfing; occasionally the cartilage cells show granular inclusions or empty spaces; in other cases the development of cartilage and bone is abnormal (Dawson 1954). The corneal opacity is due to deposition of the stored substance in the cells of Bowman's membrane. As in amaurotic family idiocy and Niemann-Pick's disease, vacuolated lymphocytes may be present in large numbers in the blood (Goodbody and Cumings 1958).

The *chemical composition* of the material stored by the neurones differs from that of the freely diffusable substances present in the liver and other organs. The latter are polysaccharides (Brante 1951), and Stacey has isolated and identified several of these complex carbohydrates from a gargoyle liver in which they were present in excess (Bishton *et al.* 1956). In the nerve cells the soluble lipid component already mentioned is probably ganglioside, but the level is not so high as in Tay-Sachs' disease (Cumings 1960). There is some variability in this finding, for in two cases analysed in the writer's laboratory the neuraminic acid in the cortex was not raised.

Gaucher's disease

In the variety of Gaucher's disease occurring in adult life the glucocerebroside kerasin is stored exclusively in the reticulo-endothelial system.

In the infantile form of the disease, which is also rare, a rapidly fatal neurological illness is characterised by opisthotonus, decerebrate rigidity and bulbar paralysis. Giampalmo (1949) has reviewed 43 cases and distinguishes an early infantile and a subacute late infantile type. In both, the neuropathological picture is that of widespread degeneration of nerve cells with chromatolysis and neuronophagia, but only in a minority of cases has neuronal lipidosis been demonstrated in some of the nerve cells. Several investigators have searched for, and have been unable to find, evidence of neuronal storage in their cases of infantile Gaucher's disease though conspicuous proliferation of adventitial cells containing P.A.S. +ve material has been demonstrated in the white matter and basal ganglia (Debré *et al.* 1951, Berard-Badier *et al.* 1962) (Fig. 6.159). Others have found limited lipid storage in some of the nerve cells (Fig. 6.155) as well as the more usual widespread degenerative lesions in brain stem, basal ganglia, cerebellum and especially the dentate nuclei (Figs. 6.156, 6.157 and 6.158). Schairer (1948) regarded this stored substance as a toxic agent which was responsible for the rapid degeneration of the neurones. A drawback to this theory is that no similar material was found in the microglial cells of the degenerating areas, for if the lipid substance had been a

6.155

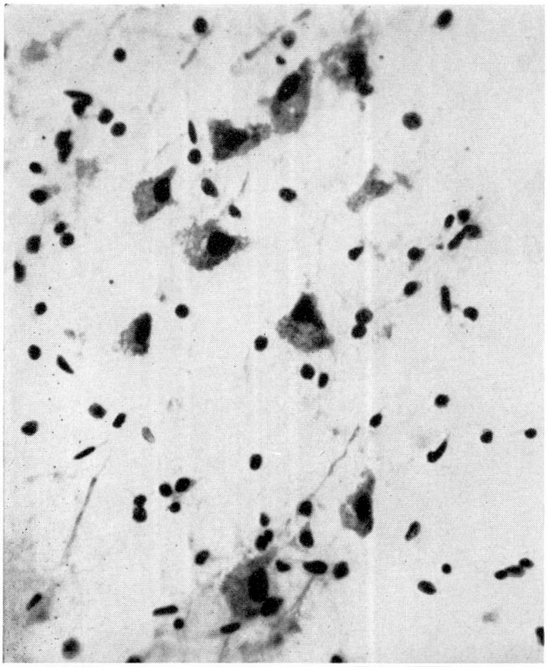

6.156

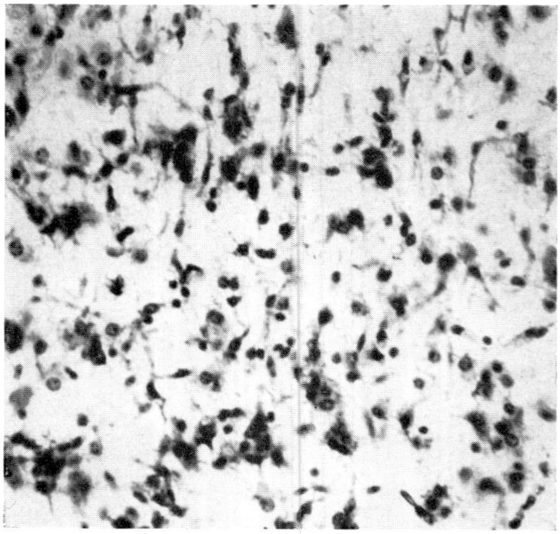

6.158

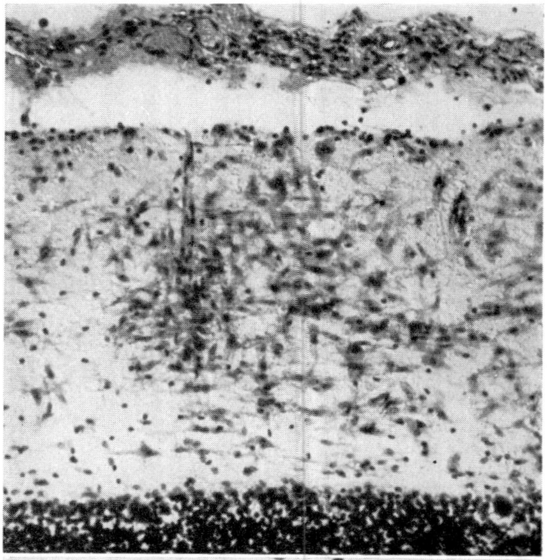

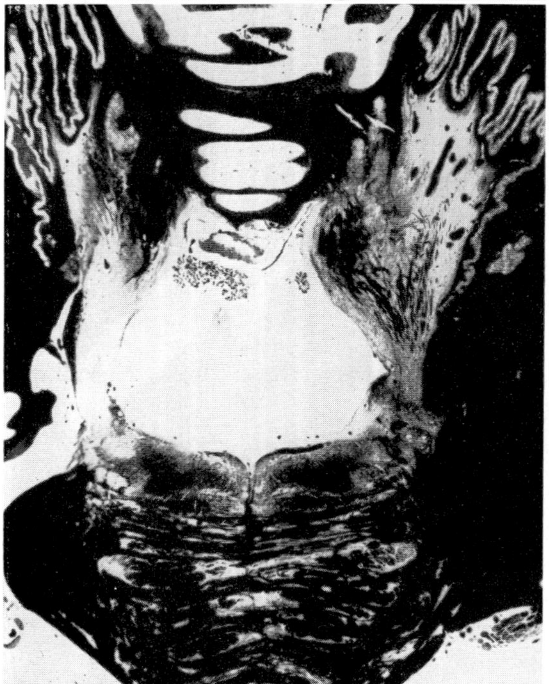

6.157

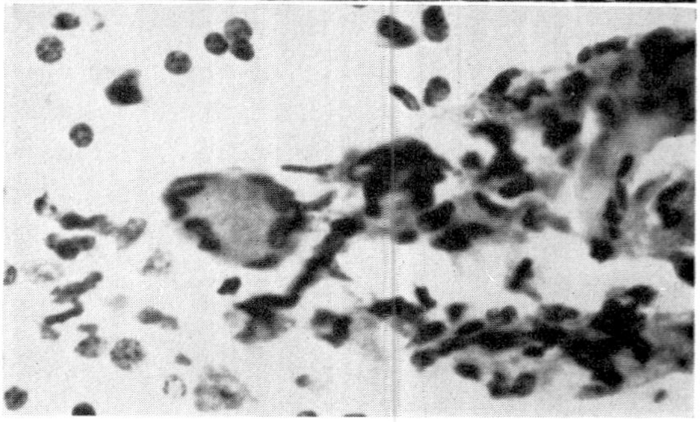

6.159

FIG. 6.155. *Infantile Gaucher's disease.* Swollen nerve cells from the uncus showing storage of lipid. (Carbol azure.)

FIG. 6.156. Acute degenerative changes and microglial proliferation in the pyramidal cell layer of Ammon's horn. (Carbol azure.)

FIG. 6.157. Demyelination of the dentate nuclei and juxta-restiform bodies. (Heidenhain's myelin.)

FIG. 6.158. A glial 'shrubbery' in the molecular layer of the cerebellum.

FIG. 6.159. A perivascular Gaucher cell from the cerebral white matter. (Carbol azure.)

prerequisite to neuronal death, it should have appeared in the local phagocytes. Norman *et al.* (1956) have suggested that both the neuronal storage and the neuronal degeneration are different aspects of the same fundamental metabolic disorder. If the metabolic upset in infantile Gaucher's disease is sufficiently severe it will lead to rapid cell death without evident storage, while a less severe process will allow the affected cells to survive for sufficient time for the products of disordered lipid metabolism to accumulate within them. Thus neuronal lipidosis was widespread in the subacute juvenile case reported by Maloney and Cumings (1960). Increased gluco-cerebroside was demonstrated in the spleen and cerebral cortex. The cases of Bird (1948) and Brain (1953) which have been classed as examples of juvenile Gaucher's disease with cerebral involvement are not regarded by Brante (1961) as belonging chemically to this group.

Glycogen storage disease

Accumulation of glycogen within nerve cells is not a feature of von Gierke's hepato-renal glycogen storage disease, but striking involvement of the nervous system has been described in the much rarer familial cardiomuscular variant of the disorder. Castaigne and Lhermitte (1953) found in the literature a group of 7 cases of this latter type of glycogen storage disease having in common the congenital or early infantile onset of a motor disability characterised by muscular hypotonia and poverty of movements. The progressive course of the illness closely resembles that of Werdnig–Hoffmann's disease and death from bulbar paralysis or respiratory infection usually occurs during the first year of life. The heart is enlarged, the liver only moderately so, and there is no hypoglycaemia and ketosis. Pathological examination of the nervous system reveals accumulation of glycogen within the nerve cells, varying from small droplets to confluent masses displacing the nucleus to the margin of the cell. The anterior horn cells are predominantly affected in this way though the cells of the posterior horns and Clarke's column also participate in the abnormal storage. In the brain stem the large motor cells may be conspicuously involved and glycogen deposits are commonly present in the neurones of the nucleus subthalamicus, globus pallidus, thalamus and dentate nuclei. The corpus striatum and cerebral cortex are usually much less affected, but in the exceptional case described by Esser and Scheidegger (1937) the nerve cells of the cerebral cortex were predominantly involved. Droplets of glycogen are found in the astrocytes, oligodendroglia and ependymal cells but not apparently in the microglia. Fibrillary gliosis is uncommon. Glycogen has also been demonstrated in the Schwann cells and in the autonomic ganglia.

In a few instances cardiomuscular storage has been combined with the classical hepato-renal hypertrophy. In Kimmelsteil's (1933) case the distinctive pathological finding was large deposits of glycogen in the central white matter of the hemispheres, situated either free in the tissues, in the perivascular spaces or in the vessel walls. Despite these examples of apparently intermediary forms it remains probable that the two types of glycogen storage disease are separate genetic entities since there is as yet no sibship in which both the hepato-renal and the cardiomuscular variants have been recorded.

Xanthomatosis of the nervous system

The brain may participate in the osseous and visceral changes of Hand-Schüller-Christian disease. The hypothalamus is commonly invaded by the granulomatous tissue present in the sella turcica, or more rarely, there may be more widely distributed discrete nodular lesions in the brain. These cerebral granulomata may be surrounded by areas of demyelination (Chiari 1933; Teilum 1942).

In a recent example recorded by Feigin (1956) numerous nodules measuring 1 mm.–3 cm. in diameter were present in the cerebral grey and white matter and also in the cerebellum. The central part of these granulomas contained dense collagen fibres, xanthoma cells and multinucleated cells. About one-third of the cells showed birefringent lipid deposits and histochemical tests indicated that most of the lipid present was in the form of cholesterol esters. The deposition of cholesterol esters in the reticulum cells is regarded as a later stage in the development of Letterer-Siwe disease and the condition should not be classed as a cerebral lipidosis.

Cerebrotendinous xanthomatosis

Van Bogaert, Scherer and Epstein (1937) described a familial disease characterised by xanthomata of tendons, xanthelasma of the eyelids, double cataract and massive deposits of cholesterol in crystalline form in the white matter of the cerebellum and cerebral peduncles. Giampalmo (1954) refers to six other examples of this condition and points out that, unlike the findings in Hand-Schüller-Christian disease, there may be hypercholesterinaemia. He regards the disorder as an inherited metabolic anomaly. There is a more controversial group of cases in which patches of demyelination associated with histiocytes containing cholesterol esters are present in the brain, without there being any manifestation of xanthamatosis. Feigin (1956) believes that the xanthoma cell found in this sort of case is distinguishable from a microglial phagocyte by virtue of its larger size and more foamy cytoplasm. The clinical picture is one of slowly progressive cerebellar disease with myoclonus starting in adolescence and terminating with bulbar paralysis in middle life. There may be pre-existing mental deficiency and signs of premature ageing are often observed. The cholesterol deposits are extracellular and there is considerable associated gliosis and demyelination with secondary atrophy of the Purkinje cells and pyramidal tracts.

V. PHENYLKETONURIA

(*Phenylpyruvic amentia*)

The discovery that certain mental defectives excrete large amounts of phenylpyruvic acid in the urine was first made by Fölling in 1934, and Jervis's (1937) analysis of 50 cases clearly established this condition as a new clinical syndrome. The patients excrete about 1 g. of the substance daily and its presence is easily detected by the green colour produced by adding 5 per cent ferric chloride to acidified urine. The associated mental deficiency is usually severe and may be accompanied by epilepsy. General physical stunting and kyphosis is common and a mild extrapyramidal syndrome has been described in some patients. A constant clinical feature is the dilution of pigment, the affected individuals having a characteristic blondness even in dark-haired families. The condition is inherited as a Mendelian recessive (Fölling *et al.* 1945).

The primary biochemical fault is a deficiency of the enzyme responsible for the oxidation of phenylalanine to tyrosine. The prospects of successful clinical treatment by a diet low in phenylalanine has stimulated biochemical studies, details of which will be found in the recent review of Knobloch and Pasamanick (1962) and of Crome and Pare (1960), but the precise factors conditioning the mental retardation have not yet been identified.

Crome and Pare (1960) have summarised the pathological features of 20 cases, adding four of their own. The occasional reports of neuronal loss in the cerebral or cerebellar cortex and of focal necrotic lesions in the grey or white matter are usually regarded as coincidental findings, particularly in view of the frequency of severe epilepsy in these patients. On the other hand, evidence of some abnormality in the myelin is accumulating. Several cases have shown large ill-defined areas of pallor of staining of the myelin sheaths, particularly in the lateral parts of the centrum ovale and in the cerebellar white matter (Fig. 6.160). Fibrous gliosis may accompany

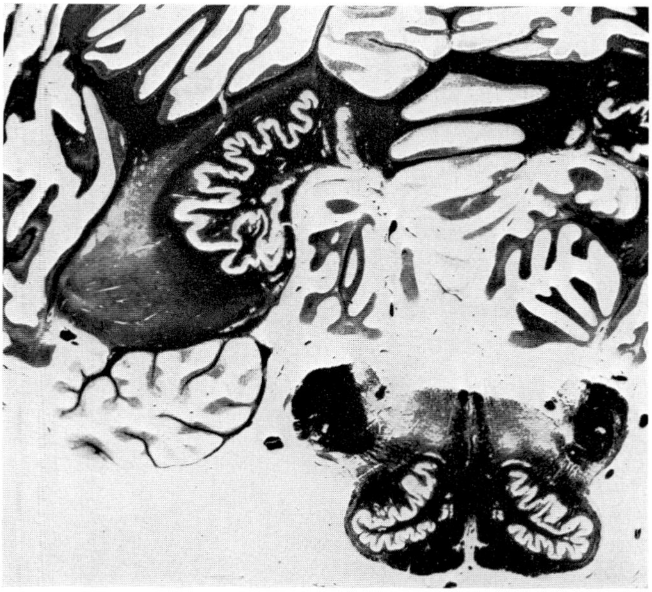

FIG. 6.160. Demyelination in lateral part of the cerebellar central white matter. (Adult untreated phenylketonuric patient.) (Heidenhain.)

these changes and is often more widespread than might have been anticipated from the myelin picture, but lipid degeneration products are absent or scanty (Poser and van Bogaert 1959). Jervis (1954) referred briefly to a phenylketonuric patient who at the age of 25 years developed a progressive neurological illness and at post-mortem showed diffuse cerebral sclerosis. In the recent case of Crome (1962) there was marked demyelination of the centrum ovale with substantial amounts of sudanophil lipid.

Chemical estimations of cerebroside and cholesterol have been made by Crome *et al.* (1962) on cases with and without visible demyelination and these myelin constituents have been found to be reduced in both types of tissue. Although it is clear that demyelination is not found in the majority of cases, the possibility cannot be ruled out that the brains of these patients are predisposed to a later breakdown of the myelin sheaths.

REFERENCES

Adams, R. D., Denny-Brown, D. and Pearson, C. M. (1953) *Diseases of Muscle*, p. 229, Cassell, London.

Addison, T. and Gull, W. (1851) *Guy's Hospital Rep.*, 2nd series, **7**, 267.

Adelmann, H. B. (1930) *Quart. Rev. Biol.*, **11**, 161 and 284.

Ajuriaguerra, J., Heuyer, G. and Lebovici, S. (1950) *Rev. Neurol.*, **83**, 312.

Alexander, G. L. and Norman, R. M. (1960) *The Sturge-Weber Syndrome*, Wright, Bristol.

Alexander, L. (1942) 'The Diseases of the Basal Ganglia,' *Proc. Ass. Res. nerv. ment. Dis.*, Baltimore, **21**, 334.

Alpers, B. (1931) *Arch. Neurol. Psychiat.* (Chicago), **25**, 469.

Alpers, B. J. (1960) *J. Nerv. ment. Dis.*, **130**, 442.
Alvord, E. C. Jr. (1961) *Disorders of the Developing Nervous System.* Edited by Fields and Desmond; Thomas, Springfield, p. 343.
Alzheimer, A. (1904) *Zentralbl. Nervenheilk.*, **27**, 497.
André-Thomas and Ajuriaguerra, J. de (1959) in *Malformations Congénitales du Cerveau*, Masson, Paris, p. 207.
Aring, C. D. (1938) *J. Neurol. Psychiat.*, **1**, 100.
Arnold, J. (1894) *Beitrag. path. Anat. u. allg., Pathol.*, **16**, 1.
Aronson, S. M., Volk, B. W. and Epstein, N. (1955) *Amer. J. Path.*, **31**, 609.
Bailey, O. T. and Hass, G. M. (1937) *Brain*, **60**, 293.
Banker, B. Q. (1961) *J. Neuropath. exp. Neurol.*, **20**, 127.
Banker, B. Q. and Larroche, J. (1962) *Arch. Neurol.*, **7**, 386.
Bargeton, E., Nezelof, C., Guran, P. and Job, J-C. (1961) *Rev. Neurol.*, **104**, 479.
Barry, A., Patten, B. M. and Stewart, B. H. (1957) *J. Neurosurg.*, **14**, 285.
Batchelor, T. M. and Mann, M. E. (1945) *Arch. Path.*, **39**, 67.
Batten, F. E. (1903) *Trans. Ophthal. Soc. United Kingdom*, **23**, 386; (1903) *Brain*, **26**, 147.
Becker, H. (1949 a) *Dtsch. Z. Nervenheilk.*, **161**, 407; (1949 b) ibid., **161**, 446; (1952) ibid., **168**, 345.
Beevor, C. E. (1902) *Brain*, **25**, 85.
Benda, C. E. (1945) *Medicine*, **24**, 71; (1947) *Mongolism and Cretinism*, London; (1952) *Developmental Disorders of Mentation and Cerebral Palsies*, New York; (1954) *J. Neuropath. exp. Neurol.*, **13**, 14.
Benda, C. E. (1949) *Arch. Neurol. Psychiat.* (Chicago), **61**, 137.
Bérard-Badier, M., Paillas, J. E., Gastaut, H. and Edgar, G. W. F. (1958) *Psychiat. Neurol.*, **135**, 50.
Bérard-Badier, M., Payan, H. and Edgar, G. W. F. (1962) *Proc. 4th International Congress of Neuropathology*, Vol. 3, Thieme, Stuttgart, p. 102.
Bertrand, I. and Bargeton, E. (1955) *Proc. 2nd International Congress of Neuropathology*, London (*Excerpta medica*, 1955, **8**, 871).
Bertrand, I. and Gruner, J. (1955) *J. Neuropath, exp. Neurol.*, **14**, 331.
Bickers, D. S. and Adams, R. D. (1949) *Brain*, **72**, 265.
Bielschowsky, M. (1914 a) *Z. ges. Neurol. Psychiat.*, **26**, 133; (1914 b) *Dtsch. Z. Nervenheilk.*, **50**, 7; (1916) *J. Psychol. Neurol.*, Leipzig, **22**, 225; (1920–1) ibid., **26**, 123; (1923–4 a) ibid., **30**, 29; (1923–4 b) ibid., **30**, 167.
Biemond, A. (1955) *Fol. psychiat. neurol. neurochirug. neerl.*, **58**, 2.
Biemond, A. and Bolhuis, J. H. van (1959) *Nederl. tydschr. geneeski*, **103**, 45.
Bird, A. (1948) *Brain*, **71**, 434.
Bishton, R. L., Norman, R. M. and Tingey, A. H. (1956) *J. clin. Path.*, **9**, 305.
Blanc, W. A. and Johnson, L. (1959) *J. Neuropath. exp. Neurol.*, **18**, 165.
Bochnik, H. (1953) *Dtsch. Z. Nervenheilk.*, **358**, 169, 382.
Borberg, A. (1951) *Clinical and Genetic Investigations into Tuberose Sclerosis and Recklinghausen's Neurofibromatosis*, Copenhagen.
Borremans, S., Dykmans, J. and Bogaert, L. van. (1933) *J. Neurol. Psychiat., Belge.*, **33**, 713.
Bouman, L. (1934) *Brain*, **57**, 128.
Bourneville, D. M. (1880–1) *Arch. neurol.*, **1**, 81; (1900) ibid., **10**, 29.
Brain, W. R. (1953) *Acta neurol. psychiat. belg.*, **54**, 597.
Brain, W. R., Greenfield, J. G. and Northfield, D. W. C. (1943) *J. Neurol. Psychiat.*, **6**, 32.
Brandt, S. (1950) *Werdnig-Hoffmann's Infantile Progressive Muscular Atrophy*, Copenhagen.
Brante, G. (1961) in *Chemical pathology of the nervous system*, edited by Folch-Pi, Pergamon Press, N.Y., p. 57.
Brante, G. (1951) *Fette u. Seifen*, **53**, 457.
Bremer, F. W. (1927) *Dtsch. Z. Nervenheilk.*, **99**, 104.
Brodal, A. and Hauglie-Hanssen, E. (1959) *J. Neurol. Neurosurg. Psychiat.*, **22**, 99.
Brouwer, B. (1936) *Proc. R. Soc. Med.*, **29**, 579; (1924) *Psychiat. en. Neurol. Bl. Amst.*, **6**, 461; (1949) *Proc. R. Soc. Med.*, **42**, 603.
Brown, N. J., Corner, B. D. and Dodgson, M. C. H. (1954) *Arch. Dis. Childh.*, **29**, 48.
Brun, R. (1917) *Schweiz. Arch. Neurol. Psychiat.*, **1**, 61; (1918 a) ibid., **2**, 48; (1918 b) ibid., **3**, 13.
Bruschweiler, H. (1927) *Schweiz. Arch. Neurol. Psychiat.*, **21**, 246; (1928) ibid., **22**, 73 and 269.
Burdick, W. F., Whipple, D. V. and Freeman, W. (1945) *Am. J. Dis. Child.*, **69**, 295.
Cameron, A. H. (1957) *J. Path. Bact.*, **73**, 213.
Carpenter, M. B. (1955) *Neurology*, **5**, 139.

Castaigne, P. and Lhermitte, F. (1953) *Proceedings of the 5th International Congress of Neurology*, Lisbon, p. 271.
Centerwall, W. R. and Miller, M. M. (1958) *A.M.A. J. Dis. Child.*, **95**, 385.
Cesaris-Demel, A. (1895) *Arch. per. le Sc. med.*, **19**, 140.
Chase, W. H. (1930) *Surg. Gynec. Obstet.*, **51**, 31.
Chiari, H. (1891) *Dtsch. med. Wschnschr.*, **17**, 1172; (1895) *Denskchr. Akad. Wissen. Wien* (Math. natur. Klasse), **63**, 71.
Chiari, H. (1933) *Virchows Arch.*, **288**, 527.
Christensen, E. and Krabbe, K. H. (1949) *Arch. Neurol. Psychiat.* (Chicago), **61**, 28.
Claireaux, A. E. (1950) *Arch. Dis. Childh.*, **25**, 51.
Clark, R. M. and Linell, E. A. (1954) *J. Neurol. Psychiat.*, **17**, 295.
Clark, W. E. le Gros. (1940) *Brit. Med. J.* (i), 476.
Clark, W. E. le Gros and Russell, D. S. (1940) *J. Neurol. Psychiat. n.s.*, **3**, 123.
Clifford, S. H. (1941) *J. Pediat.*, **18**, 567.
Cöers, C. and Woolf, A. L. (1959) *The Innervation of Muscle*, Blackwell, Oxford.
Cohn, R. and Neumann, M. A. (1946) *J. Neuropath. exp. Neurol.*, **5**, 257.
Conel, J. L. (1938) *Arch. Neurol. Psychiat.* (Chicago), **40**, 337; (1940) *Arch. of Pathology*, **30**, 153.
Courville, C. B. (1953) *Cerebral Anoxia*, Los Angeles.
Courville, C. B. and Edmondson, H. A. (1958) *Bull. Los Angeles Neurol. Soc.*, **23**, 11.
Cowen, D. and Geller, L. M. (1960) *J. Neuropath. Exp. Neurol.*, **19**, 488.
Craig, J. M. (1949) *J. Neuropath. exp. Neurol.*, **8**, 305.
Craig, W. M., Wagener, H. P. and Kernohan, J. W. (1941) *Arch. Neurol. Psychiat.* (Chicago), **46**, 36.
Craig, W. S. (1938) *Arch. Dis. Childh.*, **13**, 89.
Crigler, J. F. and Najjar, V. A. (1952) *J. Pediat.*, **10**, 169.
Critchley, M. and Earl, C. J. C. (1932) *Brain*, **55**, 311.
Crocker, A. C. and Farber, S. (1958) *Medicine*, **37**, 1.
Crome, L. (1952) *J. Path. Bact.*, **64**, 479; (1955) *J. Neurol. Psychiat.*, **18**, 17; (1958) *J. Neurol. Neurosurg. Psychiat.*, **21**, 146; (1962) *J. Neurol. Neurosurg. Psychiat.*, **25**, 149.
Crome, L. and France, N. E. (1959) *J. Clin. Path.*, **12**, 427.
Crome, L. and Pare, C. M. B. (1960) *J. ment. Sci.*, **106**, 862.
Crome, L. and Sylvester, P. E. (1958) *Arch. Dis. Child.*, **33**, 235.
Crome, L., Tymms, V. and Woolf, L. I. (1962) *J. Neurol. Neurosurg. Psychiat.*, **25**, 143.
Crosby, R. M. N., Mosberg, W. H. Jn. and Smith, G. W. (1951) *J. Pediat.*, **39**, 94.
Cumings, J. N. (1960) *Modern Scientific Aspects of Neurology*, Arnold, London.
Daniel, P. M. and Strich, S. J. (1958) *J. Neuropath. exp. Neurol.*, **17**, 255.
Danis, P., Begaux, C. and Decock, G. (1957) *J. Genet. hum.*, **6**, 91.
Davidoff, L. M. (1928) *Arch. Neurol. Psychiat.* (Chicago), **6**, 1229.
Dawson, I. M. P. (1954) *J. Path. Bac.*, **67**, 587.
Dawson, J. (1954) *Quart. J. Med.*, N.S., **23**, 113.
De Jong, R. N. and Bebin, J. (1956) *Neurology*, **6**, 208.
De, S. N. (1950) *J. Path. Bact.*, **62**, 197.
Debré, R., Bertrand, I., Grumbach, R. and Bargeton, E. (1951) *Arch. franc. pediat.*, **8**, 38.
Dekaban, A. S. (1959) *J. Neuropath. exp. Neurol.*, **18**, 621; (1962) 'Cerebral birth injury. Pathology of haemorrhagic lesions.' *Res. Pub. Assoc. nerv. ment. Dis.*, **39**, 196.
Dekaban, A. S. and Magee, K. R. (1958) *Neurol.*, **8**, 193.
Dekaban, A. S. and Norman, R. M. (1958) *J. Neuropath. exp. Neurol.*, **17**, 461.
Denny-Brown, D. (1951) *J. Neurol. Psychiat.*, **14**, 237.
Derwort, A. and Noetzel, H. (1959) *Dtsch. Z. Nervenheilk.*, **179**, 232.
Deschamps, A. and van Bogaert, L. (1948) *Acta. Neurol. Psychiat. belg.*, **48**, 480.
Dickerson, W. W. (1955) *Arch. Neurol. Psychiat.* (Chicago), **73**, 525.
Diezel, P. B. (1954) *Virchows Arch.*, **325**, 109; (1957) *Die Stoffwechselstorunges der Sphygolipoide*, Springer, Berlin.
Divry, P. and van Bogaert, L. (1946) *J. Neurol. Psychiat.*, **9**, 41.
Dominok, G. W. (1962) *Dtsch. Z. Nervenheilk.*, **183**, 340.
Druckman, R., Chao, D. and Alvord, E. C. Jr. (1959) *Neurology*, **9**, 806.
Dublin, W. B. (1949) *J. Neuropath. exp. Neurol.*, **8**, 119.
Dürck, H. (1910) *Verh. dtsch. path. Ges.*, **7**, 238.

Earle, K. M., Baldwin, M. and Penfield, W. (1953) *Arch. Neurol. Psychiat.* (Chicago), **69**, 27.

Edwards, J. H., Norman, R. M. and Roberts, J. M. (1961) *Arch. Dis. Child.*, **36**, 481.

Eicke, W. J. (1957) *In Handbuch der speziellen pathologischen Anatomie und Histologie*, edited by O. Lubarsch, F. Henke and R. Rössle, XIII (i), edited by Scholz; Springer Verlag, Berlin, Göttingen, Heidelberg.

Eicke, W. J. (1959) in *Malformations congénitales du Cerveau*, edited by Heuyer, Field and Gruner, Masson, Paris, p. 81.

Ellis, R. W. B., Sheldon, W. and Capon, N. B. (1936) *Quart. J. Med.*, **29**, 119.

Elvidge, A. R. and Jackson, I. J. (1949) *Amer. J. Dis. Child.*, **78**, 635.

Erbslöh, F. and Bochnik, H. (1958) in *Henke-Lubarsch' Handbuch der speziellen pathologischen Anatomie*, Vol. 13, pt. 11B, Springer, Berlin.

Esser, M. and Scheidegger, S. (1937) *Schw. med. Wschr.*, **67**, 970.

Feigin, I. (1956) *J. Neuropath. exp. Neurol.*, **15**, 400.

Feigin, I. and Wolf, A. (1954) *J. Pediat.*, **45**, 243.

Ferraro, A. and Barrera, S. E. (1935) *Amer. J. Psychiat.*, **92**, 509.

Fine, D. I., Barron, K. D. and Hirano, A. (1960) *J. Neuropath. exp. Neurol.*, **19**, 355.

Fischer, O. (1911) *Z. ges. Neurol. Psychiat.*, **7**, 463.

Fischer, O. (1933) *Münch. med. Wschr.*, **1**, 202.

FitzGerald, G. M., Greenfield, J. G. and Kounine, B. (1939) *Brain*, **62**, 292.

FitzGerald, P. A. M. F. (1940) *Contributions to Embryology*, No. 176, Carnegie Inst. of Washington.

Fölling, A. (1934) *Hoppe-Seyl. Z.*, **227**, 169.

Fölling, A., Mohr, O. L. and Rund, L. (1945) *Oligophrenia Phenylpyruvica*, Oslc.

Ford, C. E. (1960) in *Ciba Foundation Symposium on Congenital Malformations*, edited by Wolstenholme and O'Connor; Churchill, London, p. 32.

Ford, F. R., Livingstone, S. and Pryles, C. V. (1951) *J. Pediat.*, **39**, 33.

Ford, F. R. and Schaffer, A. J. (1927) *Arch. Neurol. Psychiat.* (Chicago), **18**, 323.

Freedom, L. (1927) *Dtschr. Z. Nervenheilk.*, **96**, 295.

Friedman, M. and Cohen, P. (1947) *Am. J. Dis. Child.*, **73**, 178.

Fuchs, A. (1909) *Wien. Med. Wschr.*, **59**, 2142.

Fünfgeld, E. (1929–30) *J. Psychol. Neurol.*, **40**, 85.

Gamper, E. (1929) *J. Psychol. Neurol.*, **39**, 39.

Gardner, W. J. (1959) *Cleveland Clin. quart.*, **26**, 206.

Gardner, W. J. (1961) *Arch. Neurol.*, **4**, 1.

Gardner, W. J., Abdullah, A. F. and McCormack, L. J. (1957) *J. Neurosurg.*, **14**, 591.

Gardner, W. J. and Goodall, R. J. (1950) *J. Neurosurg.*, **7**, 199.

Gerrard, J. (1952) *J. Laryngol. Otol.*, **66**, 39.

Giampalmo, A. (1949) *Acta. pediat.*, **37**, 6; (1954) *Acta. Neurol. Psychiat. Belg.*, **54**, 786.

Gibson, J. B. (1955) *J. Neuropath. exp. Neurol.*, **14**, 244.

Giroud, A. (1959) in *Malformations congénitales du Cerveau*, edited by Heuger, Field and Gruner; Masson, Paris, p. 15.

Giroud, A. (1960) in *Ciba Foundation Symposium on Congenital Malformations*, edited by Wolstenholme and O'Connor; Churchill, London, p. 199.

Giroud, A. and Martinet, N. (1954) *C.R. Soc. Biol.* (Paris), **148**, 1742.

Globus, J. H. (1932) *Cytology and Cellular pathology of the Nervous System*, New York, **3**, p. 1147; (1938) *Amer. J. Cancer*, **32**, 163; (1942) *J. Mt. Sinai Hosp.*, **9**, 451.

Goldstein, K. and Riese, W. (1925) *J. Psychol. Neurol. Leipzig*, **32**, 291.

Goodbody, R. A. and Cumings, J. N. (1958) *Proc. VII Congresso della Societa Internationali di Haematologia*, Roma, No. 647.

Gowers, W. R., and Taylor, J. (1899) *A manual of diseases of the nervous system*, 3rd Edition **1**, London.

Grcevic, N. and Robert, F. (1960) *J. Neuropath. exp. Neurol.*, **20**, 399.

Greenberg, M., Pellitteri, O. and Barton, J. (1957) *J. Amer. med. Ass.*, **165**, 675.

Greenfield, J. G. (1951) *Proc. R. Soc. Med.*, **44**, 686.

Greenfield, J. G. and Holmes, G. (1925) *Brain*, **48**, 183.

Greenfield, J. G. and Stern, R. (1927) *Brain*, **50**, 652.

Greenfield, J. G. and Wolfsohn, J. M. (1935) *Arch. Neurol. Psychiat.* (Chicago), **33**, 1296.

Gregg, N. McA. (1941) *Trans. Ophthal. Soc. Aust.*, **3**, 35.

Gröntoft, O. (1954) *Acta. Path. microbiol. Scand.*, suppt. C., 30.

Gross, H. and Hoff, H. (1959) in *Malformations congénitales du cerveau*, edited by Heuyer, Field and Gruner; Masson, Paris.

Gross, H. and Kaltenback, E. (1959) *Dtsch. Z. Nervenh.*, **179**, 388.

Gross, H., Kaltenback, E. and Uiberrak, B. (1957) *Dtsch. Z. Nervhlk.*, **176**, 77.

Gruenwald, P. (1945) *Anat. Rec.*, **91**, 13; (1947) *Arch. Path.*, **47**, 389, 495 and 648; (1951) *Amer J. Obstet. Gynec.*, **61**, 1285.

Gruenwald, P. (1958) *Amer. J. Path.*, **34**, 77.

Gruner, J. E. and Bargeton, E. (1952) *Rev. Neurol.*, **86**, 236.

Gunther, M. and Penrose, L. S. (1935) *J. Genet.*, **31**, 413.

Guthkelch, A. N. (1953) *Brit. Med. J.* (i), 233.

Hall, G. S. (1946) *Quart. J. Med.* (*n.s.*), **12**, 77.

Haller, E. S., Nesbitt, R. E. L. and Anderson, G. W. (1956) *Obst. & Gynea. Surv.*, **11**, 179.

Hallervorden, J. (1926) *Dtsch. Z. Nervenheilk.*, **89**, 28; (1938) *Mschr. Psychiat. Neurol.*, **99**, 78; (1939) *Z. ges. Neurol. Psychiat.*, **167**, 527; (1949) *Allg. Z. Psychiat.*, **124**, 289.

Hallervorden, J. (1930) *In Handbuch der Geisteskrankheiten*, XI, edited by O. Bumke; Julius Springer, Berlin.

Hallervorden, J. and Spatz, H. (1922) *Z. ges. Neurol. Psychiat.*, **79**, 254.

Haymaker, W., Girdany, B. R., Stephens, J., Lillie, R. D. and Felterman, G. H. (1954) *J. Neuropath.*, **13**, 562.

Haymaker, W., Margoles, C., Pentschew, A., Jacob, H., Lindenberg, R., Arroyo, L. S., Stochdorph, O. and Stowens, D. (1961) in *Kernicterus and its importance in cerebral palsy*, Thomas, Springfield, p. 21.

Helfand, M. (1935) *J. nerv. ment. Dis.*, **81**, 662.

Helmke, K. (1937) *Virchows Arch.*, **300**, 130.

Henderson, J. L. (1939) *Brain*, **62**, 381.

Henderson, J. L., MacGregor, A. R., Thannhauser, S. J. and Holden, R. (1952) *Arch. Dis. Childh.*, **27**, 230.

Herren, R. Y. and Edwards, J. E. (1940) *Arch. Path.*, **30**, 1203.

Heschl, R. (1859) *Vierteljahrschr. prakt. Heilkunde*, **61**, 59.

Hicks, S. P. (1952) *J. Pediat.*, **40**, 489; (1953 a) *Arch. Path.*, **55**, 302; (1953 b) *Amer. J. Roentgenol.*, **69**. 272; (1954) *Arch. Path.*, **57**, 363.

Hoet, J. P., Gommers, A. and Hoet, J. J. (1960) in *Ciba Foundation Symposium on Congenital Malformations*, edited by Wolstenholme and O'Connor; Churchill, London, p. 219.

Hoeve, J. van der. (1921) *v. Graefes Arch. Ophthal.*, **105**, 880.

Hoffman, J. (1893) *Deutsch. Z. Nervenhk.*, **3**, 427.

Holland, E. (1920) *Trans. Edinb. Obstet. Soc.*, **40**, 112; (1922) *J. Obstet. Gynaec, Brit. Emp.*, **29**, 549.

Holmes, G. M. (1911) *Proc. R. Soc. Med.*, **4**, 199; (1915) *Brit. Med. J.*, **2**, 769.

Hunt, J. R. (1917) *Brain*, **40**, 58.

Hunter, C. (1916–7) *Proc. R. Soc. Med.*, **10**, Sect. Dis. Child., 104.

Hurler, G. (1919) *Z. Kinderheilk.*, **24**, 220.

Hurst, E. W. (1925) *Brain*, **48**, 1.

Hutchinson, E. C. and Yates, P. O. (1956) *Brain*, **79**, 319; (1957) *Lancet*, **1**, 2.

Ingalls, T. H. (1960) in *Ciba Foundation Symposium on Congenital Malformations*, edited by Wolstenholme and O'Connor; Churchill, London, p. 51.

Ingalls, T. H., Curley, F. J. and Prindle, R. A. (1950) *Amer. J. Dis. Child.*, **80**, 34.

Inglis, K. (1946) *Brain*, **69**, 157; (1950) *Amer. J. Path.*, **26**, 521.

Ingraham, F. D. and Scott, H. W. (1943) *New Engl. J. Med.*, **229**, 108.

Jacob, A. (1927) *Normal und Pathologische Anatomie und Histological des Grosshirns*, Erster Band, Leipzig.

Jaffe, H. L. and Lichtenstein, L. (1944) *Arch. Path.*, **37**, 99.

Jakob, A. (1929) *Anatomie und Histologie des Grosshirns*, Leipzig, **1**, p. 42.

Jervis, G. A. (1937) *Arch. Neurol. Psychiat.*, (Chicago), **38**, 944; (1940) *Amer. J. Dis. Child.*, **60**, 88; (1941) ibid., **61**, 327; (1948) *Amer. J. Psychiat.*, **105**, 102; (1950 a) *Arch. Neurol. Psychiat.* (Chicago), **63**, 681; (1950 c) *J. nerv. ment. Dis.*, **111**, 398; (1954 a) *J. Neuropath. exp. Neurol.*, **13**, 105; (1954 b) ibid., **13**, 318.

Jervis, G. A. (1952) *J. Neuropath.*, **11**, 4.

Jervis, G. A. (1954) *Res. Pub. Ass. Nerv. ment. Dis.*, **33**, 259, Williams and Wilkins, New York.

Jervis, G. A. (1957) *J. Neuropath. exp. Neurol.*, **16**, 308.

Jervis, G. A. (1959) *A.M.A. Arch. Neurol. Psychiat.*, **81**, 55.

Jervis, G. A. and Schein, H. (1951) *Arch. Path.*, **51**, 640.

Johnson, F. E. (1938) *J. Pediat.*, **13**, 894.

Jonesco-Sisesti, N. (1932) *La Syringobulbie*, Masson, Paris.

Jong, H. de. (1927) *Z. ges. Neurol. Psychiat.*, **108**, 734.

Kalinowsky, L. (1927) *Mschr. Psychiat. Neurol.*, **66**, 168.

Kalinowsky, L. (1936) *In Handbuch der Neurologie*, XVI, edited by O. Bumke and O. Foerster; Julius Springer, Berlin.

Kalischer, S. (1897) *Berl. klin. Wchnschr.*, **34**, 1059; (1901) *Arch. f. Psychiat.*, **34**, 169.

Kappers, J. A. (1959) in *Malformations congénitales du Cerveau*, edited by Heuyer, Field and Gruner; Masson, Paris, p. 99.

Kass, A. (1951) *Acta. Pediat.* **40**, 239.

Kastein, G. W. (1940) *Arch.. neerl. Morph. norm. et path.*, **3**, 249.

Kautsky, R. (1949) *Dtsch. Z. Nervenheilk.*, **161**, 506.

Kimmelsteil, P. (1933) *Beitr. z. path. Anat. u.z. allg. Path.*, **91**, 1.

King, L. S. (1936) *J. comp. Neurol.*, **64**, 377.

Kirschbaum, W. (1947) *J. Neuropath. exp. Neurol.*, **6**, 78.

Klenk, E. (1953) *Proceedings of the 5th International Neurological Congress, Lisbon*, **1**, p. 253; (1955) in *Biochemistry of the Developing Nervous System*, Edited by H. Waelsch, New York, p. 397.

Knobloch, H. and Pasamanick, B. (1962) *New Eng. J. Med.*, **266**, 1045.

Koch, G. (1949) *Arztl. Forschr.*, **3**, 278.

Korein, J., Stainman, P. A. and Senz, E. H. (1961) *A.M.A. Arch. Neurol.*, **4**, 272.

Krabbe, K. H. (1934) *Arch. Neurol. Psychiat.* (Chicago), **32**, 737.

Kramer, W. (1953) *Acta. Psychiat. Neurol. Scand.*, **28**, 413; (1956) *J. Neuropath. exp. Neurol.*, **15**, 471.

Kramer, W. (1954) *Folia Psychiat. Neurol. Neurochir. Neerl.*, **57**, 298.

Kufs, H. (1925) *Z. ges. Neurol. Psychiat.*, **95**, 168; (1931) ibid., **137**, 432; (1949) *Arch. f. Psychiat. u.Z. Neurol.*, **182**, 177.

Landtman, B. (1948) *Arch. Dis. Childh.*, **23**, 237.

Lange, C. de. (1925) *J. nerv. ment. Dis.*, **62**, 449; (1937) *Acta. Pediat.*, **20**, Suppl. III, 1; (1939) *Mschr. Psychiat. Neurol.*, **101**, 350.

Lange-Cosack, H. (1944) *Arch. f. Psychiat.*, **117**, 595.

Langhans, T. (1881) *Virchows Arch. f. path. Anat.*, **85**, 1.

Laurence, K. M. (1959) *Ann. Roy. Coll. Surg. Eng.*, **24**, 388.

Lemieux, L. H. (1954) *J. Neuropath. exp. Neurol.*, **13**, 343.

Lichtenstein, B. W. (1940) *Arch. Neurol. Psychiat.* (Chicago), **44**, 792; (1942) ibid., **47**, 195; (1943) *J. Neuropath. exp. Neurol.*, **2**, 164; (1954) *Arch. Neurol. Psychiat.* (Chicago), **71**, 291.

Lindenberg, R. (1955) *J. Neuropath. exp. Neurol.*, **14**, 223.

Lindenberg, R. (1963) in C.O.I.M.S. Symposium on *Selective vulnerability of the C.N.S. in hypoxaemia*. Baden, Zurich.

Lindenberg, R. and Spatz, H. (1939) *Virchows Arch.*, **305**, 531.

List, C. F. (1941) *Arch. Neurol. Psychiat.* (Chicago), **45**, 577.

Little, W. J. (1862) *Trans. obstet. Soc., London*, **3**, 293.

Liu, M. C. and Sylvester, P. E. (1960) *Arch. Dis. child.*, **35**, 345.

Löken, A. C. and Horsdal, O. (1961) *J. Neuropath. exp. Neurol.*, **20**, 427.

Louis-Bar, D. (1941) *Confinia Neurol.*, **4**, 32; (1944) ibid., **6**, 1.

Lundström, R. (1952) *Acta. Pediat.*, **41**, 583.

Lyssenkow, N. K. (1931) *Virchows Arch., f. path. Anat.*, **280**, 611.

Magee, K. R. (1950) *Arch. Neurol. Psychiat.* (Chicago), **63**, 282.

Mair, W. G. P. (1952) *Proc. 1st. International Congress of Neuropathology*, **2**, p. 242.

Malamud, N. (1950) *J. Pediat.*, **37**, 611.

Malamud, N. (1962) *Proc. 4th International Congress of Neuropathology*, Vol. 3, Stuttgart, p. 36.

Malamud, N. and Cohen, P. (1958) *Neurology*, **8**, 261.

Mall, F. P. (1908) *J. Morphol.*, **19**, 3.

Mallory, F. B. (1896) *J. Path. Bac.*, **3**, 110.

Maloney, A. F. J. and Cumings, J. N. (1960) *J. Neurol. Neurosurg. Psychiat.*, **23**, 207.

Maresh, R. (1929) *Wien. med. Wchnschr.*, **79**, 454.

Marie, J., Lyon, G. and Bargeton, E. (1959) *Presse. méd.*, **60**, 2286.

Martin, F. (1949) *Acta. Psychiat.*, **24**, 206; (1950) ibid., **25**, 415.
Martin, J. P. (1941) *Brit. Med. J.*, **2**, 537.
Mattyus, A. (1962) *Proc. IV Internat. Congr. Neuropath.*, Vol. 3, Thieme, Stuttgart, p. 274.
McConnell, A. A. and Parker, H. L. (1938) *Brain*, **61**, 415.
Merritt, K. K., Faber, H. K. and Bruch, H. (1937) *J. Pediat.*, **10**, 374.
Meyer, A., Beck, E. and Sheppard, M. (1955) *J. Neurol. Psychiat.*, **18**, 24.
Meyer, A. and Earl, C. J. C. (1936) *J. ment. Sci.*, **82**, 798.
Meyer, A. and Jones, J. B. (1939) *J. ment. Sci.*, **85**, 206.
Meyer, J.-E. (1949) *Z. Kinderheilk.*, **67**, 123; (1953) *Arch. Psychiat. u.Z. Neurol.*, **190**, 328.
Millman, C. G. and Whittick, J. W. (1952) *J. Neurol. Psychiat.*, **15**, 253.
Miller, J. Q., Alkan, M., Pickard, E., Warner, S. and Gerald, P. S. (1962) *Amer. J. Dis. Child.*, **104**, 532
Minkowski, M. (1955) *Schweiz. Arch. Neurol. Psychiat.*, **76**, 110.
Miskolczky, O. (1931) *Arch. f. Psychiat.*, **93**, 596.
Mitchell, R. G. (1952) *Arch. Dis. Childh.*, **27**, 95.
Monakow, C. von. (1926) *Schweiz. Arch. Neurol. Psychiat.*, **18**, 3.
Morsier, G. de. (1952) *Proc. 1st International Congress of Neuropathology, Rome*, **2**, p. 213.
Morsier, G. de (1956) *Schweiz. Arch. Neurol. Psychiat.*, **77**, 267.
Morsier, G. de and Mozer, J. J. (1935) *Arch. Suisses. Neurol.*, **35**, 64 and 317.
Moschel, R. (1954) *Dtsch. Z. Nervenheilk.*, **172**, 102.
Moulton, S. L. (1942) *Arch. Int. Med.*, **69**, 589.
Muller, H. C. (1950) *Pediat.*, **5**, 320.
Murphy, D. P. (1947) *Congenital Malformations*, 2nd edition, Philadelphia.
Murphy, M. L. (1960) in *Ciba Foundation Symposium on Congenital Malformations*, edited by Wolstenholme and O'Connor; Churchill, London, p. 78.
Muskett, C. W. (1953) *Beitr. path. Anat.*, **113**, 368.
Mutrux, S., Wildi, E. and Bourquin, J. (1949) *Schweiz. Arch. Neurol.*, **64**, 369.
Naidoo, D. (1953) *J. ment. Sci.*, **99**, 74.
Nañagas, J. C. (1925) *Amer. J. Anat.*, **35**, 455.
Nathan, P. W. and Smith, M.C. (1950) *J. Neurol. Psychiat.*, **13**, 191.
Neill, C. A. and Dingwall, M. M. (1950) *Arch. Dis. Child.*, **25**, 213.
Neubürger, K. T. (1935) *Beitr. z. gerichtl. med.*, **13**, 85.
Norman, R. M. (1936) *J. Neurol. Psychopath.*, **17**, 135; (1940) *Brain*, **63**, 365; (1947) *J. Neurol. Psychiat.*, **10**, 12; (1952) *Proc 1st International Congress of Neuropathology*, Rome, **2**, 276; (1956) *Acta. Neurol. Psychiat. Belg.*, **56**, 89.
Norman, R. M. (1958) in *Temporal Lobe Epilepsy*, Thomas, Springfield, p. 203; (1961 a) *Arch. Dis. Child.*, **36**, 97; (1961 b) in *Hemiplegic cerebral palsy in children and adults*, National Spastics Society, London, p. 22; (1962) in *Modern Trends in Neurology*, edited by D. Williams; Butterworths, London; (1963) in C.I.O.M.S. Symposium on *Selective vulnerability of the C.N.S. in hypoxaemia*, Baden, Zurich.
Norman, R. M. and McMenemey, W. H. (1955) *J. Neuropath. exp. Neurol.*, **14**, 84.
Norman, R. M. and Taylor, A. L. (1940) *J. Path. Bac.*, **50**, 61.
Norman, R. M. and Urich, H. (1957) *J. Path. Bact.*, **73**, 580; (1958) *J. Neurol. Neurosurg. Psychiat.*, **21**, 159; (1960) ibid., **23**, 142; (1962) *London Conference on the Scientific Study of Mental Deficiency*, May and Baker, London, p. 299.
Norman, R. M., Urich, H. and Lloyd, O. C. (1956) *J. Path. Bac.*, **72**, 121.
Norman, R. M., Urich, H. and McMenemey, W. H. (1957) *Brain*, **80**, 49.
Norman, R. M., Urich, H. and Woods, G. E. (1958) *J. Ment. Sci.*, **104**, 758.
Norman, R. M., Urich, H., Tingey, A. H. and Goodbody, R. A. (1959 a) *J. Path Bac.*, **78**, 409.
Norman, R. M., Urich, H. and France, N. E. (1959 b) *J. Ment. Sci.*, **105**, 1070.
Onari, K. (1925) *Z. ges. Neurol. Psychiat.*, **98**, 456.
Oppenheim, H. (1900) *Mschr. f. Psychiat. Neurol.*, **8**, 232.
Orth, J. (1875) *Virchows Arch.*, **63**, 447.
Ostertag, B. (1925) *Arch. Psychiat. Nervenkr.*, **75**, 355.
Patau, K., Therman, E., Smith, D. W., Inhorn, S. L. and Picken, B. F. (1961) *Amer. J. Hum. Genet.*, **13**, 287.
Patten, B. M. (1953) *Am. J. Anat.*, **93**, 365.
Pellizi, G. (1901) *Riv. Sper. freniat.*, **27**, 265.
Penfield, W. (1954) *Brain*, **77**, 1.

Penfield, W. and Coburn, D. F. (1938) *Arch. Neurol. Psychiat.* (Chicago), **40**, 328.
Penfield, W. and Elvidge, A. R. (1932) *Cytology and Cellular Pathology of the Nervous System*, New York, **3**, p. 1203.
Penrose, L. S. (1949) *The Biology of Mental Defect.*, London, p. 180.
Pentschew, A. (1949) *Der Nervenarzt.*, **20**, 220.
Pentschew, A. and Schwarz, K. (1962) *Acta Neuropathol.*, **1**, 313.
Peter, K. (1928) *Z. ges. Neurol. Psychiat.*, **113**, 298.
Peter, K. and Schlüter, K. (1927) *Z. ges. Neurol. Psychiat.*, **108**, 21.
Peters, G. (1951) *Spezielle Pathologie der Krankheiten des zentralen und peripheren Nervensystems*, Georg Thieme, Stuttgart.
Pfeiffer, F. (1939) *Psychiat. Neurol. Wschr.*, **41**, 409.
Poser, C. M. and van Bogaert, L. (1959) *Brain*, **82**, 1.
Poser, C. M., Walsh, F. C. and Scheinberg, L. C. (1955) *Neurology*, **5**. 286.
Potter, E. L. (1953) *Pathology of the Fetus and the Newborn*, Chicago.
Probst, M. (1900) *Arch. f. Psychiat.*, **33**, 1.
Radermeker, J. (1951) *Rev. Neurol.*, **84**, 14; (1953) ibid., **89**, 368.
Raing, H. and Fowler, J. S. (1903) *Rev. Neurol. and Psychiat.*, **1**, 149.
Recklinghausen, F. von. (1862) *Mschr. Geburtskunde*, **20**, 1.
Record, R. G. and McKeown, T. (1950) *Brit. J. Soc. Med.*, **4**, 26.
Rehder, H. (1914) *Virchows Arch., f. path. Anat.*, **217**, 174.
Reye, R. D. K. (1960) *J. Path. Bact.*, **79**, 165.
Richter, R. B. (1957) *J. Neuropath. exp. Neurol.*, **16**, 281.
Richter, R. B. (1960) *J. Neuropath. exp. Neurol.*, **19**, 33.
Roback, H. N. and Scherer, H. J. (1934) *Virchows Arch.*, **294**, 365.
Rosenthal, I. M., Zimmerman, H. J. and Hardy, N. (1956) *Pediat.*, **18**, 378.
Rothman, P. E. (1931) *Amer. J. Dis. Child.*, **42**, 125.
Rothmann, M. (1915) *Neurol. Zbl.*, **34**, 44.
Rozdilsky, B. and Olszewski, J. (1961) *J. Neuropath. exp. Neurol.*, **20**, 193.
Russell, D. S. (1932) *J. Path. Bac.*, **35**, 103; (1949) *Observations on the Pathology of Hydrocephalus*, Spec. Rep. Ser. Med. Res. Coun. No. 265, London, H.M. Stationery Office.
Russell, D. S. and Donald, C. (1935) *Brain*, **58**, 203.
Sabin, A. B. and Feldman, H. A. (1948) *J. Pediat.*, **35**, 296.
Sachs, B. (1887) *J. nerv. ment. Dis.*, **14**, 546; (1896) ibid., **21**, 475.
Samuels, S., Korey, S. R., Gonatas, J., Terry, R. D. and Weiss, M. (1962) in *Cerebral Sphingolipidoses*, Academic Press Inc., New York, p. 309.
Sandbank, U. (1955) *Rev. Neurol.*, **93**, 529.
Savini-Castano, T. and Savini, E. (1913) *Z. f. Kinderheilk.*, **7**, 321.
Schaffer, K. (1930) *Arch. f. Psychiat.*, **89**, 814.
Schairer, E. (1948) *Virchows Arch.*, **315**, 395.
Schaltenbrand, G. (1951) *Die Nervenkrankheiten. Thieme*, Stuttgart.
Scherer, H. J. (1933) *Z. ges. Neurol. Psychiat.*, **145**, 335.
Schlesinger, B. and Welch, R. G. (1952) *Gr. Ormond St. J.*, No. 3, 14.
Schminke, A. (1920) *Z. ges. Neurol. Psychiat.*, **56**, 154; (1922) *Beitr. z. path. Anat. allg. Path.*, **70**, 513.
Schmorl, G. (1903) *Verh. Dtsch. path. Ges.*, **6**, 109.
Schob, F. (1921) *Z. ges. Neurol. Psychiat.*, **73**, 188; (1930) Pathologische Anatomie der Idiotie, in Bumke's *Handbuch der Geisteskrankheiten*, Berlin, **11**, part 7.
Scholz, W. (1924) *Z. ges. Neurol. Psychiat.*, **88**, 355; (1951) *Die Krampfschädigunge des Gehirns*, Berlin.
Schuster, P. (1914) *Dtsch. Z. Nervenheilk.*, **50**, 96.
Schwalbe, E. (1906) *Die Morphologie der Missbildungen des Menchen und der Tiere*, I. Teil, Fischer, Jena, p. 230.
Schwalbe, E. and Gredig, M. (1907) *Beit. path. Anat. u. allg. Path.*, **40**, 132.
Schwartz, Ph. (1924) *Z. ges. Neurol. Psychiat.*, **90**, 263; (1927) *Ergeb. inn. Med. Kinderheilk.*, **31**, 165; (1949) *Harefuah*, **37**, 168.
Schwartz, Ph. (1961) *Birth Injuries of the Newborn*, Karger, New York.
Sedgwick, R. P. and Boder, E. (1960) *Neurol.*, **10**, 705.
Seitelberger, F. and Gross, H. (1957) *Dtsch. Z. Nervhlk.*, **176**, 104.
Seitelberger, F., Vogel, G. and Stepan, H. (1957) *Arch. Psychiat. Z. Neurol.*, **196**, 154.
Sharp, O. and Hall, E. G. (1953) *Proc. Roy. Soc. Med.*, **46**, 1063.

Sherlock, E. B. (1911) *The Feebleminded*, London.
Shy, G. M. and Magee, K. R. (1956) *Brain*, **79**, 610.
Siegmund, H. (1923) *Virchows Arch.*, **241**, 237.
Sjövall, E. (1934) *Verh. Dtsch. path. Ges.*, **27**, 185.
Sjövall, E. and Ericson, E. (1933) *Acta. Path. Microbiol. Scand.*, **16**, 460.
Smith, H. A., Norman, R. M. and Urich, H. (1957) *J. Neurol. Neurosurg. Psychiat.*, **20**, 250.
Spatz, H. and Ullrich, O. (1931) *Z. Kinderheilk.*, **51**, 579.
Spielmeyer, W. (1905) *Neurol. Centralbl.*, **24**, 51; (1906) *Münch. med. Wschr.*, **53**, 1404.
Spiller, W. G. (1906) *Brit. Med. J.* (ii), 1017.
Starkman, S. P., Brown, T. C. and Linell, E. A. (1958) *J. Neuropath. exp. Neurol.*, **17**, 484.
Steegmann, A. T. and Karnosh, L. J. (1936) *Amer. J. Psychiat.*, **92**, 1413.
Steinbiss, W. (1923) *Virchows Arch.*, **243**, 22.
Stewart, R. M. (1930) *J. Neurol. Psycopath.*, **10**, 317.
Stewart, R. M. (1939) *J. Neurol. Psychiat.*, **2**, 303; (1948) *Edin. med. J.*, **55**, 488.
Stockhard, C. R. (1920) *Amer. J. Anat.*, **28**, 115.
Strumpell, A. (1884) *Jahrb. f. Kinderh.*, **22**, 173.
Suter, M. and Wichser, C. (1948) *Amer. J. Obstet. Gynec.*, **55**, 489.
Swan, C. (1949) *J. Obstet. Gynaec. Brit. Emp.*, **56**, 341 and 591.
Sylvester, P. E. (1960) *Acta. Paediat.*, **49**, 338.
Taggart, J. K., Jr., and Walker, A. E. (1942) *Arch. Neurol. Psychiat.* (Chicago), **48**, 583.
Tandon, M. S. and Harkmark, W. (1959) *Neurology*, **9**, 699.
Tay, W. (1881) *Trans. Ophthal. Soc., United Kingdom*, **1**, 55.
Taylor, J. (1905) *Paralysis and other Diseases of the Nervous System in Childhood and Early Life*, London.
Taylor, J., Greenfield, J. G. and Martin, J. P. (1922) *Brain*, **45**, 323.
Teilum, G. (1942) *Beitr. path. Anat. Allg. Path.*, **106**, 460.
Terry, R. D., Korey, S. R. and Weiss, M. (1962) in *Cerebral Sphingolipidoses*, Academic Press, New York, p. 49.
Thelander, H. E., Shaw, E. B. and Peel, J. J. (1953) *J. Pediat.*, **42**, 680.
Thieffry, S., Arthuis, M., Faure, C. and Lyon, G. (1961) *18eme Congres de l'association des Pediatres de langue française.* Rapport II, Kargar, Basle, p. 314.
Thieffry, S., Bertrand, I., Bargeton, E., Edgar, G. W. F. and Arthuis, M. (1960) *Rev. Neurol.*, **102**, 130.
Tingey, A. H. (1955) *J. ment. Sci.*, **102**, 178.
Tingey, A. H., Norman, R. M., Urich, H. and Beasley, W. H. (1958) *J. Ment. Sci.*, **104**, 91.
Tuchmann-Duplessis, H. and Mercier-Parot, L. (1960) in *Ciba Foundation Symposium on Congenital Malformations*, edited by Wolstenholme and O'Connor; Churchill, London, p. 115.
Turban. (1944) Thesis. Freiburg.
Turner, J. W. A. (1940) *Brain*, **63**, 163.
Turnham, B. and Rossler, R. (1942) *Mschr. Psychiat. Neurol.*, **105**, 228.
Uiberrack, F. (1942) *Zbl. Path.*, **80**, 187.
Ule, G. (1952) *Dtsch. Z. Nervenheilk.*, **168**, 195.
Urechia, C. J., Reteziano, A. and Maller, O. (1950) *Encéphale*, **39**, 197.
van Bogaert, L. (1939–40) *Rev. neurol.*, **72**, 448.
van Bogaert, L. (1946) *J. Neurol. Psychiat.*, **9**, 125.
van Bogaert, L. (1929) *Rev. Neurol.*, **2**, 385; (1950) *Mschr. Psychiat. Neurol.*, **120**, 169; (1951) *Acta Neurol. Psychiat. Belg.*, **51**, 621; (1952) *Dtsch. Z. Nervenheilk.* **168**, 267.
van Bogaert, L. and Borremans, P. (1937) *Z. ges Neurol. Psychiat*, **159**, 136.
van Bogaert, L., Paillas, J. E., Bérard-Badier, M. and Payan, H. (1958) *Rev. Neurol.*, **98**, 673.
van Bogaert, L. and Radermecker, M-A. (1955) *Rev. Neurol.*, **93**, 65.
van Bogaert, L., Scherer, H. J. and Epstein, E. (1937) *Une Forme Cérébrale de la Cholestérinose Généralisée*, Paris.
van Gieson, I. (1892) *New York med. J.*, **56**, 337, 365 and 421.
Verhaart, W. J. C. and Kramer, W. (1952) *Acta Psychiat. Neurol. scand.*, **27**, 181.
Verhaart, W. J. C. and van Wieringen-Rauws, G. A. (1950) *Fol. Psychiat. Neurol. Neurochir. Neerl.*, **53**, 481.
Vincent, C. and van Bogaert, L. (1936) *Rev. neurol.*, **65**, 921.
Vogel, F. S. (1958) *Amer. J. Path.*, **34**, 169.
Vogel, F. S. and McClenahan, J. L. (1952) *Amer. J. Path.*, **28**, 701.

Vogt, C. and O. (1920) *J. Psychol. Neurol.* **25,** Ergh. 3.
Vogt, C. and O. (1920) *J. Psychol. Neurol. Leipzig*, **25**, Suppl. 3, 627; (1942) ibid., **50**, 161.
Vogt, H. (1908) ibid., **24**, 106.
Vogt, M. (1929) *Encéph.*, **24**, 509.
Volland, F. (1910) *Arch. Psychiat.*, **47**, 1228.
Wachsmuth, N. and Löwenthal, A. (1950) *Acta. Neurol. Psychiat. Belg.*, **50**, 305.
Wald, A. (1930) *Z. Kinderheilk.*, **49**, 375.
Walker, A. E. (1942) *Arch. Neurol. Psychiat.* (Chicago), **48**, 13.
Walsh, F. B. and Lindenberg, R. (1961) *Bull. Johns Hopkins Hosp.*, **108**, 100.
Warkany, J. (1960) in *Ciba Foundation Symposium on Congenital Malformations*, edited by Wolstenholme and O'Connor; Churchill, London, p. 281.
Warner, F. J. (1953) *J. nerv. ment. Dis.*, **118**, 1.
Weber, F. P. (1939) *Proc. R. Soc. Med.*, **32**, 440; (1922) *J. Neurol. Psychopath.*, **3**, 134.
Weil, A. (1933) *Arch. Neurol. Psychiat.* (Chicago), **30**, 795.
Weller, S. D. V. and Norman, R. M. (1955) *Arch. Dis. Childh.*, **30**, 453.
Werdnig, G. (1891) *Arch. f. Psychiat.*, **22**, 437.
Willis, R. A. (1958) *The Borderland of Embryology and Pathology*, Butterworth, London.
Wilson, S. A. K. (1934) *J. Neurol. Psychopath.*, **14**, 193.
Windle, W. F. (1963) in C.I.O.M.S. Symposium on *Selective vulnerability of the C.N.S. in hypoxaemia*, Baden, Zurich.
Winkelman, N. W. (1932) *Arch. Neurol. Psychiat.* (Chicago), **27**, 1.
Wohlwill, F. and Yakovlev, P. I. (1957) *J. Neuropath. exp. Neurol.*, **16**, 341.
Wolf, A. and Cowen, D. (1956) 'The cerebral atrophies and encephalomalacias of infancy and childhood', *Res. Pub. Ass. nerv. ment. Dis.*, **34**, p. 199.
Wolf, A. and Cowen, D. (1959) *J. Neuropath. exp. Neurol.*, **18**, 191.
Woodhall, B. (1939) *Laryngoscope*, **49**, 966.
Woolf, A. L. (1955) *J. ment. Sci.*, **101**, 610.
Woollam, D. H. M. and Millen, D. W. (1953) *Brain*, **76**, 104; (1955) *J. Neurol. Pscyhiat.*, **19**, 17.
Woollam, D. H. M. and Millen, J. W. (1960 a) *Proc. Roy. Soc. Med. Lond.*, **53**, 711.
Woollam, D. H. M. and Millen, J. W. (1960 b) in *Ciba Foundation Symposium on Congenital Malformations*, edited by Wolstenholme and O'Connor; Churchill, London, p. 158.
Wyatt, J. P. and Tribby, W. W. (1952) *Arch. Path.*, **53**, 103.
Wyburn-Mason, R. (1943) *Brit. J. Ophthal.*, **27**, 145.
Wyllie, W. G. (1951) 'The Cerebral Palsies of Infancy' in *Modern Trends in Neurology*, edited by A. Feiling, London, p. 129.
Yakovlev, P. I. (1947) *Amer. J. ment. Def.*, **51**, 575.
Yakolev, P. I. (1959) *J. Neuropath. exp. Neurol.*, **18**, 22.
Yakovlev, P. I. and Wadsworth, R. C. (1946) *J. Neuropath. exp. Neurol.*, **5**, 116 and 169.
Yates, P. O. (1959) *Arch. Dis. Child.*, **34**, 436.
Ylppö, A. (1919) *Z. Kinderh.*, **20**, 212.
Zeman, W. and Hoffman, J. (1962) *J. Neurol. Neurosurg. Psychiat.*, **25**, 352.
Zeman, W. and Scarpelli, D. G. (1958) *J. Neuropath.*, **17**, 622.
Zülch, K. J. (1955) *Proc. 2nd International Congress of Neuropathology*, London, **2**, 613.

CHAPTER 7

TRAUMATIC LESIONS OF THE CENTRAL AND PERIPHERAL NERVOUS SYSTEMS

By J. G. Greenfield and Dorothy S. Russell

INJURIES TO THE BRAIN AND ITS COVERINGS

Introduction

The human brain is liable to trauma at all periods of life. The important group of intra- and neonatal injuries is treated in another chapter (pp. 382–397). In later life the effects of injury are conditioned by a wide range of factors, the severity of the blow and the nature of the object colliding with the skull being two of the most obvious. Not only does the normal skull vary in thickness from place to place, but there is a considerable variation in different subjects irrespective of age and sex. The unduly thin skull is manifestly more vulnerable. The adhesiveness of the dura mater to the inner table is a further factor of importance. In infancy and old age the two structures are firmly blended but, in the intervening period, they are readily separated in the normal subject. Hence epidural haemorrhage is not encountered at the extremes of life but, alternatively, an equivalent degree of trauma will more probably produce a subdural haematoma.

Cerebral injuries are said to be *open* or *closed* according to whether the dura mater is breached or intact. Open head injuries are in general the more severe, yet serious contusions may be sustained with an intact dura and skull. The lesser degrees of closed head injury are usually termed *concussion*, but recent work has disclosed so much gradation in pathological change within this group that its limits are arbitrary.

The peculiar anatomical distribution of the cerebral blood-vessels should be recalled in any consideration of the effects of trauma. The superficial ramification of these, especially the veins, over the cerebral convexities renders them vulnerable to a degree not seen in any other organ. Their inevitable implication explains the infarct-like appearances so frequently seen in the subjacent cortical lesion.

Finally, a few terms require definition. Any large deficit in the vault of the skull is liable to be followed by a *hernia cerebri*. This is a bulging of cerebral substance through the bony gap, the scalp being intact. A *traumatic cyst* (p. 455) is then often formed in the subjacent brain. Occasionally the scalp is also locally defective, thus exposing the herniated brain at the surface of the head. This condition is known as *fungus cerebri*. Though these are most often complications of craniotomy, they may be encountered wherever injury has entailed substantial loss of bone.

I. Closed head injuries

(1) **Concussion.** Since concussion is seldom fatal, our knowledge of its pathology is largely based on the results of animal experiments. Those of Denny-Brown and Russell (1941) were an important turning-point in this respect. Cats, dogs and monkeys were struck on the head by a weighted pendulum of measured velocity and mass, and loss of consciousness was

judged by loss of corneal and pinnal reflexes. The effects on respiration and on pulse rate and pressure were also studied. It was found that a blow on the occipital region by a flat object of a weight at least equal to that of the animal's head and with a velocity of more than 28 ft. per second (about 19 miles per hour) on the unsupported head regularly caused loss of corneal and pinnal reflexes. If the head were firmly supported a considerably more rapid blow, which often caused fracture of the skull, was needed to produce the same effects. If the blow had a greater velocity or were repeated several times it might cause death without producing haemorrhagic or other macroscopic lesions in the brain. Similar effects on brain-stem reflexes could be produced in the decerebrate animal, but required more severe blows. The authors named the concussion effects produced in this manner *acceleration concussion.*

Both sub-concussive and concussive blows caused an immediate rise in blood pressure due to peripheral vaso-constriction. That the cerebral arterioles did not participate in this vaso-constriction was shown by the increased flow in the jugular veins with unchanged a-v O_2 and CO_2 differential, which accompanied the rise of blood pressure. With more severe blows the blood pressure, after a small initial rise, fell progressively for up to 7 minutes, after which there might be gradual recovery or final complete heart failure associated with severe peripheral vaso-constriction. Very little increase of intracranial pressure occurred either as a direct result of the blow or following the rise of blood pressure. The authors, therefore, considered that a rise in intracranial pressure was not an essential feature of concussion. It was, however, possible to produce effects somewhat similar to those of 'acceleration concussion' by sharply striking the piston of a syringe connected by a tube with a hole in the skull, but it was not possible to cause death by this means unless the increase of pressure were prolonged sufficiently to cause herniation at the foramen magnum.

These experiments demonstrated the importance of brain-stem centres in the production of concussion. They were followed by the histological studies of Windle, Groat and Fox (1944) on the brains of guinea-pigs which had been subjected to blows on the head by a pendulum similar to that used by Denny-Brown and Russell. They found chromatolysis in the larger cells of the formatio reticularis and lateral vestibular nuclei, beginning about 14 hours after the injury and becoming more definite after 48 hours, after which it might recede or progress to a maximum in 6–8 days. By this time some of the cells had become ghosts or had disappeared completely. In experiments in which the head had been struck twice or more often, as many as 50 per cent of the cells in some nuclei might disappear in this manner. Later Groat, Windle and Magoun (1945) performed experiments on monkeys in which concussion was caused either by the piston method or by severe blows on the shielded head. In addition to similar lesions in brain-stem nuclei, these experiments produced changes in some of the large cells of the motor cortex, which were shrunken and hyperchromic with cork-screw dendrites.

Another new conception of the mechanism of head injuries is that the brain moves within the skull. This was indicated by Holbourn's (1943, 1944 a) experiments on models and more conclusively by the experiments of Pudenz and Shelden (1946) on monkeys fitted with a lucite calvarium. They studied the movements of the brain in relation to the skull during and after the impact of a blow of 6·6–7 foot-pounds, by slow-motion cinematography, and observed different effects when the impact was on different parts of the skull. Subconcussive blows on the mid-frontal or mid-occipital region produced a sliding movement of the cerebral convolutions in the direction of the blow. In both cases this movement was greatest in the parietal lobes. On the other hand blows on the temporal or parietal region caused a rotational movement in the horizontal plane.

The evidence provided by Holbourn, and by Pudenz and Shelden, suggests that the imparting to the brain of shearing strains, chiefly rotational, is likely to disrupt blood-vessels and axons;

synapses and dendrites may also be damaged. From her studies of human material Strich (1956, 1961) has implemented this concept: in a series of 20 cases in which death followed a closed head injury (a fracture was found in two cases only) the patients survived for weeks or many months in a state of dementia with severe neurological disturbances. At necropsy minimal evidence of contusion and haemorrhage was found, but histological examination revealed extensive, asymmetrical degeneration of the white matter with incomplete loss of the nerve fibres. The overlying cortex was little affected. In the degenerated areas lipid phagocytes were numerous. Degeneration of projection fibres had led to atrophy of the thalamic nuclei from which they arose and thus the dementia could be attributed to severance of thalamocortical connections. These effects, as argued by Strich, are inexplicable except as the result of stretching and tearing of the axis-cylinders at the time of the accident, as predicted by Holbourn.

It may be surmised that lesser degrees of this kind of damage are sustained in many cases of concussion. Indeed, as argued by Symonds (1962) it is doubtful whether, in concussion, the brain ever escapes some amount of irreversible damage. With increasing age residual neurological sequelae are more likely to be noted clinically and repeated incidents of this order are cumulative. This might be considered the most plausible explanation of the 'punch-drunk' syndrome in boxers: a condition on which pathology has been regrettably silent. It is, however, noteworthy that histological examination of the brain in the few cases so far recorded has revealed the changes of Alzheimer's disease (Corsellis and Brierley 1959) or of atypical Pick's disease (Neubürger *et al.* 1959).

(2) **Epidural haemorrhage** is a common result of injury in the temporal region. It results from tearing of the middle meningeal artery or vein or of both, and is usually but not invariably associated with a local crack or fracture of the skull which may involve only the inner table. The impact which causes this need not be severe since the squamous temporal and lower parts of the parietal bone are thin. For example it may result from being hit on the side of the head by a stone weighing about 100 g., thrown without great force, or by a golf ball. Blood accumulating between the skull and the dura mater strips the dura mater over a limited area and produces symptoms at first of local and later of more general compression of the brain. The rapidity with which these symptoms may increase and lead to death makes epidural haemorrhage one of the most acute emergencies of surgical practice. Epidural haemorrhages may also occur from the other vascular branches to the dura mater and bone or from tears of the veins as they enter the dural sinuses. In such cases they are usually associated with more severe, diffuse injuries which cause deformation and fracture of the skull. In Lewin's (1953) series of 1,000 cases of head injury, 31 per cent of epidural haemorrhages were in sites other than the temporal region.

(3) **Subdural haemorrhage.** (*a*) *Acute.* Variable amounts of subdural haemorrhage inevitably complicate open wounds of the brain and may, in some instances, be sufficient to contribute substantially to an increase of intracranial pressure. Gross haemorrhage in *closed* injuries results from the tearing of veins crossing the subdural space and may be attributed to forcible rotation of the brain within the skull. The inferior anastomotic vein has, in the writer's experience, been thus involved in two boxing fatalities.

(*b*) *Chronic.* These subdural haematomas are usually found in young infants and elderly subjects. In the latter the subdural space has become enlarged through atrophy of the cerebrum. In consequence the veins traversing this space are stretched, and thus specially vulnerable to shearing stresses in forcible rotation of the brain within the skull. Tearing of the veins in this way was demonstrated experimentally by Pudenz and Shelden.

In chronic subdural haematomas there is an interval of several weeks or even months between the trauma and the appearance of symptoms. They are commonly the only evident injury to the intracranial contents. The trauma which caused them may be slight and may not affect the head directly; for example, a sudden fall on to the buttocks, or a sudden jar, as in a car collision in which the head is not struck. Many are considered to be idiopathic since no history of injury can be obtained, but it is probable that in most of these there has been a sudden jar of the kind indicated, or a minor blow over the forehead or occiput. These haematomas also are most commonly situated over the convexity of the brain near the vertex and are often bilateral. They are usually completely encapsulated by a pseudo-membrane of connective tissue, but in the more recent cases the capsule may be defective on the surface in contact with the arachnoid and it is always thinner on this surface. It is adherent to the dura mater, but can be stripped from it without much difficulty (Fig. 7.1). It does not become adherent to the

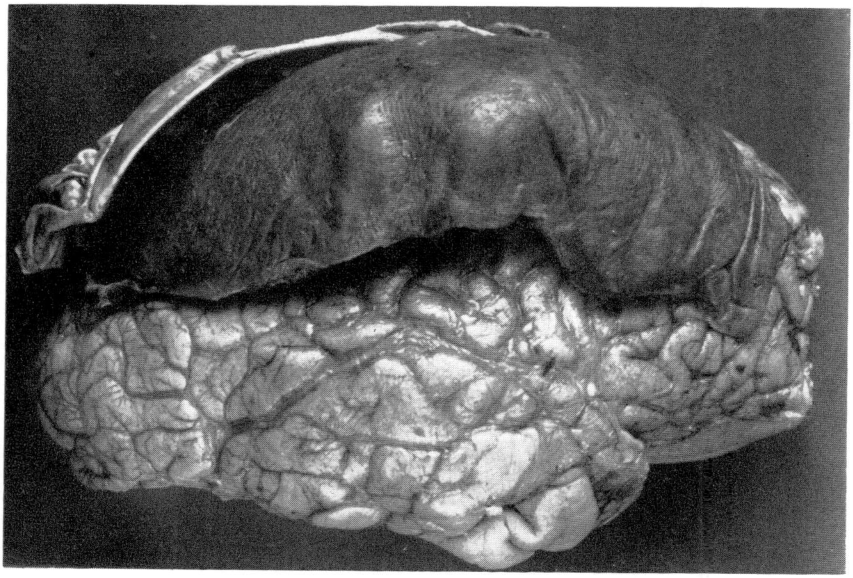

FIG. 7.1. Chronic subdural haematoma. There was no history of injury, but progressive symptoms went back for nearly a year. Note the complete encapsulation, freedom from the arachnoid and clean separation from the dura mater.

arachnoid except in rare cases where the arachnoid has been torn by the injury. This may be explained by the peculiar layer of endothelial or exothelial (del Rio Hortega 1933) cells which covers the arachnoid and which does not react to the presence of blood in the same way as the inner layer of dura mater, on which there is no true endothelium (Leary 1939). The arachnoid is, however, usually stained yellow by blood pigment. Thin-walled, sinus-like vessels are present in one or both of the layers of the capsule, most usually that in contact with the dura mater and, in time, the capsule acquires great toughness from the deposition of collagen fibres. The contents of the sac consist of dark, turbid fluid and a varying amount of apparently fresh red blood corpuscles. The brain is compressed by the haematoma which may be as much as 3 cm. in thickness, and in the more chronic cases it may not regain its normal contour for some days after surgical removal of the haematoma.

Pathogenesis. The delay in the appearance of symptoms and their subsequent progressive severity suggests that chronic haematomas increase in size after they have become encapsulated. As there is no evidence of direct communication with the vein from which the blood originated, the reason for this distension of the sac is not clear. It has been suggested that the breakdown of protein molecules in the enclosed blood increases the osmotic tension within the sac so that it tends to absorb cerebrospinal fluid (Gardner 1932). It seems, however, more probable that the thin-walled blood-vessels in the capsule may either transude plasma or may actually bleed into the sac (Putnam and Cushing 1925). This hypothesis is favoured by the constant presence of red blood cells in the contents of the sac.

(4) **Subdural hygroma.** The term is applied to the collection of clear fluid in the subdural space. At early stages it is indistinguishable from cerebrospinal fluid. Rarely seen, the condition is usually found in infants and may be associated with a depressed fracture of the temporal bone. The escape of cerebrospinal fluid into the outer space, from which it cannot be absorbed, is ascribed to tearing of the arachnoid membrane. The later stages are analogous to those in subdural haematomas: the protein of the fluid increases, and xanthochromia may develop as the cystic collection acquires a capsule of granulation tissue.

(5) **Rupture of vascular malformations.** These, especially the arterio-venous variety, may be the source of intracerebral haemorrhage after a relatively trivial blow on the head. The haemorrhage can be massive and fatal, with rapidly deepening coma from increased intracranial pressure. Sometimes, especially in children and adolescents, the malformation is so small that careful scrutiny is required for its detection (Crawford and Russell 1956).

II. Open head injuries

(1) **Penetrating wounds.** Those caused by rifle bullets or by fragments of shell or bomb casing vary chiefly according to the velocity of the object after it has perforated the skull. A high-velocity rifle bullet of 0·3-in. diameter, fired at a range up to 200 yd. causes severe disruptive effects on the brain tissue for some distance around its track, and a large exit wound in the skull through which softened brain escapes (Fig. 7.2). But a bullet of this size at long range may only damage the brain tissue along its track and unless it causes severe haemorrhage its effects may be quite local. Similarly, small shell fragments and bullets from small-calibre rifles and pistols may produce only local effects. These are complicated by the fragments of skull which may be driven into the brain. The entrance hole in the cranium is conical and the damage to the inner table may involve an area 3 or 4 times as large as the hole in the outer table, so that most of the indriven fragments of bone come from the inner table. These are sharp-edged spicules which often tear small blood-vessels and cause bleeding either on the surface or more deeply in the brain. These secondary vascular effects are often more important than the direct mechanical effects on the parenchyma. For example, a small fragment of bone may be driven into the cortex and bruise it over a very limited area, but by tearing a small artery may also produce a larger area of haemorrhage, as well as ischaemia in the territory which the vessel supplies. Thus one often finds a more superficial haemorrhagic area with an area of ischaemic softening deep to it (Fig. 7.3). In most cases of this kind, whether caused by gun-shot injuries or by blows by a pointed object, there is also the danger of infection inherent in 'open' wounds of the brain.

This danger is inherent to the penetrating wounds acquired in less violent circumstances; the writer has seen fatal cerebral abscesses incurred through the perforation of the orbital plate by a knitting needle, and of the ethmoidal air-cells by a sharp instrument. Cerebral tetanus has been reported in an airman whose brain was perforated by a splinter of wood (Lewin 1944).

(2) **Injury due to blunt forces.** *Fracture of the skull.* Although the importance of fracture of the skull in relation to these head injuries was exaggerated in the past, there are several reasons why such cases tend to be more serious and are more often fatal than those without fracture. In the first place the presence of a fracture is evidence that the impact had con-

siderable force. Secondly, it is common to find areas of cortical bruising under fractures even when they are no more than linear fissures. They are often accompanied by small haemorrhages in the underlying white matter. These areas of bruising suggest that at the moment of impact the edges of the bone impinge on the underlying cerebral cortex. Fractures of the base have a special significance; not only are they evidence of the severity of the impact, but, as they

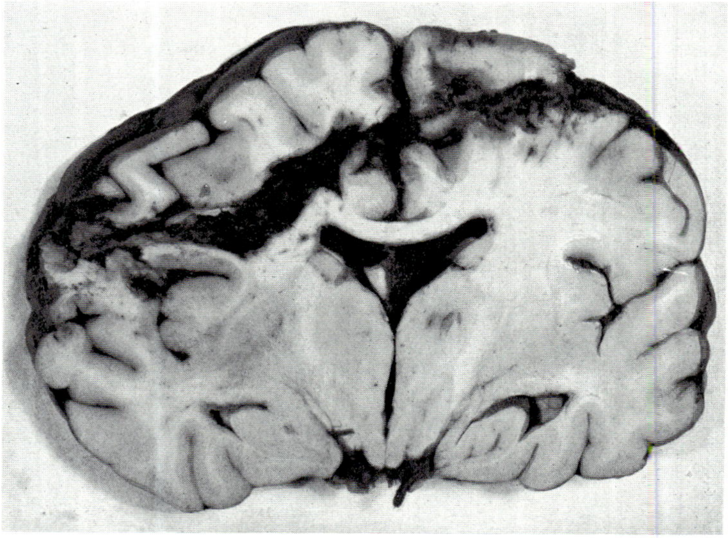

Fig. 7.2 Track of bullet wound through frontal lobes, from right to left.

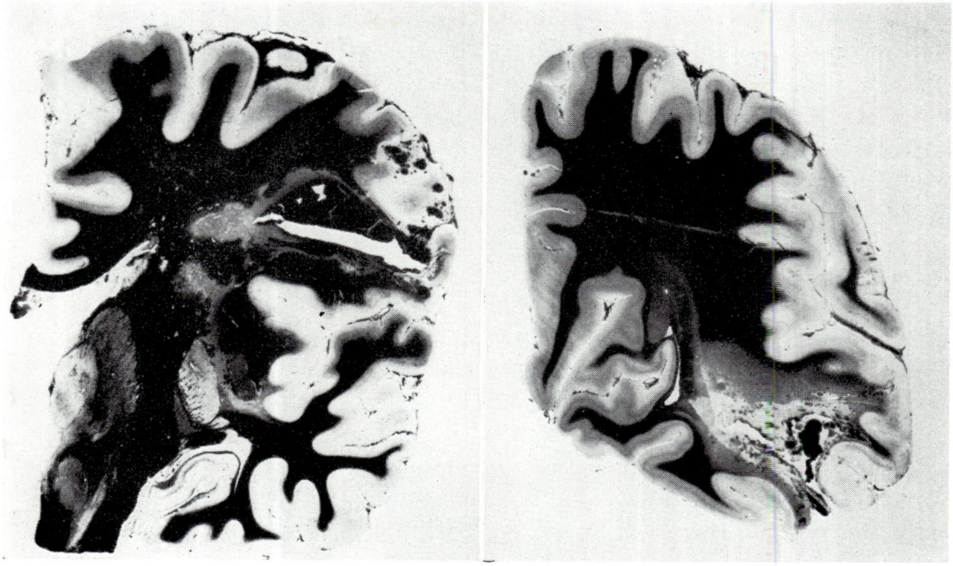

(*a*) (*b*)

FIG. 7.3. Injuries of brain due to indriven fragments of bone. (Coronal sections, myelin stain.)
(*a*) Superficial and deeper haemorrhages with a deeper area of ischaemia.
(*b*) Area of haemorrhage, ischaemia and oedema in lower temporo-occipital region.
The sharp outline of the ischaemic area in (*a*) contrasts with the indefinite outline of the oedematous area in (*b*).

often pass through paranasal sinuses or the middle ear, they may open a channel of infection from the outside air. They are also commonly associated with damage to one or more cranial nerves, especially the oculomotor and facial. The olfactory nerves and tract are also frequently damaged in injuries over the frontal region or bridge of the nose, whether or not there is fracture of the cribriform plate of the ethmoid. Fractures of the ethmoid or of the thin plates of bone which form the inner walls of the frontal or sphenoidal air sinuses may be caused by comparatively slight injuries and may allow infection to spread to the meninges. An initial rhinorrhoea of cerebrospinal fluid is a danger signal in such cases. The defect in the bone may become closed by granulation tissue which allows infection to pass to the subarachnoid space several months after the injury, and in some cases recurrent episodes of meningitis may be caused by injuries of this kind.

Contusion: coup and contrecoup. With injuries of this type the brain is damaged more widely by being made to move within the skull or by having its shape momentarily altered. Both causes may operate at the same moment. Deformation of the skull is most likely to result from blows over the vault owing to the greater rigidity of the base of the skull, whereas blows near the base of the skull, for example over the occiput, have more tendency to cause movement of the brain in relation to the skull. This movement is greater when the impact is on the frontal or occipital regions than when it is on the side of the head, as the falx prevents lateral movement. It is also likely to be greater in adults than in children since the amount of cerebrospinal fluid between the brain and the skull increases with age. On the other hand the child's skull, being thinner, is more easily deformed by a blow.

Holbourn, however, visualises shearing strains as occurring between the main mass of the brain and its more superficial areas where the latter are prevented from moving in relation to the skull by bony prominences such as the sphenoidal ridge, when the impact is on the occiput or forehead, and the cavernous sinus and crista galli in blows on the side of the head. He likens the rotation of the brain inside the skull to the movement of water in a round-bodied flask when it is suddenly turned. Because of this movement and the resistance of the sphenoidal ridges to it, the temporal poles are likely to be bruised by blows either on the occiput or frontal region. At the same time displacement of cerebrospinal fluid by the heavier brain tissue is likely to occur. If the movement of the head is suddenly arrested by impact against a solid object the momentum of the brain makes it continue to move. If on the other hand the stationary head is struck by a heavy moving object the skull moves in relation to the brain with the same eventual result. The effects in either case are due to the rate of deceleration or acceleration of the head and are essentially similar (Gillingham 1954). Blows with blunt objects of limited size, in addition to moving the skull suddenly in relation to the brain, very often produce fracture of the skull and bruising of the underlying brain at the site of impact. Denny-Brown and Russell (1941) showed that if the head is cushioned by a yielding substance, such as a crash helmet, the rate of acceleration or deceleration due to the impact and the consequent effects on the brain are reduced.

This movement of the brain within the skull may cause damage in three different ways. (1) It may tear the veins which pass from the brain to the dural venous sinuses and cause *subdural haematomas.* (2) It may produce bruising or laceration of the surface of convolutions where the brain lies on the floor of the skull. (3) It may cause moulding of brain tissue with stretching or tearing of fibre tracts and small blood-vessels.

Examination of the brain reveals a wide gradation in the extent of the injury, from examples in which large areas of the cerebrum are fragmented and haemorrhagic to those in which the damage is limited to the site of fracture with, possibly, a contrecoup lesion at the opposite pole of the brain. At the site of fracture the summits of the gyri are bruised and haemorrhagic, and may be lacerated. A wider area of the leptomeninges is suffused with blood. Such lesions seldom extend beyond the subcortical white matter, which is oedematous and stippled with small haemorrhages.

The contrecoup lesion shows similar bruising, limited to the summits of the gyri; it is most frequently observed in the region of the sphenoidal ridge, or over the convexity of a temporal lobe, and may be more spectacular than the injury at the site of impact. The pathogenesis of these contrecoup lesions is hotly argued. An excellent analysis of this controversy is given in the recent study by Lindenberg and Freytag (1960) of their large series of cases. Holbourn's theory, mentioned above, would explain the common contrecoup lesion related to the sharp border of the sphenoidal ridge, found after impact upon the occiput, and also the callosal lesions produced by the free edge of the falx. But bitemporal coup and contrecoup contusions are more difficult to explain; here the contrecoup lesion may be caused by a positive pressure, with slapping of the brain against the skull. Lindenberg and Freytag suggest that a sudden mass-shifting of the brain rather than a compression wave is responsible for this effect.

Vascular lesions

Subarachnoid haemorrhage of greater or less degree is a constant accompaniment of cerebral contusion. In some cases in which a medium-sized superficial vessel is torn it may be the chief cause of symptoms, but in most cases it arises from small vessels and is part of the surface bruising associated with fracture of the skull.

Multiple small haemorrhages in the white matter, sometimes of ring or ball type, are not uncommonly found, both in the cerebral and cerebellar hemispheres, in cases of fatal head injury. Although they are most probably caused by moulding of the brain their mechanism is not clear, since Schaller *et al.* (1937) could find no evidence of tears in the walls of the vessels in relation to them. They and others have found degenerative changes in the endothelium, hyaline changes in the media and thrombosis of vessels in haemorrhagic areas. Ring or ball haemorrhages may be due to fat-embolism (see p. 89) or be secondary to thrombosis of small vessels. Schaller *et al.* did not find them in cases of early death. Small haemorrhages or foci of softening in the midbrain and pons are most often secondary to tentorial herniation but may be found when death has been almost immediate.

Duret (1878) emphasised the importance of small haemorrhages in the walls of the 3rd and 4th ventricles and around the iter of Sylvius in cases of comparatively minor head injury which ended fatally. He considered the mechanism causing these haemorrhages to be a wave of cerebrospinal fluid which was driven from the lateral ventricles towards the spinal subarachnoid space at the moment of impact. In the writer's experience (J.G.G.), petechial haemorrhages are not uncommon in the walls of the 3rd ventricle, but are more rarely seen round the iter of Sylvius unless in association with more ventrally situated midbrain haemorrhages, and are still more uncommon under the floor of the 4th ventricle.

Lesions of arteries. Movement of the brain within the skull may also produce lesions of the superficial blood-vessels. The small perforating arteries which supply the caudate and lenticular nuclei are those most commonly affected and haemorrhages or infarctions in these nuclei may result from tearing or thrombosis of one or more of these vessels (Gillingham 1954). Thromboses of the main trunk or larger branches of the anterior or middle cerebral arteries may also occur after a head injury, especially in older subjects. De Veer and Browder (1942) described a case of traumatic thrombosis of the internal carotid and middle cerebral arteries in which microscopical examination of the latter showed the intima and elastica to be torn away from the media, which was frayed and ragged; at one point the tear extended almost through the whole thickness of the media. In other cases thrombosis of the larger arteries seems to result from the fall of blood pressure, brought on by the surgical shock of the accident, leading to thrombosis of an arteriosclerotic vessel. Occasionally occlusion of the middle cerebral artery may be caused by the pressure of an epidural or subdural haematoma which has caused tentorial herniation (Evans and Scheinker 1943). Infarctions in the territory of the posterior cerebral artery are more common sequelae of such herniations.

Arteriovenous aneurysms may be produced by fractures of the base of the skull which tear the internal carotid artery where it lies in relation to the cavernous sinus.

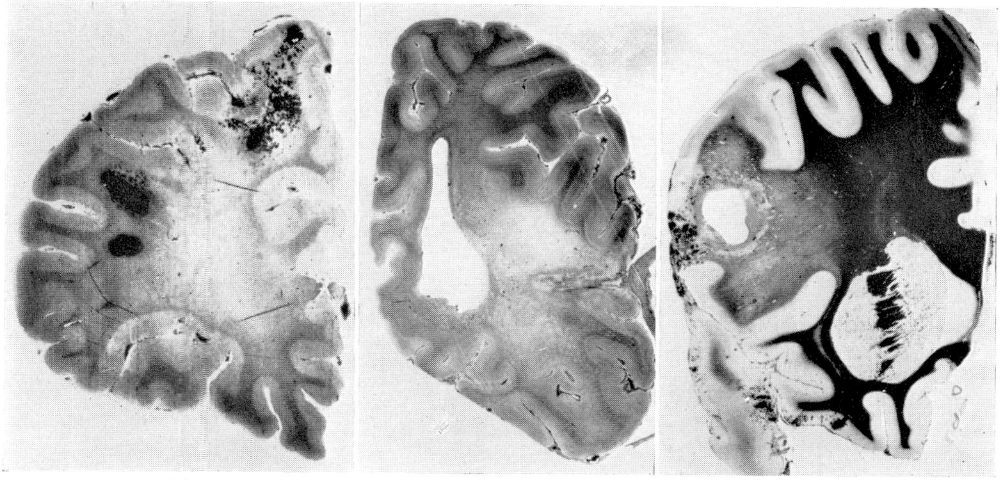

(*a*) (*b*) (*c*)

FIG. 7.4. Traumatic oedema of the brain.

(*a*) Extensive oedema of the white matter of the frontal lobe associated with multiple haemorrhages. (*b*) Oedema round the track of a shell fragment which caused a superficial abscess and left a scar of adherent meninges. There is local dilatation of the ventricle in relation to this (4 months' history). (Coronal sections, myelin stain.) (*c*) Oedema round an abscess caused by an indriven fragment of bone.

Whether or not head injuries cause vasomotor effects such as 'vasoparesis' and 'capillary prestasis' of the cerebral vessels has for long been a matter of controversy (Ricker 1919) which is not yet settled. There seems to be definite evidence that a head injury may cause temporary spasm of the smaller cerebral arteries but there is less proof that this may be followed by vasoparesis. Helfand (1939) has found zones of paling in the cortex, pallor of Sommer's sector and of the end-plate of the cornu Ammonis and hyaline changes in Purkinje cells, with glial shrubs in the molecular layer of the cerebellum. Occasionally also he found areas of white softening at a distance from the chief areas of bruising or haemorrhage. Capillary prestasis, as in other conditions, appears to depend more on respiration than on functional changes in the arterioles, since an increase of CO_2 in the blood normally causes arterial and capillary dilatation (Wolff and Lennox 1930).

Traumatic cerebral oedema. The importance of cerebral swelling or oedema as a cause of death is emphasised by some authors and discounted or denied by others. Experimental work has also given very varied results. The most careful studies (Pilcher 1937, White *et al.* 1943) indicate that injuries, which are not sufficiently severe to cause haemorrhages, may produce a minor degree of oedema which seldom increases the bulk of the brain by more than 5 per cent. An increase of this magnitude may cause a dangerous increase of intracranial pressure although it produces no evident histological change and is not easily assessed by chemical methods. White *et al.* (1942) point out that if the water content of brain tissue is reckoned as 80 per cent then 5 per cent swelling of the brain by excess of interstitial fluid would only raise the water content to 81 per cent. This difference is within the experimental error when water content is estimated by the difference between wet and dry weights. They also found that reduction of blood oxygen caused swelling of the brain which was independent of the vascular dilatations produced by an excess of blood CO_2. These experiments conform with those of Landis *et al.* (1932) who found increased capillary permeability during venous congestion of organs. Schnedorf *et al.* (1940) had found both in experiments on dogs and in human cases that after cerebral injuries the oxygen saturation in the blood might fall far below normal, and often below the critical level at which the capillaries become permeable. Nearly all their fatal cases of head injury had low O_2 levels, whereas most of those in whom the blood

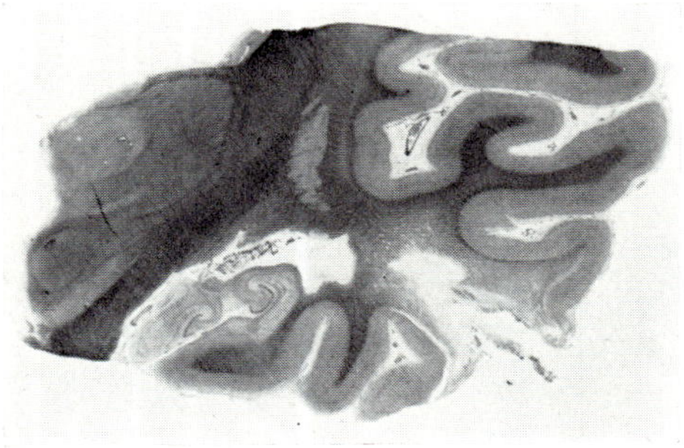

(*a*)

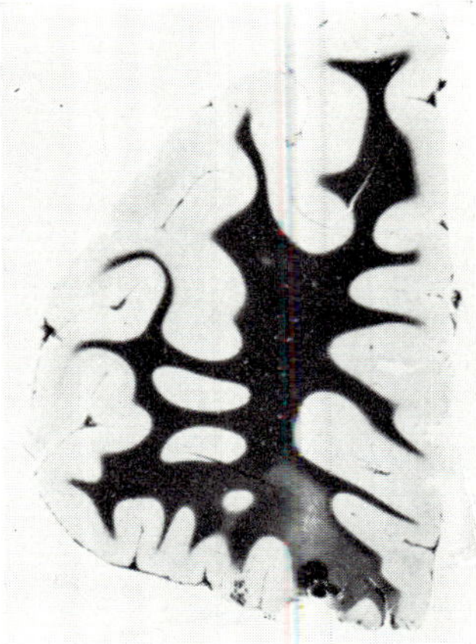

(*b*)

FIG. 7.5. Bruising of surface of convolutions. Sections stained for myelin.
(*a*) Lesion of 2nd and 3rd temporal gyri with slight oedema of underlying white matter.
(*b*) Lesion of gyrus rectus and olfactory tract.

O_2 remained above the critical level recovered. White *et al.* consider, therefore, that low O_2 levels in the blood may be an important cause of cerebral oedema following head injury.

On the other hand obvious tentorial herniation is rarely seen in fatal head injuries unless there is also an intra- or extracerebral haemorrhage. It has not always been recognised that intracerebral haemorrhages are constantly surrounded by a zone of oedema which may be quite extensive around the larger haemorrhages and in areas of multiple small haemorrhages, and brain swelling due to this combination of haemorrhage and oedema had been attributed to primary oedema (Fig. 7.4*a*). Ischaemic softening of the white matter also in its early stages is not always distinguished from oedema. Nor is there any doubt that superficial bruises of the brain are usually associated with a zone of oedema in the underlying white matter and this may extend 2 or 3 cm. from the bruised area (Fig. 7.5*a*). The writer's (J.G.G.) experience agrees with that of Connors and Wright (1934) that oedema, apart from haemorrhage, is a rare cause of death in head injuries which receive immediate hospital treatment. But White *et al.* suggest that air transport at altitudes over 11,000 ft. may cause cerebral oedema due to low O_2 pressure.

Conventional light-microscopy suggests that oedema results from the escape of fluid into the intercellular spaces of the white matter. Though electronmicroscopists have denied this, it appears that valid preparations of the white matter, as distinct from the cortex, have yet to be critically examined by this technique. Recently Rubinstein *et al.* (1962), in an experimental study, have demonstrated a rapid local response of the fibrillary astrocytes in traumatic oedema.

These cells swell up within a few hours, their fibrils become thickened, and metabolic activity is markedly increased. It is of interest that this activity persists for several months into the stage of glial scar-formation.

Injury of the pituitary body. Fractures involving the base of the skull, especially those that cross the pituitary fossa, may damage the pars nervosa which, being soft and closely adherent to the dorsum sellae, is more vulnerable than the pars distalis. Subjects who recover are liable to suffer from diabetes insipidus. Pituitary insufficiency may however be due to tearing of the stalk. Extensive infarction of the pars distalis from this cause was reported in 5 cases by Daniel *et al.* (1959). It is of interest that, in a sixth case, the pars distalis survived because the stalk was detached at its junction with the hypothalamus; the vascular supply of the gland was thus intact.

Microscopical lesions

Local lesions. In areas of bruising of the cerebral or cerebellar cortex severe lesions of nerve cells, nerve fibres and neuroglia are seen. Some of these appear to be direct mechanical effects of trauma whereas others resemble those of ischaemia. It is sometimes difficult to distinguish these effects, and they are often combined since fibrinoid necrosis of arteries and thrombosis of small vessels are common in bruised areas of cortex. The amount of haemorrhage in bruised areas varies greatly. In some it is chiefly subpial or subarachnoid, and is associated with severe ischaemic lesions in the underlying cortex, suggesting tearing of a small surface vessel. In other cases small haemorrhagic lesions in the cortex are surrounded by areas showing lesions of ischaemic or mechanical origin.

Two types of lesion of nerve cells which may be found in bruised areas are not seen in purely ischaemic lesions and, therefore, are probably directly caused by physical stresses. These are: (1) *Rapid disintegration of neurones* within a few hours of the injury. This may be associated with rupture of the nuclear membrane (Rand and Courville 1946), disappearance of the nucleus or neuronophagy by neutrophil leucocytes or microglia (Fig. 7.6*a*). (2) *Binucleated and multinucleated nerve cells* have been found on the margin of bruised areas of cortex by a number of early workers (Tigges 1863, Jolly 1870, Ceccherelli 1874, Popoff 1875) and more recently by Gaupp (1933) and Rand and Courville (1946, 1947). The latter authors did not find them in cases which were fatal in less than 10 days. In most instances the cells had two nuclei, more rarely three and very rarely four (Fig. 7.6*e*). The cell body might be relatively intact or might have an indistinct outline, as though its cytoplasm were blending with the surrounding ground substance. It is known that binucleation of nerve cells may result from stab wounds or cauterisation of the cortex and after infections such as syphilis and viral encephalitis, and it appears that mechanical trauma also can stimulate nuclear division in neurones. Various other nuclear changes are found including constriction of the nuclear membrane; Rand and Courville interpret this as a preliminary stage of nuclear division.

The ischaemic changes in bruised areas are similar to those found in other vascular lesions; pallor and eosinophilia of the cytoplasm with hyperchromia and shrinkage of the nucleus, and changes similar to homogenising cell change are commonly seen. Incrustation of the Golgi network may affect many cells in the area. Within the first few days many of the neurones in bruised areas of cortex may contain collections of birefringent, dark brown or black, haematin crystals or granules. At a later stage granules of iron-containing pigment appear in the peripheral zone of the cytoplasm of pyknotic neurones on the edges of contused areas, and still later many nerve cells are transformed into pyramidal agglomerations of strongly haematoxophilic granules and similar granules can be traced for some distance along the lines of the dendrites. These incrustations stain deeply by the Prussian blue and Turnbull's blue methods for iron.

The extent to which neurones eventually disappear from a contused area of cortex varies with the severity of the lesion. In many cases the central parts of the bruised area are completely absorbed and only a few encrusted cells or granules of blood pigment at its margin remain to indicate the nature of the lesion.

In *tâches jaunes*, in which only the summits of convolutions are bruised, the transition zone, from the margin of the gap in the cortex to the area of healthy nerve cells, may be very narrow or scarcely visible. In other cases a shrunken cortical scar containing a few pyknotic or encrusted nerve cells and gliotic tissue is invaded on the surface by collagenous fibres from the pia

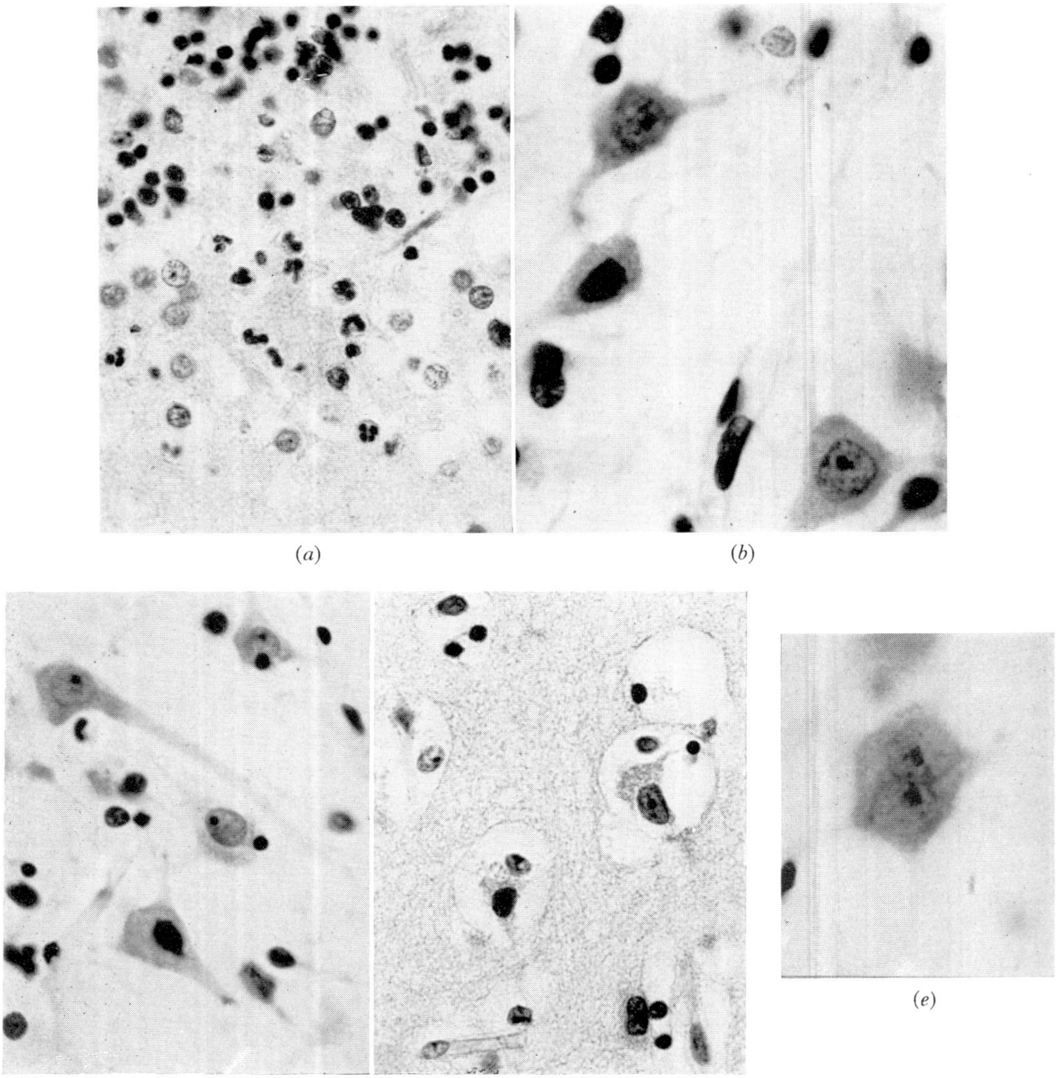

(*a*) (*b*)

(*c*) (*d*) (*e*)

FIG. 7.6. Nerve cells in or near bruised areas of brain.

(*a*) Purkinje cells 12 hours after fracture of the base of the skull. (H. and E.)
(*b*) and (*c*) Cortical nerve cells 2 days after injury. Only isolated neurones are degenerated. (H. and E.)
(*d*) Cortical nerve cells $3\frac{1}{2}$ days after injury. (H. and E.)
(*e*) Binucleated nerve cell 36 hours after injury. (Nissl $\times 750$.)

mater. These defects or cortical scars overlie areas of gliosis and demyelination in the white matter which usually extend for 1 to 3 cm. from the cortex, and after severe contusions may reach the wall of the lateral ventricle. They have the characteristics of demyelination secondary to oedema, and are no doubt chiefly produced in this manner, but end bulbs and nummular or beaded swellings on some of the axons in these areas indicate a more directly mechanical cause. To some extent also they are accounted for by the loss of axons of cortical neurones which have been destroyed. After severe local injuries of the cortex, especially after open wounds with considerable bony damage, a dense fibrous tissue scar may pass from the dura mater into the brain and merge with the deeper gliotic tissue (Foerster and Penfield 1930). Such scars are often associated with local bulging of the walls of the ventricles (Fig. 7.4 b).

Diffuse histological lesions. More widespread changes in cortical nerve cells have been described by many and are specially emphasised by Rand and Courville (1946) who divide these changes into: (1) *Chromatolysis* which is directly due to the injury and (2) *Vacuolation* which they considered to be secondary to oedema.

(1) In their series of fatal cases *chromatolysis* was seen in its early stages as soon as 1½ hours after severe head injury. In a case of death 24 hours after the injury, most of the cortical nerve cells had lost their Nissl granules and in the others the chromatic substance was irregularly distributed. In cases in which life was prolonged for 2–5 weeks the nerve cells were still chromatolytic. Similar changes were seen in the Purkinje cells, although the cerebellum showed no macroscopical lesions. Rand and Courville also found neurofibrillar changes which were visible by Cajal's reduced silver technique but not by Bielschowsky's method. The nuclear chromatin also became coarser, or was arranged in short chain-like strands. These cellular changes are in agreement with those found by Windle, Groat and Fox (1944) in the brain stem and may result from shearing strains acting on cortical and subcortical tissues. All these changes are probably reversible and in most cases transitory, but it is possible that in cases of severe head injury, especially in elderly subjects, some of the cortical nerve cells may fail to recover.

(2) *Vacuolation* of nerve cells was seen by Rand and Courville in cases of cerebral oedema. It began within a few hours of the injury in the nucleus where numerous vacuoles might displace the nuclear chromatin. At the same time two or three vacuoles, instead of the usual single one, might be seen in the nucleolus. After 24 hours small perinuclear vacuoles might appear. Cytoplasmic vacuoles were rarely found and only in cases which had survived for several days.

Lesions of the *choroid plexus* and *ependyma* were found almost constantly by Rand and Courville (1931) in a series of 61 cases of cerebral injury. In the choroid plexus there was oedema of the stroma and vacuolation of the epithelial cells. Haemorrhages into the plexus were more rarely found. Vacuolation of similar type, but usually less in degree, was seen in the ependymal cells and was often accompanied by oedema or collections of fluid in the subependymal tissues. Hoff (1930), in experimental head injuries, found evidence that the choroid plexus was unduly permeable to fluorescein and appeared to produce an excess of fluid within a few minutes of the blow. After 12 hours he found tears in the ependyma and fluorescein staining and oedema in the subependymal tissues. Gierlich (1936) also found defects in the ependyma, sometimes in association with subependymal haemorrhages. In sections stained for myelin areas of pallor may sometimes be found round the walls of the lateral ventricles especially at their frontal and occipital poles. They resemble the zones of pallor which are commonly seen in relation to defects in the ependyma in cases of subacute hydrocephalus, and appear to be caused by seepage of cerebrospinal fluid into the subependymal tissues.

In assessing the importance of these widespread microscopical lesions in relation to the

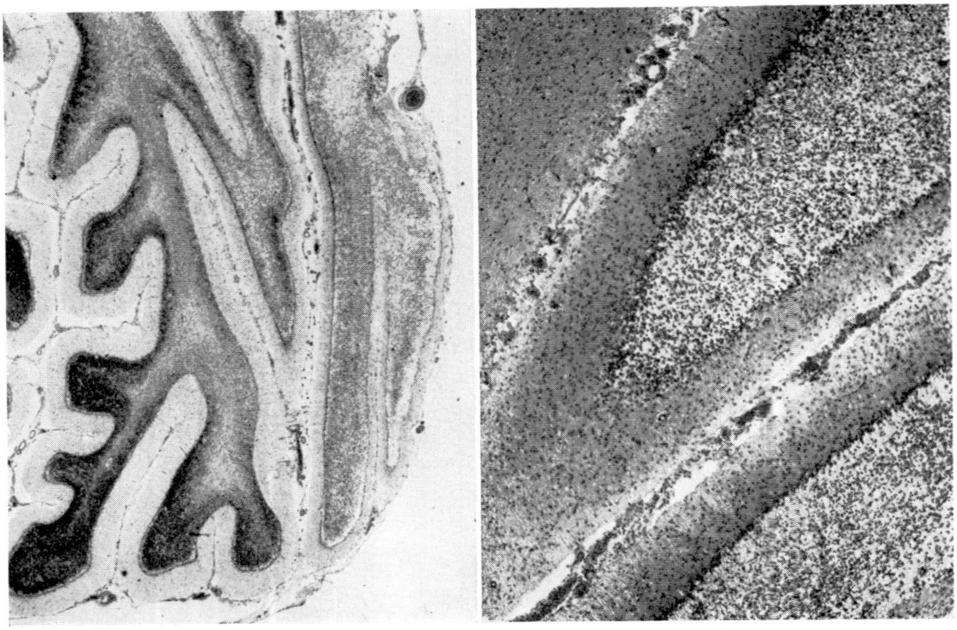

(a) (b)

FIG. 7.7. Bruising of the cerebellum, resulting from severe fracture of the skull 2 months previously in a boy of 3 years, with overriding of the edges of the fracture in the occipital bone.
(a) The degeneration is greater on the surface than more deeply.
(b) Purkinje cells are lost in areas where granule cells survive. (Haematoxylin.)

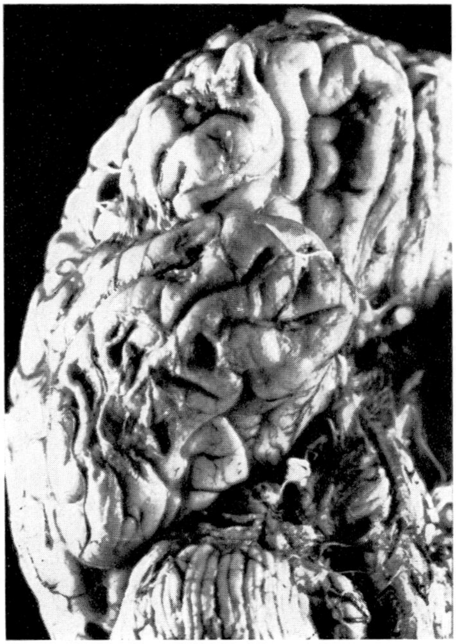

(a)

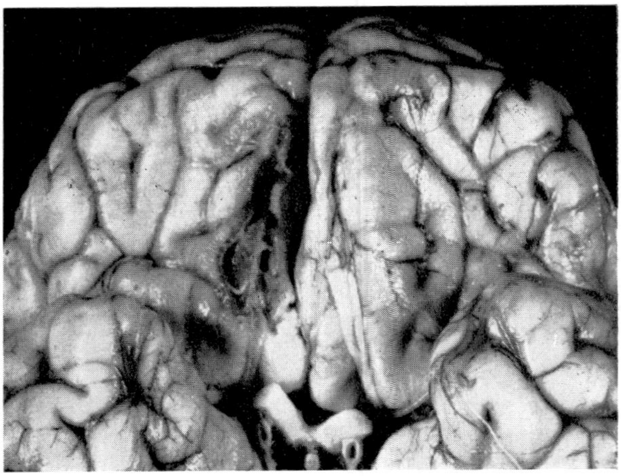

(b)

FIG. 7.8. Bruising of surface convolutions.
(a) Old traumatic lesion of lower temporal gyri.
(b) Traumatic lesion of olfactory tract and gyrus rectus. (By the kindness of Dr. S. J. Strich.)

clinical aspects of head injuries, it must be remembered that, apart from experimental work, they have been found in fatal, and therefore severe, cases. But they probably indicate that in cases which recover, even those of comparatively mild character, the cortex, subcortical white matter, periventricular tissues and brain stem may be the seat of minor disturbances which, although scarcely discernible by histological methods, may lead to disturbance of function.

Late changes (Figs. 7.7 and 7.8). The healing of cortical bruises is accompanied by shrinkage whilst the necrotic debris is removed by phagocytes and replaced by astrocytic glia. The retention of iron pigment causes a permanent yellowish staining of the area. The overlying leptomeninges are thickened by fibrosis and are often adherent to the dura mater.

Ventricular dilatation. If such an area is extensive, there is shrinkage and gliosis of the subjacent white matter, and the lateral ventricle is locally expanded; in extreme cases this has the appearance of a diverticulum (Fig. 7.4*b*). In addition Northfield (1944) has described a generalised dilatation of one ventricle, attributable to more diffuse injury of the hemisphere, with eventual shrinkage of its white matter. Symmetrical dilatation of both lateral ventricles may similarly be due to widespread lesions in both hemispheres, but is more often caused by obstruction to the flow of cerebrospinal fluid. The obstruction is usually located in the basal meninges, especially about the fourth ventricle, and is due to a low-grade inflammatory reaction provoked by extravasated blood. In some cases there is defective absorption of cerebrospinal fluid. This was found in 58 per cent of cases of head injury by Bielschowsky (1928), who used as his criterion the time interval after which NaI appeared in the urine following its injection into the ventricles or subarachnoid space. Such delay in absorption might produce external hydrocephalus along with ventricular dilatation. In a number of Bielschowsky's cases, an excess of air in the subarachnoid space was associated with delayed excretion of NaI and increased cerebrospinal pressure, but he found it difficult to assess the importance of external hydrocephalus apart from this association. In some cases of generalised ventricular dilatation in which there is also an excess of fluid in the subarachnoid space, there is at no time any increase of cerebrospinal pressure, and it is evident that in these cases there must be generalised shrinkage of the cerebral hemispheres. The cause of this is by no means clear.

Cysts and aeroceles. A cyst may form in the white matter beneath the seat of injury. This is most likely to occur when some degree of cerebral herniation has taken place.

Such cysts were observed in otherwise normal rabbits when a simple craniotomy, with opening of the dura mater, had been followed by transitory herniation (Falconer and Russell 1944). In some examples the cyst communicated with the lateral ventricle. At late stages the wall of the cyst was composed of fibrillary glia containing foci of foam-cells, some of which contained iron pigment. Though associated with marginal ecchymoses, there is no evidence that these cysts are the outcome of massive haemorrhage. Their formation was explained by Holbourn (1944 b) as the result of stresses, set up by the hernia, which tended to cause splitting at the junction of cortex and white matter: the site, in fact, at which the cysts were observed to originate.

In special circumstances, notably if the lesion is frontal and associated with rhinorrhoea, it is possible for air to enter the cavity which is then termed an *aerocele*. Bacterial infection is consequently a hazard and, should the aerocele communicate with the ventricular system, purulent leptomeningitis may ensue.

Head injury and neoplasia. The question as to whether primary intracranial neoplasms are provoked by head injuries is discussed in the companion volume (Russell and Rubinstein 1963). In brief, there is some evidence that meningiomas arise at the site of previous trauma with sufficient frequency to be significant. It is also noteworthy that certain other tumours, especially glioblastomas, may be clinically unmasked immediately after a blow on the head, not necessarily severe. The development of symptoms appears due to a spreading oedema of the white matter adjacent to the tumour.

Head injury and multiple sclerosis. After a blow on the head, which may inflict only slight trauma, or after craniotomy, patients with multiple sclerosis are apt to remain unconscious until death supervenes after a few days, or possibly weeks. Examination of the brain discloses old plaques of sclerosis, sometimes so situated that the disease was undiagnosed during life, but yields no explanation of the mysterious reaction to trauma.

Cerebrospinal fluid

In cases of head injury, in which there is damage to the brain, the cerebrospinal fluid, if examined within a few hours of the accident, always contains an admixture of blood. This is a useful criterion in distinguishing severe concussion from cerebral contusion. Although the amount of blood in the fluid is not related to the depth of coma, since this may be deep when the blood admixture is slight, large amounts of blood in the cerebrospinal fluid (e.g. over 100,000 r.b.c. per cu. mm.) are usually associated with considerable loss of consciousness which may be due in large part to the presence of blood in the ventricles and subarachnoid space (Russell 1932). Yellow coloration of the supernatant fluid appears within a few hours of the injury and deepens during the first 2 days. The blood disappears rapidly from the fluid, and unless fresh bleeding takes place, very few red cells are found after the 3rd day. In spite of the large amount of blood which may be present the fluid does not form a coagulum unless the meninges become infected.

Pressure. In the early stages the fluid is often under moderately increased pressure (between 200 and 300 mm. of water). This was found in 54 per cent of Bielschowsky's cases. Pressures above 300 mm. are more rarely found. There appears to be little relation between the intracranial pressure, as measured by lumbar puncture, and the level of consciousness. Increase of pressure is often found in conscious patients and comatose patients may show low manometric levels. However, in most, but not all, patients with pressures over 300 mm. coma is fairly deep (Russell).

Cell count. In the early stages the leucocyte count is related to blood admixture, but it may fall more slowly than the red cells disappear. A later increase in the leucocyte count suggests meningitis.

Chemical examination. The protein is also related in the early stages to the blood admixture, and falls with it. Glucose may be raised in association with the rise in blood glucose which may be caused by injury to the brain. Apart from the effects of blood admixture, the fluid usually remains otherwise within normal limits. Falls in glucose and in chlorides below normal levels occur when the meninges become infected, but are less delicate indications of meningitis than the leucocyte count.

DAMAGE BY NON-MECHANICAL FORCES

1. X-Irradiation

Several cases have been reported in which therapeutic radiation of the scalp for rodent ulcers, for intracranial tumours (Pennybacker and Russell 1948), or for mental disease (Scholz and Hsü 1938), has resulted in damage to the brain. The symptoms of this do not appear until many months or some years later, but may then progress rapidly to a fatal issue. In such cases the cortex in the damaged area is swollen, yellow or brownish, tough and poorly demarcated from the underlying white matter which also may have an unduly firm consistency or may be custic or necrotic.

Microscopically, in cases of moderate severity, there is disappearance of neurones in the cortex, especially on the summits of the convolutions, with fibrillary gliosis spreading in from the surface and involving the deeper cortical layers to a greater or less degree. Here the astrocytes are swollen, with numerous processes, and typical clasmatodendrosis may be seen in the most damaged areas. In more severe cases there may be complete loss of nuclear staining in the cortex which appears amorphous and eosinophilic. Pennybacker and Russell observed thrombosis of some of the perforating vessels with fibrinoid necrosis of their walls, and areas of fibrinous exudate were present throughout some parts of the cortex. The white matter in most of the reported cases has been more severely damaged than the cortex. Here also many of the vessels show fibrinoid necrosis or collagenous thickening of their walls. The condition of the tissues is one of severe oedema going on to necrosis. In some places the only viable elements are microglial cells which have assumed an amoeboid shape and have engulfed globules or granules of lipid. In less affected areas the astrocytes have swollen cell bodies and there is some fibrous gliosis, but the most characteristic lesion is permeation of the tissues by fibrinoid or albuminous material.

Russell, Wilson and Tansley (1949), in an experimental study, found that rabbits, whose heads had been irradiated by a single dose of 2,850 r., showed no symptoms until about the 100th day. But after the 82nd day lesions began to appear in their brains. The earliest lesions were small ring and ball haemorrhages with slight loss of definition and staining properties in the basement membrane of capillaries but without evident thrombosis. Occasional small spheroidal particles with the staining reactions of fibrin were seen in the tissues round the affected vessels. In animals killed after the appearance of symptoms, the area of necrosis and haemorrhages had spread and the lesions had become more advanced. The walls of some arterioles had undergone fibrinoid necrosis and a few were thrombosed. Gliosis, with increase in the size of the astrocytes, was now seen in the areas first affected. More severe vascular changes were found in the brains of rabbits which were given 2,440 r. and were kept alive until symptoms appeared on or about the 240th day. Cortical changes were slight and usually confined to the cerebellum where there was a patchy loss of Purkinje cells, some torpedoes in the granular layer and increase of astrocyte nuclei. After smaller doses, 2,030 r. and 1,625 r., the animals remained well and their brains showed no lesions at 15 and 24 months.

From these experiments it appears that a single dose of X-rays may initiate, in the walls of arterioles and capillaries in the white matter of the brain, progressive changes which, after a considerable interval, first cause minute foci of haemorrhage and necrosis, and later go on to increased permeability, fibrinoid necrosis and eventual thrombosis.

2. Ultra-sound

When applied through a defect in the skull ultra-sound waves may produce lesions in the brain tissue especially in the subcortical white matter. Experimentally within 12 hours there is breaking up of myelin tubes, disruption of axons and some oedema, which becomes much more evident in 24 hours. At this stage a central necrotic area is often found and in the next 24 hours this enlarges and later becomes absorbed and replaced by a cavity. These effects may be produced either partly or wholly by the rise in temperature in the tissues caused by the ultra-sound waves (Barnard *et al.* 1955). This kind of lesion has been used as an alternative to frontal leucotomy in patients. On post-mortem examination of the brains of 25 such cases Nelson *et al.* (1959) found degrees of tissue damage varying from slight astrocytic reaction and questionable myelin damage to large areas of necrosis of the white matter surrounded by a wide zone of de-myelination. In the more severe cases there was also some laminar necrosis of the cortex near the site of entry of the beam. The central core of necrosis in the white matter was sometimes remarkable in that it showed little evidence of dissolution several weeks after the treatment.

3. Atomic explosions

Uchimura and Shiraki (1952) have reported on the examination of the brains of 37 patients who died between 19 and 64 days after being near an atomic explosion. In all cases there were profound anaemia and the changes in the tissues of the body cavity which are known to follow excessive radiation by gamma rays. In general no macroscopic lesions were visible in the brain. In only 2 cases were there small haemorrhages.

Microscopically, however, small perivascular haemorrhages were found in 26 cases. Areas of paling in the cortex and in Sommer's sector of the hippocampus and small foci of softening in the white matter were found in 6 cases, and in 5 cases glial shrub formations, indicating damage to Purkinje cells, were found in the cerebellar cortex. Fibrin transudation through the walls of vessels in the white matter was found in 1 case, but there was no evidence of coagulation necrosis of vessel walls nor of the extravasation of plasma which has been found in experimental lesions of the brain by X-rays. Proliferation of endothelial cells and an excess of adventitial reticulin was commonly found in the small cortical and subcortical vessels, but lesions of nerve cells might occur without any change in the vessels of the area. The authors considered that these changes were not produced mechanically, but were secondary to the effects on the blood-vessels of gamma rays and neutrons liberated by the explosion.

TRAUMATIC LESIONS OF THE SPINAL CORD

The spinal cord is protected from injury by its bony casing and, except in the cervical region, a considerable degree of violence is needed to damage this to such an extent as to injure the spinal cord. Fracture dislocation of the lower thoracic or lumbar spine is, however, a well recognised lesion in mining accidents due to falls of the roof, and may be caused in many other ways. The cervical spine is much more vulnerable and, as in the lower animals, fracture at this level is a common cause of death. On the other hand direct injuries to the spinal cord by stab wounds, bullets or fragments of shell or bomb casing are as common at the thoracic as at the cervical level. Wounds of the spine and spinal cord by high-velocity bullets have special pathological features due to the severity of the jar to the spinal column. Traumatic lesions of the spinal cord may be classified as (1) *Direct* due to injury of the cord by stab wounds or missiles which penetrate the cord. (2) *Indirect* due to fracture dislocations, or subluxations of the spine or to acute jars to the bone which are transmitted to the spinal cord. (3) *A combination of direct and indirect violence* as in wounds with high-velocity bullets, or in cases of fracture dislocation where the cord is lacerated or pierced by a spicule of bone.

Direct injuries to the spinal cord

The spinal cord may be directly injured without obvious or serious injury to the spine by stab wounds or by bullets or fragments of explosive which pass between the vertebral laminae. *Stab wounds* are of special interest to clinicians owing to the close correlation which may be traced between the lesions and the symptoms they cause. Three of the cases showing his syndrome, in the series which Brown-Séquard published in 1868, were of this kind. Their chief interest to the pathologist is the opportunity they may give for the study of the course and termination of the longer spinal nerve tracts and the phenomena of Wallerian degeneration.

As the imbrication of the spines of the thoracic vertebrae protect the spinal canal on its dorsal surface, stab wounds must enter it dorsolaterally. The severance of nerve tracts in the spinal cord is therefore greater on one side than the other and the dorsal columns are usually more severely damaged than the ventrolateral. But in some cases the cord is more or less completely severed. There is usually little bleeding except from the epidural veins and comparatively slight bruising of the tissues of the cord. The lesion is therefore quite local and, unless complicated by sepsis or injury to the anterior spinal artery, is limited to the level of the wound and a few millimetres on either side of this where the nervous tissue is bruised and softened. Within a few hours swellings appear on the severed axons at the ends which remain in continuity with the cell body, and the softened nervous tissue becomes gradually broken up and engulfed by phagocytes. Unless the spinal cord has been completely divided the wound is eventually closed by a glio-conjunctival scar through which neurites arising from the severed axons run irregularly, chiefly along connective tissue trabeculae.

The effects of direct injuries to the spinal cord by bullets or shell fragments have been well described by Roussy and Lhermitte (1918). The degree of damage to the cord in such cases bears a relation both to the size and to the velocity of the missile. When pierced by high-velocity missiles, as a bullet fired at close range, the nervous tissue may be disintegrated over one or more segments above and below the level of entry. Shell fragments usually cause more local lesions, but may produce softening or pulping and destruction of the whole thickness of the cord. The hole in the dura mater appears small in relation to the extent of damage to the cord; it may be a longitudinal slit or a ragged tear, the edges of which tend to rejoin. It is very rare for the dura mater to be completely torn across, so that in the more severe injuries the ends of the cord are held in approximation, if not in apposition, by the dural sheath. Intramedullary haemorrhage is usually slight but there may be considerable bleeding in the epi- and subdural spaces where the blood is mixed with cerebrospinal fluid. Some subarachnoid haemorrhage is also present. When examined at an interval of weeks after the injury the dura mater is found to adhere both to the bony wall of the canal and more firmly and extensively to the pia-arachnoid, which is thickened and united with the glio-conjunctival scar tissue within the cord. The latter is shrunken and yellowish and may contain one or more cysts where tissue has been lost. Many of the nerve fibres that remain are demyelinated so that stains for myelin give an appearance of more complete destruction of nerve fibres than has actually taken place. The amount of secondary degeneration is therefore often considerably less than might be expected from the appearances at the level of the lesion.

Indirect injuries of the spinal cord

Subluxation and fracture dislocation of the spine

In civil life these are the most common form of traumatic lesion of the spinal cord. They may be caused by flying or road accidents, by diving into shallow water, by falls from horse back and by accidents in other sports and games as well as by industrial accidents. In some cases head injuries due to blows on the back of the head are complicated by fracture or subluxation of the cervical spine. Indeed, when the slenderness of the cervical spine is considered in relation to the weight of the head and the stresses to which it is commonly subjected, it is surprising that it is not more often the site of fracture dislocations or of subluxations. Sudden hyperflexion of the cervical spine in a forward direction may tear the interspinous and dorsal common ligaments of the vertebrae as well as the annulus fibrosis of one or more intervertebral discs without causing any fracture of bone. Lateral and backward hyperflexions are more likely to be associated with bony fracture but this may be limited to a pedicle or lamina or to severance of an articular process. After these slighter degrees of injury the spine returns to its normal alignment, and the fracture may not be easily visible in radiographs. Whether or not there is fracture dislocation the injury to the spinal cord is caused chiefly at the time of the accident by the sudden mechanical stresses to which the nervous tissue is subjected. But when there is dislocation with pressure on the cord, or continuous stretching of the cord over a bony or cartilaginous protrusion, the ischaemia caused in this way produces additional lesions or, at least, hinders recovery. In some cases herniation and protrusion of the nucleus pulposus, causing serious compression of the spinal cord, results immediately from an injury to the cervical spine (Schneider 1951) but in most cases injuries to cervical intervertebral discs produce symptoms of a more chronic and progressive character which differ little from those seen in cases of cervical spondylosis in which no history of trauma is obtained (*vide* Chapter 14). There appears, however, to be no doubt that in patients with existing degeneration of cervical discs paraplegia may be brought on by comparatively minor accidents, or even by voluntary flexion of the neck. In these cases the cord is subjected to abnormal stresses by being stretched over a cartilaginous or bony protrusion at the level of the degenerated disc.

Thus whether or not there is fracture of the vertebrae, sudden flexion of the neck may damage the spinal cord either (1) by immediate mechanical stresses, or (2) by compression. These effects are often combined.

Subluxation. In many cases in which paraplegia results immediately from an accident involving sudden flexion of the neck, operation or post-mortem examination shows no gross abnormality in the spine or spinal canal. The spine may, however, be unduly mobile at one intervertebral joint, or there may be fracture of a pedicle or lamina. Sometimes bleeding under the posterior common ligament of the vertebrae or the separation of a small exostosis from the upper or lower margin of a vertebral body is the only or most obvious evidence of damage to the spine. In such cases the injury to the spinal cord may be severe or slight and largely recoverable. In the early stages the cord is usually swollen over one or two segments at the level at which the greatest flexion occurred. Later it becomes shrunken at this level, but this may only be obvious when the finger is passed gently in an upward or downward direction over the cord.

On section, in early cases, the damaged area may be grossly softened. More often it is diffusely swollen and shows small haemorrhagic points in the grey columns. It is seldom very haemorrhagic. The demarcation of grey from white matter is often blurred and the tissue may appear abnormally pale. Occasionally cylindrical cores of softened tissue can be seen passing upwards and downwards from the most softened area. The usual position of these cores is the base of the dorsal horns or the ventral part of the dorsal columns. They are greyish or brownish, sometimes creamy, less often frankly haemorrhagic. The name *traumatic haematomyelia* is often given to cases of this kind, but the name is almost always a misnomer since red blood corpuscles rarely form more than a minor part of the contents of the core. These consist of softened débris of myelin and axons, sometimes contained in phagocytic cells, along with serous fluid. Cores of this kind are most commonly found when there is gross softening of the cord at one level, without tearing of the pia-arachnoid. The swelling of the tissues and outpouring of serum associated with softening is restrained by the firm pia mater and thus the softened tissue tends to track in an upward and downward direction along the grey columns or in the line of the nerve fibres. While there is no doubt, both from human and experimental observations, that these cores may exist before death, it is probable that some may be formed, or at least enlarged, by careless removal of the spinal cord at the post-mortem examination.

Microscopically in mild cases transverse sections may show only swelling of axons and myelin sheaths in the damaged segment of the cord. This may be diffuse and slight, but is usually more severe in one area which may, however, be very limited both in its transverse and longitudinal extent. The characteristic appearances are most easily recognised in longitudinal sections stained for axons which may be diffusely swollen or show beaded swellings on their course or end bulbs where they are torn across (Fig. 7.9). These appearances may persist for some weeks. The myelin sheaths show distensions conforming to those of the axons which they contain. There are also, in most cases, some changes in the nerve cells, although these may be slight and limited to a minor degree of central chromatolysis. Ghost cells are sometimes seen, and later some loss of nerve cells may be found by comparative counts. The experiments of Groat *et al.* (1945) indicate that the small internuncial neurones, both in the dorsal and ventral grey columns, suffer more than the large motor cells. Both they and Roussy and Lhermitte described agglutination of Nissl granules as a characteristic minor change in cases of this kind.

Whether or not the swelling of the spinal cord in the early stages is due to oedema is not easily determined although the spread of paralysis in an upward direction in some cases makes this probable. Although no serous transudate can be seen between the nerve fibres, it is possible that they are separated more than normally by thin unstainable fluid, as in the minor grades of cerebral oedema. On the other hand the swelling of the cord may possibly be explained by the swelling of axons and distension of myelin sheaths.

At a later stage the only obvious abnormality may be small cysts, or loss of nerve fibres in some parts of the white matter. In cases due to sudden forward flexion of the neck, loss of fibres is commonly limited to the dorsal columns and this may be compatible with a remarkable degree of clinical recovery. It would appear that the damage to nerve fibres in these cases is due to longitudinal stretching or angulation or to a combination of these two processes. These mechanical stresses probably affect a large proportion of the nerve fibres of the cord in a minor degree, which in the great majority of the fibres is recoverable. This would account for the transient nature of the paraplegia in some cases and for the remarkable degree of recovery in others.

'Blast injuries' of the spinal cord

Both in the First and Second World Wars cases were reported in which paraplegia resulted from close exposure to the blast of an explosion (Claude and Lhermitte 1915, Davison 1945). It was at first thought (Guillain 1920) that the lesions in the spinal cord were caused by sudden changes in air pressure. But when a full history could be obtained it was shown that the patient had been forcibly thrown to the ground or bruised by earth, so that subluxation of the spine, especially at the cervical level, could never be excluded and in some cases this was definitely proved. This theory of causation was confirmed by British experience during 1939–45 which showed that blast by itself had little effect on the brain or spinal cord and that lesions in either organ following bomb explosions were due to other factors, especially CO poisoning in the case of the brain and subluxation of the spine in the case of the spinal cord. Both in animals and human cases exposed to blast, death was commonly caused by the effects of sudden changes in air pressure on the lungs, but paraplegia due to this cause alone was not observed.

Fracture dislocations of the cervical spine are most common at the level of the 5th–6th vertebrae. In them the cord is stretched over a bony or cartilaginous prominence and the effects of pressure ischaemia are added to the immediate mechanical trauma. Occasionally the cord may be pierced by spicules of bone, but in most cases it is protected by the dural sheath. One or more nerve roots are also commonly compressed by the dislocation, and this may contribute to the amyotrophy caused by the destruction of motor nerve cells in the cord.

Fracture dislocations of the thoracic and lumbar spine are most common at the lower thoracic level. They are more often caused by crushing, as by an excessive weight on the shoulders in falls of the roof of mines, or by extreme forward or backward flexion of the spine in falls or road accidents. They are often therefore less sudden than fracture dislocations of the neck and the effects on the cord are due more to compression and less to the sudden jar of the accident. The degree of damage to the spinal cord varies greatly. As the space between it and the bony canal is rather greater at the thoracic than at the cervical level the cord is less

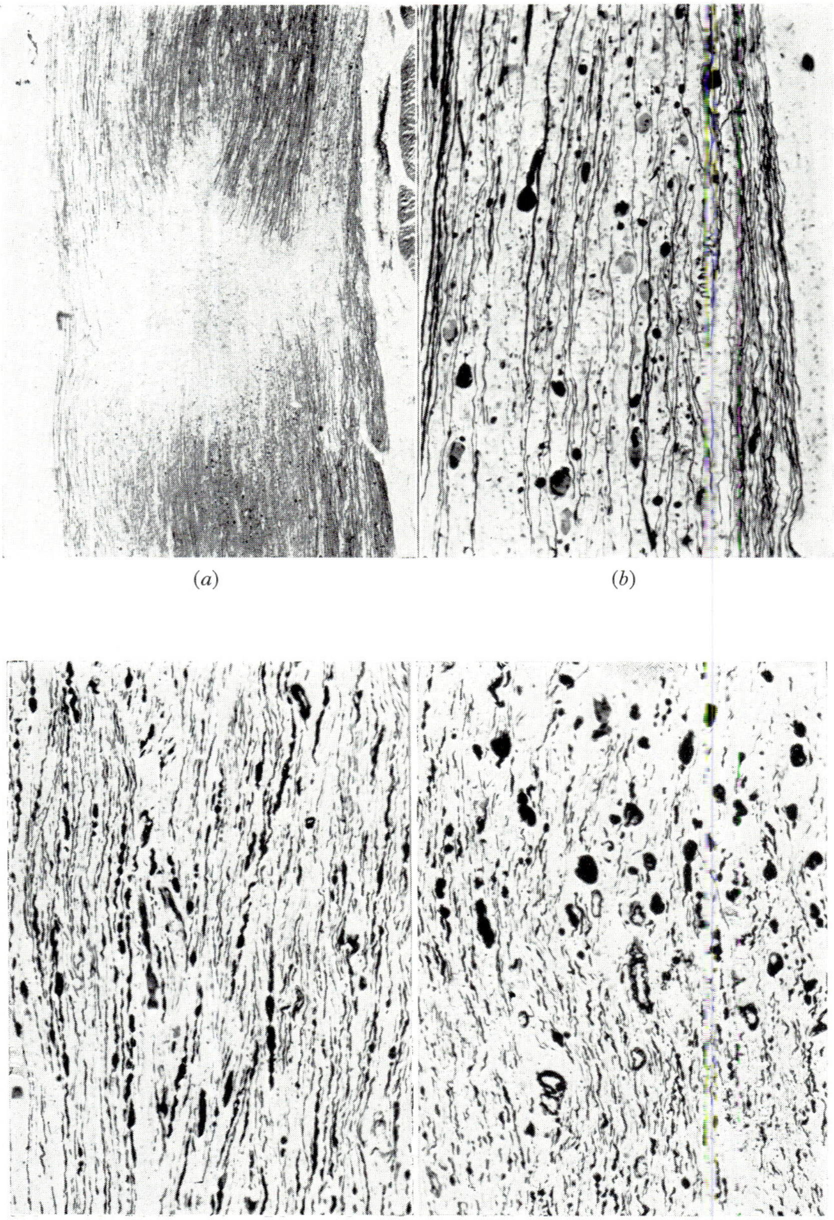

(a) (b)

(c) (d)

Fig. 7.9. Subluxation of cervical spine.
Longitudinal sections of cervical cord. (Gros-Bielschowsky method.)

(a) and (b) From a case of paraplegia due to a blow on the back of the head. (Low and high power views.)

(c) and (d) From another similar, but more recent case. (c) Beside main lesion (d) below it.

constantly damaged, and its injury is often incomplete and compatible with considerable recovery of function. In severe cases, however, there may be complete or almost complete destruction of nervous tissue at the level of the lesion. Lesions of the lumbar spine may damage the conus terminalis, with permanent effects, or may compress the less vulnerable roots of the cauda equina. In the latter case considerable recovery of function is possible.

When the spine is examined weeks or months after the injury, the canal at the level of the fracture dislocation contains dense fibrous scar tissue formed by the fusion and thickening of periosteum and dura mater. The leptomeninges are often adherent to this scar but a sub-arachnoid space may still exist either all round the cord or, more often, on one side only. The cord itself is thinned and sclerotic. In severe cases it may be represented by an ochreous fibrous band. In less severe cases it is partially or more completely demyelinated with fibrous gliosis in the degenerated areas or throughout. Sclerosis by collagenous tissue also may be present in the more severe cases.

Indirect spinal injuries from high-velocity bullets

High-velocity bullets which pass through the vertebral bodies or spines can cause severe jars to the spinal column. Even when they do not touch either the dura mater or cord they may cause complete or incomplete softening of the nervous tissue at the level of impact and minor lesions for a distance of several segments above and below this. Holmes (1915) describes small disseminated haemorrhages spread through two or more segments on either side of the wound especially in the cervical region, and moniliform or beaded swelling of axons especially near the surface of the cord. Both he and Roussy and Lhermitte also found superficial areas of necrosis in the white columns at some distance from the main lesion. These resembled the effects of thrombosis of small meningeal arteries, but although the vessels were engorged they were not thrombosed. In some the glial trabeculae were preserved and traversed the necrotic area, or the astrocytes also might be degenerated or necrotic. Holmes found these areas especially in the dorsal and ventral columns. In Roussy and Lhermitte's cases they were most common in the marginal zone of the lateral columns and the middle root zone of the dorsal columns. More rarely they were seen in the ventral horns. Lesions of nerve cells at some distance from the chief lesions were also seen by Holmes. These lesions appear to be caused by the sudden shock to the spinal column, as similar lesions have been found in experimental animals in which the spine has been struck (Schmaus 1890, Jakob 1919). In Schmaus' experiments he struck a wooden board placed against the animal's back, and the effects of the blow therefore were probably distributed over many vertebrae. It has been suggested that the shock of the blow, in these and other experiments, is transmitted by a wave of cerebrospinal fluid but this appears to be no better substantiated than Duret's similar hypothesis of the mechanics of head injury.

TRAUMATIC LESIONS OF PERIPHERAL NERVES

I. Acute lesions

Acute injuries to peripheral nerves are very common in war time but comparatively rare in civilian life. The period of both world wars saw great activity in this field both in research and clinical investigation and this added much to knowledge of the subject.

Seddon (1942–43) classified injuries of peripheral nerves in three categories, *neurapraxia*, *axonotmesis* and *neurotmesis*.

(1) *Neurapraxia* describes lesions of minor severity in which axons are injured to such a degree that their function is temporarily abolished, but there is no Wallerian degeneration in the peripheral segment. Function is therefore rapidly, and usually completely, restored.

This degree of injury is most commonly caused by pressure but may follow blows of minor severity.

(2) *Axonotmesis* describes lesions which destroy axons at the site of the injury and so cause Wallerian degeneration in the peripheral segment of the nerve; but the connective tissue sheaths of the nerve remain intact, or only slightly damaged, and guide the outgrowing fibres to the peripheral Schwann tubules. There is therefore little or no neuroma formation. Although restoration of function after axonotmesis is necessarily delayed until the outgrowing neurites can reach and make functional connection with peripheral end organs, it may eventually be remarkably complete. The most common cause of such lesions is bruising, as in fractures involving peripheral nerves. Long continued pressure or attrition, as in some ulnar nerve palsies, may have a similar effect. In them the paralysis is usually partial but the rate of recovery is of the same character as in more acute injuries.

(3) *Neurotmesis* (cutting of the nerve). This term is used to describe injuries which sever the whole or the greater part of the thickness of a nerve including its endo- and perineurium but not necessarily the epineurium. Such injuries may be caused by gun-shot wounds, by severe traction or by cuts by sharp objects such as knives or the edges of broken glass. Regeneration in such nerves occurs after the formation of a neuroma at the site of the lesion. This causes delay in re-innervation of the peripheral part of the nerve and the restoration of function is never complete.

In some cases one or the other of these terms may be applied to the whole nerve, whereas in others different fascicles have undergone different degrees of damage. More rarely an individual fascicle may show two grades of injury. It is often difficult to distinguish between *neurotmesis*, with intact epineurium, and *axonotmesis* especially in the earlier stages, but it is axiomatic that in the latter there is little or no neuroma formation and therefore eventually the nerve will show little or no swelling at the site of injury. The terms *neurotmesis*, *axonotmesis* and *neurapraxia* have therefore both a clinical and a pathological connotation. Clinically they are related to different rates and degrees of functional recovery; pathologically to differences both at the level of the injury and in the peripheral segment of the nerve.

The pathological changes which may be associated with *neurapraxia* are only known from experimental work since biopsies are not called for in such cases. The injuries concerned are caused by pressure, percussion and stretching. The resultant paralysis lasts from a few days up to two or three weeks; intervals that would not allow of restoration of function had Wallerian degeneration taken place. The temporary loss of conduction must therefore be due to changes that fall short of a break in continuity of the axon.

The experimental work of Denny-Brown and his associates Brenner and Doherty (1944 a, 1945) has illuminated this subject. They found that the effects of *stretching* small nerves depended to a large extent on the degree of damage to the perineurium and blood vessels. It appeared however that nerve fibres could be stretched to almost double their length without rupture. The ensuing paralysis from such minor degrees of stretching was slight and might disappear within 14 days. The only histological changes then were swelling and beading of the larger axons in some bundles, and beading of a few myelin sheaths. Stretching to a greater length tended to produce more widespread and severe beading of axons and myelin. In some cases rupture of small vessels caused ischaemic changes similar to those in pressure experiments (see below, p. 471). It appeared from these experiments that axons and their myelin sheaths were plastic and extensible. With increase in length up to about 100 per cent they were not irreparably damaged, but they showed little elasticity or tendency to return to their original length.

Severe *percussion* of a nerve might cause extensive local necrosis both of axons and myelin sheaths, with Wallerian degeneration of the peripheral segments. Less severe percussion produced a transient paralysis which might last for 3–4 days and pass off during the next 48 hours. In the latter a fusiform pseudoneuroma due to interstitial oedema appeared by the 3rd day and lasted for 3 weeks or more. Within this swollen area a selective damage of the largest nerve fibres was found: in these the myelin sheaths became swollen and pale, and disappeared over a short length of the fibre within a few days. At the same time the axons were swollen and distorted. The length of fibre affected did not exceed 1 mm., and was in general proportional to the size of the fibre. The smallest medullated fibres and non-medullated axons escaped damage. It was also noted that local demyelination long outlasted the paralysis induced by the blow.

Very few nerves showing *axonotmesis* have been studied for the same reason as in neurapraxia, but occasionally delay in return of function and swelling at the site of injury has induced an inexperienced surgeon to remove a piece of such a nerve. The processes by which nerves are restored, almost to their original condition, after injuries of this kind have been studied experimentally by Gutmann and Sanders (1943) and Sanders (1948).

The great majority of biopsies after lesions of peripheral nerve are made in cases of *neurotmesis*, since in almost all of these surgical union of freshly cut ends of the nerve affords the best hope of satisfactory recovery. The examination of this biopsy material has been supplemented by much experimental work based on the classical studies of Cajal (1928) and Nageotte (1932). The description which follows is based on the more recent work of Young (1954), Weiss (1943, 1944, 1945), Denny-Brown (1946), Sunderland (1947, 1948, 1950), Blackwood and Holmes (1954) and many others. The phenomena of Wallerian degeneration have already been described (Chapter 1), but as those of regeneration are most commonly seen after traumatic lesions of peripheral nerves their description has been included in this chapter.

Regeneration in peripheral nerves after acute injury

When axons in peripheral nerves are damaged in such a way as to cause their local necrosis, without destruction of the endoneurium, they degenerate back to the next node of Ranvier or to a distance of one or two internodes further. This degeneration is associated with changes in the myelin and Schwann sheaths similar to those of Wallerian degeneration. There is also separation of nerve fibres by oedema. The proximal ends of the axons swell and become frayed out giving the appearance of separation of their neurofibrils. After a short interval one or several fresh neurites sprout from each axon (Fig. 7.10*c*) and grow forwards along the endoneurial tubules at a rate which has been calculated, in human cases, at about 2·5–3 mm. a day. In their passage they become intimately associated with the band fibres formed by the cells of Schwann in the peripheral part of the nerve and in this way the young neurites are conducted to their peripheral terminations where they re-establish functional connections of motor or sensory character. Motor neurites may re-enter old end-plates on muscle fibres or may form one or more end-plates in new positions, especially when re-innervation has been delayed, as in injuries of the proximal part of the nerve. Sensory neurites may make free nerve endings in the skin, or more complex endings on muscle spindles or in Paccinian corpuscles or hair follicles. These have been less fully studied. After functional connections have thus been re-established maturation gradually takes place. The new axons increase in diameter in a centrifugal manner so that at any stage in the process they are thicker proximally than peripherally. Some may for a time exceed the normal diameter in their proximal parts. Eventually they assume a more even thickness which is usually rather less than that of the original axons. At the same time a myelin sheath forms round them. At first this is extremely thin but with the restoration of function and further maturation of the axon its thickness increases until it eventually approaches that of the original nerve fibre. This remyelination is generally considered to result from the interaction of the axon and the cells of Schwann. Brante (1952) considers that some of the lipids which are required to reform myelin, especially unsaturated lecithins and gangliosides, are provided by the axon. Although at first several neurites may lie in the same endoneurial tubule, when medullation takes place each fibre is enclosed in its own sheath cell. C fibres, however, remain unmyelinated and several of them run in a single sheath cell. As myelination becomes complete nodes of Ranvier are reformed and the nuclei of the sheath cells resume their position in the centre of the internodes.

The conception of the Schwann cell as being able to form both myelin and reticulin fibres, and the observations of Geren (1954) on the manner in which it enfolds the axon in myelination, must be related to the concept of the band of Büngner. If axons lie at first on the surface of sheath cells and gradually become enclosed in their substance, either by the enwrapping process described by Geren or more directly as in the case of the C fibres, the endoneurial tubules must form the conducting channels along which new neurites grow. Within these tubules the sheath cells persist either as a more or less continuous syncytium or as separate cells.

When lesions such as cuts and severe bruises are of such a kind as to cause both severance or local necrosis of the axon and damage to the connective tissue sheaths of the nerve the phenomena of regeneration are modified by the absence of a continuous conducting pathway for the young neurites. When a nerve is completely severed the gap between the cut ends becomes filled at first with blood and plasma. Within a few days this becomes organised by the outgrowth into it of fibroblasts many of which are oriented in the direction of the nerve and others obliquely to this (Cajal 1928). As the sprouting neurites leave the endoneurial tubules they come in contact with these fibroblasts and tend to run along them or any other tissue interfaces which they meet. Other fibroblasts soon become oriented to the neurites so as to enclose them in tubules. Later arriving neurites may enter a tubule so formed so that some tubules may contain several neurites (Denny-Brown 1946). As they pass forward through the gap between the cut ends of the nerve, the neurites become attached to other fibroblasts which are oriented in various directions and in this way a neuroma is formed in which nerve fibres are intertwined in haphazard fashion, but for the most part obliquely to the line of the nerve. In the more proximal parts of the neuroma several neurites often run close together as though enclosed in a common sheath. More peripherally the neurites run singly and are more sparsely distributed. When the gap to be bridged is narrow, the severed ends of the nerve are quickly united by fibroblastic granulation tissue and many neurites are thus directed to the peripheral stump where the great majority enter the old endoneurial tubules (Fig. 7.10*a*, *b*). When the gap is wider a similar plexiform stump-neuroma forms on the proximal cut end of the nerve and from its distal tip a few nerve fibres emerge and run along the collagen strands which join the two ends of the nerve. These nerve fibres are often oriented more directly towards the peripheral end, probably because the tensions which develop in the scar tissue tend to orient the collagen fibres in the longitudinal direction of the nerve (Fig. 7.10*d*). This appearance is most often seen in the nerves of the limbs where the movement of joints tends to separate the cut ends of the nerve. On reaching the peripheral stump the neurites enter the old endoneurial channels, but before doing so they often appear to divide, since the number of innervated tubules may be considerably greater than the number of axons in the intervening scar tissue (Nageotte 1932).

Cajal (1928) postulated some chemotactic influence which attracted neurites to the peripheral stump of the nerve but this remains uncertain. There has also been disagreement on the importance of the part played by the syncytium of Schwann in the orientation of the out-growing axons. Nageotte (1932) considered this of special importance for the reception of neurites into the peripheral stump of the nerve. He

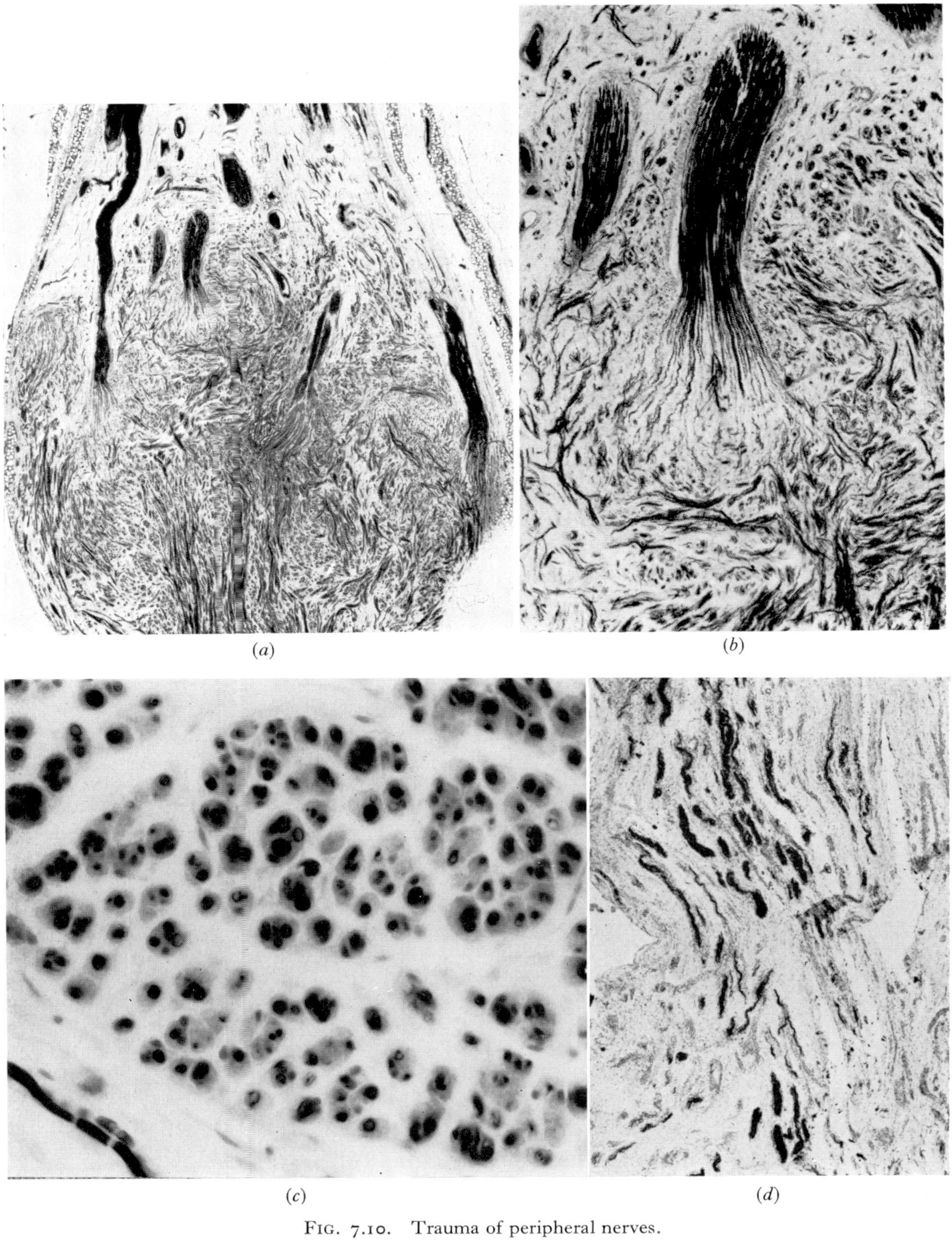

(a) (b) (c) (d)

FIG. 7.10. Trauma of peripheral nerves.

(a) and (b) Low and higher power view of traumatic neuroma. (Myelin.) Towards the lower end the fibres are again becoming longitudinally orientated.

(c) Transverse sections of sprouting nerve fibres near their origin from old nerve fibres. Note that several small fibres arise from one old fibre. (Myelin.)

(d) New nerve fibres running in scar tissue joining proximal and distal cut ends of a nerve.

described branching processes, arising from the pre-existing cells of Schwann at the distal cut ends passing out into the tissue separating the cut ends of the nerve and forming a 'plexus which invades the neighbouring tissue like an infiltrating neoplasm'. This outgrowth, which contains no nerve fibres, he called a Schwannoma. He considered that neurites which entered this Schwannoma either from the upper neuroma or from the intervening scar tissue were conducted along its processes directly to the band fibres in the old endoneurial tubules. This out-growth from the peripheral end has been frequently observed although it is not constant, but its constitution has been differently interpreted.

Denny-Brown (1946), using a differential nuclear stain, considered that the oat-shaped nuclei, which are commonly seen closely applied to young neurites, belonged to endoneurial and perineurial fibroblasts, and the thinner more elongated nuclei with blunt rounded ends were nuclei of Schwann cells. In his experiments he found only nuclei of the former type in the peripheral Schwannoma until it was entered by neurites from the central neuroma. And he found no nuclei of Schwann cell type within 0·25 mm. of the tips of young neurites. He therefore agreed with Dustin (1910) and Speidel (1935) (who studied the regeneration of living axons in the transparent tail of tadpoles) that the orientation of growing nerve sprouts was largely determined by the growth of fibroblasts. In his experiments outgrowth of Schwann syncytium appeared to follow, and to be dependent on, the outgrowth of neurites. Nageotte, who in his earlier work held that the young neurites were contained in outgrowths of Schwann syncytium throughout their course, conceded, in his later writings (1932), the possibility that their tips might be naked.

The condition found in specimens taken from the site of the lesion in cases of this kind varies very greatly. In most the two ends of the nerve are separated by a collagenous scar of varying length, and through this a few neurites have made their way and have reached and partially innervated the peripheral part of the nerve. The amount of neuroma-formation on the proximal end and of swelling of the peripheral stump varies greatly. The cut ends of the nerve may run out into scar tissue with little or no swelling at either end, but in most cases neuromas are seen at least at the proximal end. When the nerve is only partially divided, the cut ends of the divided fascicles are kept from separating by the intact fascicles and junctions by neuroma formation may be fairly satisfactory.

Lesions causing interruption of axons and Wallerian degeneration of the peripheral part of the nerve, but producing only minor degrees of damage to the connective tissue sheaths of the nerve, remain to be considered. Denny-Brown (1946) demonstrated the importance of the part played by the perineurium in preventing neurites from straying into the surrounding tissue and in orienting them towards the peripheral cut end of the nerve.

In experiments on rabbits the perineurium was slit longitudinally and the enclosed nerve fibres and endoneurium pulled out and cut across so as to remove a length of about 3 cm. The resulting tube was quickly filled by granulation tissue in which fibroblasts arising from the inner surface of the perineurium abounded. Denny-Brown considered that these cells, which he called *neural fibroblasts*, were identical with endoneurial fibroblasts but differed from fibroblasts arising from epineurium in forming a more diffuse type of collagen. In the perineurial tube they tended to become orientated longitudinally and formed a scaffolding along which young neurites could pass to the peripheral cut end of the nerve bundle. In these experiments the gap in the nerve bundle was rapidly filled with nerve fibres which were arranged more or less longitudinally, although to some extent intertwined, and showed little tendency to form nodular neuromas. In spite of a gap of about 3 cm. between the cut ends of the nerve, 30–50 per cent function was recovered after about 100 days, and even longer gaps were bridged by nerve fibres within this period.

It is clear that when there is any break in the endoneurial tubules, especially when there is neuroma-formation even of slight degree, the arrangement of the neurites when they reach the peripheral stump must be quite haphazard. Motor neurites may reach endoneurial tubules which originally carried sensory axons and vice versa. The method of selection, by which eventually motor tubules are innervated by axons arising from motor neurones and sensory tubules by those coming from dorsal root ganglia, is quite unknown. It has been suggested that several neurites of different characters compete for, or may enter, one tubule but only one eventually survives and matures in it. When the gap between the divided ends of a nerve is bridged by a well-innervated neuroma, such as may result from a successful open operation, the number of axons which arrive at the peripheral cut end may be considerably greater than the number in the proximal part of the nerve (Sanders and Young 1944). In this case the atrophy of a large number of axons would not entail an equally large reduction in the amount of function eventually regained. It seems likely that something of this kind happens in successful unions of cut peripheral nerves.

Changes in the interstitial connective tissue

Injuries of nerves, whether by bruising or cutting, are always followed by oedematous swelling which separates the nerve fibres and stretches the perineurium. As has been seen

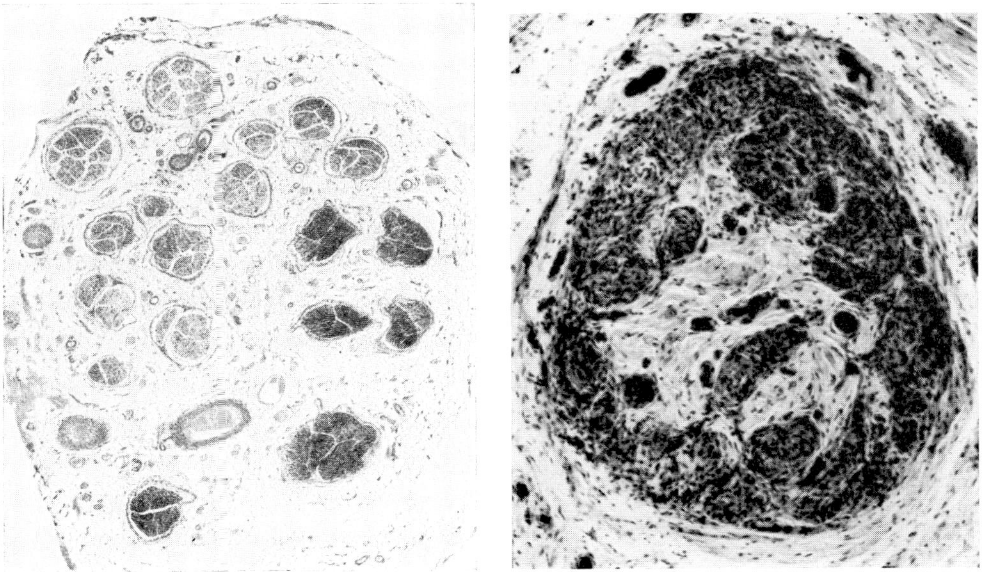

(*a*) (*b*)

FIG. 7.11 Transverse sections of peripheral ends of injured nerves.
(*a*) Re-innervation especially of bundles at one side of the peripheral stump. The bundles are separated by loose fibrous tissue. (Myelin.)
(*b*) Fibrous scarring in central part of bundle preventing neurotisation of that part. (Haematoxylin van Gieson.)

pressure on a nerve of short duration is also followed by swelling; if long continued the nerve swells above and below the compressed segment. Bruising of a nerve is also associated with haemorrhage both among the nerve fibres and in the sheaths, and by damaging the endoneurial tubules may allow neurites to wander into the surrounding tissues. It has also been shown (Johnson and Abercrombie 1946, Sunderland and Bradley 1950) that the denervated peripheral segment of a nerve undergoes a progressive increase in collagen, associated with thickening of the endoneurial tubules and reduction in their calibre which, at the end of 100 days, rarely exceeds 3μ. But, at least during the first 12 months, this shrinkage of calibre does not appear greatly to hinder either the passage of neurites down the tubules or the maturation of those which establish functional connection with end organs. It may, however, cause a reduction in the final size of the matured fibres. Sanders and Young (1944), comparing results of suture delayed for 15 months after section with those of immediate suture, found the proportion of fibres over 8μ in diameter to be 2·7 per cent in the former and 11 per cent in the latter. The normal difference between the average sizes of motor and sensory fibres was, however, still retained.

The final size of the regenerated fibres in the peripheral part of the nerve thus appears to depend both on the character of the nerve fibres from which they arise, and on the nature and state of the distal tubules which receive them. Nerve fibres which are large in the proximal part of the nerve tend to form large fibres in the distal part; small nerve fibres appear to be unable to produce regenerated fibres larger than themselves. At the same time when the neurites growing from large nerve fibres enter tubules which either are originally small or whose calibre has been reduced by fibrotic shrinkage, they are prevented from reaching the diameter which they might attain in larger tubules.

From this it is evident that the condition of the part of a nerve distal to the lesion, as seen in biopsy specimens, depends on a number of varying factors. If operation has been delayed for several weeks or some months after the injury some re-innervation of the distal segment is almost always present, but it may be confined to a few fascicles, sometimes on one side of the nerve only (Fig. 7.11*a*), or all the fascicles may be very sparsely innervated. The connective-tissue sheaths are usually thickened, sometimes very considerably, at the level of the lesion. Thickening of the epineurium and interfascicular connective tissue, and moderate thickening of the perineurium, at this level probably have little effect on the re-innervation of the fascicles. Some endoneurial thickening is also compatible with good functional recovery (Blackwood and Holmes 1954), but when the greater part of the lumen of the perineurium is filled by collagenous tissue (Fig. 7.11*b*) as may occur when there is ischaemia of the distal segment of the nerve, for example in Volkmann's contracture, satisfactory re-innervation is unlikely to occur.

II. Subacute and repeated trauma, or pressure

Whereas acute traumatic lesions of the peripheral nerves are comparatively rare in civilian life, those of a more chronic or sustained nature are a common cause of disability, especially of the upper limbs. Walshe (1951) has reviewed the important group of pressure syndromes related to the thoracic inlet and the cervico-axillary canal. A cervical rib, or rudimentary first rib, may inflict recurrent trivial injuries on roots of the brachial plexus with movements of the thorax and upper limbs. Damage may also be sustained when the related structures are normal but the subject displays sagging of the shoulder-girdle, or has undergone unwonted exertion. Motor and sensory disturbances may also be referable to degenerative changes in the cervical intervertebral discs, with consequent involvement of the nerve-roots in the intervertebral foramina (see p. 658).

Individual nerves of the upper limb may be affected, such as the musculo-spiral nerve in crutch paralysis, the ulnar nerve at the level of the elbow-joint following dislocation of the latter or fracture of the lower end of the humerus, and the median nerve in the carpal tunnel.

The sciatic nerve requires note in relation to disability of the lower limbs. Many forms of sciatica are attributable to involvement of the nerve roots in prolapse of the lumbar intervertebral discs (see p. 661). Tumours within the spinal canal are a rarer source of root-pressure. The pregnant uterus sometimes compresses the nerve within the pelvis and, in the buttock, it may be involved in severe osteoarthritis of the hip-joint.

The pathology of these nerve-lesions in the human subject has been little explored since biopsy is not requisite. It may however be noted that decompression of the median nerve in the carpal tunnel has permitted inspection of the nerve; it has been reported to be swollen and greyish pink. The ulnar nerve undergoes a palpable spindle-shaped thickening in the circumstances noted above, suggestive of fibrosis. The reversible nature of these functional disturbances in general suggests that fibrosis, if present, is largely extra- or perineural. Much of the swelling may, however, be due to oedema. Since the common cause is sustained, or repetitive, local pressure, it may reasonably be surmised that the pathogenesis of the nerve-fibre damage is a combination of ischaemia and direct trauma.

The more acute effects of such pressure have been described in the experimental studies of Denny-Brown and Brenner (1944 b). They applied spring clips of known pressure to peripheral nerves in cats for varying lengths of time. After the application for 2 hours of slighter degrees of pressure sufficient to induce loss of electrical conduction in the nerve, but with no paralysis after removal of the clip, the compressed area of the nerve swelled and became oedematous. This was associated with slight swelling of myelin and great thickening of axons. Near the nodes the myelin was pale or in partial dissolution. If the pressure were rather greater so as to cause slight residual paresis, it resulted in similar oedema with complete dissolution of myelin near some nodes over distances up to 0·1 mm., along with swelling and vacuolation of the axons. With degrees of pressure sufficient to cause paralysis for periods up to 18 days, with rapid recovery thereafter, more severe changes were seen in the nerve fibres both at the level of the clip and for a short distance below it. These outlasted the failure of conductivity in the nerve and, although sparse Wallerian degeneration was seen, most of the nerve fibres in the peripheral part of the nerve had remained intact. At the level of pressure the myelin sheaths had disappeared for some distance near the nodes, especially just peripheral to them, while over the rest of the internode they were somewhat swollen. The axons stained poorly in the demyelinated area or appeared to be thinned, but elsewhere were thickened and appeared oedematous. Thus both with myelin and axon stains the nerve fibres showed alternating thin and thick segments. These changes affected a greater proportion of the large than of the smaller fibres. They were rarely associated with Wallerian degeneration in the peripheral part of the fibre. At the level of transition to normal below the clip the chief abnormality was widening of the nodes of Ranvier with a thin myelin sheath covering the nerves as they passed through the gap. 'For the next 15 mm. distal to this point the proximal end of each myelin segment was vacuolated, thin and irregular with gradual transition to normal myelin beyond this zone' (Denny-Brown and Brenner).

When weaker clips were left on the nerve for many days the compressed segment was thinned with abrupt swelling of the nerve above and below it. This was associated with thinning and granularity of the myelin under the clip where the axons were closely packed and had an irregular outline. In the swollen parts of the nerve the myelin was swollen and the axons thickened. If stronger clips were left *in situ* for 2 or 3 weeks there was complete necrosis of the nerve in the compressed area which was extremely flattened. The myelin was in the form of narrow tubes of a finely granular structure; the axons were tortuous and irregular, and there was complete absence of nuclear staining in this area.

Effects of cold on peripheral nerves

The effects on peripheral nerves of freezing for short periods or of longer exposure to chilling have been studied experimentally for many years, but very few histological examinations have been made in human cases. In the earlier experiments (Lorrain Smith *et al.* 1915) chilling of the extremities at temperatures above freezing-point resulted only in some oedema of the nerves and swelling of axons. Freezing of the nerve for 1 minute or longer (Bielschowsky and Valentin 1922) produced dissolution of myelin and fragmentation of axons. Blackwood and Russell (1943), by keeping the tails of rats in water at a temperature of 4–5°C for 3–4 days, constantly produced degenerative changes, especially in the intramuscular branches of the nerves. Immediately after exposure there was irregularity in the outline of myelin sheaths and swelling of Schwann cells in a large proportion of the fibres and these changes progressed to disintegration of myelin and axons within 3 days after immersion had been discontinued. Some of the muscle fibres had undergone Zenker's hyaline necrosis, even in rats subjected to 1 day's immersion, and this condition affected more muscle fibres after longer exposures to wet and cold. When the animals were observed for long periods, denervation atrophy of the muscles was added to this primary degeneration.

These experiments were confirmed and amplified by Denny-Brown *et al.* (1945) who studied the sciatic nerves of rabbits both after freezing with CO_2 and after enclosing them for periods up to 2 hours in a chamber through which brine was passed at temperatures between $-4°$ and $+3°$ C. They found that they could produce lesions of different severity in the nerve according to the temperature and duration of the exposure to cold. When the nerve was frozen for 5 minutes, and sometimes after a shorter duration of freezing, all the tissue elements within the perineurium, with the exception of the capillary endothelium, underwent necrosis. This was followed after 2 or 3 days by an intense inflammatory reaction with exudation of neutrophil leucocytes, lymphocytes and plasma cells, as well as epineurial fibroblasts. The axons became segmented and coiled or swollen, and the myelin granular or amorphous with loss of its staining properties. It did not form ovoids at the level of the lesion, but there was Wallerian degeneration in the distal segment of the nerve. Regeneration from the central stump followed, as after section of a nerve, and in 3 months there was complete restitution to the normal state except for some increase in cellularity at the site of the experiment. After freezing for shorter periods there might be no necrosis of tissue, but destruction only of large and medium sized nerve fibres. The finer fibres remained intact or showed beaded swellings on their course. The nuclei of the Schwann cells became more circular and often divided by mitosis. A similar effect could be obtained by chilling the nerve for 1–2 hours to temperatures near freezing point. This never caused necrosis of the interstitial tissues but produced paralysis associated with destruction of all nerve fibres except the finest, which always escaped. Slighter degrees of chilling produced slight paralysis associated with local damage to the axons and myelin of the larger nerve fibres similar to that seen by Denny-Brown and Brenner in experimental ischaemia of nerves (p. 471). This was not always associated with Wallerian degeneration. It was, therefore, possible to produce all degrees of damage to the nerve from a condition approaching neurotmesis, but leaving the perineurium intact, through axonotmesis to neurapraxia. Denny-Brown *et al.* found that indian ink injected into the larger vessels of the nerves did not reach the necrotic part of the nerves, but with minor degrees of damage to nerves changes in the vessel walls were slight or absent. Therefore, while they considered the more severe lesions to be caused by ischaemia, they were unable to account for milder lesions on this hypothesis, and considered the possibility of a direct effect of cold on lipoproteins. The changes found in the myelin sheath immediately after the experiment appeared to favour this hypothesis.

Blackwood (1943) reported the findings in 14 cases of immersion foot, chiefly in seamen who had spent from 1 to 11 days in open boats. Except for 1 patient who died before rescue, there was an interval of from 8 weeks to 26 months between immersion and amputation or post-mortem examination. In all these cases there was degeneration of axons and myelin in the nerves of the feet, but in the cases in which immersion was of shorter duration this did not involve all the fibres in the nerves. When amputation was delayed for some months there was regeneration of nerve fibres within the nerves of the extremity. These observations agree with the experimental work cited in showing that prolonged subjection of limbs to temperatures slightly above freezing-point causes primary degeneration of axons and myelin of the nerves, a condition of axonotmesis from which very good recovery might be expected.

REFERENCES

Trauma of the Brain

Barnard, J. W., Fry, W. J., Fry, F. J. and Krummins, R. F. (1955) *J. comp. Neurol.*, **103**, 459.

Bielschowsky, P. (1928) *Z. ges. Neurol. Psychiat.*, **117**, 55.

Ceccherelli, A. (1874) *Med. Jahrb.*, p. 343.

Connors, J. F. and Wright, L. T. (1934) *Ann. Surg.*, **100**, 996.

Corsellis, J. A. N. and Brierley, J. B. (1959) *J. ment. Sci.*, **105**, 714.

Crawford, J. V. and Russell, D. S. (1956) *J. Neurol. Psychiat.*, **19**, 1.

Daniel, P. M., Prichard, M. M. L. and Treip, C. S. (1959) *Lancet* (ii), 927.

Denny-Brown, D. and Russell, W. R. (1941) *Brain*, **64**, 93.

De Veer, J. A. and Browder, J. (1942) *J. Neuropath. exper. Neurol.*, **1**, 24.

Duret, H. (1878) *Etudes expérimentales et cliniques sur les traumatismes cérébraux*, Publ. du Progrès Med.; (1920) *Traumatismes cranio-cérébraux*, **2**, Alcan, Paris.

Evans, J. P. and Scheinker, I. M. (1943) *Arch. Neurol. Psychiat.* (Chicago), **50**, 258.

Falconer, M. A. and Russell, D. S. (1944) *J. Neurosurg.*, **1**, 182.

Foerster, O. and Penfield, W. (1930) *Brain*, **53**, 99.

Gardner, W. J. (1932) *Arch. Neurol. Psychiat.* (Chicago), **27**, 847.

Gaupp, R. (1933) *Z. ges. Neurol. Psychiat.*, **149**, 122.

Gierlich, J. (1936) *Dtsch. Ztschr. ges. gericht. Med.*, **26**, 100.

Gillingham, J. (1954) *Proc. R. Soc. Med.*, **47**, 869.

Groat, R. A., Windle, W. F. and Magoun, H. W. (1945) *J. Neurosurg.*, **2**, 26.

Helfand, M. (1939) *J. nerv. ment. Dis.*, **90**, 157.

Hoff, H. (1930) *Z. ges. Neurol. Psychiat.*, **129**, 583.

Holbourn, A. H. S. (1943) *Lancet* (ii), 438; (1944 a) ibid. (i), 483; (1944 b) *J. Neurosurg.*, **1**, 190.

Hortega, P. del Rio. (1933) *Anatomia microscopica de los Tumores del Sistemo nervioso*, Blass, Madrid.

Jolly. (1870) *Studien aus dem Instit. f. exper. Pathol. in Wien*, 1869.

Landis, E. M., Jonas, L., Angevine, M. and Erb, W. (1932) *J. clin. Invest.*, **11**, 717.

Leary, T. (1939) *Arch. Path.*, **28**, 808.

Lewin, W. (1944) *Brit. Med. J.* (ii), 11; (1953) ibid. (i), 1239.

Lindenberg, R. and Freytag, E. (1960) *Arch. Path.*, **69**, 440.

Nelson, E., Lindstrom, P. A. and Haymaker, W. (1959) *J. Neuropath. exp. Neurol.*, **18**, 489.

Neubürger, K. T., Sinton, D. W. and Denst, J. (1959) *Arch. Neurol. Psychiat.* (Chicago), **81**, 403.

Northfield, D. W. C. (1944) *J. Neurol. Psychiat.*, **7**, 1.

Pennybacker, J. and Russell, D. S. (1948) *J. Neurol. Psychiat.*, **11**, 183.

Pilcher, C. (1937) *Arch. Surg.*, **35**, 512; (1941) *Surg. Gynec. Obst.*, **72**, 755.

Popoff, L. (1875) *Virchows Archiv. f. Path. Anat.*, **63**, 421.

Pudenz, R. H. and Shelden, C. H. (1946) *J. Neurosurg.*, **3**, 487.

Putnam, T. J. and Cushing, H. (1925) *Arch. Surg.*, **11**, 329.

Rand, C. W. and Courville, C. B. (1931) *Arch. Surg.*, **23**, 357; (1946) *Arch. Neurol. Psychiat.* (Chicago), **55**, 79; (1947) *J. Neuropath. exper. Neurol.*, **6**, 1.

Ricker, G. (1919) *Virchow's Arch. f. Path. Anat.*, **226**, 180.

Rubinstein, L. J., Klatzo, I. and Miguel, J. (1962) *J. Neuropath. exp. Neurol.*, **21**, 116.

Russell, D. S., Wilson, C. W. and Tansley, K. (1949) *J. Neurol. Psychiat.*, **12**, 187.

Russell, D. S. and Rubinstein, L. J. (1963) *Pathology of Tumours of the Nervous System*, 2nd edition, Arnold, London.

Russell, W. R. (1932) *Brain*, **55**, 549.

Schaller, W. F., Tamaki, K. and Newman, H. (1937) *Arch. Neurol. Psychiat.* (Chicago), **37**, 1048.

Schnedorf, J. G., Munslow, R. A., Crawford, A. S. and McClure, R. D. (1940) *Surg. Gynec. and Obst.*, **70**, 628.

Scholz, W. and Hsü, Y. K. (1938) *Arch. Neurol. Psychiat.* (Chicago), **40**, 928.

Shelden, C. H., Pudenz, R. H., Restarski, J. S. and Craig, W. M. (1944) *J. Neurosurg.*, **1**, 67.

Strich, S. J. (1956) *J. Neurol. Psychiat.*, **19**, 163; (1961) *Lancet* (ii), 443.
Symonds, C. (1962) *Lancet* (i), 1.
Tigges, W. (1863) *Allg. Ztschr. f. Psychiat.*, **20**, 317.
Uchimura, T. and Shiraki, H. (1952) *J. nerv. ment. Dis.*, **116**, 654.
White, J. C., Brooks, J. R., Goldthwait, J. C. and Adams, R. D. (1942) *Arch. Surg.*, **44**, 1; (1943) *Ann. Surg.*, **118**, 619.
Windle, W. F., Groat, R. A. and Fox, C. A. (1944) *Surg. Gynec. and Obstet.*, **79**, 561.
Wolff, H. and Lennox, W. (1930) *Arch. Neurol. Psychiat.* (Chicago), **23**, 1095.

Trauma of the Spinal Cord

Brown-Séquard, C. E. (1868) *Lancet* (ii), 593, 659, 755, 821.
Claude, H. and Lhermitte, J. (1915) *Ann. de Med.*, **2**, 479.
Davison, C. (1945) in Trauma of the central nervous system, *Proc. Ass. Res. nerv. ment. Dis.*, **24**, Williams & Wilkins.
Groat, R. A., Windle, W. F. and Magoun, H. W. (1945) *J. Neurosurg.*, **2**, 26.
Guillain, G. (1920) *Travaux neurologiques de guerre*, Paris, Masson.
Holmes, G. M. (1915) *Brit. Med. J.* (ii), 769.
Jakob, A. (1919) *Z. ges. Neurol. Psychiat.*, **51**, 247.
Roussy, J. and Lhermitte, J. (1918) *Blessures de la moelle et de la queue de cheval*, Masson, Paris.
Schmaus, H. (1890) *Virchows Archiv. f. path. Anat.*, **122**, 326, 470.
Schneider, R. D. (1951) *J. Neurosurg.*. **8**, 360.

Traumatic lesions of peripheral nerves

Bielschowsky, M. and Valentin, B. (1922) *J. f. Psychol. u. Neurol.*, **29**, 133.
Blackwood, W. (1943) *Brit. J. Surgery*, **31**, 329.
Blackwood, W. and Holmes, W. (1954) *Peripheral Nerve Injuries*, M.R.C. Special Report Series, No. 282, p. 88.
Blackwood, W. and Russell, H. (1943) *Edin. Med. J.*, **50**, 385.
Brante, G. (1952) *Proc. 1st Internat. Congress of Neuropathology*, **3**, 119.
Cajal, S. R.-y-. (1928) *Degeneration and regeneration of the nervous system*, **1**, Oxford Univ. Press.
Denny-Brown, D. (1946) *Arch. Neurol. Psychiat.* (Chicago), **55**, 171.
Denny-Brown, D., Adams, R. D., Brenner, C. and Doherty, M. M. (1945) *J. Neuropathol. exper. Neurol.*, **4**, 305.
Denny-Brown, D. and Brenner, G. (1944 a) *Arch. Neurol. Psychiat.* (Chicago), **51**, 1; (1944 b) *J. Neurol. Psychiat.*, **7**, 76.
Denny-Brown, D. and Doherty, M. M. (1945) *Arch. Neurol. Psychiat.* (Chicago), **54**, 116.
Dustin, A. P. (1910) *Arch. Biol.*, **25**, 269.
Geren, B. B. (1954) *Exper. Cell. Research*, **7**, 558.
Gutmann, E. and Sanders, F. K. (1943) *J. Physiol.*, **101**, 489.
Johnson, M. L. and Abercrombie, M. (1946) *J. Neurol. Psychiat.*, **9**, 113.
Lorrain-Smith, J., Ritchie, J. and Dawson, J. W. (1915) *J. Pathol. & Bact.*, **20**, 159.
Nageotte, J. (1932) in Penfield's *Cytology and Cellular Pathology of the Nervous System*, Hoeber, **1**, 189.
Sanders, F. K. (1948) *Proc. R. Soc. Med.*, Series B., **135**, 323.
Sanders, F. K. and Young, J. Z. (1944) *J. Physiol.*, **103**, 119.
Seddon, H. J. (1942) *Brit. Med. J.* (ii), 237; (1943) *Brain*, **66**, 237.
Speidel, C. C. (1935) *J. comp. Neurol.*, **61**, 1.
Sunderland, S. (1947) *Arch. Neurol. Psychiat.* (Chicago), **58**, 251; (1948) *Aust. N. Z. J. Surg.*, **17**, 253.
Sunderland, S. and Bradley, K. C. (1950) *J. comp. Neurol.*, **93**, 411.
Walshe, F. M. R. (1951) in *Modern Trends in Neurology*, edited by A. Feiling, Butterworth, London.
Weiss, P. (1943) *Proc. Soc. exper. Biol.*, **54**, 274, 277; *Anat. Record.*, **86**, 491; (1944) *J. Neurosurg.*, **1**, 400.
Weiss, P., Edds, McV. and Cavanaugh, M. (1945) *Anat. Record.*, **92**, 215.
Weiss, P. and Taylor, A. C. (1943) *Proc. Soc. exper. Biol.*, **52**, 326; (1944) ibid., **55**, 77.
Young, J. Z. (1954) summarised in *Peripheral Nerve Injuries*, M.R.C. Special Report Series, No. 282. H.M. Stationery Office, London.

CHAPTER 8

DEMYELINATING DISEASES

By J. G. Greenfield and R. M. Norman

In their concluding discussion of the subject of 'demyelinating diseases' at the Rome Congress (1952), Bertrand and van Bogaert limited the name to conditions in which 'injury to the myelin is the obvious lesion, without being subordinate to vascular or infiltrating lesions'. A broad definition of this sort, based on the neuropathological common denominator, is essential in view of our present state of ignorance as to the aetiology of most of these so-called primary diseases of myelin. If, in addition to damage to myelin, the definition includes the relative preservation of axis cylinders, difficulties arise in classifying perivenous encephalomyelitis and certain leucodystrophies in which the degree of axonal damage may vary considerably. In this chapter the reader will find a description of three main groups of demyelinating diseases:

(1) Acute disseminated encephalomyelitis of perivenous type. The persisting controversy as to the relationship of these probably allergic conditions to disseminated sclerosis justifies their inclusion in this chapter;

(2) A group of closely allied and often intermingled conditions comprising disseminated sclerosis, Schilder's disease, concentric sclerosis and Devic's syndrome;

(3) The leucodystrophies, which are inherited disorders presumably affecting the metabolism of the myelinated axon.

ACUTE DISSEMINATED ENCEPHALOMYELITIS

Post- or para-infectious encephalopathy. Acute perivascular myelinoclasis

Encephalomyelitis as a sequel to acute infectious disease, especially smallpox (Clifton 1724, Freind 1730) and measles (Lucas 1790, Abercrombie 1845), has been known for two centuries. Careful pathological examinations were made of cases following mild smallpox by Westphal (1874) and following measles by Barlow and Penrose (1886) but the characteristic pathological changes associated with the nervous complications of the acute exanthemata were not recognised until 1926 when Turnbull and McIntosh reported 7 cases of encephalitis which had followed vaccination against smallpox in the London area. About the same time post-vaccinial encephalomyelitis became a cause for anxiety in Holland where 139 cases with 41 deaths were reported during the 3-year period 1924–6. A full pathological report on these cases was given by Bouman and Bok (1927). Perdrau (1928) recognised perivascular zones of demyelination as the characteristic lesion in cases of this kind.

As soon as the pathological picture of post-vaccinial encephalomyelitis became recognised, cases with similar lesions following varicella (Glanzmann 1927), measles (Brock 1926, Neal and Appelbaum 1927, Wohlwill 1928), influenza (Greenfield 1930) and smallpox (Glanzmann 1927, McIntosh and Scarff 1928, Troup and Hurst 1930, Marsden and Hurst 1932) were reported. The latter cases were associated with the mild form of variola (alastrim) which was very common in Great Britain at that time. Cases with similar pathological changes were also reported following anti-rabic treatment (Bassoe and Grinker 1930, Stuart and Krikorian 1930) and mumps (Donohue 1941).

Cerebrospinal fluid. In this disease the cerebrospinal fluid does not show the cell protein dissociation which is common in encephalitis. The protein may even be slightly above normal when the cell count is low. The types of cell present are lymphocytes and larger mononuclear cells. Neutrophil leucocytes are rarely seen.

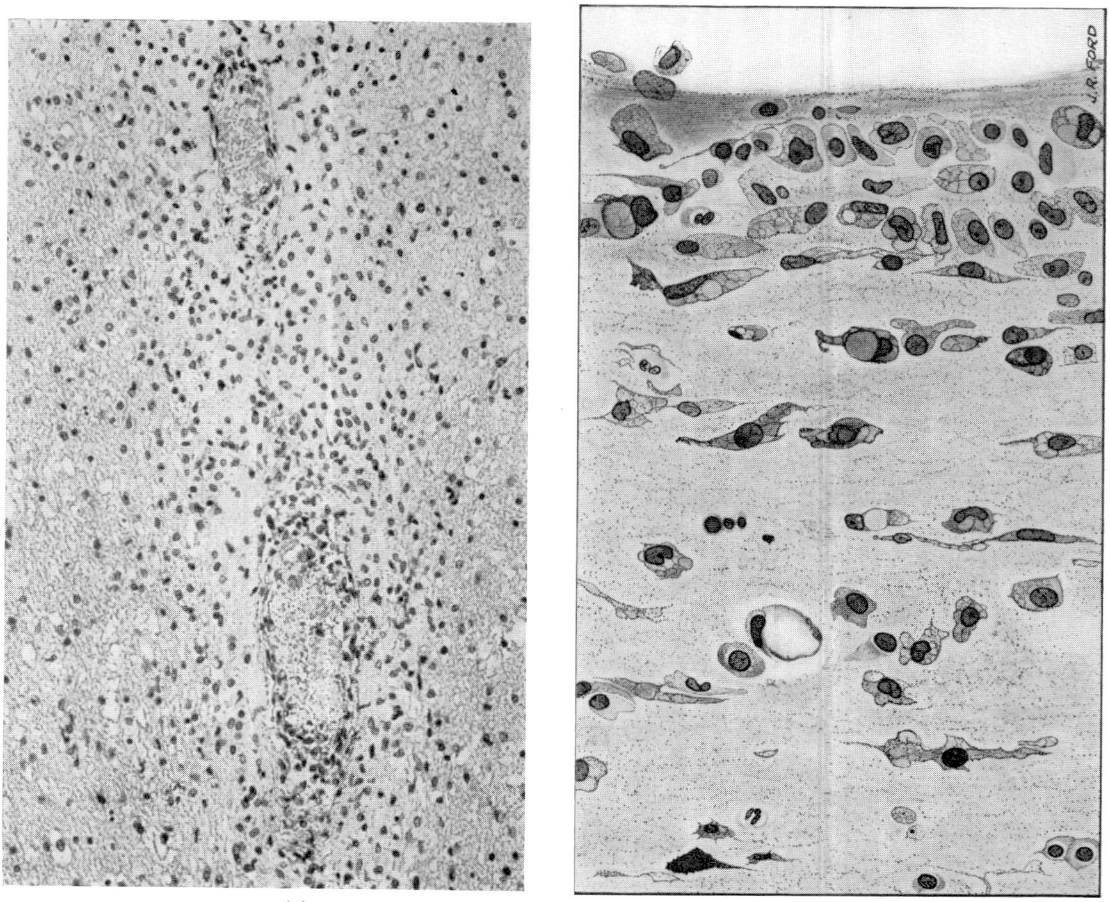

(*a*) (*b*)

FIG. 8.1. Post-morbillar encephalitis.

(*a*) A sleeve of demyelination and increase of histiocytic and microglial cells along a vein. (*b*) Details of perivascular exudate in an early case with 2 days' history. (Hortega's silver carbonate, ×490.)

Morbid anatomy and histology. Apart from congestion, the brain and spinal cord may appear normal externally, but small haemorrhages may be seen either on the surface or on section. They appear to be more common in cases following measles. The white matter appears more congested than can be accounted for by the manner of death. On the cut surface it may be possible to trace narrow greyish zones round the small venules in the white matter.

Oedema of the brain is common and is shown by increased weight, swelling of the gyri and widening of the perivascular spaces (de Vries 1959).

Histologically, in paraffin sections stained by haematoxylin and eosin or other cell stains, the most obvious lesion is an excess of cells in the nervous tissue around small veins. There may also be infiltration of the Virchow-Robin space with lymphocytes and occasional plasma cells, but in most cases this is not severe. The main cellular exudate lies external to this in a zone which is concentric with the vessel wall and usually rather less in width than the diameter of the vessel. Its outer margin is often ill-defined as the cells become more sparse at a distance from the vessel wall (Fig. 8.1*a*). These zones follow small veins for a considerable distance; sometimes those surrounding adjacent veins merge together producing a large area which may resemble a small early patch of disseminated sclerosis; but if the vessels are traced in neighbouring sections they are not found to emerge from the surrounding cellular zone as they do in disseminated sclerosis (Wohlwill 1928).

In the early stages of the disease most of the cells in this exudate have small- or medium-sized nuclei of very varied shape (Fig. 8.1*b*). Their cell body cannot be distinguished from the background of the tissue by ordinary cell stains, but with Hortega's silver carbonate method ragged, often irregularly swollen, processes can be seen running out from the nuclei, mostly tangential to the vessel wall (Fig. 8.1*b*). At a rather later stage many of the cells become early lipid phagocytes; their cytoplasm is more rounded or pear-shaped and granular or foamy and their nucleus lobed or reniform. These cells have been interpreted as microglial or histiocytic. It seems probable that many, if not all, migrate from the vessel wall, and mitoses are not uncommon in the adventitial cells of the central vessel. De Vries (1959), however, regards these cells as mainly microglial, and proposed the name 'microglial encephalitis' for the condition. A narrow, marginal subpial layer of microglial cells is also a highly characteristic feature. The astrocytes in the perivascular zone react by swelling of the cell body and nucleus but show little evidence of increase in numbers. Neutrophil leucocytes are also present in the early stages; lymphocytes and plasma cells are seen within the Virchow-Robin spaces and in the meninges, but are rare in the extra-adventitial exudate: eosinophil and mast cells have also been reported. In the grey matter the exudate may appear more diffuse than in the white matter and, owing to the greater cellularity of the tissues, may be less obvious. Late sequelae in the form of perivenous fibrous gliosis have been described by Malamud (1939).

In sections stained by Sudan IV or by haematoxylin methods for myelin, pallor of myelin staining is seen in the perivascular zones of cellular exudate. During the first day or two of the illness the outlines of this pale zone are indefinite and many of the myelin sheaths in its outer part are thin or beaded. After a few days the zones are rather wider and their outer limit more sharply defined. At this stage many of the cells in the exudate are becoming altered to lipid phagocytes containing granules or droplets of weakly sudanophilic lipid. Fusiform swelling, beading or fragmentation of axons may be seen by silver impregnation methods but the axons appear less damaged than the myelin sheaths.

The nerve cells included in the area of exudate may show mild chromatolysis but often appear quite healthy. The preservation of nerve cells in areas of myelin destruction distinguishes this condition from the perivascular necrosis which may result from thrombosis or embolism of small vessels.

Distribution of the lesions. Turnbull and McIntosh found greater involvement of the ventral half of the pons than of any other part of the brain or brainstem in all their cases, and the writer's experience agrees with this opinion. The deeper layers of the cortex, the thalamus and hypothalamus, substantia nigra and internal and external geniculate bodies, and the white matter of the hemispheres also usually show lesions of varied severity. In the striatum, globus pallidus and tegmentum of the brain stem they are usually slight, or may be absent. Zones of demyelination in the walls of the lateral ventricles are not uncommon. In the spinal cord they follow the line of the venules from the grey matter to the surface and are usually more numerous in the ventrolateral than the dorsal columns (Fig. 8·2*a*). Transverse myelitis with softening of the cord is a rare complication and may be attributed to compression of vessels following oedema. Subpial zones of demyelination independent of vessels may also be seen. Meningeal exudate is slight and often confined to the neighbourhood of veins. A few small veins in the meninges or within the brain may be thrombosed or plugged with leucocytes, but no fibrin can be seen in the majority. Small perivascular haemorrhages may also occur. Necrotic changes in the vessel walls are very rare.

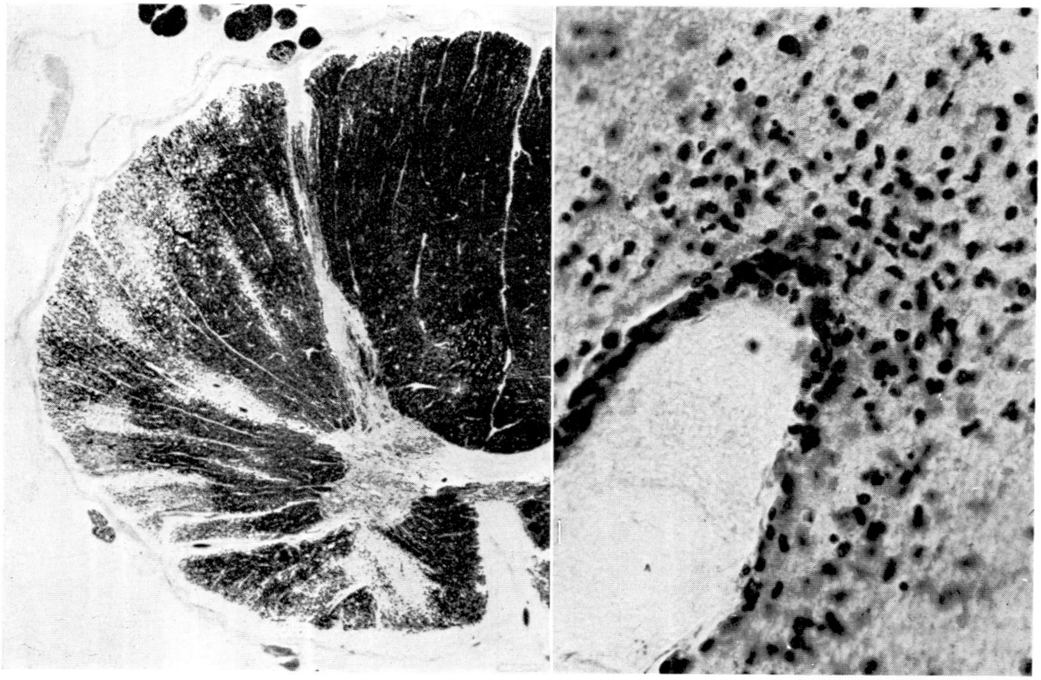

(*a*) (*b*)

FIG. 8.2. Post-infectious encephalomyelitis.

(*a*) Section of the thoracic cord in a case of post-influenzal myelitis (Case 2 of Greenfield 1930). The zones of perivascular demyelination are limited to the ventrolateral columns. (Myelin.)
(*b*) Post-morbillar encephalitis. A zone of cellular infiltration round a cerebral vessel. (Nissl.)

Turnbull and McIntosh found inflammation of the spleen in all their cases. The pulp was infiltrated with large lymphocytes and larger basophil cells which Russell (1955) interprets as plasmoblasts. Many of these were in mitosis. Neutrophil leucocytes may also be present in considerable numbers. Russell considers that these changes in the spleen may be an integral part of the disease.

Clinico-pathological studies by de Vries (1959) have shown that the characteristic perivenous lesions have in the great majority of cases an incubation period of 9–15 days. They are not found in children under 2 years. The clinical syndrome of post-infectious encephalopathy, on the other hand, is associated with very varied and non-specific pathological changes resulting from toxic and vascular disturbances, the effects of convulsions and terminal infective states.

Various theories of the *pathogenesis* of this condition have been suggested:

(1) The theory that post-vaccinial encephalomyelitis was due to a direct attack by the virus on the nervous tissue of the brain and spinal cord was supported by McIntosh (1930) but other

workers failed to find vaccinia virus in the brains of cases of this kind. When it also became clear that the lesion found in the nervous complications of other exanthemata were of the same character and that this differed in many respects from that of virus encephalitis, this theory became less acceptable.

(2) The appearance of post-vaccinial encephalomyelitis almost in epidemic form in Great Britain and Holland and the numerous cases of a similar nature following measles and other acute specific fevers which were reported at about the same time suggested the possibility that a latent, potentially neurotropic virus might be activated by the virus causing the exanthem (Wohlwill 1928, Greenfield 1930). However, Pette who carried out many experiments to test this hypothesis was unable to find any evidence to support it and none has since emerged. It now seems more probable that factors, such as increase in the strength of the vaccine used and primary vaccination of many older children and adolescents, may have been responsible for the large numbers of post-vaccinial cases in Great Britain and Holland in the years 1923–6.

(3) Glanzmann (1927) considered that the lesions of post-vaccinial encephalomyelitis had many of the characters of an antigen-antibody reaction and this theory has subsequently received strong support from the findings of experimental pathology now to be described.

Experimental allergic encephalomyelitis. Following the early work of Rivers and Schwenkter (1935) and of Ferraro and Jervis (1940), there have been numerous observations on this subject. These have been well reviewed by Wolf (1952) and by Roizin and Kolb in the volume edited by Kies and Alvord (1959). It has been shown that when brain emulsion mixed with Freund's adjuvant is injected subcutaneously in animals, perivenous demyelination is produced with great regularity after a delay of several days. There is considerable variation in the response according to the dosage, the time the animal is killed, and the species of animal used. In monkeys there is a close similarity between the experimental lesions and those of disseminated encephalomyelitis in man (Kabat *et al.* 1947). In the few human cases in which repeated injections of neural tissue have been given, as for instance in anti-rabies treatment, confluent patches very like those of multiple sclerosis have been produced (Uchimura and Shiraki 1957; Jellinger and Seitelberger 1958), although the inflammatory changes have been more intense.

The early stages of the demyelination have been studied by Waksman and Adams (1962 a) in guinea pigs and rabbits sacrificed before the onset of clinical signs. The initial lesion is a perivenous infiltration by mononuclear cells of lymphocytic type, and these cells later invade the parenchyma. Destruction of myelin occurs only after this invasion, and is sharply limited by the presence of these cells, which appear to be primary agents in the demyelinating process.

Allergic and post-infectious peripheral neuropathies

Paralysis, often local and asymmetrical, but sometimes more widespread and severe, has for long been known as an occasional sequela of serum therapy (Dyke 1918, Lhermitte 1919) and preventive inoculation against typhoid fever. Stuart and Krikorian (1933) and Getzowa, Stuart and Krikorian (1933) described cases of widespread flaccid paralysis which came on at the end of a course of anti-rabic inoculations with phenolised rabbit's spinal cord. In 2 fatal cases they could find no lesions in the brain or spinal cord except chromatolysis of ventral horn cells. Perdrau (1928), in a 14-day case of post-vaccinial encephalomyelitis, found infiltration of some of the dorsal root ganglia with lymphocytes and occasional plasma and mast cells, and Winkelman (1949) has described cases of painful paralysis, limited to the arms or involving all four limbs, after vaccination against smallpox. During the Second World War very numerous cases of paralysis of the muscles of the shoulder girdle on one or both sides were described (Spillane 1943, Parsonage and Turner 1948). The condition usually came on during convalescence from an acute specific fever or following an operation or injury. The first symptom was pain across the top of the shoulder-blade and radiating down the outside of the arm or to the neck; it might last for a few hours or for days or weeks. This was followed by atrophic paralysis of the muscles supplied by the 5th and sometimes also the 6th and 7th cervical nerve roots. Sensory loss was usually slight and confined to the area of the deltoid insertion. The authors considered these cases to resemble those following serum therapy (Kennedy 1929) but they had no pathological material. Parsonage and Turner call this condition *neuralgic amyotrophy*.

Experimental allergic neuritis. Waksman and Adams (1955, 1956) produced an allergic neuritis in rodents by the injection of homologous or heterologous peripheral nerve tissue along with Freund's adjuvants. The most severe changes were found in the central parts of the dorsal root ganglia and consisted of myelin degeneration associated with a less degree of axonal damage, and infiltration with histiocytes and variable numbers of lymphocytes and a few plasma cells and neutrophil leucocytes. Similar changes were seen in the dorsal roots but the ventral roots were slightly if at all involved and only near the inner pole of the ganglion. In the peripheral nerves there were foci of similar infiltration and degeneration. They were usually fusiform and surrounded one or several small blood vessels. They varied greatly in size and severity, the largest involving the entire transverse diameter of a nerve. In guinea-pigs more diffuse lesions with otherwise similar characteristics and infiltrations of the perineurium with lymphocytes and mononuclear cells were found in some nerves.

The almost complete absence of pathological studies of human material makes it uncertain whether the clinical symptoms which may follow acute specific fevers or allergic reactions have a similar pathological basis. The findings of Perdrau are, however, suggestive. The chief incidence on the dorsal root ganglia in the experiments of Waksman and Adams accords with the clinical observations of Winkelman, Spillane, and Parsonage and Turner who found severe pain, most often in the shoulder, to be the first symptom, heralding paralysis which was usually limited to the distribution of a few cervical nerve roots.

Acute haemorrhagic leucoencephalitis

This condition was separated by Weston Hurst (1941) from other forms of haemorrhagic encephalopathy. In one of his cases the illness came on after an attack of pharyngitis and in some cases reported later it has followed, either immediately or at an interval of a few days, an acute illness of the respiratory tract resembling influenza; in one case examined by the writer *influenza A* virus was obtained from the pulmonary lesions, but not from the brain. Other cases have followed an urticarial rash, but in some the disease has come on during a period of perfect health. The onset is often brusque with pyrexia and drowsiness or coma. Hemiplegia, sometimes with asphasia, or unilateral convulsions have been present in several cases. The disease has been fatal in from 1–6 days. It is possible that some cases recover but the clinical signs or symptoms are not distinctive enough for a diagnosis to be made during life. In most cases (Adams *et al.* 1949, Greenfield 1950, Crawford 1954) the cerebrospinal fluid has shown a leucocyte count of several hundred, or occasionally more than 1 000 cells per cu. mm. of which the great majority are neutrophil leucocytes. The protein is correspondingly increased but the glucose and chlorides retain normal levels. Occasionally, however, the fluid has been quite normal. A high or moderate leucocytosis has been found in the blood in some cases.

Morbid anatomy and histology. On naked eye examination the brain appears congested and swollen. In hemiplegic cases the swelling may be most evident in one hemisphere. The meninges are usually clear but a creamy exudate may be visible in the sulci. On section the white matter of the centrum semi-ovale shows numerous petechial haemorrhages which are most numerous in the central regions and slight or absent in the frontal, occipital and temporal poles (Fig. 8.3*a*). They may also be seen in the brain stem and the cerebellar white matter. Sometimes the haemorrhages are confluent or of larger size. Their distribution is not always symmetrical. In hemiplegic cases they may be much greater in one hemisphere, and in other cases they may be confined to a localised area of the centrum semi-ovale or to the brain stem and cerebellum (Adams *et al.* 1949). The corpus callosum shows macroscopic lesions in about half the cases. The cortex and basal ganglia are usually spared. The more affected areas of white matter are soft and oedematous, and may have a yellowish colour between the haemorrhages.

Histological examination shows that the disease extends beyond the haemorrhagic areas. The lesions are of five chief types which are associated in varying proportions. (1) Necrosis of vessel walls with fibrinous exudate into and through the wall and into the neighbouring tissue (Fig. 8.3*c*). The small veins are most often affected in this manner but small necrotic arteries are sometimes seen (Crawford 1954). This lesion is very characteristic and a diagnosis of the disease can scarcely be made in its absence. (2) Oedema which is essentially perivascular but tends to become confluent and to affect fairly large areas. It has not, however, the same diffuse character as the oedema associated with cerebral tumours. It is associated with the same degenerative changes in the astrocytes as are seen in other acute forms of oedema, such as that round cerebral abscesses. (3) Exudation of neutrophil leucocytes in the early stages and of mononuclear cells at a rather later stage. In some very early lesions the exudate of polymorphonuclear cells may be the only change. (4) Zones of perivascular demyelination (Fig. 8.3*b*). These are seen round many vessels and not only round the venules showing fibrinous exudate in their walls. There is a moderate excess of cells of microglial or histiocytic type in these zones, but this is usually less than that seen in post-infectious encephalopathy. In cases coming to post-mortem after several days of illness the majority of these cells have become lipid phagocytes. Mitoses are common in them at all stages. (5) Haemorrhages of ball or ring type or larger. Some of these are related to necrotic venules. The ring haemorrhages are usually centred on a thrombosed capillary round which there is a narrow zone of necrotic tissue. (6) Infiltration of the perivascular sheaths by neutrophil leucocytes, lymphocytes or histiocytes is often seen but may be slight. (7) Meningeal infiltration by similar cells may be quite heavy.

These lesions taken together give a very characteristic picture which has more relationship to post-infectious encephalopathy than to brain purpura. It may be mimicked by the naked-eye appearances of fat embolism, but in this condition there is neither the same wide-spread oedema nor the exudation of fibrin through the necrotic walls of venules.

Russell (1955) has reported two cases of encephalopathy following an influenza-like illness in which the pathological changes formed a connecting link between acute haemorrhagic leucoencephalitis and post-infectious encephalopathy. In one, in which the white matter of the cerebral hemispheres was most affected, perivascular foci of demyelination forming long sleeves round the venules were numerous and perivascular haemorrhages scanty. Some vessels showed fibrinous exudate and there was oedema in the more affected areas of white matter. A case reported by Jacob (1950) is somewhat similar. In Russell's second case the brain stem and spinal cord bore the brunt of the disease; in this case also zones of perivascular demyelination were much more abundant than haemorrhages. Fibrinous exudate was present round necrotic vessels in the medulla and in a lumbar root ganglion. In general it may be said that there is a remarkable constancy in the type of lesion in post-vaccinial cases, and that this is mimicked more or less exactly by the majority of the cases following other exanthemata. Cases following influenza and those which arise without any previous illness present perhaps a more varied picture, in which some of the features of acute haemorrhagic leucoencephalitis may be present.

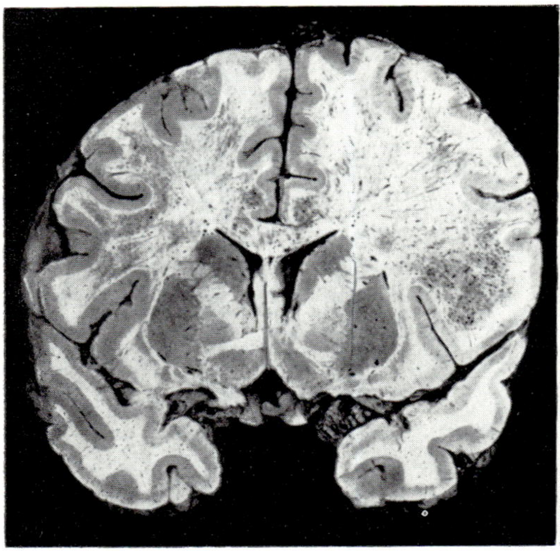

(*a*)

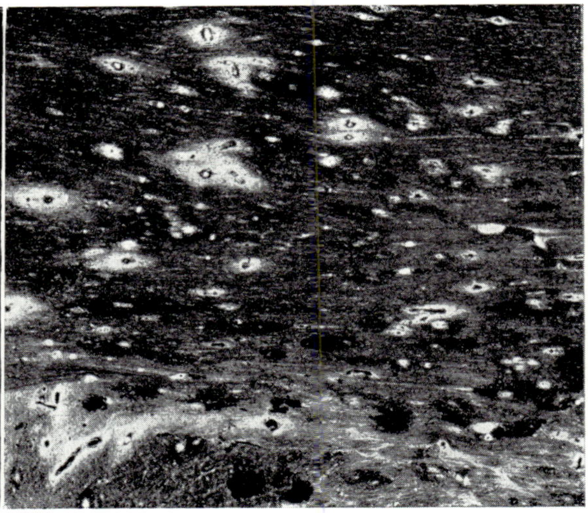

(*b*)

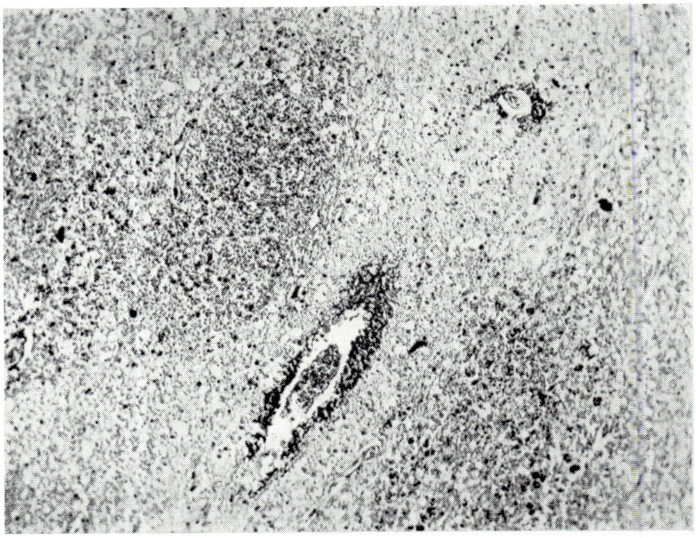

(*c*)

FIG. 8.3. Acute haemorrhagic leucoencephalitis.

(*a*) Coronal section of the brain of a case of 3 days' duration, following a respiratory infection. (Case 10, Greenfield 1950.)
(*b*) Section of corpus callosum of the same case showing perivascular demyelination and haemorrhages. (Myelin.)
(*c*) Section from a case which came on during an attack of urticaria showing fibrinous exudate through the walls of small vessels and haemorrhagic areas. (Mallory's P.T.A.H.)

DISSEMINATED SCLEROSIS

(Multiple sclerosis)

The lesions of disseminated sclerosis were recognised and illustrated by Carswell (1838) and Cruveilhier (1835–42) and were more fully described by Valentiner (1856) and Rindfleisch (1863). But to Charcot (1868) must be given the credit for first recognising the characteristic pathological feature of the disease; demyelination without destruction of axons. It is true that he was specially impressed by the sclerosis in the lesions, which he considered primary, and which prompted him to give the disease the name *sclérose en plaques*. As a result the term *sclerosis* has been universally preserved, with the descriptive adjectives, *disseminated*, *multiple* or *insular*. The term *plaque* is also commonly used to describe the lesions, although it connotes a flat object rather than the spherical, ovoid or other solid form which the lesions take. Since Charcot's description disseminated sclerosis has come to be recognised as one of the most common organic diseases of the central nervous system throughout the temperate zone. Classical descriptions of the pathology of the disease have been given by Bielschowsky (1903, 1904), Marinesco and Minea (1909), Dawson (1916), Steiner (1931) and Jakob (1929).

Lesions in typical cases

In cases which come to autopsy after an illness of several years, naked-eye examination may show little on the external surface of the *brain* that is characteristic of the disease. In some cases grey, slightly depressed areas, usually asymmetrical and sharply outlined, may be seen on the ventral surface of the pons. These are well shown in the illustrations of Carswell and Cruveilhier. In many cases there is some general shrinkage of the cerebral hemispheres with widening of the sulci and slight or moderate enlargement of the ventricles. The spinal cord more often shows characteristic lesions. These appear as greyish areas, slightly depressed from the general level, and often unilateral or involving the ventral or dorsal surface. They may be quite limited or extend over two or more segments. In some cases several segments of the cord may appear grey and be firmer than normal, but even with such extensive lesions the cord is not greatly reduced in diameter. Such severe shrinkage of the lesions as is seen, for example, in the dorsal columns in tabes and Friedreich's ataxia is rarely seen, but in severe cases the whole cord may appear more slender than normal.

In cases in which there has been temporary or more permanent amaurosis similar lesions are found in the *optic nerves*, either in their orbital course or near the chiasma, or in the optic tracts (Fig. 8.4*a*). Lehoczky (1953) in 20 autopsied cases found lesions in the optic nerves or tracts in 9 and of the chiasma in 11. In our series of 70 cases at the National Hospital, Queen Square, such lesions were much more rarely found. They may involve the whole thickness of the nerve for a length of a centimetre or more or may be limited to one side or one-half of the nerve. When the dural sheath is stripped these grey, slightly shrunken areas in the optic nerve are quite easily distinguished.

On section of the cerebral hemispheres the lesions are usually obvious. They appear as rounded, oval or irregular areas of greyish gelatinous appearance irregularly, and usually asymmetrically, scattered through the grey and white matter. In number and size they vary greatly from case to case. They may be very numerous or scanty and may be only a few millimetres or several centimetres in diameter. Their shape is equally capricious. Many are irregularly rounded or oval and many have a lobulated outline as though formed by the fusion of several plaques or by rounded extensions from a central plaque. Both modes of formation are possible but the latter is the more common. Some small lesions may lie altogether in the cortex or at the junction of cortex and white matter involving both equally, but it is not uncommon for larger plaques to stop either abruptly or more gradually as they approach the cortex, leaving a narrow subcortical band of white matter intact. In some cases lesions of the latter kind predominate, whereas in others the grey and white matter appear to be equally involved, but lesions of both kinds may co-exist. Some of the more recent lesions have a pinkish tinge before fixation. The smaller lesions are spherical or oval with sharply outlined borders. Larger lesions have a more irregular shape. Most of these also have a sharp outline, but in some the grey of the plaque shades off into the white of the surrounding tissue. Owing

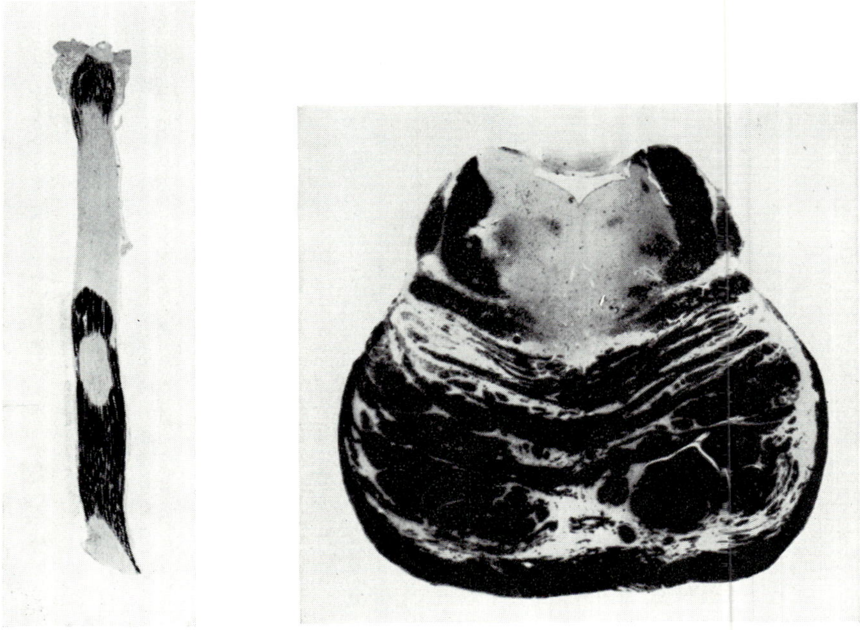

(*a*) (*b*)

FIG. 8.4. Disseminated sclerosis.

(*a*) Optic nerve from disc to optic foramen. (Myelin.) Note that the myelin towards the posterior end of the nerve is intact in spite of complete demyelination near the nerve head.

(*b*) Pons, showing a plaque of demyelination in the floor of the 4th ventricle. (Myelin.)

to their grey colour they are less easily picked out in the cortex and basal ganglia than in the centrum semi-ovale. Areas of similar appearance, but often less firm and sometimes of a spongy texture, are usually present round the walls of the lateral and 3rd ventricles. They are most common at the upper angle of the ventricles as seen in coronal sections and when thus limited may have a rounded outer margin. In severe cases the outer wall of the lateral ventricles may be entirely covered by a continuous lesion which varies in width in different parts.

In the *brain stem* similar lesions are very common. The most favoured sites are around the iter of Sylvius and under the floor of the 4th ventricle (Fig. 8.4), but they may occur in any position and often come to the pial surface over a larger or smaller area. Cerebellar lesions are not so easily seen owing to the narrowness of the white matter in the folia. They are usually small in the cortex and larger in the neighbourhood of the central nuclei.

In the *spinal cord* the most common and characteristic lesions are based on the pial surface and extend inwards as hemispherical or conical areas which involve grey and white matter equally. In severe cases the greater part of the cross-section of some segments may have this grey gelatinous appearance. But on naked-eye examination alone it may be difficult to distinguish the lesions of disseminated sclerosis in the spinal cord from the effects of other diseases or injuries, and immediate diagnosis may rest rather on the appearance of typical lesions in the brain stem and cerebral hemispheres.

Histologically the lesions or *plaques* of disseminated sclerosis are most easily demonstrated in sections stained for myelin, when they appear as demyelinated areas. Under low magnifications the outline of most plaques appears sharply defined 'as though cut out with a punch' (Gombault and Riche 1907) but with higher microscopic powers some myelin sheaths are seen to extend further into the demyelinated area than others over a zone about 50–100μ in width. In other plaques the transition zone is wider and extends over several millimetres. In addition to completely demyelinated areas, *shadow plaques* are not uncommon especially in chronic cases (Fig. 8.5*a*). In these the myelin sheaths are still present but appear thinner and less intensely stained so that the whole area has a grey colour which contrasts with the surrounding black or dark blue. These areas also are often sharply outlined. It is not unusual to see one or more crescentic or hemispherical shadow plaques on the edge of a more completely demyelinated area. Such partially demyelinated areas are common in the spinal cord. In some chronic cases in which the progress of symptoms has been gradual during the last years of life most of the lesions in the spinal cord may have this incomplete character, or they may be completely demyelinated in some areas and contain palely stained myelin sheaths in others. Such lesions may be difficult to distinguish from the Wallerian degeneration of tracts which often accompanies them.

It is characteristic of disseminated sclerosis that there is much less Wallerian degeneration in tracts which pass through demyelinated areas than might be expected. In many cases there is none or so little that it cannot be distinguished by haematoxylin stains for myelin. For example it is not uncommon to find a lesion in the pons which completely demyelinates the area occupied by one cortico-spinal tract but which causes no obvious degeneration in the corresponding medullary pyramid. In the optic nerves also a lesion may cause complete demyelination over a length of more than a centimetre without causing degeneration of the nerve near the chiasma (Fig. 8.4*a*).

In the *spinal cord*, when the number of plaques is small and in cases with a comparatively short history, no Wallerian degeneration may be seen, but in more chronic cases at least partial degeneration is seen in the corticospinal and spinocerebellar tracts and the dorsal columns. This absence or paucity of Wallerian degeneration in the parts of tracts distal to a lesion was recognised by Charcot and has since been accepted as the most distinctive feature of the lesions of disseminated sclerosis. It is not seen in any other lesion of equal severity except in some cases of long-continued pressure on the spinal cord. However, as has been said, it is not an absolute rule, since the axons may be destroyed from the beginning in the most acute lesions, and it also appears likely that they may suffer progressive damage in chronic lesions, or when they pass through several sclerotic areas or a long plaque in the spinal cord.

There have been great discrepancies between different observations as to the number of intact axons which may be found in plaques. To a large extent these have been due to differences in technique as indeed was made clear early in the history of the subject. Strähuber (1903), using an anilin blue method, saw considerable degeneration and some indications of regeneration, whereas Bielschowksy (1903) was struck by the difficulty of distinguishing the area of a plaque from its surroundings, when he applied his reduced ammoniacal silver technique. He found numerous axons in all plaques, both old and new, but confessed that the shrinkage of

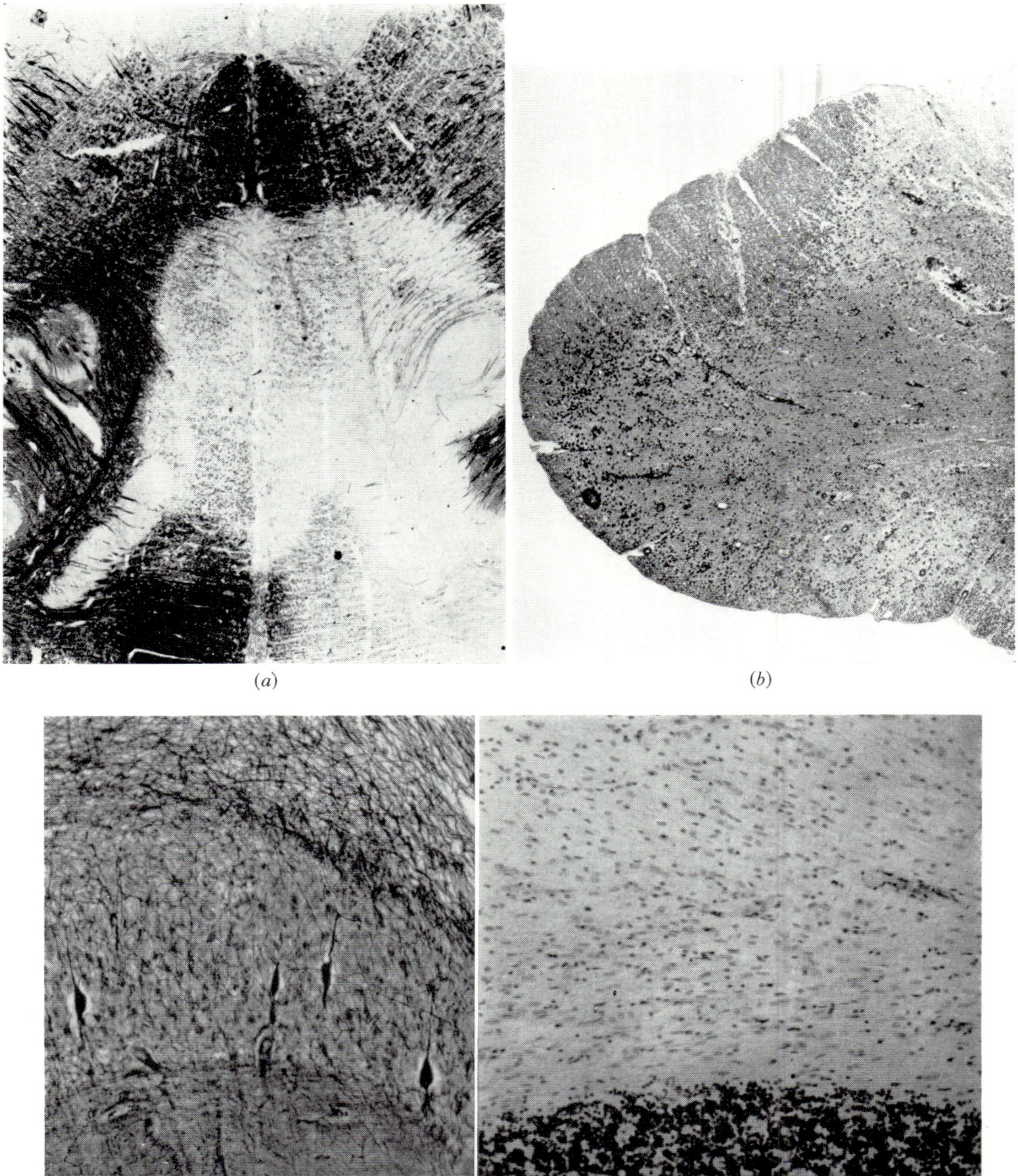

(*a*) (*b*) (*c*) (*d*)

FIG. 8.5. Disseminated sclerosis.

(*a*) Area of medulla showing various stages and degrees of demyelination in a chronic case (aet. 46). (Myelin ×20.)

(*b*) Plaque involving central area of cervical cord. (Scharlach R. Haemalum.) The demyelination is more recent towards the periphery of the plaque as shown by the larger number of lipid phagocytes.

(*c*) Torpedoes on the axons of Purkinje cells in the granular layer of the cerebellum in a shadow plaque area. Persisting axons in partially demyelinated white matter are seen at the top of the photograph. (Bielschowsky silver.)

(*d*) White matter and granular layer of cerebellum in the same shadow plaque as (*c*). Note absence of lipid phagocytes in the white matter.

(*b*), (*c*) and (*d*) from a subacute case, aet. 27 at death.

old plaques might convey a false impression of normality. Comparing his method with the older methods for axons he found that some substance which appeared to cover the neurofibrils in the axon, and which Kaplan had called axostroma, usually disappeared along with the myelin, though it might still be seen in fresh plaques which are completely demyelinated. Bartels (1904) confirmed these observations. This controversy has been carried on till more recent times, since it has not always been realised that certain silver methods (Davenport, Gros-Schulz) as well as trichrome methods stain axons as a whole rather than neurofibrils. Greenfield and King (1936) using Bielschowsky's method on frozen sections, controlled as a stain for neurofibrils, examined 125 cerebral plaques, only 10 per cent of which showed severe loss of axons, that is reduction to one-fifth or one-seventh of the normal number. Of the remaining 90 per cent half showed moderate and half little or no diminution in numbers. They were not satisfied that there was complete loss of nerve fibres in any plaque examined by them, but in two the tissue was so lax that frozen sections were impossible. It seems probable, as Bielschowsky and Bartels showed, that nerve fibres in passing through a plaque lose not only their myelin sheath but also some constituent of the axis cylinder which stains with anilin blue and with some silver impregnations.

Axons do not all pass intact through a plaque. In longitudinal sections of the spinal cord Bielschowsky found a tendency to twisting and irregularity of calibre as the most common change. Sometimes tuber-like swellings were seen, or the fibres might be beaded or frayed out to show their constituent neurofibrils over part of their course, after which they again became homogeneous darkly stained bands. Evidences of regeneration of axons in plaques have been described by several authors (Bielschowsky 1903, Marinesco and Minea 1909, Doinikow 1915, Jaburek 1931). These may take the form of collateral sprouting at acute angles or near an end bulb, or of small loop and club-shaped endings on the nerve fibres. Greenfield and King (1936) found this form of ending also in cerebral plaques, especially in those of recent date. The torpedoes on the axons of Purkinje cells (Fig. 8.2*c*), which are seen in cortical cerebellar lesions, and the large 'retraction bulbs', similar to those seen in traumatic lesions of the spinal cord, should not be interpreted as phenomena of regeneration.

When examined by cell stains such as haematoxylin eosin or by nuclear stains such as basic anilin dyes, *old plaques* of disseminated sclerosis may not be easily distinguished. In the grey matter the only abnormality is usually some increase in number of astrocyte nuclei. In the white matter this is associated with an almost complete disappearance of oligodendroglial nuclei, so that the area of the plaque appears less cellular than the surrounding tissue. This loss may be incomplete in shadow plaques. It is compensated for to a minor degree by an increase in number of astrocyte nuclei of adult type. No cell body can be seen round these. They lie in a dense feltwork of neuroglial fibres which gives most plaques a rather closer texture than normal white matter. But a few old plaques have a looser, areolar texture.

The *nerve cells* which lie within old plaques often show little abnormality. For example the cells of the cranial nerve nuclei which are included in plaques covering the floor of the fourth ventricle are usually normal in numbers and appearance. In severely sclerotic lesions in the spinal cord, Dawson (1916) found chromatolytic or atrophic changes at some levels, but a more normal condition at others. He found evidence of progressive atrophy in the cells of Clarke's column, the axons of which were involved in lesions at a higher level. However, in many cases the large motor cells of the ventral horns remain relatively normal, or show only some excess of lipofuscin. Dawson also found chromatolytic changes in the large cells of the 5th cortical layer in the neighbourhood of lesions in the white matter. Zimmerman and Netsky (1950) found considerable cell loss within plaques in the cerebral cortex and thalamus. But many of the changes in nerve cells, which have been described, may be put down to intercurrent disease or the mode of death. Loading with lipofuscin has been described especially in certain nuclei such as the inferior olives and external geniculate body, where it is very common in many diseases, and other changes which have been described, such as satellitosis of the pyramidal cells in the deeper cortical layers, are equally equivocal. In general it would appear that most of the damage which nerve cells suffer in the early stages of plaque formation are recoverable and that the changes seen in them at a later stage are secondary either to lesions of axons or to progressive sclerosis of the surrounding tissues.

Neuroglial fibre stains give the reverse of the myelin picture owing to the greatly increased density of these fibres in plaques. Some shadow plaques can be distinguished by a less intense staining from those that are more completely demyelinated but in others no such difference is evident. As a general rule plaques lying in areas poor in myelin, such as the cortex, basal ganglia and floor of the 4th ventricle, show less intense gliosis and it may be so slight that it is not evident on naked-eye examination. The arrangement of neuroglial fibres in most plaques is isomorphic and in older plaques the cell bodies of the astrocytes have usually reverted to their normal insignificance. In the grey matter the arrangement of fibres is more irregular, as it is also in plaques of looser texture in the white matter where large spider forms of astrocyte are not uncommonly seen.

The reaction of *connective tissue* in plaques of disseminated sclerosis has been much less studied. Peters (1936) and King (1937) found that many plaques, when studied by silver impregnation, showed a definite, though usually fine, network of reticulin. This varies from plaque to plaque and is usually absent in the cortex and slight or absent in shadow plaques. It is found in both young and old plaques and appears to have little relation either to the amount of perivascular cuffing, the density of the gliosis or the degree of destruction of axons. Although it probably arises from the walls of small vessels, attachment of reticulin fibres to vessel walls is not always easily traced.

Changes in the walls of *vessels* within plaques are considered common by some (Dawson 1916) but are denied by others (Erben 1898, Zimmerman and Netsky 1950). The writer agrees with Bielschowsky, Dawson and King (1937) that fibrotic thickening of the walls of vessels in old plaques is a common, although by no means a constant finding. It may be severe, going on to hyaline thickening especially in plaques of loose texture. The relationship of plaques to vessels has also been variously interpreted. Bielschowsky and Dawson emphasized the fact that small plaques were usually centred on a vessel, but found this relationship obscured in the larger plaques which they considered to be formed by the coalescence of several smaller plaques. Few dispute the observation that many small plaques contain a vessel in or near their centre, and the absence of a vessel in others may be due to the accident of sectioning the plaque parallel to the vessel it contains. But this perivascular arrangement is much less definite than in post-infectious encephalopathy and is usually completely lost in larger plaques which are probably more often formed by extension from a centre than by the coalescence of plaques.

Recent lesions

Occasional cases of disseminated sclerosis come to autopsy within a few weeks of the first symptom of the disease or during a severe relapse after mild early symptoms. In these cases it is sometimes possible to judge the age of lesions by their relation to the clinical history, or less accurately by a study of the stages of myelin katabolism. By a comparison of lesions of different ages it is thus possible to get some conception of the pathogenesis of the process of plaque formation. In more chronic cases also recent plaques, or a recent extension on the edge of an older plaque, are common.

Early studies of the breakdown of myelin were made by Marchi's osmic acid technique, but since sudan IV and similar dyes have come into general laboratory use their superiority for this purpose, especially when combined with a haematoxylin lake, has been generally recognised. More recently special histochemical methods for lipids have been used by a few workers.

In sections stained by haematoxylin-eosin or basic anilin dyes a plaque in the stage of formation can usually be distinguished from the surrounding normal tissue by its greater cellularity. The majority of the cells in it are microglia in the early stages of lipid phagocytosis. The astrocytes have swollen cell bodies and binucleated or paired astrocytes may be seen. The capillaries and small vessels are congested giving the pink colour which is seen on naked-eye examination. Often there is some loosening of tissue structure which has been interpreted as oedema. The area of increased cellularity corresponds exactly to the area of breakdown of myelin and is as sharply outlined. In many recent plaques, especially those of medium or

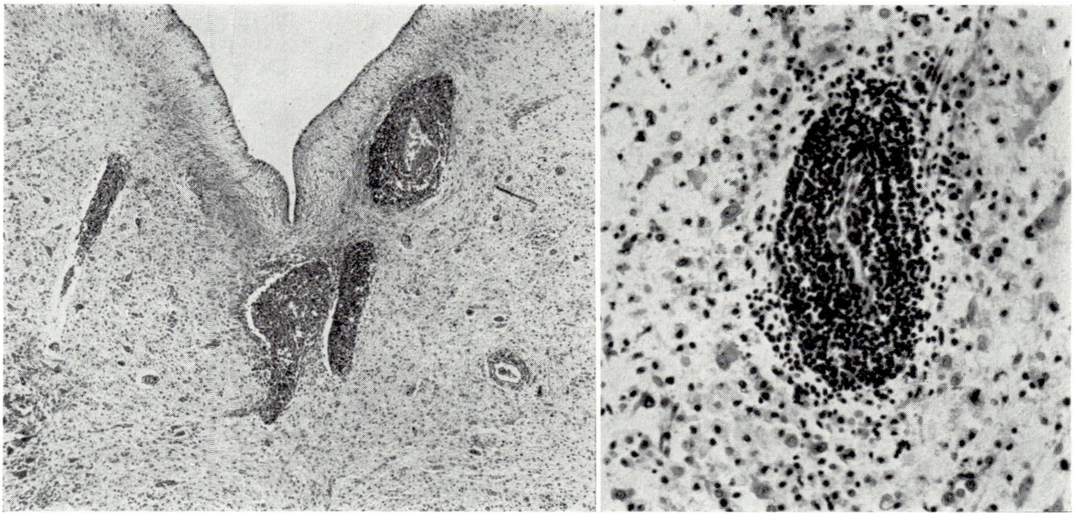

(*a*) (*b*)

FIG. 8.6 (*a* and *b*). Acute disseminated sclerosis. Bulbar paralysis came on about 3 weeks before death in a woman in whom the only previous evidence of the disease was an attack of retrobulbar neuritis 14 months previously. (*a*) Floor of 4th ventricle. (*b*) Vessel in medulla.

larger size, there is a marginal zone of still greater cell density. This 'wall-formation' stands out most distinctly in sections stained with basic anilin dyes, which stain not only the nuclei but also, more faintly, the cell bodies of the microglial phagocytes in this zone. With sudan IV and haematoxylin the intracellular lipid in these cells is found to be weakly haematoxyphilic, whereas in the more central parts of the plaque it is more sudanophilic, showing that the breakdown of myelin is of more recent date in the peripheral zone and indicating a spread of the process outwards from a central focus. In older plaques the reverse is true and lipid phagocytes are mainly found at the periphery (Fig. 8.5*b*). There are other findings which support this conception of a centrifugal spread of demyelination in the growth of the plaque. In chronic cases the average size of plaques is larger and fibrillary gliosis often confined to the central part. This more complete demyelination of the central area is also a striking feature of certain forms of shadow plaque (Lumsden 1957).

There seems to be little doubt that the increase of microglial cells in a plaque follows and is secondary to the breakdown of myelin. In very early plaques it is slight and may only show itself by the presence of a few cells in mitosis and a few early forms of lipid phagocyte (Greenfield 1952). Peters (1951) found early forms of phagocyte sometimes as early as the 2nd or 3rd day and more regularly by the 6th to 8th day. The cellular proliferation appears to be less precocious than in post-infectious encephalopathies, in which it is usually well marked within 48 hours of the onset of symptoms.

Cuffing of the Virchow-Robin spaces of vessels with lymphocytes and occasional plasma cells follows the microglial proliferation in the parenchyma. It is very variable, not only in intensity, but also in extent, as it may not be confined to vessels in or near plaques. This may be explained by the migration of the lymphocytes along the perivascular spaces towards the

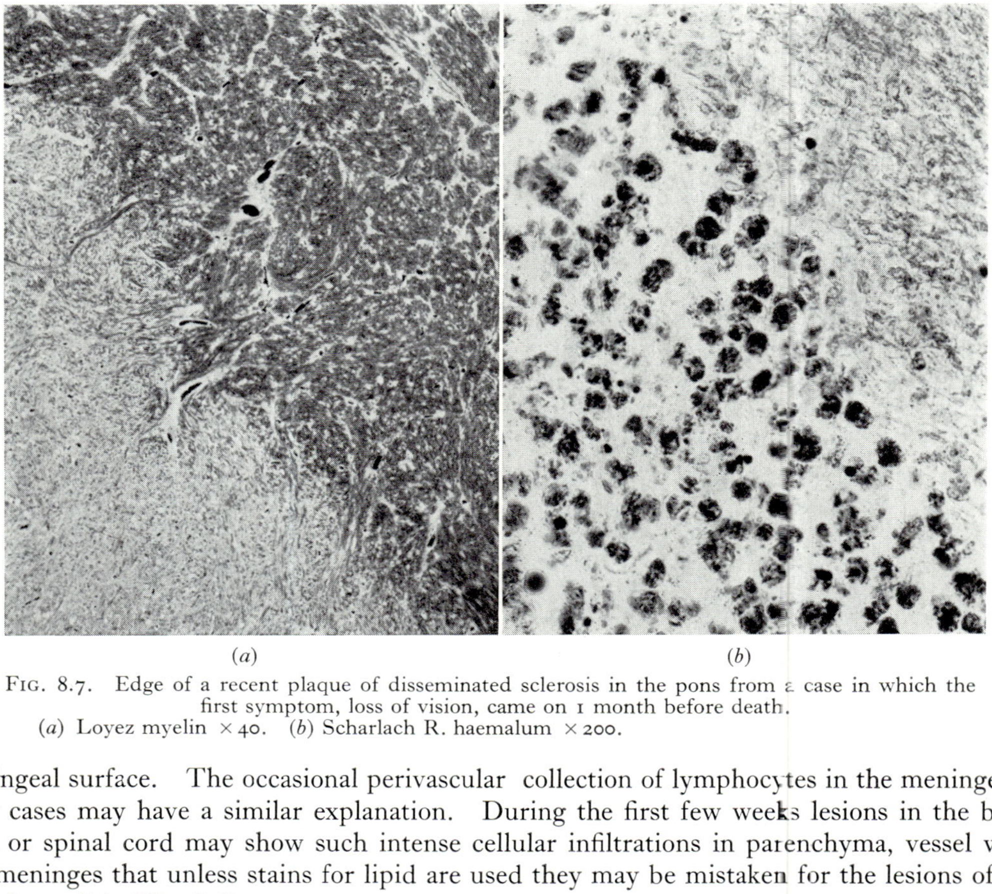

(*a*) (*b*)

FIG. 8.7. Edge of a recent plaque of disseminated sclerosis in the pons from a case in which the first symptom, loss of vision, came on 1 month before death.
(*a*) Loyez myelin ×40. (*b*) Scharlach R. haemalum ×200.

meningeal surface. The occasional perivascular collection of lymphocytes in the meninges in early cases may have a similar explanation. During the first few weeks lesions in the brain stem or spinal cord may show such intense cellular infiltrations in parenchyma, vessel walls and meninges that unless stains for lipid are used they may be mistaken for the lesions of encephalomyelitis (Fig. 8.6).

Various stages of myelin breakdown may be seen in early lesions. These are essentially the same as those of Wallerian degeneration but the process is much more rapid.

(*i*) The first sign is swelling of myelin sheaths either uniformly or irregularly, often forming rosary-like chains of spheres and ellipses which may be incompletely separated from one another. These rapidly break up into smaller globules which lie at first in rows along the line of the myelin sheath from which they were derived. During this process the property of staining with haematoxylin lakes is gradually lost and the smaller, more irregularly dispersed granules which form the next stage in the process stain only palely with this dye, but take a brighter red colour with sudan IV. These granules are engulfed by microglial phagocytes which become rounded out into typical foamy cells (Fig. 8.7). At this stage many lipid granules also lie free in the tissues. In cortical lesions it is usual to find that the majority of lipid phagocytes retain to some extent the shape of the microglial cell from which they were derived, and appear as thickened rod cells, or cells with curved or branched processes filled with sudanophilic granules.

(*ii*) In the second stage the granules of lipid become almost entirely collected within phagocytes which are gradually carried by tissue currents towards the walls of the blood-vessels. During this stage foamy cells filled with sudanophilic granules appear in increasing numbers within the Virchow-Robin spaces.

(*iii*) In the final stage the lipid gradually disappears first from the parenchyma and later from the walls of the vessels.

At all stages anisotropic lipid is present in considerable amounts. In the early stages many globules still show the characteristic myelin cross. Later some of the anisotropic lipid is stained red with sudan IV whereas some, consisting chiefly of cholesterol, remains unstained. These two forms are intermingled with isotropic lipids both outside and inside phagocytes. Seitelberger (1960) has given a detailed description of the histochemical features of these various lipid breakdown products.

Astrocyte reaction. Charcot's theory that demyelination was secondary to neuroglial sclerosis has long been disproved by the study of early plaques. When they can be examined in the earliest stages, a few days after the appearance of the symptoms to which they give rise, it can be seen that astrocytic reaction follows microglial reaction, and that this follows demyelination. While the microglia is proliferating and forming the earliest lipid phagocytes there is little astrocytic reaction, but by the time that the sudanophilic stage of lipid katabolism is reached the cell bodies of all the astrocytes in the plaque have become swollen; binucleated and paired astrocytes give evidence of proliferation and multinucleated cells can sometimes be seen. New neuroglial fibres form while the cell bodies are swollen and continue to increase in numbers as they recede to their normal small size.

In the most severe lesions, where cyst formation occurs, the astrocytes degenerate along with the myelin and axons. In some lesions, but certainly not in all, this may be due to vascular changes and the resulting ischaemia. Areolar plaques are regarded as lesions of an intermediate grade of severity. In them large binucleated and multinucleated astrocytes forming thick processes are commonly seen.

The question whether the astrocytic reaction which leads to sclerosis is primary or secondary to the stimulus of myelin katabolism seems less important when it is realised that astrocytes react to many toxic and metabolic stimuli in addition to those which appear during the breakdown of myelin. Their reaction to noxae varies with the severity of the stimulus and, as has been seen, they may degenerate and disappear early in the most severe demyelinating lesions. But in most plaques of disseminated sclerosis it would appear that the cause of demyelination, whatever it may be, is a less potent stimulus to astrocytic hyperplasia than the products of myelin katabolism.

Shadow plaques, areolar and destructive lesions

The incompletely demyelinated areas to which the name *shadow plaque* has been given have already been described. They are commonly found in the spinal cord adjoining areas of more complete demyelination. In the brain stem and the white matter of the cerebral hemispheres they are often seen on the edge of older lesions but sometimes occur independently. They have been differently interpreted by different writers. Alzheimer (1910) considered them to be young plaques or plaques in the making and his view is supported by Zimmerman and Netsky (1950). This is undoubtedly true for some shadow plaques, but others contain no lipid phagocytes and are clearly static or at least quiescent. Fibrous gliosis is often well established in plaques of this character, and may be found also in shadow plaques which still contain some lipid phagocytes. In the writer's experience these old shadow plaques are commonest in chronic cases in which during the last years of life there has been little clinical evidence of progression of the disease.

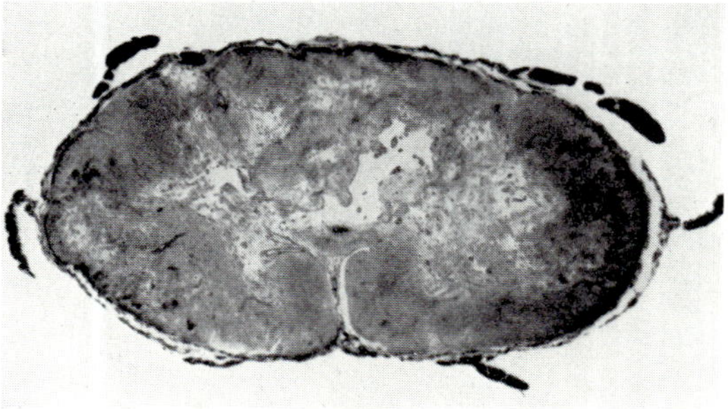

(*a*)

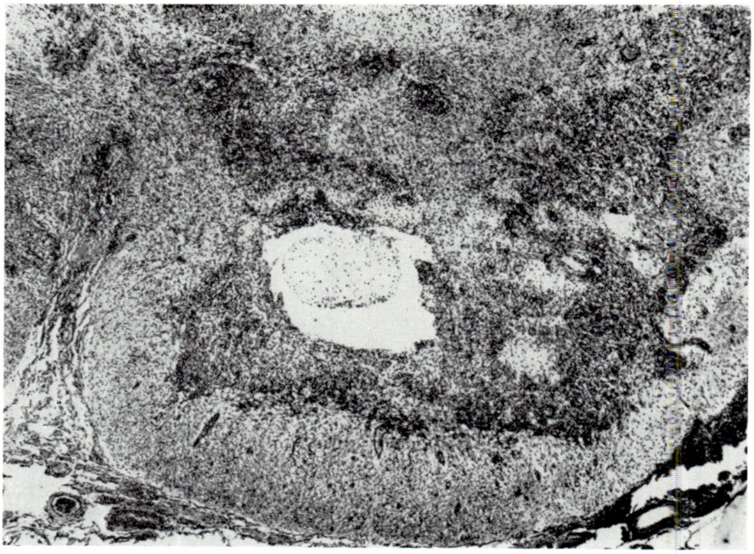

(*b*)

FIG. 8.8. Disseminated sclerosis. (Female, aet. 56).
(*a*) Low-power and (*b*) higher-power views of a severely destructive lesion in the cervical cord, associated with a previous attack of retrobulbar neuritis with residual demyelination of one optic nerve.

It would appear that the process of demyelination or plaque formation does not always proceed at the same rate or have the same intensity. In some plaques and probably also at some stages of the disease, it is subacute and fails to cause complete demyelination. It is also possible that some shadow plaques which contain a sprinkling of lipid phagocytes are formed by a slowly progressive process which might eventually produce complete demyelination, but this does not seem likely for those plaques in which no phagocytosis of lipid can be seen.

The process may also be unusually acute and severe so as to produce local destruction of the tissues and eventual *cyst formation* (Fig. 8.8). The areas of loose texture, or *areolar lesions*, which have been described are probably caused by a process which is rather less severe than that causing cystic lesions. As has been noted giant, often binucleated or multinucleated, astrocytes are not uncommon in areolar lesions. These more intense types of lesion are common in the spinal cord in cases which fall into the clinical category of neuropticomyelitis.

It has been seen that young plaques may enlarge by outward extension from a central focus. The denser marginal zone of young phagocytes often surrounds these plaques indicating a spread in all directions. Little evidence can be gleaned from histology alone as to the duration of this progressive extension. No doubt it varies greatly and in cases during childhood which fall into the category of *diffuse sclerosis* may continue without remission for months or years. In disseminated sclerosis, as judged by clinical symptomatology, it is usually of much shorter

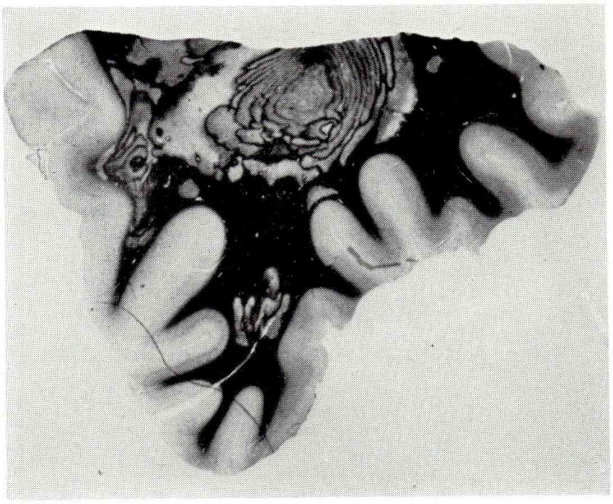

FIG. 8.9. Concentric demyelination of Balo in the subcortical white matter.

duration, but in some cases which are fatal during the first attack of the disease, the symptoms suggest steady progression of the disease for several weeks. These cases are sometimes called 'Acute disseminated encephalomyelitis' and are thus distinguished from typical disseminated sclerosis. But the lesions found in them show no differences from those often seen in cases which on both clinical and pathological grounds must be classified as disseminated sclerosis, and it seems less confusing to call them *acute disseminated sclerosis* (Peters 1951).

Concentric demyelination

In rare cases of disseminated sclerosis a concentric type of demyelination may be seen in some lesions (Fig. 8.9). In very rare cases with more extensive lesions, and which therefore resemble diffuse cerebral sclerosis, this type of demyelination forms the majority of the lesions (Balo 1928, Zeman 1949). Typical lesions appear as narrow zones of demyelination alternating with zones in which the myelin is preserved. These zones are often centred on a vessel. In early lesions the process of demyelination is evidently older in the centre than towards the periphery. In many lesions, however, the pattern is more irregular. It may be hemispherical or the zones may form smaller sectors of a circle or may follow angular or wavy lines. The similarity of these lesions to Liesegang's rings has been stressed by Hallervorden (1952) who has seen in their resemblance to the concentric foci of ringspot disease of plants a suggestion that a virus may have diffused through the tissues. Grcevic (1960) has described a unique case of diffuse cerebral sclerosis in which the demyelinated centrum ovale showed concentric septa of dense fibrous neuroglia and reticulin fibres alternating with layers of coarsely lacunated tissue composed of thin strands of glial fibres and blood vessels. Myelin was confined to the gyral cores and U-fibres.

Cerebrospinal fluid

The characteristic cerebrospinal fluid in a case of disseminated sclerosis is clear and colourless; it contains a slight or moderate excess of lymphocytes, but no polymorphonuclear cells, and a normal or slightly raised percentage of total protein with weakly positive globulin reactions. The colloidal gold curve is positive either in the first or the middle zone in a large proportion of cases. It has frequently been stated that the changes in the fluid are greatest during the more acute phases of the disease. Freedman and Houston Merritt (1950) found that although this was, to a moderate extent, true for the cell count, there was no difference in either the total protein or the colloidal gold reaction in fluids taken at various intervals after the onset or clinical relapse of the disease.

In a series of 569 cases examined at the National Hospital for Nervous Diseases during the years 1937–48, Locage and Cumings (1958) found less than 5 cells per cu. mm. in 85 per cent, 5–10 in 9 per cent and less than 25 cells in almost all the remainder. In Cuming's series the protein was below 50 mg. per 100 ml. in 52 per cent and between 50 and 110 mg. in 42·5 per cent. In the remaining 5·5 per cent it was 120 mg. or over and might rise as high as 200 mg. The colloidal gold reaction, using a citrate gold-sol, gave a first-zone curve in 17·7 per cent and a mid-zone curve in 26 per cent of cases. This figure of positive gold sol reactions is in agreement with that given by most workers who have used a reagent of moderate sensitivity. If the sensitivity is reduced so that few fluids except those from cases of syphilis cause precipitation, positive reactions in disseminated sclerosis may fall as low as 9 per cent (Freedman and Merritt 1950). On the other hand with more sensitive reagents prepared by Lange (1945) the same workers reported 73 per cent positive and the remainder doubtful. As the colloidal gold reaction depends on the balance of the precipitating action of γ globulin and the stabilising action of lower protein fractions, Kabat *et al.* (1950) examined the γ globulin directly in 100 cases of disseminated sclerosis, and found it raised in 85 per cent. This excess of γ globulin in the fluid did not appear to be related to an excess in the blood but rather to local formation within the central nervous system. Recent work on the electrophoretic fractionation of the C.S.F. globulins in disseminated sclerosis and other diseases will be found in the article by Lowenthal *et al.* (1960).

Discussion

Disseminated sclerosis may therefore be considered as due to a process which acts primarily and with varying intensity on the myelin sheaths and secondarily on other tissues in the central nervous system some of which, such as the astrocytes and microglia, it usually stimulates rather than destroys. Demyelination may be complete in a week or two or may take place more slowly. Sometimes it is partial and never becomes complete. The process may continue active for days or weeks and in the later stages of the disease sometimes appears to be continuously, although weakly, active. It may become inactive and again active in the same lesion producing new extensions of old plaques, or it may reappear in a new area. Sometimes the disease appears to relapse as a whole so that both extensions to old plaques and new plaques appear at the same time. That the disease is not always progressive is shown by the discovery of old plaques in cases in which symptoms appeared 20 or more years before death, but cleared up more or less completely. These features of the natural history of the disease must be taken into account in assessing the various theories of aetiology and pathogenesis which have been put forward.

There are superficial resemblances between the plaques of disseminated sclerosis and other focal demyelinations of a secondary type, but as Lumsden (1957) has pointed out, if vascular occlusion, venous stasis, oedema or anoxia could cause primary demyelinating disease without any other operative factor, these well studied encephalopathies would have by now provided unequivocal support to such hypotheses. Ribbert's (1882) theory that the plaques were conditioned by vascular thrombosis was restated by Putnam (1935) who found areas of demyelination and neuroglial sclerosis in the white matter of the hemispheres of dogs in which he had, some months earlier, obstructed the sagittal sinus and the large veins entering it. However, Dow and Berglund (1942), in a study of 60 plaques of disseminated sclerosis, found only 9 in relation to which venous thrombosis could be seen. In 3 it was entirely outside the plaque, in 3 partly inside and partly outside the lesion and in 3 it coincided with the lesion. In most cases it was on, or extended towards, the effluent side of the lesion. Woolf (1952) suggested that thrombosis of this kind, as well as the balls of fibrin, both outside and inside vessels, which had been observed by Putnam, may well have been due to liberation of thromboplastin from damaged nervous tissue.

Obstruction of venules and capillaries by agglutinated fatty droplets in the serum has been put forward as a theory of causation by Swank (1950). It does not account for the progressive character of the growth of plaques nor do the histological appearances of the lesions of post-traumatic cerebral fat embolism resemble those of disseminated sclerosis (Guazzi and van Bogaert 1960).

The theory that disseminated sclerosis is caused by a living micro-organism also goes back for many years. Early experiments by Kuhn and Steiner (1917, 1920) and Adams *et al.* (1923–4), in which cerebrospinal fluid from cases of disseminated sclerosis was injected into rabbits and other animals, seemed at first to give positive results in which spirochaetes were found in the infected animals. Steiner (1952) has advanced further evidence in support of this theory. By silver impregnation he found spirochaetes in about half of the cases in which recent plaques could be studied and *silver cells*, i.e. cells containing argyrophilic granules which he considers as phagocytes of spirochaetes, in 90 per cent of cases. He calls the organism *spirochaete myelophthora*. However, other workers have been unable to confirm this work.

The possibility that disseminated sclerosis may be directly or indirectly due to a *virus* has been reviewed by Innes and Kurland (1952) and Hurst (1952). Although viruses more often attack the grey than the white matter of the brain, many have an action on both. Several virus diseases of animals may be associated with a focal type of demyelination. Of these the best known and most studied is the canine encephalitis sometimes associated with distemper. From a study of the cerebral disease at all stages and in various grades of severity, Hurst, Cooke and Melvin (1943) concluded that the distemper virus, with which they were dealing, possessed a greater affinity for the white matter than that of most viruses which attack the nervous system. It might produce, in certain areas, either demyelination, accompanied or not by destruction of axons, or almost complete necrosis of the white matter. Their work has been confirmed by Koprowski *et al.* (1950). It is not known why only a minority of infected animals have lesions in the brain and it is possible that allergic mechanisms play a part in their production.

The recognition of a demyelinating disease in Icelandic sheep ('Visna') is of exceptional interest in view of its viral origin and the extraordinarily long incubation period (Sigurdsson *et al.*, 1957). In infected animals pleocytosis in the C.S.F. begins in 1–3 months but neurological signs are delayed for 1–2 years.

Waksman and Adams (1962 b) consider that the neuropathological changes in this and other viral leucoencephalitides of animals more closely resemble those of van Bogaert's subacute sclerosing encephalitis than those of multiple sclerosis, or of experimental disseminated encephalomyelitis.

The strongest evidence against a virus aetiology so far produced is given by the experiments of Lumsden (1955) who found that the inoculation of material from recent plaques of disseminated sclerosis into cultures of human nervous tissue had no adverse effect on their growth.

The view that plaques of disseminated sclerosis may be produced by an allergic reaction of some kind has gained support from the experimental production of acute perivascular encephalopathy by intramuscular injections of nervous tissue (*vide* p. 478). Ferraro (1958) considers that there are no appreciable clinical or pathological differences and recommends that disseminated sclerosis should be labelled 'a chronic variety of disseminated encephalomyelitis'. He regards demyelination as the consequence of an antigen-antibody reaction due to a number of partial antigens acting in conjunction with toxic or infectious components. In this view, a primary infection is not necessarily ruled out, but the pathogenetic mechanism of the plaque formation is essentially allergic. Lumsden (1961) expresses the opinion of many authorities in accepting the importance of the auto-immunity theory in providing a clue to the 'trigger mechanism' of the plaque, while emphasising the necessity for postulating some other factor or factors to account for the progressive character of the lesions.

Experimental allergic encephalomyelitis (*q.v.*) in monkey or man is essentially a monophasic condition and the lesions are disproportionately inflammatory compared with those of disseminated sclerosis. Although perivenous demyelination can be found in both conditions, the long sleeve-like demyelinations of encephalomyelitis are dissimilar to the more localised perivenular plaque of disseminated sclerosis (Lumsden 1957).

The primary rapid attack on the myelin sheath, leaving the axon relatively intact, cannot be explained on any simple theory of nutritional failure although this may be a contributory factor both in disseminated and diffuse sclerosis. Little is known of the mechanism, whether enzymatic or other, by which myelin is formed, preserved and nourished or of the factors which cause it to disintegrate rapidly or more gradually into its constituent lipids and proteins, and further knowledge of these processes is needed before the pathogenesis of demyelinating diseases can be understood.

NEUROPTICOMYELITIS

(Neuromyelitis optica, Devic's Syndrome)

These names are given to the association of rapid bilateral loss of vision with an equally rapid onset of paraplegia. Their clumsiness has led to the common use of the eponymic *Devic's syndrome*, since Devic (1894) and his pupil Gault (1895) collected a number of cases. The first clinical report was given by Clifford Allbutt (1870). Gault collected 16 cases of which 7 had recovered more or less completely, 7 had died and in 2 the outcome was not known. Full pathological examinations of cases had at that time been made by Dreschfeld (1882), Sharkey and Lawford (1884), Achard and Guinon (1889) and Fuchs (1893), and Gault added the clinico-pathological examination of a case of Devic's. Since then about 200 cases have been reported. The condition is not rare if cases are included in which there is an interval of weeks or months between the attacks of blindness and of paraplegia. Less frequently these come on within a few days of one another and all variants are found between these modes of onset. Sometimes the disease begins by an attack of blindness or of paraplegia which clears up temporarily but relapses when the other component of the syndrome makes its appearance. The loss of vision is usually severe and may be complete. It is commonly associated in the early stages with papillitis or papilloedema but in relapses optic atrophy is more often found. The paraplegia also is usually severe; it is often heralded by pain or paraesthesiae in the area to be involved and is associated with more sensory loss than is usual in disseminated sclerosis. This often ascends to involve the chest and arms. An initial pyrexia may be present. Both loss of vision and paraplegia may remain severe or one or both may clear up more or less completely. Scott (1952) collected a series of 10 cases, in the milder of which sensory loss over the trunk or lower limbs was the chief evidence of lesion to the spinal cord. In most of these cases vision returned and there was no relapse during the 9–14 years for which they were followed up. Stansbury (1949) collected 5 cases with autopsy, but his cases were not typical as loss of vision was not always severe and in some cases was unilateral. In a full review of the literature

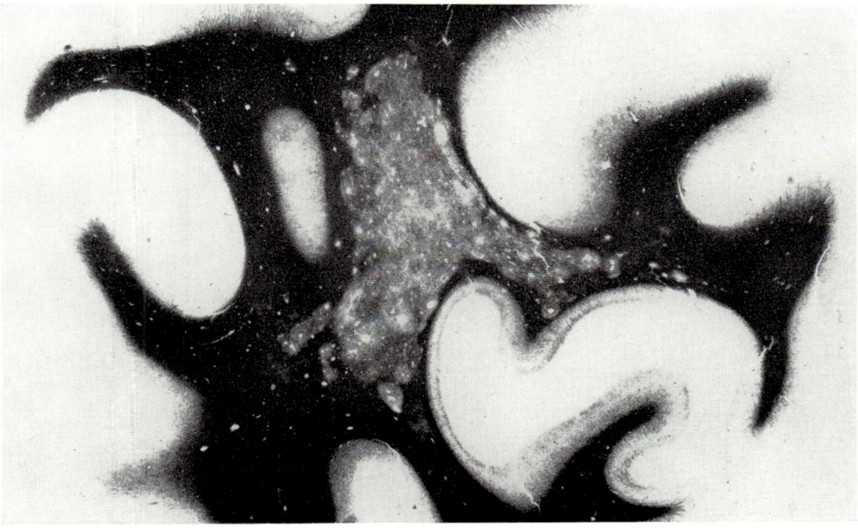

FIG. 8.10. Area of acute demyelination in the occipital pole made up of confluent perivascular zones. The areas in the occipital poles were symmetrical and were associated with similar lesions in the pons, cervical cord and optic nerves. (Case 3 of Stewart, Greenfield and Blandy 1927.)

he found about 200 cases. The age incidence in these was 9–60 years with the majority occurring between the ages of 30 and 50. McAlpine (1938) gives it as from 5 to over 60 years. Stansbury found that death occurred most often either during the first 3 months or the second year after the onset of symptoms. Remissions occurred in about half of the cases. Apart from McAlpine's identical twins, no familial tendency has been observed.

Pathologically the lesions causing this syndrome may be predominantly of one of three types. But these are not sharply separated from one another and lesions which resemble more than one type may be present in the same case.

(1) In some cases typical recent plaques of *disseminated sclerosis* are found in the optic nerves and spinal cord as well as elsewhere in the cerebrum and brain stem. These cases differ from acute disseminated sclerosis only in the severity of the lesions in the optic nerves.

(2) In other cases the lesions are essentially *perivascular*, but where they are most abundant, as in the optic nerves and in some part of the spinal lesion, they fuse together to form larger

areas of demyelination or more severe destruction of tissue (Fig. 8.10). In less confluent areas, and in less affected regions such as the brain stem or cerebral hemispheres, the appearances resemble closely those of post-infectious encephalomyelitis, and indeed severe confluent lesions in the spinal cord, similar to those seen in these cases, may sometimes be seen in post-vaccinial myelitis. These lesions are commonly associated with inflammatory infiltration of a rather more acute type than is common in post-infectious encephalopathy. Neutrophil leucocytes and sometimes fibrinous exudate may be seen in or near the vessel walls. As in post-infectious encephalomyelitis the initial loss of function may be greater than the extent of the lesions would suggest, and it seems likely that many cases which recover completely or almost completely and have no recurrence are of this type. Some cases, however, with lesions predominantly of this kind, have a history of remissions and relapses.

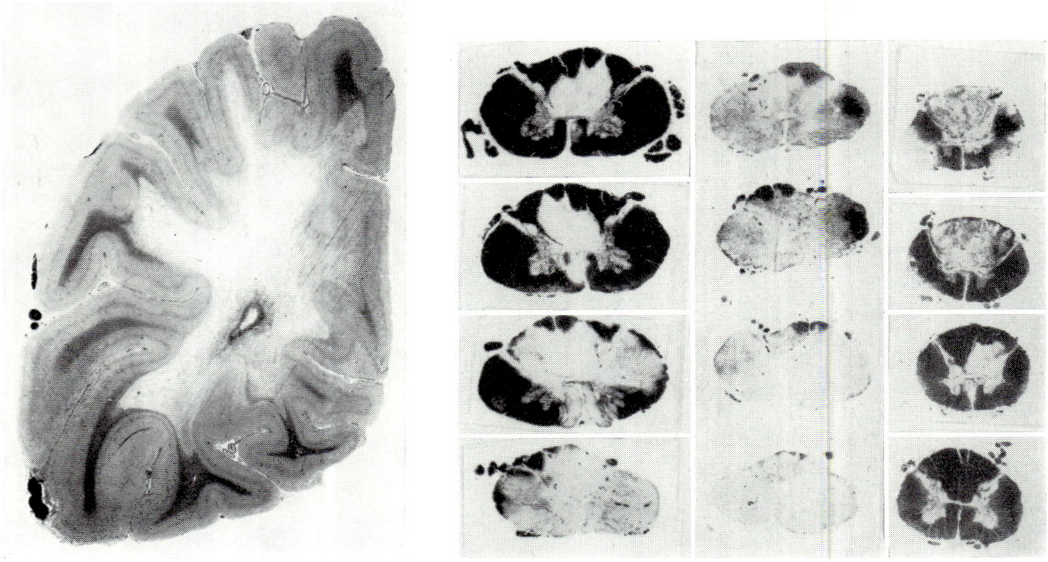

(*a*) (*b*)

FIG. 8.11. Diffuse cerebral sclerosis with diffuse myelitis.
(*a*) Section of the left occipital lobe. (Mallory's P.T.A.H.)
(*b*) Diffuse demyelination of the cord from C6 to L1. Segments Th.6–10 have been omitted as they were as completely demyelinated as Th.5. (Myelin.) (Case reported by Greenfield 1950.)

(3) In the majority of cases coming to autopsy the lesions are *diffuse* involving many segments of the spinal cord in one large lesion, or in two or more lesions (Fig. 8.11). The optic nerves and chiasma are usually involved in a similar extensive lesion which may also include part of the optic tracts. But in some cases only the central part of the optic nerves is affected causing central or para-central scotomas. Lesions may be found also in the brain stem or white matter of the cerebral hemispheres. These lesions have less sharply defined margins than plaques of disseminated sclerosis, and may resemble very closely the lesions of diffuse cerebral sclerosis. In fact several cases have been reported in which the differentiation between acute diffuse sclerosis of the brain and neuropticomyelitis has been difficult (Stewart, Greenfield and Blandy [case 3] 1927 (Fig. 8.9), Marinesco, Draganesco, Sager and Grigoresco 1930). Balzer (1936) described a case in which two large lesions in the spinal cord extending from C2 to C8, and from Th3 to L2, were associated with a small lesion in the optic tracts which had caused no impairment of vision during life. There was, however, slight papilloedema. A

similar case, with very extensive and severe spinal lesions and a small lesion in the right optic nerve which had caused no visual symptoms, has more recently been examined by the writer. These cases fall into the syndrome of neuropticomyelitis on pathological, if not on clinical grounds. Necrotic lesions which later become cystic are common and may be present in the optic nerves or chiasma as well as in the spinal cord (Beck 1927) (Fig. 8.8). These severe lesions result from an acute inflammatory process in which astrocytes and nerve cells, as well as nerve fibres, are destroyed. In some cases lesions of this severity extend over several or many segments of the spinal cord causing gross softening and loss of definition between the grey and white matter. But in many cases the lesions are less severe and the external and internal configuration of the cord are preserved.

Histologically these lesions in the early stages usually show severe inflammatory reactions with lymphocytic cuffing of vessels and with plasma cells and neutrophil leucocytes both in and around the vessel walls. Myelin is rapidly broken down and there is considerable destruction of axons which show irregular swellings, fragmentation and end bulbs. Around the more severe lesions it is common to find a zone of lacunar degeneration, with distension of the individual myelin sheaths, similar to that seen round necrotic areas due to vascular occlusion. This is sometimes referred to as oedema. The astrocytes and oligodendroglia in the central parts of the lesions may show more regressive than progressive changes, and in some areas they succumb leaving only connective tissue and microglia viable. In cases of longer duration scarring with reticulin and collagen fibres and some degree of cavitation are commonly found, but for the most part the lesions undergo neuroglial sclerosis. Thickening of vessel walls is commonly seen in old lesions as in the more severe lesions of disseminated sclerosis.

In many cases it is difficult both on clinical and pathological grounds to draw any sharp dividing line between neuropticomyelitis and disseminated sclerosis. In the former condition the lesions certainly tend to be more destructive than in most cases of disseminated sclerosis. There is more inflammatory reaction in the early stages, more necrosis of tissue and more scarring with connective tissue. The severity and bilateral character of the loss of vision and the rapid onset of severe paraplegia in most of the fatal cases, many of which terminate from respiratory paralysis, agrees with the histological evidence of acuteness and severity. But the condition may be merely an especially acute and extensive form of disseminated sclerosis which differs from the cases with very diffuse cerebral lesions chiefly in the distribution of the disease. The tendency to remission and relapse which is considered typical of disseminated sclerosis is also found in the history of many cases which have been called neuropticomyelitis and indeed the earliest symptoms, whether visual or paraplegic, often lead to the diagnosis of the more common disease. On the other hand, from the ophthalmological standpoint, there is a group of these cases having much more in common clinically with acute encephalomyelitis than with disseminated sclerosis (Scott 1961). There seems little doubt that the syndrome does not comprise a uniform clinico-pathological entity.

Diffuse myelitis

In the literature of last century the name *diffuse myelitis* was used to distinguish cases with extensive lesions in the spinal cord from cases of *transverse myelitis* in which only one or two segments of the spinal cord were involved. Thus Gault 'on the advice of Dr. Devic' proposed the name *acute diffuse neuromyelitis* for the syndrome which he described. Further study showed that diffuse myelitis might be due to a variety of causes including syphilis and subacute phlebitis of spinal veins (subacute necrotic myelitis of Foix and Alajouanine). The term therefore fell into disuse. But when these two conditions and the effects of thrombosis of the anterior spinal artery are excluded the great majority of cases of diffuse myelitis show lesions like those of neuropticomyelitis. It is possible that, if a careful examination of the optic nerves had been made, it would have revealed an inflammatory or demyelinating lesion which had caused no symptoms. But it must not be assumed that diffuse myelitis is always associated with lesions in the optic nerves. Kahle and Schaltenbrand (1955) have called cases of this kind *myelitis necroticans diffusa*. In 3 of their 5 cases paraplegia was associated with blindness, but in the other 2, in which there was a similar history of rapidly progressive paralysis, no visual symptoms were present. In all 5 cases the spinal cords showed very extensive demyelination which had gone on to necrotic softening of tissues in the most affected segments. In some cases the lesions tapered at their upper and lower ends so as to involve only the central parts of the cord, especially the base of the dorsal columns. The 2 cases without amaurosis had counts of 60 and 315 cells in their cerebrospinal fluids. In 1 case with visual loss the count reached the unusual figure of 635 cells. These authors point out that it is impossible to distinguish cases with, from those without, blindness by the character of the lesions in the spinal cord. The writer's experience is in full agreement with this view, but in some of his cases there has been less tendency to necrosis even in extensive lesions (Greenfield 1950, Fig. 8.8). The addition of the word *necroticans* to the older name will therefore exclude some cases which are of an essentially similar nature. It is also liable to cause confusion with the name *subacute necrotic myelitis*, which is still in general use for cases due to subacute phlebitis of spinal veins. There appears to be little objection to the use of the term *diffuse myelitis* or *myelopathy* for cases of this kind, but their possible relationship to Devic's syndrome should be borne in mind and the optic nerves and chiasma examined for lesions even when no visual symptoms have been present during life.

Cerebrospinal fluid. A difference between disseminated sclerosis and neuropticomyelitis is evident in the examination of the cerebrospinal fluid. In the latter syndrome the cell count varies greatly but often exceeds 100 cells per cu. m.m., and includes a considerable percentage of polymorphonuclear leucocytes, as well as plasma and other large mononuclear cells. The fluid may form a fine coagulum as in tuberculous meningitis. The percentage of protein is often considerably raised even when the cell count is low. On the other hand Lange's gold sol and the benzoin reactions are constantly negative or very weak. As the examination of the fluid has usually been made during the early and acute stages of the disease these negative colloidal reactions, which are often associated with high cell counts, are significant, since at this stage positive reactions of greater or less strength are found in at least 35 per cent of cases of disseminated sclerosis. This difference does not appear to be due to the acuteness of the process, since subacute and relapsing cases show the same feature, but it may be due to differences in the reactions of the protective tissues of the body.

SCHILDER'S DISEASE

The generic term 'diffuse cerebral sclerosis' is applied to a variety of conditions in which widespread demyelination and gliosis occurs mainly in the centrum ovale. It is still useful as a macroscopic diagnosis, but histological examination enables a more precise classification to be made. Schilder (1912, 1913, 1924) described three cases of diffuse cerebral sclerosis, the second of which would now be classified as a familial leucodystrophy, and the third probably as an adult form of subacute sclerosing leucoencephalitis (Lumsden 1951). The eponymic 'Schilder's disease' is now commonly limited to the first type of case described in 1912 (Lhermitte 1950; Poser and van Bogaert 1956).

There has been confusion between Schilder's disease proper and leucodystrophies with purely sudanophil breakdown-products, the latter cases having in the past been called 'familial

Schilder's disease' or simply included in the main group of sudanophil diffuse sclerosis without any attempt at subdivision. As will be seen from the following account, the over-all neuropathological features of a leucodystrophy are different from those of Schilder's disease, and the limited definition of the term Schilder's disease proposed by van Bogaert and others brings into focus the close relationship of this condition with disseminated sclerosis.

Pathological changes. External examination of the brain shows no abnormality unless the disease has been present for several years, in which case there may be general shrinkage of the cerebral hemispheres with some widening of sulci and ventricular enlargement. On section large areas in the white matter of the hemispheres appear brownish and softer than normal in cases with a history of a few months, or greyish, gelatinous and firm in cases with a history of a year or more. These areas are usually irregularly rounded and include the walls of the ventricles, but on approaching the cortex they cease either before reaching the deeper sulci or at the subcortical layer of U fibres (arcuate fibres) which are preserved as a thin white line. The lesions are most common in the occipital lobes but may be seen in any situation in the centrum semi-ovale. The writer has never seen a case in which every part of this was involved. They do not usually involve the internal capsule but may spread under the insula into the external capsule sparing the basal ganglia. They are by no means always symmetrical, indeed, symmetry between the two hemispheres is the exception in early cases, but may be found in advanced cases in which all the white matter of the occipital lobes, except the arcuate fibres, is involved. These large bilocular foci are often connected by continuous demyelination of the posterior part of the corpus callosum (Heernu *et al.* 1945). In many cases the lesions are discontinuous or appear so on section. In early cases the outline of the lesions is much less definite than in the plaques of disseminated sclerosis, but shades off into normal white matter over a zone 5–10 mm. in width. Some early lesions are not easily distinguished on naked-eye examination. Their colour is little changed, but they are softer and appear more granular than normal white matter. The cerebellar white matter may contain focal, or, more rarely, diffuse lesions (Poser 1956). They may be of similar age or more recent than those in the cerebral hemispheres. Focal lesions may also occur in the brain stem as in Schilder's (1912) original case. In very chronic cases, or cases which have come to a standstill, shrinkage of the lesions may lead to local dilatations of the ventricles.

In addition to the large hemispheric lesion, aptly called the 'giant Schilder plaque' by McAlpine *et al.* (1955), there are often smaller, focal lesions in the centrum ovale, cerebellum or brain stem, which are indistinguishable from those of disseminated sclerosis. Such cases are sometimes classified as 'transitional sclerosis' or 'diffuse-disseminated sclerosis', and they have the same age distribution as those of disseminated sclerosis proper (Poser 1956).

Microscopically, all the forms of myelin degeneration which have been described in disseminated sclerosis may be seen especially towards the periphery of the lesion, the central parts being completely demyelinated.

Stains for *axons or neurofibrils* show a very considerable loss and often complete disappearance in the more central parts of the lesions with many end-bulbs and much beading of axons in the outer zones. The degree of axonal damage varies but is usually much greater than that seen in most plaques of disseminated sclerosis.

Cell stains show swelling and proliferation of fibrous astrocytes, many of which are binucleated, along with excess of microglial cells in various stages of lipid phagocytosis. There is the same type of glial wall formation as in disseminated sclerosis, but the central parts of the white matter appear less cellular than normal because of the disappearance of oligodendroglial nuclei. Some degree of lymphocytic infiltration of the Virchow-Robin spaces is commonly, but not constantly, present. In the cortex overlying large lesions the majority of the nerve cells are usually normal but some chromatolysis (axonal reaction) or atrophic change may be seen in the large pyramidal cells of the deeper layers. An important distinguishing feature from subacute sclerosing leucoencephalitis is the absence of inflammatory reactions in the grey matter (van Bogaert *et al.* 1956).

Stains for *neuroglial fibres* show a degree of fibrous gliosis which varies with the duration of the disease. It is often rather lax and irregular with abnormally thick fibres arising from giant, sometimes binucleated, astrocytes running in all directions among finer fibres. Isomorphic gliosis is less common.

Stains for *lipid* show all the usual stages of myelin katabolism (Seitelberger 1961). Most of the lipid is contained in microglial phagocytes but some appears as extracellular granules and the swollen cell bodies of astrocytes also may contain a few granules at or near their margin. The amount of anisotropic lipid is usually less than in plaques of disseminated sclerosis. Phagocytes containing neutral fat fill the perivascular spaces of many small vessels where they may be mixed with lymphocytes. In long standing cases the neutral fat remains mainly at the periphery of the lesions, as in disseminated sclerosis.

THE LEUCODYSTROPHIES

The name 'leukodystrophia' was introduced by Bielschowsky and Henneberg (1928) to denote a familial and progressive degeneration of the cerebral white matter. Since that time, sufficient cases have accumulated to enable a classification to be made on a neuropathological basis. Most of these diseases appear to be inherited as Mendelian recessives and in some types the presumed metabolic defect is reflected in the presence of large amounts of lipids which fail to stain or stain only feebly with Sudan dyes. The term 'prelipoid', originally used by Alzheimer (1910) to designate the material found in the nerve cells of amaurotic idiocy, is still commonly used to describe these lipid substances. Irrespective of whether the preponderant lipids present are sudanophil or non-sudanophil, all leucodystrophies have over-all neuropathological features which distinguish them from Schilder's disease (Poser and van Bogaert 1956). In the majority of cases of leucodystrophy the demyelination is much more diffuse and symmetrical throughout the centrum ovale, the gyral cores and the cerebellar white matter. The brain stem is often severely involved. The demyelination does not have the circumscribed focal character of the Schilder-disseminated sclerosis type of case, nor is there histological evidence of the centrifugal spread of the lesions. The gliosis is isomorphic and inflammatory reactions are usually minimal or absent. In most forms of leucodystrophy the loss of axis cylinders is commensurate with the demyelination.

The leucodystrophies form an extremely complex group of disorders and there has been much discussion about their relationship with the lipidoses (Poser 1961; Einarson and Strömgren 1961). A few cases have additional features of malformation (Hallervorden 1957: Norman *et al.* 1962), cerebral calcification (*q.v.*) or system-like tract degenerations (van Bogaert *et al.* 1961), but only the better recognised types will be described in this chapter.

Krabbe type. (*Epithelioid or globoid cell type*)

The first description of this condition was given by Bullard and Southard (1906) in a boy dying at the age of 6½ years after an illness lasting one year. Krabbe's (1916) paper on diffuse cerebral sclerosis in infancy included an account of two siblings suffering from the disease, but it was not until Collier and Greenfield (1924) described their infantile case with its perivascular cell packets, and coined the name 'globoid' for the characteristic large multinucleated histiocytes, that a clear-cut pathological picture emerged. Since that time about 30 cases have been

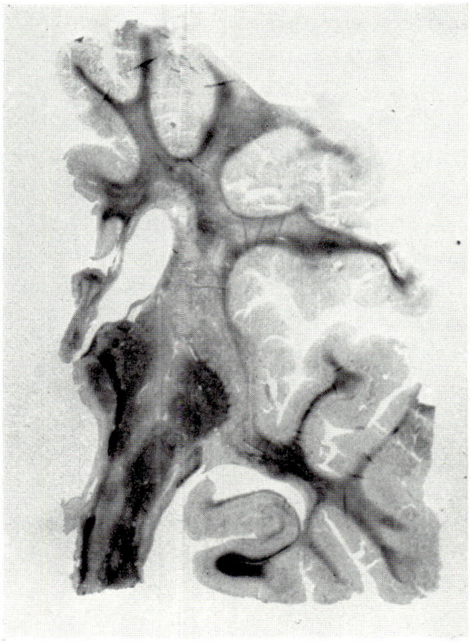

(a)

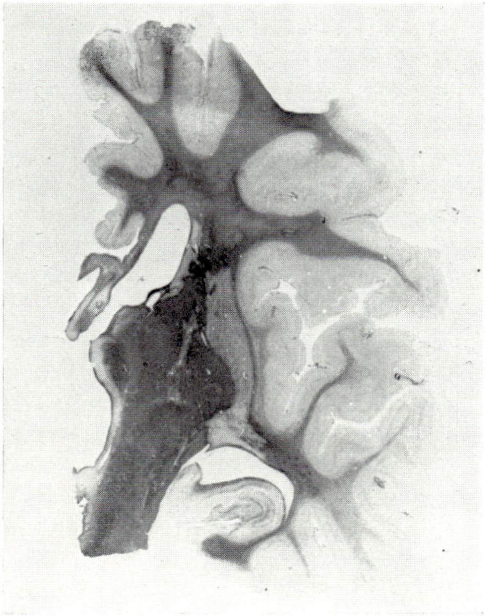

(b)

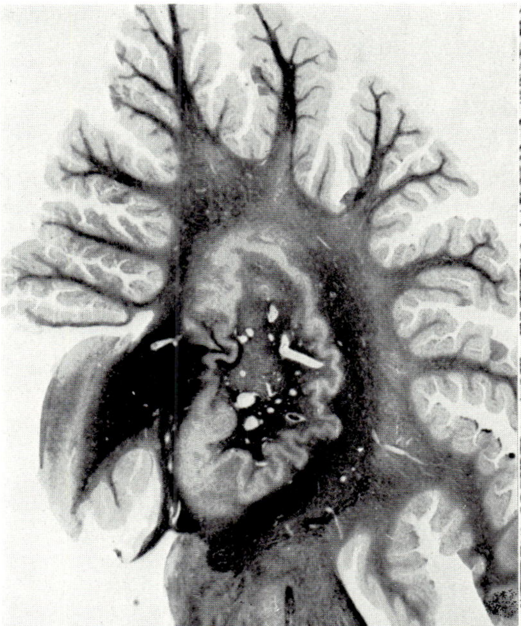

(c)

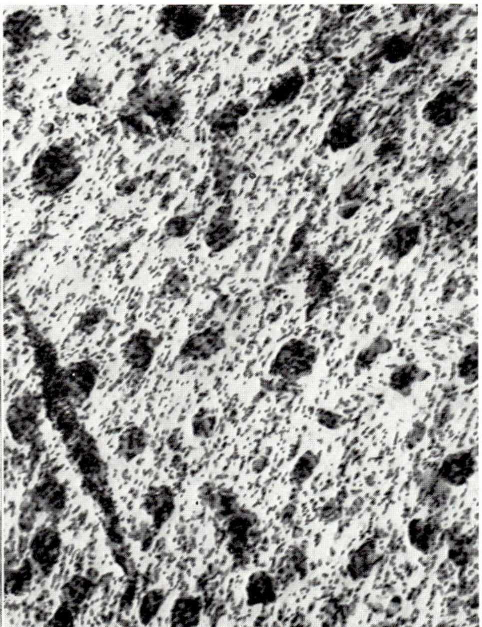

(d)

FIG. 8.12. *Krabbe type.* (*a*) Diffuse demyelination of the centrum ovale. (Kultschitsky-Pal (frozen section).) (*b*) Corresponding section showing dense gliosis of demyelinated and relatively preserved areas. (Holzer.) (*c*) Demyelination in the cerebellum. (Kultschitsky-Pal (frozen section).) (*d*) Packets of globoid and epithelioid cells in the fully demyelinated cerebellar white matter. (Carbol azure.)

recorded, in the majority of which signs of a rapidly progressive neurological illness have begun in the first year of life. It is very doubtful if an adult form of the disease exists. The condition appears to be inherited as a Mendelian recessive. A comprehensive review of the subject has recently been given by Bignami *et al.* (1961).

Pathology. The brain is reduced in weight and appears normal externally, but on section the white matter is obviously demyelinated and sclerosed. Sections stained for myelin show the characteristic widespread lesions of a leucodystrophy in the centrum ovale, cerebellum and brain stem (Figs. 8.12*a* and *c*). There is, however, considerable variation from case to case in the distribution of the demyelination, certain tracts or fibre systems being sometimes relatively intact. The loss of axis cylinders is commensurate with the demyelination. Fibrillary and astrocytic gliosis is intense and not confined to areas showing the greatest loss of myelin (Fig. 8.12*b*). The astrocytic nuclei are unusually large and pleomorphic and the cell bodies are often swollen and stain faintly with P.A.S. This cellularity of the white matter is markedly increased in some of the more degenerated areas, notably in the internal capsule and crura, because of the presence of numerous histiocytes (Fig. 8.12*d*). The majority of the cells in these areas are medium-sized, round or oval mononuclear cells with a matt or finely granular cell body and an oval nucleus which is larger and less hyperchromic than that of the lipid phagocytes, of which a few are also present. In some places these mononuclear *epithelioid* cells are collected in packets of 20 or more, often surrounding a small vessel. In addition there are larger cells which may lie singly or in groups or larger packets (Fig. 8.13*a*). These measure from 20μ to 50μ, and are always spherical unless compressed by neighbouring cells. They may have from 2 to 15 nuclei, which are similar in size and character to those in the smaller epithelioid cells, and almost always lie on the surface of the cell, often appearing to be flattened against the cell membrane. The cytoplasm stains faintly blue and appears clear with basic blues or with haematoxylin eosin; with polychrome stains it is finely granular. It may contain one or two vacuoles but is never foamy. To these cells Collier and Greenfield gave the name *globoid cells* owing to their spherical shape and superficially placed nuclei. In some places it is possible to see all transitions between epithelioid and globoid cells and both types may occur together in one packet. These cell packets are often rounded or oval with a smooth outer boundary. They are commonly seen around or close to a vessel of precapillary type, as judged by the presence of scanty reticulin fibres in their walls.

The staining reactions of the epithelioid and globoid cells are similar and have been studied by several authors, notably Diezel (1955) and Stammler (1956). The strong staining with P.A.S., the feeble staining with Sudan Black, and the insolubility of the intracellular material with powerful lipid solvents has led to the conclusion that the substance is a cerebroside bound to protein. Chemical analysis has also shown a surprisingly normal level of neutral cerebroside in two cases (Norman *et al.* 1961) and an actual increase of glycolipids in another (Blackwood and Cumings 1954). Neutral cerebroside is also present in larger amount in tissues containing a higher proportion of cell packets (Bignami *et al.* 1961).

It seems likely, both from their position and character, that these abnormal cells arise from histiocytes in the walls of vessels. The problem of the origin of the globoid cells has been discussed in detail by Peiffer (1957). This author believes that while all the glial and mesenchymal cells contain glycolipid, only the microglia change into multinucleated globoid cells. Blackwood also derives some from microglia which he found surrounding, rather than engulfing, masses of lipid material with similar staining reactions to those in the cells. The idea that globoid cells might be of neuroglial origin (Collier and Greenfield, de Lange) is disproved by the constant absence of neuroglial fibres and by the smaller size and darker staining of the nuclei. It seems probable that they appear first as mononuclear epithelioid cells which migrate outwards and by fusing together, or by dividing incompletely as they absorb lipoprotein material, form the large multinucleated globoid cells. These may later break down and be absorbed by microglial phagocytes.

The experimental work of Austin *et al.* (1961) is of considerable interest in this connection. Cells closely resembling globoid and epithelioid cells were produced in the white matter of rats by the intracerebral injection of cerebroside, but not of other lipids. However attractive this theory of the phagocytic action of the histiocytes may be, it must be pointed out that a primary storage of lipid by the adventitial cells is not to be ruled out. Spindle-shaped adventitial cells of the larger vessels may also store a similar substance, and the globoid cell packets have a striking resemblance to the cerebral perivascular formations of infantile Gaucher's disease (Norman 1962) (Figs. 8.13*a* and *b*).

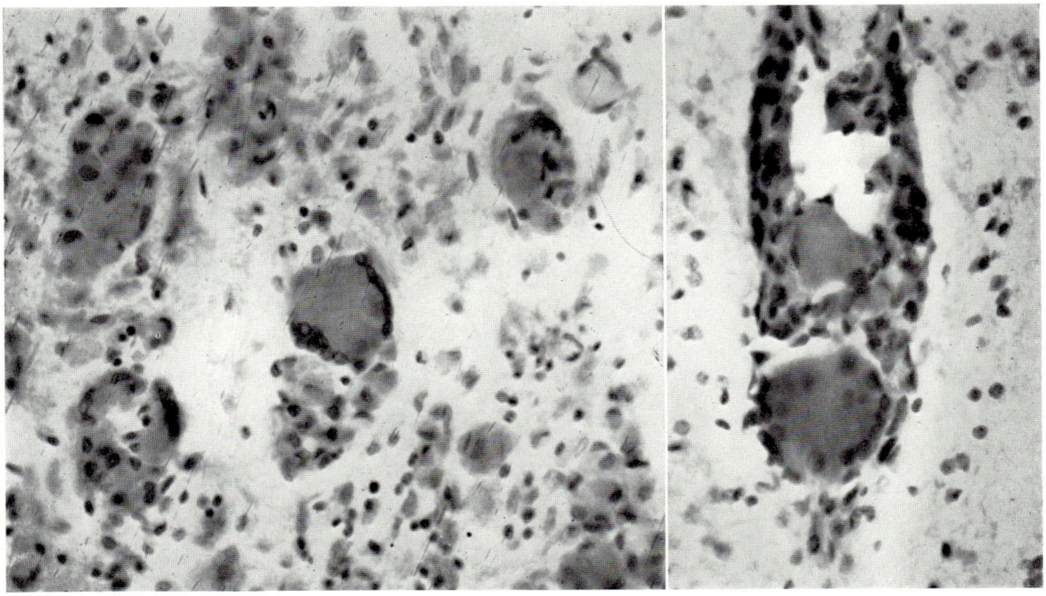

(*a*) (*b*)

FIG. 8.13. The globoid cell packets of Krabbe's leucodystrophy (*a*) are closely similar to the vascular adventitial storage cells present in the cerebral white matter in infantile Gaucher's disease (*b*). (Carbol azure. Same magnification.)

Microglial phagocytes containing neutral fat may be present in some areas, but in most cases this is an insignificant feature.

The neurones often show varying degrees of chromatolysis and cell losses have been reported in the striatum. A unique case apparently belonging to the Krabbe type but with widespread destruction of nerve cells in the cerebral cortex and other regions has been reported by de Vries (1958). No neuronal lipidosis has been observed in any case.

Metachromatic leucodystrophy

Some metachromatic lipids can always be demonstrated among early breakdown products of myelin, but in the type of leucodystrophy considered here they dominate the histological picture, while neutral fat can only be seen in small amounts around a few of the vessels. The first typical description of the disease was recorded in an adult by Einarson and Neel (1938) but by far the commonest variety is the late infantile form, clearly delineated by Brain and Greenfield (1950) and rightly called 'Greenfield's disease' by Jervis (1960). Lyon *et al.* (1961) have reviewed the clinical and pathological features in 30 cases in the majority of which the disease had started in the second year of life and had progressed to a fatal termination during the third or fourth year. The familial character of the condition is well established.

Pathology. In the late infantile form the brain is often larger and heavier than normal. The ventricles are not usually dilated. On section the white matter may not show the patchy greyish discoloration so often found in other degenerative conditions, and in the siblings described by Norman *et al.* (1960) it was noted to have a peculiar chalky white colour.

Sections stained for myelin show the diffuse distribution of lesions in the centrum ovale, cerebellum and brain stem characteristic of a leucodystrophy, though demyelination is often intensified around blood vessels (Fig. 8.15*a*). The cortical U-fibres may or may not be involved. Greenfield was impressed by the relative sparing of tracts and areas which myelinate early, in particular the optic radiations (Figs. 8.17*a* and *b*), white matter of the vermis and the middle portion of the crus, but these findings have not always been substantiated in later cases. The demyelinated areas usually show a severe loss of axis cylinders and there is well-marked fibrous gliosis which may be intensified around blood vessels. Lymphocytic cuffing of vessels has not been observed.

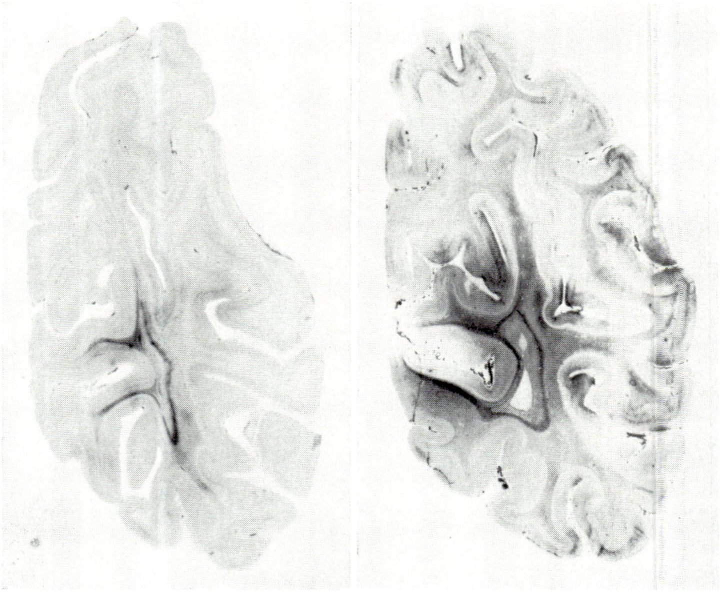

(*a*) (*b*)

FIG. 8.14. Late infantile metachromatic leuco-encephalopathy. (*a*) Myelination of occipital lobe in normal infant at 3 months. (*b*) Weigert-Pal myelin stain in child of 3 years with metachromatic leuco-encephalopathy.

The pathognomonic feature of the white matter, whether fully or only slightly demyelinated, is the presence of a metachromatically staining lipid, characteristically in the form of irregularly spherical granular masses measuring about 15–20μ in diameter (Fig. 8.15*d*). This substance is also found in histiocytes or dispersed in diffuse form in the tissues. The densest aggregations are always seen in the most demyelinated areas. Sudanophil lipid, on the other hand, is extremely scanty and only found in small amount in the walls of a few vessels. The metachromatic staining can be properly appreciated only in frozen sections and the early difficulties in deciding what particular shade of metachromasia with polychrome dyes was characteristic of the condition have now been resolved by the introduction of the Hirsch-Peiffer stain (cresyl violet in 1% acetic acid) which colours the material a golden brown (von Hirsch and Peiffer 1955; Peiffer 1959 a). A re-examination of several of the early cases of 'prelipoid leucodystrophy', including the original juvenile case of Scholz (1925), have proved these to belong to the metachromatic variety. Stam (1960) has described a more sensitive method for demonstrating metachromasia but this has not as yet been widely applied, and as matters stand at present the finding of brown metachromasia is considered to be essential in diagnosis. The metachromatic masses also stain strongly with P.A.S. and this latter property persists after celloidin embedding or the application of powerful lipid solvents to the sections.

A peculiar feature of the degenerated white matter is that another type of lipid substance is found in granular form, scattered freely between the brown metachromatic masses. This material was regarded by Brain and Greenfield (1950) as phospholipid and has the same staining properties as myelin. It may be present in such large amount as to give Kultschitsky-Pal preparations the appearance of relatively normal myelination when viewed by the naked eye, though when the sections are examined microscopically the fields are found to contain only scanty myelinated axons lying amid abundant darkly stained granules (Norman *et al.* 1960) (Figs. 8.15*b* and *c*).

In all areas showing loss of myelin, even when this is slight and recent, there is a considerable and in some places complete loss of the nuclei of the interfascicular oligodendroglia. This may be evident in isolated tracts or fibre systems, such as the fibres traversing the globus pallidus, the hilum of the olive, and the pyramidal tract in the cord. This loss is not secondary to loss of myelin but appears to occur at the same time. With cell stains the deserted, acellular appearance of the white matter of the cerebral hemispheres, in which nuclei are very scanty except in the vessel walls, is very striking (Fig. 8.16*a*).

The peripheral nerves show mild demyelination of segmental type with abundant metachromatic lipid in Schwann cells and phagocytes. The electronmicroscopic changes have been described by Webster (1962). Sural nerve biopsy has been found to be a valuable diagnostic procedure (Hagberg *et al.* 1962) (Fig. 8.15*e*). The examination of the myenteric plexus for metachromasia in rectal biopsies has also proved useful (Nakai and Landing 1960).

The changes in the grey matter may be equally distinctive in that groups of neurones containing metachromatic lipid are commonly found in certain sites (Fig. 8.16*b*). This neuronal lipidosis is far from being ubiquitous and the cerebral cortex is usually exempt, though in one or two cases scattered neurones and the Betz cells with their satellite glia have shown metachromasia. The nuclei of the brain stem may be widely affected and storage of the lipid is also very commonly seen in the dentate nuclei, globus pallidus, corpus Luysii and thalamus. The ganglion cells of the retina have been found to be involved in two cases (Lyon *et al.* 1961). A further link with the lipidoses is found in the occasional selective atrophy of the cerebellar granular layer, but in such cases neither the remaining granular cells nor the Purkinje cells store the lipid (Fig. 8.16*c*).

Metachromatic lipid has also been frequently found in the epithelium of the renal tubules, the gall bladder and the intra-hepatic bile ducts (Fig. 8.16*e*). The finding of metachromatic sediment in the urine, however, cannot be regarded as diagnostic of this disease (Helfant *et al.* 1962).

The rarer cases with onset in later childhood or adult life (van Bogaert and Dewulf 1939;

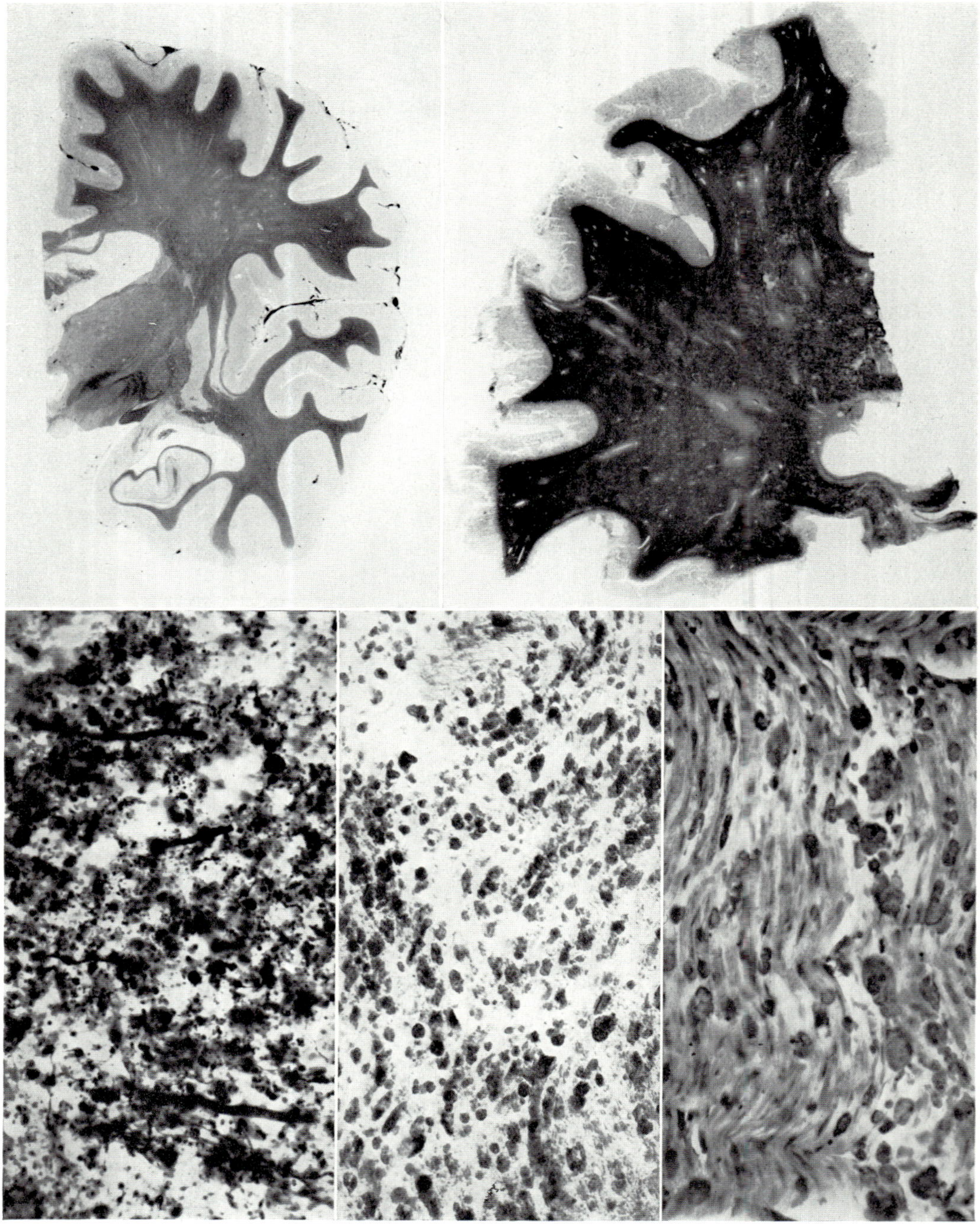

(a) (b)

(c) (d) (e)

FIG. 8.15. *Late infantile metachromatic leucodystrophy.* (*a*) Coronal section of the hemisphere showing diffused pallor of myelin staining. (Heidenhain.) (*b*) Frozen section showing the much darker staining which is largely due to granular material rather than myelin sheaths. The obvious demyelination is perivascular. (Kultschitsky-Pal.) (*c*) Higher power view of (*b*) showing poverty of myelin sheaths and much granular material. (*d*) Metachromatic bodies in the demyelinated white matter. (Hirsch-Peiffer stain.) (*e*) Sciatic nerve: metachromatic lipid is present in Schwann cells and in macroplages. (Toluidin blue.)

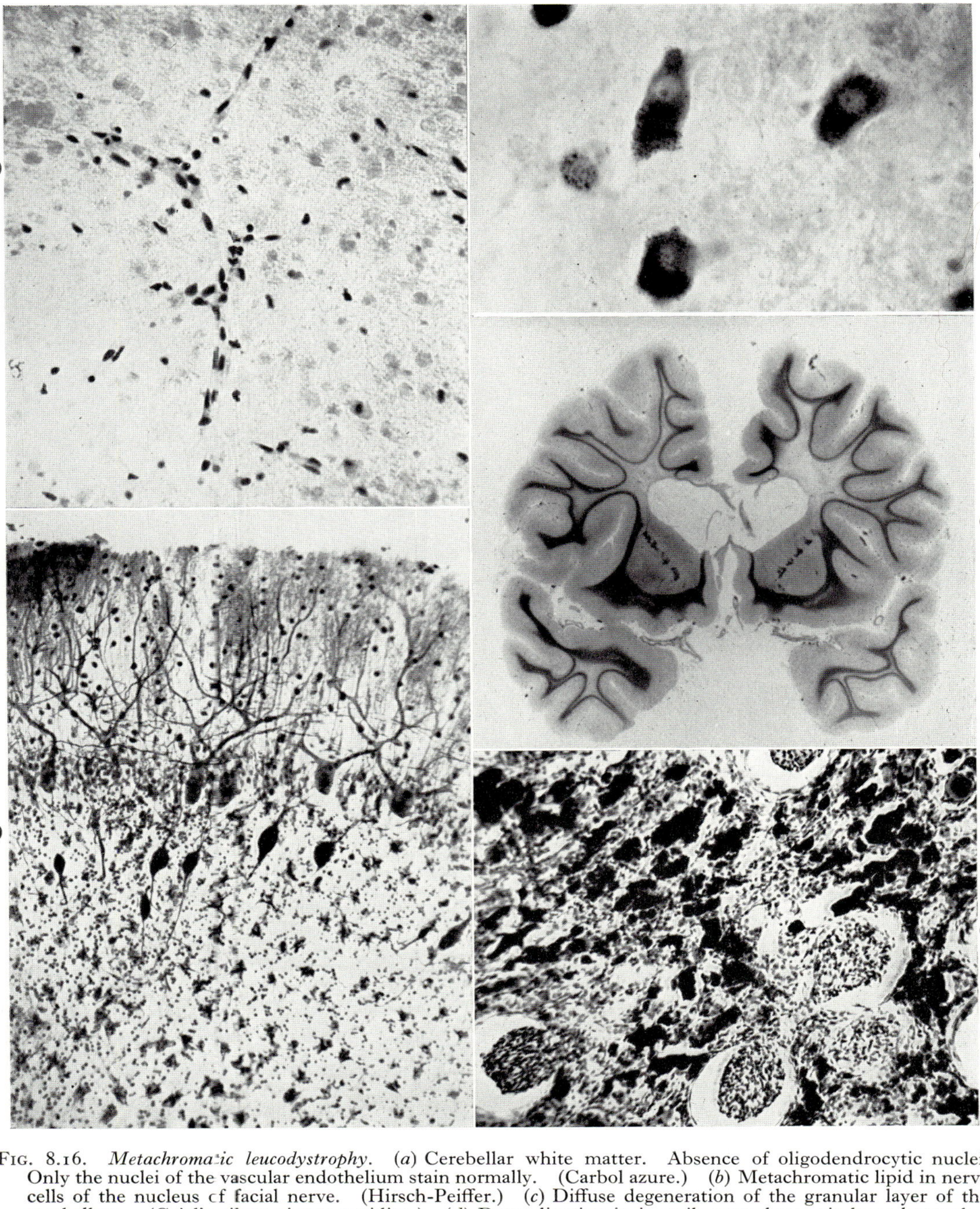

FIG. 8.16. *Metachromatic leucodystrophy.* (*a*) Cerebellar white matter. Absence of oligodendrocytic nuclei. Only the nuclei of the vascular endothelium stain normally. (Carbol azure.) (*b*) Metachromatic lipid in nerve cells of the nucleus of facial nerve. (Hirsch-Peiffer.) (*c*) Diffuse degeneration of the granular layer of the cerebellum. (Cajal's silver nitrate-pyridine.) (*d*) Demyelination in juvenile metachromatic leucodystrophy. (Heidenhain.) (*e*) Metachromatic lipid deposits in the kidney. Sclerosis of glomeruli. (Cresyl violet.)

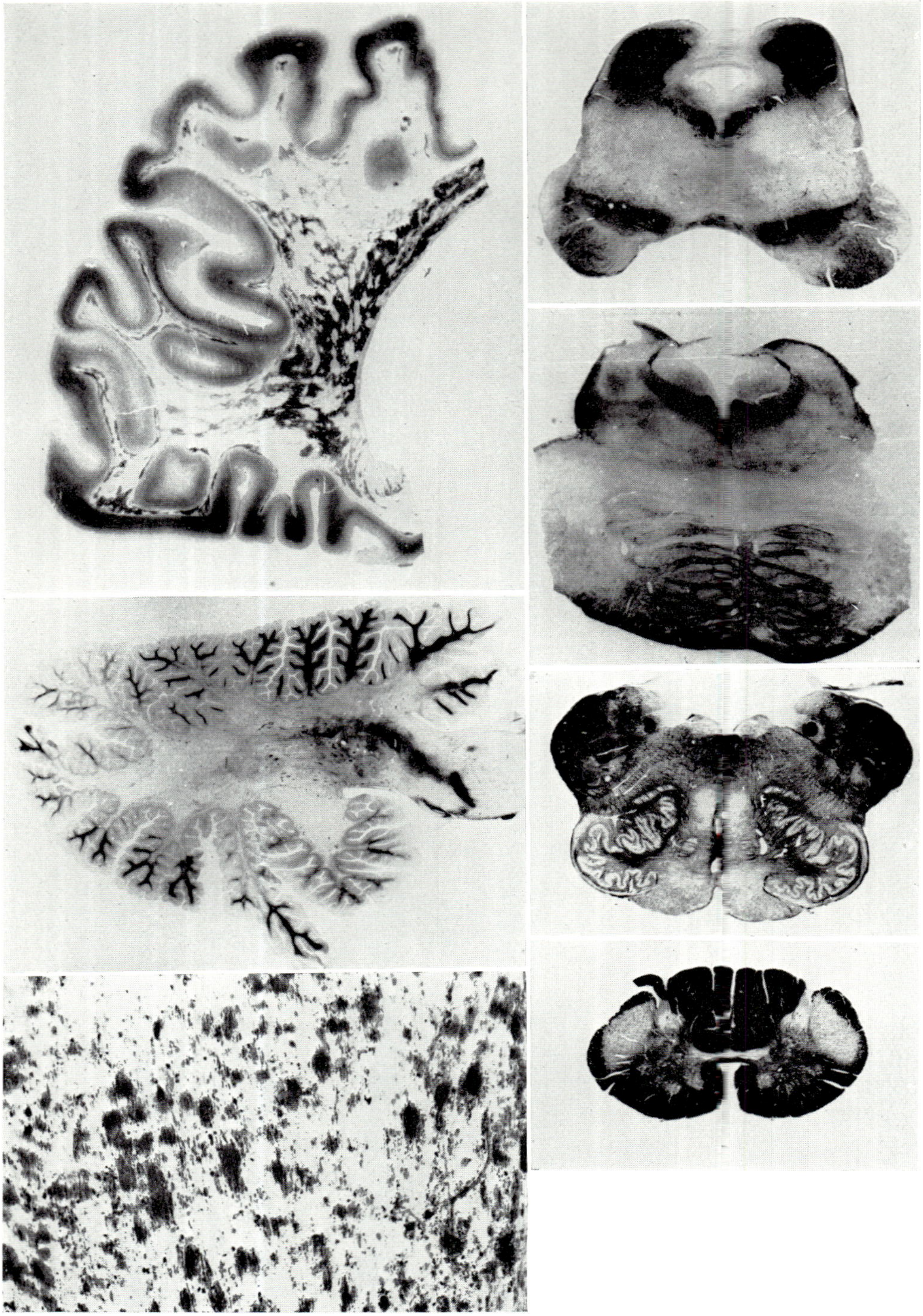

(a) (b) (c) (d) (e) (f) (g)

FIG. 8.17. *Pelizaeus-Merzbacher disease.* (*a*) Demyelination of centrum ovale with exception of myelin islands near the ventricle. The cortex is well myelinated. (Kultschitsky-Pal (frozen section).) (*b*) Cerebellum showing partial preservation of myelin in the gyral cores. (Kultschitsky-Pal (frozen section).) (*c*) Extracellular sudanophil lipid in demyelinated white matter near a myelin island. (Scharlach R and Haematoxylin.) (*d*)–(*e*) Brainstem showing demyelination. (*f*) Spinal cord: degeneration of the crossed pyramidal tracts. (Kultschitsky-Pal (frozen section).)

Sourander and Svennerholm 1962) differ from the late infantile form only in a quantitative way. The demyelination tends to spare the U-fibres, and the deposition of metachromatic lipid may not be so massive (Fig. 8.16*d*). Neuronal lipidosis has been reported in several cases and the cerebral cortex may be more involved than in the early cases. Einarson and Strömgren (1961) make the point that widespread disappearance of the oligodendrocytes is not a feature of the older cases.

Chemical findings. The metachromasia of the abnormal lipid had suggested the presence of sulphuric acid esters to Brain and Greenfield (1950), but several years elapsed before chemical proof was obtained by Jatzkewitz (1958) that this substance was sulphatide (cerebroside sulphate). Several recent papers have confirmed the large excess over normal of sulphatide in the white matter and also in the kidney of the late infantile cases (Austin 1960). Neutral, or 'true' cerebroside, on the other hand, is substantially reduced, as in most other demyelinating diseases. This accumulation of sulphatide indicates a primary disturbance in the metabolism of cerebroside.

The non-lipid hexosamines are also increased (Tingey 1959; Hagberg *et al.* 1960; Cumings 1962), a finding which supports the histochemical conclusions of Urich (1962) who has suggested that mucopolysaccharides form part of the non-metachromatic deposits in the tissues.

Cerebrospinal fluid. Cases of the late infantile metachromatic type have, in several instances, shown a considerable excess of protein to between 100 and 200 mg. per 100 ml. without other change. In some cases the association of high protein with a rise in pressure has suggested the diagnosis of cerebral tumour.

Relationship to the lipidoses. The abnormal accumulation of sulphatide in the white matter, its presence within nerve cells, and perhaps the additional feature of localised visceral deposits, justify Austin's (1959) suggestion that this condition should be renamed 'sulphatide lipidosis'. It is retained in this chapter on the grounds that the over-all picture is that of a leucodystrophy, the brunt of the metabolic disturbance falling upon the myelinated axon.

Sudanophil leucodystrophy

The separation of Schilder's disease from the main group of the sudanophil diffuse cerebral scleroses leaves behind a complex collection of familial and sporadic cases having in common the features of an apparently primary demyelinating process accompanied by myelin breakdown products of predominantly sudanophil type. Such cases have been classified as 'neutral fat leucodystrophy' (Poser and van Bogaert 1956), 'simple degenerative diffuse sclerosis' (Hallervorden 1957) and 'simple orthochromatic leucodystrophy' (Peiffer 1959 b). Cases previously called 'familial Schilder's disease' come into this group.

There is considerable variation from case to case in the extent of the lesions. Demyelination and gliosis, with abundant sudanophil lipid, were present in the cases of Einarson *et al.* (1944, case 14) and Jervis (1955). In that of Peiffer (1959 b) demyelination was slight, but gliosis and fatty products obvious. In the familial cases of van Bogaert *et al.* (1961) the cerebellum and brain stem were more affected than the centrum ovale.

This group of sudanophil leucodystrophies is enlarged if the logical step is taken to include cases previously classified as 'Pelizaeus-Merzbacher disease'. In the members of the original family this disease started in infancy and ran an extremely long course, often of about 20 years. This slow tempo was reflected in the partial or discontinuous character of the demyelination, islands of preserved or partially degenerated fibres being a striking feature in otherwise devastated areas. Norman (1962) has suggested that the name may be usefully retained to describe those rare cases which conform in broad outline to the classical ones. The name is best avoided in adult forms with mottling of the degenerated white matter due to partial preservation of patches of fibres, such as the case of Lowenberg and Hill (1933) which was later shown to be familial (Camp and Lowenberg 1941). Had the term 'chronic sudanophil leucodystrophy' been available it is doubtful whether the name 'Pelizaeus-Merzbacher' disease would have been applied to this and other cases of late onset, in view of their obviously different clinical and genetic features. A type of case with prenatal onset, hitherto called P-M disease, may also with advantage be removed from the category and renamed the 'Seitelberger form of sudanophil leucodystrophy' since it has distinctive pathological features. These last two forms, which occur in early life, will now be considered in more detail.

Pelizaeus-Merzbacher type. In the original family (Pelizaeus 1885, 1899) the condition was transmitted as a sex-linked recessive. Pathological descriptions were given by Merzbacher (1910) and Liebers (1928). The demyelination and gliosis were diffuse and symmetrical in the cerebral and cerebellar white matter, and the brain stem and spinal cord were also affected (Figs. 8.17*a–e*). Axis cylinders were relatively intact and sudanophil lipid scanty. Conspicuous residual 'islands' of preserved or partially degenerated myelinated fibres remained in the otherwise degenerated white matter (Fig. 8.17*a*). Another instance of the disease in a member of a family showing sex-linked inheritance has recently been reported by Norman and Tingey (1961). The tempo of the illness was more rapid, the neurological disorder having started insidiously at about the age of 6 years, and most of the affected males dying at about 12 years. The main differences from the classical cases were the more extensive demyelination of the cortical U-fibres and basal ganglia, a substantial loss of axis cylinders in the centrum ovale, and considerably more neutral fat in the cerebellum where the degeneration was evidently of more recent date. Myelin-axonal dissociation was present, however, in the brain stem, and in other respects there was a close similarity to the previous cases. Seitelberger (1954) in his review of the literature refers to other examples of slowly developing sudanophil leucodystrophy which have started in childhood.

The congenital type of Seitelberger

Seitelberger (1954) has given a detailed description of three male siblings, with congenital idiocy, dying in the 2nd, 3rd and 8th years of life. Neurological abnormalities had been noted at birth or in early infancy, and had shown some tendency to progress. The distinctive neuropathological feature is the virtual absence of stainable myelin throughout the whole C.N.S., even the spinal nerve roots being sometimes pale (Fig. 8.18*a* and *b*) Here and there a few poorly staining fibres may be found, as in Norman and Tingey's (1961, case 2) example, where sparse myelinated axons were present in the floor of the fourth ventricle. The axis cylinders, on the other hand, are remarkably well preserved. There is a diffuse fibrillary gliosis throughout the white matter. Neutral fat is mainly extra-cellular and rarely present in fat granule cells except in the internal capsule where larger deposits may sometimes be found. The case of Bargeton *et al.* (1962) and Jacobi's (1947) case 2 belong to this type, though rather more feebly staining myelin was present in the latter. In this condition there is evidently a combination of defective myelin formation and later degeneration of partially myelinated sheaths. Chemical analysis of the completely demyelinated white matter in a 2-year-old patient (Norman and Tingey 1961) showed neonatal levels of true cerebroside and cholesterol.

Leucodystrophies with mixed sudanophil and 'prelipoid' material

The adult cases of Ferraro (1927) and the juvenile case of Meyer and Pilkington (1936) are examples of familial variants in which substantial amounts of these differently staining lipids were present in the demyelinated areas. The presence of multinucleated cells in the former cases is not, in itself, a sufficient criterion to class the condition as Krabbe's disease.

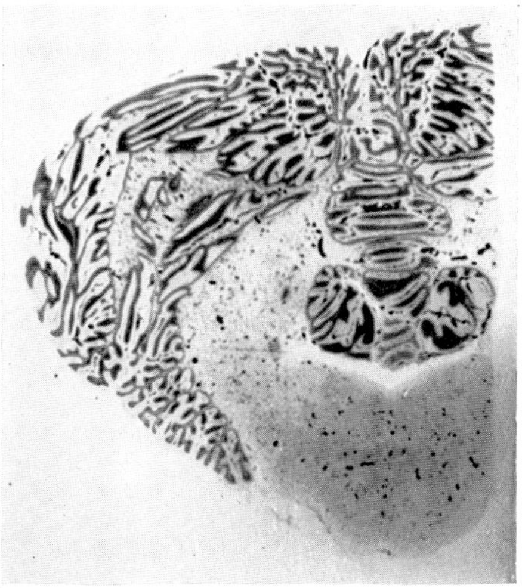

(*a*)

FIG. 8.18. *Seitelberger type.* Complete absence of stainable myelin in the cerebral hemisphere (*a*) and in cerebellum and brain stem (*b*). (Heidenhain.)

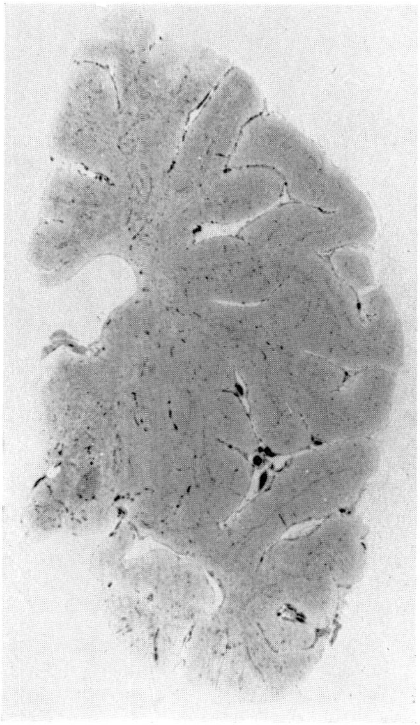

(*b*)

In the leucodystrophy described by Divry and van Bogaert (1946) there was the additional feature of a leptomeningeal angiomatosis of Sturge-Weber type, but without intracerebral calcifications. Lichtenstein and Rosenbluth (1959) have reported the case of a child with Addisonian melanoderma and diffuse cerebral demyelination. Sudanophil and P.A.S. + ve lipids were present, the latter predominating, but there were no true globoid cells or pericapillary cell packets. In the children described by Norman *et al.* (1963) severe demyelination was mainly confined to the optic pathways, cerebellum and brain stem. Dense perivascular rings of mononuclear histiocytes contained an insoluble, P.A.S. + ve, non-metachromatic lipid. A remarkable feature was the presence of similar material in certain groups of nerve cells, chiefly in the brain stem. Chemical analysis showed no increase in sulphatide or lipid hexosamine in the demyelinated tissue and a sharp distinction could be drawn from Krabbe's disease.

A distinctive sub-group is formed by the adult cases of van Bogaert and Nyssen (1936), Diezel and Richardson (1957), Diezel (1957) and Peiffer (1959). In addition to varying amounts of sudanophil and non-metachromatic 'prelipoid' material, the characteristic feature is a light brown pigment, sometimes staining positively for iron, which is found in the branched microglial cells or less frequently in compound granular corpuscles throughout the degenerated white matter.

Leucodystrophy with deposits resembling Rosenthal fibres (Alexander type)

Clinically, this is a form of congenital idiocy which may be familial, and which is usually associated with megalencephaly. The white matter shows varying degrees of defective myelin staining, slight in Alexander's (1949) original case, severe and diffuse in others. In Crome's

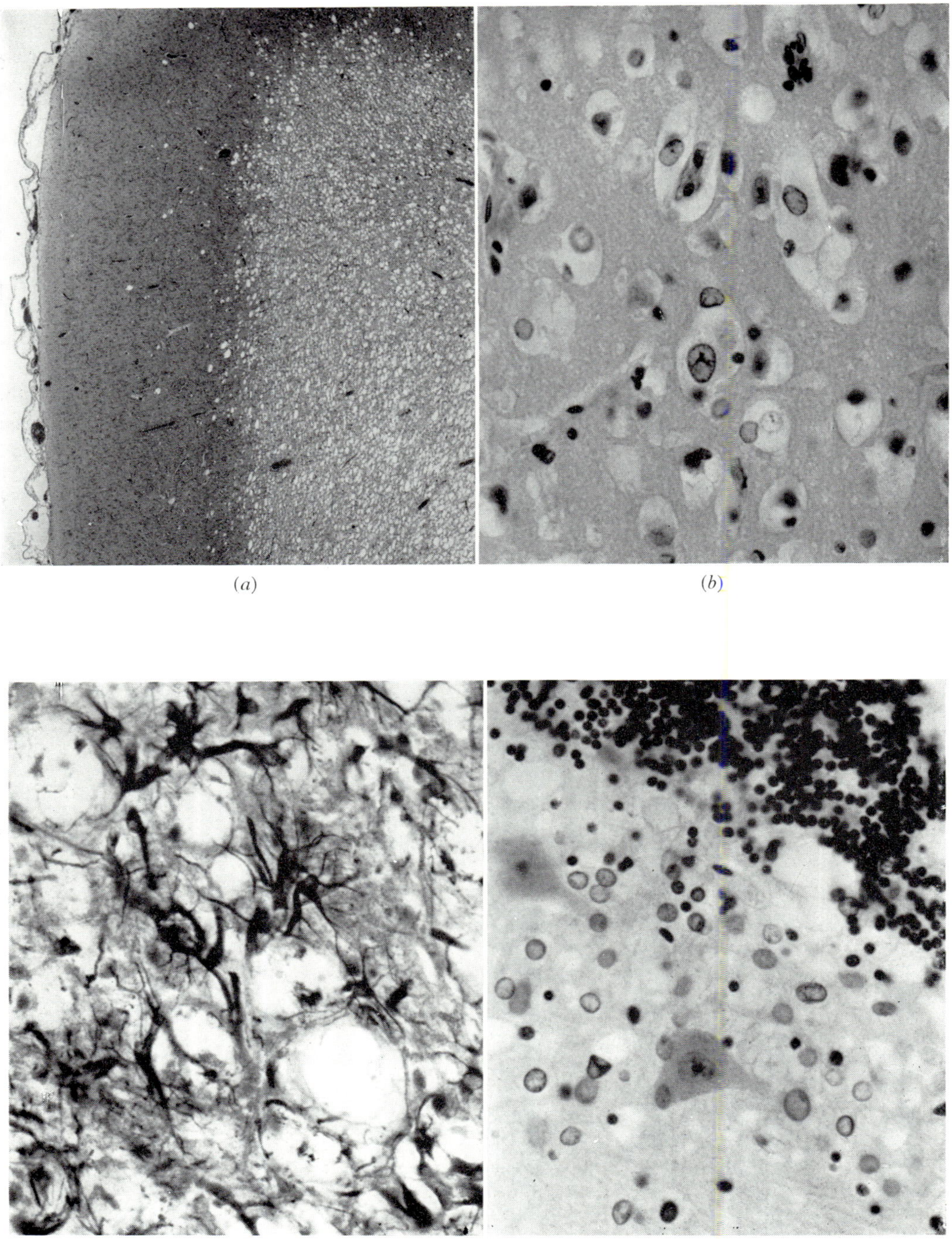

(a) (b) (c) (d)

FIG. 8.19. Spongy degeneration of the white matter in a child of 23 months. (Case of Blackwood and Cumings, 1954.)

(a) Low-power view of the cortex and white matter. (b) Deeper layers of cortex. (Haematoxylin van Gieson.) (c) White matter of the parietal region. (Cajal's gold sublimate × 400.) (d) Cerebellar cortex. Note large vesicular astrocyte nuclei. (Haematoxylin van Gieson × 400.)

(1953) case there was status spongiosus in the centrum ovale and parts of the cerebral cortex. Axis cylinders are well preserved and neutral fat is usually absent or very sparse, though in the case of Wohlwill *et al.* (1959) fat granule cells were abundant in circumscribed areas in the medulla. The characteristic feature, which necessitates classifying this disorder as a special type of leucodystrophy, is the presence in the tissues of dense accumulations of vermiform or spherical bodies which stain black with myelin methods and purple with P.T.A.H. These bodies are found in greatest concentration at the sub-pial and ependymal surface of the neuraxis and also around blood vessels, where they congregate outside the Virchow-Robin space. The designation 'fibrinoid' was given to these bodies by Alexander (1949) who considered them to be degenerated astrocytes. Their resemblance to the Rosenthal fibres of glioma has recently been noted by Hallervorden (1961) and by Vogel and Hallervorden (1961). These authors suggest that they are derived from the spongioblasts present in large numbers during the early phase of myelination. If this process of myelination is inhibited or disturbed, the glial cells degenerate and remain as Rosenthal fibres. Wohlwill *et al.* (1959), on the other hand, regard these bodies as glycolipid substances deposited in the course of faulty myelination.

Spongy degeneration of the white matter

In the earlier reports this condition was grouped with diffuse cerebral sclerosis, but more recently the difference in its pathogenesis has been recognised and it has been described as a separate entity. The cases which have been recorded are very similar both clinically and pathologically (Globus and Strauss 1928, case 4, Canavan 1931, van Bogaert and Bertrand 1949 (2 brothers, 1 with autopsy), Meyer 1950 (2 cases), Blackwood and Cumings 1954, de Vries *et al.* 1958; Wolman 1958, Rhein *et al.* 1960). In these cases signs of the disease were noticed between the 3rd and 9th month of infancy. There was progressive dementia, initial hypotonia followed by spasticity of the limbs, blindness and sometimes deafness. Convulsions occurred in some cases but not in all. In most cases the head became progressively enlarged with separation of sutures and increased pressure of cerebrospinal fluid. Death occurred at ages varying from 6 months to 2 years.

Post-mortem examination. In most cases it has been noticed that there is an excess of subarachnoid fluid which was yellow in Canavan's case. The convolutions were flattened in some cases but rather shrunken in others. The brain as a whole felt very soft. In Canavan's case, aged 16½ months at death, it weighed 1890 g. after 3 days' fixation in formalin, and in the case of Blackwood and Cumings', aged 23 months at death, 1595 g. On section the cortex looked thin but normal. The white matter was described as pearly or greyish. In the familial case reported by de Vries *et al.* (1958) death occurred at the age of 12 months. The brain weighed 1720 g. and the convolutional pattern was simple, with gyri larger than the normal adult size.

Histologically there is little evidence of myelin in the centrum semi-ovale but the more compact fibre bundles such as the corpus callosum, optic radiations, internal capsule, and the tracts of the brain stem and cord, are usually at least partially myelinated; the optic nerves and tracts and the brain stem and spinal cord are fairly well myelinated. The white matter of the cerebral hemispheres, and, to a less extent, that of the cerebellum consists of a fine meshwork in which naked axons and neuroglial fibres surround and enclose small cystic spaces (Fig. 8.19). In some cases the subcortical U-fibres are mainly affected by the spongy state. There is little excess of neuroglial fibres and no loss of oligodendroglial nuclei. This finely cystic, spongy appearance may extend into the deeper layers of the cerebral cortex and here many of the astrocytes have large pale, naked nuclei resembling Alzheimer's Type II cells. A similar cystic condition may be seen in the basal ganglia especially the lenticular nucleus. Some vacuolation is also seen in many of the fibre tracts in the brain stem and spinal cord, but without evident demyelination.

In the *cerebellum* there is a cystic zone between the granular layer and the layer of Purkinje cells, the latter being displaced outwards into the molecular layer. These cells are otherwise normal. The nuclei of Bergmann glial cells are enlarged and pale and increased in number (Fig. 8.19*d*). Some vacuolation is also seen in the granular layer and the white matter of the cerebellum where there may be fibrous gliosis. Fat stains show no lipid phagocytes in the white matter except a few in the perivascular sheaths. De Vries *et al.* noted granules of neutral fat in the oligodendroglia lying in the tissue separating the cavities.

Chemical analysis in the case of Blackwood and Cumings showed very low percentages of the myelin lipids and suggested that the disease might be due to an arrest in myelination. The fully myelinated medullary pyramids in the case of de Vries *et al.* is not in accord with this theory and one has to conclude that the disease is one of gradual demyelination following an oedematous process of unknown origin. Van Bogaert (1962) has recently suggested that the disease should be named 'Progressive cerebral degeneration from serous inbibition of the nervous centres'. The condition has been described in this chapter because of the diffuse degeneration of myelinated fibres and the familial character of the disorder, not because there are grounds for believing that it is a primary disease of lipid metabolism.

REFERENCES

Abercrombie, J. (1845) *Diseases of the Brain and Spinal Cord*, 4th ed., Edinburgh.

Achard, C. and Guinon, L. (1889) *Arch. de Med. exper.*, **1**, 696.

Adams, D. K., Blacklock, J. W. S., Dunlop, E. M. and Scott, W. H. (1923–4) *Quart. J. Med.*, **17**, 129.

Adams, R. D., Cammermeyer, J. and Denny-Brown, D. (1949) *J. Neuropathol. exp. Neurol.*, **8**, 1.

Alexander, W. S. (1949) *Brain*, **72**, 373.

Allbutt, C. (1870) *Lancet* (i), 76.

Austin, J. H. (1959) *Proc. Soc. exp. Biol.*, N.Y., **100**, 361; (1960) *Neurology*, **10**, 470.

Austin, J., Leyfeldt, D. and Maxwell, W. (1961) *J. Neuropath. exper. Neurol.*, **20**, 284.

Balo, J. (1928) *Arch. Neurol. Psychiat.* (Chicago), **19**, 242.

Balzer, B. H. (1936) *Brain*, **59**, 353.

Bargeton, E., Lyon, G., Ribierre, M. and Joseph, R. (1962) *Arch. franç. Pédiat.*, **19**, 495.

Barlow, T. and Penrose, (1886) *Med-chir. Trans.*, **70**, 77.

Bartles, M. (1904) *Dtsch. Z. Nervenheilk.*, **24**, 403.

Bassoe, P. and Grinker, P. R. (1930) *Arch. Neurol. Psychiat.* (Chicago), **23**, 1138.

Beck, G. (1927) *Brain*, **50**, 687.

Bielschowsky, M. (1903) *Neurol. Centralbl.*, **22**, 770; (1904) ibid., **23**, 59.

Bielschowsky, M. and Henneberg, R. (1928) *J. Psychol. Neurol.*, **36**, 131.

Bignami, A., Tingey, A. H. and Torre, C. (1961) *Riv. Neurol.*, **31**, 712.

Blackwood, W. and Cumings, J. N. (1954) *J. Neurol. Neurosurg. Psychiat.*, **17**, 33.

Bouman, L. and Bok, S. K. (1927) *Z. ges. Neurol. Psychiat.*, **111**, 495.

Brain, W. R. and Greenfield, J. G. (1950) *Brain*, **73**, 291.

Brock, J. (1926) *Z. f. Kinderheilk.*, **40**, 552.

Bullard, W. N. and Southard, E. E. (1906) *J. nerv. ment. Dis.*, **33**, 188.

Camp, C. and Lowenberg, K. (1941) *Arch. Neurol. Psychiat.*, **45**, 261.

Canavan, M. M. (1931) *Arch. Neurol. Psychiat.* (Chicago), **25**, 299.

Carswell, R. (1838) *Pathological Anatomy, Illustrations of the Elementary Forms of Disease*, London.

Charcot, J. M. (1868) *Gaz. des Hôp.*, 405, 409, 554, 557, 566.

Clifton, F. (1724) *Dissertatio inauguralis de distinctis et confluentibus variolis*, Leyden (Lugduni Batavorum).

Collier, J. and Greenfield, J. G. (1924) *Brain*, **47**, 489.

Crawford, T. (1954) *J. clin. Path.*, **7**, 1.

Crome, L. (1953) *Brain*, **76**, 215.

Cruveilier, J. (1835–42) *Atlas d'anatomie pathologique du corps humain*, **2**, Ballière, Paris.

Cumings, J. N. (1953) *Brain*, **76**, 551; (1957) in *Modern Trends in Neurology*, edited by Denis Williams; (1962) *Proc. London Conference on the Scientific Study of Mental Deficiency*, Vol. 2, May and Baker, Dagenham, p. 449.

Dawson, J. W. (1916) *Trans. Roy. Soc. Edin.*, **50**, 517.

de Vries, E. (1958) *J. Neuropath. exp. Neurol.*, **17**, 501; (1959) *Post vaccinal perivenous encephalitis*, Elsevier, Amsterdam.

de Vries, E., van Bogaert, L. and Edgar, G. W. F. (1958) *Rev. Neurol.*, **98**, 271.

Devic, C. (1894) *Congrès français de Med.*, **1**, 139.

Diezel, P. B. (1955) *Virchows Archiv. f. path. Anat.*, **327**, 206.

Diezel, P. B. and Richardson, E. P. (1957) *J. Neuropath. exp. Neurol.*, **16**, 130.

Divry, P. and van Bogaert, L. (1946) *J. Neurol. Neurosurg. Psychiat.*, **9**, 41.

Doinikow, B. (1915) *Z. ges. Neurol. Psychiat.*, **27**, 151.

Donohue, W. L. (1941) *J. Pediat.*, **19**, 42.

Dow, R. S. and Berglund, G. (1942) *Arch. Neurol. Psychiat.* (Chicago), **47**, 1.

Dreschfeld, J. (1882) *Lancet* (i), 52.

Dyke, S. C. (1918) *Lancet* (i), 570.

Einarson, L., Neel, A. V. and Stromgren, E. (1944) *Acta Jutland*, **16**, No. 1, 1.

Einarson, L. and Neel, A. V. (1938) *Acta Jutlandica*, **10**, 2.

Einarson, L. and Stromgren, E. (1961) *Acta Jutland*, **33**, 1.

Erben, S. (1898) *Neurol. Centralbl.* **17**, 626.

Ferraro, A. (1927) *J. nerv. & ment. Dis.*, **66**, 329, 479 and 616; (1958) *J. Neuropath. exp. Neurol.*, **17**, 278.

Ferraro, A. and Jervis, G. A. (1940) *Arch. Neurol. Psychiat.* (Chicago), **43**, 195.

Freedman, D. A. and Merritt, H. H. (1950) in Multiple Sclerosis, *A. Res. nerv. ment. Dis. Proc.*, **28**, p. 428 Williams & Wilkins, Baltimore.

Freind, J. (1730) *Nine commentaries upon fevers and two epistles concerning smallpox*, Cox, London.

Fuchs. (1893) *Dtsch. Z. Nervenheilk.*, **4**, 155.

Gault. (1895) *De la neuromyélite optique aigue*, Thèse de Lyon.

Gauzzi, G. C. and van Bogaert, L. (1960) *Acta Neurol. Psychiat. Belg.*, **60**, 333.

Getzowa, S., Stuart, G. and Krikorian, K. S. (1933) *J. Path. Bact.*, **37**, 483.

Glanzmann, E. (1927) *Schweiz. med. Wschr.*, **57**, 145.

Globus, J. H. and Strauss, I. (1928) *Arch. Neurol. Psychiat.* (Chicago), **20**, 1190.

Gombault, A. and Riche, A. (1907) in Cornil and Ranvier, *Manuel d'histologie pathologique*, **3**.

Grcevic, N. (1960) *A.M.A. Arch. Neurol.*, **2**, 266.

Greenfield, J. G. (1930) *J. Path. Bact.*, **33**, 453; (1933) *Volume Jubilaire de Marinesco and J. Neurol. Psychopath.*, **13**, 289; (1950) *Folia Psychiat. Neurol. et Neurochir. Neerlandica*, **53**, 255; (1950) *Brain*, **73**, 141; (1952) *Proc. 1st Internat. Congress of Neuropathology*, Rome, **1**, 107.

Greenfield, J. G. and King, L. S. (1936) *Brain*, **52**, 445.

Hagberg, B., Sourander, P., Svennerholm, L. and Voss, H. (1960) *Acta Paediat.*, **49**, 135.

Hagberg, B., Sourander, P. and Thoren, L. (1962) *Acta Paediat., Suppl.*, **135**, 63.

Hallervorden, J. (1952) *Proc. 1st Internat. Cong. of Neuropathology*, Rome; (1957) in Henke, F. and Lubarsch, *O. Hanbuch der speziellen pathologischen Anatomie und Histologie.* Band 13, Teil 1, Banteil A, p. 716; (1961) *Dtsch. Z. Nervenheilk.*, **181**, 547.

Heernu, J., Martin, P. and van Bogaert, L. (1945) *Monatschr. Psychiat. Neurol.*, **110**, 68.

Helfant, M. H., Borgeson, M. and Hellstrom, B. (1962) *Acta Paediat.*, **51**, 49.

Hurst, E. W. (1941) *Med. J. Australia* (ii), 1; (1942) *Austral. J. exper. Biol. & med. Sci.*, **20**, 297; (1952) *Amer. J. Med.*, **12**, 547.

Hurst, E. W., Cooke, B. T. and Melvin, P. (1943) *Austral. J. exper. Biol. & Med. sci.*, **21**, 115.

Innes, J. R. and Kurland, L. T. (1952) *Amer. J. Med.*, **12**, 574.

Jaburek, L. (1931) *Arbeit. Neurol. Inst. Wien*, **33**, 93.

Jacob, H. (1950) *Arch. Psychiat. Nervenkr.*, **184**, 522.

Jacobi, M. (1947) *Virchows Arch. path. Anat.*, **314**, 460.

Jakob, A. (1929) *Specielle Histopathologie des Grosshirns*, Deuticke, Wien.

Jatzkewitz, H. (1958) *Hoppe-Seyl. Z.*, **311**, 279.

Jellinger, K. and Seitelberger, F. (1958) *Klin. Wschr.*, **36**, 437.

Jervis, G. A. (1955) *J. Neuropath. exp. Neurol.*, **14**, 376; (1960) ibid., **19**, 323.

Kabat, E. A., Freedman, D. A., Murray, J. P. and Knaub, V. (1950) *Amer. J. M. Sc.*, **219**, 55.

Kabat, E. A., Wolf, A. and Bezer, A. E. (1947) *J. Exp. Med.*, **85**, 117.
Kahle, W. and Schaltenbrand, G. (1955) *Dtsch. Z. Nervenheilk.*, **173**, 234.
Kennedy, F. (1929) *Amer. J. med. Sc.*, **177**, 555.
Kies, M. W. and Alvord, E. C. (1959) *Allergic Encephalomyelitis*, Springfield, Ill.
King, L. S. (1937) *Arch. Pathol.*, **23**, 338.
Krabbe, K. (1916) *Brain*, **39**, 74.
Kuhn, P. and Steiner, G. (1917) *Med. klinik.*, **13**, 1007; (1920) *Z. Hyg. u. Infectionskrankh.*, **90**. 417.
Lange, C. (1945) *J. lab. & clin. Med.*, **30**, 1006.
Lehoczky, T. (1953) *Acta Morphologica. Acad. Sci. Hungaricae*, **4**, 395.
Lhermitte, F. (1950) *Les leuco-encéphalites*, Editions med. Flammarion, Paris.
Lhermitte, J. (1919) *Gaz. des Hop.*, **92**, 1053.
Lichtenstein, B. W. and Rosenbluth, P. R. (1959) *J. Neuropath. exp. Neurol.*, **18**, 384.
Liebers, M. (1928) *Z. Neurol. Psychiat.*, **29**, 1232.
Lowenberg, K. and Hill, T. S. (1933) *Arch. Neurol. Psychiat.*, **29**, 1232.
Lowenthal, A., van Sande, M. and Karcher, D. (1960) *J. Neurochem.*, **6**, 51.
Lucas, J. (1790) *London med. J.*, **11**, 325.
Lumsden, C. E. (1951) *Brit. Med. J.* (i), 1035; (1955) *Proc. 2nd Internat. Cong. of Neuropathology*, London; (1957) *Proc. 3rd International Congress of Neuropathology*, Brussels, p. 27; (1961) *Proc. Roy. Soc. Med.*, **54**, 11.
Lyon, G., Arthuis, M. and Thieffry, S. (1961) *Rev. Neurol.*, **104**, 508.
McAlpine, D. (1938) *Brain*, **61**, 430; (1955) *Multiple sclerosis* by McAlpine, D., Compston, N. D. and Lumsden, C. E., Livingstone, Edinburgh.
McIntosh, J. (1930) *Lancet* (i), 618.
McIntosh, J. and Scarff, R. W. (1928) *Proc. roy. Soc. Med.*, **21**, 705.
Malamud, N. (1933) *Arch. Neurol. Psychiat.*, **41**, 943.
Marinesco, G., Draganesco, S., Sager, O. and Grigoresco, D. (1930) *Rev. Neurol.*, **2**, 193.
Marinesco, G. and Minea, J. (1909) *Rev. Neurol.*, **17**, 957.
Merzbacher, L. (1910) *Z. ges. Neurol. Psychiat.*, **3**, 1.
Meyer, A. and Pilkington, F. (1936) *J. ment. Sc.*, **82**, 812.
Meyer, J. E. (1950) *Arch. Psychiat. Nervenkr.*, **185**, 35.
Nakai, H. and Landing, B. H. (1960) *Pediat.*, **26**, 225.
Neal, J. B. and Appelbaum, E. (1927) *J. Amer. med. Ass.*, **88**, 1552.
Norman, R. M. (1962) in *Modern Trends in Neurology*, edited by D. Williams, Butterworth, London.
Norman, R. M. and Tingey, A. H. (1961) *7th International Congress of Neurology, Neurochemistry Symposium*, Rome.
Norman, R. M., Tingey, A. H. and Oppenheimer, D. H. (1961) *J. Neurol. Neurosurg. Psychiat.*, **24**, 223.
Norman, R. M., Tingey, A. H., Valentine, J. C. and Danby, T. A. (1962) *J. Neurol. Neurosurg. Psychiat.* **25**, 363.
Norman, R. M., Urich, H. and Tingey, A. H. (1960) *Brain*, **83**, 369; (1963) *Acta Neuropath.* (in the press).
Parsonage, M. J. and Turner, J. W. A. (1948) *Lancet* (i), 973.
Peiffer, J. (1957) *Arch. Psychiat. Z. Neurol.*, **195**, 446; (1959 a) ibid., **199**, 386; (1959 b) ibid., **199**, 417.
Pelizaeus, F. (1885) *Arch. psychiat.*, **16**, 598; (1899) ibid., **31**, 100.
Perdrau, J. F. (1928) *J. Path. Bact.*, **31**, 17.
Peters, G. (1936) *Z. ges. Neurol. Psychiat.*, **155**, 178; (1951) *Spezielle Pathologie des Nervensystems*, Thieme, Stuttgart.
Poser, C. M. (1956) *J. Neuropath. exp. Neurol.*, **16**, 61; (1961) *A.M.A. Arch. Neurol.*, **4**, 323.
Poser, C. M. and van Bogaert, L. (1956) *Acta Psychiat. Neurol. scand.*, **31**, 285.
Putnam, T. J. (1935) *Arch. Neurol. Psychiat.* (Chicago), **33**, 929.
Rhein, G. M. Zu, Eichman, P. L. and Puletti, F. (1960) *Neurology*, **10**, 998.
Ribbert. (1882) *Virchows Archiv.*, **90**, 243.
Rindfleisch. (1863) *Virchows Archiv.*, **26**, 474.
Rivers, T. M. and Schwenkter, F. F. (1935) *J. Exp. Med.*, **61**, 689.
Roizin, L. and Kolb, L. C. (1957) *3rd International Congress of Neuropathology*, Brussels, p. 57.
Russell, D. S. (1955) *Brain*, **78**, 369.
Schilder, P. (1912) *Z. ges. Neurol. Psychiat.*, **10**, 1; (1913) *Arch. Psychiat. Nervenkr.*, **15**, 359; (1924) ibid.. **71**, 327.

Scholz, W. (1925) *Z. ges. Neurol. Psychiat.*, **99**, 651; (1933) *Monatsschr. Psychiat. u. Neurol.*, **86**, 111.
Scott, G. I. (1952) *Amer. J. Ophthal.*, **35**, 755; (1961) *Proc. Roy. Soc. Med. J.* (i), 1151.
Seitelberger, F. (1954) *Wiener Zeit. f. Nervenheilk. u. deren Grenzgebiete*, **9**, 228; (1960) in *Modern Scientific Aspects of Neurology*, edited by Cumings, Arnold, London, p. 146.
Sharkey, S. J. and Lawford, J. B. (1884) *Trans. Ophthal. Soc. U.K.*, **4**, 232; *Brit. Med. J.* (i), 1151.
Sigurdsson, B., Palsson, P. A. and Grinsson, H. (1957) *J. Neuropath. exp. Neurol.*, **16**, 389.
Sourander, P. and Svennerholm, L. (1962) *Acta Neuropath.*, **1**, 384.
Spillane, J. D. (1943) *Lancet* (ii), 532.
Stam, F. C. (1960) *Psychiat. Neurol. Neurochir.*, **63**, 237.
Stammler, A. (1956) *Dtsch. Z. Nervenheilk.*, **174**, 505.
Stansbury, F. C. (1949) *Arch. Ophthal.*, **42**, 292, 465.
Steiner, G. (1931) *Krankheitserreger und Gewebsbefund bei Multipler Sklerose*, Springer, Berlin; (1952) *Proc. 1st Internat. Congress of Neuropathology*, Rome.
Stewart, T. G., Greenfield, J. G. and Blandy, M. A. (1927) *Brain*, **50**, 1.
Strähuber, A. (1903) Zieglers *Beitr. path. Anat. u. allg. Path.*, **33**, 409.
Stuart, G. and Krikorian, K. S. (1930) *Lancet* (i), 1123; (1933) *Brit. Med. J.* (i), 501.
Swank, R. L. (1950) *Am. J. M. Sc.*, **220**, 421.
Tingey, A. H. (1959) *J. Neurochem.*, **3**, 320.
Troup, A. G. and Hurst, E. W. (1930) *Lancet* (i), 566.
Turnbull, H. M. and McIntosh, J. (1926) *Brit. J. exper. Pathol.*, **7**, 181.
Uchimura, I. and Shiraki, H. (1957) *J. Neuropath. exp. Neurol.*, **16**, 139.
Urich, H. (1962) *Proc. 4th Internat. Congress Neuropathology*, **1**, 42.
Valentiner, W. (1856) *Dtsch. Klinik.*, **8**, 147.
van Bogaert, L. (1962) *Proc. London Conference on the Scientific Study of Mental Deficiency*, Vol. 2, May and Baker, Dagenham, p. 444.
van Bogaert, L. and Bertrand, I. (1949) *Acta neurol. et psychiat. belg.*, **49**, 572.
van Bogaert, L. and Dewulf, A. (1939) *Arch. Neurol. Psychiat.* (Chicago), **42**, 1083.
van Bogaert, L., Edgar, G. W. F. and Karcher, D. (1961) *Acta Neuropath.*, **1**. 289.
van Bogaert, L. and Nyssen, R. (1936) *Rev. Neurol.*, **65**, 21.
van Bogaert, L., Radermecker, J. and Thivry, S. (1956) *Rev. Neurol.*, **95**, 185.
Vogel, F. S. and Hallervorden, J. (1961) *Proc. 4th International Congress of Neuropathology*, Vol. 3, Thieme, Stuttgart, p. 108.
von Hirsch, T. and Peiffer, J. (1955) *Arch. Psychiat.*, **194**, 88.
Waksman, B. H. and Adams, R. D. (1955) *J. exper. Med.*, **102**, 213; (1956) *J. Neuropathol. exper. Neurol.*, **15**, 293; (1962 a) *Amer. J. Path.*, **41**, 135; (1962 b) *J. Neuropath. exp. Neurol.*, **21**, 491.
Webster, H. de F. (1962) *J. Neuropath. exp. Neurol.*, **21**, 534.
Westphal, C. (1874) *Arch. Psychiat. Nervenkr.*, **4**, 335.
Winkelman, N. W. Jr. (1949) *Arch. Neurol. Psychiat.* (Chicago), **62**, 421.
Wohlwill, F. (1928) *Z. ges. Neurol. Psychiat.*, **112**, 20.
Wohlwill, F. J., Bernstein, J. and Yakovlev, P. I. (1959) *J. Neuropath. exp. Neurol.*, **18**, 359.
Wolf, A. (1952) *Proc. 1st International Congress of Neuropathology*, Rome, Vol. 1, p. 121.
Wolman, M. (1958) *Brain*, **81**, 243.
Woolf, A. L. (1952) *J. Path. & Bact.*, **64**, 385.
Zeman, W. (1949) *Arch. Psychiat. Z. Neuro.*, **182**, 187.
Zimmerman, H. M. and Netsky, M. G. (1950) 'Multiple Sclerosis and the Demyelinating Diseases', *Proc. Ass. Res. nerv. & ment. Dis.*, **28**, Williams & Wilkins, Baltimore.

CHAPTER 9

THE DEMENTIAS AND PROGRESSIVE DISEASES OF THE BASAL GANGLIA

By W. H. McMenemey

Dementia

Many of the causes of dementia have been dealt with in other chapters. Here we shall confine our attention to 'primary' dementias, which are most commonly met with in middle and old age, and arteriopathic dementia.

Although Webster (1843, 1845, 1849) made careful post-mortem observations on many cases of dementia developing in middle and old age, scientific knowledge of the subject did not develop until the advent of improved histological techniques in the latter half of the nineteenth century. It then became apparent that general paralysis was not the only disease that could cause dementia, and one of the major tasks which confronted investigators was to enquire into the possibility of there being an organic background to other forms of mental illness. The work of Virchow and his school had stimulated interest in arteriosclerosis with the result that the neuropathologists of the 1880s and '90s were absorbed in its contribution to the problem of the insanity of the aged. Binswanger (1894) described what became known as the sub-cortical, or white matter, form of cerebral arteriosclerosis. Alzheimer (1898, 1902) confirmed the importance of arteriosclerotic changes in the brain but concluded that they did not account for all cases of insanity in the aged. He therefore separated arteriosclerotic dementia from senile dementia.

Apart from Huntington's chorea, no example of familial dementia seems to have been known at the turn of the century, but a form of dementia which was later to be assigned to the group of heredo-degenerative diseases had been observed by Pick (1892)* and was investigated subsequently by Alzheimer (1911). By 1903, general paralysis, arteriosclerosis and lobar atrophy (of Pick) had already been split off from the generic group of 'senile dementia', while certain intoxicants were known to be a cause of organic dementia and to account for at least some instances in the senile group. It remained for Alzheimer and his pupils to describe the pathology of what still remained under the name of senile dementia, and so, for the last fifty years the primary dementias have been intimately associated in the minds of clinician and pathologist alike with the process of senile involution. This outlook has been strengthened by the occurrence of certain histological stigmata, notably the 'senile plaque' and the lipochrome-laden nerve cell, common to 'normal' ageing and to certain pathological states.

Meanwhile, Gowers (1902) had postulated the theory of abiotrophy, by which he implied a premature degeneration or ageing of certain tissues or systems of the body, and especially of the nervous system. He mentioned, among other examples, paralysis agitans as a possible instance of a localised failure of the nervous system to withstand the strain of life, and also Friedreich's ataxia, some cases of spastic paraplegia and 'simple mental failure'. The same concept had been accepted by several medical writers long before his time; thus Cheyne (1725)

* Case 24 of Webster (1845) may have been an instance of Pick's disease.

was aware that 'some chronical distempers are such . . . by being Hereditary and interwoven with the principle of life as never to be overcome'. Indeed, Aristotle was aware in certain persons of the lack of 'the inborn capacity of easy resistance to unhealthy influences' (Garrod 1927).

While other interpretations might now be advanced to explain some of Gowers' examples, all are agreed that there are individuals whose nervous systems in part or whole are endowed with a 'grave defect of vital endurance' (Gowers 1899). Schaffer (1913) held that all the heredo-degenerations had this in common and that the explanation for this premature failure of vitality might lie in a constitutional and chemical anomaly in the hyaloplasm. There is, however, lack of agreement in defining what constitutes a pure degeneration. Some workers will accept as instances of abiotrophy only those diseases which pathologically appear as a simple neuronal degeneration. Friedreich's ataxia is a generally accepted instance of an abiotrophy. But in Parkinson's and Pick's diseases the microscopical evidence does not suggest a simple degeneration; in the former, cytoplasmic inclusion bodies appear in the pigmented cells of the brain stem, and in the latter there may be the ballooned cells of Pick or other evidence of a more complicated form of neuronal degeneration. It is, however, reasonable to assume that the concept of abiotrophy will be narrowed as time goes on and as more reasons for cellular degeneration are discovered. The unusual chemical constitution of the pigmented cells of the brain stem may increase the susceptibility to a peculiar form of cell degeneration. Such vulnerability due to minor chemical differences in cells is the main idea behind the Vogts' term *pathoklisis.* The failure of particular enzymes may perhaps explain some atrophies; others may be due to intoxications or infections.

While we can conceive of 'pure abiotrophies' in which external factors do not operate, it has to be remembered that the longer the patient lives the more likelihood is there that environmental factors will make themselves felt. There is more justification for assigning a disease to the group of abiotrophies if there is evidence of a familial character (the so-called heredo-degenerations), but family incidence of a disease does not exclude the possibility that external factors are concerned in its aetiology because members of families so commonly share the same environment. When Cooke (1685) talked of 'the antecedents of a disease which though at present they act not yet they may generate a disease', he was expressing the view that an abiotrophy may be 'lit up' by some environmental cause. Thus both intrinsic and extrinsic factors may be concerned in the aetiology of presenile diseases.

Rothschild (1937, 1942, 1956) has drawn attention to the variety of factors which may influence the process of ageing and has shown, in a study of 28 cases of arteriopathic psychosis, that there is often a discrepancy between the pathological findings and the duration and degree of intellectual impairment. Individuals, faced with either organic disease of the body or of the brain, vary greatly in their liability to develop mental symptoms, and it would appear that the brain, like other organs, has both reserves and powers of compensation. In some individuals organic changes in the brain can seemingly be far advanced before there is derangement of mental function. Physical or psychical trauma often appears to determine the onset of mental symptoms (Eitinger 1954). In the study of the presenile and senile dementias, knowledge of the prepsychotic personality and the symptoms are of prime importance.

Arteriopathic Dementia

Cerebral arteriosclerosis is among the more common causes of mental symptoms in later life and occasionally may produce profound dementia. Multiple softenings so situated as to destroy cortical connections may be evident in some such cases; in others no gross changes may be seen but only microscopic lesions indicating poor nutrition of the grey matter Fine changes involving the smaller vessels are often more important than grosser vascular lesions in giving rise to mental symptoms (Marchand 1949).

The high rate of metabolism of the brain demands the maintenance of a generous supply of blood and serious reduction of the lumen of vessels due to atheroma, unless compensated by hypertension, may impair the nutrition of the parenchyma. Measures which improve the oxygen supply to the brain may therefore in some arteriopathic cases succeed in controlling such mental symptoms as confusion and agitation (Weberitsch 1955). Dementia of a temporary character may occur in elderly patients with hypertension and be followed by a remarkable degree of recovery; a likely explanation of such instances is a temporary derangement of the cerebral circulation giving rise to some degree of stagnant anoxia. Psychotic reactions in patients who are subsequently proved to have cerebral arteriosclerosis may be precipitated by such factors as alcohol, malnutrition, accidents, debilitating illnesses, a failing cardiovascular system and emotional factors (Raskin and Ehrenberg 1956 b) all of which may be explained on the basis of an inadequacy of blood flow to the brain. The location of the responsible arteriosclerosis is not always intracranial, for Fisher (1951) and Hutchinson and Yates (1956) have stressed the importance of carotid and vertebral arteriosclerosis respectively in reducing the flow of blood to the brain. Cerebral arteriosclerosis commonly begins before the advent of senescence, often anticipating the latter by as much as 25 years.

Clarke and Murphy (1956) found some degree of mental disturbance in 23 per cent of 190 cases of malignant hypertension. Mental changes were noted in 9 cases with focal softenings in the brain and of these 3 had developed progressive dementia. They noticed that the average age of those showing mental abnormalities was 57·7 years whereas that of the whole series was 47·3. Dementia was more noticeable when the dominant hemisphere was involved.

Multiple softenings usually involve the grey matter of the cortex and basal ganglia, but Binswanger (1894) described a form of arteriosclerosis which involved the arterioles supplying the subcortical white matter, giving rise to widespread softening and demyelination (*vide* Chapter 2). Alzheimer (1902) was impressed with its localised character in the occipital and temporal lobes. Multiple slit-like haemorrhages and granular atrophy of the cortex (*vide* Chapter 2) may also be associated with dementia.

Alzheimer (1895) described a form of atrophy due to arteriosclerosis in which the smaller blood-vessels were thickened and the nerve cells had degenerated, often in groups; this was associated with glial proliferation especially around the blood-vessels. Wildi (1951) studied the capillaries of the cortex in 167 cases of cerebral arteriosclerosis. He noted nests of astrocytes surrounding capillaries especially in laminae 3 and 5; they tended to be more numerous in the crowns of the convolutions than in the depths of sulci. He found this condition in 50·8 per cent of cases of cerebral arteriosclerosis but in only 12 per cent of controls. Of the cases in which he found these nests, arteriosclerosis was present in 43 per cent.

Cerebral arteriosclerosis is so common a finding in later life that it is often difficult to assess its importance when some other disease is also present. Raskin and Ehrenberg (1956 a) indeed hold that it is a commoner post-mortem finding in the elderly hospitalised patient than are the changes of senility. It may for instance co-exist with Alzheimer's disease or any other of the diseases referred to in this chapter but the effect one has on the other and the relative importance of each in bringing about the initial symptoms is uncertain. It has to be remembered too that a fall in neuronal population could be a reason for a compensatory reduction in the calibre of the supplying arteriole. The problem is further complicated by the fact that we have to reckon with the probability of functional disturbances of blood vessels preceding any of the organic changes that we can recognise after death.

Changes in the brain with ageing

In old age the brain, in company with all other organs of the body, tends to atrophy, while the leptomeninges become thickened, more opaque and adherent. An excess of fluid collects both in the surface leptomeningeal space and in the ventricles, which latter show a slight to moderate degree of dilatation, more especially of the horns. The convolutions become narrower as age advances, particularly those of the frontal and temporal lobes, so that the Sylvian fissures appear to be widened. This gyral atrophy which was well detailed by Esquirol (1838) is most noticeable when the leptomeninges are removed. On cutting the brain coronally, the ventricular dilatation, the gaping of the Sylvian fissures and a general deepening of the sulci will be obvious. But the naked eye often fails to detect the slight degree of cortical and central grey matter atrophy although the shrinkage of the white matter, which largely accounts for the general atrophy, will be at once apparent. It is because of this excess of fluid, and of the potential space it provides (Fig. 9.1), that a tumour or subdural haematoma may, in elderly subjects, grow to some size before it produces symptoms. Thus while the free space between brain and skull represents 7·4 per cent in man and 6·1 per cent in women at the age of 20, these values are increased at the age of 70 to 12·7 per cent and 11·3 per cent respectively. In old age the grey matter tends to acquire a deeper shade of grey.

The weight of the brain begins to decline from the fourth decade onwards, at first very slowly but more noticeably in the eighth, ninth and tenth decades. For instance, while the average weight of the male brain at 20 is 1,399·8 g., it is 1,360·8 between the ages of 41 and 50, 1,337·6 between 51 and 60, 1,306·4 between 61 and 70, 1,265·9 between 71 and 80, and 1,170·9 over the age of 80. The corresponding weights in women are 1,260·3, 1,240·2, 1,253·6, 1,209·7, 1,150·2 and 1,061·2 (von Braunmühl 1957).

According to Alexander and Looney (1938), whose studies concerned especially subjects with senile dementia or cerebral oedema, the water content of grey matter varies from 83–87 per cent and that of white matter from 66–80 per cent. They found that the water content of white matter showed no positive correlation with that of grey matter, nor was either positively correlated with oedema or atrophy. For instance, their highest values for grey matter were found in a case of Pick's disease but their lowest value was in an unaffected part of the cortex of the same case. It is now generally admitted that brain weight is seldom of value as an indication of either atrophy or oedema: this is partly due to the wide range of normality. But Alexander and Looney found that atrophy or oedema can be measured quantitatively if use is made of the differential ratio of skull capacity to either the volume or weight of the brain. The normal differential ratio of skull capacity to brain volume (i.e. the difference between these two measurements expressed as a percentage of the former) varies between 4 and 9 per cent. Oedema is associated with values under 4 per cent, whereas atrophy provides figures over 9 per cent. The extremes noted by Alexander and Looney were −7·8 per cent (nephrosclerosis with oedema) and +29·31 per cent (Pick's disease). The range was less when use was made of the differential ratio of skull capacity to brain weight, normality varying from 0 to 5·5 per cent: the minimum was −8·29 (oedema) and the maximum +10·4 per cent (Alzheimer's disease).

Morel and Wildi (1952), who estimated the ventricular capacity in subjects with 'pure degenerative processes', find that it tends to increase until about the age of 80 in men and 85 in women, thereafter decreasing rather markedly. The capacity of men's ventricles is greater than that of women of the same age while in both sexes the left ventricle tends to be greater than the right.

Changes take place in both nerve and glial cells with advancing years. Nerve cells tend to get smaller and show pallor of the cytoplasm, reduction in the amount of Nissl substance and increase of basophilia within the nucleus.

True sclerosis of nerve cells is not a normal accompaniment of age. An almost constant finding, however, is the appearance of lipochrome in the pyramidal cells of the cortex including the Betz cells, and an excess of it in those cells where it is normally seen before or by middle age, i.e. olivary and dentate nuclei and anterior horn cells. Campbell (1894) noted that the most striking and constant finding in senile insanity was pigmentary or "fuscous" degeneration. It seems likely, however, that the lipochrome of old age differs from that in the younger nerve cells, the lipid portion predominating in the latter and the pigment portion in the former. Hydén and Lindstrom (1950) have shown that ribonuclease is inactive in areas of cytoplasm containing the yellow pigment, which chromatographically they find contains pterine. As the yellow pigment appears, so does the ribonucleic acid content of the cell diminish. The subject of fatty changes in nerve cells was reviewed by Lansing (1951).

Some of the nerve cells disappear altogether but the degree of loss is often difficult to determine. It tends to be greatest in the 3rd cortical lamina. Critchley (1942) mentions that the

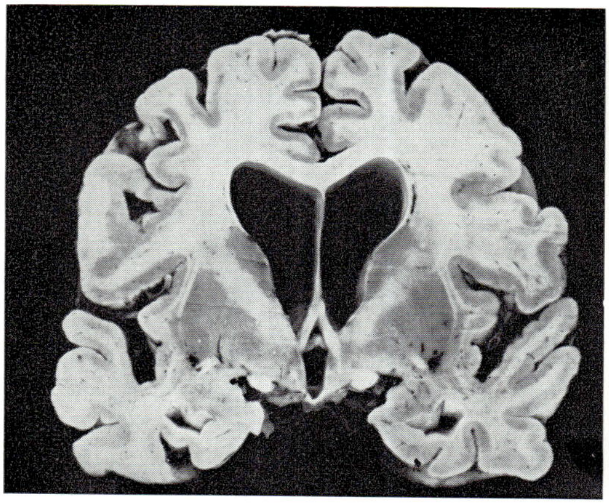

FIG. 9.1. '*Senile dementia*'.

Section of the brain of a woman aged 78 showing general atrophy and dilatation of anterior horns of ventricles.

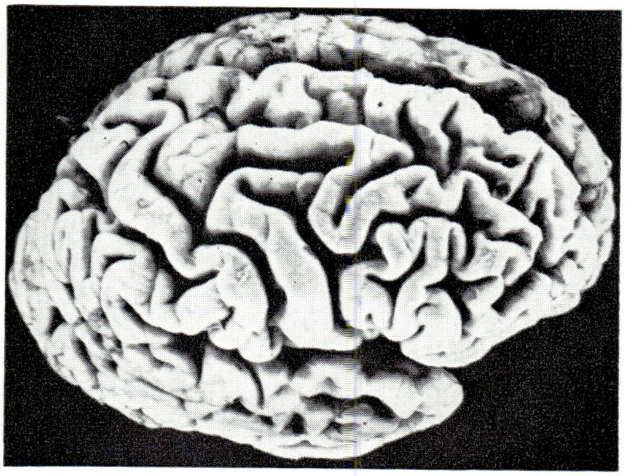

FIG. 9.2. *Alzheimer's disease.*

Showing atrophy of brain greatest in the frontal lobes.

loss often occurs in strips suggesting a vascular dysfunction. C. and O. Vogt claim that there is a loss of cells in the thalamus. Some evidence in favour of a progressive reduction in nerve-cell population was supplied by Andrew and Cardwell (1940), who found neuronophagia in the senile cortex, especially in the polymorphic cells. They found too an increase of satellitosis around the large pyramidal cells. Riese (1946), in a study of the very old human brain, observed some degree of cortical atrophy in the majority of them, either diffuse or regional, but it was by no means proportional to age. In a case of senile dementia believed to be 107 years old, Riese and Zfass (1944), for instance, found minimal cortical atrophy and cellular changes only moderate in degree. They noted the presence of binucleated ganglion cells and suggested that in old age there might be an attempt at nerve-cell regeneration, a view which has not gained acceptance.

The changes in the astrocytes are comparable to those found in nerve cells. Some of the protoplasmic astrocytes tend to become fibrous in old age, especially those in the basal ganglia, and their cytoplasm is often seen to contain a yellow and rather granular pigment. There is an increase of glial fibres in the subpial zone spreading into the second layer, but this extends even deeper when it is in relation to the perforating vessels of the cortex. An accentuation of glial fibres can be seen round the blood-vessels of the striatum and to an even greater extent in the globus pallidus where the vessels are notoriously prone to undergo a degeneration of the elastic layers with the deposition of calcium and iron. With advancing years there is also a general increase in glial fibres throughout the striatum and globus pallidus. Simma (1949), however, commented on an increase of glial nuclei in the thalamus without a corresponding increase in the glial fibres.

No changes are seen in oligodendroglia or in the microglia, although it has been suggested, but with little evidence, that the capacity of the latter to react is neither so rapid nor so complete in old age. Corpora amylacea are common in the elderly brain, especially near to the ventricles.

The blood-vessels tend to become thicker and less pliable with increasing age. Binswanger and Schaxel (1917) showed that the elastic lamina of the cerebral arteries ceases to grow by middle life but that the muscle continues to develop until the age of 60, after which the collagenous tissue alone continues to grow. The relative paucity of both elastic and muscle fibres in the media of small cerebral arteries and the predominance of collagenous fibres even in the young and healthy was commented on by Baker (1937) and by Eros (1951). Very small arteries may indeed be composed almost entirely of collagenous tissue and so may be mistaken for a pathological state of fibrosis. According to Baker, therefore, the so-called medial fibrosis of small cerebral arteries is not a pathological change. As age advances, the elastic lamina of the arteries becomes reduplicated and frequently loses its normal staining properties, while the media undergoes fibrosis and may appear hyalinised or more rarely there may be calcification. Calcareous material is often noticed in the walls of arterioles and precapillaries.

Congophilic degeneration of the arterioles of the leptomeninges and cerebral cortex is sometimes seen in the brains of very old persons and, exceptionally, it may be noted at a younger age. A thin layer of congo red-positive material is found within the wall of the vessel, the adventitial surface being free (Pantelakis, 1954).

Scholz (1938) has studied a special type of *plaque-like degeneration of blood vessels* which had been previously observed by Bielschowsky (1911) and Bouman (1925), and to which he has given the name *drüsige Entartung*. It is most likely to be found in area 17 of Brodmann, and its presence seems to be unrelated to arteriosclerosis. It was noted by Scholz in 12 per cent of persons over the age of 69. The material which surrounds the vessels consists of amyloid embedded in an argyrophilic granular matrix. In such vessels the lamina elastica is lacking, having been destroyed. Morel and Wildi, who prefer to call the condition *dyshoric angiopathy*, claim that there are several factors in the production of these bodies; there must be first a paraproteinaemia and secondly an alteration of the vascular permeability to allow of this substance transuding. In their view these structures result when the amyloid substance diffuses through the wall of a vessel. They are found in many of the brains showing argyrophilic plaques but they are never seen in their absence.

In the aged there are minimal increases in the amount of non-haemic iron in the motor cortex which roughly correlate with the lipo-fuscin content of the nerve cells. To a somewhat lesser extent a similar increase is apparent in the occipital, sensory and parietal cortex (Hallgren and Sourander 1958).

Argyrophilic ('Senile') plaques

An interesting but inconstant feature of the elderly brain is the presence of *argyrophilic plaques*. They are most usually found in the frontal cortex and in the hippocampus. These strange bodies were first noticed by Blocq and Marinesco (1892) in an epileptic, and afterwards by Redlich (1898) in 2 cases of 'senile epilepsy'. They were subsequently studied by Fischer

(1907), and named 'senile plaques' by Simchowicz (1910). Most of the studies on them have been made in cases of Alzheimer's disease, in which condition they are very numerous.

They are only occasionally noticeable in Nissl or haematoxylin and eosin preparations and for certain demonstration require methods which make use of silver impregnation. The rapid method described by von Braunmühl is more reliable than that of Bielschowsky by which they are sometimes obscured. They are readily shown with Davenport's method on celloidin. In paraffin sections the method of Dixon (1953) has been recommended (Sim and Smith 1953). There are many varieties of plaques, but in general they consist of masses of argyrophilic particles of varying size, sometimes granular but occasionally more definitely filamentous, scattered in halo fashion around an indefinite centrum which often contains sudanophilic fat or amyloid. Plaques measure on the average 50–60μ in diameter, but they may be as small as 5–10μ or may exceed 100μ. The larger appear sometimes to be the result of fusion of two or more smaller ones. The smallest of all are to be found in the outer layers of the cortex, Ammon's horn and the Purkinje layer of the cerebellum (Ferraro 1931). Astrocytes tend to collect round the periphery, while microglial cells may be seen either round the periphery or in the centre, the more mobile ones seeming to approach the plaque from without whilst those replete with fat are to be found in the centre. The important part believed to be played by the microglia and the astrocytes in the formation of these masses has been stressed by Timmer (1925) and by many since then. Margolis (1953) recognises four elements in the senile plaque, the amorphous, the fibrillary, the cellular and the reticular.

In the centres one occasionally finds, in Nissl-stained preparations, the ghost-like form of an effete cell. Liss (1960) claims that they are nerve cells and this is undoubtedly true sometimes. The earlier workers mostly believed that senile plaques had their origin in disintegrating glial reticulum (Blocq and Marinesco 1892, Redlich 1898, Alzheimer 1907, Simchowicz 1910, Bielschowsky 1911), but some including Bonfiglio (1908) claimed that they originated in nerve cells. Soniat (1941) believed that cells showing Alzheimer's neurofibrillary change might disintegrate and the resulting debris become the centre of a plaque, a view that was shared by Liss (1960). King (1942) doubted this possibility and observed that while plaques occasionally developed in relation to cells which showed this particular type of degeneration, more usually they appeared to arise independently. Fuller (1911) thought that the presence of plaques in the outer molecular layer of the cortex and in the white matter argued against their origin from degenerated ganglion cells and followed Fischer (1907) in believing that they might have their source in degenerating nerve fibres. Rothschild (1934) noted that plaques were most plentiful in the 3rd cortical lamina and in the outer molecular zone of the gyrus dentatus both of which are rich in unmyelinated nerve fibres. On the other hand Neumann (1960) thought that an origin from axis cylinders was more likely. Urechia and Elekes (1925) believed that oligodendroglial and microglial elements were responsible for plaque formation and that only later did the axis cylinders become implicated. Ferraro (1931) concluded that oligodendroglia and microglia might degenerate and give rise to very small plaques or constitute the origin of large ones: some of them he thought could even originate in nerve cells, as for instance the so-called monocellular plaques found in the place of Purkinje cells. Others have subscribed to the view put forward by Lowenberg (1925) that plaques may originate sometimes in degenerate neuroglia and sometimes in nerve cells and axis cylinders, but von Braunmühl (1931) believed that neither nerve nor glial cells had anything to do with the origin of plaques. Instead he thought that they were the result of a condensing of the intercellular ground substance, a view originally put forward by Marinesco (1911). Present day interpretation of this view would site the change within the cytoplasm of astrocytes but electronmicroscopical confirmation of the fact is lacking. Occasionally the plaques present a pattern suggesting a vascular distribution (see Fig.

9.4*d*) but it is noteworthy that Friede and Magee (1962) in their study were impressed with the fact that 92 per cent of them lacked a capillary. It would seem best to support the pluralistic view that they may originate in a nerve or glial cell or their processes, in relation to a capillary, or sometimes in the intercellular ground substance (for an account of which see Chapter 1). Many factors may determine the pattern and extent of plaques and account for the presence within them of reactive microglial cells, astrocytes and nerve cells and their processes, which may have become 'caught up'. Argyrophilic plaques may be a manifestation of age or they may result from disease. Schenk (1955) maintains that the most classical plaques (i.e. those with a centre and a surrounding halo) are to be found in the parts of the cortex least affected by parenchymatous changes and that they represent a relatively early stage in the life history of the plaque.

Opinions differ greatly as to the frequency with which argyrophilic plaques are found in 'normal old age'. Critchley (1929) found only a very few in two subjects aged 99 and 102, where they were most noticeable in the precentral gyrus. Shükrü-Aksel (1936) found none in the brain of a man reported to be 130 years old when he died. Gellerstedt (1933) found them in 84 per cent of 50 brains from subjects who had died at the age of 65, but sometimes they were scanty in number. Rothschild (1937) in a study of 50 'healthy' brains between the ages of 55 and 86 found plaques in 25 (very scanty in 12): they were more readily found as age advanced. Neumann (1960) reported finding numerous plaques in a 45-year-old woman whose illness was not characterised by significant mental changes. They have been seen, too, in a variety of conditions, but whether or not in excess of the numbers to be expected on the basis of Gellerstedt's studies it is difficult to say. Corsellis (1962) has compared the incidence of plaque formation at different ages under the psychiatric groupings of 'organic' and 'functional', finding it substantially greater in the former. The structures reported by Neubürger and Rosch (1935) as being present in the brains of 32 per cent of patients dying with cancer in the 40–60 age group are probably identical with these so-called senile plaques.

Alzheimer (1907), who upheld the theory that plaques originate in a disturbance of the glial reticulum, noted the deposition in them of what appeared to be an abnormal metabolic substance, which was later identified by Divry (1927) as amyloid on the basis of its birefringent property when stained with congo red and examined with polarised light. This proteose, however, is not present in all plaques and to explain this fact Divry (1952) postulates that there are two principal stages in their formation. First there is the *primitive plaque* (called *substance trichosique* by Divry), believed to be simply a condensing of the ground substance of the brain. It consists of amorphous argyrophilic material in the form of a halo round a paler centre. The halo, according to Liss (1960), consists of microglial and oligodendroglial elements which can be demonstrated by suitable techniques. Sometimes, however, these primitive or 'essential' plaques have a laminated appearance suggesting a Liesegang phenomenon. Blood-vessels and cells are seldom found inside these halos and histochemical studies at this stage are completely negative for amyloid, fat or any other abnormal metabolite. The primitive plaque is found in the elderly brain in most parts of the cortex, but is rare in the occipital lobe. It can also be found in the striatum, pallidum, thalamus, cerebellar cortex, the superficial white matter of the cerebrum and even in the centrum semi-ovale.

The second stage in the formation of the senile plaque, according to Divry, is the deposition in the centre of this primitive plaque of amyloid or hyalin-amyloid. This substance appears to act as a foreign body and attracts the microglial cells, many of which contain amyloid, fat, and occasionally iron. These replete cells sometimes give the impression of being imprisoned for life within the plaque though doubtless numbers of them escape to find their way eventually into the bloodstream. The astrocytes adjacent to the plaques tend to proliferate and in this way the plaque becomes virtually walled off. These 'senile plaques' *sensu stricto* are found in all the places where one expects to find the primitive plaques but they seem to have a special predilection for layers 5 and 6. They differ from the primitive plaques in that they are often found in the occipital cortex.

While Divry's view on the aetiology of the senile plaque proper provides a useful working hypothesis, it is difficult to prove. Indeed it is not yet known if the primitive plaque is a natural accompaniment of colloid ageing and the deposition of amyloid due to a superimposed metabolic disturbance. Many authors in fact do not distinguish between the primitive and the more mature plaque. One may find occasional deposits of an amyloid material in a brain independent of any primitive plaque. It should be added that Dias (1930) believed that amyloid could only be found in 'old' material and Vraa-Jensen (1955) seems inclined to accept this possibility. Amyloid has been reported absent from plaques in the cases of Benedek and McGovern (1949) and Reiss and Staemmler (1950).

The stainability of plaques with haematoxylin and eosin and with Nissl's method may depend upon the pH, for Bülow (1956) found that methylene blue is effective only in the limited range of 4·49 to 4·17. Hiroisi and Lee (1936) occasionally found mucin in plaques, to demonstrate which material Alcian blue can be recommended. Young plaques exhibit marked acid phosphatase activity but as the argentaffinity increases so does their enzyme activity decrease (Morel and Wildi 1952). Friede and Magee (1962) in a biopsy study on a case of Alzheimer's disease found that the early plaques were characterised by a marked activity of diphosphopyridine nucleotide diaphorase (DPNH) and succinic dehydrogenase. The activity varied from plaque to plaque but within each plaque it was remarkably uniform. In older plaques there was a loss of oxidative enzyme activity and of mitochondria in the centre but the microglia attracted in by the fat showed a marked acid phosphatase activity. Smith (1961), in a study of five cases, found that the mitochondrial respiratory enzymes were most marked at the periphery, particularly DPNH and TPNH. It should be added that birefringency is not specific for amyloid, even when stained with congo red; neither is all congophilic material optically active. The amyloid substance is normally PAS positive (Margolis 1953; Bülow 1956; Fabiani 1957). Sim and Smith (1955) found in biopsy specimens that the PAS-positive material was amylase-fast.

Because they are not constant in the brains of ageing man, Bonfiglio (1952) is not prepared to accept argyrophilic plaques as evidence of senility. It is of interest to note that von Braunmühl (1956) found argyrophilic plaques in small numbers in 6 out of 20 senile dogs examined, but so far their presence has not been recorded in wild animals.

Neurofibrillary degeneration

The *neurofibrillary degeneration* first described by Alzheimer (see Chapter 1) may exceptionally be found in the brains of apparently healthy old persons, especially in the pyramidal cells of the hippocampus. Hirano and Zimmerman (1962) found this change in 28 out of 36 'senile patients' over the age of 70, the two areas of predilection being the glomerular formation and Sommer's sector. In general it may be stated that neurofibrillary degeneration is indicative of chronic disease of the neurone rather than of ageing, for it has been found in many different conditions (see p. 37). The cytochemistry of cells showing this peculiar form of degeneration has been studied by Morel and Wildi (1952): they find that the acid phosphatase disappears but the metabolism of desoxyribonucleic acid continues with a diminished content of ribonucleic acid. With the PAS stain there appears to be a normal component of polysaccharides. Such cells therefore should be regarded as incapable of function but not necessarily dead. Morel and Wildi do not regard this form of cell degeneration as being closely related to old age as are the argyrophilic plaques and the perivascular plaques of Scholz. Soniat (1941), in a study of 100 brains showing argyrophilic plaques, found neurofibrillary changes in 75 per cent of those which exhibited numerous plaques, in 50 per cent of those with a moderate number of plaques and in 25 per cent of those with few plaques only.

King (1942) notes that many of the cells exhibiting the 'Alzheimer change' are to be seen in close contact with extracellular argyrophilic material. This suggests to him that not only is the cell involved, but also the interstitial tissue which forms its immediate environment, and he likens this state of perineuronal argyrophilia to the spread of crystal formation in a supersaturated solution. Studying the development of Alzheimer's neurofibrillary degeneration in the hippocampus he finds that the fibrils here are in general much less coarse than in the cells of the neocortex. He is in agreement with Bielschowsky (1911) that argyrophilia may begin in parts of cells in which no neurofibrils exist, so it would appear that amyloid may sometimes be laid down on neurofibrils and sometimes not.

Pathogenesis of Cerebral Amyloidosis

Divry (1955) has noted the presence of amyloid in the cells of the choroid plexus; it is usually confined to the free margins of the cell and is quite commonly found in elderly brains. With increasing age there is therefore a tendency for the separation out of amyloid. Whether it is preformed in the nervous system or is a complication of a para-amyloidaemia is not certain. In conditions of atypical, or primary, amyloidosis it is believed that amyloid is deposited in or about altered reticulum.

Cerebral amyloidosis is rarely a component of generalised amyloidosis (Krücke 1950), whether of the primary or secondary variety, and when it does occur it is not in the form met with in Alzheimer's disease. Jones and Frazier (1950), for instance, found no evidence of amyloid in the cerebral vessels of 15 cases of primary cardiovascular amyloidosis, although 6 of them had died of cerebrovascular accidents. Nor does one find Alzheimer's disease in association with systemic amyloidosis. Therefore, a dietetic origin for cerebral amyloidosis seems unlikely although this possibility cannot be lost sight of in amyloidosis of the peripheral nerves (*vide* p. 646) However Horta (1955), in one of his 4 cases of amyloidosis of peripheral nerves studied *post mortem*, found amyloid deposits resembling 'senile' plaques in the cerebral cortex together with small doubly refractile crystal aggregates.

As age increases there is in the blood an alteration in the albumin-globulin ratio, so that the former tends to decrease and the latter to increase. At the same time there is a tendency for the colloids of the body generally, including the bloodstream, to become less dispersed. To this phenomenon Ružička (1922) gave the name *protoplasma-hysteresis** by which he meant the condensation of living substance within the ageing organism caused by the progressive decrease of the electric potential of the colloids (1924). This same change within the cell could presumably be expedited by disease.

Alzheimer's Disease

In 1907 Alzheimer reported the case of a 51-year-old woman whose illness consisted of memory defects, disorientation, hallucinations and delusions. Within 5 years the disease had progressed to a profound dementia and death. The brain was found at necropsy to be generally atrophied but more particularly in the frontal and occipital lobes. Throughout the cerebral

* Hysteresis (ὑστέρησις 'a coming late'), the lagging of magnetic effects behind their causes S.O.E.D., 1936, **1**, 947.

cortex he found numerous plaques similar to those originally described by Blocq and Marinesco and by Redlich together with a type of nerve cell degeneration* which we now know as Alzheimer's neurofibrillary change. Alzheimer was clearly impressed with the severity of the pathological lesions and also with the unusual age of onset of this presumed instance of senile dementia. Bonfiglio (1908) described another case in a 60–year-old male with physical signs and histology suggestive of coexisting neurosyphilis and Perusini (1910) four others, the latter claiming them as an independent disease and urging that they be separated out from the category of senile dementia. This view was shared by Kraepelin (1910) who suggested that this particular type of presenile dementia, which he regarded as a premature form of cerebral senility, should be named after Alzheimer. In Italy it is known as the Alzheimer-Perusini disease.

Fischer (1910) described 19 cases of psychosis in which he found 'senile' plaques and the neurofibrillary change of Alzheimer, but because of their advanced ages did not regard them as examples of Alzheimer's presenile psychosis. Instead he preferred to call them *presbyophrenic dementia*, which disease he attempted to establish on the basis of histological lesions. He did not, however, relate the neurofibrillary change *per se* to senility. In the following year Alzheimer recorded the case of a woman aged 59 at death whose illness lasted 5 years: in this brain miliary plaques were plentiful but neurofibrillary degeneration was absent.† He concluded that these cases were simply instances of senile dementia, the pathological process of ageing having begun particularly early. The clinical picture could, he said, be found as late as the seventieth year; on the other hand, the pathological process of senility might occur as early as the fortieth year. Miskolczy (1959) appears to take the view that Alzheimer's disease is but a transition to senile dementia.

However, the view that Alzheimer's disease was rather more than precocious senile dementia gained support from Barrett (1913) when he reported the findings in a woman of 37 whose illness started 2 years before death. He did not think it justifiable to lower the limit of senility still further in order to include this case in the category of senile dementia. Thus while the term 'presenile' was used originally to connote premature senility it is now employed in respect of a period of life which is arbitrarily fixed between 40 and 60 or 65. The term presenile dementia is used by some as synonymous with Alzheimer's disease, although others would include also Pick's disease and the Creutzfeldt-Jakob group of diseases. Alzheimer's disease is undoubtedly the commonest of the 'primary' dementias of the presenile period of life.

Alzheimer's disease appears typically between the ages of 50 and 60. In several cases the age of onset has been below 40. Nine cases have been reported in the fourth decade of life and 1 in the third decade; Perusini (1910) at 37, Urechia and Danetz (1924) at 37, Schottky (1932) at 38, Lowenberg and Waggoner (1934) at 32, Jervis and Soltz (1936) at 38, Kufs (1937) at 28, Ferraro and Jervis (1940) at 33 and at 38, Orlando and Arndt (1947) at 31 and Marchand *et al.* (1956) at 38. Malamud and Lowenberg (1929) described the disease in a boy of 15 whose illness had begun at the age of 7 following an attack of scarlet fever. During the course of this illness there was an unexplained remission lasting 4 years, but when he died at the age of 23 the post-mortem findings were typical of Alzheimer's disease. Løken and Cyvin's (1954) patient was only 6 when a progressive dementia appeared and proved fatal at the age of 17. Clinically the condition was regarded as amaurotic idiocy but histologically there were the classical lesions of Alzheimer's disease. There appears to be no upper age limit if one accepts the view that senile dementia is but a senile variant of Alzheimer's disease.

It is not so rare as was at one time imagined. In mental hospital necropsies it has varied considerably; 1·2 per cent (McMenemey 1940), 1·5 per cent (English 1942), 4 per cent (Roths-

* Bielschowsky and Brodmann (1905) illustrate what appears to be this alteration in a case of senile dementia.
† Mansvelt (1954) has suggested that this may have been an instance of Pick's disease.

child and Kasanin 1936), 4 per cent (Bini 1948), 5·8 per cent (Schenk 1955), 10 per cent (Newton 1948), but differences in frequency are to be expected according to the population sample and to where the observers draw the line, if any, between Alzheimer's disease and senile dementia: in the first series, for instance, only those cases which began at the age of 60 or under were accepted, while in the last series no age limit was imposed. It is commoner in females than in males.

Clinically Alzheimer's disease shows a slowly progressive mental degeneration characterised by failure of memory, disorientation and confusion leading eventually to a profound dementia. Focal symptoms such as aphasia, agnosia, apraxia and seizures are not uncommon, while both pyramidal and extrapyramidal systems may provide evidence of impaired function. Cortical blindness has been reported by Grünthal (1936) and Parkinsonian symptoms by Rothschild and Kasanin (1936). These symptoms point both to the widespread nature of the pathology in the brain and to its severity. Commonly the illness passes through an early phase of restlessness and excitement with hallucinations and delusions; but sometimes the mood is one of apathy throughout.

The progress of the disease is usually slow with an average duration of 2 to 5 years but the patient may die of an intercurrent malady, commonly a respiratory infection, before the clinical picture and pathological process have run their full course; this may happen within 8 months or even less of the initial symptoms. Abely, Guiraud, Dechosal and Jeanneau (1958) have described a case coming on acutely in an epileptic aged 63 with death three months later. At the other extreme a case has been reported lasting for as long as 21 years (Newton 1948). Although the course is usually regular in its march there are sometimes phases when the disease appears to be stationary (Rothschild's case 3, 1934), although it is always possible in such an instance that Alzheimer's disease has been superimposed on a recurring affective psychosis. In the final stage there is often profound emaciation and the last weeks of existence may be spent in a state of complete decortication, but seldom, if ever, are the patients described as appearing prematurely old. Indeed on one of their cases, aged 45, Rothschild and Kasanin (1936) comment that he seemed young for his years. Pregnancy has been known to occur in the course of the disease. No significant changes have to date been reported in the cerebrospinal fluid.

The brain at post-mortem shows naked-eye atrophy but this is not always obvious, especially if death has occurred early in the course of the disease. More usually, however, the atrophy is of a severe degree and the weight of the brain is below 1,000 g. But convolutional atrophy is never so striking as the 'knife-blade' type of atrophy seen in advanced cases of Pick's disease. The characteristic feature of the atrophy in Alzheimer's disease is that it is general and this distinguishes it from the essentially focal lobar atrophy of Pick. However, the gyral wasting, while it is widespread, is apt to be most obvious in the frontal and occipital lobes and to a less extent in the temporal poles, and sometimes this accentuation may be so striking as to suggest the possibility of Pick's disease. Moreover, both diseases can occur in the same patient (Berlin 1949). The hippocampus and the fornix are particularly apt to show atrophy (Schenk 1955). The leptomeninges may be thickened but they are not normally adherent to the underlying brain surface as is the case in general paralysis. The major cerebral blood vessels are mostly within the limits of normal. When the brain is sectioned in the coronal plane the ventricles are usually found to be dilated, while the cortex is noticeably reduced in size (Fig. 9.3*a*). Disease is confined to the brain. Other organs, both grossly and microscopically, show no departure from what is usual for the age in question.

Histologically there are two striking features, although they are by no means the only features: firstly the plethora of argyrophilic plaques which are found in the cerebral cortex and often too in the basal ganglia, and secondly the neurofibrillary degeneration of the nerve cells.

In a severe case, that is to say one that has run its course, the destructive process may be so complete that few if any healthy nerve cells can be seen. In the silver preparations grossly swollen and distorted neurofibrils stand out starkly in relief. These argyrophilic tangles, often likened to tennis racquets, skeins of wool or to pretzels, and the plaques which so constantly accompany them, have a haphazard arrangement. In Nissl preparations the cells may still retain a relatively orderly pattern and even the lamination may be recognisable, but a severe loss of cells is noticeable especially in layers 3 and 5. Apart from the obvious cell loss a characteristic grouping of cells may be seen with many clear areas between them. It is in these spaces that the plaques are to be sought. Their presence may be indicated by a palely staining and sometimes metachromatic mass of substance which is the amyloid component of the plaque. With silver impregnation methods such plaques are found in enormous numbers in the cerebral cortex, sometimes so numerous that little room appears to be left for nerve and glial cells and blood-vessels: they are, however, infrequent in the external granular layer. They are to be found in most profusion in the frontal and occipital lobes, the insula and especially in the hippocampus, but are less plentiful in the pre-central and post-central gyri. Mutrux (1947) claims that they occur most in the association areas. They are also commonly found in small numbers in the corpus striatum, substantia nigra, periaqueductal grey matter, hypothalamus, corpora mamillaria and especially the amygdaloid nucleus. They are less usually seen in the thalamus, while in the globus pallidus, pons and medulla they are rare. The cerebellum is relatively immune to plaque formation but they may feature in the Purkinje cell layer and in the molecular layer. Plaques may be found in white matter but then they are usually adjacent to grey matter: an exception seems to be a case reported by Strauss (1956) and commented upon by Roizin (1956). Grünthal (1926) has provided a useful chart showing the anatomical distribution of the lesions in 13 cases. They occur haphazardly; they may be seen in largish numbers in one part of the convolution yet nearby they will be few or even absent: in general they tend to be most plentiful in the depth of a sulcus. Plaques are always present in Alzheimer's disease and, provided the disease has run its natural course, they are plentiful. An exception seems to be one of siblings reported by Grünthal and Wenger (1940).

The perivascular plaques of Scholz have seldom been reported except in the older age groups and in some familial cases (*quod vide*).

The neurofibrillary changes are also widespread affecting especially the pyramidal cells of the frontal and temporal cortex. A particularly vulnerable area is the cornu Ammonis. The cortical areas of projection, both afferent and efferent (areas 1, 4, 17 and 42), tend to be spared (Morel and Wildi 1952; Schenk 1955). They occur with greatest frequency in layers 3 and 5. They are not infrequently found in the putamen, while they have been noted in the thalamus, corpora mamillaria, substantia nigra, pons and medulla. The larger motor cells, such as the Betz and anterior horn cells, seem to escape this form of degeneration although swelling and vacuolation of the former has been observed. The Purkinje cells too are not afflicted with neurofibrillary degeneration, although some of them may disappear. In general the neurofibrillary change runs parallel with plaque formation, and the longer the course of the disease the more prolific will they be and the scarcer the intact neurones.

In Nissl and haematoxylin-eosin stained sections neurofibrillary degeneration can seldom be recognised in the cerebral cortex but the majority of the nerve cells will be seen to be pathological. The changes are varied but very evident is an excess of lipochrome, sometimes causing the cell to adopt a globular outline. Various degrees of chromatolysis and chronic cell change are common, but the latter finding in a biopsy specimen needs to be interpreted with caution. The seemingly degenerating neurones are, paradoxically enough, associated with an increased activity of DPNH and TPNH in the perikarya and proximal parts of the axons. This seems to be more than can be accounted for by reason of cell shrinkage (Smith 1961). Friede and Magee (1962) are cautious in attributing to the 'Alzheimer cell' a strong oxidative enzymatic activity because certain identification of these cells proved impossible. Korey, Scheinberg, Terry and Stein (1961) in their electronmicroscopic studies noted an increase of lipid in these cells with

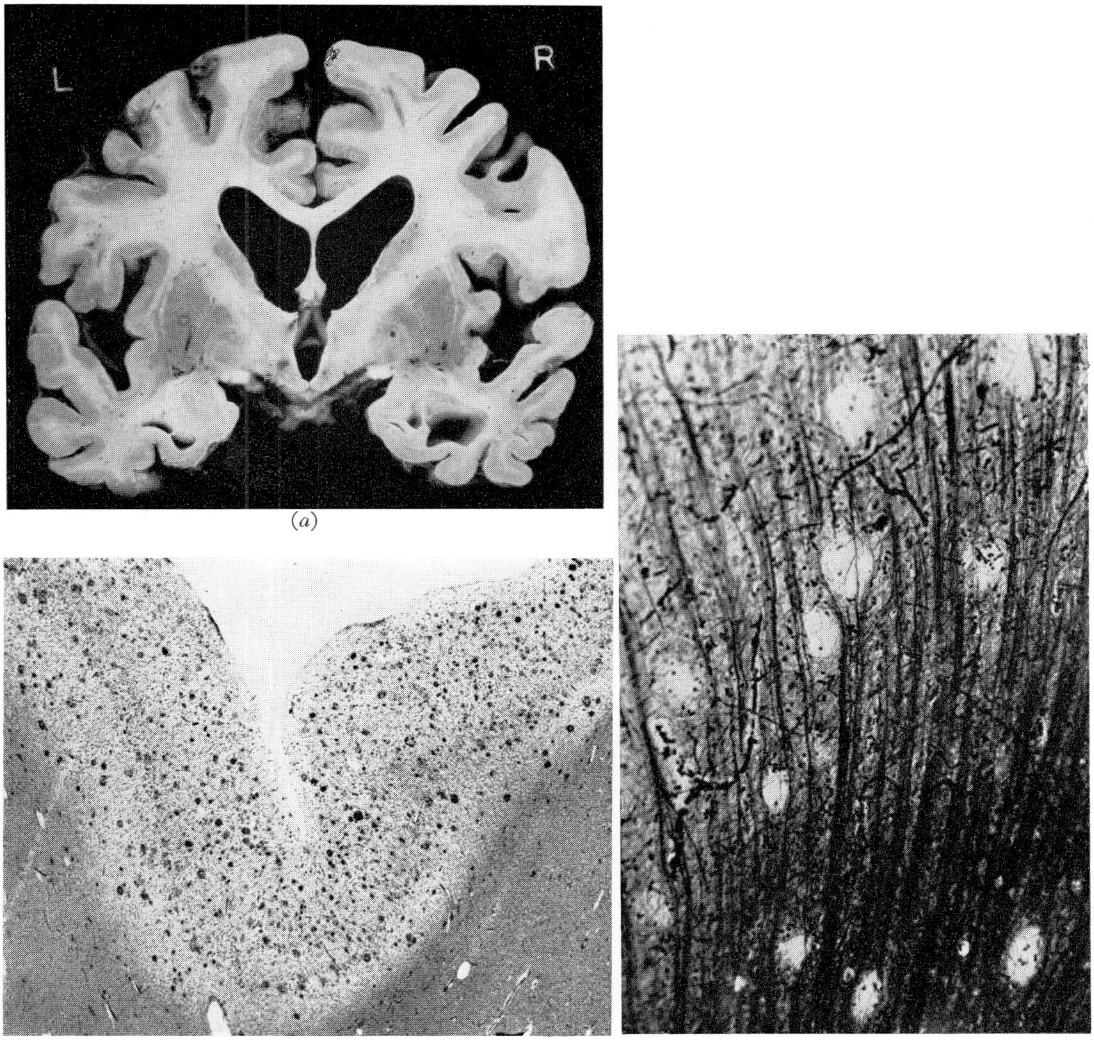

(*a*) (*b*) (*c*)

FIG. 9.3. *Alzheimer's disease.*

(*a*) General shrinkage of brain.
(*b*) Numerous argyrophilic plaques in cortex (King's silver method for amyloid.)
(*c*) The same (Heidenhain's myelin stain).

neurofilaments which were increased in number and coarser than normal. In a later study Terry (1962) concluded that these presumed neurofilaments were in fact tubules of 200 Å diameter. Kidd (1963) has identified similar structures in biopsy specimens of Alzheimer's disease as double helices of some 150 Å in diameter and 1600 Å per turn: these appear not to be present in normal cells. Kreindler, Hornet and Appel (1959) have noted the presence of binucleated nerve cells.

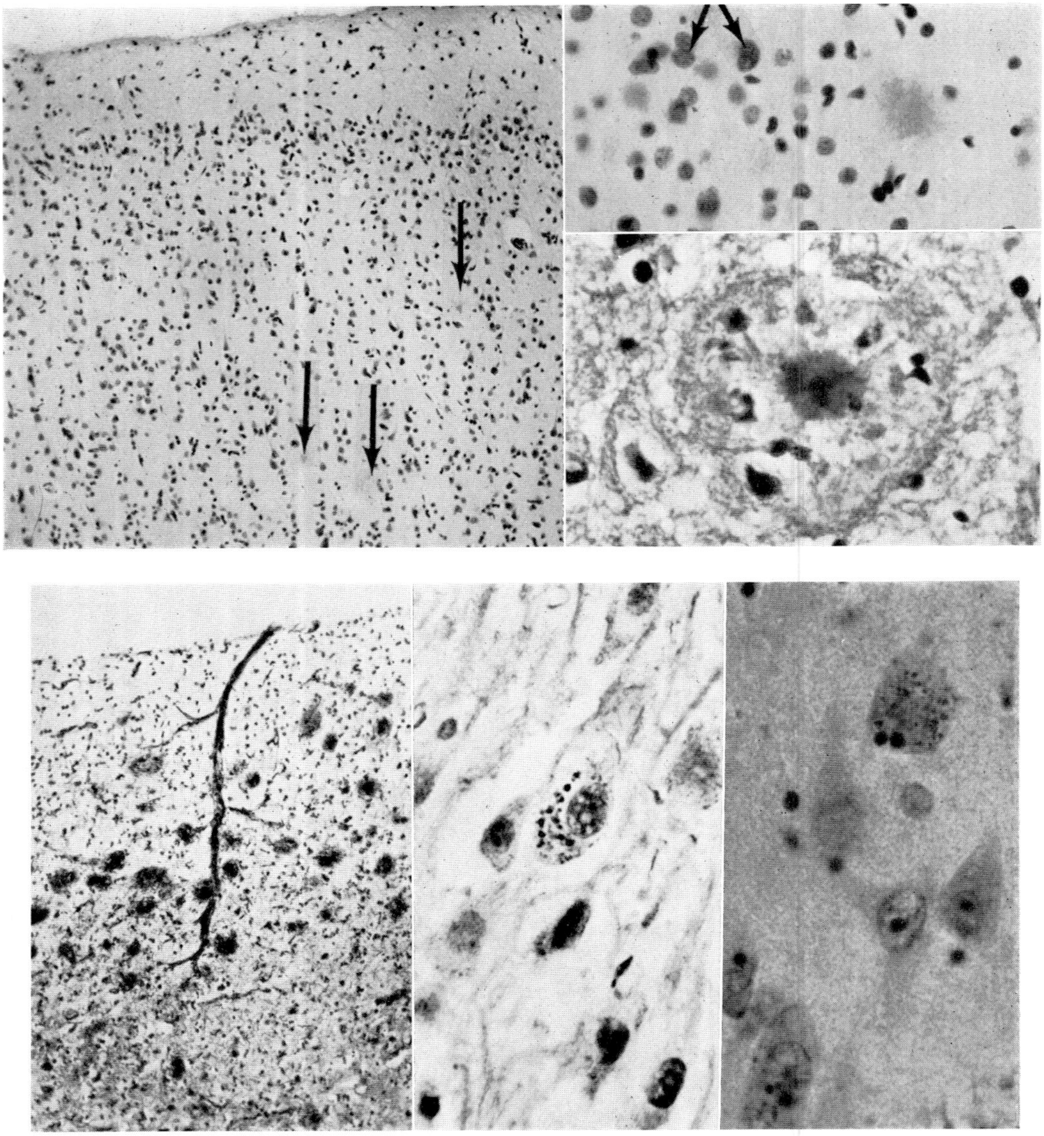

(*a*) (*b*) (*c*)

(*d*) (*e*)*i* (*e*)*ii*

FIG. 9.4. *Alzheimer's disease.*

(*a*) Superior frontal gyrus showing widespread loss of cells in all laminae, degenerative changes in surviving nerve cells and increase in astrocytes. Some argyrophilic plaques are recognisable (arrows). (Celloidin. Cresyl violet, ×90.)

(*b*) Argyrophilic plaque as seen in Nissl's stain: note surrounding microglia, also recently divided astrocytes (arrow). (Celloidin. Cresyl violet, ×400.)

(*c*) The ring of this plaque is just discernible with this routine stain but the central core is prominent. Microglial nuclei, disposed as here in ring form, may lead one to suppose the presence of a plaque. (Paraffin. Haematoxylin-eosin, ×400.)

(*d*) Biopsy from right middle frontal gyrus. The plaques in this instance suggest a perivascular distribution. (Frozen. von Braunmühl, ×50.)

(*e*) Pyramidal cells in area H_1 showing granulo-vacuolar degeneration (Simchovicq) : (i) chronic cell change is noticeable in the neurone immediately below the cell showing the granules (Celloidin. Davenport, ×400): (ii) the cell in the bottom left-hand corner is also slightly involved (Celloidin. Haematoxylin-eosin, ×400).

The nuclei of astrocytes are present in excess and are often seen in pairs with palely-staining yellowish granules in the perikarya concentrated against the nuclear membrane, usually on one side. Sim and Smith (1955) found PAS-positive granules in the glial cells of white matter in one of these biopsy specimens and Smith (1961) has commented on their high activity. Sometimes microglial nuclei will be seen in increased numbers. Ferraro and Jervis (1941) commented on the resemblance of these cell changes to those seen in senility.

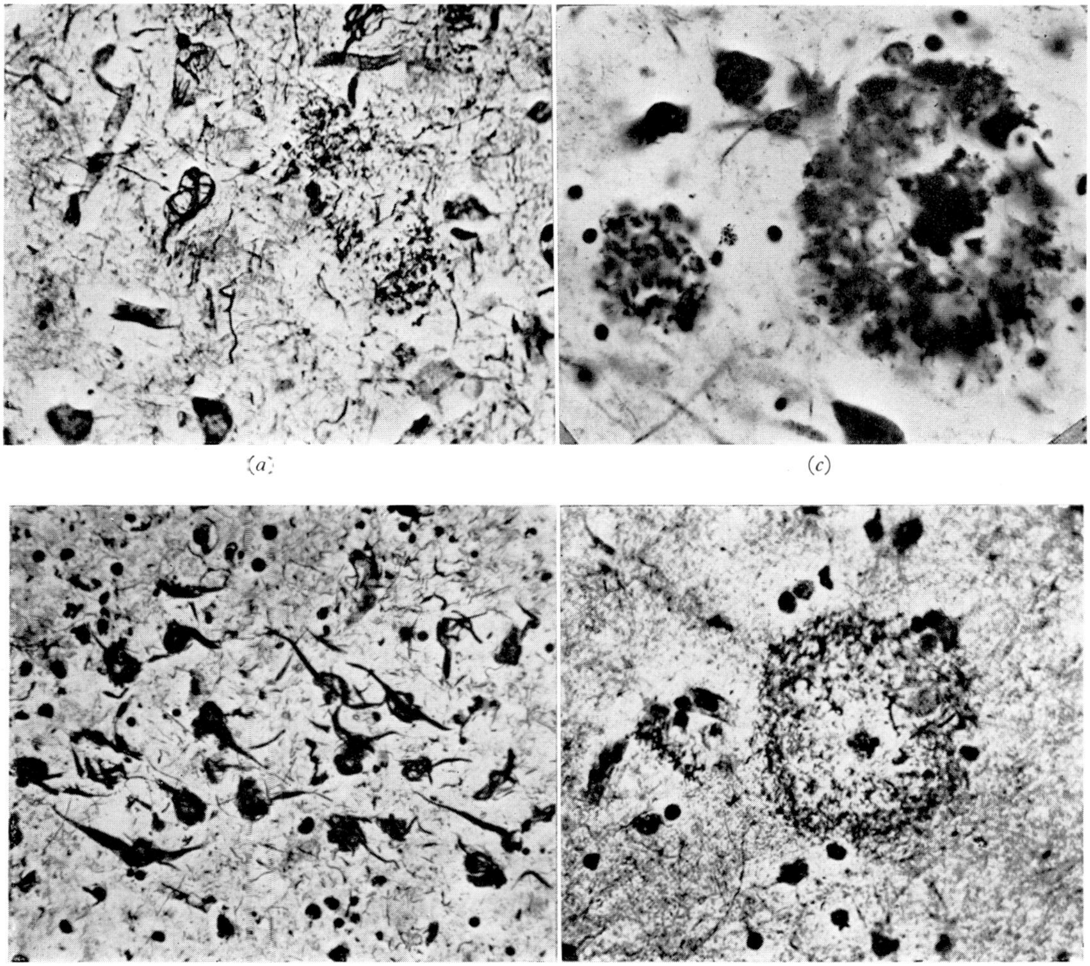

FIG. 9.5. *Alzheimer's disease.*

(*a*) Cortex showing Alzheimer nerve cells round an argyrophilic plaque.
(*b*) Cornu Ammonis showing neurofibrillary changes in all the nerve cells.
(*c*) and (*d*) Argyrophilic plaques in the cortex. (Bielschowsky's silver impregnation.)

Opinions differ as to whether the 'Alzheimer change' in nerve cells is an invariable finding in this disorder. Cases have been reported in which they have been noticeably absent, but these cannot be accepted as typical examples of the disease. Fuller and Klopp's (1912) patient was ill for only 7 months following a streptococcal infection of her throat and rheumatism. Plaques were not plentiful, a fact which could be attributed to the short course of the illness but the nerve cells were rich in lipid and some were atrophic. Lowenberg and Rothschild's

(1931) case, aged 37, developed late in pregnancy an acute toxic psychosis which after a partial remission proved fatal on relapse 8 years later. Plaques were very limited in their distribution. A case described by Stern and Reed (1945) as the abiotrophic type of Alzheimer's disease should not be accepted as such because, although the brain was very atrophic (864 g.), neither plaques nor neurofibrillary degeneration were found. We therefore consider that the neurofibrillary degeneration constitutes an essential part of the pathology of this disease. It may contribute substantially to the dementia, although cells as yet unaffected by this form of degeneration may be diseased in other ways. The view that greater importance is to be attached to neurofibrillary degeneration than to senile plaques is further substantiated by Morel and Wildi (1952) who find, especially under 60, that an abnormally great dilatation of ventricles and enlargement of the pericerebral space occurs much earlier when neurofibrillary degeneration is a prominent feature of a case. Such structural changes, they believe, may have appreciably antedated symptoms; however, with increasing age of onset and with increasing duration of the illness, both the pericerebral space and the ventricles tend to diminish in volume in those cases in which neurofibrillary degeneration is prominent, whereas in those unaffected by this change they tend to increase. The importance of changes in the corpora mamillaria, Ammon's horn and the hippocampal gyrus in causing amnesia is discussed by Brierley (1961).

Granulo-vacuolar degeneration of nerve cells (*vide* Chapter 1), which was first noted by Alzheimer and described by Simchovicz, is commonly found in the pyramidal cell layer of the cornu Ammonis. Morel and Wildi (1952), on the basis of histochemical studies, believe it to be an early stage in the process of 'Alzheimerization', a view which is supported by Agostini (1958).

As the nerve cells die their axons and myelin sheaths degenerate too and this has been held to account for the retrograde degeneration of the thalamus which may be observed. Axons are noticeably few in number in diseased parts of the cortex. Myelin destruction, however, is seldom appreciable, for sudanophilic material is not found and compound granular corpuscles are not a feature of this disease: nor are microglial cells present in excess in the white matter. Sections stained for myelin may show some rarefaction, and the plaques bordering on the white and grey matter are sometimes revealed as clear-cut areas of pallor (Fig. 9.3*c*). In some cases the cortex may show a severe status spongiosus (von Braunmühl 1957).

Goodman (1953) has found much free iron in the nerve cells, in the oligodendroglia and in the walls of capillaries and arterioles. He believes that the disease may be essentially a disorder of iron metabolism giving rise to a devitalisation of the microglia with a gradual accumulation of waste products. Hallgren and Saunders (1960) also find stainable iron in the cortex but there is no overall increase in iron content. They assume therefore that in this disease there has been a redistribution of iron as a result of altered binding.

The astrocytes are not conspicuously active in the early stages of Alzheimer's disease but, as in general paralysis, they play a role in producing the final cortical scar. Large astrocytes grouped in pairs or more, indicative of recent division, form a marginal ring round many of the older plaques. In addition they are diffusely scattered throughout the cortex and the underlying white matter in numbers in excess of normal and with much increase of fibres.

In a proportion of cases the blood-vessels of the cortex and leptomeninges show no significant alterations; in others pathological changes involving especially the arterioles may be striking. Cerebrovascular amyloidosis, a manifestation of the ageing brain and rare under the age of 70, can occur for instance in younger subjects afflicted with Alzheimer's disease; also when it occurs it is a more widespread process than the *drüsige Entartung* of Scholz, affecting especially the muscle layer of the vessels of the leptomeninges and cortex. It would appear not unlikely that the amyloid material sited between the muscle fibres or on the adventitial surface of the muscle layer is the result of a dyshoric phenomenon (Mandybur and McMenemey 1963) as has been advocated in the instance of *drüsige Entartung* (Scholz 1938, Morel and Wildi 1952).

Amyloid degeneration of the blood vessels associated with numerous argyrophilic plaques has been described by Newman (1961) in a woman aged 49 with neurological symptoms but no significant degree of dementia; in this case there was no change in the neurofibrils. The occurrence of cerebrovascular amyloidosis in Alzheimer's disease is not necessarily associated with the presence of amyloid in plaques (Benedek and McGovern 1949). The pathological changes of Alzheimer's disease may also co-exist with severe cerebral arteriosclerosis, so that diagnosis of this latter disease, even when accompanied by multiple softenings, should not preclude the investigation of a brain for the parenchymatous lesions of the former.

Familial cases

The few familial and hereditary cases of Alzheimer's disease which have been recorded stress the likely importance of genetic factors in its aetiology. Schottky (1932) described the disease in father and daughter with 7 presumed cases in four generations, while von Braunmühl (1932) found it in twins. English (1942) reported it in four sibs and in the daughter of one of them. Wheelan (1959) recorded in a family of ten, two proven and three presumed cases; the mother of this family was thought also to have been a victim of the disease. The parents of the juvenile case described by Løken and Cyvin (1954) were first cousins. Lowenberg and Waggoner (1934) described a case of what was believed to be Alzheimer's disease beginning in a male at the age of 32: he had five children and four of them developed the same clinical condition at the ages of 31, 32, 33 and 34 respectively. One of them came to necropsy and was found to be a typical instance of Alzheimer's disease: the father's parents were first cousins. A first cousin marriage was reported also in a family examined by McMenemey, Worster-Drought, Flynd and Williams (1939): in this instance three of four siblings and the child of one were affected but only one necropsy was obtained. Grünthal and Wenger (1939, 1940) described 4 cases in two generations with post-mortem findings in a sister and brother, while Essen-Möller (1946) described a family in which a father, a son and a daughter developed the disease; a remaining son was mentally defective. Davidson and Robertson (1955) described a case in one of identical twins: this patient, whose symptoms began at the age of 50 and whose death occurred 19 years later, had spent her life in Edinburgh, while the sister, still in good health at the age of 73, had lived mostly in Australia. In searching for environmental factors which might have explained this difference in health of the twins the authors noted that the patient, after contending with the dietetic restrictions of the First World War from which her sister was free, had had a febrile delirium during the 1918–19 influenza epidemic. Bini (1948) reports, in his series of 20 patients with Alzheimer's disease, 2 unrelated cases, one a male and the other a female, whose mothers suffered from a like form of dementia. Other familial cases are reported by Goodman (1953), Josephy (1956) and Marchand *et al.* (1956).

In the two families in which the disease appeared as the result of first cousin marriages, a recessive gene can be held responsible. In the other cases transmission could be by means of an autosomal dominant gene. Sjögren, Sjögren and Lindgren (1952), as a result of their study of 26 cases, came to the conclusion that a multifactorial inheritance was likely, whereas in Pick's disease a dominant major gene with modifying genes appeared more acceptable. To account for the preponderance of females over males in both diseases they thought a totally or partially sex-linked inheritance unlikely and favoured instead a monohybrid autosomal dominant gene combined with either reduced manifestations and a certain sex limitation or a sex-controlled inhibiting factor. In other cases there may be inheritance by dominant genes (Essen-Möller 1946).

Apart from these familial instances of Alzheimer's disease, it is not unusual to obtain a history of neuropsychiatric disorders in the families of patients. Schenk (1955), for instance, found a history of dementia in a near relative in 10 out of 35 cases and of severe disease of the nervous system in 15.

It will be seen therefore that only in recent years has a genetic background for Alzheimer's disease gained any support. The case of Davidson and Robertson, however, raises the possibility that environmental factors may precipitate a disease, the liability to which is genetically determined. In this particular patient there was also acne rosacea but again not in the twin. Davidson and Robertson explain this double discordance on the basis of somatic mutation occasioned by environmental factors. Further observations of this nature are clearly needed; meanwhile it is noteworthy that Alzheimer's disease is much commoner in Gothenburg than in Stockholm whereas Pick's disease is more common in Stockholm than in Gothenburg (Sjögren, Sjögren and Lindgren 1952). Also it is interesting to learn that Alzheimer's disease and senile dementia have not so far been recognised in the Chinese and Malayan populations of Indonesia whereas Pick's disease is known there (Verhaart 1936).

Atypical cases

In the literature there are several unusual cases which are seemingly related to Alzheimer's disease and which have sometimes been claimed as such.

Schnitzler (1911) described the case of a woman of 32 who died at the age of 37. Neurofibrillary changes were plentiful but there were no senile plaques. In this case an associated dysthyroidism was sufficient to suggest a thyrogenic disturbance, comparable with that present in senility, as a basis for the production of the histological changes. Weimann (1921) described a case of a male aged 37 who had neurofibrillary changes but no senile plaques. There was a marked degree of arterial degeneration of the brain vessels together with diffuse calcinosis. Other cases without plaques have been reported by Goodman (1953) and Raskin and Ehrenberg (1956 a).

Hemphill and Stengel (1941) described the histological findings of Alzheimer's disease in a woman of 41 whose illness began after pregnancy and proved fatal at the age of 59. The case was unusual also in that there was an asymmetry in the involvement of the disease, the right cerebral hemisphere being affected more than the left while there were changes in the left cerebellum.

Liebers (1933) recorded the 5-year illness of an engineer who died aged 52 with the atrophy and histological features of Alzheimer's disease but with a marked accentuation of the atrophy (described by the author as 'Pick-like') in the parieto-occipital region.

Other examples of focal atrophy in Alzheimer's disease, usually fronto-temporal, have been described (Divry, Ley and Titeca 1935, Rothschild and Kasanin 1936, Seitelberger and Jellinger, 1958): a case reported by Creutzfeldt (1922) was complicated by the fact that the Wassermann reaction in both blood and cerebrospinal fluid was positive thus raising the question of a coexisting Lissauer's type of dementia. Berlin (1949) has described 2 cases of Alzheimer's disease in which the histological changes as well as the gross focal atrophy of Pick's disease have been present. They are generally accepted as examples of the double disease. A case reported by Kreindler, Hornet and Appel (1959) could be another instance. Liebers (1939) has reported the case of a 61-year-old woman with a circumscribed bilateral frontotemporal atrophy of the Pick type with numerous argyrophilic plaques and neurofibrillary alterations in the relatively unaltered parietal and occipital lobes. No Pick cells were identified. Liebers claims it as a case of Alzheimer's disease but Mansvelt regards it as an instance of Pick's disease: it too could be regarded as an instance of the double disease. Other cases which have sometimes been considered as variants of Alzheimer's disease (Moyano 1932) are more appropriately included as variants of Pick's disease.

Reference will now be made to several cases in which features of Alzheimer's disease have been found in association with amyloid disease of the cerebral blood vessels. In some instances there has been a marked inherited susceptibility to the disease.

Marinesco (1931) described the case of a 55-year-old man with a 9 years' history of pyramidal and extrapyramidal disease with nystagmus, inco-ordination, disorientation and loss of memory. At necropsy he was found to have massive cholesterol stone formation in the biliary tracts with amyloidosis of blood-vessels in the liver, kidney, spleen and in the white matter of the brain, more especially the brain stem. Closely associated with the amyloidosis of blood-vessels (which in illustration resembles the perivascular plaques of Scholz) were typical 'senile' plaques with microglia encircling them. Marinesco considered that in this case the plaques were secondary to the amyloid changes in the vessels.

Worster-Drought, Greenfield and McMenemey (1940, 1944) reported the pathological findings in two patients belonging to a family (previously described by Worster-Drought, Hill and McMenemey 1933) in which nine females and two males in three generations were affected with a progressive dementia associated with spastic paraplegia. In both cases areas of demyelination were found in the subcortical white matter and especially the corpus callosum, associated with patchy but gross swelling of the arterioles (Scholz's perivascular plaques). The pathological material has been found to give the reactions for amyloid. The same abnormal state of the arterioles was noted in the cerebellum and cornu Ammonis and was associated with the presence of classical 'senile' plaques and, in the latter situation, neurofibrillary degeneration also. These cases if accepted as coming within the category of Alzheimer's disease must be deemed very atypical for the cerebral cortex was mostly not involved. Indeed, in its distribution, the condition bore more resemblance to Binswanger's disease.

Van Bogaert, Maere and de Smedt (1940) described a family in which two out of four offspring and four of six of the second generation were affected, like the original parent, with progressive dementia and spastic paraplegia. Although the findings were more characteristic of Alzheimer's disease than the family to which we have previously referred, in that argyrophilic plaques and neurofibrillary degeneration were widespread, the perivascular plaques of Scholz were present in spite of the fact that the patient was only 39 at death. Two siblings, who in life had been diagnosed as multiple sclerosis, were described by Luers (1947), with brains conforming rather more to those of the family recorded by Worster-Drought *et al.* than to that of the family of van Bogaert *et al.*

Corsellis and Brierley (1954) described the post-mortem findings of 2 unrelated cases aged respectively 54 and 65 at death, the former possibly familial, which were typical of Alzheimer's disease apart from the severity of the perivascular plaques of Scholz and the presence of patches of myelin loss, especially in the first. The abnormal substance, whether in plaques, in blood-vessel walls and/or in free-lying masses was obvious in routine stains. It gave a positive reaction with the P.A.S. technique but negative with Feigl's reaction, thus indicating a mucopolysaccharide (Figs. 9.7 and 9.8).

A 31-year-old woman who died of a cerebellar disorder with psychotic symptoms was possibly of the same order. Gerstmann, Straussler and Scheinker (1936), who reported the case, found an atrophy of the cerebellum with an abundance of large plaques in the molecular layer together with some degree of atrophy of the cerebral cortex in association with atypical ganglion cells. Three previous generations were concerned in this disease and the trait was believed to be dominant. Von Braunmühl (1954) has reported the findings in a sister of this

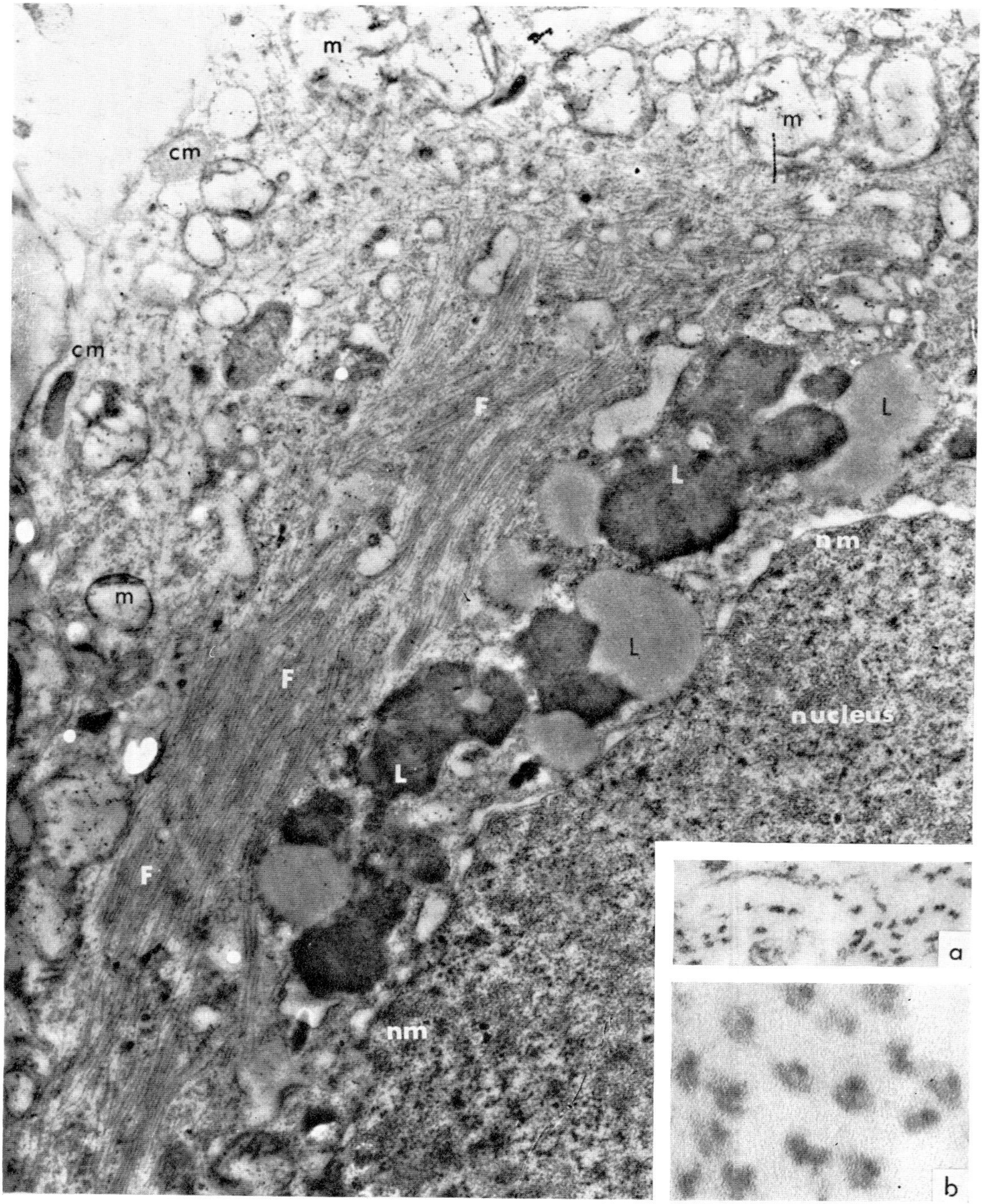

FIG. 9.6. Electron micrograph of part of an affected nerve cell in a case of Alzheimer's disease. A bundle of the characteristic filaments (F.) is seen running in the cytoplasm. ×22,000. (cm = nerve cell membrane; nm = nuclear membrane; m = mitochondrion; L = lipochrome). Inset a. A region in the neuropil showing a longitudinal helix above and a number of helices in transverse section. ×60,000. Inset b. Higher magnification of helices in transverse section. ×224,000. (Biopsy preparation by Dr. Michael Kidd.)

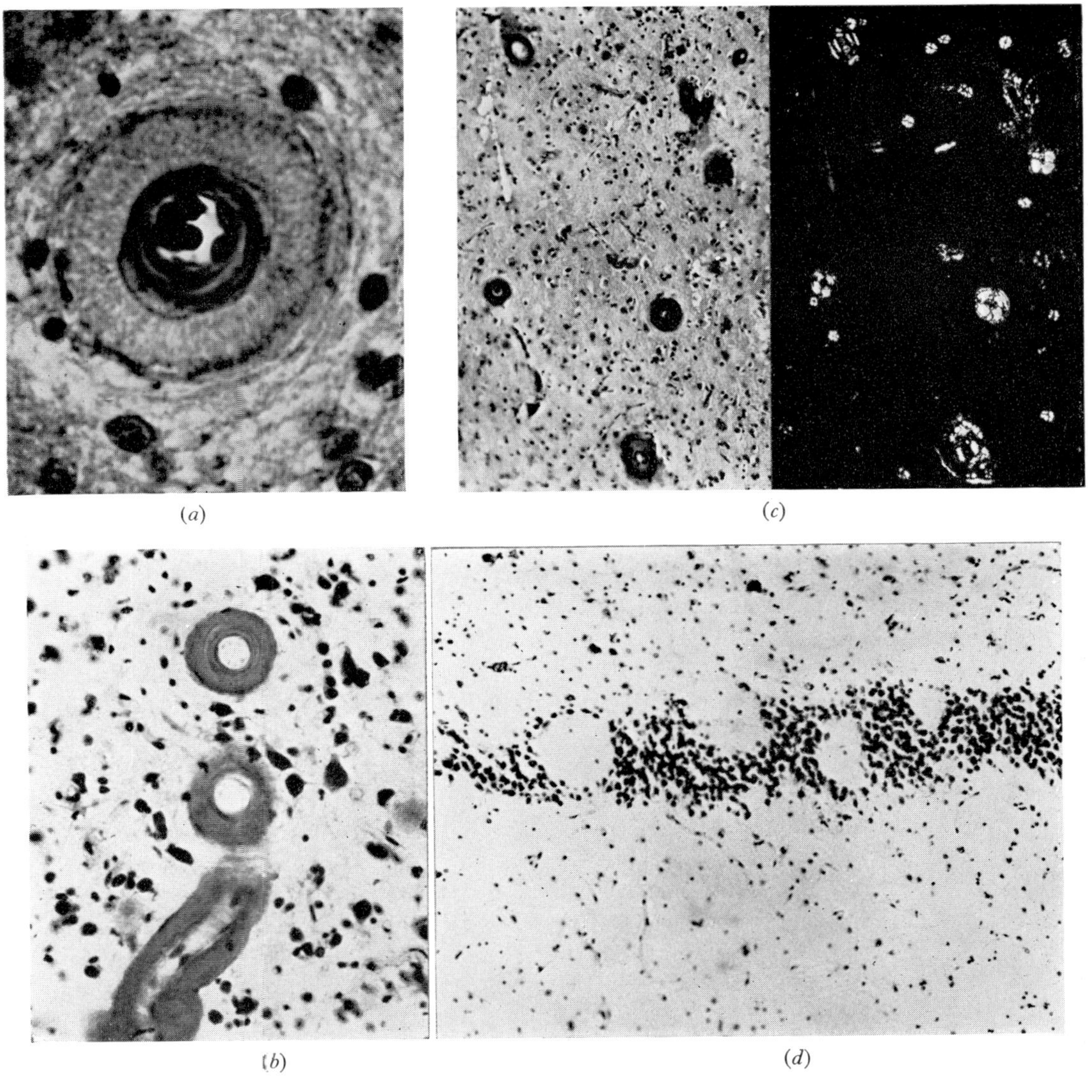

FIG. 9.7. *Atypical Alzheimer's disease.* (Case of Corsellis and Brierley 1954.)

(*a*) Cortical arteriole showing gross thickening of middle coat with a radial fibrillar structure.
(*b*) Cortical arterioles with homogeneous appearance of wall.
(*c*) Small vessels stained by Congo red. The photograph on the right is taken under polarised light.
(*d*) Plaques in fascia dentata. (Cresyl violet, ×90.)

patient and found that the amyloid substance in the large plaques which characterised this brain was not dissolved by dichlordiphenyltrichlormethylmethane (D.D.T.) in contradistinction to the typical argyrophilic plaques of Alzheimer's disease.

Neumann (1960) has reported the case of a 45-year-old woman with abundant large plaques in the cerebral cortex staining readily with aniline dyes as well as with silver and associated with marked hyaline-like changes in the walls of the smaller arterioles. This patient had no significant degree of mental deterioration and there were no neurofibrillary alterations.

Familial cerebellar disorders associated with neurofibrillary degeneration in parts of the cerebral cortex have been recorded by Schaffer (1922, 1926) and by Bielschowsky, Boumann and Smitt (1934).

Ritama (1954) reports the case of a 64-year-old painter who was a mild diabetic and who for the last 2 years of his life was troubled with nocturia. His terminal illness which lasted only a few weeks consisted of weariness, increasing somnolence and slight mental derangement. At autopsy he was found to have amyloidosis of the secondary type in the spleen, adrenals, pancreas and kidney, this last organ showing lesions of the Kimmelstiel-Wilson variety. Amyloid deposits in relation to the capillaries were found on the under-surface of the cerebellum and similar lesions were found in the vessels of the posterior commissure, of the spinal cord and in the periphery of the medulla. Missmahl and Hartwig (1954) have found amyloid substances in the bone marrow, spleen and kidneys in Alzheimer's disease, while Krücke (1950) reported their presence in heart muscle and in veins.

Of great interest are those cases of post-traumatic dementia which show the histological changes of Alzheimer's disease. Claude and Cuel (1939) described the case of a woman who became demented following a fractured skull at the age of 50: she died 5 years later with the histological changes of Alzheimer's disease. Corsellis and Brierley (1959) report the histological findings of Alzheimer's disease in a 55-year-old man who five years earlier was involved as a passenger in an automobile accident. Another instance was reported by Grosch (1959) ten years after an injury which at the time caused unconsciousness and later a proneness to syncopal attacks, with personality changes and dysarthria two years before death. Neubürger and von Braunmühl (1930) record the presence of abundant plaques in a 56-year-old man who died of traumatic dementia 34 years after an injury. Brandenburg and Hallervorden (1954) describe the case of a demented boxer who died at the age of 38 with senile plaques and neurofibrillary changes. They suggest that repeated episodes of commotio cerebri may suffice to disturb the permeability of the brain vessels and so produce organic changes comparable to those seen in Alzheimer's disease. They prefer not to regard their patient as an example of Alzheimer's disease but of a traumatically induced example of what von Braunmühl calls 'the syneretic syndrome'. Corsellis and Brierley (1959) refer to two other cases in boxers with the histological findings of Alzheimer's disease; the first had also a scar in the corpus callosum, the second, who died at the age of 67 after a severe memory defect dating back 24 years, had a considerable degree of hyaline thickening of the cerebral blood vessels and a pallidal haemorrhage. Grahmann and Ule (1957) found neurofibrillary degeneration but no plaques in a boxer aged 48.

It will be seen therefore that, in the course of time, the view, propounded originally by Perusini (1910) and affirmed by Barrett (1913) that Alzheimer's disease is a pathological condition independent of senility, has gained ground. It was upheld by Grünthal in 1930 and gained considerable support as a result of the juvenile cases described by Malamud and Lowenburg (1939) and Løken and Cyvin (1954). There is indeed justification for entertaining von Braunmühl's conception of the *syneretic syndrome* (synäretisches Syndrom). According to this author (1932) there are probably many reasons, both endogenous and exogenous, to account for the appearance of argyrophilic plaques and of cells exhibiting neurofibrillary degeneration. While the process of normal senility itself may induce these changes in the course of time, other factors including trauma, constitution and possibly environment may precipitate them at an earlier age. The occurrence of 'senile' plaques in Mongolian idiots in early adult life (Struwe 1929, Bertrand and Koffas 1946, Jervis 1948, Verhaart and Jelgersma 1952) may be related to the lack of thyrotropic hormone reported by Benda (1949), but Jervis suggests a disorder of the corticotropic hormone of the pituitary and of the adrenal cortical hormone. In 2 of Jervis's 3 cases neurofibrillary degeneration was also found and he has called the condition 'senile dementia'. Similar changes were noted by Jelgersma (1958) in a mongol who at the age of 53 lost interest in his favourite game of dominoes and died six years later. This author comments on the fact that the lipofuscin content of the cortical nerve cells was high and many of them were in addition sclerotic. Schob and Guntz (1932) describe a case of Alzheimer's disease in association with Simmonds disease. In this connection it is interesting to recall Schnitzler's (1911) suggestion that thyrogenic disturbance may furnish a basis comparable with that found in senility for the production of the characteristic histological process of Alzheimer's disease. However, Lotmar (1929, 1933) found only slight argyrophilia but no true thickening of the neurofibrils in thyreoaplasia and cretinism, while the experimental work of Balli (1907), Lewy (1923), Rasdolsky (1926), Alexander (1934) and Stern and Elliott (1949) has failed to reproduce true neurofibrillary degeneration of Alzheimer after thyroidectomy. Biemond (1955) found the changes of cerebral oedema with giant astrocytes in a case of coma due to myxoedema but makes no mention of thickened neurofibrils.

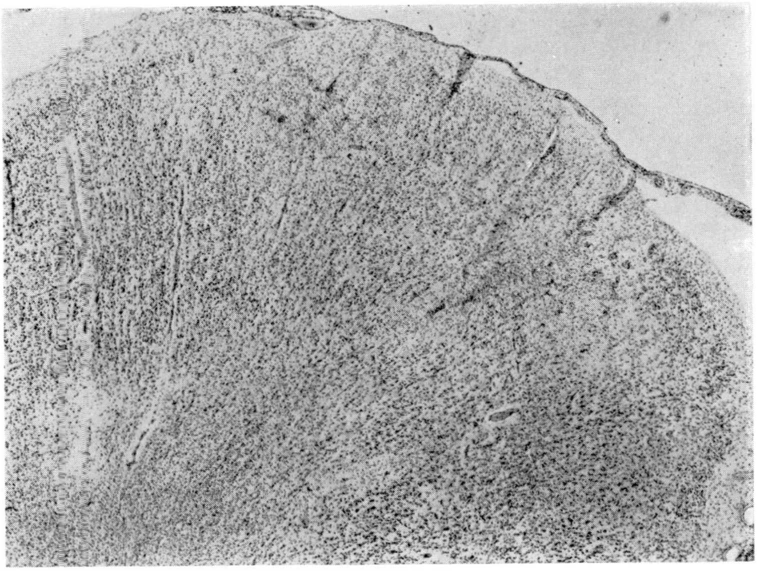

FIG. 9.8. *Atypical Alzheimer's disease.* (Case of Corsellis and Brierley.) Showing irregular areas of ischaemic degeneration of nerve cells due to amyloid disease of small vessels (Nissl × 25).

'Senile dementia'

The term senile dementia is not synonymous with senile psychosis for the latter includes a large group of affective disorders which are not associated with visible organic changes in the brain. A diagnosis of senile dementia is commonly reserved to denote an organic dementing process originating in a person over the age of 65 which is not attributable to Pick's disease, arteriosclerosis, syphilis or any other established condition, and which is regarded as being too old for consideration as Alzheimer's disease. The bulk of these cases will be found to present atrophied brains with neuronal atrophy, argyrophilic plaques and Alzheimer neurofibrillary changes. If one accepts them, in spite of their late age of onset, as instances of Alzheimer's disease, then few cases remain to be labelled senile dementia.

There have been two schools of thought up to now, those who believe in the identity of Alzheimer's disease with senile dementia and those who believe that they are separate. The latter school adduces certain evidence both clinical and pathological. On the clinical side, it is held that in Alzheimer's disease there is much overactivity: the patients are restless, irritable and show stereotyped movements. However, cases of "senile dementia" may show motor unrest.

On the other hand, some authors have reported instances of Alzheimer's disease which, far from manifesting unrest, were characterised by depression and apathy (Hemphill and Stengel 1941, English 1942). Grünthal (1930 b) who favoured the individuality of both diseases, admitted that clinically they might be almost the same, the only difference being a tendency in Alzheimer's disease to more focal symptoms, such as aphasia, apraxia or epilepsy. Mutrux (1958) claims that aphasia, agnosia and apraxia occur in Alzheimer's disease but not in senile dementia. King (1960) has attempted a statistical comparison of Alzheimer's disease with 'senile brain disease' and, because he observed the former more often than was to be expected, he regards them as not the same. However the incidence of mental disorders in the relatives of patients with Alzheimer's disease is of an order comparable to that found in senile dementia. Meggendorfer (1926) found an incidence of 33 per cent in the relatives of patients with senile dementia and Cresseri (1948) gives a figure of 34 per cent. Schenk (1955) reported a family history of insanity in 28·6 per cent of his cases of Alzheimer's disease.

On the pathological side it has been claimed that the changes in Alzheimer's disease are more severe than those in senile dementia (Rothschild and Kasanin 1936) and that the atrophy of the brain and loss of neurones is greater (Mutrux 1947, 1953), but these findings may be due to the fact that the presenile patient is better able to withstand the disease and to survive longer with it as compared with the senile patient. Certain observers (Simchowicz 1910, 1914, 1924; Mayer-Gross 1938) have claimed that in Alzheimer's disease the brunt of the pathological process tends to fall more on the occipital than on the frontal cortex whereas the opposite is true of senile dementia. This is not supported by Rothschild (1934), Jervis (1937) and our own observations. Critchley (1930) believes that senile plaques may be considered characteristic of senile dementia and neurofibrillary degeneration of Alzheimer's disease. Mutrux (1947) found that the neurofibrillary changes were rarely seen in Heschl's gyrus and its vicinity in senile dementia, an area constantly involved in Alzheimer's disease. Mutrux (1953) also claims that in the areas of projection the changes are always greater in Alzheimer's disease. He states too that the plaques tend to occur in the outer four layers in senile dementia and in the inner four layers in Alzheimer's disease. More recently (1958) he has reported finding significant differences between them in (von Economo) areas FAγ, FC and FE, neurofibrillary degeneration being virtually absent in instances of 'senile dementia'.

Some authors have attempted to establish a qualitative difference between the plaques of Alzheimer's disease and 'senile dementia'. Hannah (1936), for instance, thought that the plaques were larger in the former disease and that there was no microglial reaction around them. Others, on the contrary, hold that the microglial reaction is greater in Alzheimer's disease than in senile dementia. Verhaart (1930 a) believed that the plaques developed slowly in senile dementia and quickly in Alzheimer's disease and that the astroglial cicatrice was greater in the latter than in the former. He claimed that in Alzheimer's disease the plaques were of irregular shape whereas in senile dementia they tended to be concentric. Simma (1951) noted retrograde cell degeneration in the thalamus in Alzheimer's disease but not in senile dementia: this, however, may be yet another example of the fact that the younger patient has the greater expectation of survival and can tolerate more injury than the older one. The perivascular plaques of Scholz, found especially in the fourth lamina in area 17 (Brodmann), have, be it noted, been reported much more frequently in senile than in presenile dementia.

Many workers agree with Grünthal (1936), Jervis and Soltz (1936), Wilson (1940 b) and Newton (1948) that it is impossible to distinguish between Alzheimer's disease and senile dementia. Mutrux (1953) for instance concludes that such differences as he has noted between them are purely quantitative and he leaves open the question of the unity or duality of the diseases. Schenk (1955) regards any such distinction between a presenile and senile form of Alzheimer's disease as arbitrary and untenable but he does recognise all gradations between Alzheimer's disease and a benign form of senile dementia characterised by few plaques and by only a few cells exhibiting neurofibrillary degeneration. A similar view is expressed by Miskolczy (1959) when he asserts that the clinical picture of senile dementia is caused not only by Alzheimer's disease but by other processes too.

Neumann and Cohn (1953) tackled the problem from another viewpoint. They found in a mental hospital study that, irrespective of age, the clinical picture associated with widespread plaque formation and neurofibrillary degeneration was remarkably consistent. They prefer to regard all such cases as examples of Alzheimer's disease. Twenty-two out of 50 patients between the ages of 58 and 94 with a clinical diagnosis of senile psychosis had the clinico-pathological features of Alzheimer's disease, that is to say argyrophilic plaques and neurofibrillary changes, while an additional 10 had plaques only. Only those with both lesions exhibited the history and symptomatology of Alzheimer's disease. They further found that 49 out of 100 patients diagnosed as suffering from arteriopathic psychosis presented the pathological picture of Alzheimer's disease and, on review, the typical personality changes and behaviour disorders of Alzheimer's disease.

Newton (1948), in a series of 150 consecutive autopsies on psychotics, found that 54 per cent of males and 77 per cent of females over the age of 65 exhibited plaques: the corresponding figures in the age group 50–64 were 11 per cent and 29 per cent respectively. He found that in the senile age group 4 times as many females as males showed miliary plaques and 6 times as many in the presenile age group. Twenty-three out of his 150 consecutive mental hospital necropsies showed the histological changes of Alzheimer's disease. These included 15 out of 37 cases diagnosed as organic dementia. Raskin and Ehrenberg (1956), in an histological study of 270 patients aged 60 to 97 in a state hospital, found 24 with numerous cells exhibiting neurofibrillary degeneration, all but one of them with argyrophilic plaques. Because the dementia in all instances was profound they classified them retrospectively as Alzheimer's disease irrespective of age of onset. Only 5 of them had been diagnosed as such in life.

Simchowicz (1910), Fischer (1910), Uyematsu (1923) and Grünthal (1927, 1936) all claim that plaques occur in all cases of senile dementia. According to Rothschild (1956) the phylogenetically older parts of the cortex are least affected. He states that, while the pathology of senile dementia is characteristic, it is not specific for that disease, because there may be a lack of correlation between the histological changes and the degree of intellectual impairment and sometimes equally severe alterations are found in normal old age. He attributes these inconsistencies to differences in the capacity of individuals to compensate for cerebral damage, a capacity which, rather than the pathological changes themselves, is in his opinion the determining factor in the origin of a senile psychosis. Rothschild (1937), Rothschild and Sharp (1941), Jacob (1952), Fattovich (1955 (i) and (ii)) and Sjögren (1956) believe that senile dementia may occur without the presence of miliary plaques. These last three authors, for instance, have reported classical instances of the clinical disease in which both plaques and neurofibrillary changes have been absent. One woman reported by Fattovich was 92 when she died after an 18-year history. The brain showed simple atrophy with fatty granules in the nerve cells. Another died aged 76 in a marasmic state after a 5-year history. There was widespread and diffuse atrophy of the convolutions with a marked loss of cells sometimes showing hypertrophic and pyknotic nuclei.

Reference has already been made to the fact that Mutrux (1958) regards agnosia, aphasia and apraxia as symptoms characteristic of Alzheimer's disease and lacking in senile dementia. Sjögren (1956) and Sjögren and Sourander (1961) on the other hand, distinguish a group of cases which display this same triad of symptoms but differ from Alzheimer's disease in a later age of onset, a lack of spontaneity, akinesis, Parkinsonism and seizures, a liability to psychomotor restlessness and, pathologically, a paucity or even an absence of argyrophilic changes in the brain: to this condition they give the name 'atrophia cerebri simplex'.

There are many factors which require further elucidation and which may have a bearing on the determination of dementia in the elderly. Reference has already been made to the importance of an adequate blood circulation. Impaired oxygenation due to lack of exercise, progressive stooping and anaemia, as well as the insidious onset of malnutrition, can be remedied and so help to distinguish functional brain disorder from organic disease. Stern, Hinds and Askonas (1945), making use of the hippuric acid synthesis test, found that evidence of faulty detoxication by the liver was 3 times as common in psychotics over 60 as compared with healthy individuals, while 5 cases of senile dementia had conspicuously low values even when compared with those of the same age group with affective disorders.

It would seem that in considering the pathogenesis of Alzheimer's disease and senile dementia we have to reckon with both endogenous and exogenous factors. Some latitude must be permitted in the histological criteria of diagnosis, more especially in those cases which by their family histories may be considered to be abiotrophically determined, but in general it may be stated that the term Alzheimer's disease should be reserved for those cases, irrespective of age, which show an abundance of senile plaques and neurofibrillary changes, and that a diagnosis of *atrophia senilis simplex* should be made in those cases over the age of 60 in which the histological criteria of Alzheimer's disease are incomplete. In this way the term 'senile dementia' is confined to cases awaiting an histological diagnosis.

If the diagnosis of Alzheimer's disease be restricted to cases which show an abundance of plaques and neurofibrillary changes then the following classification is possible:

(A) *Alzheimer's disease (sensu stricto)*
- (*a*) Infantile (Malamud and Lowenberg 1929; Løken and Cyvin 1954);
- (*b*) Adult ('presenile'), described also with focal accentuation (Liebers 1933);
- (*c*) Senile.

(B) *Alzheimer's disease in association with or complicating other conditions*
- (*a*) Post-traumatic (including some cases of dementia pugilistica);
- (*b*) Cerebrovascular disease (especially arteriolar amyloidosis);
- (*c*) Mongolism (Jervis 1948);
- (*d*) Simmond's disease (Schob and Guntz 1932);
- (*e*) Syphilis (Creutzfeldt 1922);
- (*f*) Pick's disease: (i) involving the atrophied parts only (Moyano 1931, 1932); (ii) the so-called 'double disease' (Berlin 1949).

Pick's disease

Pick's disease is a progressive and focal atrophy involving the frontal and temporal, and less often the parietal, lobes of the brain, with a course varying from 2 to 10 years. It occurs most frequently in middle-aged persons, and about twice as often in women as in men. It has, however, been described in early adult life. Guillain, Bertrand and Mollaret's patient (1934), for instance, was an engine driver aged 24, while Lowenberg, Boyd and Salon (1939) described a case at the age of 21. It may be met with in old age. Pick himself described a case at the age of 75, fatal 4 years later; Moyano's (1932) patient was aged 91. Schenk (1955) found that the age incidence curve of Pick's disease paralleled that of Alzheimer's disease but was about 10 years earlier.

It is rare; Neumann (1949) found that it constituted only 0·2 per cent of necropsies at a mental hospital; Bini (1948) found 5 cases (0·6 per cent), diagnosed by biopsy or necropsy, amongst 8,500 patients as against 20 cases of Alzheimer's disease.

The symptoms are varied, as one might expect from the fact that the atrophy may begin in either the frontal or temporal lobe only or in both simultaneously. In spite of this variation in location of the disease, in most cases the story is one of insidious intellectual deterioration, characterised by difficulty in concentration and loss of memory for recent events and, when marked, giving rise to such symptoms as disorientation in time and place, disorderliness in dress, lapses in social conduct and general lack of normal restraint. These symptoms are associated with a rather characteristic lack of initiative, and apathy. There is blunting of affect and insight is lost early. Malamud and Boyd (1940) however note that, in those cases in which the disease involves only the temporal lobe, memory, orientation and active attention are well preserved in the early stages. Disturbance of speech occurs in about two-thirds of cases and takes the form either of an amnesic or a sensory aphasia (Mayer-Gross, Slater and Roth 1954) and, except in those patients whose apathy is sufficient to make them more or less mute—and they constitute the majority—the result is sometimes a logorrhoea of peculiar jargon. According to Mansvelt logorrhoea has been found in about half of the cases of predominantly temporal lobe atrophy but never in a case of purely frontal lobe atrophy. Polylalia, echolalia, dysarthria and logoclonia are occasionally found but the patient may continue to be able to answer simple questions until the disease is well advanced. Dyspraxia, dysgraphia, dyslexia or agnosia are present not infrequently and are attributable to lesions in the parietal lobes. Disturbances of gait are not uncommon especially towards the end of the illness, but Parkinsonian symptoms are rarely met with. Akelaitis (1944) described such a case in which the substantia nigra and the nucleus subthalamicus were atrophied but which was otherwise typical of Pick's disease. Epileptic seizures are rare, as are also disturbances in tone, while choreiform and athetotic movements are very unusual.

The disease is slowly but relentlessly progressive. There are occasional bursts of excitement and over-activity but in general, after the initial phase of disinhibition, which may be attended by anti-social and sometimes surprising behaviour, the patient becomes more and more apathetic, losing much weight and ending up in a state of almost complete decortication. Boulimia, gluttony and rubbish-eating sometimes occur during the course of the disease.

Sometimes there are variations in the rate of progress and apparent periods of temporary arrest. A patient reported by Marchand, Bessière, Lelion and Marty (1955), for instance, showed a slow progress for 10 years and then a rapid evolution previous to death from pulmonary tuberculosis in the 14th year of the disease. The immediate cause of death is usually a complicating infection.

Occasionally the symptoms are masked. Winkelman and Book's (1949) patient, for instance, who died at the age of 34, was thought to have schizophrenia. De Boor, Spiegelhoff and Stammler (1952) describe an atypical and unsuspected case in a 63-year-old woman with an hypophyseal-diencephalic syndrome associated with gross obesity and a compulsion neurosis.

In 1930 Grünthal described the occurrence of Pick's disease in two brothers, of whom the younger by 2 years fell ill 1 year before the elder. This was the first familial case to be described although the family history of a case of a patient of von Braunmühl's (1928) was suggestive but unproven, while a possible instance of the disease having occurred in sisters was noted by Reich (1927). In the following year Grünthal described a case in the son of one of his patients. Three other examples of mental disease had occurred in this family over a period of four generations. As a result of his study, Grünthal concluded that a dominant autosomal gene was concerned.

Since then other familial examples have been reported; Schmitz and Meyer (1933) in three sisters and possibly in a cousin, Hăskovec (1934) in three sisters, probably the paternal grandfather and possibly the son of one of them, and von Braunmühl and Leonhard (1934) in two sisters and possibly their mother. In a remarkable family investigated by Sanders, Schenk and van Veen (1939) there were 4 proven cases and 13 presumed cases in four generations. In the Swedish survey by Sjögren, Sjögren and Lindgren (1952), further familial instances are described and another is reported by Friedrich (1940). There was a suggestive family history in the patient described by Lowenberg, Boyd and Salon (1939), the youngest in the literature, and in other recorded cases (Entres 1931, Murray 1958).

In addition to these instances of familial lobar atrophy there are several cases reported in which insanity or alcoholism has occurred in parents or siblings. In one interesting pair of sisters described by Korbsch (1933), Pick's disease was confirmed at necropsy in one, while a clinical diagnosis of Huntington's chorea was established in the other. It seems clear therefore that, even though they constitute a minority of the reported cases of Pick's disease, there are now sufficient examples in the literature to justify the assumption that this disease can be classified with the heredo-degenerations.

Little is known as yet of the geographic incidence of this disease but it is probably worldwide. Sjögren and his associates (1952) have commented on its relative frequency in Stockholm as compared with Gothenburg. Verhaart (1936) described the disease in Chinese and Malays in Indonesia.

Gross appearances

At necropsy it is usual to find a striking degree of atrophy of the frontal and temporal lobes but sometimes it is not obvious at post-mortem: possibly these are cases which have not run the normal course, life being brought to a close on account of interrcurrent illness. Delay, Brion and Sadoun's (1954) patient, for instance, died of pneumonia after a mental illness of 6 months; histological lesions were marked and characteristic but there was no gross atrophy. If the atrophy is unilateral, as it sometimes is, any wasting is at once apparent. When the wasting is equal on both sides and its degree is slight it may readily be overlooked. Frontal and especially temporal lobe atrophy is often most noticeable when the brain is viewed from in front. If the leptomeninges, which in this condition are often a little thickened and yellow though not adherent, are removed, the gyral wasting is always more obvious. In extreme cases of this disease the name has been given of 'knife-edge atrophy' of the convolutions (Fig. 9.9).

While the atrophy is in general temporal or frontal or, more usually, both, the distribution and confines of the atrophy conform to certain recognised patterns which have been studied by Spatz (1952). When the frontal lobe is involved there are two sub-types (*a*) a more usual frontobasal sub-type in which there is involvement of the gyrus rectus and Brodmann's area 11, with maximal atrophy in the gyrus frontalis inferior, extending as far backwards as the oral part of the insula. This is associated with atrophy in the operculum and area 44 and sometimes in areas 45 and 46, and (*b*) a frontal convexity sub-type which is rarer than the former; in this form the focus of shrinkage is believed to be caudad to the operculum and may extend into the gyrus precentralis. If the temporal lobe is involved the focus is always in the pole and spreads to involve the whole of the middle and inferior temporal gyri and the anterior third of the superior temporal gyrus. The escape of the posterior two-thirds of this gyrus is highly characteristic of Pick's disease and allows diagnosis to be speedily made. On the rare occasions when the parietal lobe is involved it usually concerns the inferior parietal lobule consisting of the supramarginal and angular gyri. All these areas have one feature in common: they represent parts of the brain which are ontogenetically and phylogenetically the latest to develop.

Certain parts of the brain appear to be relatively and sometimes absolutely resistant, as for instance the paracentral lobule (except the caudal part), the posterior two-thirds of the superior temporal gyrus, the gyrus transversus including the auditory convolution of Heschl, the superior parietal lobule, the post-central gyrus and the whole of the occipital lobes. These parts are all phylogenetically and ontogenetically early in development. Pick (1906) also noted, but not in such detail, that the atrophy in general was confined to the association areas of Flechsig. While the view of Pick, supported by Spatz and others, is generally held today, it is recognised that exceptions to the rule occur. Spatz, for instance, accepts the fact that the rhinencephalon and cornu Ammonis may sometimes be severely involved, but does not agree with the view held by some that the occipital lobes may be implicated.

Mansvelt (1954), in a detailed thesis, has analysed the incidence of the various locations of atrophy of all the cases in the literature. Some of his findings may be summarised as follows. The atrophy was symmetrical in 36·4 per cent of cases; it was most marked on the left in 46·2 per cent and on the right in 17·4 per cent of cases. Only in 1 case was the discrepancy very marked and this was in a patient whose disease began after a head injury (Reich 1927). The lobe

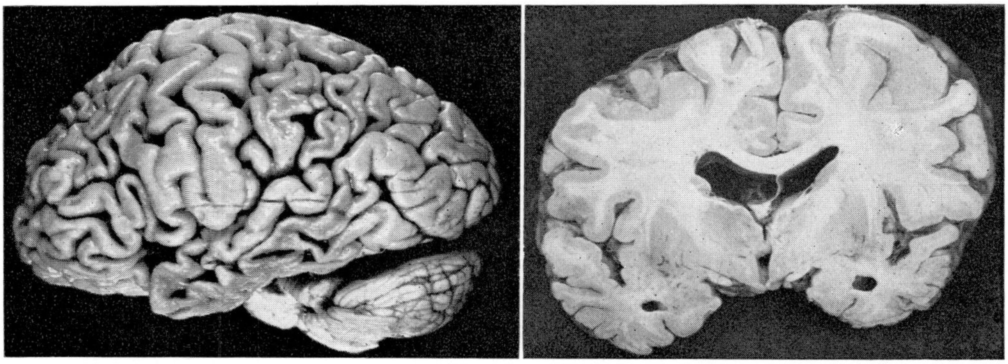

(*a*) (*b*)

FIG. 9.9. *Pick's disease.* In (*a*) there is atrophy in the parietal, as well as in the frontal and temporal lobes. The sparing of the posterior two thirds of the superior temporal gyrus is noteworthy.

distribution was as follows: frontal 24·8; temporal 16·8; parietal 1·2; frontal and temporal 54·3; frontal and parietal 1·7; others 1·2. Although there are reports in the literature of the occipital lobe being implicated (Horn and Stengel 1930, Urechia, Dragomir and Elekes 1935, Korbsch 1933, Bouton 1940, von Bagh 1941 and Sjögren, Sjögren and Lindgren 1952, Jakob 1960) the changes are mostly slight or even indefinite and appear to be at the most an extension from a focus of atrophy in the temporal lobe. In Urechia's case, however, the occipital lobe was heavily involved.

Involvement of the hippocampal gyrus or of the cornu Ammonis, and sometimes both together, occurred in 30% of the cases in the literature. In 6·7% of cases the degree of atrophy was greater than that noted in the second and third temporal convolutions suggesting the probability of their being primary shrinkage areas. Mansvelt sees in the relatively frequent appearance of the disease in these areas an objection to the view that differences in zones of atrophy are based on differences in myelogenesis.

The average weight of brains in Pick's disease, according to the compilation of Mansvelt, was 900–1,000 g. for women and 1,100–1,200 g. for men. The lightest reported brain was 690 g. and the heaviest 1,430. The lowest brain weights occurred in the group of mixed

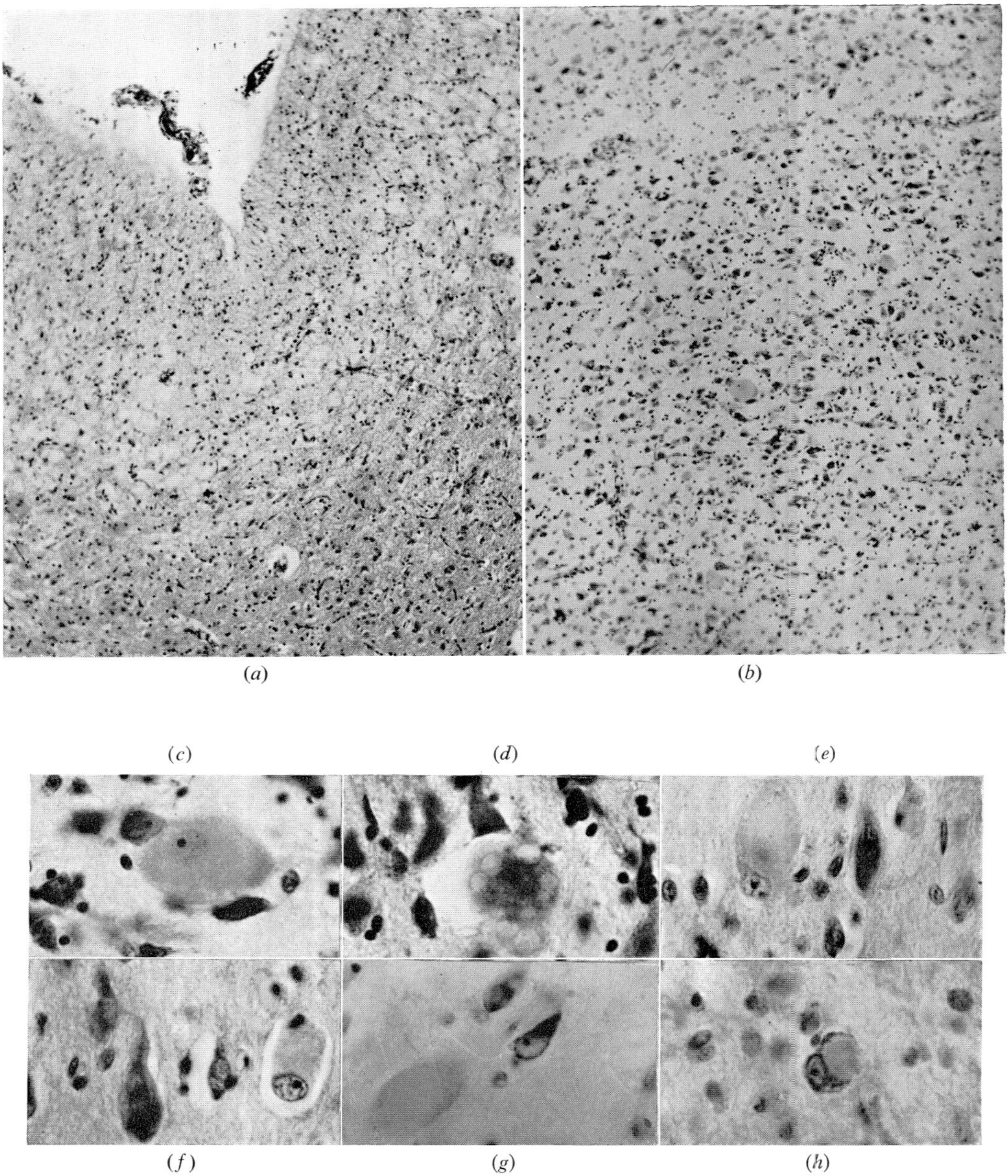

FIG. 9.10. *Pick's disease.*

(*a*) Second temporal gyrus showing widespread atrophy of the cortex with resulting status spongiosus. The section is taken in the depth of a sulcus. (Celloidin. Haematoxylin-eosin, ×90.)
(*b*) Superior temporal gyrus. There is widespread neuronal degeneration with disalignment of neurones: note pale globose forms (Pick's cells). Near the top is the line of a sulcus. (Cresyl violet, ×90.)
(*c*) is an enlargement of the cell seen in the centre of (*b*). (*d*), (*e*), (*f*), (*g*) and (*h*) are nerve cells in various stages of degeneration. The nucleus is not visible in the large cell in (*g*). (Cresyl violet, ×400.)

atrophies and there appeared to be a distinct relation between the duration of the disease and the degree of atrophy.

The atrophy is by no means confined to the cortex: indeed shrinkage of the subcortical white matter is so constant a feature of the disease as to have warranted the earlier workers referring to the condition as *lobar sclerosis*. But in addition the central grey matter may be involved and frequently is so. There are several instances in the literature in which atrophy of the caudate nucleus has been of such a degree as to raise the question of the alternative diagnosis of Huntington's chorea. Von Braunmühl (1930) has discussed their clinical and anatomical similarities. Whereas involvement of the caudate nucleus to some degree is common (apparently in about two-thirds of cases), it is less usual to find atrophy of the putamen (46·5 per cent) and still less so of the globus pallidus (34·1 per cent) and in each instance it is of a lesser degree of severity (Mansvelt 1954). In a case reported by Akelaitis (1944), however, the caudate nucleus had almost disappeared and the globus pallidus was severely involved although the putamen was fairly well preserved. The involvement of the phylogenetically older pallidum cannot be explained on the basis of retrograde degeneration. The thalamus often shows a degree of atrophy such as could be accounted for, and as one would expect, after destruction of large parts of the frontal and temporal lobes, but there are occasional reports in the literature of intact thalami in the face of marked frontal lobe atrophy (von Bagh 1941). The nucleus subthalamicus (Luysii) may occasionally be involved in this disease and also the substantia nigra. Such changes as occur in the pons, medulla and spinal cord are believed to be mostly of a secondary character, but Guillain, Bertrand and Mollaret (1934) described atrophic changes in the olives. Jakob (1960) found atrophy of the lateral part of the pontine nuclei in 6 out of 12 cases and swelling of the nerve cells in the medulla of all of them. Verhaart (1930 b) found degeneration of the cerebellar cortex and Lowenberg (1936) reported atrophy in the vermis and quadrangular and semi-lunar lobules; several authors have described minor changes in this organ. Bruetsch (1947) has described central cystic degeneration of the optic nerves, tracts and chiasm in a male negro whose dementia began at the age of 58 and lasted 10 years. Blindness developed in the 5th year of the illness.

Histology

The first histological account was given by Alzheimer (1911). The findings consist essentially of a loss of nerve cells in the affected areas with an accompanying cortical and subcortical gliosis which some believe to be secondary to the nerve cell loss. Others, however, hold that the gliosis is primary (Sanders, Schenk and van Veen 1939, Malamud and Waggoner 1943). The last of these authors have noted that neuroglial changes were present in parts of the brain where no changes in the neurones were apparent, while Yano, Nishina and Kumano (1960) claim that proliferative changes in the microglia are widespread throughout the cortex and basal ganglia.

The cell loss is greatest in the outer three layers. Schenk and Mansvelt (1955) were unable to substantiate the contention of M. Vogt (1928) that there is a predilection for the large cells of layer III and layer V. Many of the nerve cells which have not as yet disappeared show the characteristic swellings and argyrophilic inclusions (see Chapter 1) which were first described by Alzheimer (1911). These cells are often displaced out of their proper alignment. These *Pick cells* are found in most but not all cases which are actively progressing, and may be widespread and plentiful in the atrophying areas. They have a striking appearance especially when they are seen, as is so often the case, alongside normal cells. The demarcation between normal and abnormal cortex is very sharp. The granulo-vacuolar type of cell degeneration seen in

Alzheimer's disease is also found in Pick's disease. Again it is most commonly seen, although not exclusively so, in the pyramidal cells of the cornu Ammonis. The astroglial proliferation is often very marked and may be associated with status spongiosus. Scharenberg (1958), with the aid of silver techniques, has demonstrated the presence of inclusions within the astrocytes. Divry, Titeca and Vermeylen (1935) found sudanophilic and birefringent material around the blood-vessels.

In the atrophied parts of the brain in Pick's disease one may find both 'senile' plaques and neurofibrillary changes. This was described by Liebers (1939) who regarded his case as one of Alzheimer's disease. The 5 cases of Pick's disease from Argentina described by Moyano (1931, 1932) all had this association of the lesions of Alzheimer's disease confined to the atrophic areas. Such cases, and there are other examples in the literature, are not the same as those rare instances of combined Alzheimer's and Pick's diseases such as have been reported by Berlin (1949): in his 2 cases not only were argyrophilic plaques and neurofibrillary changes widespread but there were focal atrophies in the 'primary shrinkage areas' with swollen cells containing argyrophilic cytoplasmic inclusions. Nor are they to be confused with cases of Alzheimer's disease which show a particularly severe involvement of one part of the brain (commonly the frontal lobes). Whatever be the essential mechanism of Alzheimer's disease it seems that its changes may occur in the focally atrophic parts of the brain in some instances of Pick's disease, and von Braunmühl's conception of the syneretic syndrome is consistent with this finding. The constancy of this association in Moyano's cases suggests that there may be some genetically or environmentally determined reason for it.

Buchanan, Overholt and Neubürger (1947) describe the findings of Pick's disease associated with parenchymatous cerebellar cortical atrophy in a woman of 45. Symptoms which had lasted for 5 years were thought to be due to multiple sclerosis. She died rather suddenly of a carcinoma of the bronchus with intracranial metastases. The focal cerebral atrophy involved the right insula, the hippocampi, temporal lobes and the caudate nuclei: the cerebellar atrophy concerned the entire dorsal surface and was associated with degeneration of the inferior olives. Argyrophilic plaques were found in the hippocampal gyrus, maximal in the atrophic part; they were also present in the frontal cortex which was not concerned in the atrophy.

Akelaitis (1944) commented on the presence of iron in his case, maximal in the globus pallidus and subthalamic nucleus, although there was none in the very atrophied caudate nucleus. The iron was contained in the oligodendroglia, the astrocytes and the nerve cells.

Onari and Spatz (1926) recognised the resemblance of Pick cells to cells undergoing axonal degeneration and Spatz (1952) has reaffirmed his belief that the degeneration in Pick's disease begins in the periphery of the neurone, in the white matter. This is in keeping with the view of Freeman (1933) who states that the white matter is the first part of the brain to be involved. Williams (1935) held that in order to produce Pick cells the site of axonal injury had to be near the cell of origin and it had also to be recent. It is wise in considering a case of this disease always to attempt to explain atrophy as secondary to disease elsewhere in the brain before assuming that it constitutes a primary shrinkage area.

The cause of this peculiar and systematic degeneration of nerve cells still remains conjectural. Ferraro and Jervis (1936) were impressed with the abrupt transitions between normal and pathological cortex and postulated that the disease might be the result of angiospasm, probably in predisposed tissue. Reich (1907) was the first to suggest that Pick's disease was a systemic atrophy and should be reckoned independent of senility. Richter (1918), reporting a case in a woman aged 37, commented on a histological resemblance, which however is only superficial, to amaurotic familial idiocy: he suggested that the disease was in the nature of an heredo-degeneration. The role of trauma in bringing out this condition has been noted by several authors (Reich 1907, Crezée 1949, Mansvelt 1954). This last author in his exhaustive monograph has stressed the importance of exogenous factors in many cases of the disease.

Arteriosclerosis is not a feature in this disease though naturally in later life it may be met with as a co-existing factor.

There are no associated post-mortem findings in the other organs of the body.

Huntington's Disease

In 1872, the year after his qualification, George Huntington described a mother and daughter with a familial disorder characterised by chorea, progressive mental deterioration and suicidal tendencies He had observed them in the family practice for twelve years but his grandfather, Abel Huntington, had known the family since his arrival in East Hampton, Long Island, in 1797. Huntington's now classical paper appeared 9 years after that of Lyon, who in 1863 described chronic hereditary chorea, including one family in which the disease had been known for five generations. Hereditary chorea is, however, also mentioned by Waters (1841) and by Bernt (1810) but it is not clear from the latter's account if he had met with Huntington's chorea or if he was referring to an hereditary tendency in some instances of Sydenham's chorea. Meynert (1871) too was familiar with progressive chorea in its gross pathological appearances but made no mention of its hereditary character.

The disease lasts on the average 13·7 years (Bell 1934) but it may prove fatal in 5 years or last as long as 30. Death is commonly the result of respiratory or other intercurrent illness. The onset is usually in the fourth decade but it may be delayed till into the eighth decade. In a series of 47 cases, however, Lyon (1962 a) found the average age of onset to be 52. In fact, it often begins in a family for the first time at a late age. It is often stated to exhibit the phenomenon of anticipation, but this has sometimes been doubted: however, this seems to have occurred in a Chinese family reported by Singer (1962). If, as Huntington showed, a generation escapes, the disease does not usually return. Falstein and Stone (1941) recorded 2 cases beginning just under the age of 17 but according to Bell (1934), who has collected together the family trees, 4 out of the 460 cases were reported to have begun under the age of 4. The disorder is believed to be transmitted by a single dominant gene (Entres 1931), so that children of an afflicted parent have a 50 per cent chance of inheriting it. Associated disorders such as mental deficiency and psychopathic tendencies are often met with in siblings, but seem to have been even commoner in the days when these poor victims of disease suffered persecution. Pleydell (1954) observes that choreic families appear to be drawn mainly from group IV of the Registrar-General's social classification, but two siblings in one of the families reported by him were decorated in the First World War, one of them twice and the other 3 times, prior to developing the disease.

It is a rare disorder. Pleydell however found an incidence of about 5 cases per 100,000 of the population in Northamptonshire, while Bickford and Ellison (1953) estimate its frequency in the rather static population of the Duchy of Cornwall as at least 5·57 per 100,000. A focus of disease in the Moray Firth area producing 47 cases has been reported by Lyon (1962 a). In the United States it is perhaps rather more frequent than in Great Britain (Vessie 1932). The disease is known in most countries.

The choreiform movements, which include the characteristic grimacing movements of the face, usually appear before the mental deterioration sets in and indeed in some cases mental changes do not develop. Wilson (1954) believed that the motor restlessness is due to the changes in the cerebral cortex rather than to those in the striatum. Occasionally, however, the derangement of mental function antedates the chorea while there are several cases on record

(Davenport and Muncey 1916, Worster-Drought and Allen 1929, and Curran 1930) in which the disease appears to have been 'sine chorea' throughout. Pohlisch (1941) found that the presenting symptoms tended to vary according to the age of onset and that while chorea was characteristic at the age of 35, it was more usual to find striatal rigidity when the disease began in the twenties and intention tremor when the age of onset was delayed until the sixties. An example of this is the report by Lindenberg (1960) of finding the changes of Huntington's disease in a man and his daughter, the latter having died at the age of 29 with a diagnosis of 'juvenile Parkinsonism'. Davenport and Muncey went so far as to suggest that there may be two essential components of the disease which may be inherited independently. Certainly one may find rare examples of senile chorea in which the atrophy is confined to the striatum (Alcock 1936) but which have not the hereditary character of Huntington's disease. Allegedly sporadic cases are difficult to substantiate, but Lyon (1962 b) reported two presumed examples beginning in women aged 45 and 47 respectively. In some families the disease has a characteristic pattern (Davenport 1915). Dyslalia, for instance, usually a late symptom, was often the first to appear in one of the families reported by Pleydell (1954) and rigidity has characterised others (Schob 1927, Hallervorden 1957 and Campbell, Corner, Norman and Urich 1961). Marchand, Achalle, Achalle and Fadenilke (1958) describe seven instances of psychosis in three generations of a family but only five of them had chorea. Korbsch (1933) records the histological findings of Pick's disease in the sister of a patient with Huntington's chorea.

The mental derangement is ushered in with disturbances of emotion, irritability and personality changes going on to apathy and dementia. Insight is usually lost. Minski and Guttmann (1938) have studied the prepsychotic personality of these patients and it would appear that early diagnosis may be facilitated by a careful study of members of afflicted families. Of great interest is their observation that a particular physique and physiognomy may accompany the disease through a family.

The pathological atrophy of the striatum was noted by Meynert (1871), and a brief account of the histology was given by Jelgersma (1908). Alzheimer (1911) gave a short but excellent description of the pathology of 3 cases, drawing attention not only to the striatal atrophy but also to that in the cerebral cortex and in the subthalamic nucleus. Ramsay Hunt (1917), too, found that the atrophy of the caudate nucleus and putamen was the conspicuous finding. A posthumous paper by Dunlap (1927) gives the pathological findings in 17 certain cases, 12 less certain and 30 controls. Like Kiesselbach (1914) he counted the cells in sample areas. Usually the brain shows a moderate degree of gyral atrophy especially in the frontal lobes and bordering on the Sylvian fissures. The ventricles usually show a moderate or even severe degree of dilatation but, because of the focal atrophy of the caudate nuclei which border on their lateral surfaces, the anterior horns may appear more dilated than the rest. Stone and Falstein (1938) found dilatation of ventricles mentioned in just over half the cases in the literature. With the atrophy of the caudate nucleus is an associated shrinkage of the putamen. Both these areas of grey matter may present a brownish discoloration. The corpus callosum is usually thinned (Fig. 9.11).

The essential feature of the disease is a primary loss of nerve cells in the caudate nucleus and in the putamen, especially of the smaller cells. With the loss of cells the neurofibrils become very scarce (Marie and Lhermitte 1914). Several authors have commented on the fact that the large cells of the striatum may be spared: but it is not unusual to see in them shrinkage and excess of lipochrome while neuronophagia has been reported (Davison *et al.* 1932). In all probability the large cells are more resistant than the smaller ones and only when the disease is well advanced are they seriously affected. It is essentially in the middle and posterior parts of the putamen that the atrophy is to be found and the extent of disease here is nearly always greater than in the caudate nucleus (Dunlap 1927). The anterior quarter of the putamen and the head of the caudate, especially in their most inferior parts (McCaughey 1961), are not so seriously involved. In spite of the fact that the neurones are numerically reduced the caudate nucleus, although shrunken in size, may give a superficial impression of increased cellularity because of the marked proliferation of astrocytes. Jelgersma (1908), in fact, speaks of 'colossal' increase in neuroglial elements. These cells can often be seen in clusters suggesting that repeated division has taken place. The nuclei are large and the cytoplasm is sometimes abundant. Alzheimer made no mention of the astrocytes showing fibrous processes but Marie and Lhermitte (1914) and Dunlap (1927) commented on their abundance, as also did Alcock (1936) in his account of the changes in senile chorea. Dunlap found, however, that in three brains which had been in formalin for 12 years, the processes stained imperfectly and he was inclined to blame the formalin for previous failures to demonstrate the fibrous processes. On the other

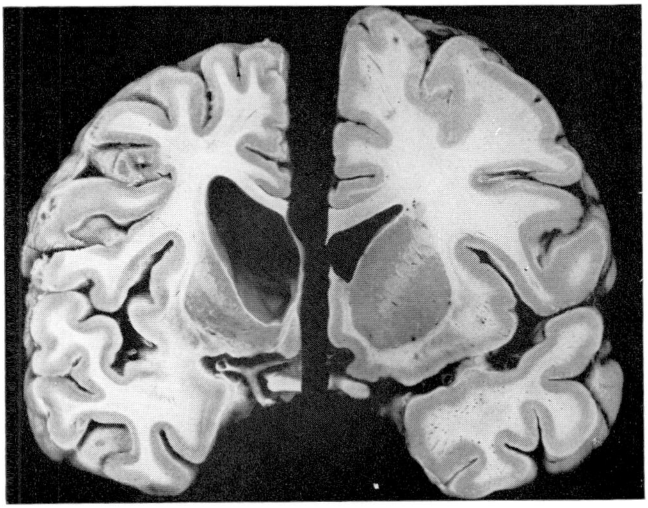

FIG. 9.11. *Huntington's disease.* The hemisphere on the left is from a case of this disease in a woman aged 49. (Brain weight 1,065 g.) That on the right is from a normal woman aged 69. (Brain weight 1,415 g.)

hand glial proliferation is sometimes reported as being slight (Hassin 1948). In our experience fibre formation is not a conspicuous feature of the astrocytes in the atrophic striatum, probably because the astrocytes here are normally protoplasmic (Fig. 9.12(*b*) and 13). Fibre formation, however, seems to be well developed just immediately deep to the ependyma and when astrocytes are found in relation to blood-vessels, a fact which has been commented upon by several authors. Sometimes the nerve cell loss in the caudate nucleus is so great as to cause a status spongiosus similar to that which is sometimes seen in the cortex in Pick's disease. With the loss of nerve cells there is a loss of nerve fibres, the surviving fibres tending to run together in bundles (status fibrosus of Vogt). Cell changes do not usually occur in the globus pallidus although this centre may be severely involved: the same is true of the subthalamic nucleus. Changes may occur in the substantia nigra and thalamus but in the red nucleus they are only minimal. Peters (1951) mentions atrophic changes in the cells of the dentate nucleus, while Davison *et al.* (1932) illustrate patchy cell loss in the granular layer of the cerebellum, which is not however convincing.

The blood-vessels in the affected ganglia often show secondary degenerative changes with, in more actively progressive cases, fat-filled histiocytes in the perivascular spaces. In general, however, microglial activity is not conspicuous. Iron pigment can sometimes be found, most often in relation to the adventitia of blood-vessels. Corpora amylacea are not uncommonly seen in great numbers especially in the subependymal layers.

Degeneration in the cerebral cortex has been noted by most workers and especially by Alzheimer (1911) who believed, however, that it was not the cause of the motor unrest. It amounts to a general reduction in neuronal population especially of layers 3, 5 and 6 with inconspicuous changes in some of those which survive, amounting to chromatolysis, excess of

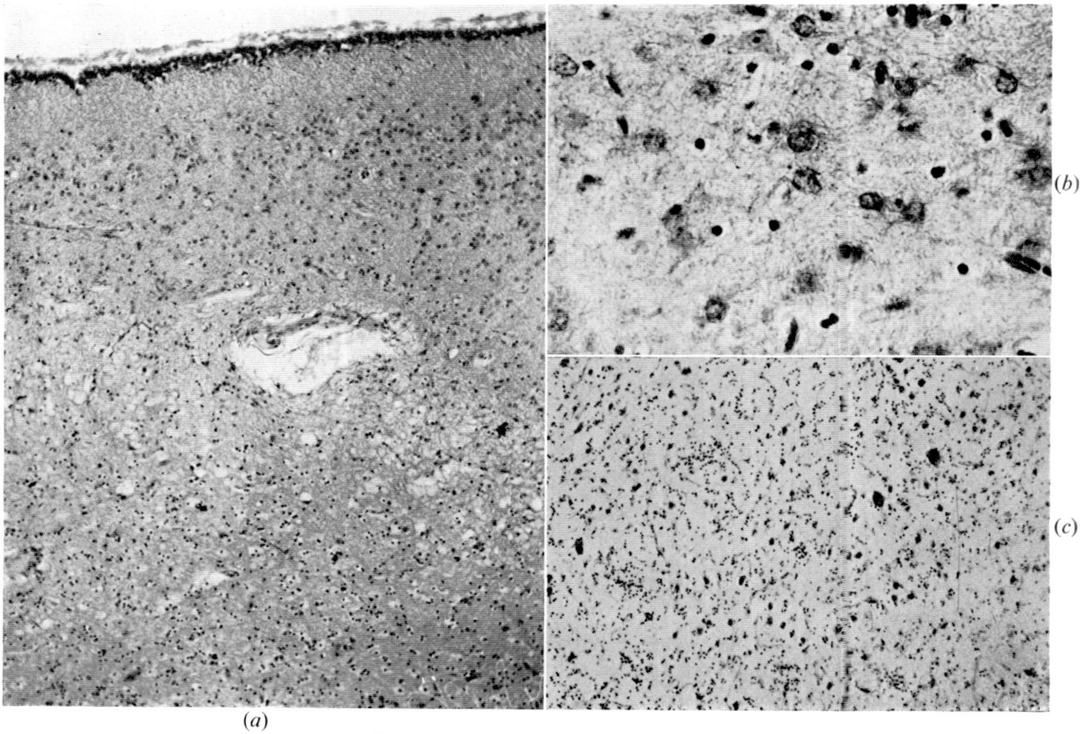

FIG. 9.12. *Huntington's disease.*

(*a*) Caudate nucleus showing a spongiose state due to almost complete disappearance of neurones: proliferation of astrocytes is most noticeable deep to the subependymal layer. (Celloidin. Haematoxylin-eosin, ×90.)

(*b*) Proliferating astrocytes near ventricular surface of caudate nucleus showing only scanty fibre formation. (Celloidin. Mallory's Phosphotungstic acid haematoxylin, ×400.)

(*c*) Putamen. The small neurones have largely disappeared but occasional large ones are to be seen. (Celloidin. Cresyl violet, ×90.)

lipochrome and chronic cell disease. C. and O. Vogt, however, commented on the vulnerability of layer 4 (Hallervorden 1930). Stone and Falstein (1938) found that the frontal and precentral cortex are especially involved. Dunlap (1927), however, believed that the cortical cells might not be reduced in numbers but only shrunken: he did not study the cortex quantitatively. McCaughey (1961) described the changes as those of 'simple, senile atrophy'. Glial changes are inconspicuous and there seems to be little compensatory reaction on the part of these cells: on the other hand there may be astroglial proliferation in the white matter. The myelin may be well preserved but Davison *et al.* (1932) illustrate extensive demyelination in the frontal and parietal lobes and also in the posterior two-thirds of the internal capsule of 1 of their cases. The leptomeninges are usually a little thickened.

It is commonly stated that the changes in the cortex are secondary to the cell loss in the striatum, but this is difficult to understand as these nuclei have so few connections with the cortex. Moreover Alcock (1936) has described the striatal changes of Huntington's chorea without cortical changes in 2 cases of non-hereditary senile chorea. It would rather appear that the cerebral cortex, and more particularly the frontal lobes, are involved as well as the caudate nucleus and putamen and that further studies may even lend confirmation to the contention of Davenport and Muncey (1916) that the cortical and central components of the disease may be inherited independently. A complicating feature in the study of this disease is that the symptomatology does not always tally with the pathological findings. The first of Davison's, *et al.* (1932), patients for instance had no mental symptoms when she died after an illness of $7\frac{1}{2}$ years but the cortex was involved from the frontal pole to the post-central gyrus. Their second patient, however, had mental symptoms but the cortical changes were slight. The patient with the rigid form of the disease reported by Campbell, Corner, Norman and Urich (1961) was found after death to have fibrillary gliosis of the putamen but not of the caudate nucleus, suggesting that the former centre was the first to be involved.

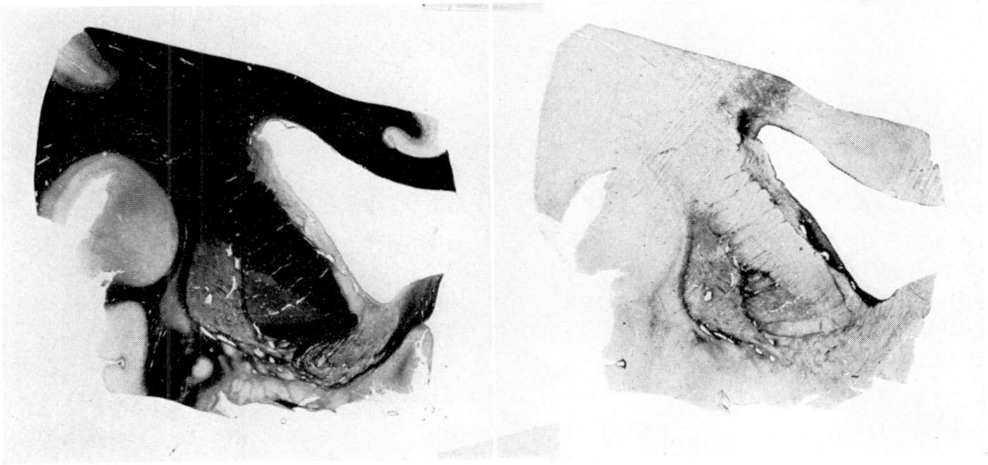

(*a*) (*b*)

FIG. 9.13. *Huntington's disease.* Coronal sections of the corpus striatum.
(*a*) Myelin stain.
(*b*) Holzer's neuroglial fibre stain.

Of recent years there has been a tendency to locate the basis of choreiform and other involuntary movements at a lower level than the corpus striatum (Mettler 1957), and the lesions which have been described in the subthalamic nucleus in Huntington's disease may be specially important in this respect. Cases of progressive chorea, in which the lesions were severe in this centre but were minimal in the striatum, have been reported by Casper (1930), Titeca and van Bogaert (1946) and others. Malamud (1960) has described marked atrophy and gliosis of the subthalamic nucleus as the predominant finding in two siblings dying in late childhood with choreiform movements and behaviour disorders: he reports similar findings in a 36-year-old woman with chorea and mild dementia whose mother may have had the same condition.

Huntington's disease, which is generally regarded as essentially abiotrophic in character, bears a close pathological resemblance to Pick's disease when the latter involves the striatum, as it sometimes does, and the two conditions have once been reported in the same family (Korbsch).

Simma (1952) attempted to set out the essential differences between the two diseases so far as the striatum is concerned but they are not as clear-cut as he suggests. In Pick's disease, however, the large cells of the striatum are involved as well as the small ones, whereas in Huntington's disease the large cells tend to be spared or involved late; also in Pick's disease the caudal half of the putamen tends to be spared, which is not the case in Huntington's disease. In both diseases, if the striatum is at all heavily involved, the globus pallidus, the centromedial nucleus of the thalamus, the subthalamic nucleus, the substantia nigra, and the superior olivary nucleus may be atrophied. A loss of cells was noted in the dentate nucleus by McCaughey (1961) in 9 out of 21 cases: it was marked in 3. In general the atrophy of the basal ganglia in Huntington's disease appears to be more localised and selective in its choice of cell than in Pick's disease.

Van der Eecken, Adams and van Bogaert (1960) have described a condition characterised clinically by extrapyramidal rigidity with minimal tremor and pathologically by pronounced shrinkage and brownish discoloration of parts of the putamen and globus pallidus and depigmentation of the substantia nigra. There was a virtual disappearance of the small cells of the caudate nucleus and putamen. While this condition appears to have affinities with Huntington's disease, the authors prefer to call it *striopallidal-nigral degeneration.*

Difficulty is seldom experienced in distinguishing between Huntington's chorea and the striatal variety of the Creutzfeldt-Jakob disease. In general the former disease is chronic and focal while the latter is subacute and widespread.

Pathological changes in other organs have seldom been reported and there is no clue, as there is in Wilson's disease, to any extracerebral associated disorder. Lhermitte and Porak (1914), however, noted hyperplasia of the parathyroids in a 52-year-old subject whose disease had lasted 8 years. The first patient of Davison *et al.* (1932) died of a severe secondary anaemia while a patient of Jakob's had a macrocytic anaemia, but in these cases a fortuitous association of diseases cannot be excluded.

It is not clear if trauma can precipitate this condition but Claude, Lhermitte and Meignant (1930) report an interesting case of mild chorea in a male aged 36, an observer in a military balloon who in 1916 made a faulty parachute landing. Following this he suffered a recrudescence of his chorea and developed dementia and rigidity. At necropsy the small cells of the putamen and caudate nucleus had gone and the large cells were reduced in number. Posteriorly, at the junction of the putamen with the globus pallidus the vessels were cuffed with leucocytes and there was proliferation of the microglia.

The Creutzfeldt-Jakob disease

This name is given to a progressive dementia with pyramidal and extrapyramidal signs, often with amyotrophy, associated with widespread nerve cell degeneration in the brain and spinal cord. The condition has several synonyms including *spastic pseudosclerosis* and *cortico-striato-spinal atrophy*. Many regard it not as a disease but as a group of diseases and recently there have been attempts to separate them. The number of cases adequately studied is still too few to form any conclusions especially in view of the diversity of symptoms and the widespread nature of the pathology. It is probably a commoner condition than is generally imagined but as the pathological changes, unlike those of Alzheimer's and Pick's diseases, are sometimes non-spectacular and difficult to demonstrate and still more difficult to interpret, the study of these brains is often shelved.

In 1920 Creutzfeldt described the first case in a woman of 23 with motor, sensory and psychical disturbances. The illness proved fatal in 6 weeks. In the brain he noted focal destruction of cortical nerve cells with neuronophagia, reparative changes in the glia and some vascular proliferation. The illustrations show a convincing loss of cells in the 3rd cortical layer with reactive changes which include the presence of rod cells and glial rosettes in the thalamus. In the following year Jakob reported 3 cases of progressive dementia with focal neurological signs associated at necropsy with a widespread degeneration of nerve cells especially in the frontal and temporal lobes, the corpus striatum, the ventromedial nucleus of the thalamus, the substantia nigra, the Purkinje cells and the motor cells of the medulla and cord. The pallidum was little affected as were also the parietal and occipital cortex. Jakob likened his cases to that of Creutzfeldt and called the condition *spastic pseudosclerosis* (because of a resemblance of the neurological findings to those of multiple sclerosis) or *encephalomyelopathy with disseminated degenerative lesions*. The apathy, depression, catatonia and epileptiform seizures with eventual dementia, in addition to the neurological symptoms and a relentless and rapid course sometimes lasting under a year, provide a distinctive pattern of disease.

In 1929 Meyer reported the case of a disease resembling amyotrophic lateral sclerosis but with psychical disorders which he believed to be 'a bridge' between amyotrophic lateral sclerosis and the Creutzfeldt-Jakob disease. Davison (1932) described 2 similar cases. The acceptance of these cases as variants of the Creutzfeldt-Jakob disease has tended to cause confusion and, in the opinion of some, to widen the nosological concept too much, but Jakob did comment on involvement of the anterior horn cells in his cases.

In 1938 Jansen and Monrad-Krohn reviewed the disease as it was then known and drew attention to the rigidity, to the coarse tremor and to the occasional presentation in the form of a psychosis. They commented on a histological resemblance to Pick's disease but regarded the involvement of the anterior central gyrus as typical of the Creutzfeldt-Jakob disease.

Jakob (1923) provided two further cases and kept in mind the possibility of the disease being a complication of the von Economo encephalitis which was then still endemic. Kirschbaum (1924), who described two additional cases from Jakob's laboratory, commented on fatty degeneration in some of the surviving cells.

Hallervorden (1930) and Jansen and Monrad-Krohn (1938) considered many unusual cases of rapid dementia with neurological symptoms which had accumulated in the literature but were not prepared to accept more than a few of them into the group.

Wilson (1940 a) stressed the amyotrophy and gave the name of *cortico-striato-spinal degeneration* to a condition characterised by degeneration in various motor centres associated with dementia and sometimes with extrapyramidal symptoms. According to Meyer, Leigh and Bagg (1954), about a third of the reported instances of the Creutzfeldt-Jakob group fall into this category. Jervis, Hurdum and O'Neill (1942), in reporting a case, reviewed the literature up to that time.

The essential features of the Creutzfeldt-Jakob disease, as now understood, are the extrapyramidal symptoms in association with psychic disorders and amyotrophy. The course varies from 3 months to about 3 years. Most cases have occurred in middle-aged persons but it has been described at the age of 20 (Stender 1930). There is no special sex incidence. After an initial period of undue fatiguability, with loss of memory, strange behaviour and a mood of general apathy, neurological symptoms develop including ataxia, dysarthria, spasticity of the limbs, choreo-athetosis and muscular wasting. A Parkinsonian syndrome may occur (Stengel and Wilson 1949). The march of symptoms varies according to whether the brunt of the disease is cortical, striatal or spinal, but in typical cases all three functional levels are involved simultaneously to lesser or greater degree. An instance of this disease occurring with extraordinary frequency in a family named Backer has been reported (Kirschbaum 1924, Meggendorfer 1930, and Jacob, Pyrkosch and Strube 1950).

At post-mortem the brain usually appears normal. There is seldom any obvious atrophy and there is no thickening of the leptomeninges. The ventricles may be dilated but most often

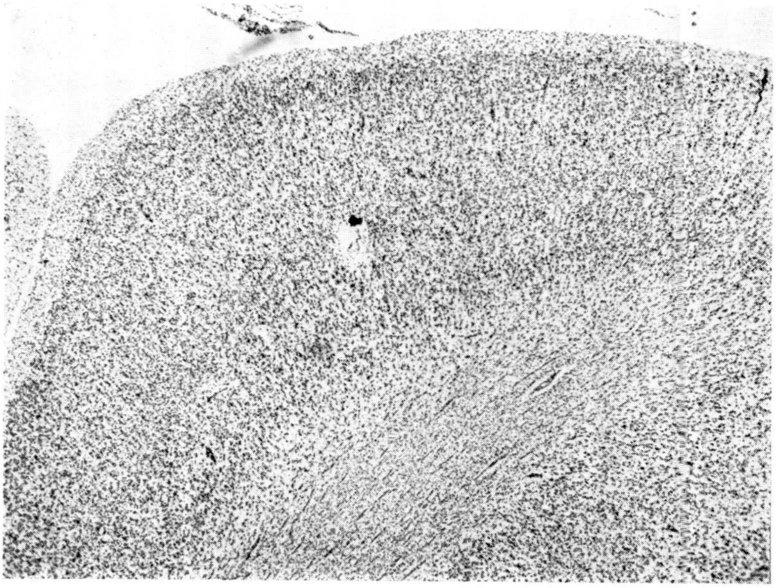

(a)

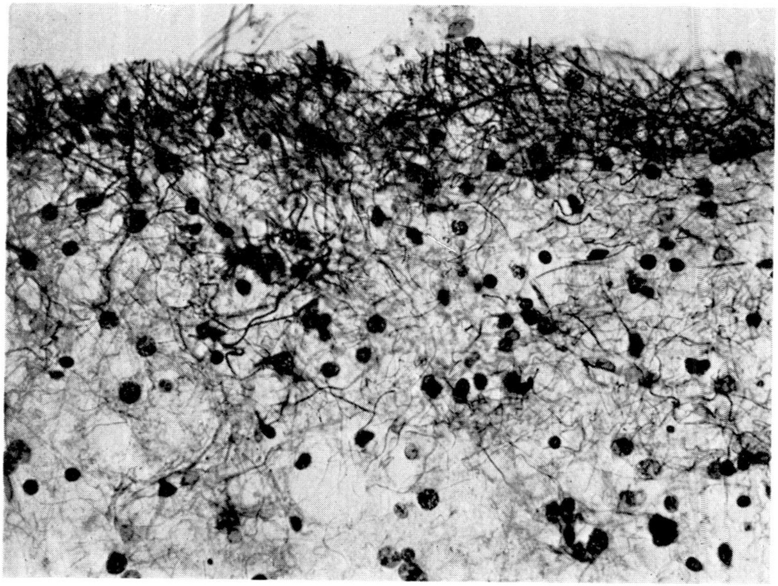

(b)

FIG. 9.14. *Creutzfeldt-Jakob disease.*

(a) Frontal cortex showing almost complete disappearance of large pyramidal cells. (Nissl ×20.)
(b) Subpial layer of frontal cortex (Holzer ×350).

they are not and the blood-vessels appear healthy. The nerve-cell loss, however, is widespread and may be considerable throughout the brain and cord. The line of Baillarger may disappear. Neuronophagia is sometimes observed. Most of the nerve cells are shrunken but often there is a relative excess of lipochrome. The larger cells, including the Betz cells and the cells of the anterior horns, may be swollen with lipochrome and even larger than normal but they too are liable to degeneration. The cell loss is maximum in the deeper layers but it is patchy. The frontal and temporal lobes seem to be affected most. Neurofibrils become rarefied and in some instances the typical neurofibrillary alterations of Alzheimer have been found (Jervis *et al.* 1942). Stengel and Wilson (1949) observed a few 'senile' plaques in the

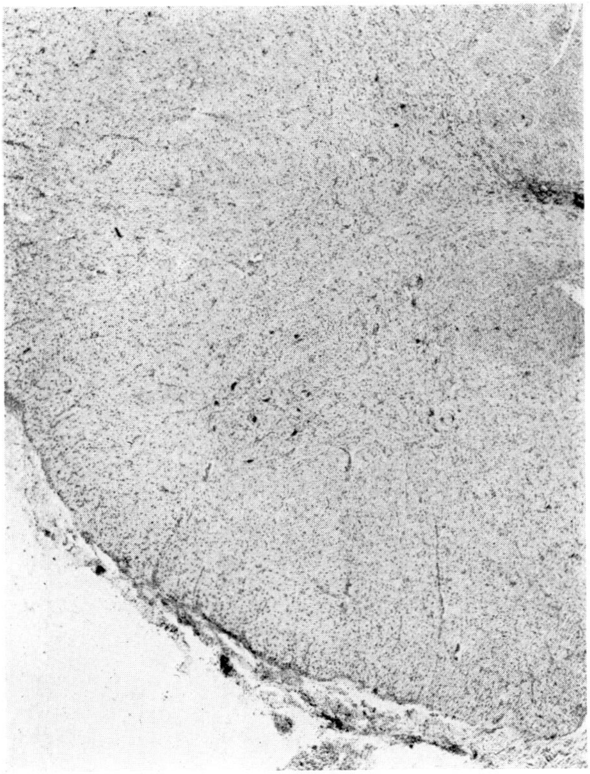

FIG. 9.15. *Creutzfeldt-Jakob disease.* Section of spinal cord at level L.3 showing almost complete disappearance of motor nerve cells. (Nissl ×25.)

depths of sulci but they failed to find any neurofibrillary tangles. The latter however have been noted by Jervis, Hurdum and O'Neill (1942). The astrocytes undergo considerable proliferation and form some fibrous processes. Glial rosettes in the cortex and basal ganglia are a feature of this disease: they tend to be found around acellular areas from which it is presumed that nerve fibres have disappeared. These glial scars may be seen also in the superficial layers of the white matter.

The white matter usually appears normal with no loss of myelin and no gliosis but diffuse degeneration of the centrum semi-ovale has been reported. The blood-vessels look blameless in the majority of cases and compound granular corpuscles are not normally found in the perivascular spaces. Only in the case of Teichmann (1935) has perivascular cuffing been noted.

In the spinal cord there can be seen, in addition to atrophy of some of the anterior horn cells (Fig. 9.15), degeneration of the tracts but with no particular pattern. Korey, Scheinberg, Terry and Stein (1961) in their electronmicroscopical study of a biopsy specimen noted a distortion of the protein synthesis apparatus of the neurones and—an observation of considerable interest—a distension of the presynaptic process with numerous small laminated bodies interspersed among the synaptic vesicles, suggesting a fault at the synapse.

A resemblance between this condition and pellagra has often been commented upon while Jervis *et al.* (1942) and Stengel and Wilson (1949) have suggested that nutritional deficiency may be a factor in its aetiology. Several of the earlier case reports of the Creutzfeldt-Jakob disease may, in point of fact, have been instances of cerebral pellagra. Plumbism, barbiturate intoxication and alcoholism are other conditions which may need to be considered in the differential diagnosis. It has been described in its classical form following an accident (Behrman, Mandybur and McMenemey 1963). The extraordinary Backer family, which now claims 14 cases in four generations and to which reference has already been made, suggests that a genetic factor can at times be responsible. Davison and Rabiner's (1940) is the only other record of this disease being a familial disorder, two brothers and one sister being concerned. Nevertheless a few authors like Jakob (1923) and Marchand and Abély (1948) have tended to put this disease in the group of abiotrophies, the latter seeing a link between it and Pick's disease: but the evidence so far is not convincing.

The most likely cause would seem to be one or more enzyme deficiencies induced perhaps by toxic factors which affect a wide range of nerve cells bringing about their death. The age of onset and the occasional familial incidence would be in keeping with an endogenous deficiency. The resemblance to cerebrospinal pellagra is sufficient to warrant further studies along the line of enzyme dysfunction.

Conditions possibly allied to, but at present distinguished from, the Creutzfeldt-Jakob disease

In 1928 Heidenhain described 3 cases of progressive parenchymatous degeneration of the cerebrum, 2 of them rapid, which had several features in common with the Creutzfeldt-Jakob disease. In 2 of Heidenhain's cases, however, a predominant symptom was amaurosis and the incidence of the disease was particularly heavy on the occipital cortex. In his first case there was no involvement of the frontal cortex and dementia was not a symptom. There was, however, permanent tonic tension of all muscles and athetoid movements of the upper limbs. Histological changes in the occipital lobe consisted of shrinkage and loss of nerve cells, most marked in the 4th lamina, with proliferation of the protoplasmic and fibrous astrocytes. Changes were less severe in the parietal cortex and insula and very slight in the frontal and precentral regions. Status spongiosus was present in 2 of the cases in the more severely affected areas. Meyer, Leigh and Bagg (1954) have described a further instance of what they name *Heidenhain's syndrome*, and have suggested that the first 2 cases of Heidenhain's and their own justify consideration as a separate syndrome in that the course in each instance varied between 4 and 6 months, the disease had a peculiar predilection for, although it was not always confined to, the occipital and especially the calcarine cortex, and the basal ganglia were not apparently involved. Cortical blindness in association with dementia were the symptoms. The ages of the 3 patients were 55 (Heidenhain, case I), 53 (Heidenhain, case II) and 38 (case of Meyer *et al.*) respectively. Meyer, Leigh and Bagg did not accept Heidenhain's 3rd case, presumably because the history extended over a period of 6 years and also because blindness was not a symptom. However, the occipital cortex was heavily involved and it is possible that amaurosis may have existed terminally but was obscured by the profound dementia (Fig. 9.16).

Rauch (1948) has described a condition which Peters (1951) regards as half way between the classical disease of Creutzfeldt-Jakob and the syndrome of Heidenhain. Although this patient's memory was not appreciably impaired (his symptoms were restlessness and loss of consciousness) the nerve cells of the frontal lobe as well as of the inferior temporal convolution, the gyrus fusiformis and the spinal cord were involved. The affected cells were mostly swollen. The glia was only a little proliferated but some rosettes and clusters of proliferated glia were seen. They regard the condition as a primary disease of the neurones, probably toxic in origin.

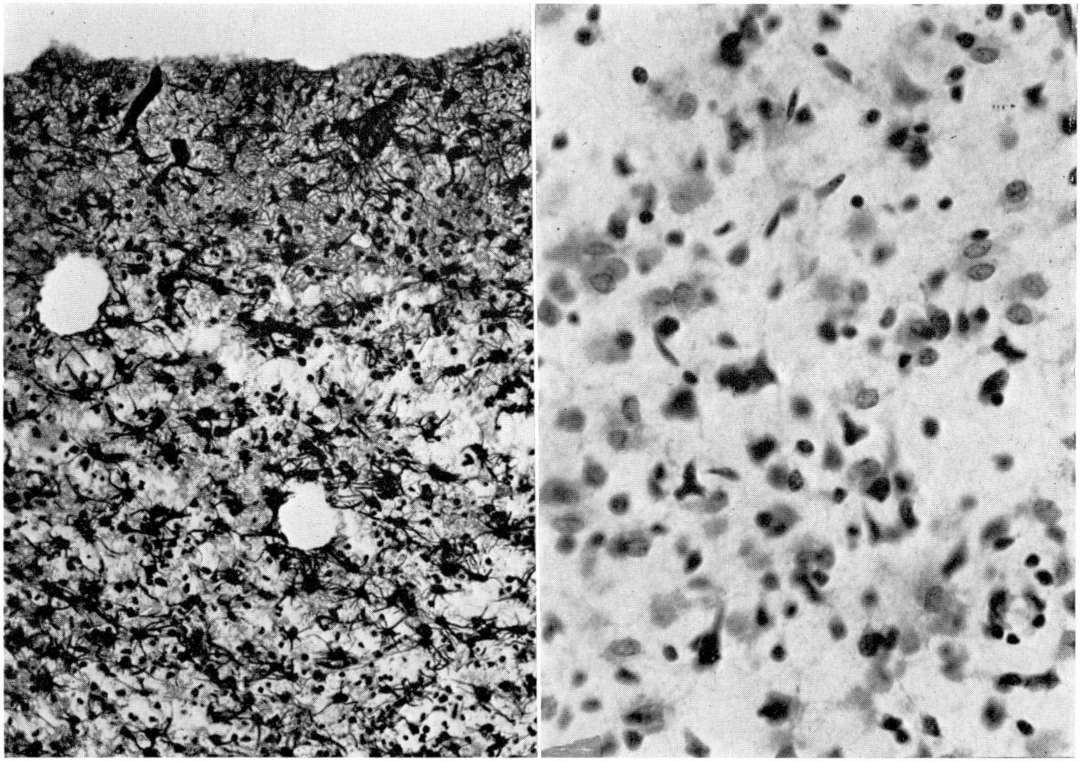

(*a*) (*b*)

FIG. 9.16. *Subacute cortical atrophy* of Heidenhain type. (Case of Meyer, Leigh and Bagg 1954.) Occipital cortex.

(*a*) Stained by silver carbonate. ×150.
(*b*) Nissl stain, showing degeneration of nerve cells and astrocytic hyperplasia. ×500.

Claude, Lhermitte and Baruk (1932) described the case of a 57-year-old man who was suddenly overcome with generalised trembling while visiting a parent. He rapidly developed a catatonic syndrome, pseudobulbar lesions and a widespread mental disturbance. He had an extreme degree of bulimia, ate rubbish and became profoundly emaciated. The brain showed atrophic changes in the thalamus with loss of small cells in the striatum, and degeneration of ganglion cells in the second frontal convolution. The integrity of the pyramidal system and of the cerebellum was a striking feature. The authors believed that only a toxin could cause so rapid and peculiar a picture but they noted that 2 years previously he had suffered a serious head injury. This case appears to have an affinity with the Creutzfeldt-Jakob group.

Alajouanine and van Bogaert (1950) have described two instances of a subacute disease associated with diffuse tetanoid contractures, hyperkinesis and visual hallucinations. Histologically they found areas of cell loss with gliosis especially in the striate cortex, but in general were impressed with the relative paucity of anatomical findings to account for such a striking clinical picture. They postulated a functional disorder of the cerebral blood-vessels possibly due to the action of toxins. Such cases do not necessarily have dementia but their relationship to the condition under discussion cannot be doubted. Three somewhat similar cases are described by Pallis and Spillane (1957) under the heading of *subacute progressive encephalopathy with rigidity, hypokinesia, mutism and myoclonus*. The third of their cases had a slight amount of cortical scarring suggestive of disease of some of the penetrating arterioles. Garcin and his co-workers (1950) reported two cases of extrapyramidal rigidity, involuntary movements and psychic disorder in two patients in late middle age that proved fatal in 3 and 2 months respectively. There was widespread loss of cells in the striatum and thalamus as well as in various parts of the cerebral cortex. The proliferating astrocytes were characterised by '*noyaux nus*'. More recently they have described three further cases (Garcin *et al.* 1962).

Under the name *subacute vascular encephalopathy*, Jones and Nevin (1954) have described 2 cases of rapidly progressive cerebral degeneration characterised by mental disorder, focal disturbances and myoclonic epilepsy. There was no hypertension. An unusual pattern of electro-encephalographic changes was noted in each of their patients. The changes were similar in the two brains but more marked in the first, which showed a general loss of cortical neurones, marked glial overgrowth and a peculiar status spongiosus in the most severely involved parts (Fig. 9.17). They liken their cases to those of Heidenhain and attribute the condition, in the absence of any evidence of organic disease of the cerebral blood-vessels, to their abnormal function. They base their contention on the facts that there was no evidence of any toxic or infective element but that, on the contrary, several acute softenings were found. Into this same group they are prepared to accept the cases of Fischer (1910) and Hallervorden (1930 (ii)).

Foley and Denny-Brown (1955) have given, under the heading of *subacute progressive encephalopathy with bulbar myoclonus*, 3 case reports, with two necropsies, which they regard as a unique disease. Amaurosis is not mentioned as a symptom but in the necropsy report of their third case the occipital cortex was one of the most severely damaged areas. In their first patient, whose illness lasted for 13 months, macroscopic atrophy of the cerebral and cerebellar cortices with dilatation of the ventricles was found at necropsy. There was an extreme degree of cell loss in the granular layer but many Purkinje cells survived. They attributed this disease to a primary degeneration of the protoplasmic astroglia: the status spongiosus which was present they regarded as a measure of the acuteness of the process.

Jacob, Eiche and Orthner (1958) described 4 further instances of this condition under the title of *Subacute Presenile Spongiform Atrophy with a Dyskinetic Endstage* and Nevin, McMenemey, Behrman and Jones (1960) 8 additional cases. Both groups of authors regard it as probably distinct from the Creutzfeldt-Jakob disease. In the latter series previous brain damage had occurred in half of the cases. Other instances of what appear to be the same condition have been reported by Alema and Bignami (1959), Kramer (1959), and Garcin, Brion and Khochneviss (1962). A case of Pick's disease with rapid evolution reported by Schmidt (1959) appears to be another instance.

Nevin *et al.* (1960) have set out the ways in which subacute spongiform encephalopathy differs from the Creutzfeldt-Jakob disease of classical type. In the former any part of the cerebral cortex may be involved but there is a predilection for the occipital lobe: in the latter the emphasis of the cortical component is characteristically temporo-central. Fragmentation of the affected neurones with the appearance of small darkly staining and often triangular fragments is characteristic of the former disease whereas in the latter shrinkage of the whole cell

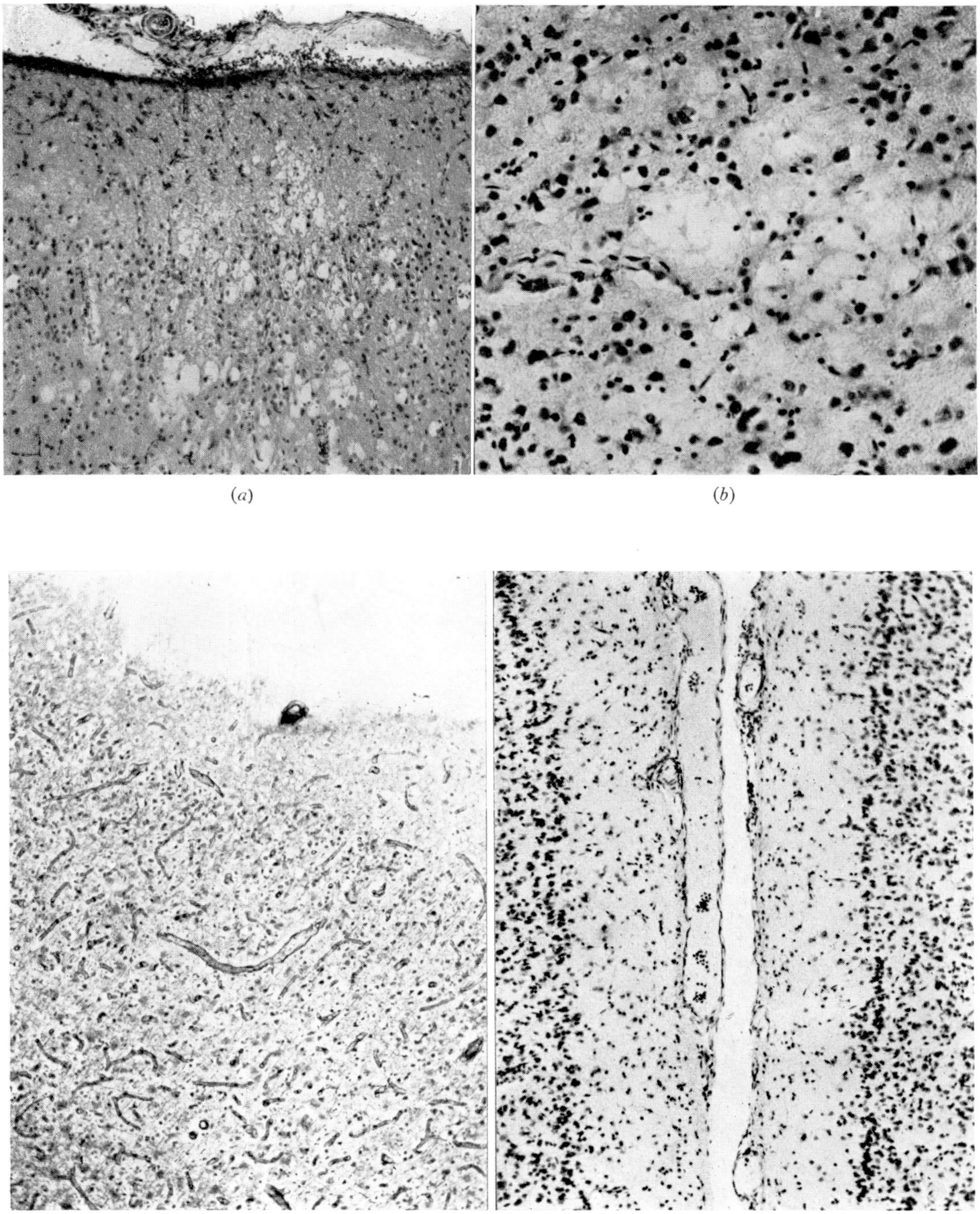

(a) (b)

(c) (d)

FIG. 9.17. *Subacute cortical atrophy.* (Cases of Jones and Nevin 1954.)

(*a*) and (*b*) show cortical atrophy of spongy type (Case 1).
(*c*) An area of more severe degeneration in the frontal cortex, showing hyperplasia of the capillaries (Case 1).
(*d*) Neuroglial hyperplasia at junction of molecular and external granular layers (Case 2).

occurs, often with a corkscrew apical dendrite. The glial rosettes and neuronophagia seen in the Creutzfeldt-Jakob disease are not characteristic of the other condition, in which the astrocytes tend to be gemistocytic. Brain-stem and spinal cord involvement is characteristic of Jakob's disease but in subacute spongiform encephalopathy death seems to occur before significant changes in these areas can take place. Finally, status spongiosus is rare in the former condition and common although not invariably constant in the latter disease. Khochneviss (1962) who recognises 4 clinical and pathological types of the Creutzfeldt-Jakob disease, namely the classical (33 cases), the amyotrophic (14 cases), the thalamic (6 cases) and the Heidenhain (9 cases) will not accept all of the cases of Nevin and his co-workers as coming within the as yet ill-defined group of subacute spongiform encephalopathy.

Status spongiosus, it will be noted, has been reported in Heidenhain's syndrome, and was found in the cases of Jones and Nevin, Foley and Denny-Brown and in some of those reported by Nevin and his colleagues. It has also been described in several cases of the Creutzfeldt-Jakob disease. It was observed by von Stender in the deeper layers of the cortex in his case of spastic pseudosclerosis, while Marchand and Abély (1948) refer to an 'aspect areolaire' in the deeper layers of the cortex and in the central grey matter. Perhaps, as appears to have been the case with their patient, it may be looked for especially in those examples of the disease which have a rapid course. The significance of this condition is not understood, but it has been reviewed by Spielmeyer (1922), Bielschowsky (1911) and Sträussler and Koskinas (1926). Status spongiosus is unlikely to be always the result of the same process. A spongy state of the cortex may occur in Pick's disease and in Alpers' disease ('progressive degeneration of the grey matter') but in these conditions the cell loss is so profound that the spaces formerly occupied by the cells remain empty, the fibrous glia being inadequate to fill in the vacuum. In the conditions we now describe the status spongiosus is patchy as if an exudate were forcing bubbles between the cells. Indeed normal nerve cells and proliferated glia may be identified on the periphery of the bubbles. Sträussler and Koskinas (1926) suggest that status spongiosus may result if there is obstruction to the flow of cerebrospinal fluid within the brain but they appear to have associated the disorder with arteriosclerosis. Jones and Nevin, however, believe that their patients had disordered function of the cerebral vessels: one of their patients had in the early stage of the illness a right-sided hemiplegia with oedema of the left hemisphere evidenced angiographically. In the case reported by Schmidt (1959) oedematous infiltration of the cortical arterioles with transudations is illustrated in Figure 3.

Stern (1939) studied the brain of a 41-year-old man with a severe dementia associated with drowsiness, thirst and polyuria. He displayed a marked inertia and a loss of pupillary reflexes. At necropsy he was found to have a severe parenchymatous degeneration of the thalamus with a consecutive glial response. Changes of a rather less degree were present in the cerebral cortex and in the inferior olives. This case has sometimes been regarded as an unusual form of Pick's disease, but Stern regarded it as a pure system degeneration involving the thalamus. Schulman (1956) reported a case of bilateral symmetrical degeneration of the thalamus, especially of the dorsal medial and lateral posterior nuclei, in a 50-year-old male who died after a 6-months history of progressive intellectual deterioration, with choreic and clonic movements in the last weeks of life. The cell loss was accompanied by a moderate gliosis. In the cortex and white matter there was a mild to moderate gliosis. Khochneviss (1962) has included the cases of Stern and Schulman under the heading of the thalamic form of the Creutzfeldt-Jakob disease.

There is clearly a need for futher analysis and categorisation of these cases which sometimes have been assigned to the Creutzfeldt-Jakob group of diseases. Bornstein and Jervis (1955), in reporting 2 cases of *presenile dementia of the Jakob type*, recognise one parent disease with three clinicopathological sub-groups, namely spinostriocortical, striocorticospinal and corticostriospinal. This view is shared by Schwarz and Barrows (1958) who under the title of *Polioencephalomyelopathy reminiscent of the Creutzfeldt-Jakob syndrome* report finding conspicuous lymphocytic cuffing of blood vessels in the upper half of the cord and cell changes there and also in the brain-stem and cerebellum. This patient had first noted unsteadiness while walking and one week later had developed diplopia and emotional lability. He died after an illness of 18 months characterised by episodes of nausea and vomiting, myoclonus and finally wasting of all muscles. Jones and Nevin and Foley and Denny-Brown have attempted to explain the disease, the one on the basis of vascular insufficiency, the other as a dyscrasia of the astrocytes. Silberman, Cravicoto and Feigin (1961), impressed with the intense activity of the astrocytes in three cases of rapid evolution, refer to the likelihood of noxious factors being responsible and draw an analogy with hepatic encephalopathy.

Until more is known about the nature of these conditions it would seem best to regard them for the time being as constituting a group of disorders of like character but not necessarily all caused by the same agent. The peculiar predilection for the occipital cortex, which characterises the cases of Heidenhain and others and for the thalamus, striking features in the cases of Stern, Schulman and of Garcin *et al.*, justifies their recognition as distinct patterns within the group. The relentless march of symptoms, the frequency with which cases prove fatal in from eight to sixteen weeks, and the behaviour of the glia suggest the possibility that drug intoxication may be the prime cause in some of them although an infective agent should always be sought. Such topographical and cytological differences as distinguish the classical form of the Creutzfeldt-Jakob disease from these several conditions may have to do with interference of varying enzyme systems according to the nature of the intoxicant and the stability of the individual's blood brain barrier. Whatever the cause the mechanism of the encephalopathy would appear to be dyshoric.

'Parkinsonism—Dementia Complex of Guam'

Under this title Hirano and his associates (1961) describe a disease clinically resembling the Creutzfeldt-Jakob syndrome, often familial and responsible for the deaths of 70 per cent of the adult Chamorro population on the island of Guam. It is sometimes associated with that form of amyotrophic lateral sclerosis which has been reported by Kurland and Mulder (1954) as being common in this race: the two conditions are to be regarded as variants of the same process. Pathological examinations on 17 cases (Hirano, Malamud and Kurland 1961) revealed widespread ganglion cell degeneration with neurofibrillary degeneration and granulovacuolar degeneration, abundant in the hippocampus but present also in frontal and temporal cortex, amygdaloid nucleus, hypothalamus, periaqueductal grey matter, thalamus, pallidum, tegmentum, substantia nigra and locus caeruleus. Reactive glial proliferation was noted in the affected areas with gliosis of the mamillary bodies. Conspicuous by their absence were argyrophilic plaques, Lewy bodies and inflammatory reaction. The visual cortex seemed to be largely spared.

Except for its peculiar racial incidence within the Mariana islands and the frequency with which neurofibrillary degeneration is found there is nothing inconsistent with the view that this is a form of the Creutzfeldt-Jakob disease. It appears premature to exclude a toxic factor as being in part at least responsible.

Kuru

This fatal disease was first recognised by McArthur in 1954 and has since been extensively studied (Gajdusek and Zigas 1957, 1959; Simpson, Lander and Robson 1959; Fowler and Robertson 1959; Klatzo, Gajdusek and Zigas 1959). It appears to be confined to members of the

Fore tribe in the Eastern Highlands of New Guinea and amongst them it has a morbidity rate of 1 per cent and claims the lives, it has been estimated, of more than half the women and 10 per cent of the males. About three-quarters of the cases occur in women and the remaining quarter in children, boys and girls being equally affected. It has not been reported in infancy and it is rare in men. Epidemiological studies today suggest that it is a genetically determined disease with a dominant trait and incomplete penetration: but the influence of toxic factors has by no means been excluded.

Clinically the disease first shows as a cerebellar type of ataxia (hence the Fore name of *Kuru*, meaning 'the shakes') which before long renders walking and speech impossible. Euphoria and convergent strabismus follow, then finally dysphasia, incontinence and some degree of intellectual deterioration. Death usually occurs in six to nine months but it may be delayed for three years.

Pathologically the disease has been thought by Klatzo and his colleagues to approximate most to the Creutzfeldt-Jakob group but there are many differences. There are varying neuronal changes which because of the field conditions under which the necropsies are conducted require care in their interpretation. They include amongst others cytoplasmic vacuolation, excessive lipochrome content, neuronophagia and binucleation of nerve cells. The parts most affected are the brain stem, striatum, thalamus, dentate nucleus, cerebellar cortex and olives. Neuronal changes in the cerebral cortex are not marked and perhaps not significant but an astrocytosis is noticeable here as indeed it is almost everywhere in the brain. Demyelination is to be seen in the corticospinal and spino-cerebellar tracts and in the cerebellum. Perivascular cuffing with lymphocytes was noted by Klatzo and his associates in many cases, and in about half of them anisotropic plaque-like bodies in the cerebellum which lack the well-defined halo of the classical argyrophilic plaques. In the mamillary bodies astroglial proliferation with cyst formation has been noted. The widespread astrocytosis suggests the operation of a toxic substance.

Kraepelin's disease

Kraepelin (1910) first described a rare form of dementia, which now bears his name; 17 cases have been reported to date. It consists of rapidly progressive mental deterioration with restlessness, anxiety, depression, speech defects, and sometimes catatonia, and lasts 1 or 2 years. Oksala (1923) reported post-mortem findings in three patients from Kraepelin's clinic, aged 47, 59 and 48 respectively. Catatonia was present in the first 2 cases, diagnosed as *pernicious presenile psychosis*, with symptoms lasting respectively 9 and 3 months. The illness of the third patient also lasted 3 months and was associated with delusions, rapid loss of weight and eventually paralysis of one half of the face. In each case the essential feature appeared to be a phased destruction of the Nissl substance and consequent breaking up of the ganglion cells. Fat could be demonstrated in the cells and around the blood-vessels and there was neuronophagia and evidence of axis cylinder degeneration. The most affected areas were the frontal, the central and Ammon's horn, and the least, the occipital. The 3rd lamina was most concerned in this change with the 5th next: there was not much involvement of the 6th lamina. The changes were patchy in distribution. The father of the third patient was insane.

Best (1941) reported the necropsy findings of a further case of Kraepelin's presenile dementia in a man aged 34. The illness began as an acute catatonic psychosis leading to an expansive type of organic dementia and it proved fatal in 5 months. There was a family history of mental instability on the maternal side. She describes and illustrates swollen ganglion cells with an homogeneous, pale and glassy cytoplasm sometimes obscuring the nucleus, but sometimes associated with swelling of the nucleoli. This change appeared to affect the larger cells, including the Betz cells, but other neurones showed the severe cell change of Nissl. Fat was not identified in the swollen cells but was present around the blood-vessels. Neuronal degeneration was most evident in layers 1, 2 and 3, but it also involved the cells of the striatum, pallidum and dentate nucleus. Caution is necessary in interpreting these changes for the mode of death was asphyxiation due to the inhalation of vomitus induced by scopolamine and morphia medication for the alleviation of catatonic excitement.

A further case was reported by Grünthal (1936) and 11 others by Grünthal and Kuhn (1959), all with post-mortem findings. They stress the catatonic-like features which accompany the psychosis, the shrunken pyknotic appearance of the neurones and the involvement of both the dentate nucleus and the large cells of the striatum. The age of onset was most commonly in the fourth decade but three were first affected in adolescence, while one appears to have been only 6 years old. The duration varied from under 1 year to 23, some of the histories being recurrent.

The infrequency with which the disease has been reported, its variable duration and the fact that the nerve cell changes, genuine although they may appear to be, are unassociated with any significant changes in the glia renders this condition as a pathological entity still *sub judice*.

Unclassified pathological conditions associated with dementia

Okazari, Lipkin and Aronson (1961) have described the occurrence of Lewy type intracytoplasmic inclusion bodies in the medium-sized neurones of the cerebral cortex and in the pigmented cells of the brain stem in two elderly patients with progressive dementia and tetraparesis in flexion. One patient had shown evidence of mental deterioration for one year, the other for only one week. In neither case was there atrophy of the substantia nigra or any inflammatory feature.

Glees and Griffith (1952) report the post-mortem findings on a woman aged 58 who had a severe dementia of 15 years' duration. She eventually developed seizures and showed evidence of bilateral pyramidal impairment. At autopsy the hippocampus was found to be largely atrophied and both the gyrus hippocampus and gyrus fusiformis were completely destroyed. The fibres of the fornix were depleted to 25 per cent of their normal number. This is possibly a case of Pick's disease, for in 13 cases out of 196 in the literature there is evidence of a primary shrinkage area in the hippocampus and gyrus hippocampus. They observe that the hippocampal formation of the adult seems to be essential for the retention of recent memory.

Greenfield (1954) has discussed the association of mental deterioration with hereditary ataxia and progressive cerebellar degeneration. Mental changes have been noted in several cases of cerebellar atrophy, more especially in those of the primary parenchymatous type (Greenfield 1934, Akelaitis 1938, and Richter 1940). Akelaitis, for instance, found a diffuse loss of nerve cells in the cerebral cortex most evident in the 3rd and 5th layers. Schroeder and Kirschbaum (1928) describe and illustrate cerebral atrophy in olivocerebellar atrophy: the duration of the illness in the third case was only 18 months. The cell loss was most noticeable in layers 3 and 4 in the temporal lobe, layers 3 and 5 in the parietal lobe and layers 2, 3 and 4 in Broca's area. (The occipital lobe was involved in the two other brains they examined.) In a case of primary cerebellar atrophy beginning at the age of 41 reported by Kirschbaum and Eichholz (1932), the whole brain was grossly atrophic but the pathology appears to have been essentially that of cerebral arteriosclerosis. Neuronophagia and glial rosettes were observed. This patient was an alcoholic. Maas and Scherer (1933) report the post-mortem findings in 3 cases of cerebellar disease. Their second patient had olivopontocerebellar atrophy and died at the age of 45 with minimal changes in the cerebral cortex; the third patient, aged 73 at death, showed patchy loss of nerve cells in the cortex, but fresh vascular lesions were present. The case described by

Buchanan, Overholt and Neubürger (1947), of parenchymatous cerebellar degeneration in a woman of 45 who also had Pick's disease, is referred to on page 552.

Hassin and Levitin (1941) described a case of progressive dementia of some 2 years' duration or more in a 58-year-old woman. At necropsy there was found to be a widespread but slight degree of parenchymatous atrophy involving the entire brain and cord, associated with a diffuse proliferation of the astrocytes in the subcortex, especially of the frontal lobes which showed gross atrophy. The glial overgrowth was marked in the substantia nigra and medulla where the nerve cell changes were slight. Although this case was regarded by the authors as an example of Pick's disease they noted a resemblance in their findings to those seen after experimental metrazol intoxication.

Neumann (1949) has described three interesting cases of dementia in which the characteristic lesion has been a diffuse gliosis of the subcortical white matter associated with a varying degree of pallor of the myelin. Parenchymatous changes have been slight. The histories varied from 1 to 2½ years but the brain weights of the first and third cases were reduced to 900 g. and 720 g. The second died of a teratoma of the testis. The atrophy tended to be general but in the second there was an accentuation of the atrophy in the left frontal lobe, while in the third case the atrophy was maximum in the motor cortex. It is interesting to note that the third patient, who was 46 years of age, was described as looking at least 15 years older than her years. Neumann regarded her cases and that of Hassin and Levitin as constituting a special variety of Pick's disease, which she has called Type II. As the atrophy appears to have been in the white matter with relative sparing of the cortex, and as the process has been more diffuse than is normal in Pick's disease, it would seem best to regard these as belonging to some other condition. Perhaps they are of the same order as the second of two patients reported by Stern and Reed (1945), who died at the age of 48 after an illness lasting just over 6 years: she is described as looking old for her years. The brain weighed 846 g. and the atrophy was general but especially marked in Broca's area. There was loss of nerve cells especially in the middle layers of the cortex with lipoid atrophy of the survivors and an increase of astrocytes. Although neither senile plaques nor the neurofibrillary changes of Alzheimer were present, the authors regarded their case as an example of the abiotrophic type of Alzheimer's disease. The possibility of Alzheimer's disease occurring exceptionally in the absence of plaques and neurofibrillary alterations must be kept in mind, because the second familial case of Grünthal and Wenger was characterised by an absence of plaques; nevertheless no useful purpose is served by admitting to the category of Alzheimer's disease cases which lack both of the striking histological characteristics of this disease and which have no familial history to justify their consideration as exceptions. It would seem best, therefore, for the time being to regard the cases of Hassin and Levitin, of Neumann, and Stern and Reed as constituting one or more special forms of presenile dementia. The case reports are still too few to justify classification.

REFERENCES

Abely, X., Guiraud, P., Dechosal (Mme.), Jeannau. (1958) *Ann. méd. psychol.*, **116**, 294.

Agnostini, L. (1958) *Psychiatria* (Basel), **136**, 1.

Akelaitis, A. J. (1938) *Amer. J. Psychiat.*, **94**, 1115; (1944) *Arch. Neurol. Psychiat.*, **51**, 27.

Alajouanine, T. and van Bogaert, L. (1950) *Rev. Neurol.*, **82**, 21.

Alcock, N. S. (1936) *Brain*, **59**, 376.

Alema, G. and Bignami, A. (1959) *Revista Sperimentale di Freniatria Suppl. Fasc.* IV, **83**, 1492.

Alexander, L. (1934) *Arch. Neurol. Psychiat.*, **32**, 933.

Alexander, L. and Looney, J. M. (1938) *Arch. Neurol. Psychiat.*, **40**, 877.

Alzheimer, A. (1895) *Allg. Z. f. Psychiat.*, **51**, 809; (1898) *Mschr. Psychiat. Neurol.*, **3**, 101; (1902) *Allg. Z. Psychiat.*, **59**, 695; (1907) *Neurol. Zbl.*, **18**, 177; ibid., **30**, 891; (1911) *Z. ges. Neurol. Psychiat.*, **4**, 356.

Andrew, W. and Cardwell, E. (1940) *Arch. Path. (Lab. Med.)*, **29**, 400.
Bagh, K. von. (1941) *Arch. Psychiat. Nervenkr.*, **114**, 68.
Baker, A. B. (1937) *Amer. J. Path.*, **13**, 453.
Balli, R. (1907) *Riv. sper. Freniat.*, **32**, 803.
Barrett, A. M. (1913) *J. nerv. ment. Dis.*, **40**, 361.
Behrman, S., Mandybur, T. and McMenemey, W. H. (1963) *Rev. Neurol.*, **107**, 453.
Bell, Julia. (1934) *The Treasury of Human Inheritance*, Cambridge, **4**, 1.
Benda, C. E. (1949) *Mongolism and Cretinism*, 2nd ed., N.Y.
Benedek, S. and McGovern, V. J. (1949) *Med. J. Aust.* (ii), 429.
Berlin, L. (1949) *Arch. Neurol. Psychiat.*, **61**, 369.
Bernt, J. (1810) *Monographia Choreae Sti Viti*, Prague.
Bertrand, I. and Koffas, D. (1946) *Rev. Neurol.*, **78**, 338.
Best, Christiane-Ruth. (1941) *Mschr. Psychiat. Neurol.*, **103**, 308.
Biagini, G. (1933) *Riv. Neurol.*, **6**, 141.
Bickford, J. A. R. and Ellison, R. M. (1953) *J. ment. Sci.*, **99**, 291.
Bielschowsky, M. (1911) *J. Psychol. Neurol. Lpz.*, **18**, 273, 513.
Bielschowsky, M., Bouman, L. and Smitt, W. G. S. (1934) *Jb. Psychiat. Neurol.*, **51**, 1.
Bielschowsky, M. and Brodmann, K. (1905) *J. Psychol. Neurol. Lpz.*, **5**, 173.
Biemond, A. (1955) *Folia Psychiat. Neurol. Neurochir. Neerlandica.*, **58**, 217.
Bini, L. (1948) *Le Demenze Presenili*, Rome.
Binswanger, O. (1894) *Berl. klin. Wochenschr.*, **31**, 1180; (1895) *Z. für Psychiat. von Laehr.*, **51**, 804.
Binswanger, O. and Schaxel, J. (1917) *Arch. Psychiat. Nervenkr.*, **58**, 141.
Blocq, P. and Marinesco, G. (1892) *Sem. Méd. Paris.*, **12**, 445.
Bogaert, L. van, Maere, M., and de Smedt, E. (1940) *Mschr. Psychiat. Neurol.*, **102**, 249.
Bonfiglio, F. (1908) *Riv. sper. Freniat.*, **34**, 196; (1952) *Proc. 1st Int. Cong. Neuropath*, **2**, 297.
de Boor, W., Spiegelhoff, W., and Stammler, A. (1952) *Arch. Psychiat. Nervenkr.*, **188**, 51.
Bornstein, S. and Jervis, G. A. (1955) *Arch. Neurol. Psychiat.*, **74**, 598.
Bouman, L. (1925) *Z. ges. Neurol. Psychiat.*, **94**, 267.
Bouton, S. M. (1940) *J. nerv. ment. Dis.*, **91**, 9.
Brandenburg, W. and Hallervorden, I. (1954) *Virchow's Arch.*, **325**, 680.
Braunmühl, A. von. (1928) *Virchow's Arch.*, **270**, 448; (1930) *Z. ges. Neurol. Psychiat.*, **124**, 214; (1931) ibid., **133**, 391; (1932) ibid., **142**, 1; (1954) *Arch. Psychiat. Nervenkr.*, **191**, 419; ibid., (1956) **194**, 396; (1957) *Handbuch der speziellen pathologischen Anatomie und Histologie* (Lubarsch-Henke-Rössle), Berlin **13** (i), 347.
Braunmühl, A. von and Leonhard, K. (1934) *Z. ges. Neurol. Psychiat.*, **150**, 209.
Brierley, J. B. (1961) *Geront. Clin.*, **3**, 97.
Bruetsch, W. L. (1947) *Trans. Amer. Neurol. Ass.*, **72**, 28.
Buchanan, A. R., Overholt, L. C. and Neubürger, K. T. (1947) *J. Neuropath. exper. Neurol.*, **6**, 152.
Bülow, I. C. (1956) *Arch. Psychiat.*, **195**, 1.
Cameron, D. E., Himwich, H. E., Rosen, S. R., and Fazekas, J. (1940) *Amer. J. Psychiat.*, **97**, 566.
Campbell, A. M. G., Corner, Beryl, Norman, R. M. and Urich, H. (1961) *J. Neurol. Neurosurg. Psychiat.*, **24**, 71.
Campbell, A. W. (1894) *J. Ment. Sc.*, **40**, 638.
Casper, J. (1930) *Z. Neurol. Psychiat.*, **57**, 855.
Cheyne, G. (1725) *An Essay on Health and Long Life*, London, p. 174.
Clarke, E. and Murphy, E. A. (1956) *Brit. med. J.* (ii), 1319.
Claude, H. and Cuel, J. (1939) *Ann. Méd. lég.*, **19**, 173.
Claude, H., Lhermitte, J. and Baruk, H. (1932) *Encéphale*, **27**, 177.
Claude, H., Lhermitte, J. and Meignant, P. (1930) *Encéphale*, **25**, 417.
Cooke, J. (1685) *Mellificium Chirurgiae.*, London, p. 360.
Cooper, G. W. (1955) *J. Amer. Geriat. Soc.*, **3**, 488.
Corsellis, J. A. N. (1962) *Mental Illness and the Ageing Brain*, London, p. 38.
Corsellis, J. A. N. and Brierley, J. B. (1954) *Brain*, **77**, 571; (1959) *J. Ment. Sc.*, **105**, 714.
Cresseri, A. (1948) *Boll. Soc. ital. biol. Sper.*, **24**, 200.
Creutzfeldt, H. G. (1920) *Z. ges. Neurol. Psychiat.*, **57**; (1922) *Zbl. Neurol. Psych.*, **29**, 249.
Crezée, P. (1949) *Ned. Tijdschr. Geneesk.*, **93**, 2871.
Critchley, M. (1929) *J. Neurol. Psychopath.*, **10**, 124; (1930) *Proc. R. Soc. Med.*, **23**, 533; (1942) *Problems of Ageing*, ed. by Cowdry, E. V., Baltimore.

Curran, D. (1930) *J. Neurol. Psychopath.*, **10**, 305.

Davenport, C. B. (1915) *Proc. nat. Acad. Sci.*, Wash., **1**, 283.

Davenport, C. B. and Muncey, Elizabeth, B. (1916) *Amer. J. Insan.*, **73**, 195.

Davidson, Esther A. and Robertson, E. Elizabeth. (1955) *J. Neurol. Psychiat.*, **18**, 72.

Davison, C. (1932) *Brain*, **55**, 247.

Davison, C., Goodhart, S. P. and Schlionsky, H. S. (1932) *Arch. Neurol. Psychiat.*, **27**, 906.

Davison, C. and Rabiner, A. B. (1940) *Arch. Neurol. Psychiat.*, **44**, 578.

De Jong, R. N. (1953) in *The Founders of Neurology*, ed. by Webb Haymaker, Springfield, Ill., p. 305.

Delay, J., Brion, S. and Sadoun, R. (1954) *Rev. Neurol.*, **91**, 81.

Delay, J., Desclaux, P., Perrin, J. and Buvat, J. F. (1945) *Rev. Neurol.*, **77**, 85.

Dias, A. A. (1930) *Z. Neurol. Psychiat.*, **128**, 23.

Divry, P. (1927) *J. Belge Neurol.*, **27**, 643; (1952) *Proc. 1st Int. Cong. Neuropath.* (Rome), Turin, **2**, 312; (1955) *Acta Neurol. Belg.*, **49**, 282.

Divry, P., Ley, J. and Titeca, J. (1935) *J. belge Neurol.*, **35**, 495.

Divry, P., Titeca, J. and Vermeylen, G. (1935) *J. belge Neurol.*, **35**, 486.

Dixon, K. C. (1953) *J. Path. Bact.*, **66**, 539.

Dunlap, C. B. (1927) *Arch. Neurol. Psychiat.* **18**, 867.

Eitinger, L. (1954) *Acta psychiat. neurol. Scand.*, **29**, 411.

English, W. H. (1942) *Psychiat. Quart.*, **16**, 91.

Entres. (1931) *Allg. Z. Psychiat.*, **94**, 222.

Eros, G. (1951) *J. Neuropath. exper. Neurol.*, **10**, 257.

Esquirol, E. (1838) *Des Maladies Mentales*, Paris, **2**, 44.

Essen-Möller, E. (1946) *Acta. psychiat. Kbh.*, **21**, 233.

Fabiani, F. (1957) *Riv. pat. nerv.*, **78**, 1154.

Falstein, E. I. and Stone, T. T. (1941) *Arch. Neurol. Psychiat.*, **1**, 151.

Fattovich, G. (1955) *Cervello*, **31**, 1; (1955) *G. Psychiat. Neuropat.*, **83**, 1.

Ferraro, A. (1931) *Arch. Neurol. Psychiat.*, **25**, 1042.

Ferraro, A. and Jervis, G. A. (1936) *Arch. Neurol. Psychiat.*, **36**, 739; (1940) *Psychiat. Quart.*, **14**, 17. (1941) ibid., **15**, 3.

Fischer, O. (1907) *Mschr. Psychiat. Neurol.*, **22**, 361; (1910) *Z. ges. Neurol. Psychiat.*, **3**, 371.

Fisher, C. M. (1951) *Canad. med. Ass. J.*, **65**, 1.

Foley, J. M. and Denny-Brown, D. (1955) *Excerpta Med. Neurol. Psychiat.*, **8**, 782.

Fowler, M. and Robertson, E. G. (1959) *Australasian Ann. Med.*, **8**, 16.

Freeman, W. (1933) *Neuropathology*, Philad., 263.

Friede, R. and Magee, K. R. (1962) *Neurology*, **12**, 213.

Friedrich, G. (1940) *Z. ges. Neurol. Psychiat.*, **170**, 311.

Fuller, S. C. (1911) *Amer. J. Insan.*, **68**, 147.

Fuller, S. C. and Klopp, H. I. (1912) *Amer. J. Insan.*, **69**, 17.

Gajdusek, D. C. and Zigas, V. (1957) *New England J. Med.*, **257**, 974; (1959) *Amer. J. Med.*, **26**, 442.

Garcin, R., Bertrand, I., van Bogaert, L., Gruner, J. and Brion, S. (1950) *Rev. Neurol.*, **83**, 161.

Garcin, R., Brion, S. and Khochneviss, A. (1962) *Rev. neurol.*, **106**, 506.

Garrod, A. E. (1927) *Lancet*, **2**, 1113.

Gellerstedt, N. (1933) *Uppsala LäkFören. Förh.*, **38**, 193.

Gerstmann, J., Straussler, E. and Scheinker, I. (1936) *Z. ges. Neurol. Psychiat.*, **154**, 736.

Glees, P. and Griffith, H. B. (1952) *Mschr. Psychiat. Neurol.*, **123**, 193.

Goodman, L. (1953) *J. nerv. ment. Dis.*, **118**, 97.

Gowers, W. R. (1899) *Lancet* (ii), 1591; (1902) ibid. (i), 1003.

Grahmann, H. and Ule, G. (1957) *Psychiat. et Neurol.* (Basel), **134**, 261.

Greenfield, J. G. (1934) *Brain*, **57**, 161; (1954) *The spino-cerebellar degenerations*, Oxford.

Grosch, H. (1959) *Deut. Z. Nervenh.*, **179**, 217.

Grünthal, E. (1926) *Z. ges. Neurol. Psychiat.*, **101**, 128; (1927) ibid., **111**, 763; (1930 a) ibid., **129**, 350; (1930 b) in *Handbuch der Geistenkrankheiten*, ed. by O. Bumke, Berlin, **11**, 638; (1931) *Z. ges. Neurol. Psychiat.*, **136**, 464; (1936) in *Handbuch der Neurologie*, ed. by O. Bumke and O. Foerster, Berlin, **11**, 497; (1942) *Mschr. Psychiat. Neurol.*, **107**, 114.

Grünthal, E. and Kuhn, R. (1959) *Psych. et Neurol.*, **137**, 1.

Grünthal, E. and Wenger, O. (1939) *Mschr. Psychiat. Neurol.*, **101**, 8; (1940) ibid., **102**, 302.

Guillain, G., Bertrand, I. and Mollaret, P. (1934) *Ann. Méd.*, **36**, 249.

Hallervorden, J. (1930) in *Handbuch der Geistenkrankheiten*, ed. by O. Bumke, Berlin, **11**, 1019; (1930) ibid., **11**, 1094.
Hallgren, B. and Sourander, P. (1958) *J. Neurochem.*, **3**, 41; (1960) ibid., **5**, 307.
Hannah, J. A. (1936) *Canad. med. Ass. J.*, **35**, 361.
Haškovec, V. (1934) *Zbl. ges. Neurol. Psychiat.*, **73**, 345.
Hassin, G. B. (1948) *Histopathology of the Peripheral and Central Nervous Systems*, 3rd edition, Chicago.
Hassin, G. B. and Levitin, D. (1941) *Arch. Neurol. Psychiat.*, **45**, 814.
Heidenhain, A. (1928–9) *Z. ges. Neurol. Psychiat.*, **118**, 49.
Hemphill, R. E. and Stengel, E. (1941) *J. Neurol. Psychiat.*, **4**, 97.
Hirano, A., Kurland, L. T., Krooth, R. S. and Lessell, S. (1961) *Brain*, **84**, 642.
Hirano, A., Malamud, N. and Kurland, L. T. (1961) *Brain*, **84**, 662.
Hirano, A. and Zimmerman, H. M. (1962) *Neurology*, **7**, 227.
Hiroisi, S. and Lee, C. C. (1936) *Arch. Neurol. Psychiat.*, **35**, 827.
Horn, L. and Stengel, E. (1930) *Z. ges. Neurol. Psychiat.*, **128**, 673.
Horta, J. da S. (1955) *Acta Neuroveget.*, **12**, 105.
Hunt, J. Ramsay. (1917) *Brain*, **40**, 58.
Huntington, G. (1872) *Med. Surg. Reporter* (Philadelphia), **26**, 317.
Hutchinson, E. C. and Yates, P. O. (1956) *Brain*, **79**, 319.
Hydén, H. and Lindstrom, B. (1950) *Disc. Faraday Soc.*, **9**, 436.
Jacob, H. (1952) *Proc. 1st Int. Cong. Neuropath.* (Rome), Turin, **2**, 422; (1960) *Arch. Psychiat. u Zeit. Neurol.* **201**, 17.
Jacob, H., Eicke, W. and Orthner, H. (1958) *Deut. Z. Nervenh.*, **178**, 330.
Jacob, H., Pyrkosch, W. and Strube, H. (1950) *Arch. Psychiat. Nervenkr.*, **184**, 653.
Jakob, A. (1921) *Z. ges. Neurol. Psychiat.*, **64**, 147; (1923) *Monographic über die extrapyramidalen Erkrankunger* mit besonderem. Berüchsichtigung der anatomischen Pathologie und Histologie und der Pathophysiologie der Bewegungstorüngen. Springer, Berlin.
Jansen, J. and Monrad-Krohn, G. H. (1938) *Z. ges. Neurol. Psychiat.*, **163**, 670.
Jelgersma, G. (1908) *Neurol. Zbl.*, **27**, 995.
Jelgersma, H. C. (1958) *Folia Psychiat. Neurolog. Neurochirug., Neerl.*, **61**, 501.
Jervis, G. A. (1937) *Psychiat. Quart.*, **11**, 5; (1948) *Amer. J. Psychiat.*, **105**, 102.
Jervis, G. A., Hurdum, H. M. and O'Neill, F. J. (1942) *Amer. J. Psychiat.*, **99**, 101.
Jervis, G. A. and Soltz, S. E. (1936) *Amer. J. Psychiat.*, **93**, 39.
Jones, D. and Nevin, S. (1954) *J. Neurol. Psychiat.*, **17**, 148.
Jones, R. S. and Frazier, D. B. (1950) *Arch. Path. Lab. Med.*, **50**, 366.
Josephy, H. (1956) *J. Neuropath. exp. Neurol.*, **15**, 234.
Katzman, R., Kagan, E. H., Zimmerman, H. M. (1961) *J. Neuropath. exp. Neurol.*, **20**, 78.
Khochneviss, A. (1962) *Thèse de Paris.*
Kidd, M. (1963) *Nature*, **197**, 192.
Kiesselbach, G. (1914) *Mschr. Psychiat. Neurol.*, **35**, 525.
King, L. S. (1942) *Arch. Neurol. Psychiat.*, **48**, 241.
King, P. D. (1960) *J. clin. exp. Psychopath.*, **21**, 31.
Kirschbaum, W. (1924) *Z. ges. Neurol. Psychiat.*, **92**, 175.
Kirschbaum, W. and Eichholz, A. (1932) *Dtsch. Z. Nervenheilk.*, **125**, 21.
Klatzo, I., Gajdusek, D. C., Zigas, V. (1959) *Lab. Invest.*, **8**, 779.
Korbsch, H. (1933) *Arch. Psychiat.*, **100**, 326.
Korey, S. R., Scheinberg, L., Terry, R. and Stein, A. (1961) *Trans. Amer. Neurol. Ass.*, **86**, 99.
Kraepelin, E. (1910) *Klinische Psychiatrie*, Leipzig, **2**, 624.
Kramer, D. W. (1959) *Nederl. tijdschr. geneesk.*, **103**, 1662.
Kreindler, A., Hornet, Th. and Appel, E. (1959) *Rum. Med. Rev.*, **3**, 43.
Krücke, W. (1950) *Arch. Psychiat. Z. Neurol.*, **185**, 165; (1952) *Proc. 1st Int. Cong. Neuropath.* (Rome), Turin, **3**, 237.
Kufs, H. (1937) *Arch. Psychiat. Nervenkr.*, **107**, 431.
Kurland, L. T. and Mulder, D. W. (1954) *Neurology*, **4**, 355, 438.
Lansing, A. I. (1951) *Physiol. Rev.*, **31**, 224.
Lewy, F. H. (1923) Cited by Alexander, L. (1934).
Lhermitte, J. and Porak, R. (1914) *Rev. Neurol.*, **22**, 45.
Liebers, M. (1939) *Arch. Psychiat.*, **109**, 363; (1933) ibid., **100**, 100.
Lindenberg, R. (1960) *J. Neuropath. exp. Neurol.*, **19**, 160.

Liss, L. (1960) *J. Neuropath. exp. Neurol.*, **19**, 559.
Løken, A. Christie and Cyvin, K. (1954) *J. Neurol. Neurosurg. Psychiat.*, **17**, 211.
Lotmar, F. (1929) *Z. ges. Neurol. Psychiat.*, **119**, 491; (1933) ibid., **146**, 1.
Lowenberg, K. (1925) *Z. ges. Neurol. Psychiat.*, **98**, 549; (1936) *Arch. Neurol. Psychiat.*, **36**, 769.
Lowenberg, K., Boyd, D. and Salon, D. D. (1939) *Arch. Neurol. Psychiat.*, **41**, 1004.
Lowenberg, K. and Rothschild, D. (1931) *Amer. J. Psychiat.*, **11**, 269.
Lowenberg, K. and Waggoner, R. W. (1934) *Arch. Neurol. Psychiat.*, **31**, 737.
Luers, Thea. (1947) *Arch. Psychiat. Nervenkr.*, **179**, 132.
Lyon, I. W. (1863) *Amer. med. Times*, **7**, 289.
Lyon, R. L. (1962a) *Brit. med. J.* (i), 1301; (1962b) ibid. (i), 1306.
McCaughey, W. T. E. (1961) *J. nerv. ment. Dis.*, **133**, 91.
McMenemey, W. H. (1940) *J. Neurol. Psychiat.*, **3**, 211.
McMenemey, W. H., Worster-Drought, C., Flind, J. and Williams, H. G. (1939) *J. Neurol. Psychiat.*, **2**, 293.
Maas, O. and Scherer, H. J. (1933) *Z. ges. Neurol. Psychiat.*, **145**, 420.
Malamud, N. (1960) *J. Neuropath. exp. Neurol.*, **19**, 161.
Malamud, N. and Boyd, D. A. (1940) *Arch. Neurol. Psychiat.*, **43**, 210.
Malamud, N. and Waggoner, R. W. (1943) *Arch. Neurol. Psychiat.*, **50**, 288.
Malamud, W. and Lowenberg, K. (1929) *Arch. Neurol. Psychiat.*, **21**, 805.
Mandybur, T. and McMenemey, W. H. (1963) Not yet published.
Mansvelt, J. van. (1954) *Pick's Disease, A syndrome of lobar cerebral atrophy*, Enschedes.
Marchand, L. (1949) *Ann. méd. psychol.*, **107(i)**, 433.
Marchand, L. and Abély, X. (1948) *Ann. méd. psychol.*, **106**, 30.
Marchand, L., Achalle, J. Y., Achalle, P. and Fadeuilhe, A. (1958) *Ann. méd. psychol.*, **116**, 290.
Marchand, L., Bessière, R., Lelion, R. and Marty, R. (1955) *Ann. méd. psychol.*, **113**, 232.
Marchand, L., Le Conte, M., and Halpern, B. (1956) *Presse méd.* **64**, 1412.
Margolis, G. (1953) *Amer. J. Path.*, **29**, 588.
Marie, P. and Lhermitte, J. (1914) *Ann. méd.*, **1**, 18.
Marinesco, G. (1911) *C. R. Soc. biol.*, **70**, 606; (1931) *Arch. roum. Path. exper. Microbiol.*, **4(i)**, 41.
Mayer-Gross, W. (1938) *Proc. R. Soc. Med.*, **31**, 1443.
Mayer-Gross, W., Slater, E. and Roth, M. (1954) *Clinical Psychiatry*, London.
Meggendorfer, F. (1926) *Z. ges. Neurol. Psychiat.*, **101**, 387; (1930) ibid, **128**, 337.
Mettler, A. (1957) *Proc. 1st Intern. Congr. Neurol. Sciences*, **1**, 11.
Meyer, A. (1929) *Z. ges. Neurol. Psychiat.*, **121**, 107.
Meyer, A., Leigh, D. and Bagg, C. E. (1954) *J. Neurol. Psychiat.*, **17**, 129.
Meyersburg, H. A. (1945) *New Engl. J. Med.*, **233**, 173.
Meynert, T. (1871) *Wien. med. Pr.*, **12**, 1135.
Minski, L. and Guttman, E. (1938) *J. ment. Sci.*, **84**, 21.
Miskolczy, D. (1959) *Rum. Med. Rev.*, **3**, 62.
Missmahl, H. P. and Hartwig, M. (1954) *Deut. Z. Nervenh.*, **171**, 173.
Morel, F. and Wildi, E. (1952) *Proc. 1st Int. Cong. Neuropath.* (Rome), Turin, **2**, 347.
Moyano, B. A. (1931) *Sem. méd.*, **2**, 1921; (1932) *Arch. arg. de neurol.*, **7**, 231.
Mutrux, S. (1947) *Mschr. Psychiat. Neurol.*, **113**, 100; (1953) ibid., **125**, 19.
Neubürger, K. T. and Braunmühl, A. von. (1930) *Handbuch der Geisteskrankheiten*, ed. by O. Bumke, Berlin, **11**, 347.
Neubürger, K. T. and Rösch, A. (1935) *Virchow's Arch.*, **294**, 537.
Neumann, M. A. (1949) *J. Neuropath. exp. Neurol.*, **8**, 255; (1960) ibid., **19**, 370.
Neumann, M. A. and Cohn, R. (1953) *Arch. Neurol. Psychiat.*, **69**, 615.
Nevin, S., McMenemey, W. H., Behrman, S. and Jones, D. P. (1960) *Brain*, **83**, 519.
Newton, R. D. (1948) *J. ment. Sci.*, **94**, 225.
Okazaki, H., Lipkin, L. E. and Aronson, S. M. (1961) *J. Neuropath. exp. Neurol.*, **20**, 237.
Oksala, O. (1923) *Z. ges. Neurol. Psychiat.*, **81**, 1.
Onari, K. and Spatz, H. (1926) *Z. ges. Neurol. Psychiat.*, **101**, 470.
Orlando, R. and Arndt, M. (1947) *Rev. Neurol. de B.A.*, **12**, 135.
Pallis, C. and Spillane, J. D. (1957) *Quart. J. Med.*, **26**, 349.
Pantelakis, St. (1954) *Mschr. Psychiat. Neurol.*, **128**, 219.
Perusini, G. (1910) *Histol. histopath. Arb.*, **3**, 297.
Peters, G. (1951) *Spezielle Pathologie des Nervensystems*, Stuttgart, p. 152.

Pick, A. (1892) *Prag. med. Wschr.*, **17**, 165; (1901) *Wien klin. Woch.*, **14**, 403; (1906) *Mschr. Psychiat. Neurol.*, **19**, 97.
Pleydell, M. J. (1954) *Brit. Med. J.*, **2**, 1121.
Pohlisch, K. (1941) *Proc. 7th Int. Genet. Congress (Edinburgh)*, Cambridge, p. 239.
Rasdolsky, J. (1926) *Z. ges. Neurol. Psychiat.*, **106**, 96.
Raskin, N. and Ehrenberg, R. (1956 a) *Amer J. Psychiat.*, **113**, 133; (1956 b) *Amer. Practit.*, **7**, 1095.
Rauch. (1948) Cited by Peters, G. *Spezielle Pathologie des Nervensystems*, Stuttgart, 1951, p. 215.
Redlich, E. (1898) *J. Psychiat. Neurol.*, **17**, 208.
Reich, F. (1907) *Allg. Z. Psychiat.*, **64**, 380; (1927) *Z. ges. Neurol. Psychiat.*, **108**, 803.
Reiss, E. and Staemmler, M. (1950) *Arch. Psych. Zsch. Neurol.*, **183**, 481.
Richter, H. (1918) *Z. ges. Neurol. Psychiat.*, **38**, 127.
Richter, R. (1940) *J. nerv. ment. Dis.*, **91**, 37.
Riese, W. (1946) *J. Neuropath. exp. Neurol.*, **5**, 160.
Riese, W. and Zfass, I. S. (1944) *Arch. Neurol. Psychiat.*, **51**, 78.
Ritama, V. (1954) *Ann. Med. intern. Fenn.*, **43**, 51.
Roizin, L. (1948) *J. Neuropath. exp. Neurol.*, **7**, 216.
Rothschild, D. (1937) *Amer. J. Psychiat.*, **93**, 757.
Rothschild, D. (1934) *Amer. J. Psychiat.*, **91**, 485; (1942) *Arch. Neurol. Psychiat.*, **48**, 417; (1956) *Mental Disorders in Later Life*, ed. by O. J. Kaplan, Oxford, p. 289.
Rothschild, D. and Kasanin, J. (1936) *Arch. Neurol. Psychiat.*, **36**, 293.
Rothschild, D. and Sharp, M. L. (1941) *Dis. nerv. System*, **2**, 49.
Ružička, V. (1922) *Pflüg. Arch. ges. Physiol.*, **194**, 135; (1924) *Arch. mickr. Anat.*, **101**, 459.
Sanders, J., Schenk, V. W. D. and van Veen, P. (1939) *Proc. Acad. Sc. Amst.*, **38**, 1.
Schaffer, K. (1913) *Z. ges. Neurol. Psychiat.*, **21**, 49; (1926) *Über die morphologischen Wesen und die Histopathologie der hereditar-systematisch Nervenkrankheiten*, Berlin; (1922) *Dtsch. Z. Nervenheilk.*, **73**, 101.
Scharenberg, K. (1958) *J. Neuropath. exp. Neurol.*, **17**, 346.
Schenk, V. W. D. (1955) *Folia Psychiat. Neurolog. Neurochirurg. Neerl.*, **58**, 422.
Schenk, V. W. D. and Mansvelt, J. van. (1955) *Folia Psychiat. Neurolog. Neurochirurg. Neerl.*, **58**, 42.
Schmidt, H. (1959) *Arch. Psychiat.*, **199**, 519.
Schmitz, H. A. and Meyer, A. (1933) *Arch. Psychiat.*, **99**, 747.
Schnitzler, J. G. (1911) *Z. ges. Neurol. Psychiat.*, **7**, 34.
Schob and Güntz. (1932) *Allg. Z. Psychiat.*, **97**, 242.
Schob, F. (1927) *Mschr. Psychiat. Neurol.*, **65**, 286.
Scholz, W. (1938) *Z. ges. Neurol. Psychiat.*, **162**, 694.
Schottky, J. (1932) *Z. ges. Neurol. Psychiat.*, **140**, 333.
Schrœder, A. H. and Kirschbaum, W. (1928) *Z. ges. Neurol. Psychiat.*, **114**, 681.
Schükrü-Aksel, I. (1936) *Arch. Psych.*, **106**, 260.
Schulman, S. (1956) *J. Neuropath. exp. Neurol.*, **15**, 208.
Schwarz, G. A. and Barrows, L. J. (1958) *J. Neuropath. exp. Neurol.*, **17**, 352.
Seitelberger, F. and Jellinger, K. (1958) *Deut. Z. Nervenh.*, **178**, 365.
Silberman, J., Cravioto, H. and Feigin, I. (1961) *J. Neuropath. exp. Neurol.*, **20**, 105.
Sim, M. and Smith, W. T. (1955) *J. ment. Sc.*, **101**, 604.
Simchowicz, T. (1910) *Hist. histopath. Arb.*, **4**, 267; (1914) *Encéphale* **9**, 218; (1924) *Rev. neurol.*, (i), 221.
Simma, K. (1949) *Mschr. Psychiat. Neurol.*, **118**, 44, (1951) ibid. **122**, 156; (1952) ibid., **123**, 205.
Simpson, D. A., Lander, H. and Robson, H. N. (1959) *Australasian Ann. Med.*, **8**, 8.
Singer, K. (1962) *Brit. med. J.* (i), 1311.
Sjögren, H. (1956) *Acta Psychiat. neurol. Scand.*, **106**, 9.
Sjögren, H. and Sourander, P. (1961) *Svenska Lakartidningen*, **58**, 3448.
Sjögren, T., Sjögren, H. and Lindgren, A. (1952) *Acta Psychiat. neurol. Scand.*, Suppl. 82.
Smith, B. (1961) Personal communication.
Soniat, T. L. L. (1941) *Arch. Neurol. Psychiat.*, **46**, 101.
Spatz, H. (1952) *Proc. 1st Int. Cong. Neuropath. (Rome)*, Turin, **2**, 375.
Spielmeyer, W. (1922) *Histopathologie des Nervensystems*, 335, Springer, Berlin.
Stender, A. (1930) *Z. ges. Neurol. Psychiat.*, **128**, 528.
Stengel, E. and Wilson, W. E. J. (1949) *J. ment. Sci.*, **92**, 370.
Stern, K. (1939) *Brain*, **62**, 157.
Stern, K. and Elliott, K. A. C. (1949) *Amer. J. Psychiat.*, **106**, 190.

Stern, K., Hinds, E. G. and Askonas, Brigitte. (1945) *Amer. J. Psychiat.*, **102**, 325.
Stern, K. and Reed, G. E. (1945) *Amer. J. Psychiat.*, **102**, 191.
Stone, T. T. and Falstein, E. I. (1938) *J. nerv. ment. dis.*, **88**, 602 and 773.
Strauss, E. E. (1956) *J. Neuropath. exp. Neurol.*, **15**, 233.
Sträussler, E. and Koskinas, G. (1926) *Z. ges. Neurol. Psychiat.*, **105**, 55.
Struwe, F. (1929) *Z. ges. Neurol. Psychiat.*, **122**, 291.
Teichmann, E. (1935) *Z. ges. Neurol. Psychiat.*, **154**, 34.
Terry, R. (1962) Abst. meeting of Amer. Neuropathol. Assoc., June.
Timmer, A. P. (1925) *Z. Neurol. u. Psych.*, **98**, 43.
Titeca, L. and van Bogaert, L. (1946) *Brain*, **69**, 251.
Urechia, C. I. and Danetz, C. (1924) *Encéphale*, **19**, 382.
Urechia, C. I., Dragomir, L. and Elekes, N. (1935) *Arch. int. neurol.*, **54**, 55.
Urechia, C. I. and Elekes, M. (1925) *Bull. Acad. med.*, **94**, 795.
Uyematsu, S. (1923) *J. nerv. ment. Dis.*, **57**, 1, 131 and 237.
van der Eecken, H. V., Adams, R. D. and van Bogaert, L. (1960) *J. Neuropath. exp. Neurol.*, **19**, 159.
Verhaart, W. J. C. (1930 a) *Nederl. tijdschr. geneesk.*, **74** (i), 2114; (1930 b) ibid., **74** (ii), 5586; (1936) *Meded. Dienst Volksgezdh, Nederl. Indie*, **25**, 341.
Verhaart, W. J. C. and Jelgersma, H. C. (1952) *Psychiat. Neurol. Neurochir. Neerland*, **55**, 453.
Vessie, P. R. (1932) *J. nerv. ment. Dis.*, **76**, 553.
Vogt, C. and O. (1920) *J. Psychol. Neurol. Lpz.*, **25**, 627.
Vogt, M. (1928) ibid, **36**, 124.
Vraa-Jensen, G. (1955) *Acta Psychiat. Neurol. Scand.*, **30**, 375.
Waters, C. O. (1841) in R. Dunglison's *The Practice of Medicine*, Philadelphia 1848, **2**, 216.
Weberitsch, W. (1955) *Nord. Med.*, **54**, 1525.
Webster, J. (1843) *Med. Chir. Trans.*, **26**, 374: *Ibid.*, **28**, 427: (1849) *Ibid.*, **32**, 115.
Weimann, W. (1921) *Zbl. Neurol.*, **23**, 355.
Wheelan, L. (1959) *Ann. Human Genet.*, **23**, 300.
Wildi, E. (1951) *Confinia Neurol.*, **2**, 139.
Williams, H. W. (1935) *Arch. Neurol. Psychiat.*, **34**, 508.
Wilson, S. A. K. (1940 a) *Neurology*, 1st ed., London, **2**, 907; (1940 b) ibid, **2**, 919; (1954) ibid, 2nd ed., **2**, 981.
Winkelman, N. W. and Book, M. H. (1949) *J. Neuropath. exper. Neurol.*, **8**, 30.
Worster-Drought, C. and Allen, I. M. (1929) *Brit. Med. J.*, **2**, 1149.
Worster-Drought, C., Greenfield, J. G. and McMenemey, W. H. (1940) *Brain*, **63**, 237; (1944) ibid., **67**, 38.
Worster-Drought, C., Hill, T. R. and McMenemey, W. H. (1933) *J. Neurol. Psychopath.*, **14**, 27.

Hepatolenticular degeneration (Wilson's disease)

By J. G. Greenfield

The name hepatolenticular degeneration was given by Hall of Copenhagen (1921) to a familial metabolic dyscrasia in which cirrhosis of the liver is associated with degeneration of the corpus striatum; in both situations there is a great excess of copper, and brown granules containing copper are also present in most cases in the outer zone of the cornea (Kayser-Fleischer ring). The symptoms usually appear towards the end of the second decade but a few cases have begun in the first decade and onset in the third and fourth decade is not unusual. In untreated cases the duration of the disease is usually between 3 and 10 years but it may be considerably longer. The onset of nervous symptoms occasionally follows, at an interval of months or years, an attack of febrile jaundice which may be transient, but in many instances the cirrhosis of the liver remains silent throughout the course of the disease. There may, however, be some ascites or swelling of the ankles and the spleen may be enlarged, firm and palpable. A heavy urinary excretion of amino-acids, including some types which are not usually found in cirrhosis of the liver, has been noted in the great majority of cases.

Clinically there is progressive rigidity and coarse tremor of the limbs, a spastic condition of the face, mouth and pharynx, causing dysarthria and dysphagia and, in the closing stages of the disease, some degree of dementia.

Historical. Kinnier Wilson (1912) reported 6 cases with 3 post-mortem examinations and collected 8 more from the literature. Two or three members of some families were affected but there was no other evidence of hereditary transmission. Hoesslin and Alzheimer (1912) reported a case with full post-mortem examination under the diagnosis of *pseudosclerosis*. In addition to cirrhosis of the liver, they found degenerative changes widespread in the brain, but especially in the striatum; they emphasised the presence in all the degenerated areas of large astrocytes with swollen, vesicular and sometimes multiple nuclei which are now called by Alzheimer's name (*vide* page 52). Fleischer (1909, 1912) found the ring of brown corneal pigmentation, which had first been described by Kayser (1902) and himself (1903), in cases of pseudosclerosis associated with cirrhosis of the liver. These various observations were brought together by Hall (1921) who added 53 further cases from the literature and 4 personal cases. In some of these the disease was widespread in the brain, involving the cerebral cortex, the other basal ganglia and brain stem nuclei and the nucleus dentatus and superior cerebellar peduncle; but it was always most severe in the striatum. Opalski (1930) added to the microscopic picture of the disease the large phagocytic cells which bear his name, and Haurowitz (1930) and Lüthy (1931) found an excess of copper both in the corpus striatum and liver. By 1948 Denny-Brown had found over 150 case reports in the literature and, with Uzman, described the amino-aciduria which is a usual feature of the disease.

Pathology. The brain shows no external abnormality except some sinking in of the insular cortex. On section the corpus striatum appears shrunken, especially in its middle third, so that on horizontal section the outline of its external border is sinuous, resembling a Cupid's bow. This is less obvious in coronal sections in which the outline is flatter than normal and at some levels may even be concave. The corpus striatum, and sometimes also the nucleus subthalamicus, have a brownish or brick-red colour according to the duration of formalin fixation. Cavitation is often, but not constantly, found in the putamen. In milder form it is chiefly perivascular, but when severe may involve most of the central and anterior parts of the putamen and spread into the caudate nucleus. Very rarely it has been found in other nuclei such as the thalamus and red nucleus (Howard and Royce 1919).

Microscopic examination of the putamen shows, in most cases, an increased cellularity due chiefly to large numbers of astrocyte nuclei. Many of these are larger and more vesicular than normal with one or more basophilic nucleoli, so that they may resemble the nuclei of small nerve cells. Some are considerably larger than this, up to 15μ in their longer diameter, and are surrounded by fine yellow-brown granules which appear to be enclosed in tenuous processes. They do not form neuroglial fibres. These nuclei belong to cells of Alzheimer Type II. Multi-nucleated cells of Alzheimer's Type I are much rarer and are not present in every case. Both in the putamen and nucleus caudatus there is a general reduction in the number of nerve cells in which both the large and small cells share. In some cases this loss falls most heavily on the large cells, in others on the small cells, and it varies greatly in degree. There is also a diffuse reduction in the number of myelinated fibres in the corpus striatum. When cavities are present they have ragged edges which show little attempt at scarring either by neuroglial or collagen fibres. Lüthy (1931) and Lichtenstein and Gore (1955) found pericapillary concretions which stained heavily for copper in the putamen.

The globus pallidus usually shows little change except a reduction in the number of myelinated fibres which traverse it, but Alzheimer Type II nuclei, Opalski cells and phagocytic cells containing haemosiderin are usually seen in it. In the nucleus subthalamicus also Alzheimer and Opalski cells may be present and there is often degeneration of neurones and reduction in their number. Focal degenerations of the cerebral cortex are not uncommon especially in the frontal lobes. There may be areas of hyper-myelination, status spongiosus or diffuse loss of nerve cells and fibres, both in the cortex and the white centres of the convolutions (Barnes and Hurst 1926). In the thalamus and the nuclei of the brain stem Alzheimer nuclei and Opalski cells may be found. Phagocytes containing iron pigment are commonly found in the globus pallidus and substantia nigra. In the latter nucleus Lichtenstein and Gore (1955) found unilateral scarring but this is unusual. Degeneration of the nucleus dentatus, often associated with Marchi or sudanophilic degeneration of the superior cerebellar peduncle, has been found in a number of cases (Greenfield *et al.* 1924).

Opalski cells. Opalski (1930) described a special form of cell which he found only in cases of hepatolenticular degeneration. These were large cells with a cell body 'three to five times the size of a cell of the substantia nigra'. They were oval or rounded without processes, and had a finely granular or slightly foamy cytoplasm which stained a light rose colour by Nissl's method. The oval nucleus was usually central. It was smaller and more darkly stained than in cells of Alzheimer's Type II. Very rarely a larger nucleus was present, and very occasionally the cells were multi-nucleated. Regressive changes in the nucleus and cytoplasm, in which the nucleus might come to lie peripherally and the cytoplasm became vacuolated, were frequently seen. These cells were very much rarer than those of Alzheimer's Type II. Opalski found them especially in the thalamus, globus pallidus and zona reticulata of substantia nigra but very rarely in the striatum. The presence of these cells in hepatolenticular degeneration has been confirmed by numerous subsequent writers. We have found similar cells measuring up to 35μ in the globus pallidus and nucleus subthalamicus in a typical case. They stood out prominently in sections stained by van Gieson's counterstain by the bright orange-brown colour and rounded outline of the cell body. Like Opalski, we were unable to find them in the striatum. There is no evidence that they are derived from astrocytes; the character of the nucleus suggests rather an origin from histiocytes (Fig. 9.19).

Kayser-Fleischer ring. Sections of the cornea show a row of granules of brown pigment in Descemet's membrane near the limbus of the cornea. In some cases the granules appear to lie almost on the inner surface of the membrane but they usually spread into it and never into the endothelial cells covering it. They do not give a Prussian blue reaction for iron and do not bleach like melanin granules with oxidising agents. Brand and Takatz (1951) found that they gave the staining reactions of copper with rubeanic acid (black on a greenish background) and rhodanin (reddish-brown) and they have been shown to contain copper by spectroscopic analysis (Gerlach and Rohrschneider 1934). In some cases a sunflower cataract, such as is seen when fragments of copper enter the eye, is found in cases of hepatolenticular degeneration (Steger 1954) (Fig. 9.18). The electronmicroscopic appearances are described by Uzman and Jakus (1957).

The liver may be enlarged in the early stages of the disease, but is usually smaller than normal at its termination. It is coarsely cirrhotic with lobules which may vary in size from 1 mm. to 2 cm. or more. In some cases most are of small size, in others they are coarser than in alcoholic cirrhosis. The colour varies in different cases and the individual lobules in a liver may also vary, some being yellow, others brick red, greenish or brown. This appears to be due to differences in the amount of copper storage, fatty degeneration or bile staining. Microscopically the characteristic appearances of multilobular cirrhosis are seen, but the fibrous septa are often less heavily collagenous than in most chronic cirrhotic livers, and may contain perivascular collections of lymphocytes and numerous small bile ducts. In some early cases the appearances have been those of subacute hepatitis. Okinawa *et al.* (1954) found granules in the liver cells which gave the reactions of copper with rubeanic acid and rhodanin; they varied in number in different lobules. Iron-containing pigment and bile pigment are often also present.

The spleen is often enlarged, congested and firmer than normal, with fibrous tissue hyperplasia due to back pressure, but in many cases, in which hepatic cirrhosis has been clinically silent, it has shown no abnormality. Böttiger and Möllerberg (1959) describe cardiomegaly in this disease with coarse dark intracellular pigment, which failed to give the staining reactions for iron, around the nuclei of the muscle cells. Various forms of skeletal disease may occur in association with Wilson's disease including osteoporosis (Rosender and Michell 1959).

Biochemistry. The chief metabolic abnormality in heptatolenticular degeneration is failure to bind the copper absorbed from the intestines to the serum globulins. Normally copper is taken up from the intestine in loose combination with albumin and after about 24 hours is transferred to globulin, to which it is more firmly bound (Earl *et al.* 1954, Bearn and Kunkel

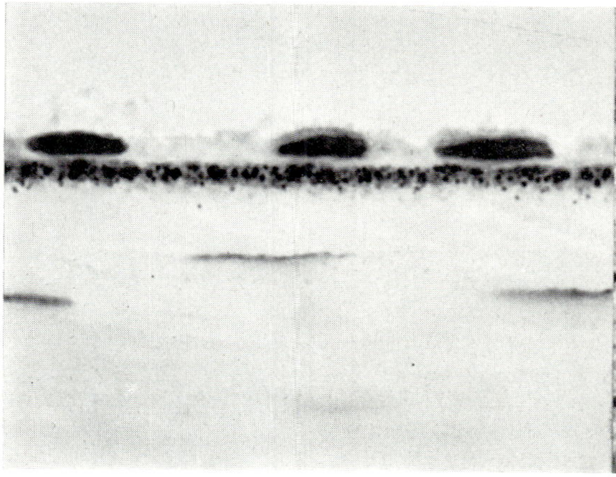

9.18

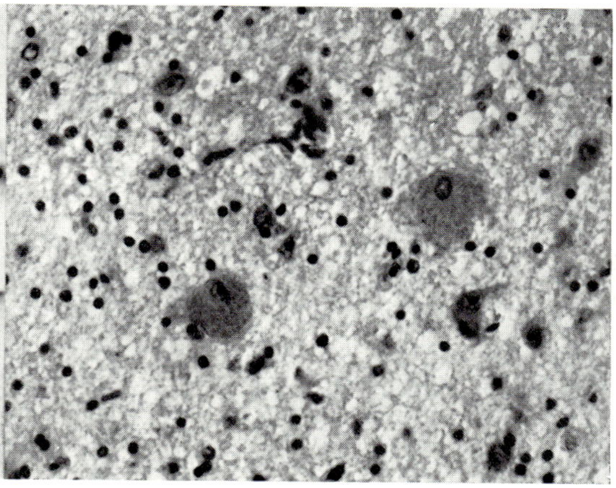

9.19

FIG. 9.18. Kayser-Fleischer zone of pigment in Descemet's membrane. The pigment lies in the inner layer of the membrane with a few granules more deeply. (×1,200.)

FIG. 9.19. Opalski cells in subthalamic nucleus. Their cytoplasm is stained a light brown in iron haematoxylin–van Gieson preparations. (×250.)

1954). In the blood serum, copper is attached to the α, β and γ globulins in proportions of about 25 per cent, 50 per cent and 20 per cent and only 2–5 per cent remains attached to albumin. In hepatolenticular degeneration, on the other hand, only 40–60 per cent of the total serum copper is bound to globulin, chiefly to the β and γ fractions; in 4 out of 5 cases Cumings *et al.* (1955) found only traces of copper in combination with α globulin. The remainder is loosely attached to albumin from which it more easily becomes detached and is either taken up by the proteins of the brain and liver or excreted by the kidneys. The urinary excretion therefore rises from the normal 10–100 μg. of Cu per diem to amounts of 400–600 μg. or even higher. Under treatment with BAL these figures may be greatly exceeded. Holmberg and Laurell (1948) isolated from human serum a blue protein substance in which copper was combined with α globulin. They called this substance *caerulo-plasmin* and found that, using *p*-phenylenediamine as a substrate, it could act as an oxidase. In hepatolenticular degeneration caeruloplasmin is normally absent or present in very small amounts and has no oxidase activity (Scheinberg and Gitlin 1952, Bearn and Kunkel 1954). In 2 out of 40 cases, however, Cumings (1962) found it present in normal quantity. The serum copper level was normal in 4 out of the 40 cases. The amount of serum caeruloplasmin may also be diminished in a patient's siblings who themselves show no sign of the disease (Turpin *et al.* 1953, Bush *et al.* 1955).

The increase of amino-acids in the urine, which may reach 300–800 mg. of amino-acid nitrogen per diem (about 4–6 times normal), affects all those normally present and the abnormal amino-acids proline and citralline also have occasionally been found. As there is no corresponding rise in the amino-acids of the blood serum it is probable that the increased excretion is related to defective re-absorption in the convoluted tubules of the kidneys. The relation of amino-aciduria to the abnormal copper metabolism is not clear. Excess of amino-acids appears in the urine in other diseases of the liver, but only when its function is gravely disturbed as in acute yellow atrophy, and it is rarely seen in cases of hepatic cirrhosis without jaundice. In hepatolenticular degeneration the amino-aciduria is therefore quite out of proportion to the disturbance of liver function, which is usually slight and in many cases is not evident on routine testing.

(Revised by W. H. McMenemey.)

REFERENCES

Barnes, S. and Hurst, E. W. (1925) *Brain*, **48**, 279; (1926) ibid., **49**, 36.

Bearn, A. G. and Kunkel, H. G. (1954) *Proc. Soc. exper. Biol. (N.Y.)*, **85**, 44.

Böttiger, L. E. and Möllerbers, H. (1959) *Acta Med. scand.*, **165**, 413.

Brand, I. and Takats, I. (1951) *Arch. f. Ophthal.*, **161**, 391.

Bush, J. A., Mahoney, J. P., Markowitz, H., Gubler, C. J., Cartwright, G. E. and Wintrobe, M. M. (1955) *J. clin. Invest.*, **34**, 1766.

Cumings, J. N. (1948) *Brain*, **71**, 410; (1957) *Modern Trends in Neurology*, 2nd Edition; (1962) *Proc. Nutrition Soc.*, **21**, 29.

Cumings, J. N., Goodwin, H. J. and Earl, C. J. (1955) *J. clin. Path.*, **8**, 69.

Earl, C. J., Moulton, M. J. and Selverstone, B. (1954) *Amer. J. Med.*, **17**, 205.

Fleischer, B. (1903) *Klin. Monatsbl. f. Augenheilk.*, **41**, 489; (1909) *Münch. med. Wschr.*, **56**, 1120; (1912) *Dtsch. Z. Nervenheilk.*, **44**, 179.

Gerlach, W. and Rohrschneider, W. (1934) *Klin. Wschr.*, **13**, 48.

Greenfield, J. G., Poynton, F. J. and Walshe, F. M. R. (1924) *Quart. J. Med.*, **17**, 385.

Hall, H. C. (1921) *La dégénérescence hépato-lenticulaire*, Masson, Paris.

Haurowitz, F. (1930) *Z. physiol. Chemie*, **190**, 72.

Hoesslin, C. von and Alzheimer, A. (1912) *Z. ges. Neurol. Psychiat.*, **8**, 183.

Holmberg, C. G. and Laurell, C. B. (1948) *Acta chem. Scand.*, **2**, 550; (1951) *Scand. J. clin. Invest.*, **3**, 103.

Howard, C. P. and Royce, C. E. (1919) *Arch. Int. Med.*, **24**, 497.

Kayser, B. (1902) *Klin. Monatsbl. f. Augenheilk.*, **40**, 22.

Lichtenstein, B. W. and Gore, I. (1955) *Arch. Neurol. Psychiat. Chicago*, **73** 13.

Lüthy, F. (1931) *Dtsch. Z. Nervenheilk.*, **123**, 101.

Okinawa, S., Yoshikawa, M., Toyoda, M., Mozai, T., Toyokura, Y. and Kamiyama, M. (1954) *Arch. Neurol. Psychiat. Chicago*, **72**, 573.

Opalski, A. (1930) *Z. ges. Neurol. Psychiat.*, **124**, 140.

Rosenoer, V. M. and Michell, R. C. (1959) *Brit. J. Radiol.*, **32**, 105.

Scheinberg, I. H. and Gitlin, D. (1952) *Science*, **116**, 484.

Steger, J. and R. (1954) *Dtsch. Z. Nervenheilk.*, **172**, 321.

Turpin, R., Jerome, H. and Schmitt, H. (1953) *Proc. Roy. Soc. Med.*, **46**, 1061.

Uzman, L. L. and Denny-Brown, D. (1948) *Amer. J. med. Sc.*, **215**, 599.

Uzman, L. L. and Jakus, M. A. (1957) *Neurology*, **7**, 341.

Wilson, S. A. K. (1912) *Brain*, **34**, 295.

CHAPTER 10

SYSTEM DEGENERATIONS OF THE CEREBELLUM, BRAIN STEM AND SPINAL CORD

By J. G. Greenfield

The diseases in this group are characterised clinically by progressive disturbance of equilibrium and motion and pathologically by lesions of nuclei and tracts subserving these functions. All have an hereditary tendency. Some were first described as affecting several members of a family and have always been regarded as familial or hereditary; others have usually occurred in isolated cases, and their hereditary nature has therefore not been so apparent. In amyotrophic lateral sclerosis the hereditary tendency has a curious geographical distribution since in Europe and America the disease has rarely appeared in this guise, but in Guam and other islands of the Mariana group it has been found to affect many members of the Chamarro race, but no members of other races inhabiting these islands (Kurland and Mulder 1955). The rate of progress in most of the diseases in this group is usually slow, to be measured in years rather than in months, but occasionally they assume subacute form and cause severe incapacitation or death within a year of their onset. The cause of this exacerbation is often obscure, but in some cases appears to be related to general metabolic disturbances, especially those due to bronchial or ovarian carcinoma. (See p. 314.)

It is characteristic of this group of diseases that the dividing line between the more closely related forms tends to be blurred by the occurrence of borderline and transitional cases. These may be found even in one family if several branches or many members can be examined, but in such cases the differences are often more clinical than pathological and depend on an earlier or greater incidence of lesions on one or the other tract or nucleus. The characteristic lesions of the disease in the cerebellum, brain stem and spinal cord are often associated with lesions at a higher level, and these may reveal themselves clinically by such symptoms as dementia, epilepsy or blindness. But in spite of these tendencies to wider spread of the disease, both clinical signs and pathological lesions are commonly stereotyped and it is possible to assign most cases to one or another category.

Certain of these diseases tend to appear in a pure form while others are more often transitional or mixed. Among the former are paralysis agitans, cerebello-olivary degeneration and amyotrophic lateral sclerosis. Into the latter group fall olivo-ponto-cerebellar degeneration and the various forms of spinocerebellar degeneration; in these there is a greater tendency towards spread of the lesions from tracts or neuronal systems which are primarily affected to other tracts with which they make important synaptic connections. Trans-synaptic degeneration of this kind has been seen to occur as a consequence of any form of lesion, especially in certain tracts and nuclei, but in this group of diseases it appears to be more common and widespread. Indeed some authors consider the pathogenesis of these diseases to be largely *a chain degeneration.* It must, however, be recognised that in each form of disease the incidence falls chiefly on a small number of tracts and nuclei and that the degeneration of other neuronal systems to which these are anatomically and functionally related is usually slight and may not appear until late in the course of the disease.

The type of lesion in all the diseases in this group is *simple neuronal atrophy*. Its chief characteristics have already been described (Chapter 1) and are especially well illustrated in the more subacute forms. (1) The nerve tracts containing fibres of large diameter are especially liable to be affected. (2) The nerve fibres in these tracts are affected first at their periphery: later the whole fibre atrophies and disappears. (3) The cell body of the affected neurones tends to shrink and eventually to disappear without showing the chromatolysis of axonal reaction. In *paralysis agitans*, however, atrophy of neurones is associated, especially in the melanin pigmented cells of the brain stem, with the hyaline cytoplasmic inclusions which have been described, but what proportion of the affected neurones undergoes this type of degeneration is not known. Neurofibrillary changes in cortical neurones have also been described in some systemic diseases of the spinal cord.

Paralysis agitans (Parkinson's disease)

In his *Essay on the Shaking Palsy* Parkinson (1817) gave the first full clinical description of the disease which often bears his name. The Latin equivalent *paralysis agitans* came into use during the latter half of the nineteenth century. This is a disease of the second half of life, often coming on in the sixth or seventh decade, with slowly progressive rigidity of the limbs, trunk and face and constant, rapid tremor of the hands and, to a less degree, of the arms and legs, which is present at rest and usually diminishes rather than increases on movement. Either symptom may be the first to appear and in many cases the disability is confined to one limb in the early stages of the disease, but as it progresses both sides of the body are involved in tremor and rigidity. The course of the disease is usually slow and many cases last for 20 years or more, but it may eventually become extremely disabling. It is an idiopathic disease in the sense that no causative factor is known except hereditary tendency, and this is less evident than in many progressive system diseases of the spinal cord. Denny-Brown (1949) puts familial cases as between 4 and 16 per cent of the total.

During the last 50 years there has been a tendency to consider Parkinsonism as a symptom complex which may be due to a variety of causes, among which premature senility, vascular disease and antecedent encephalitis lethargica are the most important, while trauma, syphilis and certain metabolic or inorganic poisons, especially manganese, have been blamed for other cases. But as Walshe (1955) points out, typical paralysis agitans, as described by Parkinson (1817), differs in its clinical features from the results of vascular disease or of metallic or other forms of poisoning and also from most cases in which the symptoms follow an attack of encephalitis lethargica. Nor does the presence of a positive Wassermann reaction in a patient's blood prove that his disease is due to syphilis. At least the pathology in syphilitic patients may differ in no respect from that found in idiopathic cases (Greenfield and Bosanquet 1953).

Pathology. Until Trétiakoff's (1919) study of the substantia nigra, idiopathic paralysis agitans remained a disease without a characteristic pathology. Previous workers, of whom the most important were Jelgersma (1908) and Lewy (1913), appear to have neglected this nucleus, but described minor changes in the basal ganglia and the tracts arising in them. For the most part these were changes common in brains of similar age, but Lewy's description of concentric hyaline cytoplasmic inclusions in cells of the nucleus substantiae innominatae and dorsal vagal nucleus was an important exception. Trétiakoff found similar inclusions in the pigmented cells of the substantia nigra in 6 cases of typical paralysis agitans. In all his 9 idiopathic cases these cells were reduced in number and some of the remainder showed such lesions as neurofibrillary change, binucleation or grumose degeneration.* He considered (1921) that lesions of the substantia nigra were always associated with Parkinsonism unless damage to important motor pathways prevented the appearance of the characteristic signs of the disease but after sudden vascular lesions these might not appear for several weeks or months. This fact, which had previously been observed by Holmes (1904), may explain the difficulty which experimentalists have had in producing Parkinsonian symptoms by local lesions in the neighbourhood of the substantia nigra (Carpenter *et al.* 1950).

The first complete description of the pathology of idiopathic paralysis agitans was given by Foix and Nicolesco (1925). They found very widespread lesions in the brain and brain stem with more involvement of nerve cells than of fibre tracts. Severe lesions were constantly seen in the zona compacta of the substantia nigra which, on naked-eye examination, appeared smaller and less uniformly pigmented than normal. The other pigmented nuclei of the brain stem, the globus pallidus and the substantia innominata of Reichert, also habitually showed

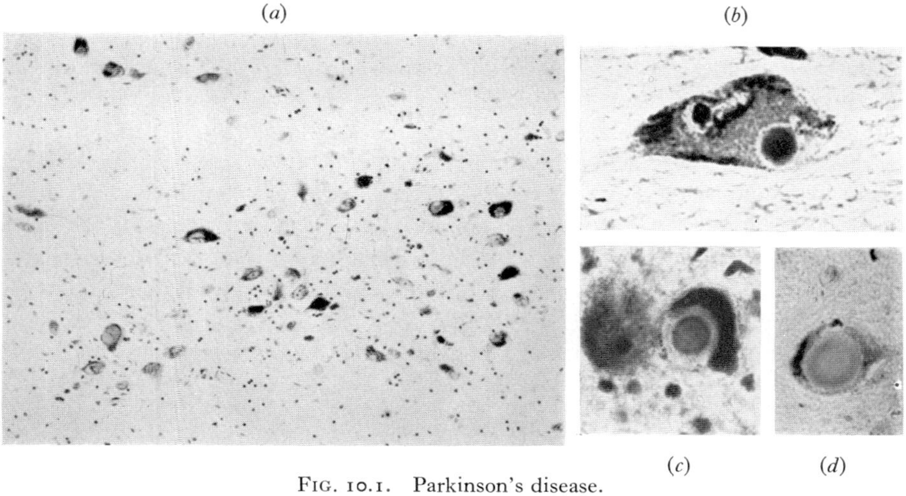

FIG. 10.1. Parkinson's disease.

(*a*) Substantia nigra showing loss of pigmented cells and increase in glial nuclei. Note the poverty of melanin in some of the remaining cells and the small vacuole in one of the cells. Nissl stain × 100.

(*b*) Pigmented cell which still retains some of its melanin with an intracytoplasmic inclusion body (Lewy body). Nissl stain × 300.

(*c*) Intracytoplasmic inclusion body at the periphery of a cell. Note the small amount of pigment over its stretched surface. Nissl stain × 280.

(*d*) Pigmented cell, the cytoplasm of which is greatly distended by a laminated inclusion body. Nissl stain × 280.

lesions. Less constant lesions were seen in the hypothalamic nuclei and reticular formation of the brain stem. The nucleus dentatus and thalamus also were frequently affected, less often the cerebral and cerebellar cortex.

The lesions in the substantia nigra varied in intensity and topography from one case to another. The chief lesion was a simple atrophy and destruction of nerve cells especially in the ventro-external and medial small-celled groups. Shrinkage of the cell body was often at first associated with swellings on the dendrites and increase in size of the nucleus. Later the nucleus became eccentric and the dendrites shrunken and finally only a ghost cell remained. This process was often associated with the presence in the cytoplasm of vacuoles, as seen in sections stained by basic blues, or argyrophilic spherical bodies resembling corpora amylacea

* 'Dégénérescence grumeleuse.' In this the cells are filled with colourless, ill-defined granules of unknown nature.

in silver impregnations. These were probably Lewy's hyaline bodies, but the special staining methods by which Lafora (1913) and Trétiakoff (1919) differentiated them were not used and little emphasis was therefore placed on their presence. Irregularities in the endocellular neurofibrillar network were also seen in silver impregnations. Neuroglial scarring was present in the islands from which nerve cells had disappeared. It was especially dense around vessels, but the vascular lesions were slight. Changes similar to those in the substantia nigra were found in the other melanin-pigmented cells of the brain stem such as the locus coeruleus and the pigmented cells in the reticular formation and dorsal nucleus of the vagus; in the latter inclusions were especially prominent. Similar inclusions, sometimes almost filling the cell body, were seen in some cells of the substantia innominata; in others there was disorganisation of the endocellular neurofibrils, corkscrew dendrites or a glassy appearance of the cell body. The hypothalamic nuclei showed very similar lesions. In the less affected nuclei of the brain stem, such as the reticular formation and nucleus dentatus, the nerve cells were shrunken with an excess of lipofuscin pigment.

The lesions in the globus pallidus, which in their cases were constant and sometimes severe, were essentially those of senility. They consisted of atrophy, with excess of lipofuscin, and rarefaction of nerve cells and zones of état criblé or pré-criblé around some of the vessels. The lesions in the nerve cells were rarely generalised but usually involved either the antero-internal or the dorso-external part of the nucleus. État criblé, which is normally greater in the striatum than in the globus pallidus in senile cases, had the reverse distribution in their cases. The changes in the blood-vessels corresponded with the age of the brain and had no distinctive features. The striatum showed similar but, in general, slighter lesions than the globus pallidus. The special incidence of atrophy on the large nerve cells, described by Ramsay Hunt (1917), was not observed, as the small cells were equally affected. Excess of lipofuscin and some atrophy was found in the ventro-external part of the *subthalamic nucleus*, especially when the globus pallidus was severely damaged. The nucleus ruber and the middle and ventral parts of the thalamus might show similar changes.

In the cerebral cortex the lesions of senility were present in varying degree, especially in the frontal lobes. In the cerebellar cortex of some cases there was disappearance of Purkinje cells with torpedoes on the axons of some of those that remained and preservation of pericellular baskets. These changes were similar to those seen in late cortical cerebellar atrophy. Tract lesions were slight, but the ansa lenticularis, fasciculus lenticularis (H^2), zona incerta and posterior commissure were diminished in size in certain cases.

Summing up, they emphasised both the diffuse and the localised character of the lesions. The diffuse lesions differed little from those of senility, whereas the localised lesions, especially those in the melanin-bearing cells of the brain stem and in the globus pallidus, were not found in the same intensity in any other disease of the nervous system.

Hassler (1937–8) studied the normal anatomy of the substantia nigra and the changes which are seen in this nucleus in paralysis agitans. He found the most severe lesions in the central part of the zona compacta where some groups of pigmented cells had almost disappeared and others had lost about half of their neurones. The medial and lateral cell groups were less affected. Some cell loss was found also in the nucleus substantiae innominatae and in 1 case this was severe. Inclusions of Lewy type were seen both in the substantia nigra and locus coeruleus. In some cases lesions were also present in the striatum where they appeared to be related to the severity of the tremor, but in other cases both this nucleus and the globus pallidus were intact. The special incidence of the disease on the central cell groups of the substantia nigra has been confirmed by Klaue (1940). In the cases examined by Greenfield and Bosanquet (1953) hyaline inclusions of Lewy type were almost constantly found in the melanin-bearing cells of the substantia nigra and locus coeruleus, and occasionally in the substantia innominata, the pigmented cells of the dorsal vagal nucleus and the oculomotor nucleus. They might also be present in postencephalitic cases but in these, as Hallervorden (1933–5) had shown, neurofibrillary changes were more usual. Both types of degeneration appear to be more common, or at least more easily found, in the locus coeruleus than in the substantia nigra. In the former situation Beheim-Schwarzbach (1952) found hyaline inclusions also in cases of senile dementia and in a few other senile brains. In her cases of true paralysis agitans they were constantly found and were combined with cells showing neurofibrillary changes in 25 per cent (1954). Greenfield and Bosanquet also confirmed Trétiakoff's observation of binucleated nerve cells and cells undergoing grumose degeneration in the substantia nigra. Cells containing an excess of lipofuscin pigment, lying either between the nucleus and the melanin granules or among the latter, were very common.

Lipkin (1959) found Lewy-type inclusions in 25 out of 29 cases of idiopathic paralysis agitans, in 4 out of 9 instances of post-encephalitic Parkinsonism and in 4·9 per cent of controls. In no instance did he find an inclusion in an otherwise normal neurone. Bethlem and den Hartog Jager (1960) found them in all of 15 cases of paralysis agitans but in none of 4 cases of post-encephalitic Parkinsonism and of 20 controls. In Parkinson's disease they may be found elsewhere than in the pigmented nuclei of the brain stem. Lipkin (1959) found them in the inferior olive and in the cerebral cortex and den Hartog Jager and Bethlem (1960) in a variety of centres in the diencephalon and brain stem, in the lateral and posterior horns of the spinal cord and in sympathetic ganglia of 5 out of 6 cases. Intracytoplasmic inclusion bodies in the cells of sympathetic ganglia had been previously noted (Herzog 1928; Wohlwill 1928) and argyrophilic bodies in these cells are illustrated by Hechet and Nussbaum (1931).

These more recent studies on the pathology of idiopathic paralysis agitans agree in considering it as a nosological entity in which the most important lesions are found in the substantia nigra. These lesions, although more discrete and usually less severe than those seen in post-encephalitic Parkinsonism, are equally constant and very characteristic. They are always associated with similar, but less severe, lesions in the other melanin-bearing nerve cells in the brain stem. The less constant but sometimes severe lesions which may be found in the globus pallidus and substantia innominata, and the changes in the hypothalamic nuclei, described by Foix and Nicolesco, may also have some bearing on the symptomatology of the disease. Indeed, Denny-Brown (1961) has stressed the likely importance of the pallidal lesions which include the 'paravascular degeneration' in the outer segments and the paucity of finely myelinated fibres giving rise to a pallor, which he regards as characteristic. This loss of fibres is more apparent in sections stained for axons. He regards the common feature as a breakdown of the blood-brain barrier in the capillaries of the globus pallidus and less frequently in the substantia nigra and dentate nucleus.

The atrophic changes in the nerve cells of the globus pallidus may well be secondary to the lesions in the substantia nigra, in the sense of trans-synaptic degenerations, since the substantia nigra has an important projection on this part of the basal ganglia (Ranson and Ranson 1941).

Spino-cerebellar atrophies

This term is used for the diseases in which the cortex and peduncles of the cerebellum and the long motor and proprioceptive tracts of the spinal cord undergo neuronal degeneration and atrophy. Various forms have been distinguished by the distribution of the lesions, which may be confined to the cerebellum and one or more of its afferent systems of neurones, or to the long tracts and nerve roots of the spinal cord, or may extend widely over both regions and even involve the retina and optic nerves and the cerebral cortex. These diseases have been reviewed by Greenfield (1954). They are true *abiotrophies* and were indeed used by Gowers to illustrate what he meant by this term. The pathogenesis of all is *primary neuronal atrophy* as already described (p. 26). In most cases this is a slow process, and even in long-standing cases the cell body and proximal part of the nerve fibre may survive, but in many cases the whole neurone atrophies and disappears. Occasionally the rate of degeneration is more rapid so that there may be severe loss of nerve cells and tract degenerations within a few months of the onset of symptoms. In such cases the appearances may closely resemble Wallerian degeneration.

This group of degenerative, often familial or hereditary, diseases is linked to *paralysis agitans* on the one hand, since many cases of *olivo-ponto-cerebellar atrophy* develop Parkinsonian rigidity and tremor, and to *amyotrophic lateral sclerosis* on the other, by the amyotrophy and spastic paraplegia which is seen in some families of hereditary ataxia. Among the varieties of disease included in this group the *cerebello-olivary degeneration* of Holmes (sometimes called *late cortical cerebellar atrophy*) stands out as having little tendency to vary from case to case in a family, or for its lesions to spread from the areas usually attacked to others with which they make synaptic connection. The other members of the group form a continuous chain linked by border-line cases, from olivo-ponto-cerebellar atrophy to familial spastic paraplegia and Friedreich's ataxia which also is linked to peroneal atrophy. There is, however, a tendency for the disease in each affected family to keep to a similar pathology, although the order and severity with which it attacks the different nuclei and tracts may cause considerable variations in the clinical picture. In most families the disease appears at about the same age in different siblings and even in successive generations. Some of the variations from this rule may be explained by environmental factors such as febrile illness or malnutrition which may hasten or even precipitate the onset of nervous symptoms. Many varieties of hereditary transmission have been found. As is usual the forms which begin in childhood appear as recessives while those with onset in later life may be either recessive or dominant. In a few families there is a tendency to sex linkage.

This group of diseases is also linked, in varying degree, to hereditary degenerations of the eye and ear and to dementia. In Friedreich's ataxia the incidence of blindness, which is usually due to optic atrophy and less often to cataract, has varied from 9 to 12 per cent in different surveys and is still higher in cases of spastic ataxia with a later age of onset. In almost all families blindness has occurred only in ataxic members, but in the large family collected by Franceschetti and Klein in Switzerland (1948) and in one reported by Ferguson and Critchley (1928) retinal or macular degeneration was also found in members with no evidence of spinal disease. The incidence of dementia is even higher. In cases of hereditary ataxia Bell and Carmichael (1939) found dementia associated with ataxia in 13·5 per cent of the 242 families included in their survey, and, in a further 9·5 per cent of the families, non-ataxic members showed some degree of dementia. In Sjögren's (1943) smaller series of 91 cases of Friedreich's ataxia 14 or 15·5 per cent were oligophrenic. Cases of subacute cerebellar and spinocerebellar degeneration commonly show severe dementia and more chronic cases of cerebellar ataxia may show mental regression towards their termination.

Classification of spino-cerebellar ataxias

(A) Spinal forms

(1) *Friedreich's ataxia.*
- (a) Pure forms.
- (b) Associated with peroneal atrophy. (*Hereditary areflexic dystasia* of Roussy and Levy or *familial claw foot with absent tendon jerks* of Symonds and Shaw.)
- (c) *Posterior column ataxia* of Biemond.

(2) *Hereditary spastic ataxia.* (In some families associated with 3.)

(3) *Hereditary spastic paraplegia.*

(B) Spino-cerebellar forms

(1) *Menzel type of hereditary ataxia.* (*Olivo-ponto-cerebellar degeneration.*)
(2) *Subacute spino-cerebellar degeneration.* (Carcinogenic and sporadic.)

(C) Cerebellar forms

(1) *Holmes type of hereditary ataxia.* (*Cerebello-olivary*, or *late cortical cerebellar atrophy* of Marie Foix and Alajouanine. Subacute familial type of Akelaitis.)
(2) *Diffuse atrophy of Purkinje cells.* (Toxic and carcinogenic.) (See pp. 262 and 315.)

Spinal forms of hereditary ataxia

Friedreich's ataxia

It is convenient to retain this eponym which derives from Friedreich of Heidelberg who in 1861, 1863 and 1876 described a familial form of progressive ataxia affecting children under the age of 20. Since then the disease has come to be recognised as one of the most common hereditary diseases of the nervous system. Bell and Carmichael were able to analyse over 400 cases occurring in 242 families and very numerous sporadic cases have also been described. In the great majority of cases the disease begins before the age of 20, and as often during the first as the second decade. The chief early symptoms are ataxia of gait and pes cavus; these are followed later by clumsiness of the hands, dysarthria of speech and nystagmus. The knee and ankle jerks are lost early and kyphosis, often with much deformity of the chest, comes on as the disease progresses. The first symptoms often appear after one of the acute infectious fevers of childhood and may come on earlier in such cases than in other siblings, but in many families the onset is at about the same age in all affected members. The course of the disease is relentless and most patients become unable to walk within 5 years of its onset. Death, to which deformity of the chest or dysphagia may contribute, or which may be caused by cardiac failure, usually occurs during the third decade if not earlier. In some cases the course of the disease is subacute, leading to death within a year of the onset (Fig. 10.3).

Pathology. The main brunt of the atrophy falls on the long ascending and descending tracts of the spinal cord, i.e. the dorsal columns, direct and indirect spinocerebellar tracts and pyramidal tracts (Fig. 10.2). There is also loss of the larger fibres in the dorsal roots, especially in the lumbosacral enlargement. In the dorsal columns the earliest degeneration is seen in the middle-root zone. This is most often evident in the fasciculus cuneatus in the cervical region, as this tract is involved later and less than the fasciculus gracilis which is usually degenerated throughout at most levels. Clarke's column shows atrophy and loss of nerve cells and fibrous gliosis, and the spinocerebellar tracts are usually atrophied throughout their course. On the other hand the pyramidal tracts may be relatively or completely intact at the level of the brain stem, and show progressive pallor on descending through the cord. Fibrous gliosis, which is often intense, replaces the atrophied fibres but does not compensate for their bulk, so that there is always considerable shrinkage in the cross-section of the cord. Shrinkage and loss of cells is seen also in the dorsal root ganglia. Atrophy or degeneration of nuclei or tracts at the lower brain-stem levels has been frequently reported. These include the fasciculus solitarius and the lower cranial nerves, especially the sensory roots of the trigeminal and the vestibular, glossopharyngeal, vagus and hypoglossal. In many cases degeneration has been found in the median fillet and its nuclei of origin (nuclei gracilis and cuneatus). Loss of Purkinje cells in the superior folia of the cerebellum or atrophy of the nucleus dentatus and superior cerebellar peduncle have been found by some observers. Other fibre systems which may undergo atrophy are the median longitudinal fasciculus, central tegmental fasciculus, middle cerebellar peduncle and the decussations of Meynert and Forel.

Atrophic sclerosis of the superior olive and ventral cochlear nucleus were found by Urich *et al.* (1957) in a patient without evident loss of hearing. In a few families Friedreich's ataxia has been associated with deaf mutism or progressive deafness. In Hunt's (1921) case degeneration of the nucleus dentatus and superior cerebellar peduncle was associated clinically with myoclonus, but this is exceptional. In the case of Urich *et al.* there was also degeneration of the nucleus ventralis lateralis of the thalamus in which many of its fibres end. Degeneration of the nucleus ventralis posterior of the thalamus, and of the external segment of the globus pallidus and external two-thirds of the subthalamic nucleus was also found. The association of the lesions of Friedreich's ataxia with degeneration of the zona compacta of the substantia

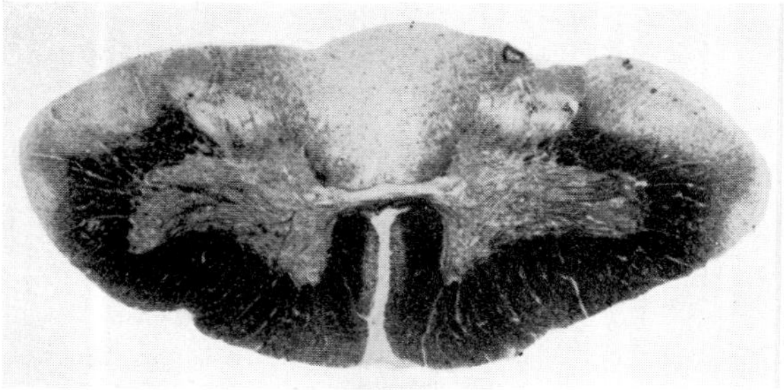

10.2

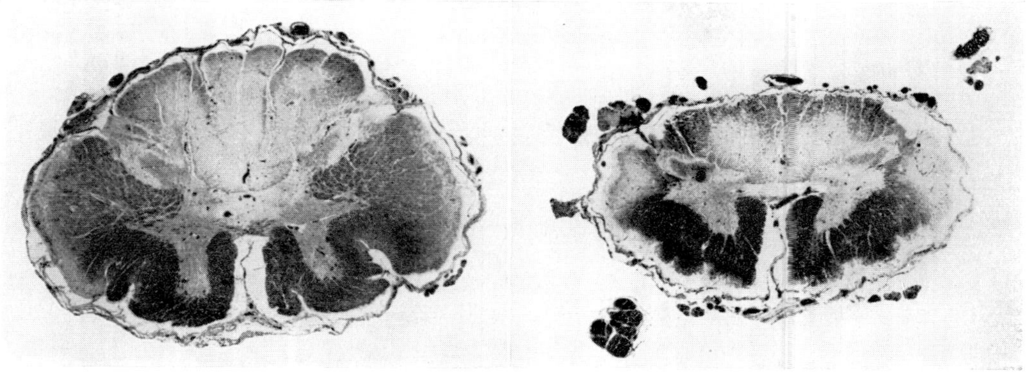

10.3 (*a*) 10.3 (*b*)

FIG. 10.2. Section of the lower cervical cord from a case of Friedreich's ataxia. (Weigert-Pal.)
FIG. 10.3. Sections of (*a*) upper cervical and (*b*) thoracic cord from a case of subacute spinal ataxia (aet. 50) fatal in less than 1 year. (Myelin.)

nigra has been described by Biemond and Sinnege (1955). In the three members of their family whom they examined, Parkinsonian symptoms predominated over ataxia. No Lewy inclusions were found.

Retina and optic nerves. The forms of optic atrophy which may occur in Friedreich's and other forms of hereditary spinal ataxia were classified by André-Van Leeuwen (1949) as belonging to three types: (1) Retro-bulbar neuritis with central loss of vision; these cases are rare. (2) Optic atrophy of rapid onset with reduction either of peripheral or central vision. (3) A slow diminution of vision with loss of peripheral vision. In the last two forms the ophthalmoscopic appearances might be those of retinitis pigmentosa. In some cases the clinical picture has resembled the Leber or Stargardt (Rayner Batten) type of retinal atrophy. Pathological evidence of the changes in the retina is lacking. Degeneration of the papillomacular bundle in the optic nerve, as in the case described by André-Van Leeuwen and van Bogaert (1942), may be due, as in Leber's atrophy, to primary degeneration of the ganglion cell layer of the retina. In the cases with pigmentary change the degeneration probably affects chiefly the outer nuclear layer.

Heart. In many cases the heart is enlarged and there are some pericardial adhesions. Microscopical examinations by a number of observers from Friedreich to Russell (1946) have shown interstitial myocarditis with necrosis or granular degeneration of some muscle fibres and hypertrophy of others. This may be associated with diffuse or focal cellular infiltrations. Valvular lesions of congenital or acquired type are much less common. The tachycardia and arrhythmia which often usher in death in Friedreich's ataxia may be due to myocardial degeneration or may depend, in greater or less degree, on degeneration of the vagus nerve. The restricted capacity of the chest due to kyphoscoliosis may also contribute to cardiac failure.

Association of Friedreich's ataxia with peroneal atrophy

In several families (Biemond 1928, Spillane 1940) some siblings show the signs of Friedreich's ataxia and others those of peroneal atrophy. In other families pes cavus, ataxia of gait and absence of knee and ankle jerks, usually of mild degree and showing little tendency to progress, are combined in some members with amyotrophy of the muscles below the knee and in the hands and forearms. To this syndrome Roussy and Levy (1926) gave the name 'hereditary areflexic dystasia'. Symonds and Shaw and Rombold and Riley described similar families in the same year. In some of these families the disease was transmitted as a dominant, in others as a sex-linked recessive. As the disease causes only slight disability very few post-mortem examinations have been made. Spiller (1910) found lesions in the cord similar to those of Friedreich's ataxia.

Biemond's posterior column ataxia

Biemond (1951) described a family in which the father, his brother and 4 of his children showed signs of degeneration of the dorsal columns of the cord without other evidence of hereditary ataxia. Post-mortem examination in 1 case showed severe degeneration of the dorsal columns throughout their length and of the larger fibres in the dorsal roots. Loss of Purkinje cells in some folia of the cerebellum was also found.

Hereditary spastic ataxia

There are records of a large number of families in which ataxia came on later than in Friedreich's disease and in which the knee jerks were preserved or increased. In some cases, but not in all, some degree of spasticity was present in the lower limbs. The feet are not usually deformed in these cases. The average age of onset in 259 cases collected by Bell and Carmichael was 26·2 years. It was higher in families in which the disease was transmitted as a dominant and lower (14·7 years) when transmitted as a recessive. Post-mortem examinations have been made in a few cases and have shown lesions of the long tracts of the cord, not always including the pyramidal tracts (Adolf Meyer 1897, Barker 1903, Guillain *et al.* 1941) or the indirect spinocerebellar tracts, with little or no abnormality in the brain stem or cerebellum.

Spino-cerebellar forms of ataxia

Menzel type of hereditary ataxia (Olivopontocerebellar degeneration)

Menzel (1891) described a form of generalised ataxia affecting three generations of a family. In Menzel's patient, who was one of 4 affected siblings of the second generation, the disease began at the age of 28 and he died aged 46. Post-mortem examination showed degeneration of the pyramidal and direct spinocerebellar tracts and of Clarke's column and the dorsal columns of the cord. At the level of the medulla there was loss of cells in the nuclei cuneatus and gracilis and the nuclei of the hypoglossal, facial and trigeminal nerves. There was also atrophy of the inferior olivary nuclei, nuclei pontis and cerebellum, including poverty of myelin in the white matter, rarefaction of the granular layer and great loss of Purkinje cells. The cerebellar lesions were least in the vermis, flocculus, uvula and amygdaloid lobes.

Since then a large number of similar cases, both isolated and familial, have been reported. A very large family has been examined in the United States by Schut and Haymaker (1951) and Book (1953) with 8 post-mortem examinations. In these familial cases the age of onset has varied from 12 to 52 years with a mean of 38 years. The lesions which have been found have varied in intensity and extent in different cases and include atrophy of the middle cerebellar peduncle, nuclei pontis, inferior olives and olivocerebellar tracts, cerebellar white matter and cortex in that order of constancy. The dorsal columns, pyramidal tracts and one or both of the spinocerebellar tracts are usually degenerated, and atrophy of motor neurones in the lower brain stem and spinal cord is also commonly found. As in Menzel's case the atrophy in the cerebellum is greatest in, or may be limited to, the phylogenetically newer parts of the cerebellum, and spares the flocculonodular lobe and parts of the vermis. In some familial cases there is loss of myelin staining in the cerebellar hemispheres with little damage to the cortex and preservation, sometimes in shrunken form, of the nuclei pontis. This may be considered as an early stage of the condition.

The name *olivo-ponto-cerebellar atrophy* was given to an isolated case of this disease by Dejerine and Thomas (1900). The distinction which they made between isolated and familial cases, and between cases with and without spinal involvement, has not been supported by later experience. Peters (1951) considers that some degeneration of spinal tracts, especially of the dorsal columns and the spinocerebellar tracts, is present in almost every case whether familial or isolated, but the examination of the spinal cord is not always reported. Scherer (1933) and Rosenhagen (1943) found loss of nerve cells in the substantia nigra and cell loss and fibrous gliosis in the corpus striatum in a considerable proportion of their cases, especially those in which Parkinsonian symptoms had appeared either early or later in the course of the disease. In Rosenhagen's view cases with lesions in the spinal cord have more tendency to be familial than those in which the lesions are limited to the cerebellum and brain stem, and Parkinsonian symptoms were more common in cases of the latter type: but this rule is not always followed.

The naked-eye appearances in this condition are often striking and may be diagnostic. There is great shrinkage of the ventral part of the pons which appears wedge-shaped (Fig. 10.4*a*), and the olives are less prominent than usual. The atrophy of the cerebellum affects the hemispheres and in most cases is of moderate degree. The long tract lesions in the spinal cord are rarely severe enough to be macroscopically evident. The extent and severity of the disease is well demonstrated in sections stained for myelin. At the level of the pons the tegmentum appears normal or almost so, but there is pallor, which may amount to complete loss of staining, of the transverse fibres in the ventral half, among which the pyramidal tract fibres stand out by their normal staining (Fig. 10.4*a*). In the medulla, along with shrinkage and loss of cells in the inferior olives, the olivocerebellar fibres are pale or unstained both in the hila of the olives and in the inferior peduncle (Fig. 10.5*b*). The atrophy of these two chief afferent tracts to the cerebellum, along with the loss of many Purkinje cells, leads to pallor of the white matter of the cerebellar hemispheres. That of the vermis and floccular lobules is usually well stained (Fig. 10.4*b*). The degree of cell loss in the cerebellar cortex varies from case to case. While both granules and Purkinje cells are usually affected to some extent, there is rarely complete

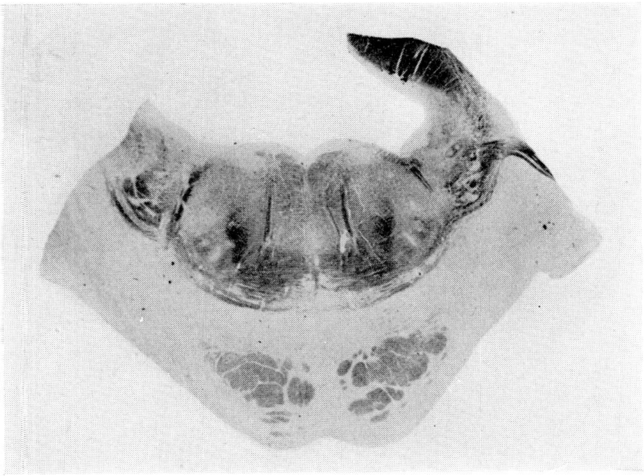

(*a*)

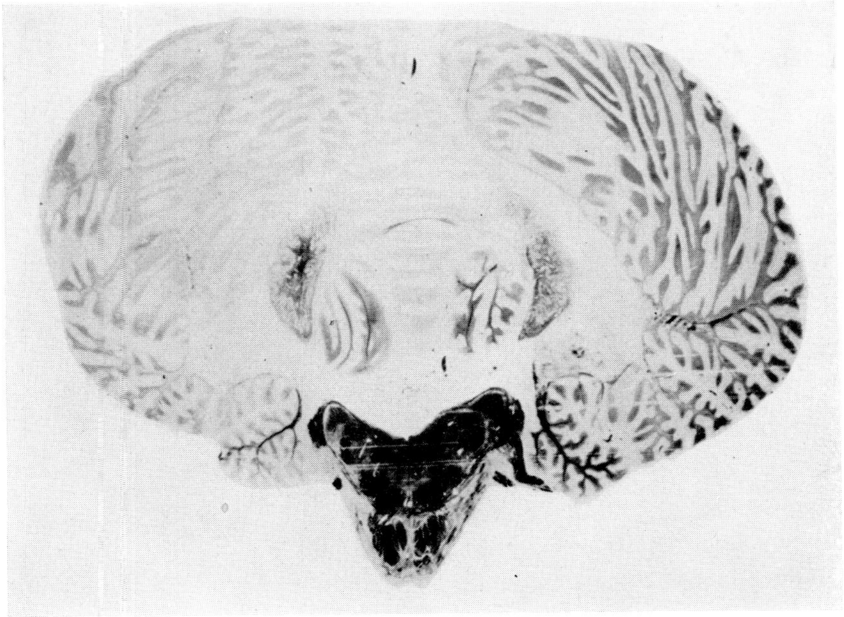

(*b*)

Fig. 10.4. Olivopontocerebellar atrophy.

(*a*) Section of pons, showing complete loss of transverse pontine fibres and of myelin staining in the middle cerebellar peduncle. (Case 1 of Critchley and Greenfield, 1948.)

(*b*) Section at the pontobulbar level, showing loss of staining of the white matter of the cerebellar hemispheres but preservation of the white centre of the flocculus. The granule cells of the cerebellar cortex are well preserved. (W.P. alum carmine.) (Case 2 of Critchley and Greenfield, 1948.)

loss of either and it is not uncommon to find almost complete loss of myelin staining in the cerebellar hemispheres associated with preservation of most of the granule cells (Fig. 10.4*b*). Where Purkinje cells have disappeared empty baskets with hypertrophied fibres are commonly seen and a few torpedo-like or more rounded swellings may be found in the molecular layer on the axons of degenerated Purkinje cells.

Pathogenesis. Scherer (1933) and others have considered the primary lesion in the cerebellar hemispheres to be demyelination with relative preservation of axons. Certainly the pallor of myelin staining in the middle peduncle may in some cases seem disproportionate to the comparatively slight loss of neurones in the nuclei pontis, but this anomaly is probably explained by the tendency, common to all system diseases and well illustrated in the spinocerebellar atrophies, for the nerve fibres to degenerate before their cells of origin show marked changes. It is also not improbable that loss of myelin may be the earliest obvious stage in the atrophy of nerve fibres. This question has also arisen in relation to the peripheral neuropathies.

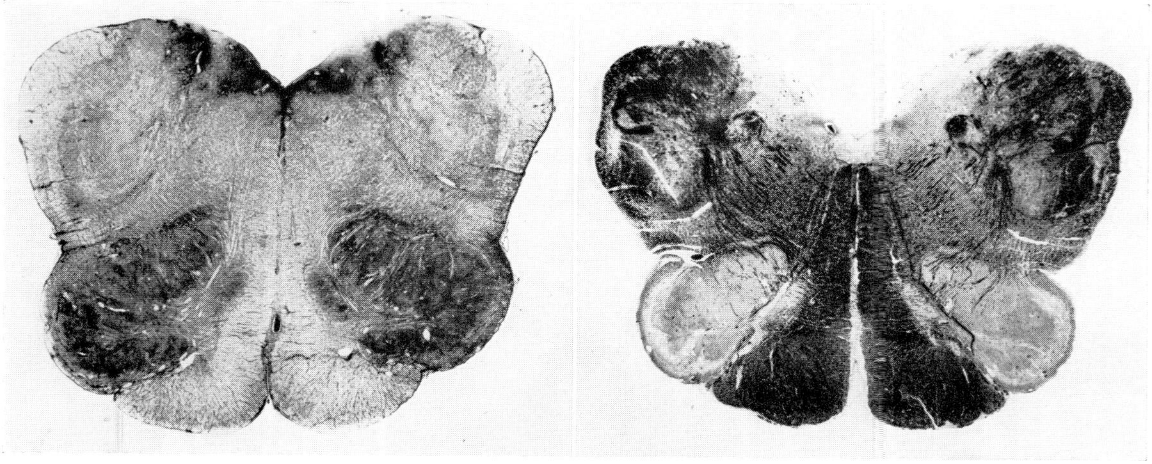

(*a*) (*b*)

FIG. 10.5. (*a*) Normal medulla, stained by Prof. Carl Weigert by his last, unpublished, method for neuroglial fibres, showing the normal heavy gliosis in the inferior olives and the floor of the 4th ventricle. (By the courtesy of Sir Gordon Holmes.)
(*b*) Medulla in olivopontocerebellar atrophy, showing loss of olivocerebellar fibres. (Myelin.) (Case 2 of Critchley and Greenfield, 1948.)

Cerebellar forms of ataxia

Cerebello-olivary degeneration

Gordon Holmes (1907) reported a family in which three brothers and one sister became ataxic between the ages of 35 and 40. Four siblings remained well. Gait was first affected, then the finer hand movements. Dysarthria of speech and tremor of the head and limbs appeared later. There was little alteration of deep or superficial reflexes. A post-mortem examination on one patient who reached the age of 70 showed considerable atrophy of the cerebellum, greatest in the superior parts of the vermis and hemispheres and sparing the amygdalae, uvula, nodulus and part of the lobulus centralis (Fig. 10.5).

Histologically there was almost complete disappearance of Purkinje cells in the most affected areas with proliferation of Bergmann nuclei and fibrous gliosis of the molecular layer. The granule cells were less damaged. There was some loss of myelinated fibres in the folia proportionate to the loss of Purkinje cells, and the amiculus of the nucleus dentatus was less deeply stained than the surrounding white matter, but no degeneration of the superior or middle cerebellar peduncles was present and there was little loss of myelin staining in the white matter of the cerebellum. The inferior and accessory olives had also undergone atrophy (Fig. 10.7) associated with loss of olivocerebellar fibres. This spared to some extent the medial half of the ventral layer and the caudal end of the medial accessory olive. The latter parts of the olivary nucleus were found (Stewart and Holmes 1908) to project to the less affected parts of the cerebellum, whereas the dorsal folia projected to the superior surface. Holmes therefore considered that the olivary degeneration was secondary to atrophy of the cerebellar cortex.

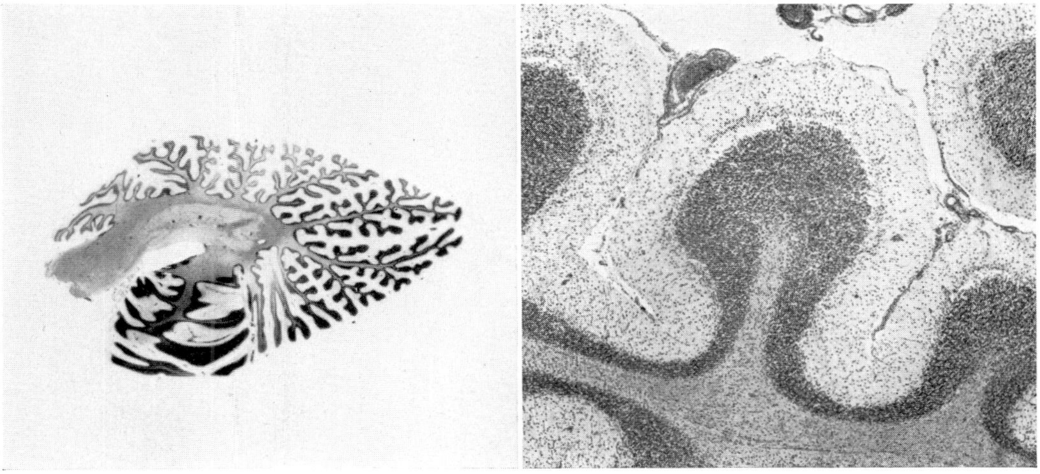

(*a*) (*b*)

FIG. 10.6. Familial cerebello-olivary degeneration. (Case of Greenfield and Weber, 1942.)
(*a*) Parasagittal section of cerebellum showing atrophy greatest in the superior folia.
(*b*) Higher-power section of less atrophied folia, showing complete disappearance of Purkinje cells. (Haematoxylin van Gieson.)

An isolated case of progressive ataxia with a similar distribution of cerebello-olivary atrophy had been described by Murri (1900) and a number of similar, isolated cases were collected by Marie, Foix and Alajouanine (1922) under the name of *late cortical cerebellar atrophy*. In these the onset of the disease was usually later, with an average of 57 years. In some the cerebellar atrophy was less widespread than in Holmes' case, and was greatest in the lobulus quadrangularis, superior vermis and flocculus. It thus contrasted with the distribution of olivo-ponto-cerebellar atrophy which tends to spare the vermis and flocculus. There was also much less pallor of myelin staining in the central white matter than in that disease. When the distribution of atrophy in the inferior olives was reported it usually corresponded to that found in Holmes' case in being greater in the dorsal laminae.

Since this report there have been about 20 further pathological descriptions of similar cases and in approximately half of these the disease has been familial. Therefore more familial than isolated cases have now been put on record, but this is probably due to the special interest taken in familial diseases. Hall *et al.* (1941, 1945) reported on a large family in which 9 members in two generations were known to have been affected. Post-mortem examination in two members of the older generation, who died aged 80 and 82, showed the atrophy to be limited to the cerebellar cortex and medullary olives. In these and other familial cases the average age of onset was 45·5 years and the average duration of the disease 17·7 years. In most cases it does not shorten life, but in a family recorded by Akelaitis (1938) the course of the disease was rapid and accompanied by mental confusion and led to death in less than 2 years. Whereas in many cases the distribution of the cerebellar and olivary atrophy has resembled that in the cases of Holmes and Marie *et al.*, in others it has been rather more widespread. In this form of cerebellar atrophy the spinal cord is either entirely normal or there is slight degeneration of the fasciculus gracilis or the spinocerebellar tracts. In the case of Blackwood *et al.* (1957) cerebello-olivary degeneration was associated with the hereditary sensory radicular neuropathy of Denny-Brown (1951) (Fig. 10.6). Cerebello-olivary degeneration has therefore more tendency

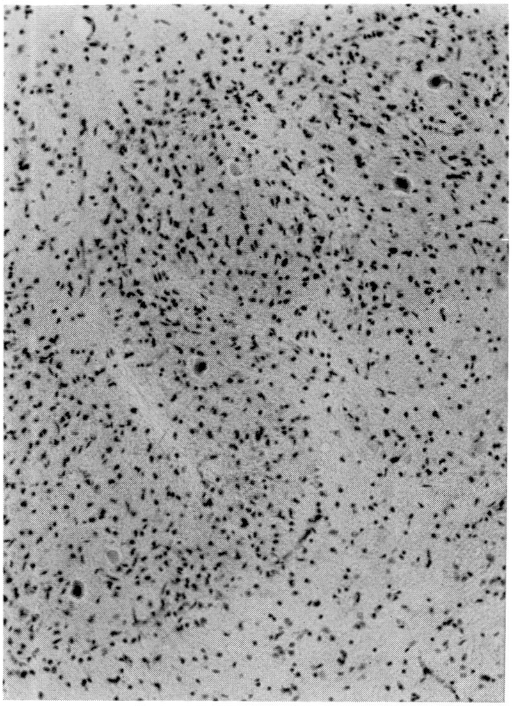

FIG. 10.7. Atrophy of cells of the inferior olive associated with loss of Purkinje cells. (× 150.) (From a case of hereditary posterior radicular neuropathy. Blackwood *et al.* 1957.)

than olivo-ponto-cerebellar atrophy to appear as an hereditary disease and less tendency to involve higher or lower nerve centres or tracts. Apart from these features the two diseases are not easily distinguished by clinical examination and it is therefore difficult to assign to one or the other group many large families of ataxia on which only clinical reports have appeared. There is, however, the distinction that the pyramidal tracts are commonly involved in cases of olivo-ponto-cerebellar atrophy, but never in those of cerebello-olivary degeneration. Extra-pyramidal symptoms also point towards the former type of disease.

Devos (1957) has described the association of late cortical cerebellar atrophy with oculomotor paralysis and a sex linked dominant form of inheritance. A necropsy revealed that the oculomotor nucleus including the nucleus of Perlia had gone: the distribution of the cerebellar atrophy was unusual, however, in that the lateral lobes were more involved than the vermis.

Familial spastic paraplegia

Strümpell (1880) reported the cases of two brothers in whom spastic paraplegia, with very little involvement of the arms or face, came on in middle life. On post-mortem examination of the younger case (1886) he found degeneration of the pyramidal tracts which began below their decussation and was most definite in the lower thoracic and lumbar segments. Degeneration of the dorsal columns was slight at the lumbar level but became more evident in the upper thoracic and cervical segments where the fasciculus gracilis was extensively, and the fasciculus cuneatus slightly, involved. Degeneration of the spinocerebellar tracts was also evident at these levels. Strümpell (1904) described the examination of another familial case in which the first symptoms appeared at the age of 35 and progressed slowly till death at the age of 69. The lesions in the cord in this case were almost identical with those in the first case.

Many families with spastic paraplegia have been put on record since then. In some the onset of the disease has been in childhood or infancy so that some siblings were never able to walk properly or to run, whereas in others the first signs appeared later in the first or during the second decade (Dick and Stevenson 1953). In other families the disease has come on during middle age. The age of onset may vary widely in different members. For example in three families put on record by Schwartz (1952) it ranged in the first family (six generations) from 8 to 25 years, in the second from 5 to 35 years and in the third from 10 to 60 years. In most cases in which the disease appears during childhood there is pes cavus with some degree of talipes equinus but usually less than is common in Friedreich's ataxia. The knee and ankle jerks are exaggerated and the plantars are usually of extensor type. Wasting of the muscles below the knee and sometimes also of the muscles of the hands and fore-arms (Holmes 1905) in some families links the condition to the Roussy-Levy syndrome. In spite of the pathological findings ataxia of gait and clumsiness of the hands are not usually evident, but some dysarthria of speech, possibly due to spasticity, has been present in several cases. Dick and Stevenson (1953) have drawn attention to the presence of extrapyramidal signs in some members of families in which other members have a pure spastic paraplegia. Retinal degeneration (Jéquier and Streiff 1947), retrobulbar neuritis (Bickerstaff 1950) and other causes of optic atrophy may occur occasionally but are less common in association with spastic than with ataxic paraplegia (Bell and Carmichael 1939). No pathological evidence of the basis of these unusual complications is so far available.

The disease does not shorten life and few post-mortem examinations have been made. These have shown degeneration in the cord, either involving all the long tracts (Strümpell, Kahlstorf 1937, Schwarz and Liu 1956) or limited to the pyramidal tracts and dorsal columns (Bischoff 1902, Newmark 1904, 1907, Appel and van Bogaert 1951). In very few cases has it been possible to trace the degeneration of the pyramidal tract into or above the medulla. In a patient who had been paraplegic for 38 years Schwarz and Liu found shrinkage without evident pallor in the medullary pyramids. By fibre count there appeared to be only half the normal number of fibres at this level, but the normal proportions of large, medium and small fibres were not altered. In the cerebral cortex there was loss of about one-third of the Betz cells, as compared with counts made on normal subjects by Lassek. Similar loss of Betz cells has been described by others and Appel (1949) found some loss of cells also in layers III and IV of the precentral gyrus. Abnormalities in the cerebrum or cerebellum of apparently developmental origin have also been found in a few cases.

Amyotrophic lateral sclerosis

The credit of separating this disease from other forms of muscular wasting must be given to Charcot who with Joffroy (1869) gave the first good pathological description. The name *amyotrophic lateral sclerosis* which he gave is sufficiently comprehensive to include all the clinical varieties and is more correct than the suggested alternative *motor neurone disease*, since degeneration is not confined to motor neurones. The name Charcot's disease is often used in France but has never become popular in English terminology. This common disease is linked to other systemic diseases of the brain stem and spinal cord through cases of hereditary spastic ataxia with amyotrophy, but its course is usually much more rapid and its pathology, which is remarkably stereotyped in spite of clinical variations, differs from that of other forms.

Clinical features. The disease may begin with wasting and weakness in almost any muscle of the body, but usually appears in one of three forms: (1) The most common is the classical association of wasting in the upper limbs with spasticity of the lower limbs. (2) Less commonly the first signs are those of bulbar palsy, and in many cases these lead on to death before there is evidence of limb involvement. (3) In a minority of cases signs of pyramidal tract degeneration appear before there is any muscular wasting. These motor symptoms may be preceded or accompanied by subjective sensory symptoms such as stiffness, pains or cramps in the parts of the limbs where wasting first appears, but there is never any cutaneous anaesthesia.

The disease may begin at any age from the second decade onwards, but most often during the fourth and fifth decades. In the Mariana islands the age incidence is slightly later with the peak between 45 and 54 years (Kurland and Mulder 1954). Its course is usually subacute. Many cases, especially those with predominantly bulbar symptoms, prove fatal in less than a year, and in the majority of all forms the interval from first symptoms to death is less than 3 years. In the writer's experience of more than 30 verified cases, the longest period of survival was $3\frac{1}{2}$ years. But more slowly progressive cases, and cases with a temporary standstill of the disease, may last for 5 or 10 years.

Aetiology. Although many factors have been blamed as predisposing to the disease, nothing is known of its aetiology. The great majority of cases have no obvious cause but in some cases weakness and wasting appear first in a limb soon after it has received an injury. As has been said familial incidence has been recorded in a few American and European families. These have been reviewed by Kurland and Mulder (1955) who also found 5 familial cases among 58 cases examined at the Mayo Clinic. In the Chamarro natives of the Mariana Islands 8–10 per cent of all deaths are due to this disease and familial cases are very common (Kurland and Mulder 1956). The cerebrospinal fluid rarely shows any abnormality nor have any deviations from normal in the blood chemistry been described.

Pathology. On removal of the spinal cord grey atrophy of the ventral roots of the cervical enlargement is usually the most obvious abnormality. In the brain the hypoglossal nerve is similarly affected and there may be evident atrophy of the precentral gyrus, especially in the upper third.

Microscopically the widespread sclerosis of the lateral columns, which was observed by Charcot and Joffroy, is found to be associated with a diffuse pallor of myelin staining, usually greatest in the pyramidal tracts but by no means confined to them. The spinocerebellar tracts may be less involved than other parts of the lateral columns (Fig. 10.7*b*) but usually suffer to some extent (Holmes 1909). The anterior columns stain in a similar manner to the lateral columns and may be especially pale in the area occupied by the direct pyramidal tract. There is no distinction, except for this, between the more superficially and the more deeply placed fibres and even the area of the pyramidal tract may be no paler than the surrounding white matter, at least at the cervical level (Fig. 10.7*a*). The degeneration evidently affects some fibres and spares others intermingled with them and it is tempting to suppose that descending fibres are degenerated and ascending fibres spared. Certainly the absence of any superficial sensory loss indicates that the spinothalamic fibres at least escape. But the spinocerebellar tracts are undoubtedly degenerated in many cases although not as severely as the pyramidal tracts. Probably there is also degeneration of other ascending systems such as the spinoreticular fibres. The degeneration in the pyramidal tracts can usually be traced through the medullary pyramids into the pons but becomes less evident in the crus and internal capsule. By stains for myelin degeneration products Kojewnikoff (1883) traced degeneration as far up as the white centre of the precentral gyrus, but this varies in different cases. Davison (1941) in 37 cases found 15 in which degeneration extended up to or above the internal capsule; in 9 of the remainder it was seen at the level of the pons; in 12 it did not extend above the medullary pyramids and in 4 was confined to the spinal cord. On the other hand, Smith (1960) found degenerated myelin fibres from the cortex downwards in all of 7 cases. She found that not only were they present in the precentral gyrus and paracentral lobule but they were abundant in the postcentral gyrus and occurred in considerable numbers in the adjacent parietal and frontal gyri. All authors agree that the amount of degeneration diminishes on passing upwards from the medulla and often becomes more complete on passing downwards through the spinal cord. There is also

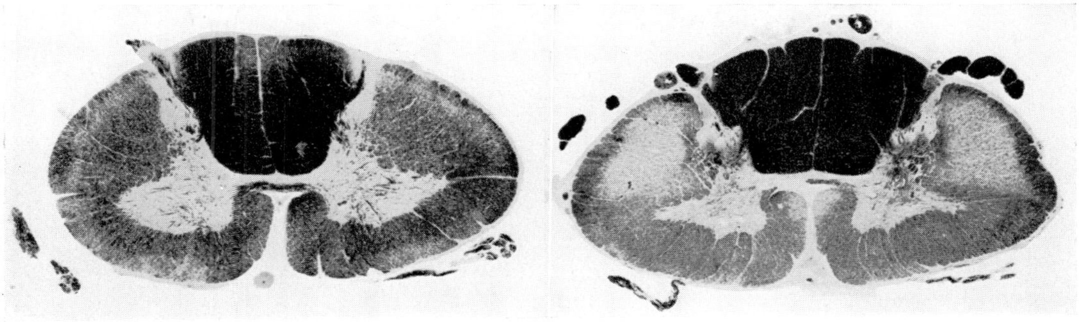

(*a*) (*b*)

FIG. 10.8. Amyotrophic lateral sclerosis. Sections from the cervical enlargement. (Myelin.)
(*a*) From a case with 9 months' history of bulbar palsy. No abnormal physical signs in the arms or legs.
(*b*) From a typical case with wasting of the small hand muscles and spastic paraplegia.
Note the diffuse pallor of the anterolateral tracts which in (*b*) is greatest in the pyramidal tracts. The spinocerebellar tracts are relatively well-preserved.

considerable loss of myelinated fibres in the ventral horns, and in the anterior (white) commissure, which may suffer as severe a loss of fibres as the pyramidal tracts. The atrophied ventral roots of the cervical enlargement, and of other segments which supply atrophied muscles, contrast with the normal dorsal roots. The dorsal columns usually escape completely and their dark staining contrasts with the diffuse pallor of the ventrolateral columns. But in some cases there is slight pallor in the fasciculus gracilis (Fig. 10.8*a*): this may be no greater than is sometimes seen in clinically normal subjects of similar age.

In the brain stem degenerated fibres can be traced in the direct and indirect spinocerebellar tracts as far as the cerebellar vermis, and degenerated fibres can also be seen going to or from the lateral reticular formation of the medulla and the median longitudinal fasciculus. These diminish rapidly on passing up to the level of the pons. The degenerated fibres which are often seen at the latter level in the median fillet are probably pyramidal fibres going to the lower cranial nerve nuclei. The transverse fibres of the pons may show some degeneration but the corticopontine fibres are usually intact. Bertrand and van Bogaert (1925) found the rubrospinal tract to be constantly degenerated and, at the mid-brain level, the ansa lenticularis showed pallor of myelin staining. In the internal capsule degeneration is usually confined to the anterior two-thirds of the posterior limb. The middle third of the corpus callosum also often contains degenerated fibres.

These tract degenerations are found with equal constancy in cases which begin with muscular wasting and even in those of clinically pure bulbar palsy or progressive muscular atrophy, although in these the degeneration of the pyramidal tract may be less evident (Fig. 10.7*a*). Gowers stated that he had never seen a case of progressive muscular atrophy in which the

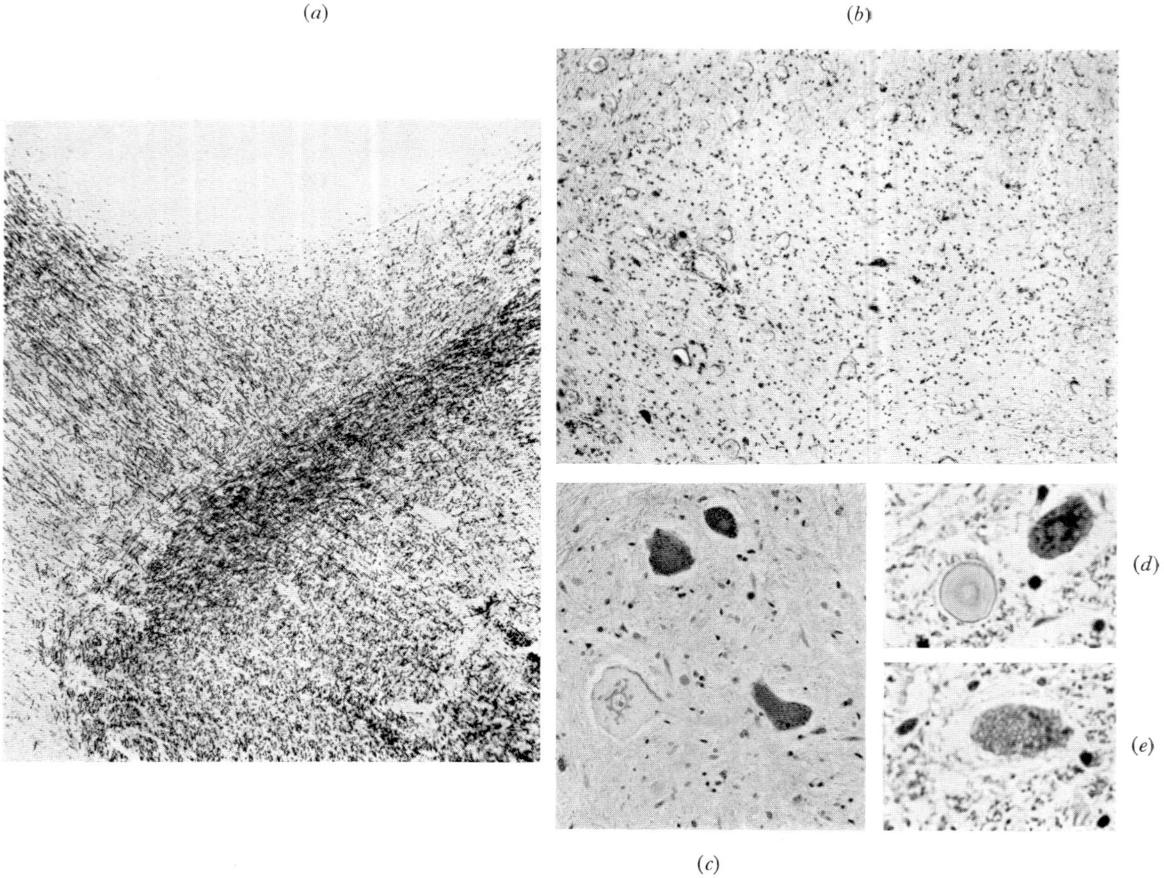

FIG. 10.9. Amyotrophic lateral sclerosis.

(*a*) Adjoining basal parts of post-central gyrus (on left) and pre-central gyrus (on right) showing degenerating fibres (stained black in both gyri). Marchi preparation. × 7 (Dr. Marion Smith's case).

(*b*) Anterior horn in cervical enlargement showing almost complete depletion of motor cells. Celloidin, Nissl, × 100.

(*c*), (*d*), (*e*) Anterior horn cells undergoing degeneration. In (*c*) the cell at the bottom left is unusual: there is almost complete loss of structure in the perikaryon. The oval form, top right, and also the cells in (*d*) and (*e*) are very characteristic of this disease. Note the corpora amylacia in the bottom left-hand corner of (*d*). Celloidin, Nissl, × 280.

pyramidal tracts were unaffected and this agrees with the writer's experience of this disease. Progressive muscular atrophy from other causes, for example peroneal muscular atrophy and post-encephalitic cases, are, of course, exceptions to this rule.

In sections stained by the Nissl method there is obvious loss of neurones in the ventral horns of the cervical enlargement and degeneration or atrophy of many of those that remain, but the shape and size of the horns of grey matter is little affected. In this way amyotrophic lateral sclerosis differs from amyotrophic spinal syphilis and from the effects of protrusion of cervical discs as in both these conditions there is often gross shrinkage of the anterior horns. In general the loss of neurones is greatest in the dorso-lateral cell column and least in the ventro-mesial column. The remaining nerve cells show various degenerative changes, many are shrunken and contain an excess of lipofuscin (pigmentary atrophy). In others the cell body is more rounded than normal with apparent loss of dendrites, and the Nissl granules are conglomerated into large masses which lie either at the periphery of the cell body or near the nucleus. Typical central chromatolysis is rare but may be seen in very acute cases (Holmes 1909). Owing to the paucity and smaller size of the motor neurones at the thoracic level their loss is less easily recognised, but atrophied and degenerated neurones may be seen in any of the thoracic segments, as well as in the lumbosacral enlargement in cases with muscular atrophy in the legs. The cells of Clarke's column show only slight changes. The lesions in the ventral horns, as in the anterolateral white columns, are accompanied by marked fibrous gliosis, and perivascular infiltration may be seen in the more acute cases.

Of the cranial nerve nuclei the hypoglossal is most constantly and most severely affected. Holmes found the nucleus of Roller intact. In the nucleus facialis he saw the greatest changes in the ventral and lateral cells, that is in those cells which supply the muscles of the mouth and lower face. The nucleus ambiguus may escape or may show changes of varying severity. The abducens and other oculomotor nuclei are very rarely affected.

In the cerebral cortex the greatest cell loss is among the giant cells of Betz in the precentral gyrus, and in old-standing cases very few of these can be recognised. Many of those that remain have undergone pigmentary atrophy and occasional cells show Nissl's atrophic sclerosis. Other pyramidal cells in the 3rd and 5th cortical layers may have disappeared or undergone atrophic changes. Degenerated cells are also occasionally seen in the 5th layer in the posterior wall of the Rolandic fissure.

Although in some of the familial Mariana Island cases the pathological changes resembled the classical picture of amyotrophic lateral sclerosis, in others there was more degeneration than usual of the dorsal columns. And in some familial American cases, with the usual short duration of illness, the degeneration in the dorsal columns and spinocerebellar tracts is at least as early and severe as that in the pyramidal tracts. In these cases, as in Friedreich's ataxia, the degeneration in the dorsal columns may be confined to the middle-root zone, especially in the lumbar segments, so that at the cervical level the fasciculus gracilis shows little evidence of degeneration. Degeneration in the fasciculus cuneatus also tends to have a similar distribution. These cases link amyotrophic lateral sclerosis to cases of familial spinocerebellar degeneration with amyotrophy (Schut and Haymaker).

(Revised by W. H. McMenemey.)

REFERENCES

Akelaitis, A. J. (1938) *Amer. J. Psychiat.*, **94**, 1115.

André Van-Leeuwen, M. (1949) *Brain*, **72**, 340.

André-Van Leeuwen, M. and van Bogaert, L. (1942) *Monatschr. f. Psych. u. Neur.*, **105**, 314; (1949) *Brain*, **72**, 340.

Appel, L. (1949) *Acta. Neurol. et Psychiat. Belg.*, **49**, 415.

Appel, L. and van Bogaert, L. (1951) *Acta. Neurol. et Psychiat. Belg.*, **51**, 129.

Barker, L. F. (1903) *Trans. Amer. Ass. Physicians*, **18**, 637.

Battaquer-Ferré, L. and Barraquer-Bordas, L. (1951) *Acta Neurol. et Psychiat. Belg.*, **51**, 264.

Beheim-Schwarzbach, D. (1952) *J. nerv. & ment. Dis.*, **116**, 619; (1954) *J. für Hirnforschung*, **1**, 61.

Bell, J. M. and Carmichael, E. A. (1939) *Treasury of human inheritance*, **4**, part 3.

Bertrand, I. and van Bogaert, L. (1925) *Rev. Neurol.* (ii), 779.

Bethlem, J. and den Hartog Jager, W. A. (1960) *J. Neurol. Neurosurg. Psychiat.*, **23**, 74.
Bickerstaff, E. R. (1950) *J. Neurol. Psychiat.*, **13**, 134.
Biemond, A. (1928) *Dtsch. Z. Nervenheilk.*, **104**, 113; (1951) *Folia Psychiat. Neurol. et Neurochir. Neerl.*, **54**, 216.
Biemond, A. and Sinnege, J. L. M. (1955) *Confinia Neurologica*, **15**, 129.
Bischoff. (1902) *Jahrbuch. f. Psychiat.*, **22**, 109.
Blackwood, W., Carmichael, E. A. and Hallpike, C. (1957) unpublished.
Brain, W. R., Daniel, P. M. and Greenfield, J. G. (1951) *J. Neurol. Psychiat.*, **14**, 59.
Carpenter, M. B. and Mettler, F.A. (1950) *J. Comp. neurol.*, **93**, 1.
Charcot, J. M. and Joffroy, A. (1869) *Archiv. de Physiol.*, **2**, 354, 629, 744.
Critchley, M. and Greenfield, J. G. (1948) *Brain*, **71**, 343.
Davison, C. (1941) *Arch. Neurol. Psychiat.* (Chicago), **46**, 1039.
Dejerine, J. and Thomas, A. (1900) *Nouv. Icon. de la Salpêt.*, **13**, 330.
Denny-Brown, D. (1949) *Diseases of the basal ganglia and subthalamic nuclei* in *Oxford Loose-leaf Medicine*, Oxford Univ. Press, New York; (1951) *J. Neurol. Psychiat.*, **14**, 237; (1961) *Int. J. Neurol.*, **2**, 25.
Devos, J. (1957) *Psychiat. Neurol.*, **133**, 46.
Dick, A. P. and Stevenson, C. J. (1953) *Lancet* (i), 921.
Ferguson, F. R. and Critchley, M. (1928) *J. Neurol. Psychopath.*, **9**, 120.
Foix, C. and Nicolesco, J. (1925) *Les noyaux gris centraux et la région mésencéphalo-sous-optique*. Masson, Paris.
Franceschetti, A. and Klein, D. (1948) *Rev. oto-neuro-ophthal.*, **20**, 109; (1941) *Arch. der Julius-Klaus-Stiftung*, **16**, 469; (1947) ibid., **22**, 93.
Freeman, W. and Dumoff, E. (1944) *Arch. Neurol. Psychiat.* (Chicago), **51**, 67.
Friedreich, N. (1861) *Versammlung deutsch. Naturforsch. u. Arzte*; (1863) *Virchows Archiv. path. Anat.*, **26**, 391, 433; **27**, 1; (1876) ibid., **68**, 145.
Gowers, W. R. (1899) *A Manual of Diseases of the Nervous System*, Vol. 2, 2nd edition, Churchill, London.
Greenfield, J. G. (1934) *Brain*, **57**, 161; (1954) *The spino-cerebellar degenerations*, Blackwell, Oxford.
Greenfield, J. G. and Bosanquet, F. D. (1953) *J. Neurol. Psychiat.*, **16**, 213.
Guillain, G., Bertrand, I. and Godet-Guillain, J. (1941) *Rev. Neurol.*, **73**, 609.
Hall, B., Noad, K. B. and Latham, O. (1941) *Brain*, **64**, 178; (1945) *Med. J. Austral.* (i), 101.
Hallervorden, J. (1933) *Klin. Wschr.*, **12**, 692; (1935) *Dtsch. Z. Nervenheilk.*, **136**, 68.
Hartog Jager, W. A. den and Bethlem, J. (1960) *J. Neurol. Neurosurg. Psych.*, **23**, 283.
Hassler, R. (1937) *J. Psychol. Neurol.*, **48**, 1. (1938) *ibid* **48**, 387.
Hechst, B. and Nussbaum, L. (1931) *Arch. Psychiat. Nervenkr.*, **95**, 556.
Herzog, E. (1928) *Deut. Z. Nervenh.*, **107**, 75.
Holmes, G. (1904) *Brain*, **27**, 327; (1905) *Rev. Neurol. Psychiat. Edin.*, **3**, 256; (1907) *Brain*, **30**, 466; (1909) *Rev. Neurol. Psychiat. Edin.*, **7**, 693.
Hunt, J. R. (1917) *Brain*, **40**, 58; (1921) ibid., **44**, 490.
Hunter, D. and Russell, D. S. (1954) *J. Neurol. Psychiat.*, **17**, 235.
Jelgersma. (1908) *Neurol. Zbl.*, **27**, 995.
Jéquier, M. and Streiff, E. B. (1947) *Archiv. der Julius Klaus-Stiftung*, **22**, 129.
Kahlstorf, A. (1937) *Z. ges. Neurol. Psychiat.*, **159**, 774.
Klaue, R. (1940) *Arch. Psychiat. Nervenkr.*, **111**, 251.
Kojewnikoff, A. (1883) *Arch. de Neurol.*, **6**, 356.
Krainer, L. (1949) *Arch. Neurol. Psychiat.* (Chicago), **51**, 441.
Kurland, L. T. and Mulder, D. W. (1954) *Neurology*, **4**, 356. (1955–6) *Neurology*, **5**, 182. *Ibid.*
Lafora, G. R. (1913) *Trab. del lab. invest. biol. Madrid.*, **11**, 43.
Lewy, F. W. (1913) *Dtsch. Z. Nervenheilk.*, **50**, 50; (1923) *Die Lehre vom Tonus und der Bewegung*, Springer, Berlin.
Lichtenstein, B. H. and Levinson, S. A. (1946) *J. Neuropath.*, **5**, 29.
Lipkin, L. E. (1959) *Amer. J. Path.*, **35** ii, 1117.
Marie, P., Foix, C. and Alajouanine, T. (1922) *Rev. Neurol.*, **38**, 849, 1082.
Menzel, P. (1891) *Arch. Psych. Nervenkr.*, **22**, 160.
Meyer, A. (1897) *Brain*, **20**, 276.
Murri, A. (1900) *Riv. Crit. di clin. Med.*, **1**, 593, 609.
Newmark, L. (1904) *Dtsch. Z. Nervenheilk.*, **27**, 1; (1907) ibid., **31**, 224.

Parkinson, J. (1817) *An Essay on the Shaking Palsy*, London, reprinted in Critchley's *James Parkinson*, 1955, Macmillan, London.
Peters, G. (1951) *Spezielle Pathologie der Krankheiten des zentralen und peripheren Nervensystems*, Thieme, Stuttgart.
Ranson, S. W. and Ranson, S. W., Junr. (1941) *Trans. Amer. Neurol. Ass.*, **67**, 168.
Rombold, C. R. and Riley, H. A. (1926) *Arch. Neurol. Psychiat.* (Chicago), **16**, 301.
Rosenhagen, H. (1943) *Arch. Psychiat. Neurol.*, **116**, 163.
Roussy, G. and Levi, G. (1926) *Rev. Neurol.* (i), 427; (1934) ibid., (ii), 763.
Russell, D. S. (1946) *J. Path. Bact.*, **58**, 739.
Scherer, H. J. (1933) *Z. ges. Neurol. Psychiat.*, **145**, 406.
Schut, J. W. and Book, J. A. (1953) *Arch. Neurol. Psychiat.* (Chicago), **70**, 169.
Schut, J. W. and Haymaker, W. (1951) *J. Neuropath. & Clin. Neurol.*, **1**, 183.
Schwarz, G. A. (1952) *Arch. Neurol. Psychiat.* (Chicago), **68**, 655.
Schwarz, G. A. and Liu, C. N. (1956) *Arch. Neurol. Psychiat.* (Chicago), **75**, 144.
Sjögren, T. (1943) *Klinische und erbbiologische Untersuchungen uber die Heredoataxien*, Munskgaard, Copenhagen; (1950) *Confinia neurol.*, **10**, 293.
Smith, Marion C. (1960) *J. Neurol. Neurosurg. Path.*, **23**, 269.
Spillane, J. D. (1940) *Brain*, **63**, 275.
Spiller, W. G. (1910) *J. nerv. and ment. Dis.*, **37**, 411.
Stender, A. and Lüthy, F. (1931) *Dtsch. Z. Nervenheilk.*, **119**, 604.
Stewart, T. G. and Holmes, G. (1908) *Brain*, **31**, 125.
Strümpell, A. (1880) *Arch. Psychiat. Neurol.*, **10**, 711; (1886) ibid., **17**, 217; (1904) *Dtsch. Z. Nervenheilk.*, **27**, 291.
Symonds, C. P. and Shaw, M. E. (1926) *Brain*, **49**, 387.
Trétiakoff, C. (1919) *Contribution a l'étude de l'anatomie du locus niger*, Thèse de Paris; (1921) *Rev Neurol.*, 592.
Urich, H., Norman, R. M. and Lloyd, O. C. (1957) *Confin. Neurol.*, **17**, 360.
de Villaverde, J. M. (1927) *Trab. del lab. invest. biol. Madrid*, **25**, 41.
Walshe, F. M. R. (1955) in Critchley's *James Parkinson*, Macmillan, London.
Weber, F. P. and Greenfield, J. G. (1942) *Brain*, **65**, 220.
Wohlwill, F. (1928) *Deut. Z. Nervenh.*, **107**, 124.
Zülch, K. J. (1948) *Dtsch. Z. Nervenheilk.*, **159**, 501.

CHAPTER 11

EPILEPSY

By A. Meyer

The great interest which the problems of epilepsy have attracted during the last few decades has been mainly due to the introduction of electro-encephalography, the increasing refinement and boldness of neurosurgical intervention and the information, almost of a physiological nature, which has accrued in these ways.

Advances have been made in several directions. The demonstration of the electrophysiological concomitants has provided confirmation of Hughlings Jackson's early concept of the epileptic seizure as a discharge of nerve cells within the grey matter of the brain, the grand mal attack being associated with spikes of very high frequency and the petit mal with a three-per-second wave and spike discharge. Collaboration of the neurosurgeon with the electro-encephalographer has resulted in remarkable concrete advances in the localisation and surgical treatment of focal epileptic attacks. The category of focal attacks has been considerably enlarged. Penfield and Kristiansen (1951) now regard the majority of cases in which loss of consciousness is the initial sign as being caused by focal lesions in the anterior frontal region. Where initial unconsciousness is associated with adversive features, the focal lesion was found to be in the intermediate frontal region (area 6). Evidence has accumulated that seizures may also take their origin in the temporal lobe. This type of focal epilepsy has been known since Jackson and Beevor (1890) described their 'uncinate' fits or 'dreamy states'. Interest in temporal lobe epilepsy has been recently revived. This group will be treated in greater detail later.

The extension of our knowledge of epileptic foci has resulted in the tempting concept that all seizures are at least potentially focal. Penfield and Kristiansen tentatively distinguish between: (1) Focal cortical seizures with lesion in the cerebral cortex; (2) Highest level seizures with focus in the higher brain stem (diencephalon and mesencephalon). This group would comprise both petit mal and the grand mal seizures of the so-called idiopathic or essential group. (3) Myoclonic seizures with focus in lower brain stem and spinal cord. (4) A provisional group of seizures often caused by extracerebral disease such as hypoglycaemia.

However, classification of this kind is at present a distant goal as Penfield and Kristiansen fully realise. From the point of view of morbid anatomy it still remains necessary to present the pathological data under the old headings of: (1) symptomatic epilepsy; (2) cryptogenic epilepsy, a term preferable to the often synonymously used 'idiopathic' and 'essential' epilepsy; and (3) special forms of epilepsy. Recent developments which will be mentioned later are likely to modify this classification mainly by restricting the cryptogenic group by the exclusion of temporal lobe epilepsy.

Even if all epilepsies were proved to be focal in origin, it would nevertheless still be doubtful whether a lesion would be the only factor. It is likely that several factors whose nature is still little known must combine with those lesions which can at present be demonstrated to cause epileptic manifestations (Williams 1950). Familial inheritance is frequent in the cryptogenic (idiopathic) group and it is not absent in the symptomatic and overtly focal epilepsies. Cortical dysrhythmia as revealed by the E.E.G. is found to be 6 times more frequent in the relatives of sufferers from 'cryptogenic' epilepsy than in a normal control group (Lennox, Gibbs and Gibbs 1940). The nature of the predisposing factor is not known. It has been considered either as a failure to prevent the spread of epileptic discharge (Williams) or as cortical disinhibition in the Pavlovian sense (Crome 1954).

Symptomatic epilepsies

Almost any disease of the brain may be associated with epilepsy. Brain (1951) has listed the most important local and general causes; the local factors range from raised intracranial pressure, inflammatory disease, trauma, and congenital abnormalities to degenerative and vascular disease. The list of general causes includes intoxication, anoxia, disturbances of metabolism, endocrine disorders and allergy. Epilepsy associated with childhood fevers (teething, rickets, acute infections) are listed as a special group.

Brain gives no indication of the relative frequency of the various causes, but relevant figures based upon a material of 742 epileptic children have been presented by Bridges (1949). In this author's material, birth and neonatal injuries accounted for 22·8 per cent; congenital malformation for only 0·3 per cent; vascular accidents for 12 per cent; head injuries for 7·1 per cent; encephalitis for 2·8 per cent. In 21 per cent there was brain injury of uncertain cause and in 30 per cent no evidence of brain disease was obtained.

Penfield and his associates, mainly from their experience in *traumatic epilepsy*, have devoted much work to the elucidation of the local mechanism through which anatomical lesions may give rise to convulsions (Penfield 1927, Penfield and Ericson 1941, Penfield and Bridgers 1942). These authors found evidence of progressive ischaemic destruction of grey matter in an intermediate zone surrounding the lesion. Penfield and Bridgers had, however, to admit that the same type of progressive ischaemic lesion occurred in traumatic cases without epilepsy.

The incidence of traumatic epilepsy varies greatly in different statistics. This variation depends on several factors, in particular on the percentage of penetrating wounds and on the duration of the follow-up. In a material of 820 cases of penetrating brain wounds suffered during the Second World War, Russell (1951) and Russell and Whitty (1952) found that the incidence 5 years after the injury already approached 43 per cent. This rate agrees fairly closely with other statistics based on similar material. It is of interest that there does not seem to be a significant difference in the incidence of epilepsy in statistics of the First and Second World Wars, despite the great improvement in débridement and combat of infection during the latter war. This fact, in Russell and Whitty's view, militates against Penfield and his associates' hypothesis of progressive ischaemia in the vicinity of the lesion, since this should occur far less frequently after successful primary treatment of the wound.

A figure of over 40 per cent is too high to be accounted for by a genetic factor; it comes near to a one-to-one ratio between cases that do or do not develop epilepsy. This, according to Russell and Whitty, suggests that the balance between two equally important factors has been disturbed. The normal equilibrium, for example, of excitatory and inhibitory impulses acting upon neurones, might be upset by the loss, through brain damage, of inhibitory stimuli, resulting in excessive neuronal discharges. Admittedly, this explanation is, at present, largely hypothetical and, owing to the complex and variable pattern of impulses, is difficult to prove in any individual case.

In an earlier communication Russell (1947) had been impressed by a rather striking distribution of epileptogenic lesions in the vicinity of suppressor bands (areas 8, 4s, 2s). This view was later abandoned, since the existence of suppressor bands, never proven in the human brain, had become doubtful. Lesions, however, in the motor and premotor area (55 per cent) and the parietal cortex (65 per cent) have a definite epileptogenic preponderance over those in the prefrontal and inferior frontal (39 per cent), temporal (38 per cent) and occipital lobes (38 per cent). This result of Russell and Whitty (1952) is in general agreement with previous investigations; they made, however, a new observation—that medial wounds within 5 cm. of the sagittal line are significantly less epileptogenic than more laterally situated lesions.

Walker (1949) attached some importance to the distortion of the ventricular system and its displacement towards the scar, as described by Foerster and Penfield (1930), in head injuries. Although this is also found in cases without epilepsy, distortion was significantly greater in Walker's epileptic material.

Cryptogenic (idiopathic or essential) epilepsy

There still remains a formidable group of epilepsies in which neither the focal nor the general causes enumerated above have been recognised. The absence of clear-cut causative lesions in this group does not mean, however, that pathological changes do not occur. On the contrary, the presence of such changes has been noted for a long time and the literature on these phenomena has been so extensive that only a broad outline can be given here. A full historical review is found in Scholz's (1930, 1951) publications.

Ammon's horn sclerosis. This is the oldest and most familiar lesion. The first macroscopic description of the phenomenon was given by Bouchet and Cazauvieilh (1825); the finding of the French authors was confirmed by several French and German workers. Sommer (1880) published the first histological description of the lesion and demonstrated the special vulnerability of what has become known as the Sommer sector which approximately corresponds to Rose's (1927) field h^1. Subsequently Bratz (1899) described the additional vulnerability also of the end-plate (Rose's h^3–h^5); he stressed that the intermediate zone (Rose's h^2) usually displays greater resistance (Fig. 11.1).

It had already been noted by the older investigators that Ammon's horn sclerosis occurred in approximately 50 per cent of epileptic brains, that it was usually unilateral, or if bilateral more marked in one hemisphere. It was observed not only in cases of 'idiopathic', but also of symptomatic, epilepsy and had even been found in the brains of patients who had not suffered from epileptic convulsions.

Interest in the sclerosis of Ammon's horn was lively as long as this area could be regarded as a possible motor centre but, when Ammon's horn was included in the so-called rhinencephalon, interest waned.

Spielmeyer (1927) and his disciples, especially Scholz, have confirmed and extended the earlier findings and have provided clear evidence that the sclerosis is due to vascular disturbances and/or anoxia. In its initial stages, the nerve cells are seen undergoing ischaemic or homogenising degeneration, to be followed by microglial and macroglial proliferation which finally results in dense gliosis (Fig. 11.2). While the fields h^1 and h^3–h^5 are particularly susceptible, all the areas of the pyramidal band and even the cells of the dentate gyrus may be affected in severe cases. The shrinkage in the latter type of lesion is usually very marked (Fig. 11.3). In most instances the nerve cells alone are affected, the glia cells are preserved and proliferated: the lesions present what has been referred to as incomplete infarction or selective parenchymatous degeneration. Total infarction with ultimate cyst formation has, however, also been described.

No further descriptive detail is necessary here, as the lesion in the epileptic brain corresponds

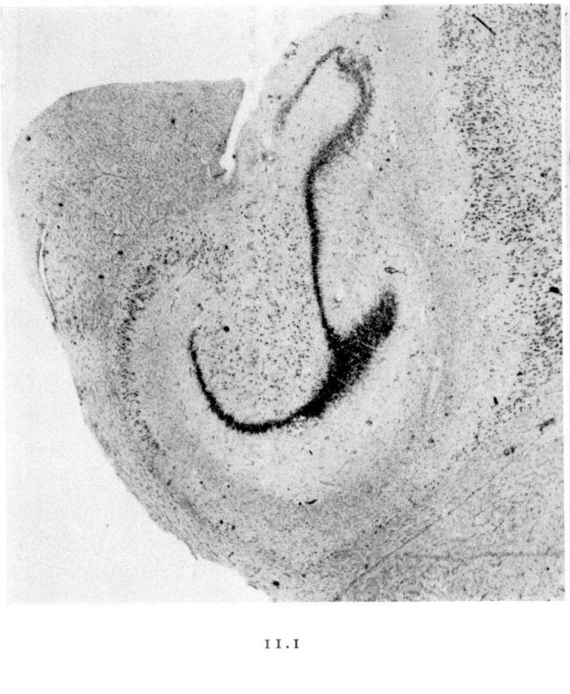

11.1

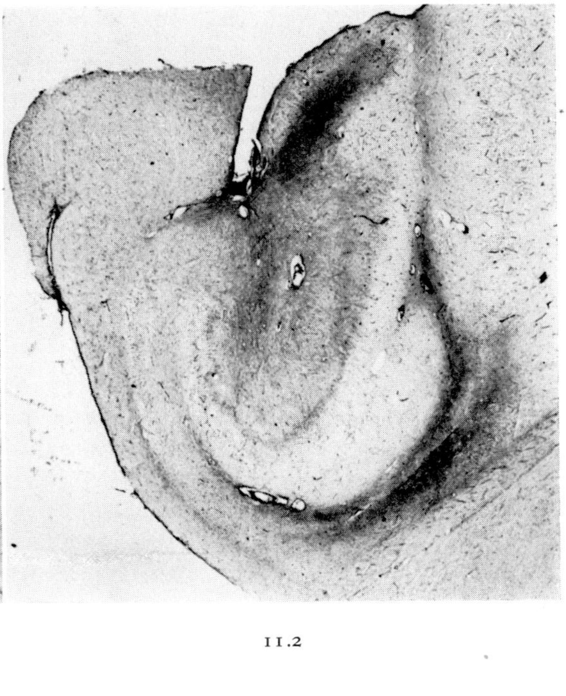

11.2

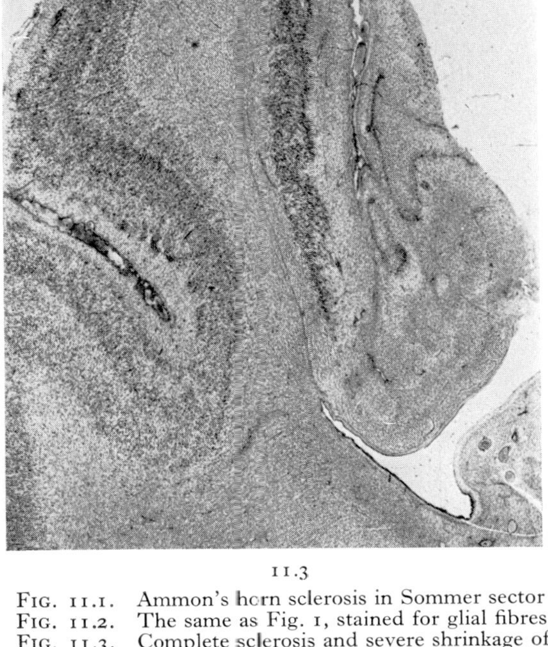

11.3

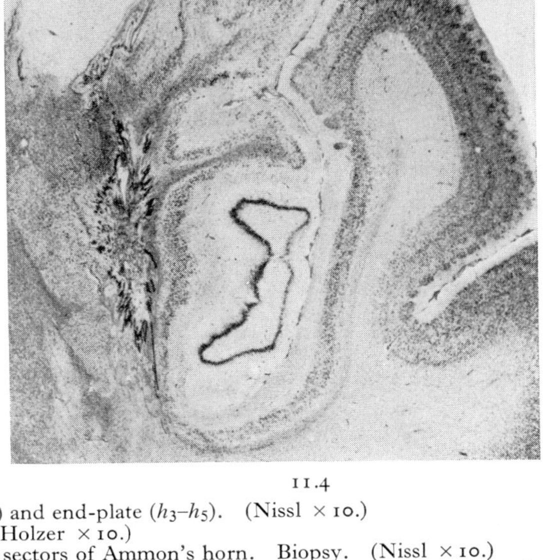

11.4

FIG. 11.1. Ammon's horn sclerosis in Sommer sector (h_1) and end-plate (h_3–h_5). (Nissl × 10.)
FIG. 11.2. The same as Fig. 1, stained for glial fibres. (Holzer × 10.)
FIG. 11.3. Complete sclerosis and severe shrinkage of all sectors of Ammon's horn. Biopsy. (Nissl × 10.)
FIG. 11.4. Severe degeneration of uncus and basal part of amygdaloid nucleus with considerable glio-mesodermal proliferation. (Nissl × 5·5.)

in every detail to that which commonly occurs in anoxia and related conditions of non-utilisation of oxygen, such as hypoglycaemia (*vide* pages 237, 252).

Sclerosis of the hippocampus extends most frequently rostrally into the uncus (Bodechtel 1930, Meyer and Beck 1955). Sano and Malamud (1953), Meyer and Beck, Norman (1958) and others have also described in particularly severe cases an extension of the uncal sclerosis into the basal parts of the amygdaloid complex (Fig. 11.4). Amygdaloid necrosis and sclerosis, similar to that of Ammon's horn and uncus, has been reported also in non-epileptic cases of anoxia.

Lesions of the cerebral cortex

Abnormal cells. Gross developmental abnormalities have been dealt with in Chapter 6. Here we shall confine ourselves to those abnormal cells which have been recognised to occur frequently in otherwise not greatly malformed cortical tissue. The best known are the so-called 'Cajal-Retzius' cells. These are elements of nerve cell origin which often present a bipolar appearance and are usually arranged horizontally within the tangential layer. In addition Turner (1907) described neuroblast-like cells in the tangential layer. The occurrence of these and other abnormal cells has been confirmed by many subsequent writers as occurring frequently, though not consistently, in brains of epileptic patients. Ranke (quoted from Scholz 1930) found such cells in the tangential cortical layer of normal foetuses. These tend to disappear with normal development.

The cells which Norman (1954) has described seem to constitute still another variety. They are large cells of disproportionate size which occur in all layers of the cortex and even within the white matter. Norman considered the possibility that they may be of significance as epileptogenic foci.

Chaslin's gliosis. This was first described by Chaslin (1889) as a considerable densification of the usually delicate horizontal glial fibres which are normally found within the tangential layer immediately beneath the pial surface. If severe, it may fill the entire 1st layer and even extend into the 2nd and 3rd layer (Fig. 11.5). Chaslin himself regarded the lesion as primary, congenital and related to glial tumour, but this view was soon superseded by the assumption that it is the consequence of the convulsions. Bleuler (1895) made a full study of the phenomenon in 80 epileptic cases, 26 of which showed marginal gliosis. He correlated its presence with the dementia exhibited by these patients, a view which was shared by Alzheimer (1898) and subsequent workers. Alzheimer, however, regarded the marginal gliosis as a reaction to loss of cortical nerve cells which was often so slight that it could be identified only by careful comparison with normal control material. Alzheimer's interpretation of Chaslin's gliosis as a secondary phenomenon has been widely accepted and is, for example, shared by Scholz.

Chaslin's gliosis is usually ubiquitous although it often exhibits varying intensity in different regions, e.g. the hippocampal gyrus and the surface of Ammon's horn, which even under normal conditions have a more than usually dense glial covering. It is more frequent than Ammon's horn sclerosis and may be seen in patients suffering from periodic grand mal or in those who have undergone prolonged chemical or electrical convulsive treatment (Corsellis and Meyer 1954).

The marginal gliosis seems in many cases to extend also to subependymal regions: it is often accompanied by a glial fibrosis within the white matter, which is usually slight, but particularly marked around the blood-vessels.

Severe cortical damage. In most cases of epilepsy no loss of nerve cells severer than that concealed behind the marginal gliosis is found. Severe cortical lesions may occur, however, and they have been described with particular frequency following serial convulsions in infancy

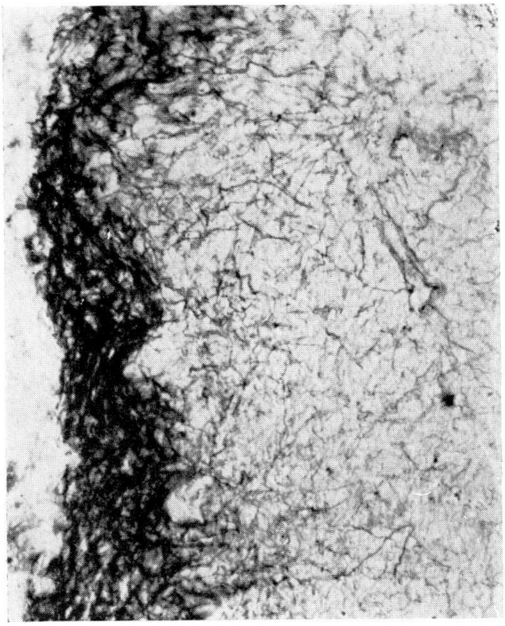

11.5

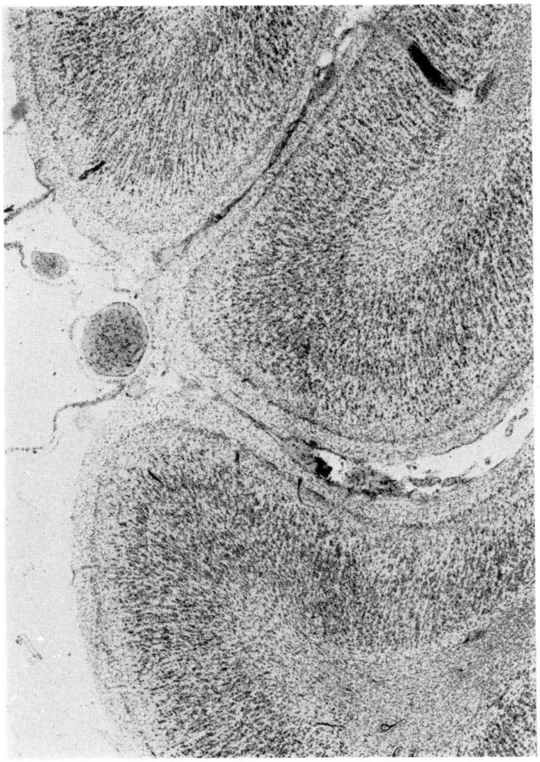

11.6

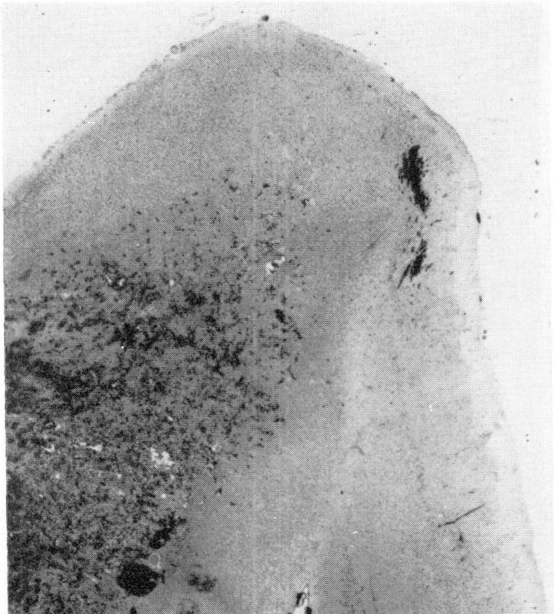

11.8

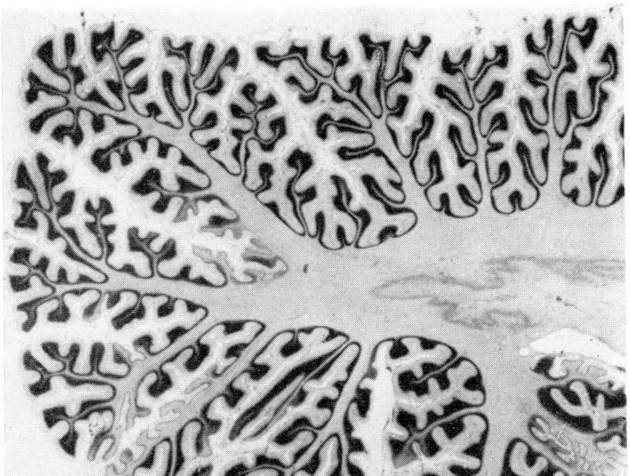

11.7

FIG. 11.5. Marginal gliosis of cerebral cortex. (Holzer ×470.)
FIG. 11.6. Temporal lobe. Severe laminar loss of nerve cells mainly within 3rd layer. Dense gliosis of white matter. (Nissl ×25.)
FIG. 11.7. Disseminated lobular sclerosis of cerebellar cortex. (Nissl ×2·5.)
FIG. 11.8. Atypical glioma in the region of uncus and amygdaloid complex. (Haematoxylin and eosin ×8.)

and early childhood (Scholz 1951, Zimmerman 1940). Such status-like convulsions occur often in the course of acute, but not necessarily severe, childhood fevers, gastro-intestinal infections and acute allergic reactions. The present writer has seen among other examples status epilepticus developing in the course of Still's syndrome in a boy aged 8 (Meyer, Beck and Shepherd 1955).

The lesions are either focal or, more characteristically, affect the 3rd and less frequently the 2nd layer in a laminar fashion. The cortex in the depth of sulci is particularly vulnerable. In the early stages the lesions betray the signs of ischaemic necrosis, later they present laminar atrophy and gliosis as illustrated in Fig. 11.6. In addition to the cortical lesions, heavy gliosis of the white matter may be found. Laminar necrosis and atrophy may be circumscribed; the occipital area surrounding the calcarine region is a favourable site. On the other hand they may be so extensive that they give rise to lobar, total or hemi-atrophy of the brain. Apparently all lobes may be affected, but in a few cases the temporal lobe has been described as particularly severely involved (Meyer, Beck and Shepherd, Norman).

Subcortical lesions. Lesions of the *cerebellar cortex* have been described by Spielmeyer. These occur as disseminated atrophies of cerebellar lobules. In the earlier stages they are identical with the disseminated ischaemic necrosis of the Purkinje cells and their dendrites and the characteristic microglial shrub formations within the molecular layer, described by Spielmeyer and his school in many types of anoxias and anoxic intoxication (*vide* page 258). The depth of the sulci and consequently the vicinity of the cerebellar white matter are preferential sites (Fig. 11.7). In some cases cerebellar lesions may be so extensive as to approximate to the histological picture of the hereditary systemic degenerations. Cases of this kind have been described by Scholz (1951) and van Bogaert and Colle (1955). According to Scholz, the focal vascular genesis is even then clearly recognizable and serves as a guide in differential-diagnosis. In van Bogaert and Colle's case the cerebellar symptomatology was progressive.

Scholz was the first to describe ischaemic necrosis in the *thalamus* following severe convulsions. This author considers necrosis and atrophy of the thalamus and particularly of its lateral nucleus as a lesion occurring almost as frequently as Ammon's horn sclerosis and disseminated lobular atrophy of the cerebellum.

Of other subcortical centres, the dentate nucleus (von Braunmühl 1938), the inferior olives (Minkowsky 1930) and the corpus striatum (Scholz 1951) may be affected. As regards the dentate nucleus and the inferior olives, the circumscribed vascular damage in epileptic brains must be distinguished from the pigment atrophy which usually affects all the nerve cells of the two grey centres. The glial scars of the corpus striatum often become hypermyelinised and present the appearances of status marmoratus. Occasionally the motor cortex and the insula may be selectively affected (Scholz 1959).

General remarks. While, in general, the distribution of lesions follows the anoxic pattern, there are important differences: as Scholz has repeatedly pointed out, the globus pallidus, and the subthalamic nucleus are damaged very rarely indeed. Some of the centres which are predominantly affected, such as Ammon's horn and other rhinencephalic centres, are known to have a low threshold for after-discharges (Jung 1949, 1950, Kaada 1951; Andy and Akert 1955, among others). This would make for increased oxygen requirement which should bring about 'consumptive' anoxia, but almost certainly this is not the whole explanation. The problem will be taken up again in the discussion of temporal lobe epilepsy.

Miscellaneous

Traumatic lesions are frequent findings in symptomatic epilepsies. They are, however, also encountered in the 'cryptogenic' group and, here, are probably caused by injury during grand mal attacks. These lesions are often of the contre-coup type, bruising the base of the frontal and temporal lobes and resulting in superficial irregular lesions (état vermoulu, tâches jaunes). This type of lesion has been fully described on page 452. It is mentioned here because of its relevance to the problem of so-called 'psychical' seizures and in particular of temporal lobe epilepsy.

At one time fibrosis of the choroid plexus (de Allende-Navarro 1926) and Pacchionian granulations (Winkelman and Fay 1930) have attracted attention because of their possible significance in the production and absorption of the cerebrospinal fluid. These findings and their interpretation have not been generally accepted.

Necrosis of heart muscle. Neubürger (1933) found in 14 among 34 epileptic patients below the age of 40 areas of recent necrosis of the heart muscle side by side with older fibrotic foci. According to this author, these lesions are caused by spasm of coronary arteries during grand mal seizures.

Pathogenic considerations

Most of the findings reported above are clearly the consequence of the disturbance of the blood circulation and/or lack of oxygen, and they are identical with those which have been considered in detail under the heading of anoxia. Only a few remarks are therefore necessary on specific points which arise from the pathology of epilepsy.

Spielmeyer, using Ammon's horn sclerosis as a test case, suggested that disturbance of vasomotor regulation, and in particular angiospasm, caused the necrosis and he therefore postulated angiospasm as a possible cause of the convulsion. Scholz (1951) and his collaborators Dreszer and Jötten have provided evidence in support of an angiospastic theory by means of blood corpuscle staining methods (benzidine stain) in cat brain tissue obtained during progressive stages of epileptic convulsions which were evoked either chemically or electrically. There is, however, no proof that the areas of anaemia which they clearly demonstrated are in fact due to spasm of blood-vessels. Penfield (1936) in contradistinction to earlier impressions failed to observe blanching of the brain and the meninges *preceding* convulsions which occurred during surgical exposure. Likewise the present writer and his associates (Meyer 1939), using a histological technique similar to that of Scholz, were unable to confirm the finding of anaemia *preceding* the onset of the fit. There seems to be general agreement, however, that during the convulsions and particularly in their later stages, profound disturbances of the circulation occur, anaemia alternating with stasis. Scholz has demonstrated that these disturbances are prolonged for some time beyond the termination of the convulsion. Measurement of cerebral blood flow also does not indicate decrease before and at the beginning of the seizure (Gibbs, Lennox and Gibbs 1934); during subsequent stages of the convulsions it is, however, definitely increased. Although these facts do not absolutely exclude the occasional significance of angiospastic abnormalities in the pathogenesis of epileptic seizures, they suggest that angiospasm does not play the very significant rôle attributed to it previously.

Biochemical changes. Since the frequency of the electrical discharges of motor nerve cells and probably of other nerve cells during convulsions is a multiple (up to 1,000 per second) of the normal rate (Adrian and Moruzzi 1939, Jung 1949), metabolic requirements are correspondingly increased. This increase is at least partially met by a considerable acceleration of cerebral blood flow, tissue respiration and glycolysis. The tissue content of high energy substances (adenosine triphosphate, phosphocreatine, etc.) is decreased while inorganic phosphate and lactic acid appear in greater amounts. Convulsions can be prolonged by administration of oxygen and glucose.

Acetylcholine appears in the cerebrospinal fluid, both during and following convulsions. When applied locally to the cortex or injected intracisternally, convulsions or their electro-encephalographic concomitants appear. These findings have led to investigations (in both human and animal brains) into the acetylcholine metabolism of tissue obtained from epileptogenic cortical foci. No significant difference has been found between epileptogenic and normal tissue, either in total acetylcholine content or in the rate of synthesis of free acetylcholine, except that the epileptogenic tissue showed a failure to produce *bound* acetylcholine (Tower and Elliott 1952; Tower 1961).

An abnormal metabolism of glutamic acid appears to be involved also. Ammonia, whose close relationship to convulsive states has been demonstrated by Richter and Dawson (1948), may be derived from this aminoacid. During seizures induced in animals, glutamic acid has been found depleted. In the presence of pyridoxal phosphate as a coenzyme, glutamic acid is decarboxylated to γ-aminobutyric acid (Gaba) which was finally identified by Bazemore, Elliott and Florey (1957) and is now known to be present in considerable amounts in grey matter, mostly, as Tower points out, in the mitochondrial fraction. There is also substantial evidence that it acts as an inhibitory transmitter; its decrease or abnormal function may thus be an important factor in lowering the threshold of convulsive discharges. It will be remembered (page 301) that pyridoxine deficiency leads to convulsions in experimental animals, and that spontaneous convulsions in human infants may be relieved by this vitamin. Deficiency of γ-aminobutyric acid may be caused by depletion of glutamic acid, by failure of glutamic decarboxylase or by increased utilisation of Gaba itself.

Abnormality of electrolytes may also be involved in seizure activity since, in experimental animals, the intracellular potassium content of neurones decreases and is replaced by sodium. 'Epileptogenic' slices of human brains are incapable of regaining lost potassium (Tower).

Precipitating factors such as hyperventilation, hydration, ethanol, etc., have been much investigated in the past. The exact mechanism of their action is not yet fully understood, although pH, electrolyte distribution and cell membrane permeability are all likely to play a part.

Temporal lobe epilepsy

The first observations of temporal lobe epilepsy were made by Hughlings Jackson and Beevor (1890). These workers described attacks with an olfactory, gustatory or visceral aura; furthermore the characteristic feelings of unreality or familiarity (jamais vu, déjà vu), dream-like experiences, illusions or hallucinations (visual or auditory) which occurred before or during the attack. Visual hallucinations often display an organised scenic character in contrast to hallucinations related to lesions in the occipital region. In cases showing such symptomatology, small focal lesions were found, usually in the anterior part of the temporal lobe and, in particular, in the hippocampal (uncinate) gyrus. Hughlings Jackson's observations have been re-examined by a number of workers who have confirmed this localisation of the lesions.

Although Hughlings Jackson's findings were accepted as a new focal variety of epilepsy, for a long time this had no wider repercussion on the problem of epilepsy in general. It is historically interesting that to all appearances nobody saw the interesting relationship of the lesion within the uncinate gyrus with the hippocampal and uncal sclerosis in other epileptic brains. The reason probably was that no important functional significance was attributed to a lesion of centres which were at that time regarded as serving olfactory function.

The situation has perceptibly changed within the last two decades. With the advent of electro-encephalography, diagnosis of what has been called by Gibbs, Gibbs and Lennox (1937) psychomotor epilepsy was put upon a broader and safer basis. It has been estimated that

50 per cent or more of all institutionalized epilepsies fall into this group (Gastaut 1954), but this figure depends on definition, as has been pointed out in a thoughtful paper by Margerison and Liddell (1961). Several varieties with varying localisation of lesions have been described. Gastaut distinguishes within the temporal lobe a superficial (lateral) from the far more frequent hippocampal variety. Psychomotor epilepsies of similar symptomatology may also be caused, however, by lesions outside the temporal lobe, for example by lesions situated in the insula, orbital cortex, anterior olfactory centres and in the diencephalon. Diencephalic epilepsy, an earlier term coined by Penfield (1929), to describe attacks presenting mainly with autonomic disturbances, seems to have been absorbed into this wider concept. No consistent anatomical lesions have ever been described. Penfield (1954) speaks of temporo-insular epilepsy and he subdivides this, similarly, into an uncinate variety responsible for automatism, a variety affecting the superior and lateral convolutions of the temporal lobe resulting in hallucinations and illusions, and an insular variety responsible for seizures with alimentary and respiratory aura. In patients suffering from temporal lobe attacks Penfield and Rasmussen (1950) were able to elicit similar phenomena by electrical stimulation of the superior and lateral convolutions of the temporal lobe, of the adjacent cortex in the insula and parietal region and of the deep structures within and near the hippocampal gyrus. Neither Penfield nor Gastaut was able to elicit temporal lobe seizures by stimulation of Ammon's horn proper, but succeeded after stimulation of the cortex of the hippocampal gyrus and of the uncus and amygdaloid complex.

With the increase of surgical intervention the scope of pathological investigations has increased. The first large-scale report was that of Earle, Baldwin and Penfield (1953) who claimed that 'incisural sclerosis' was the most common cause of temporal lobe epilepsy. This change was noted in 100 out of 157 patients who were submitted to operation. The extent of this sclerosis ranged from involvement of a single gyrus to that of the entire temporal lobe, but the apex and the anterior part of the hippocampal gyrus with the uncus and amygdaloid nucleus were most frequently involved. The lesion was presumed to be the result of herniation of the temporal lobe, or more strictly its most medial and inferior parts, into the tentorial opening during the head moulding phase of parturition. Such herniation occurs at a time when the temporal lobe is poorly developed and particularly susceptible to damage through local anoxia, following the compression of the anterior choroidal and posterior cerebral arteries against the tentorial edge. These statements on pathology were mainly based on macroscopic inspection which often revealed gross atrophy and/or increase of consistency to the touch. No systematic histological investigations were carried out, however, and the medial structures were not included in the biopsy tissue.

In the remaining 57 cases, Penfield and his associates found a postnatal pathology usually in the form of tumours or the sequelae of head injury or of infection.

Sano and Malamud's (1953) clinico-pathological post-mortem studies were published almost at the same time. Twenty-nine of their 50 cases of epilepsy were found to have Ammon's horn lesions. After excluding severely demented cases unsuitable for clinico-pathological analysis, these authors found that all cases with clinical temporal lobe symptoms had Ammon's horn sclerosis and/or traumatic fronto-temporal lobe lesions. Nine cases, in which Ammon's horn sclerosis was the only appreciable focal lesion in the brain, showed ictal phenomena of a temporal type, while in 5 cases without cerebral changes no clinical signs of temporal lobe affection had been present.

Sano and Malamud's results in essence agree with a similar analysis by Stauder, which is remarkable because of its early date (1935). This author found Ammon's horn sclerosis in 36 of 53 cases of epilepsy. Thirty-three of these 36 cases had shown clinical signs suggestive of temporal lobe lesion; a number had, in addition or as an alternative, traumatic scars in the fronto-temporal basal region as a result, probably, of contrecoup bruising. None of the 17 cases with normal Ammon's horn had shown clinical signs of temporal lobe involvement.

Such a high incidence of Ammon's horn sclerosis has not been reported by other workers. Combined clinical, electroencephalographic, radiological and pathological investigations have been carried out by a team of workers at the Maudsley Hospital in London. The pathological findings in biopsy tissue of temporal lobes (resected by Falconer) have been communicated in a number of publications (Meyer, Falconer and Beck (1954), Cavanagh and Meyer (1956) and Cavanagh, Falconer and Meyer (1958), among others). The 1958 report covered 50 cases which were divided into two groups: a group of focal lesions (14 cases); and another of diffuse lesions (36 cases) which would roughly compare with the 'incisural sclerosis' group of the Montreal workers. In the focal group, small tumours and glial hamartomas formed the majority (Cavanagh 1958). They could be found in any of the excised regions, but were more frequent near the apex and in the medio-inferior aspects, and occasionally almost exclusively confined to the uncal and amygdaloid region (Fig. 11.8); involvement of Ammon's horn was, however, negligible. In the second group, Ammon's horn sclerosis was recorded in about two-thirds of the total of 36 cases and frequently extended into the uncus and, less often, into the basal parts of the amygdaloid complex. Extension into more anterior structures may facilitate a possible 'trigger' action (Cavanagh and Meyer 1956) of the Ammon's horn lesion, although this latter may not be directly involved in the mechanism of temporal lobe seizures. Sometimes Ammon's horn sclerosis was the only noteworthy pathological change; often, it was accompanied by moderate to severe sclerosis of cortex and/or white matter. In the remaining 15 cases glial proliferation, mainly in the molecular layer of the cortex and in the white matter, was usually slight. It is certainly justifiable to doubt its value as a substrate of the psychomotor attacks, and, in not a few cases, it was of doubtful pathological significance altogether.

Other workers have reported even lower figures for the presence of Ammon's horn sclerosis or of other lesions. Haberland (1958) observed histopathological changes in only 19 of 47 temporal lobes resected for relief of psychomotor epilepsy; these changes included 6 instances of typical Ammon's horn sclerosis. Morris (1956) found macroscopic or microscopic changes present in only 50 per cent of temporal lobe biopsies, although in two-thirds of his operated cases a lasting and significant improvement was recorded. It is possible, as has been pointed out by Falconer *et al.* (1955) and Dell (1958), that improvement may be achieved by removal of histologically normal centres and pathways, of importance to the mechanism of the psychomotor seizure.

Only one instance of trauma was found in the Maudsley material of 1958: a small scar occupying the fusiform and inferior temporal convolutions. Courville (1958), reviewing a material of 113 cases with old traumatic lesions of the temporal lobe, found seizures recorded in 33, of whom 18 had grand mal, 11 combined grand mal and psychomotor attacks; only 3 had pure psychomotor epilepsy. Psychomotor attacks occurred even when the lesion was remote from the medial aspects and, conversely, were absent in some cases with localisation in the hippocampal region.

Encephalitis (absent in the Maudsley series of 1958) was common in Malamud's (1958) material. Haymaker *et al.* (1958) recorded epileptic convulsions in 30 and psychomotor attacks in only 5 of their 46 cases of infantile acute herpetic inclusion encephalitis (mostly of short survival), with marked histological involvement of the temporal lobe, and especially of the medial centres. The same authors failed to record any signs of epilepsy in 21 cases of infantile kernicterus (also of short survival) in all of whom varying degrees of Ammon's horn lesion were present at post-mortem. In another series of 200 cases selected at random, 20 in whom no symptoms of epilepsy had been shown during life, had some involvement of the hippocampal region.

Peiffer (1962), reviewing a material of 439 epileptic brains, recorded a lesion of Ammon's horn in 39·6 per cent. Cases which had presented with psychomotor attacks during life showed only a slightly increased incidence of Ammon's horn sclerosis, while the number of other lesions, such as angiomas and tumours within the pararhinal region, was significantly higher.

These contradictory observations have led Percival Bailey (1958) to a rather reserved assessment of the role of the hippocampal centres (including Ammon's horn) in the aetiology of temporal lobe epilepsy. One should not forget, however, that, as in other forms of focal epilepsy, lesions in the temporal lobe give rise to epileptic manifestations in only a limited percentage and after a sufficiently long survival period. Clearly, other 'epileptogenic' factors, to some extent genetically determined, are necessary for overt epilepsy to become manifest. Different criteria for the selection of cases submitted to temporal lobectomy may also account for some of the contradictory findings. Present uncertainties should not obscure the significant and intriguing advance (the 'new look' of Scholz 1959) brought about by experimental work on the rhinencephalon and by the introduction of the concept of incisural sclerosis. Clarification will eventually result from a widening of observations on biopsy material and—especially—from statistically valid series of cases in which clinical, electroencephalographic and post-mortem investigations are adequate.

Experimental investigations may also assist in clarifying the pathogenesis of Ammon's horn sclerosis (Green *et al.* 1957; Gastaut, Bérard-Badier *et al.* 1958; Gastaut, Toga and Naquet 1958; Gastaut, Meyer *et al.* 1959). Though differing in their technical approach, all these authors stressed local vascular factors as operative in the pathogenesis of Ammon's horn sclerosis. In Gastaut, Meyer *et al.* experiments, for example, alumina cream applied to the temporal pyriform cortex of cats escaped into the ventricles; secondary anoxic damage (including Ammon's horn necrosis) was found to occur in several cats, predominantly on the side to which this spread and its concomitant inflammatory reaction and tissue herniation was more or less confined. In several cats granulation tissue was found in the vicinity of the basal (posterior cerebral and anterior choroidal) arteries, which may have acted as a mechanical irritant to the vessels, resulting in temporary compression or constriction. In Green *et al.* experiments, anoxic damage to Ammon's horn only occurred in those 23 cats in which epileptic convulsions had been recorded; it is difficult entirely to exclude the possibility that there may have been a causal relationship inverse to that accepted by the authors. Severe generalised convulsions were not recorded in about half of the animals of Gastaut, Meyer *et al.*, that showed secondary anoxic damage; but, again, it cannot be excluded that their occurrence may have escaped notice. For these reasons, the authors emphasised the need for 'more cogent evidence concerning the relationship between epileptic seizures and anoxic lesions'.

Gastaut, Toga and Naquet, producing convulsions by agenised flour, concluded that the lesions in the temporal pyriform cortex and in the cerebellum had preceded the convulsions. It is of considerable interest, however, that Tower and Olszewski (1958) were unable to find any histological abnormality in Ammon's horn or elsewhere (apart from slightly pale staining of nerve cells in Deiter's nucleus) in the brain of a cat, fixed 8 hours *after* the onset of methionine sulfoximine induced seizures. This design of experiment may eventually supply the decisive evidence, so far still lacking.

The concept of incisural sclerosis of Penfield and his associates seems to challenge the hypothesis of the Munich school, particularly of Scholz, that Ammon's horn sclerosis is caused by severe grand mal seizures. This contradiction is, however, not as unreconcilable as it might appear at first glance, particularly if on both sides the viewpoint is widened. Lindenberg

(1955), whose views have been discussed more fully elsewhere (*vide* pages 260 and 396), has suggested that compression of arteries occurs in a number of conditions in the course of which supratentorial pressure increases suddenly through oedema or otherwise enlarged volume of the brain. Penfield and his associates have dealt with one aspect of raised supratentorial pressure by the moulding of the infant's head during parturition. If one accepts Lindenberg's hypothesis or some modification of it, there is no reason why other conditions resulting in sudden increase of pressure, such as, for example, anoxia at birth or at a later period, should not have similar effects. From what has been said above about the considerable relative anoxia which occurs during the cyanotic stage of convulsions, one may safely assume that the same chain of events will take place in them and may lead to the damage described by Scholz, provided that the convulsions are of particular severity and occur in the form of status. Such a wider view will, in the opinion of the present writer, more readily conform to the statistical facts than the exclusive theory of birth injury of the Montreal workers. Scholz (1959) remarks that, as a whole, post-epileptic damage is not as severe as the anoxic damage described by Lindenberg and by Pia (1957). This, he considers, may be because increase of intracranial pressure and oedema during severe epileptic attacks is more evenly distributed and not confined to either the supratentorial or to the infratentorial spaces.

It has been shown by Cavanagh and Meyer (1956), and confirmed by Corsellis (1957), that in the majority of cases which showed Ammon's horn sclerosis and other lesions of anoxic type, the onset of the epileptic disease was in the first decade of life. This confirms observations made by Pfleger, as long ago as 1880, and for which this author quotes an even earlier authority, Hemkes. In about 50 per cent of the Maudsley material (second group) a history of difficult or protracted birth was recorded. In the majority of the remainder the disease was initiated a few years after a normal birth by a severe status epilepticus, which was frequently associated with a not necessarily severe febrile condition such as teething fevers, chicken pox, whooping cough, Still's syndrome, etc. Why these febrile convulsions should have such grave sequelae is not yet understood. Lennox (1953), discussing their significance, considers them innocuous in the overwhelming majority of cases, but should cyanosis and coma be protracted, then they are followed by irreversible damage. Among 392 cases which had suffered brain injury during the first decade of life, febrile seizures were blamed as the cause of injury and continuing epilepsy in 5·4 per cent. The febrile seizure is, according to Lennox, almost invariably the child's initial seizure; a striking number of such cases present with psychomotor features. Genetic traits are also unduly high.

Millichap (1960) and his associates, who approached the problem experimentally, found that the threshold to febrile seizures in young rats rose with increasing age, and was associated with changes in balance of water and electrolytes. In adult animals, the threshold could be lowered by bringing about similar chemical changes. A labile salt and water metabolism, due to upset of the blood-brain barrier, has been implicated by Radermecker (1956, 1958) for the disorders which follow hyperthermic episodes. The difficulty remains, however, of explaining why this should have grave consequences in only a tiny minority of cases. Gardner (1958) suggests the possibility that aspiration of food and vomit may be of pathogenic importance, since 40 per cent of infants vomit during or after fits; he estimates that at least half the fatalities occur through inhalation which is often overlooked at post-mortem: Small and Woolf (1957), on the other hand, stressed the pathogenic importance of respiratory embarrassment during the epileptic convulsion. Clearly some such factor, at present unknown, seems to determine the outcome of the convulsions. Some cases may belong to the category of 'symptomatic' epilepsy, rather than of the 'cryptogenic' variety. The febrile primary disease may give rise to encephalitis. That certain viral encephalitides may predominantly affect the temporal lobe and rhinencephalic centres has been already mentioned. It is known that thrombosis of venous channels may follow trivial head injury or fever and may easily be overlooked at post-mortem (Martin 1955, Lindenberg). Small and Woolf, however, found no such morphological bridge between the trivial trauma and the fatal anoxia in their case.

Myoclonus epilepsy

Myoclonic contractions are common in epileptics; Muskens (1909) observed them in approximately two-thirds of all patients suffering from epileptic convulsions, but such figures are misleading as there is no generally accepted agreement of what constitutes a myoclonic phenomenon.

Myoclonus epilepsy is common in cases of lipidosis affecting the cerebellum (Greenfield 1954); it is a prominent feature also in the sclerosing type of subacute leuco-encephalitis, in which however the cerebellum is affected to a lesser degree than the diencephalon, midbrain and other parts of the brain stem. In epilepsia partialis continua, called after Kojevnikow, myoclonic twitching is confined to one segment of the body. The pathology of the myoclonic component in this condition is not yet known; in most of the pathologically investigated cases of the literature emphasis has been placed on the cortical lesions.

Foix *et al.* (1926) have described another variety: myoclonus of the soft palate, pharynx, larynx, eye muscles and diaphragm (syndrôme myoclonique de la calotte); further cases of this category have been published by van Bogaert (1926), Lhermitte *et al.* (1935) and Guillain (1938). Foix *et al.* and van Bogaert first attributed this variant of myoclonus to a lesion of the central tegmental tract, but later attention shifted to the inferior olives and the dentate nucleus and their respective connections.

The most fully investigated form of myoclonus epilepsy is the progressive, familial and often hereditary variety first described by Unverricht (1891) and Lundborg (1903). Cases of this kind have been reported by Lafora and Glück (1911), Westphal and Sioli (1921), Ostertag (1925), Hodskins and Yakovlev (1930), van Bogaert (1949), Harriman and Millar (1955) and many others. Lafora described the amyloid intracellular inclusions which have been named after him, and of which a full description will be found on page 42. These inclusions may be ubiquitous, but Westphal and Sioli found them with particular frequency in the dentate nucleus, red nucleus and thalamus, while Ostertag stressed their predominance in the substantia nigra. In Harriman and Millar's case they were found in heart and liver, in addition to their presence in the central nervous sytem. However, they are not present in all cases of familial Unverricht disease. Hodskins and Yakovlev found them reported in the literature in only 7 of 19 cases with post-mortem reports; they were, for example, absent in the case described by van Bogaert (1949), to whom we owe a critical review of the whole problem. In the advanced stage of the disease van Bogaert's case showed, in addition to the myoclonic and epileptic phenomena, an extrapyramidal syndrome recalling that of post-encephalic or idiopathic Parkinsonism. The histological changes, which consisted of nerve cell loss and consequent gliosis, were most marked in the inferior olives, the compact zone of the substantia nigra and the centromedian nucleus of the thalamus, followed in the degree of severity by lesions in the dentate nucleus and cerebellar cortex. Cerebral cortex, Ammon's horn and corpus striatum were not involved. The lateral aspects of the substantia nigra were more severely affected than the medial ones. Van Bogaert is inclined to attribute the Parkinsonian-like symptoms in his case to the lesion of the substantia nigra, while he relates the myoclonic features to olivary and dentate involvement.

Myoclonus epilepsy (familial or sporadic) may combine with spinocerebellar system degenerations: dentato-rubral atrophy, to which Greenfield has given the name of 'the Ramsay

Hunt syndrome', is an important example. In Hunt's (1921) case, the cerebellar cortex was intact, the dentate nucleus atrophic and there was rarefaction of myelin in the superior cerebellar peduncle. In a similar case of Louis-Bar and van Bogaert (1947) there were, among other changes, slight loss of granule cells, and severe cell loss in the nuclei dentatus, emboliformis, globosus and fastigii. The superior olives, the superior vestibular nuclei and the spinal root of the trigeminal nucleus were also atrophic, and the superior cerebellar peduncle showed pale staining. In an earlier case of Hänel and Bielschowsky (quoted from Greenfield) the cerebellar cortex and medullary olives were more severely affected than either the dentate nucleus or the superior cerebellar peduncle.

While the problem of the pathological 'substrate' of myoclonus still awaits a final answer, these examples show how frequently the dentate nucleus, the olives and other centres and pathways of the brain stem are affected. A similar localisation is suggested by the results of electrophysiological experiments: Penfield and Kristiansen place the origin of myoclonic seizures in the lower brain stem and the spinal cord. The thalamus and more caudal centres figured prominently in the experimental observations of Gastaut *et al.* (1951, 1952).

Convulsive treatment

The wide employment of convulsive therapy in psychiatry calls for a description of its pathology. In recent years the provocation of convulsions by chemical substances such as cardiazol and related drugs has been almost universally superseded by electroconvulsive treatment.

Fatalities from both chemical and electroconvulsive treatment have been in the main due to complications, particularly independent disease of the cardiovascular system. This emerges clearly in the review by Maclay (1953) and in the more recent reports of Paarmann and Veltin (1955), Madow (1956), Gaitz *et al.* (1956) and Stensrud (1958). A rare complication is fat embolism following bone fracture or mobilisation of other fat depots (Meyer and Teare 1945, Paarmann *et al.*). In electrically induced convulsions death may be due to faulty placing of the electrodes allowing the current to flow through the hind brain (Alexander and Lowenbach 1945). These same authors do not believe that the current, if used in therapeutic strength, is itself strong enough to cause irreversible damage of an appreciable degree. The prior injection of muscle relaxants may in certain circumstances act cumulatively with the anoxia resulting from the convulsions and thus prove dangerous or fatal (Maclay).

Much discussion and experimental work has been directed to the question whether uncomplicated convulsive therapy, particularly electroconvulsive therapy, causes brain damage. The problem has been recently reviewed by Corsellis and Meyer (1954). Most reviewers, including Alpers (1946) and Will, Rehfeldt and Neumann (1948) consider that irreversible damage in such uncomplicated cases is unlikely. Where experimental conditions approximated to 'therapeutic' dosage histological findings in the brains of animals were either negative or negligible (Cerletti and Bini 1940, Barrera *et al.* 1942, Winkelman and Moore 1944, Alexander and Lowenbach 1944, Sickert, Williams and Windle 1950), or they were not severe (Neubürger *et al.* 1942, Lidbeck 1944, Ferraro and Roizin 1949). The problem has been recently investigated and comprehensively discussed also by Hartelius (1952) who found significant changes in nerve cells, blood-vessels and glia, although by far the greater proportion of these seemed to be reversible. This does not preclude the possibility that occasionally, particularly after a large number of convulsions or after intensive treatment, mild changes of the kind seen after spontaneous convulsions may occur both in human patients and in experimental animals (Ferraro and Roizin 1949, Corsellis and Meyer 1954). Such changes may take the form of a marginal gliosis and astrocytic proliferation within the white matter. In a large material of brains of patients who had previously undergone electric shock treatment and had died from intercurrent disease, Ammon's horn sclerosis and lobular sclerosis of the cerebellum was never seen by the present writer. In the literature only one worker, Zeman (1950), has observed necrosis in Ammon's horn and the cerebellum, but in the few cases he studied the effect of the convulsions was aggravated by serious complications (endocarditis and pneumonia). Corsellis and Meyer concluded that the absence of appreciable neuronal loss in Ammon's horn, cerebellum and cerebral cortex was a further indication of the mildness of the sequelae which rarely may follow electrically induced convulsions. It is possible that the slight memory defect, which not infrequently lasts for some time, may in some cases be associated with these minimal changes.

The mechanism of the lesions seems in principle to be the same as in other forms of epilepsy; it consists of relative anoxia followed by disturbances of the circulation and increased vascular permeability (Hartelius 1952). Scholz and Jötten (1951), with their technique of blood corpuscle staining in experimental animals, observed areas of anaemia alternating with hyperaemia, similar to those which they had seen after other types of experimental convulsions. The disturbances of circulation were noticeable up to 40 minutes after the termination of the tonic-clonic convulsions.

Discussion of the therapeutic rationale of convulsive therapy is outside the scope of this book. Various hypotheses have been promulgated varying from a general effect of shock through anoxia and other metabolic events of the convulsion, to a more specific stimulating effect upon the hypothalamus and the pituitary-adrenal system (Gellhorn 1953) or the reticular system (Roth 1950). Irreversible damage is too infrequent to provide an explanation of the therapeutic effect in general.

REFERENCES

Adrian, E. D. and Moruzzi, G. (1939) *J. Physiol.*, **97**, 153.

Alexander, L. and Lowenbach, H. (1944) *J. Neuropath.*, **3**, 139.

Alpers, B. J. (1946) *Dig. Neurol. Psychiat.*, **14**, 136.

Alzheimer, A. (1898) *Mschr. Psychiat. Neurol.*, **4**, 345.

Andy, O. J. and Akert, K. (1955) *J. Neuropath.*, **14**, 198.

Bailey, P. (1958) in *Temporal Lobe Epilepsy*, edited by Baldwin, M. and Bailey, P., Springfield, Ill., p. 503.

Barrera, S. E., Lewis, N. D. C., Pacella, B. L. and Kalinowsky, L. B. (1942) *Trans. Amer. neurol. Ass.*, **68**, 31.

Bazemore, A. W., Elliott, K. A. C. and Florey, E. (1957) *J. Neurochem.*, **1**, 334.

Bleuler, E. (1895) *Münch. med. Wschr.*, **42**, 769.

Bodechtel, G. (1930) *Z. ges. Neurol. Psychiat.*, **123**, 485.

Bouchet and Cazauvieilh. (1825) *Arch. gen. de méd.*, Paris, **9**, 510.

Brain, W. R. (1951) *Diseases of the Nervous System*, 4th edition, Oxford University Press, London, New York, Toronto.

Bratz, E. (1899) *Arch. Psychiat. Nervenkr.*, **31**, 820.

Bridges, E. M. (1949) *Epilepsy and Convulsive Disorders in Childhood*, McGraw Hill, New York.

Cavanagh, J. B. (1958) *Brain*, **81**, 389.

Cavanagh, J. B., Falconer, M. A. and Meyer, A. (1958) in *Temporal Lobe Epilepsy*, edited by Baldwin, M. and Bailey, P.; Springfield, Ill.

Cavanagh, J. B. and Meyer, A. (1956) *Brit. Med. J.* (ii), 1403.

Cerletti, U. and Bini, L. (1940) *Riv. sper. Freniat.*, **64**, 311.

Chaslin, P. (1889) *C.R. Soc. Biol.*, Paris, **1**, 169.

Corsellis, J. A. N. (1957) *Brain*, **80**, 193.
Corsellis, J. A. N. and Meyer, A. (1954) *J. ment. Sci.*, **100**, 375.
Courville, C. B. (1958) in *Temporal Lobe Epilepsy*, edited by Baldwin, M. and Bailey, P.; Springfield, Ill., p. 220.
Crome, L. (1954) *Proc. R. Soc. Med.*, **47**, 850.
de Allende-Navarro, F. (1926) *Schweiz. Arch. Neurol. Psychiat.*, **16**, 57.
Dell, M. B. (1958) in *Temporal Lobe Epilepsy*, edited by Baldwin, M. and Bailey, P.; Springfield, Ill., p. 497.
Earle, K. M., Baldwin, M. and Penfield, W. (1953) *Arch. Neurol. Psychiat.* (Chicago), **69**, 27.
Falconer, M. A., Hill, D., Meyer, A., Mitchell, W. and Pond, D. A. (1955) *Lancet* (i), 827.
Ferraro, A. and Roizin, L. (1949) *Amer. J. Psychiat.*, **106**, 278.
Foerster, O. and Penfield, W. (1930) *Brain*, **53**, 99.
Foix, C., Chavaux, J. A. and Hillemand, P. (1926) *Rev. neurol.*, **33**, 942.
Gaitz, C. M., Pokorny, A. D. and Mills, M. (1956) *A.M.A. Arch. Neurol. Psychiat.*, **75**, 493.
Gardner, A. M. N. (1958) *J. Quart. Med.*, **27**, 227.
Gastaut, H. (1954) in *Colloque sur les problèmes d'anatomie normale et pathologique posés par les décharge epileptiques*, Les Editions, 'Acta Medica Belgica,' Bruxelles.
Gastaut, H., Bérard-Bardier, M., Darraspen, M. and van Bogaert, L. (1958) ibid., p. 243.
Gastaut, H., Meyer, A., Naquet, R., Cavanagh, J. B. and Beck, E. (1959) *J. Neuropath.*, **18**, 270.
Gastaut, H. and Rémond, A. (1952) *Rev. neurol.*, **86**, 596.
Gastaut, H. and Roger, A. (1951) *Rev. neurol.*, **84**, 94.
Gastaut, H., Toga, M. and Naquet, R. (1958) in *Temporal Lobe Epilepsy*, edited by Baldwin, M. and Bailey, P.; Springfield, Ill., p. 268.
Gellhorn, E. (1953) *Physiological Foundations of Neurology and Psychiatry*, University of Minnesota Press, Minneapolis.
Gibbs, F. A., Gibbs, E. L. and Lennox, W. G. (1937) *Brain*, **60**, 377.
Gibbs, F. A., Lennox, W. G. and Gibbs, E. L. (1934) *Arch. Neurol. Psychiat.* (Chicago), **32**, 257.
Green, J. D., Clemente, C. D. and de Groot, J. (1957) *A.M.A. Arch. Neurol. Psychiat.*, **78**, 259.
Greenfield, J. G. (1954) *The Spino-Cerebellar Degenerations*, Blackwell Scientific Publications, Oxford.
Guillain, G. (1938) *Proc. R. Soc. Med.*, **31**, 1031.
Haberland, C. (1958) *Psychiatria et Neurologia*, **135**, 12.
Harriman, D. G. and Millar, J. H. (1955) *Brain*, **78**, 325.
Hartelius, U. (1952) *Acta psychiat.*, Kbh., suppt. 77.
Haymaker, W., Pentschew, A., Margoles, C. and Bingham, W. G. (1958) in *Temporal Lobe Epilepsy*, edited by Baldwin, M. and Bailey, P.; Springfield, Ill., p. 166.
Hodskins, M. B. and Yakovlev, P. I. (1930) *Amer. J. Psychiat.*, **9**, 827.
Hunt, J. R. (1921) *Brain*, **44**, 490.
Jackson, J. Hughlings and Beevor, C. E. (1890) *Brain*, **12**, 346.
Jung, R. (1949) *Arch. Psychiat. Nervenkr.*, **183**, 206; (1950) ibid., **184**, 261.
Kaada, B. R. (1951) *Acta Physiol. scand.*, **23** (Suppl. 83), 1.
Lafora, G. R. and Glück, B. (1911) *Z. ges. Neurol. Psychiat.*, **6**, 1.
Lennox, W. G. (1953) *Pediatrics*, **11**, 341.
Lennox, W. G., Gibbs, F. A. and Gibbs, E. L. (1940) *Arch. Neurol. Psychiat.* (Chicago), **44**, 1155.
Lhermitte, J., Lévy, G. and Trelles, J. O. (1935) *Rev. neurol.*, **63**, 238.
Lidbeck, W. J. (1944) *J. Neuropath.*, **3**, 81.
Lindenberg, R. (1955) *J. Neuropath.*, **14**, 223.
Louis-Bar, D. and van Bogaert, L. (1947) *Mschr. Psychiat. Neurol.*, **113**, 215.
Lundborg, H. (1903) *Die Progressive Myoklonus-Epilepsie (Unverrichts Myoklonie)*, edited by Almquist and Wiksells, Uppsala.
Maclay, W. S. (1953) *Proc. R. Soc. Med.*, **46**, 13.
Madow, L. (1956) *Amer. J. Psychiat.*, **113**, 337.
Malamud, N. (1958) in *Temporal Lobe Epilepsy*, edited by Baldwin, M. and Bailey, P.; Springfield, Ill., p. 149.
Margerison, J. H. and Liddell, D. W. (1961) *J. Ment. Sci.*, **107**, 909.
Martin, J. P. (1955) *Brit. Med. J.* (ii), 467.
Meyer, A. (1939) *J. ment. Sci.*, **85**, 927.
Meyer, A. and Beck, E. (1955) *Proc. R. Soc. Med.*, **48**, 457.

Meyer, A., Beck, E. and Shepherd, M. (1955) *J. Neurol. Psychiat.*, **18**, 24.
Meyer, A., Falconer, M. A. and Beck, E. (1954) *J. Neurol. Psychiat.*, **17** 276.
Meyer, A. and Teare, D. (1945) *Brit. Med. J.* (ii), 42.
Millichap, J. G. (1960) *Neurology*, **10**, 312.
Minkowsky, M. (1930) *Dtsch. Z. Nervenheilk.*, **116**, 68.
Morris, A. A. (1956) *A.M.A. Arch. Neurol. Psychiat.*, **76**, 479.
Muskens, L. J. J. (1909) *Epilepsia*, **1**, 161.
Neubürger, K. T. (1933) *Frankfurt. Z. Path.*, **46**, 14.
Neubürger, K. T., Whitehead, R. W., Rutledge, E. K. and Ebaugh, F. C. (1942) *Amer. J. med. Sci.* **204**, 381.
Norman, R. M. (1954) in *Colloque sur les problèmes d'anatomie normale et pathologique posés par les décharges epileptiques*, Les Editions 'Acta Medica Belgica,' Bruxelles. (1958) in *Temporal Lobe Epilepsy*, edited by Baldwin, M. and Bailey, P.; Springfield, Ill., p. 203.
Ostertag, B. (1925) *Arch. Psychiat. Nervenkr.*, **73**, 633.
Paarmann, H. F. and Veltin, A. (1955) *Nervenarzt*, **26**, 106.
Peiffer, J. (1962) *Dtsch. Z. Nervenheilk.*, **183**, 245.
Penfield, W. (1927) *Brain*, **50**, 499; (1929) *Arch. Neurol. Psychiat.* (Chicago), **22**, 358; (1936) ibid., **36**, 449; (1954) in *Colloque sur les problèmes d'anatomie normale et pathologique posés par les décharges epileptiques*, Les Editions 'Acta Medica Belgica,' Bruxelles.
Penfield, W. and Bridgers, W. H. (1942) *Trans. Amer. Neurol. Ass.*, **68**, 158.
Penfield, W. and Ericson, I. C. (1941) *Epilepsy and Cerebral Localization*, Baillière, Tindall & Cox, London.
Penfield, W. and Kristiansen, K. (1951) *Epileptic Seizure Patterns*, Charles C Thomas, Springfield.
Penfield, W. and Rasmussen, T. (1950) *The Cerebral Cortex of Man*, Macmillan, New York.
Pfleger, L. (1880) *Allg. Z. Psychiat.*, **36**, 359.
Pia, H. W. (1957) *Acta Neurochir.* (Vienna), Suppl. **4**.
Radermecker, J. (1956) *Electroenceph. Clin. Neurophysiol.*, Suppl. 5; (1958) *Acta Neurol. Psychiat.*, Belg., **58**, 50.
Richter, D. and Dawson, R. M. S. (1948) *J. biol. Chem.*, **176**, 1199.
Rose, M. (1927) *J. Psychol. Neurol.*, Lpz., **34**, 261.
Roth, M. (1950) Premier Congrès Mondial de Psychiatrie, Paris, *Comptes Rendus*, **4**, 229.
Russell, W. R. (1947) *Brain*, **70**, 225; (1951) *J. Neurol. Psychiat.*, **14**, 35.
Russell, W. R. and Whitty, C. W. M. (1952) *J. Neurol. Psychiat.*, **15**, 93.
Sano, K. and Malamud, N. (1953) *Arch. Neurol. Psychiat.* (Chicago), **70**, 40.
Scholz, W. (1930) *Epilepsie, Handbuch der Geisteskrankheiten*, **XI**, edited by O. Bumke, Julius Springer, Berlin; (1951) *Die Krampfschädigungen des Gehirns*, Springer-Verlag, Berlin.
Scholz, W. (1959) *Epilepsia*, **1**, 36.
Scholz, W. and Jötten, J. (1951) *Arch. Psychiat. Nervenkr.*, **186**, 264.
Sickert, R. G., Williams, S. C. and Windle, W. F. (1950) *Arch. Neurol. Psychiat.* (Chicago), **63**, 79.
Small, J. M. and Woolf, A. L. (1957) *J. Neurol. Neurosurg. Psychiat.*, **20**, 293.
Sommer, W. (1880) *Arch. Psychiat. Nervenkr.*, **10**, 631.
Spielmeyer, W. (1927) *Z. ges. Neurol. Psychiat.*, **109**, 501.
Stauder, K. H. (1935) *Arch. Psychiat. Nervenkr.*, **104**, 181.
Stensrud, P. A. (1958) *Acta psychiat. neurol. scand.*, **33**, 115.
Tower, D. B. (1961) in *Chemical Pathology of the Nervous System*, edited by Folch-Pi, J., New York, London.
Tower, D. B. and Elliott, K. A. C. (1952) *J. appl. Physiol.*, **4**, 669.
Tower, D. B. and Olszewski, J. (1958) in *Temporal Lobe Epilepsy*, edited by Baldwin, M. and Bailey, P.; Springfield, Ill., p. 291.
Turner, W. A. (1907) *Epilepsy: a Study of the Idiopathic Disease*, Macmillan, London.
Unverricht, H. (1891) *Die Myoklonie*, Franz Deuticke, Leipzig and Vienna.
van Bogaert, L. (1926) *Rev. neurol.* (i), 977; (1949) *Mschr. Psychiat. Neurol.*, **118**, 170.
van Bogaert, L. and Colle, G. (1955) *Acta psychiat.*, Kbh., **30**, 55.
von Braunmühl, A. (1938) *Z. ges. Neurol. Psychiat.*, **161**, 292.
Walker, A. E. (1949) *Post-traumatic epilepsy*, Blackwell, Oxford.
Westphal, A. and Sioli, F. (1921) *Arch. Psychiat. Nervenkr.*, **62**, 1.

Will, O. A., Rehfeldt, F. C. and Neumann, M. A. (1948) *J. nerv. ment. Dis.*, **107**, 105.
Williams, D. (1950) *Brit. Med. J.* (i), 685.
Winkelman, N. W. and Fay, T. (1930) *Arch. Neurol. Psychiat.* (Chicago), **23**, 44.
Winkelman, N. W. and Moore, M. T. (1944) *J. Neuropath.*, **3**, 199.
Zeman, W. (1950) *Arch. Psychiat. Nervenkr.*, **184**, 440.
Zimmerman, H. M. (1940) *J. Pediat.*, **13**, 859.

CHAPTER 12

PSYCHOSES OF OBSCURE PATHOLOGY

By A. MEYER

This group includes the commonly designated 'functional psychoses' which, among others, comprise the schizophrenias, the manic-depressive group, the involutional psychoses and some of the symptomatic psychoses. Some histological investigations have been made on all of these, but attention has been concentrated on the schizophrenias, probably because from the beginning Kraepelin's concept of dementia praecox suggested a disease entity of organic and progressive type. Some of the earlier histological observations were made by well-known authorities, including Alzheimer (1897, 1913), Klippel and Lhermitte (1909 and earlier papers), Buscaino (1920–21), the Vogts (1922), Mott (1922a) and Josephy (1923).

The histological changes in the brain described by these earlier workers were rather slender. They consisted of nerve cell changes, particularly increase of lipids and shrinkage (Schwunderkrankung) with the formation of miliary areas of loss of neurones (Lückenfelder). Compensatory proliferation of the glia was not consistent. Other changes described included the well known and frequently discussed grape-like degeneration of the white matter called after Buscaino and changes in the choroid plexus. It should be remembered that these findings were recorded soon after the great advances made by Nissl and Alzheimer in the field of the organic dementias. The limitations of interpretation of histological changes were at that time little understood and critical reassessment of these earlier findings by Dunlap (1928), Spielmeyer (1930), Peters (1937) and others established that changes of this kind might well be due to misjudgement of normal variation and to coincidental factors such as age, complicating disease and terminal illness. Dunlap, in carefully selected cases in which coincidental factors could as far as possible be excluded, saw no changes in schizophrenic brains which were beyond the normal range. Spielmeyer and Peters detected changes (increase of lipids and small areas of neuronal loss) in young executed criminals mentally and physically normal, with fixation of the brain under optimal conditions.

For a time these critical reinvestigations of the problem restricted further attempts, so that the Werthams (1934) felt justified in stating that with the histological methods available at that time there was no proof that schizophrenia has a demonstrable substrate in the brain.

More recently, however, claims have been renewed which are, perhaps, more definite than the earlier ones. This new wave of optimism found its expression in a discussion on the histopathology of schizophrenia at the first International Congress of Neuropathology held in Rome in 1952. A majority of speakers, among whom were Lhermitte, the Vogts and Buscaino, either revived the earlier positive claims or gave new evidence for a histological substrate in the brain or other organs. It is therefore necessary to describe these findings in some detail.

Cerebral Pathology

Post-mortem findings. The more recent studies include those by Winkelman and Book (1949), the Vogts (1949, 1952), the Vogts' disciples (Beheim-Schwarzbach, Braitenberg, Hopf, Bäumer, Fünfgeld, Wahren); Lhermitte, Marchand and Guiraud; Buscaino, de Vries, Bolsi and Longo, all in 1952. Of these Lhermitte *et al.*, Buscaino, de Vries and Longo in general maintained the earlier findings. The Vogts and their disciples based the pathology of schizophrenia on the 'Schwunderkrankung' and fatty degeneration of the nerve cells, but also introduced some new points into the discussion. First, they used extensive control material, although this was not published in detail. Secondly, they insisted that it is the persistence of diseased cells rather than the loss of nerve cells which causes the schizophrenic symptomatology. Furthermore, they maintained that certain regions are predominantly involved: these were, within the cortex, the prefrontal, anterior cingular region and the cortex of the third temporal convolution; among subcortical centres the striatum and particularly the globus pallidus, the anterior and medial nuclei of the thalamus, while the hypothalamus and the corpus mammillare showed no consistent specific changes. As far as the medial nucleus of the thalamus is concerned, Heyck (1954), in Grünthal's laboratory, has submitted the recent findings of the school of Vogt to critical re-examination, with negative result.

While the Vogts' material was controlled, this does not appear to be the case in Winkelman and Book's material. In this series case 9 had been submitted to 111 electric shocks; case 8 had likewise undergone considerable electroconvulsive treatment and had died from starvation following escape from hospital. Case 7 had bilateral pyelonephritis, case 6 several episodes of congestive heart failure; cases 2 and 3 early arteriosclerosis. It is, thus, perhaps not surprising that these authors found changes such as heavy fibrous gliosis, demyelination and large areas of focal cortical nerve cell loss, which surpassed the findings of the earlier workers as well as the more recent ones of the Vogts and their disciples.

Some writers consider that in schizophrenia we are dealing not with one clear-cut disease, but with different syndromes, and that it is for this reason that in some cases no histological changes are found in the brain and organs, while in others there are gross changes. Ferraro (1943), for example, has described cases diagnosed clinically as schizophrenia, in which post-mortem investigation revealed extensive demyelination particularly in the white matter of the frontal lobe. The posterior frontal region and the corpus callosum were the seat of tumours (one a glioblastoma, the other an oligodendroglioma), described by Symonds (1960) in an interesting observation in a brother and sister, both of whom developed psychotic attacks indistinguishable from schizophrenia. In other cases of schizophrenia-like psychoses, following epidemic encephalitis, diffuse sclerosis, CO poisoning, etc. (for references *vide* Peters 1956), the localisation was quite different. Hillbom (1951) found schizophrenia-like psychosis developing with particular frequency after injury of the temporal lobes, and Beard and Slater (1962) drew attention to the occurrence of such psychoses in epilepsy, preponderantly of the temporal lobe variety. It is also of considerable interest in this connection that the response of chimpanzees to lysergic acid is abolished by previous bilateral ablation of the outer temporal convolutions, but not by that of the prefrontal cortex (Baldwin *et al.* 1959). Bruetsch, in a series of papers summarised at the Rome Congress in 1952, has reported histological changes in 9 of 100 'schizophrenic' brains which were sometimes gross, and which were the consequence of rheumatic occlusive endarteritis of the small meningeal and cortical arteries, usually in the presence of rheumatic valvular heart disease. Similar cases have been reported by van der Horst (1952) and by Bini and Marchiafava (1952). All these authors concur that the brains of other schizophrenic patients may be histologically normal. Bini and Marchiafava have scrutinised the large material of the psychiatric hospital in Rome and found no cases clinically labelled as schizophrenia with evidence of rheumatic pathology. They point out that the definition of schizophrenia in the United States is wider than that used by most European psychiatrists.

A statistical investigation by Feuchtwanger and Mayer-Gross (1938) established that schizophreniform syndromes occurred in about 1 per cent of 1,554 cases of war head injuries, i.e.

only double the percentage of 'idiopathic' schizophrenia whose incidence in this material was the same as in the average population. Manfred Bleuler (1951a) observed schizophreniform, manic-depressive and hysterical traits in only 5 per cent of 600 cases of cerebral tumour with signs of psychosis. He considered that in such cases familial predisposition accounted for the specific symptomatology of these organic psychoses. While these statistical series do not disprove that schizophrenia-like conditions may be precipitated by organic disease of the brain, they must have a sobering effect on any interpretation of their numerical and nosological importance in the problem of schizophrenia as a whole. In neither survey was there in the brain a consistent localisation which might have been implicated for the schizophreniform manifestations.

Biopsy investigations. The advent of neurosurgical therapy in mental disease has given greatly increased opportunity for studies of this kind. Elvidge and Reed (1938) have reported swelling of the oligodendroglia in the cerebral white matter in biopsy material from patients showing mental symptoms (no distinction was made between schizophrenia and other types of functional psychoses). This claim was not confirmed in investigations by Wolf and Cowen (1952) and Meyer (1952). Kirschbaum and Heilbrunn (1944) described degenerative changes of the nerve cells and of the glia in 10 of 11 schizophrenic brains. Hydén and Hartelius (1948) investigated biopsies from 10 schizophrenic patients with the aid of ultra-violet microspectroscopy. They described 2 types of abnormal cortical nerve cells, one narrow and shrunken with corkscrew-shaped processes, the other swollen and hypochromatic; both were lacking in nucleoprotein. Both teams of workers, however, used post-mortem material as controls, and they do not appear to have been sufficiently aware of the artefacts peculiar to all biopsy material of the human and animal brain (Meyer and Meyer 1949). The findings of Messimy *et al.* (1951) are also open to criticism because of the absence of suitable controls. The present writer described similar findings in biopsies taken from non-schizophrenic psychoses and neuroses and is inclined to explain them by coincidental factors.

Macroscopic abnormalities. Abnormality of the meninges and apparent cortical atrophy has been reported by a number of neurosurgeons who have performed neurosurgical operations on schizophrenics and other psychotics (Puech 1949, Pool 1949, Palma and Sotelo 1952). These findings have been supported by pneumo-encephalographic evidence indicating cortical atrophy (Donovan, Galbraith and Jackson 1949, Meschan and Scruggs 1951, Huber 1953). It is difficult to reconcile these findings with macroscopically negative post-mortem observations. Broser (1949) failed to find differences in weight between a large series of schizophrenic brains and those from mentally normal patients of corresponding age groups. In interpreting these findings, physiological range, age and complications must be carefully considered. It is possible that we are dealing with functional fluctuations of brain volume and it would certainly be of great value to clarify their significance (Meyer and McLardy 1950).

Extracerebral changes

There have been numerous reports of histological findings in organs other than the brain. These include a small heart and small calibre of blood-vessels, capillaroscopic abnormalities, gastro-intestinal changes, damage of the liver, changes in the reticulo-endothelial system, gonadal atrophy and pathological changes in other endocrine glands.

Aplasia of the heart and blood-vessels has been described in catatonic patients by Lewis (1923). Shattock (1950 a and b), among others, confirmed Lewis' findings of small heart and small calibre of limb vessels in all the catatonic subjects in her series of post-mortem examination of 25 schizophrenics. The auricular wall was found to be reduced in thickness almost to the consistency of tissue paper. Some of the disturbances of the circulation in catatonics such as acrocyanosis and vasoconstriction may, according to Shattock, be reversible phenomena which should be understood as part of a physiological mechanism for conserving heat in circumstances of reduced general metabolism.

Capillaroscopy. The history of this interesting approach in relation to psychiatry has been reviewed by Lovett Doust (1950, 1955). Lombard (1911) seems to have been the first to show that the capillaries of the skin could be observed microscopically after treatment of the skin with a refractile oil and suitable illumination. Lewis (1927) among many others described the arrangement of the hairpin-shaped normal capillaries of the nailfold within a semicircle. He also noted considerable variation in their number between individual persons. Jaensch (1930) studied and illustrated the maturation of the capillaries. Subsequent studies have demonstrated that the capillary pattern of the nailfold varies little once it reaches maturity which according to Lovett Doust takes place within a period ranging from 6 months to 8 years. The similarity of the pattern is strikingly more similar in identical than in binovular twins.

The first attempt to apply the method to problems of psychiatry was made by Parrisius (1921) who found abnormalities in neurotics with labile vasomotor system. Subsequently marked differences were found between mentally healthy persons and physically normal mental defectives, epileptics, schizophrenics, those with affective disorders, psychoneurotics and criminal psychopaths. Large series of psychotics were investigated by Olkon (1939, 1945), Hauptmann (1946) and Hauptmann and Myerson (1948). The main distinction between the capillary pattern inmental health and in disease is the lack of maturation in the latter. Immaturity is particularly marked in feeble-minded children, myxoedema, psychoneurosis, epilepsy and schizophrenia. However, signs of immaturity are not entirely lacking among healthy controls. Lovett Doust (1955), who in the main confirms the results of earlier work, distinguishes nine categories of capillary structure (*vide* his Table 3 and Fig. 2). Only Type 1 and 3 are fairly consistently found in healthy controls. There also seem to be differences in the capillary pattern, though perhaps in a less striking degree, in the various forms of mental disease.

Although considerable evidence has accumulated and there is a fair degree of agreement between various groups of contributors, much remains to be done. The accuracy of the method has been questioned by several critics; it is admittedly exposed to subjective error. The results so far obtained are, however, of considerable interest as a contribution to the constitutional aspects of mental disease. It is likely that capillaroscopy and related investigations will take their place with other constitutional investigations such as the Kretschmerian and Sheldonian types of physique. It is, however, questionable whether, from the appearance of the capillaries of the nailfold, conclusions can be drawn as to the intracranial capillaries. No comparable abnormalities have been reported after ordinary histological investigations of the brains of neurotics, epileptics and schizophrenics.

Gastro-intestinal tract, liver, reticulo-endothelial system. The literature on the pathology of these organs and systems in schizophrenia is extensive. Buscaino (1952) and his school have carried out perhaps the most systematic histological and biochemical investigations. In their opinion pathological changes in the intestines were found to be common, and were most frequent in the small intestines, with the stomach and the colon next in order of incidence. They may be inflammatory or haemorrhagic, or consist of sclerosis of the mucosa.

The weight of the liver was found by Buscaino and others in large series of cases to be subnormal: the most commonly reported histological changes were fatty degeneration, albuminous swelling, and foci of loss of liver cells, commonly in the centre of the lobules. The reticulo-endothelial cells in both liver and spleen are also affected.

From these and biochemical findings Buscaino has developed the hypothesis that schizophrenia is a somatic disease due to amine intoxication: he considers changes in the brain and in particular the grape-like degeneration of the cerebral white matter and basal ganglia as the end result of this intoxication.

Scheidegger (1952) among others has questioned the liver findings reported by Buscaino. In his opinion, it is not possible to prove the existence of any particular disease of the liver which can be attributed to schizophrenia.

Endocrine glands. Histological changes have been claimed in the gonads, adrenal glands and thyroid. The best-known finding is that of Mott (1922 b) in testes and ovaries. Mott's findings, which were never generally accepted as significant, have found recent support in investigations by Hemphill, Reiss and Taylor (1944). The histological appearances in the testicular biopsy specimens examined by them were similar to those described by Mott and in certain aspects resembled the secondary atrophy caused by hypophysectomy in animals. The validity of these biopsy findings has been severely criticised by Blair *et al.* (1952).

While it is difficult to judge these organic findings without wide personal experience, it is probably true to say that most have remained controversial at least as far as their causal significance for schizophrenia is concerned. Some may be primarily associated with the body build and thus be parallel manifestations; many may be the consequence rather than the cause of the psychotic manifestations, of the difficulty of adequate nutrition and hygiene, and of prolonged institutionalisation.

Conclusions and outlook

When Spielmeyer (1930) reviewed the problem of the histopathology of schizophrenia he carefully abstained from passing a negative judgment. He only stated that what changes there may be in the brain and, one might add, in other organs are so subtle that with the available histological methods they cannot be clearly distinguished from the normal and that, where they are more marked, they are likely to be due to coincidental causes such as age, complicating disease, etc. The present writer believes that Spielmeyer's view is to-day still substantially correct and in this cautious attitude he is in general agreement with the conclusions of Wolf and Cowen (1952), Peters (1956), David (1957) and Dastur (1959), who have all given valuable and comprehensive reviews of previous work. The array of more positive claims, impressive as it appeared at the Conference in Rome, loses some of its significance when it is remembered that many were recapitulations or developments of earlier claims by the older investigators and their disciples. Findings, of which the Vogts' and Buscaino's were the most comprehensive, will need further confirmation with careful controls before they can definitely be accepted. Vogt's suggestion, for a total serial investigation of schizophrenic brains and similarly comprehensive cytological study of the cellular elements, has much justification, although it is difficult to achieve in view of the labour involved. Again Scholz (1936), and the Vogts (1937) have recommended the study of individual variability of cerebral architecture in relation to normal and abnormal mental function. This variability, which is apparent not only in cortical architecture but also in subcortical centres, may not be haphazard. If facilities were given for such time-consuming investigations, one might well arrive at interesting correlations between abnormal personality and brain morphology.

A sober appreciation of the situation will have to take into consideration our ignorance of the anatomy and function of many parts of the brain, and in particular of phylogenetically old regions in the brain stem, diencephalon and the so-called 'rhinencephalon'. Much recent research into the cerebral substrate of emotion and emotional expression has concentrated upon the experimental exploration of these regions. Because of its importance, a brief account of this line of research will be given later.

The possibility has, however, to be faced that our present staining methods may not be adequate to demonstrate a structural substrate for the subtle and reversible mental aberrations which underly the 'functional' psychoses. New histochemical and microchemical techniques and the ultramicroscope will play a part of increasing importance. These methods are still in their infancy, and present considerable difficulties of both technique and interpretation.

Biochemical and physiological aspects

In these circumstances it is not surprising that emphasis of research has shifted to the biochemical and physiological aspects of pathology. A considerable volume of work has been carried out on the chemical pathology of the body fluids and on special aspects—glucose tolerance, liver function, hippuric acid synthesis, defective oxygen consumption by the brain and hormones, to mention only a few. Most recent reviewers (Manfred Bleuler 1951 b, Richter 1957, McIlwain 1959, Kety 1961, for example) express a very reserved and often a negative opinion on the primary significance of the claims that have been made. Many of the chemical findings may be attributable to secondary factors, especially prolonged institutionalisation, difficulty of adequate nutrition, etc. (Richter). Fleischhacker (1960), who from long continued investigations, claims a diagnostic significance for a positive glyoxylic acid reaction and for increase of γ-globulins in the serum and CSF of undoubted 'idiopathic' cases, feels unable to consider these findings as specific or to give an adequate explanation for them. Bleuler concludes that, at most, biochemical and physiological findings in schizophrenics, show a wider range and a lesser reactivity to normal stimuli than is found in a normal series. This concept of hypo-reactivity or 'physiological withdrawal' has been fully investigated by Hoskins (1946), although it may apply also to chronic psychoses other than schizophrenia. It may manifest itself, for example, in a greater stability of the rhythm in schizophrenics submitted to stress than is apparent in normal individuals (Hill *et al.* 1951). The latter finding has been interpreted as indicating reduced excitability of the sympathetic-adrenal system. Thus, the problem of hypo-reactivity links up with the adaptation syndrome of Selye (1946), in which the pituitary-adrenal system plays a central role.

The disturbances of nitrogen metabolism in the phases of stupor and excitement of recurrent catatonia (Gjessing 1938) have aroused great interest and have been confirmed by subsequent investigators, but the findings in this rare condition cannot be applied to schizophrenia in general. Gjessing's painstaking work serves, however, as a model for biochemical research in mental patients.

Recent interest has focused on the so-called neurohormones, i.e. acetylcholine, sympathin (adrenaline and noradrenaline), serotonin (5-hydroxytryptamine), substance *P* and γ-aminobutyric acid. Some of these have an interesting relationship to 'hallucinogenic' substances, for example, mescal and lysergic acid. γ-Aminobutyric acid is of special interest to epilepsy and has been discussed on page 610.

Acetylcholine has a characteristic distribution in the C.N.S. which has been studied in detail by Feldberg and Vogt (1948). The enzyme choline acetylase which is essential for its formation was found to be present in significantly greater amounts in motor than in afferent pathways; its amount was particularly high in anterior horns, the motor nuclei of the cranial nerves and the ventral roots, while the pyramidal tract had low values. Its presence in the striate body was more striking than in any other centre. Injection of acetylcholine into the lateral ventricle of experimental animals (cats) produces stupor and catatonia-like postures, and with larger doses generalised convulsions (Feldberg and Sherwood 1955 a, Feldberg 1958). Drugs injected into the lateral ventricle will, according to these authors, easily reach the 3rd and 4th ventricle and there is reason to believe that much of the response is due to an effect on the periventricular grey matter, which would include the hypothalamus. Catatonic stupor was a typical late effect, as one would expect, of intraventricular injection of anti-cholinesterases (eserine, di-isopropylfluorophosphonate (D.F.P.)). In cats Feldberg and Sherwood (1955 b) also observed stupor after intraventricular injection of bulbocapnine which, since De Jong's original observations (reviewed by him in 1945), had been known to cause catatonic symptoms. The effect of intraventricular injection again seems to indicate the action of the drug on the hypothalamus and its immediate anterior and posterior neighbourhood.

Sympathin is found in the dog's brain in greatest amounts in the hypothalamus and in slightly lesser amounts in the tectum of midbrain, pons and medulla (Vogt 1954). This distribution seems approximately to coincide with the arousal areas of the ascending reticular formation. The values obtained from hippocampus, amygdaloid nucleus, anterior cingular region and orbital region did not exceed the low values found in the rest of the cortex: they were high, however, in the dorso-medial and anterior nuclei of the thalamus as well as in the area postrema even though neurones are absent in the latter. The amount of sympathin in the hypothalamus has been found to be reduced after injection of reserpine which is the active principle of Rauwolfia serpentina and which is used as a hypotensive and 'tranquillising' drug (Holzbauer and Vogt 1956). Intraventricular injection of adrenaline produces a condition of impaired consciousness resembling light nembutal anaesthesia (Feldberg and Sherwood 1955 a). Adrenochrome and adrenolutin, both being derivatives of adrenaline, are, according to Hoffer, Osmond and Smythies (1954) 'hallucinogenic' drugs producing in man schizophrenia-like psychoses; recent re-examinations, however, have produced considerable doubt on this claim (Smythies 1960 and others).

Serotonin (5-hydroxytryptamine) has been known to cause constriction of the smooth muscle of the vascular wall. Amin, Crawford and Gaddum (1954), among others, have shown that its distribution in the brain is much the same as that of noradrenaline, i.e. predominating in the hypothalamus and in and near the regions where the reticular formation ascends in the brain stem. Lysergic acid is a potent inhibitor of hydroxytryptamine and from this fact Woolley and Shaw (1954) have suggested that some functional psychoses may be due to deficiency or abnormal metabolism of serotonin, but this has not been confirmed.

For a brief period much interest was centred on the investigation of the level of *copper* and *caerulo-plasmin* in the blood, reported to be increased in schizophrenia (Akerfeldt 1957). It was found, however, that it may be raised also in conditions other than schizophrenia, and may be related to deficiency in ascorbic acid (*vide* Kety 1961).

While the idea that the blood serum, cerebrospinal fluid and urine of schizophrenics may be toxic to experimental animals and human volunteers is not new (Keup 1954), renewed interest in such *taraxeins* has recently followed systematic studies initiated at Tulane University by Heath and his associates (1957, 1958). Despite some encouraging experimental results, however, 'the possibility, remote as it may be, that the reported effects of taraxein are a result of a combination of suggestion, non-specific toxic reaction from ammonium sulphate or other contaminants, and reinforcement of these cues by biases of subject and observer . . . is one which has not been ruled out' (Kety). It is noteworthy that in his review on these recent biochemical developments, Kety has come to conclusions which, in their cautious yet constructive appraisal of the situation, much resemble those expressed earlier by Spielmeyer on the morphological aspects. Only a sizeable minority of workers will regard these—so far—disappointing results as indicating that schizophrenia and the other functional psychoses are purely psychogenic in origin. The majority, while not neglecting the importance of psychological and psychosocial factors, will continue their patient search for an organic, probably chemical substrate.

The cerebral substrate of emotion and emotional expression

While the search for a substrate for the so-called functional psychoses has not yet led to unequivocal success, it has nevertheless stimulated clinico-pathological and experimental research into those parts of the brain which appear to be involved in the elaboration of emotion and emotional expression. It is going too far to speak of *localisation* of emotion in the brain; for example, Freeman and Watts (1947) at one time pronounced the thalamus as the seat of emotion. Modern thought is inclined to conceive of the function of the brain, and indeed of the organism and its environment, as a whole; and the most that may be attributed to individual parts of the brain is to specialising more than other parts in a particular function (Critchley 1953). In this sense one may be justified in saying that the organic dementias are caused mainly by disease or destruction of the cerebral cortex. As far as the emotional processes are concerned, attention has been focused among others on the prefrontal region, the diencephalon (thalamus, hypothalamus and its vicinity) and the rhinencephalon and their connections. It is with these centres that the following remarks are principally concerned.

The frontal lobe syndrome. The history of this syndrome has been exhaustively treated by Rylander (1939), Freeman and Watts (1950), Fulton (1951) and Denny-Brown (1951), and, as regards the anatomical aspects of leucotomy and related operations by Meyer and Beck (1954). There is now general agreement that, in man, bilateral frontal lesions cause flattening of emotional depth, loss of higher sublimations in the social, aesthetic and ethical spheres and that these characteristics are associated with hyperactivity or apathy, euphoria or depression. Perhaps the most satisfactory definition, so far, is that of Freeman and Watts, who consider the prefrontal region to be concerned with consciousness of the self and its projection into the future, and their view is in general agreement with the physiological analysis of Denny-Brown. The frontal region seems necessary for such general functions as attention, learning, imagination and phantasy. If sufficient substance of the prefrontal region is destroyed the general attitude towards the future is lost; the patient becomes a victim of concrete stimuli, loses his initiative and becomes shallow in his emotional reactions. Bilateral lesion of the frontal lobe will, therefore, not only blunt the emotional sphere but lead to (perhaps secondary) impairment of intellectual performance although memory is unimpaired and there is no dementia in the accepted sense.

Similar changes have been described in primates. The prefrontal lobectomies carried out by Jacobsen (1935), under Fulton's direction, are particularly well known. A film demonstrating behaviour changes in these animals, which was shown at the Second International Neurological Congress in London in 1935, was attended by Egaz Moniz, who had been planning the operation of prefrontal leucotomy for some time and performed the first prefrontal leucotomy only a few months later. Since then, observations made on mental patients submitted to neurosurgical treatment have become a new and important source of information on the frontal lobes. The original 'blind' leucotomies (Fig. 12.1) have been partially superseded by more selective operations, usually carried out under vision and designed to ablate or undercut circumscribed areas of the frontal region.

Kleist (1931, 1937) has assigned separate function to almost every architectonic area: initiative to area 9; motor skill to area 10; constructive thought to area 46; sentiment to area 47; 'social' ego to area 11 and 'visceral' ego to area 24 of Brodman. Although Kleist's chart has not been generally accepted, there is little doubt that his views have had considerable influence on the recent concept of the 'visceral brain'. Moreover, most workers in the field (Freeman and Watts, Scoville 1949, Le Beau 1954 and Meyer and Beck 1954) accept a difference in symptomatology at least between orbital and convexity lesions, although the nature of this difference is still controversial. The most posterior agranular parts of the orbital cortex, including area 13 of Walker (1940), seem to be rather more concerned with autonomic function than the rest of the orbital cortex.

Spatz (1937) has introduced the concept of the basal neocortex to designate those parts of the frontal and temporal neocortex, recognisable by view from below. These parts are most markedly developed in the adult human brain, to a lesser degree in non-human primates, and may be entirely missing in lower mammals, for example in the hedgehog. In early hominides (for example, homo rhodensiensis), the basal neocortex is relatively little developed as far as one can judge from endocranial casts of their skulls. These comparative facts, together with experiences in pathological brains, led Spatz to the view that the basal cortex is concerned with specific human mental activities (Spatz 1955).

Much experimental work, as well as anatomical study in the human brain after prefrontal leucotomy and other frontal lesions, has been done on the connections of the frontal lobes. The results of this work demonstrate the intimate relation of both the prefrontal and cingular cortex with the diencephalic region: Le Gros Clark (1948) is inclined to regard the frontal region as the projection area of the hypothalamus. The afferent pathways arising from the dorsomedial nucleus and anterior nucleus of the thalamus to the prefrontal and cingular region respectively are extensive and highly organised: their severance results in retrograde degeneration which is easily demonstrated in Nissl stained sections, even on naked-eye inspection (Figs. 12.2 and 12.3).

The diencephalic syndromes. In the last decades extensive anatomical and physiological work has been carried out on the hypothalamus by many workers including Hess (for references *vide* 1954), Le Gros Clark (1938), Ranson and Magoun (1939), Bard (1928), the Scharrers (1945). Its rôle as autonomic 'headganglion,' as a centre for the control of consciousness and the sleep-waking rhythm, and of the metabolism of water, protein, carbohydrate and fat has been established. It exercises neural control also over the pituitary and thus indirectly over the whole endocrine system (Harris 1955). Recently the hypothalamus has to a large extent been incorporated into the wider system of the ascending reticular formation or diffuse thalamic system first described by Jasper (1949) and subsequently elaborated by Magoun (1952). At present this is still mainly an electrophysiological concept, whose anatomical basis is not yet fully established, but is assumed to depend on the medially situated groups of the reticular cells in the medulla, pons, midbrain and hypothalamus, on so far unestablished cell groups and fibre connections within the subthalamus, and on the intralaminary (including the centromedian) and the reticular nuclei of the thalamus. How impulses conveyed in this system reach the cerebral cortex is not yet definitely known. What is known is that electrical stimulation along this route influences cortical electrical activity and this influence is exercised over the whole cerebral cortex, although usually beginning in the frontal region. Stimulation of the caudal part of the reticular system up to the hypothalamus produces activation or the arousal reaction, while stimulation of the intralaminary region in the thalamus has a recruiting effect on sleep spindles.

The significance of the hypothalamus, the medially situated nuclei of the thalamus and the ascending reticular formation for autonomic activity is underlined by the high content of this whole region in several neurohormones, including adrenaline and noradrenaline.

In the light of this physiological background, it is not surprising that experimental lesions and disease in this region should give rise to psychopathological reactions. Bard in 1928 produced what he called sham rage reaction in cats by ablation of the neocortex and the cranial half of the hypothalamus including, possibly, the most ventral and caudal portion of the corre-

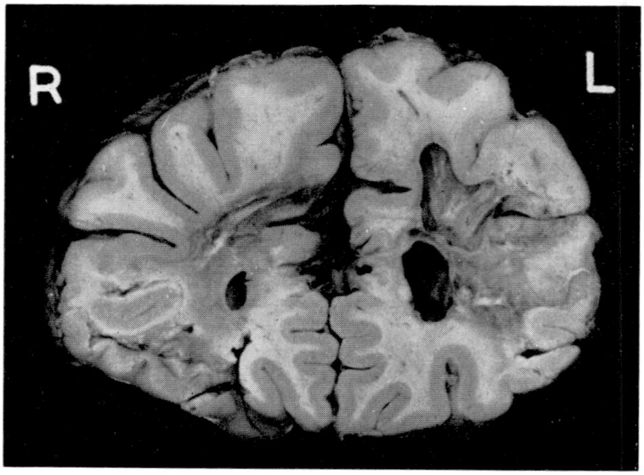

12.1

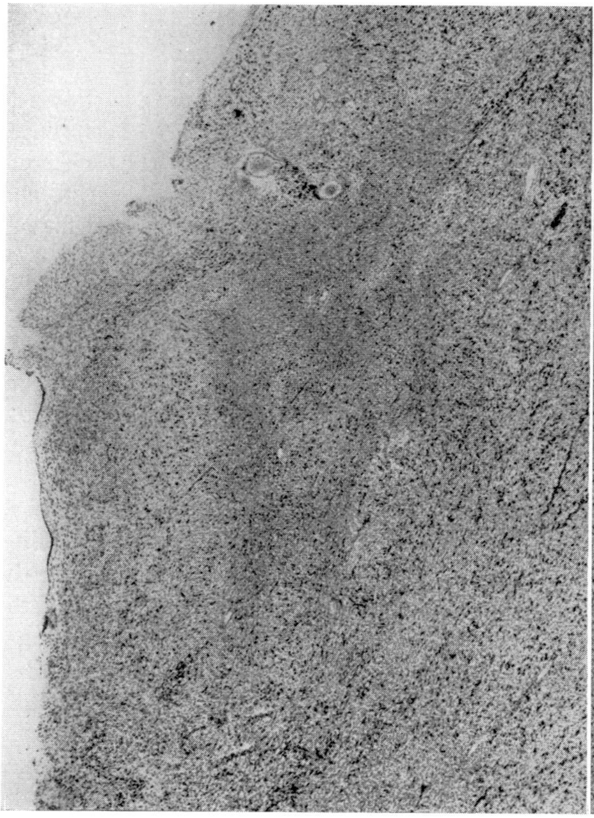

12.2

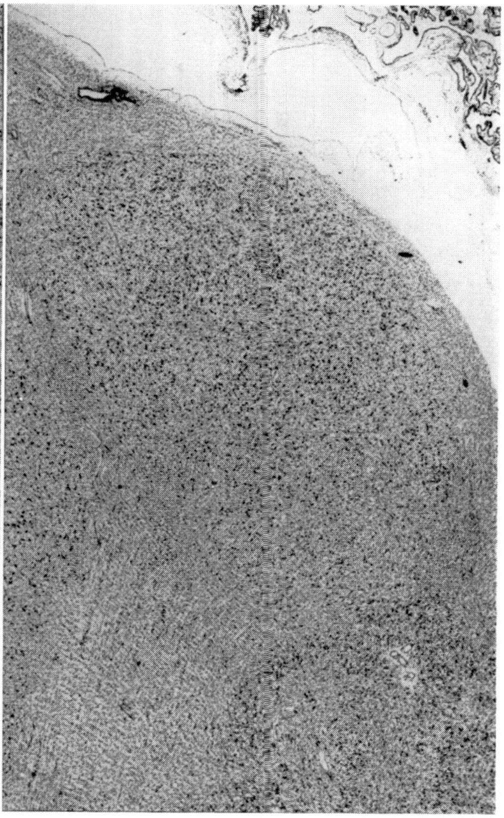

12.3

FIG. 12.1. Fairly full and symmetrical prefrontal leucotomy lesion.
FIG. 12.2. Retrograde degeneration and gliosis in the lateral aspects of the dorsomedial nucleus of the thalamus. (Nissl × 15.)
FIG. 12.3. Retrograde degeneration in ventral half of anterior nucleus of thalamus. (Nissl × 15.)

sponding segment of the thalamus. These experiments have been confirmed by Fulton and Ingraham (1929) and Ranson and Magoun, who concluded that it was the isolation and stimulation of a mechanism located in the posterior part of the lateral hypothalamus which was responsible for the rage reaction. Since then it has been found that a bilateral lesion of the ventromedial nucleus produces rage reactions in monkeys (Wheatley 1944). Rage has resulted also from experimental bilateral lesions of the amygdaloid complex of, at least, cats (Bard and Mountcastle 1948) and of the olfactory tubercles (Spiegel, Miller and Oppenheimer 1940). There has been much discussion as to whether hypothalamic rage is associated with true feeling or is only a sign of disturbed emotional expression. Present opinion supports Masserman's (1942) contention that the hypothalamus is to be regarded as an effector organ of emotional expression.

Mania-like syndromes have been reported in human cases of hypothalamic lesion. In most of these the lesion was a tumour or cyst and precise localisation was difficult. Meyer (1944) reported a manic syndrome in a case of atypical Wernicke syndrome in which the lesion was predominantly in the chiasmatic part of the hypothalamus, leaving the mamillary bodies and the posterior hypothalamic nucleus intact.

Lesions in the *posterior* hypothalamic nucleus and the region of the mamillary nucleus result in hypersomnia and disturbances of consciousness, phenomena well known through experience of epidemic encephalitis, the Wernicke syndrome, etc. The occurrence of akinetic mutism or stupor has aroused special interest. In the case of Oldfield, Cairns, Pennybacker and Whitteridge (1941) a precise localisation was not possible, since the lesion was a cyst of the 3rd ventricle. Jefferson (1944), however, has described 2 cases of traumatic stupor, in which the anterior hypothalamus was found intact. Disturbance of consciousness in cases showing post-mortem lesions in the brain stem has also been reported by Cairns (1952), M. Jefferson (1952) and Brain (1958). The last-mentioned author has reviewed the physiological problems of consciousness and sleep, especially in relation to recent work on the ascending reticular formation. According to Brain, conscious sensory perception is a complex process in which cerebral cortex, reticular formation and the sensory inflow all appear to be involved. The relationship between diencephalic and cortical function is not so much that of a hierarchy as of an integrative unity.

The concept of the visceral brain. Hypothalamus and thalamus are anatomically connected with another system of centres: the cingular (limbic) gyrus, amygdaloid nucleus, the hippocampus and its rostral uncal formation. These centres form a sort of circuit. From the mamillary body arises the tract of Vicq d'Azyr to the anterior thalamic nucleus which in turn relays to the cingular gyrus. This, then, sends fibres via the fasciculus cinguli to the vicinity of the hippocampus from which the fornix reconnects with the mamillary body (and the septal nuclei). There is also an important afferent connection from the septal nuclei to the hippocampus. The amygdaloid nucleus connects via the stria terminalis with not yet definitely established nuclei of the anterior hypothalamic and, possibly, septal region. Evidence has been accumulating that all these centres are also electrophysiologically well interconnected (Kaada 1951). They are considered to be part of the rhinencephalon, but there is now considerable evidence that, although they have developed in close proximity to the olfactory system, most of them have little to do with (at least direct) olfactory function. In experimental animals and, as far as experience goes, in the human, lesions in most of these centres lead to changes in emotional behaviour either in the direction of rage or of tameness. Papez (1937), in his 'proposed mechanism of emotion' linked mamillary body, anterior nuclei of the thalamus and the anterior cingular region with the hippocampus. This functional linkage has been developed by MacLean (1949) and his collaborators Kaada and Pribram in Fulton's laboratory into the wider concept of the 'visceral brain' to include, besides hypothalamic and thalamic nuclei, the cingular region, the posterior orbital cortex, the temporal pole, insula, amygdala, uncus and hippocampus.

It is not possible to give a full account of the wealth of experimental data accumulated on this subject during the last few years. The interested reader will find a full critical evaluation in the reviews by Pribram and Kruger (1954), MacLean (1958) and Adey (1959). The relation of this region to sexual function has been especially studied, among others, by Olds (1958) and Maclean and Ploog (1962). Obviously the whole problem is still in considerable flux. Pribram and Kruger have expressed doubts about the uniformity of function in this system. They also criticise the term 'visceral' brain which, they consider, may give rise to the erroneous impression that control of autonomic acitivity and of emotion is its exclusive function.

Almost certainly the function of the rhinencephalic centres in the temporal region seems to differ from the more anterior parts of which the activity is similar to that of the frontal lobe. In monkeys, Klüver and Bucy (1939) described the appearance of visual agnosia, oral tendencies and hypersexuality together with greater tameness after bilateral temporal lobectomy, provided that it included the hippocampus and amygdaloid complex. The inability of the ablated monkeys to discriminate visually, may well have been due to loss of memory. In Maclean's definition memories, feelings and actions, in relation to the oral senses and to the sexual sphere, are the concern of what he calls the fronto-temporal aspect of the visceral brain. In Grünthal's (1947) case, bilateral Ammon's horn sclerosis was the only morphological abnormality in an elderly patient who became demented after hypoglycaemic coma; this author, in a more recent publication (1959), regards the mental change in this patient as a modified Klüver-Bucy syndrome. Reviewing 23 cases (which included several new observations of his own), he found that of 15 cases with bilateral Ammon's horn loss, a modified 'Klüver-Bucy' syndrome developed in 3, while the remaining 12 showed a Korsakoff syndrome. In 8 cases with only unilateral Ammon's horn loss, disturbances of recent memory, when present, were slight and transient. Defect of recent memory was the main change observed by Scoville and Milner (1957), after bilateral removal of the hippocampal gyrus, including Ammon's horn, uncus and amygdaloid nucleus. In view of the recent emphasis on memory function, it is of historical interest that, as early as the second decade of the nineteenth century, G. R. Treviranus (who, according to Neubürger (1897), was an active member of the German school of 'natural philosophers' and also the first to introduce the term 'Biologie'), associated Ammon's horn with memory function, because he was impressed by the importance of smell in evoking past events.

While a cautionary attitude must thus at present be maintained, there is no doubt that this whole sphere of exploration is of considerable potential importance to the understanding of mental function and indirectly to the pathology of the 'functional' psychoses.

REFERENCES

Adey, W. R. (1959) *Int. Rev. Neurobiol.*, **1**, 1.

Akerfeldt, S. (1957) *Science*, **125**, 117.

Alzheimer, A. (1897) *Mschr. Psychiat. Neurol.*, **2**, 82; (1913) *Z. ges. Neurol. Psychiat.* (Referate, etc.), **7**, 621.

Amin, A. H., Crawford, T. B. B. and Gaddum, J. H. (1954) *J. Physiol.*, **126**, 596.

Baldwin, M., Lewis, S. A. and Bach, S. A. (1959) *Neurology*, **9**, 469.

Bard, P. (1928) *Amer. J. Physiol.*, **84**, 490.

Bard, P. and Mountcastle, V. B. (1948) *Proc. Ass. Res. nerv. ment. Dis.*, **27**, 362.

Bäumer, H. (1952) *1st Int. Congr. Neuropath.*, **3**, 636.

Beard, A. W. and Slater, E. (1962) *Proc. Roy. Soc. Med.*, **55**, 311.

Beheim-Schwarzbach, D. (1952) *1st Int. Congr. Neuropath.*, **3**, 609.
Bini, L. and Marchiafava, G. (1952) *1st Int. Congr. Neuropath.*, **1**, 670.
Blair, J. H., Sniffen, R. C., Cranswick, R. H., Jaffe, W. and Kilme, N. S. (1952) *J. ment. Sci.*, **98**, 464.
Bleuler, M. (1951 a) *Brit. Med. J.* (ii), 1233; (1951 b) *Fortschr. Neurol. Psychiat.*, **19**, 385.
Bolsi, D. (1952) *1st Int. Congr. Neuropath.*, **1**, 533.
Brain, W. R. (1958) *Brain*, **81**, 426.
Braitenberg, V. (1952) *1st Int. Congr. Neuropath.*, **3**, 621.
Broser, K. (1949) *Arch. Psychiat. Nervenkr.*, **182**, 439.
Bruetsch, W. L. (1952) *1st Int. Congr. Neuropath.*, **1**, 486.
Buscaino, V. M. (1920/21) *Riv. pat. nerv. ment.*, **25**, 197. (1952) *1st Int. Congr. Neuropath.*, **1**, 548.
Cairns, H. (1952) *Brain*, **75**, 109.
Clark, W. E. Le Gros. (1938) in *The Hypothalamus*, Oliver & Boyd, Edinburgh; (1948) *Lancet* (i), 353.
Critchley, M. (1953) *The Parietal Lobes*, Edward Arnold, London.
Dastur, D. K. (1959) *A.M.A. Arch. Neurol. Psychiat.*, **81**, 601.
David, G. B. (1957) in *Schizophrenia: Somatic Aspects*, edited by Richter, D., London.
Denny-Brown, D. J. (1951) *Modern Trends in Neurology*, edited by A. Feiling, Butterworth, London.
de Jong, H. H. (1945) *Experimental Catatonia*, Williams and Wilkins.
de Vries, E. (1952) *1st Int. Congr. Neuropath.*, **1**, 579.
Donovan, J. F., Galbraith, A. J. and Jackson, H. (1949) *J. ment. Sci.*, **95**, 655.
Dunlap, C. B. (1928) *Proc. Ass. Res. nerv. ment. Dis.*, **5**, 371.
Elvidge, A. R. and Reed, G. E. (1938) *Arch. Neurol. Psychiat.* (Chicago), **40**, 227.
Feldberg, W. S. (1958) *Proc. Ass. Res. nerv. ment. Dis.*, **36**, 401.
Feldberg, W. and Sherwood, S. L. (1955 a) *Proc. R. Soc. Med.*, **48**, 853; (1955 b) *Brit. J. Pharmacol.*, **10**, 371.
Feldberg, W. and Vogt, M. (1948) *J. Physiol.*, **107**, 372.
Ferraro, A. (1943) *J. Neuropath.*, **2**, 84; (1952) *1st Int. Congr. Neuropath.*, **1**, 217.
Feuchtwanger, E. and Mayer-Gross, W. (1938) *Schweiz. Arch. Neurol. Psychiat.*, **41**, 17.
Fleischhacker, H. H. (1960) *Arch. Psychiat. Z. ges. Neurol.*, **201**, 1.
Freeman, W. and Watts, J. W. (1947) *J. comp. Neurol.*, **86**, 65; (1950) *Psychosurgery in the Treatment of Mental Disorders and Intractable Pains*, Blackwell, Oxford.
Fulton, J. F. (1951) *Frontal Lobotomy and Affective Behaviour*, Chapman & Hall, London.
Fulton, J. F. and Ingraham, F. D. (1929) *Amer. J. Physiol.*, **90**, 353.
Fünfgeld, E. W. (1952) *1st Int. Congr. Neuropath.*, **3**, 648.
Gjessing, R. (1938) *J. ment. Sci.*, **84**, 608.
Grünthal, E. (1947) *Mschr. Psychiat. Neurol.*, **113**, 1. (1959) *Psychiatria et Neurologia* (Basel), **138**, 145.
Harris, G. W. (1955) *Neural Control of the Pituitary Gland*, Edward Arnold, London.
Hauptmann, A. (1946) *Arch. Neurol. Psychiat.* (Chicago), **56**, 631.
Hauptmann, A. and Myerson, A. (1948) *J. nerv. ment. Dis.*, **108**, 91.
Heath, R. G., Martens, S., Leach, B. E., Cohen, M. and Angel, C. (1957) *Amer. J. Psychiat.*, **114**, 14.
Heath, R. G., Martens, S., Leach, B. E., Cohen, M. and Feigley, C. A. (1958), ibid., 917.
Hemphill, R. E., Reiss, M. and Taylor, A. L. (1944) *J. ment. Sci.*, **90**, 681.
Hess, W. R. (1954) *Diencephalon: Autonomic and Extrapyramidal Function*, William Heinemann, London.
Heyck, H. (1954) *Mschr. Psychiat. Neurol.*, **128**, 106.
Hill, D., Loe, P. St. J., Theobald, J. and Waddell, M. (1951) *J. ment. Sci.*, **97**, 111.
Hillbom, E. (1951) *Acta psychiat. scand. Suppl.*, **60**, 36.
Hoffer, A., Osmond, H. and Smythies, J. (1954) *J. ment. Sci.*, **100**, 29.
Holzbauer, M. and Vogt, M. (1956) *J. Neurochem.*, **1**, 8.
Hopf, A. (1952) *1st Int. Congr. Neuropath.*, **3**, 627.
Hoskins, R. G. (1946) *The Biology of Schizophrenia*, W. W. Norton, New York.
Huber, G. (1953) *Arch. Psychiat. Nervenkr.*, **190**, 429.
Hydén, H. and Hartelius, H. (1948) *Acta psychiat.*, Kbh., **58**, 1.
Jacobsen, C. F. (1935) *Arch. Neurol. Psychiat.* (Chicago), **33**, 558.
Jaensch, W. (1930) *Z. ärztl. Fortbild.*, **27**, 323.
Jasper, H. (1949) *Electroenceph. clin. Neurophysiol.*, **1**, 405.
Jefferson, G. (1944) *Brit. med. J.* (i), 1.
Jefferson, M. (1952) *Brain*, **75**, 55.

Josephy, H. (1923) *Z. ges. Neurol. Psychiat.*, **86**, 391.
Kaada, B. R. (1951) *Acta. physiol. scand.*, **23**, suppt. 83.
Kety, S. S. (1961) in *Chemical Pathology of the Nervous System*, edited by Folch-Pi, J., New York, London.
Keup, W. (1954) *Mschr. Psychiat. Neurol.*, **128**, 56.
Kirschbaum, W. R. and Heilbrunn, G. (1944) *Arch. Neurol. Psychiat.* (Chicago), **51**, 155.
Kleist, K. (1931) *Z. ges. Neurol. Psychiat.*, **131**, 442; (1937) ibid., **158**, 159.
Klippel, M. and Lhermitte, J. (1909) *Rev. Neurol.*, **17**, 157.
Klüver, H. and Bucy, P. C. (1939) *Arch. Neurol. Psychiat.* (Chicago), **42**, 979.
Le Beau, J. (1954) *Psycho-chirurgie et fonctions mentales*, Masson, Paris.
Lewis, N. D. C. (1923) *The Constitutional Factors in Dementia Precox*, Nervous and Mental Disease Publishing Company, New York and Washington.
Lewis, T. (1927) *The Blood Vessels of the Human Skin and their Responses*, Shaw & Sons, London.
Lhermitte, J., Marchand, L. and Guiraud, P. (1952) *1st Int. Congr. Neuropath.*, **1**, 465.
Lombard, W. P. (1911) *Zbl. Physiol.*, **25**, 157.
Longo, V. (1952) *1st Int. Congr. Neuropath.*, **1**, 584.
Lovett Doust, J. W. (1950) in *Recent Progress in Psychiatry*, **II**, edited by G. W. T. H. Fleming, Churchill, London; (1955) *J. nerv. ment. Dis.*, **121**, 516.
MacLean, P. (1949) *Psychosom. Med.*, **11**, 338. (1958) *J. Nerv. Ment. Dis.*, **127**, 1.
MacLean, P. D. and Ploog, D. W. (1962) *J. Neurophysiol.*, **25**, 29.
McIlwain, H. (1959) *Biochemistry and the Central Nervous System* (1st edition 1955), London.
Magoun, H. W. (1952) in *The Biology of Mental Health and Disease*, Hoeber, New York.
Masserman, J. H. (1942) *Amer. J. Psychiat.*, **98**, 633.
Meschan, I. and Scruggs, J. B. (1951) *Arch. Neurol. Psychiat.* (Chicago), **65**, 60.
Messimy, R., Berdeth, H., Feld, M., Geuyer, G. and Petit-Dutaillis, D. (1951) *Rev. neurol.*, **84**, 230.
Meyer, A. (1944) *J. Neurol. Psychiat.*, **7**, 66; (1952) *1st Int. Congr. Neuropath.*, **1**, 649.
Meyer, A. and Beck, E. (1954) *Prefrontal Leucotomy and Related Operations: Anatomical Aspects of Success and Failure*, Oliver & Boyd, Edinburgh.
Meyer, A. and Meyer, M. (1949) *J. ment. Sci.*, **95**, 180.
Meyer, A. and McLardy, T. (1950) in *Recent Progress in Psychiatry*, **II**, edited by G. W. T. H. Fleming, Churchill, London.
Mott, F. W. (1922a) *J. Ment. Sci.*, **68**, 333. (1922b) *Brit. Med. J.* (i), 463.
Neubürger, K. T. (1897) *Die historische Entwicklung der Experimentellen Gehirn-und Rückenmarksphysiologie vor Flourens*, Stuttgart.
Oldfield, R. C., Cairns, H., Pennybacker, J. R. and Whitteridge, D. (1941) *Brain*, **64**, 273.
Olds, J. (1958) in *Neurological Basis of Behaviour* (Ciba Foundation Sympos.) edited by Wolstenholme, G. E. W. and O'Connor, C. M., London.
Olkon, D. M. (1939) *Arch. Neurol. Psychiat.* (Chicago), **42**, 652; (1945) *Essentials of Neuropsychiatry*, Henry Kimpton, London.
Palma, E. C. and Sotelo, J. R. (1952) *1st Int. Congr. Neuropath.*, **1**, 637.
Papez, J. W. (1937) *Arch. Neurol. Psychiat.* (Chicago), **38**, 725.
Parrisius, W. (1921) *Dtsch. Z. Nervenheilk.*, **72**, 310.
Peters, G. (1937) *Z. ges. Neurol. Psychiat.*, **160**, 361; (1956) *Dementia Praecox and Manisch-Depressives Irresein* in *Handb. Speciell. Pathol. Anat. Histol.*, 13/4 Berlin.
Pool, J. L. (1949) *Lancet* (ii), 776.
Pribram, K. H. and Kruger, H. (1954) *Ann. N. Y. Acad. Sci.*, **58**, 109.
Puech, P. (1949) *Presse méd.*, **57**, 115.
Ranson, S. W. and Magoun, H. W. (1939) *Ergebn. Physiol.*, **41**, 56.
Richter, D. (1957) in *Schizophrenia: Somatic Aspects*, edited by Richter, D., London.
Rylander, G. (1939) *Personality Changes after Operation on the Frontal Lobe*, Einar Munksgaard, Humphrey Milford, Copenhagen and London.
Scharrer, E. and Scharrer, B. (1945) *Physiol. Rev.*, **25**, 171.
Scheidegger, S. (1952) *1st Int. Congr. Neuropath.*, **1**, 603.
Scholz, W. (1936) *Allg. Z. Psychiat.*, **105**, 64.
Scoville, W. B. (1949) *J. Neurosurg.*, **6**, 65.
Scoville, W. B. and Milner, B. (1957) *J. Neurol. Neurosurg. Psychiat.*, **20**, 11.
Selye, H. (1946) *J. clin. Endocrin.*, **6**, 117.
Shattock, F. M. (1950 a) *J. ment. Sci.*, **96**, 32; (1950 b) *Proc. R. Soc. Med.*, **43**, 625

Smythies, J. R. (1960) *Lancet* (i), 1287.
Spatz, H. (1955) Nachr. Giessen, Hochsch. Gesellsch., **24**, 52; (1937) *Z. ges Neurol. Psychiat.*, **158**, 208.
Spiegel, E. A., Miller H. R. and Oppenheimer, M. J. (1940) *J. Neurophysiol.*, **3**, 538.
Spielmeyer, W. (1930) *J. nerv. ment. Dis.*, **72**, 241.
Symonds, C. P. (1960) *Brit. med. J.* (ii), 1.
Van der Horst, L. (1952) 1st *Int. Congr. Neuropath.*, **1**, 670.
Vogt, C. and O. (1922) *J. Psychol. Neurol.* (*Lpz.*), **28**. (1937) *Sitz und Wesen der Krankheiten im Lichte der topistischen Hirnforschung*, Part I, Ambrose Barth, Leipzig; (1949) *Ärztl. Forsch.*, **4**, 141; (1952) 1st *Int. Congr. Neuropath.*, **1**, 515.
Vogt, M. (1954) *J. Physiol.*, **123**, 451.
Wahren, W. (1952) 1st *Int. Congr. Neuropath.*, **3**, 660.
Walker, A. E. (1940) *J. comp. Neurol.*, **73**, 59.
Wertham, F. and Wertham, F. L. (1934) *The Brain as an Organ*, Macmillan, New York.
Wheatley, M. D. (1944) *Arch. Neurol. Psychiat.* (Chicago), **52**, 296.
Winkelman, N. W. and Book, M. H. (1949) *Amer. J. Psychiat.*, **105**, 889.
Wolf, A. and Cowen, D. (1952) in *The Biology of Mental Health and Disease*, Hoeber, New York.
Woolley, D. W. and Shaw, E. (1954) *Brit. Med. J.* (ii), 122.

CHAPTER 13

DISEASES OF THE LOWER MOTOR AND SENSORY NEURONES
(OF UNCERTAIN PATHOGENESIS)

By J. G. Greenfield

Diseases which were originally thought to affect wholly or predominantly the lower motor and/or sensory neurones have been classified in various ways by various authors following the historical pattern of dividing 'peripheral neuritis' first on a clinical, then on a histological and lastly on an aetiological basis. Limited advances, first in one direction then in another, have led to many classifications, none of which was entirely satisfactory. Often one group would be separated from the rest on the basis of symptoms and signs (mononeuritis multiplex); another on what is known or thought to be the histological basis (parenchymatous neuropathy): and another upon aetiological factors (ischaemic neuropathy or traumatic neuropathy or metabolic disorders of nerve). The main groups, and sometimes even the subgroups in such a classification, have had varying bases for their differentiation and were therefore not mutually exclusive. Such a classification is a mixed classification and leads in pathology to confusion, as Cathcart pointed out in 1896.

Recent advances in microscopical and biochemical techniques and knowledge are at present adding so much to our small amount of knowledge of the pathology of neuropathies that it is considered unwise, even if it were possible, to attempt to produce another classification. Instead, where the pathology of a particular neuropathy is known with some degree of certainty, it is not discussed in this chapter, but elsewhere in the book in its appropriate chapter. Those which remain have been divided anatomically into (1) *parenchymatous* and (2) *interstitial* groups, depending on whether the evidence suggests that the process is chiefly one of disturbance of (1) the bodies of the nerve cells in the cord or posterior nerve root ganglia and their axons, particularly the peripheral parts of their axons, or segmental demyelination of the axons in part of their course, or (2) the interstital connective tissue and blood vessels.

PARENCHYMATOUS NEUROPATHY

Peroneal atrophy. (*Charcot-Marie-Tooth type of neuropathy*)

Charcot and Marie (1886) and Tooth in the same year collected 39 cases from personal observations and reports in the literature of a slowly progressive, often familial, type of amyotrophy which usually began in the anterior muscles of the lower leg. Later the calf muscles, the lower third of the thigh and the small muscles of the hands became atrophied. As the peroneal group was usually the first to be affected Tooth named the disease the *peroneal type of progressive muscular atrophy*. In common parlance this is shortened to *peroneal atrophy*, but it must be recognised that atrophy never remains limited to the peroneal muscles. The onset of the disease is usually in the first or second decade, but in some families it has been considerably later. When it begins before the age of 10 years the disease is transmitted as a recessive, sometimes sex-linked as in Herringham's (1888) large family. More often it has appeared as a dominant. Although atrophy and weakness are the most prominent symptoms throughout the disease its onset may be heralded by pains in the legs and there is usually some sensory loss to touch and position. There is little ataxia except in the Roussy-Levy type of case.

At the time of the descriptions by Charcot and Marie and Tooth post-mortems had been made by Virchow (1855), Oppenheimer and Friedreich (1873). In two of these there was degeneration of the dorsal columns of the cord, but in the other two the spinal cord appeared normal. The peripheral nerves showed an excess of interstitial connective tissue. From these reports the disease was recognised as a form of peripheral neuropathy. Owing to its slowly progressive character and long duration few post-mortem examinations have been made and its pathogenesis has not yet been established. Its strongly familial character and its association in some families with mild degrees of Friedreich's ataxia (the Roussy-Levy syndrome) place it among the abiotrophies.

The few more recent post-mortem examinations which have been made add little to the original descriptions by Virchow and Friedreich. There is some loss of fibres in the peripheral nerves especially in the muscular branches, but many fibres, especially those of finer diameter, are preserved. Both in the medium and fine branches there is some excess of interstitial connective tissue which may well be secondary to the degeneration of nerve fibres. It is scarcely evident in the larger nerves of the limbs. Degeneration of the dorsal columns is associated with loss of neurones in the dorsal root ganglia. In many cases it is limited to the fasciculus gracilis, and in some cases no tract degeneration can be seen. The ventral horn cells in the lumbo-sacral enlargement may be smaller than normal though not much reduced in number (Marinesco 1894) or there may be considerable loss of these cells (Sainton 1899), but without comparative cell counts this may be difficult to establish.

Most observers have found in the muscles only the changes of neurogenic atrophy, but Brodal *et al.* (1953) found also evidence of sarcoplasmic degeneration. These changes, which were seen in fibres of all sizes, consisted of granular degeneration, cloudy swelling, fragmentation and cleavage. They seemed to be related to the intensity of the disease. Changes were also seen in the muscle spindles but these did not differ from those of neurogenic atrophy.

Hereditary sensory radicular neuropathy

Under this title Denny-Brown (1951) described the findings in the post-mortem examination of a member of a family which Hicks (1922) had reported from the clinical side. Of 34 members in four generations 11 suffered from perforating ulcers on the feet, shooting pains about the body and deafness. English and Continental literature contains clinical records of several similar families and a large family, in which 26 members in four generations were affected, was reported from Australia by Jackson (1949). He adopted the diagnosis of *familial lumbosacral syringomyelia* which has been that most commonly made, but for this there has been no pathological confirmation (Jughenn *et al.* 1949). Other suggested diagnoses have been leprosy, tabes dorsalis and polyneuritis.

In Hicks' family the age of onset was usually in the third or fourth decade but cases beginning in the second decade were reported by him and were common in Jackson's and other families. The first symptom was usually the appearance of ulcers on the pressure-bearing areas of the feet. In Jackson's and van Bogaert's (1953) families these were preceded or immediately followed by absorption and necrosis of the heads of the metatarsal bones with the extrusion of sequestra through the ulcers and gross deformity of the feet. These symptoms were found to be associated with loss of sensibility to temperature and pain in the feet and later in the lower parts of the legs. Touch was only slightly impaired in the earlier stages in all cases, and at the time of examination most authors found considerable dissociation of sensory loss. It was less evident in Denny-Brown's case. A similar analgesia and thermanaesthesia often spread to the hands and fore-arms after a few months or years, and ulcers might develop on the fingers. The tendon reflexes, especially those in the legs, were lost. There was no thickening of the peripheral nerves. Deafness appears to have been a symptom only in the families reported by Hicks and Denny-Brown, and by Blackwood (1952). It is probable that certain familial cases of congenital indifference to pain, resulting in ulceration and destruction of the toes and fingers, are related to this disease.

Pathology. In the case reported by Denny-Brown the most obvious lesion was degeneration and disappearance of many of the nerve cells in the dorsal root ganglia. This was most marked in the lower lumbar and upper sacral ganglia but was also severe in the 8th cervical and 1st thoracic ganglia. The dorsal roots of the cauda equina were grey and atrophic and the peripheral nerves thinner than normal. In the affected ganglia many neurones showed proliferation of capsule cells and some were represented by clumps of spindle-shaped nuclei. In the most severely affected ganglia very few nerve cells remained and subcapsular dendritic outgrowths or convolutions of the axon were very common. In these ganglia hyaline bodies containing pale distorted nuclei were seen between the surviving neurones just under the capsule of the ganglion. Some of them seemed to be formed in relation to the walls of capillaries. The hyaline material stained variably with Congo Red but gave no other reaction for amyloid, and no amyloid infiltration was found in the organs of the body cavity. An occasional ganglion cell showed a small accumulation of similar material under its capsule. The dorsal roots had lost many of their myelinated fibres and degeneration was also present in the dorsal columns of the spinal cord. In the lumbar segments this was greatest in Flechsig's posterior root zone and it could be traced in the fasciculus gracilis up to the medulla. The ventral roots were intact. Examination of the acoustic nerve and petrous temporal bone showed a marked reduction in the number of cells in Scarpa's ganglion and degenerative changes and cell loss also in the cells of the spiral ganglion. The cochlear nerve was, however, fairly well myelinated.

In Blackwood's case, Hallpike found severe degeneration of the peripheral sensory ganglia of the cochlear and vestibular nerves. In addition to a degeneration in the dorsal columns of similar distribution to that found by Denny-Brown (Fig. 13.1b), there was also extensive loss of Purkinje cells in the cerebellar cortex associated with a loss of neurones, of at least equal severity, in the inferior olives.

In van Bogaert's case hyaline material giving no reactions for amyloid was present under the capsule of the affected dorsal root ganglia and in the walls of the vessels of the ganglia and dorsal roots. It also ensheathed the nerve fibres in the cauda equina and lay between the pia mater and the parenchymatous tissue of the spinal cord. In the latter situation it was associated with lymphocytic infiltration. The lesions in the dorsal root ganglia, nerve roots and dorsal columns were otherwise similar. Several small neuromata were found alongside the vessels near the central canal of the cord. These were also found in the case of Jughenn *et al.* Their resemblance to those commonly seen in association with lesions of the dorsal roots in cases of protrusion of intervertebral discs suggests that they were due to regeneration of dorsal root fibres.

It seems probable that the hyaline material found in the ganglia and nerve roots in this case, as in that of Denny-Brown, may have resulted from the chronic suppuration and osteomyelitis in the feet. Its complete absence in Blackwood's case, in which, however, the capsule of the ganglia was considerably thickened, also favours the view that it is not the cause but rather is the indirect result of the degeneration of sensory neurones. This disease should therefore be clearly distinguished from cases in which amyloid infiltration is the primary cause of degeneration of peripheral nerves. The hereditary incidence of the disease and its early age of onset suggest that it should be grouped along with other familial systemic degenerations of the nervous system, such as Friedreich's ataxia and peroneal atrophy. Its association with olivo-cerebellar degeneration in the case of Blackwood points in the same direction. That it should sometimes be associated with spina bifida occulta (Tocantins and Reimann 1939, Jackson 1949) does not invalidate this thesis, since this common deformity has also been described in the Roussy-Levy syndrome (Jéquier 1948).

For the dissociation of sensory loss in this disease Denny-Brown and van Bogaert favour the explanation that it is due to the small number of dorsal root ganglia attacked in the early stages, since damage to one dorsal root or ganglion produces an area of sensory loss which is more extensive to thermal and painful stimuli than to touch. But it seems more likely that in these families the degeneration tends to involve especially the smaller nerve fibres and neurones of

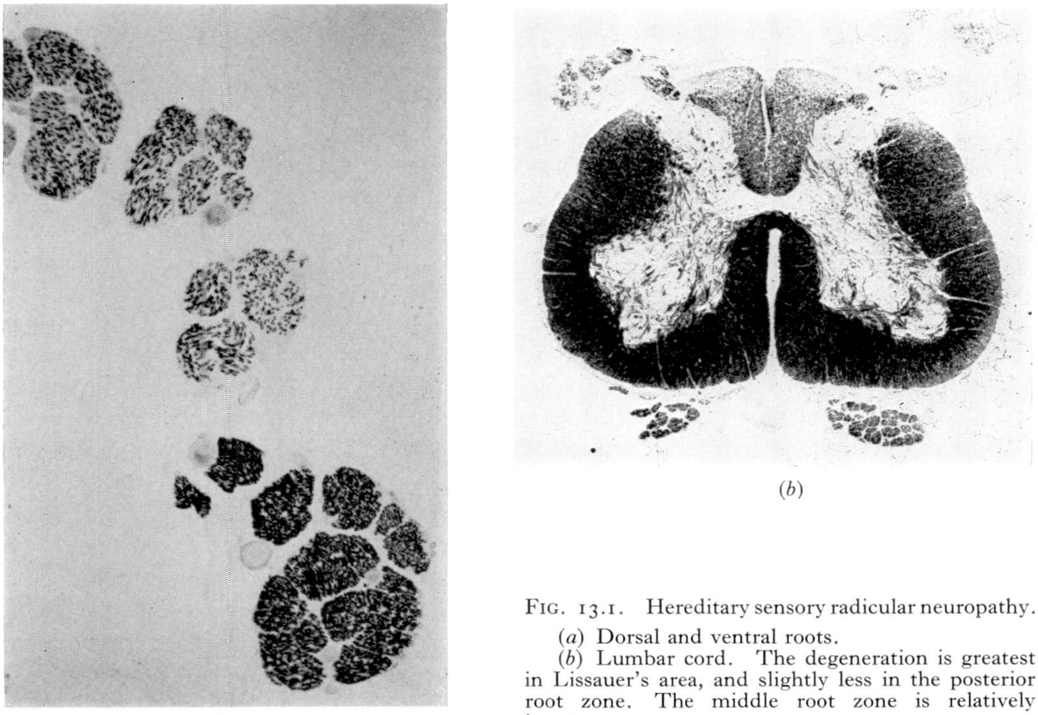

(a) (b)

FIG. 13.1. Hereditary sensory radicular neuropathy.
(a) Dorsal and ventral roots.
(b) Lumbar cord. The degeneration is greatest in Lissauer's area, and slightly less in the posterior root zone. The middle root zone is relatively intact.

the dorsal roots and ganglia. The peculiar incidence of the degeneration on the fibres entering the cord from the dorsal roots points in this direction. In both Denny-Brown's and Blackwood's cases it was considerably greater in the posterior than in the middle-root zone of Flechsig, but the degeneration of these tracts of large fibres was evidently much less than that of the fibres going directly to the dorsal horns, as judged by the profound analgesia and thermanaesthesia. At no level did the distribution of the degeneration suggest a complete, or almost complete, lesion of one or two dorsal roots. A selective degeneration of fibres carrying one modality of sensation is not unusual in familial diseases of the nervous system, since it is seen both in Friedreich's ataxia and in Biemond's hereditary posterior column ataxia (1951).

INTERSTITIAL FORMS OF PERIPHERAL NEUROPATHY

Acute infective polyneuritis. Landry's paralysis. (*Guillain-Barré syndrome*)

A form of acute or subacute polyneuritis of unknown aetiology, sometimes occurring in small groups of cases, has been recognised since the second half of the nineteenth century. Landry (1859) described 5 personally observed cases and collected a further 5 from the literature. He called the condition *acute ascending paralysis*, using the word *ascending* as synonymous with *centripetal*. He noted that the paralysis might come on during convalescence from an acute illness. In the case which he described fully weakness spread from the feet and hands to the trunk and thence to the cranial and intercostal nerves and was associated, towards the end of the disease, with loss of sensation to touch and posture in the feet and hands. Pain and temperature sensibility was preserved. Although he described the paralysis as *ascending or centripetal*, he noted that, along with the toes and feet, the hamstrings and muscles of the pelvic girdle were affected in the first stage of the disease. Later weakness spread to the anterior and internal muscles of the thighs. Similarly in the arms the scapular muscles were affected before those of the forearm. In some cases the sensory and motor systems were equally affected. Of the 10 cases which he collected only 2 were fatal, and in these post-mortem examination showed no lesions in the spinal cord. Osler (1892) used the name *acute febrile polyneuritis* for cases which corresponded clinically to Landry's description, and this name was used by Holmes (1917) for a small number of cases which he saw in British soldiers in France in the winter of 1916–17. He emphasised the early weakness in the proximal muscles of the limbs, and found some degree of facial paralysis as a constant symptom. In his, as in Landry's series, the death rate was 20 per cent. Bradford, Bashford and Wilson (1918) saw 20 further cases during the following year in soldiers in France. They found that it followed, at an interval of a few days or weeks, a febrile illness, often so mild as not to take the soldier off duty, but there might be no rise of temperature with the onset of paralysis. They claimed to have transferred the disease to monkeys by inoculation of spinal cord, but these claims were later withdrawn, and in spite of repeated trials no successful transfer of the disease to animals has since been made (Sabin and Aring 1941). Because of the apparently successful transfer of the disease, they adopted the name *acute infective polyneuritis*. Foster Kennedy (1919) describing cases in the American army used the name *infective neuronitis*.

The death-rate has varied greatly from 67 per cent (Lassen and Fog 1943) to 9 per cent (Baker 1943) but in most reported series it has been in the neighbourhood of 20 per cent. Although in most cases death has been due to respiratory paralysis or bronchopneumonia, many patients die suddenly from heart failure.

Similar cases, in which the cerebrospinal fluid contained a great excess of protein, with no increase in the cell count, were described by Donath (1905), Roemheld (1908), Claude (1909), Renon and Monier-Vimard (1909) and Guillain, Barré and Strohl (1916). The name *Guillain-Barré syndrome* came into general use about the year 1925 to describe cases of acute or subacute peripheral neuropathy, with recovery, in which the cerebrospinal fluid showed similar cell-protein dissociation, and it has since been more loosely used as a clinical name for the disease. But, if an eponymic is preferred to a descriptive name, credit for the description of the disease should be given to Landry.

Pathology. In this form of polyneuritis the lesions vary with the stage at which the disease is fatal. Haymaker and Kernohan (1949), in a series of 50 fatal cases, most of which occurred in soldiers, were able to trace all stages from 2 to 21 days and had 1 case with a duration of 46 days. They found the chief incidence of the disease to fall on the proximal part of the peripheral nerves, just beyond the dorsal root ganglia. In the earliest stages (2 days) there is little change except oedema. At 5 days, degeneration of axons and myelin begins and increases during the following days. About the 9th day cellular infiltration appears in the form of scattered groups of lymphocytes. During the next few days these increase in number and numerous phagocytes and early activation of Schwann cells are also seen. In cases which were fatal during the 3rd week the degenerative changes in the nerve fibres had become severe and were often associated with considerable accumulation of coagulated fluid between the nerve fibres in the fascicles. At all stages oedema was more prominent than cellular infiltration. Wallerian degeneration occurs in many nerve fibres, and the view that this may account for most of the changes which are seen in peripheral twigs is supported by the electronmicroscopic findings of Finean and Woolf (1962).

In the *dorsal root ganglia* the lesions varied in severity from case to case, but some degree of chromatolysis was usually found in a considerable number of the nerve cells. Slight lymphocytic infiltrations and proliferation of capsule cells round degenerating neurones were sometimes seen (Fig. 13.2*c*). The cranial and spinal nerve roots were less affected, but degeneration of the dorsal roots and columns was present in some cases which died after 10 days or more of illness (Fig. 13.2*a* and *b*). Degeneration of ventral roots was less common and in only 2 cases could it be traced back to their intramedullary course. Lymphocytic infiltration in the meninges and nerve roots was rare.

In the central nervous system the only important lesion is central chromatolysis (axonal reaction) of varying degree in the neurones of the anterior horns and motor cranial nerves. In the writer's experience this is usually minimal in cases which are fatal within the first 7 days of illness or in motor neurones supplying muscles which have been paralysed for less than a week. It is therefore clearly secondary to the lesions in the nerve fibres. Acutely fatal cases may therefore show no lesions within the dura mater, except some congestion of vessels, which may be interpreted as due to the respiratory embarrassment or cardiac failure which caused death, and oedema of nerve roots. The lesions in the peripheral nerves may also be minimal at this stage.

The most evident lesions in the organs of the body cavity, in Haymaker and Kernohan's cases, were swelling of the spleen and lymph nodes and this was greatest in early cases. In 6 of their cases the cellular infiltrations in these organs suggested infectious mononucleosis, and in 2 other cases this diagnosis was confirmed. Interstitial myocarditis was present in 7 of their cases and in the 3 cases examined by Roseman and Aring (1941). In the liver focal necrosis with intralobular collections of lymphocytes were found in 2 cases and the lesions of subacute hepatitis in 1. The changes in the skeletal muscles are usually only those of early neurogenic atrophy.

Aetiology and pathogenesis. The relationship of this form of neuritis to a preceding febrile illness, which was noted by Landry and Bradford *et al.*, is also emphasised by Roseman and Aring and by Haymaker and Kernohan. Some of their cases followed influenza, measles, varicella or smallpox vaccination, or came on in the course of infectious mononucleosis; and most of the other cases were ushered in by mild infections of the respiratory tract. The great variety of the types of infection which may be followed by polyneuritis, and the long interval which sometimes elapses between the febrile illness and the onset of paralysis, suggest that the latter is not due to direct attack of a virus or other infectious agent on the nerves, but is more probably related to the infection in a manner similar to that of post-infectious encephalomyelitis. There may therefore be a similarity between cases of Landry's paralysis and some of the neuro-paralytic accidents following anti-rabic injections (Stuart and Krikorian 1933, Getzowa, Stuart and Krikorian 1933). The changes in the peripheral nerves are not those of an acute infection; inflammatory exudate appears late, is always slight and may well be explained as a concomitant of the neuronal degeneration. The most obvious change at all stages is oedema of the nerve fascicles which is suggestive of an allergic reaction. The rapidity with which

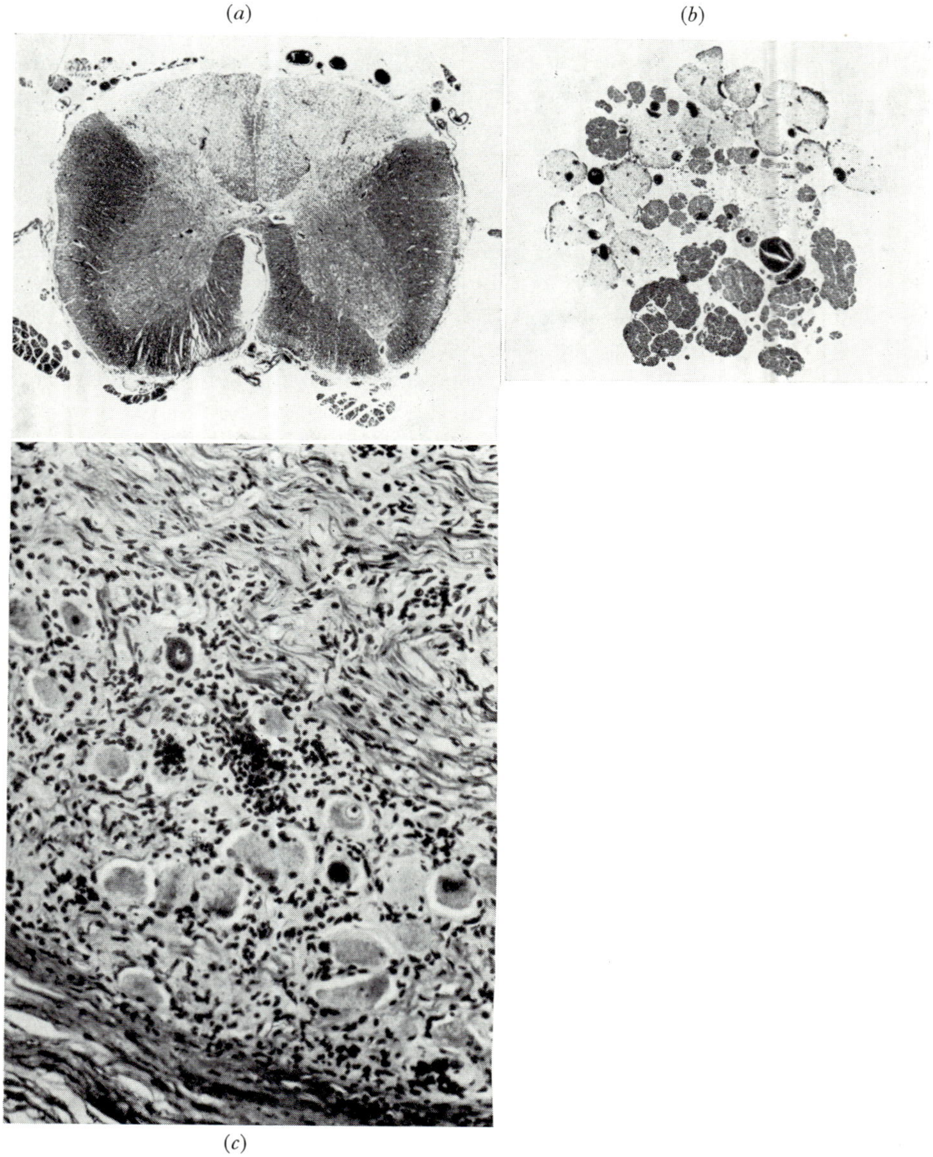

FIG. 13.2*a*, *b* and *c*. Subacute peripheral neuropathy of unknown aetiology.
(*a*) Section of lumbar cord, showing severe degeneration of the dorsal columns. (Myelin.)
(*b*) Lumbar nerve root showing degeneration chiefly of the dorsal components.
(*c*) Dorsal root ganglion showing small celled infiltration.

symptoms may appear and disappear indicates that the lesion in the nerve fibres is at first more functional than structural, but in severe cases this goes on to destruction of myelin and to changes in the axons which, in some, may be severe enough to cause Wallerian degeneration in the peripheral part of the nerve fibre. But the rapidity and completeness of recovery, in a large proportion of cases, indicate that, in most nerve fibres, the lesion stops short of this stage.

Cerebrospinal fluid. The separation of cases with high protein and normal cell count in the cerebrospinal fluid from cases with more normal fluids which are otherwise similar has been found to be unjustified. In many cases the protein has been found to be normal during the early stages of the disease and to rise with its progress but it may also rise at a fairly early stage and fall rapidly. The fluid may be yellow and clot spontaneously (Donath 1905, Claude 1909). The cell count is equally capricious. Although it is usually within normal limits, cell counts of 100 per c.mm. or over have been found in some cases (Haymaker and Kernohan 1949) and a moderate increase of cells is not unusual. The protein excess appears to be limited to the spinal fluid since in several cases the cisternal fluid has had a much lower protein content. It probably reflects the vascular congestion and oedema of the nerve roots and proximal parts of the peripheral nerves. Gold-sol reactions of mid- or first-zone type have also been found in some cases, but they appear to bear little relation to the stage or course of the disease. The glucose may rise or fall to a moderate extent. The chlorides are normal or slightly reduced.

Hypertrophic interstitial neuropathy of Dejerine and Sottas. (*Heredopathia atactica polyneuritiformis, Refsum*)

The name 'progressive hypertrophic interstitial neuritis of childhood' was given by Dejerine and Sottas (1893) to a condition found in a brother and sister in whom disorder of gait appeared as the first symptom at the ages of 15 and 12 years. Later there was progressive weakness of the legs and arms, with ataxia, deformity of the feet and atrophy of the hand muscles, diminution of all forms of sensibility of glove and stocking distribution and loss of tendon reflexes. A similar case with onset at the age of 7 years had previously been described by Gombault and Mallet (1889). Since then many similar cases have been described and the disease is now recognised as a well-defined pathological entity, with a clinical picture of weakness and ataxia of the limbs, loss of tendon and plantar reflexes, and a variable degree of sensory loss. The disease is commonly familial and occasionally hereditary. Refsum (1955) considers that it is usually transmitted as a recessive, but occasional families have been reported in which it has appeared as a dominant (Russell and Garland 1930). In many cases the first symptoms appear in adult life and the sub-title 'of childhood' is therefore no longer used. Although usually progressive, in several well-authenticated cases it has run a relapsing course in which as many as five attacks of paralysis have been followed by complete remissions (Harris and Newcomb 1929). When the nerves are not easily palpable there may be clinical confusion with Friedreich's ataxia, especially in cases beginning during childhood with deformity of the feet, kyphoscoliosis, ataxia and intention tremor, but there is little pathological evidence of any relationship between the two diseases. Fresh interest in the condition was aroused by Refsum's (1946) clinical description of 5 cases from two Norwegian families under the title *Heredopathia atactica polyneuritiformis* and by the full pathological descriptions of the peripheral nerves in 4 of these cases (Cammermeyer, Haymaker and Refsum 1954, Cammermeyer 1956). Atypical retinitis pigmentosa is usually present and abnormalities may be present in the electrocardiogram. In one of the cases described by Gordon and Hudson (1959) there were widespread non-specific degenerative changes in the myocardium of the greatly enlarged heart.

Pathology. The peripheral nerves are swollen throughout their course from the spinal cord and brain stem to their peripheral terminations. The swelling of nerve roots may be obvious throughout the neuraxis or most evident in the cauda equina. The dorsal root ganglia do not share in the swelling and appear relatively small. In some cases the peripheral nerves are more than twice their normal size, but in others the hypertrophy is less marked. It is usually uniform but may produce fusiform or beaded swellings on the course of some nerves. On cross-section the individual fascicles may be more separated from one another than normal, and appear as firm, tough gelatinous rods in which the finely fibrillar structure of normal nerve is completely lost.

Microscopically the epineurium is normal. There may be an excess of fibroblastic, collagenous or mucoid tissue between the fascicles. The perineurium may be of normal or increased thickness. In the former case it is usually thrown into folds, especially in paraffin sections, by the shrinkage of its contents during the processes of fixation and section (Fig. 13.3*a*). Beneath it and separating the individual nerve fibres from one another is a thin fluid which stains metachromatically with toluidin blue and is P.A.S. (leucofuchsin) positive. It is usually most abundant immediately under the perineurium but varies greatly in amount in different nerves and even in different fascicles of the same nerve. It is not so evident in the spinal nerve roots. The individual nerve fibres are reduced in number and their myelin sheaths are thinned. Each fibre is invested by a rather cellular connective tissue which either forms cords of considerable thickness round single myelinated fibres (Fig. 13.3*b* and *d*) or ensheaths a group of fine non-myelinated fibres. Occasionally a thicker myelinated fibre and several thin naked axons are enclosed in one cord. Sparse longitudinal collagen fibres also run in the fluid which separates these cords. In transverse sections the sheath enclosing the nerve fibre has an appearance of concentric lamellae which was aptly termed 'onion-bulb' by Dejerine and Sottas. The lamellae are closely set near the nerve fibre and more loosely towards the outer surfaces of the cords where they appear to form overlapping sectors like the leaves of a leek. The innermost lamellae are often highly refractile and eosinophilic but with polychrome stains (Mallory, Masson, Azan) the sheath throughout takes the neutral, blue or green dye (Wolf *et al.* 1932). With silver methods a few strands of reticulin may appear to run in a circular or spiral manner round the nerve but the majority are cut transversely. Three to six or more nuclei are usually seen lying between the lamellae in the cross-section of each cord.

In longitudinal sections the appearances are much less characteristic as now the great majority of the collagen and reticulin fibres are seen to run longitudinally. The nuclei also are seen to be oriented in the longitudinal axis of the nerve. Degenerative changes in the myelin, in the form of clubs or globules are common, and Wallerian degeneration is seen in some fibres. Many of the axons are swollen but there are also very many fine unmyelinated axons. These have been interpreted by most authors following Bielschowsky (1922) as evidence of regeneration.

In addition to changes in the peripheral nerves degeneration of the primary sensory neurones can be traced in the dorsal columns of the cord as far as the medullary nuclei. The median fillet may also show degeneration which may perhaps be regarded as trans-synaptic. The inferior olives and the circumamicular tracts of the cerebellum may also show degenerative changes (Cammermeyer 1956). In a few cases the disease has been associated with disseminated sclerosis (Schob 1912, 1923) or other disease of the central nervous system (Greenfield and Bosanquet 1953).

The pathogenesis of the disease process and the nature of the cells taking part in it are still unknown and must remain so until the character and potentialities of the sheath of Schwann are better understood. There appears to be little doubt that, in spite of the onion-bulb appearance, the majority of the fibres ensheathing the nerve fibres run longitudinally. Bielschowsky (1922) described them as fine fibrils, developing in the cytoplasm of the Schwann syncytium and splitting into cylindrical layers. Others (Dejerine and Thomas 1906) regard them as

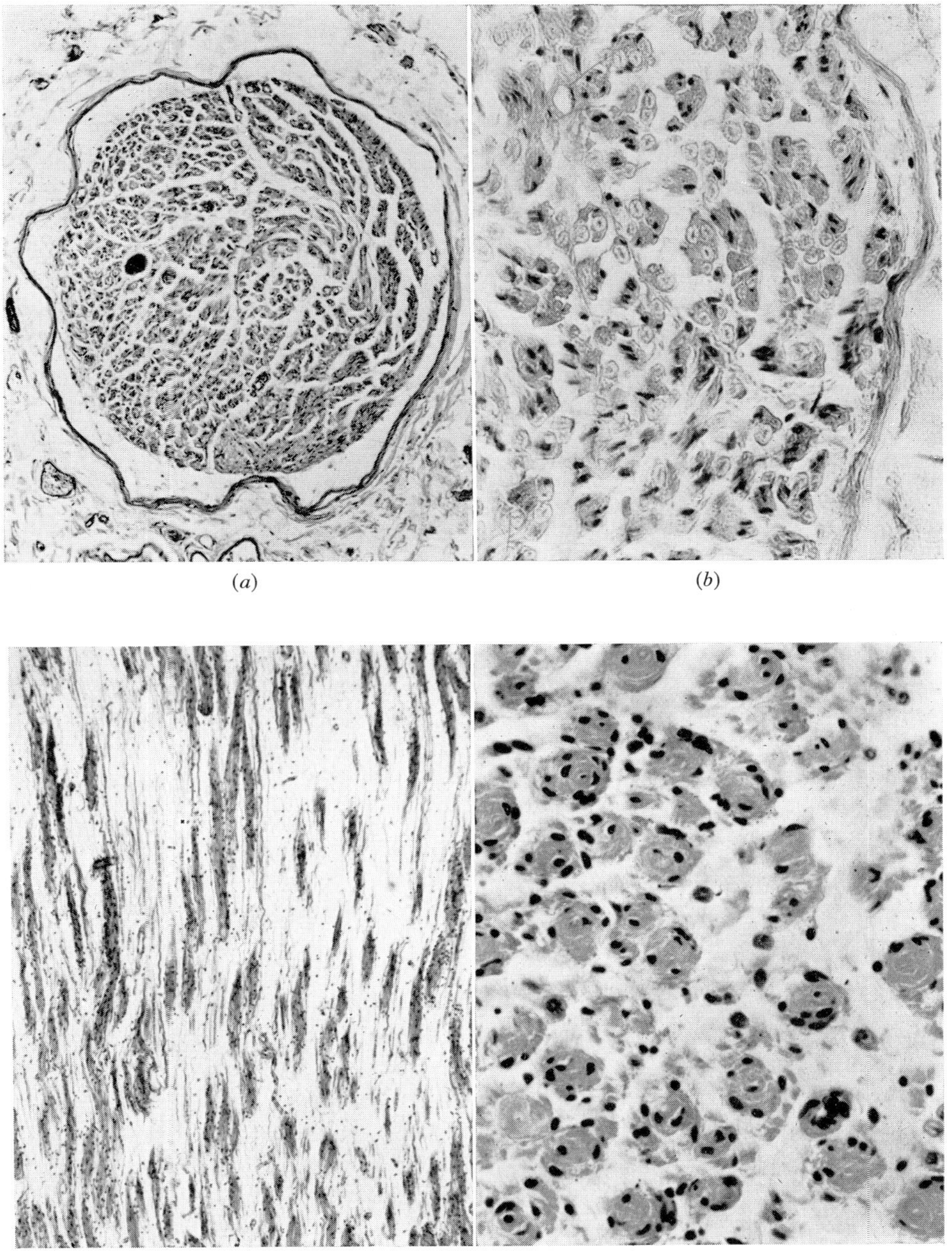

(*a*) (*b*)

(*c*) (*d*)

FIG. 13.3. Hypertrophic neuritis of Dejerine-Sottas.

(*a*) Low-power view of a nerve bundle to show the loose, wrinkled perineurium and the space under it. (×75.)

(*b*) Transverse section of nerve. Many axons are still seen surrounded by myelin (unstained). (Haematoxylin van Gieson.)

(*c*) Longitudinal section of nerve showing great separation of fibres. (By the courtesy of Dr. Bosanquet.)

(*d*) Transverse section of a nerve with considerable collagenous thickening round the individual fibres.

arising from the endoneurium, and this view is supported by modern staining methods. Cammermeyer (1956) found increase in number of Schwann nuclei only round nerve fibres which had undergone Wallerian degeneration. All authors agree that along with disappearance of many myelinated fibres and thinning of myelin sheaths there are many evidences of regeneration of fine unmyelinated fibres which may arise at any level where the axon has been damaged. This damage appears to be caused by pressure, but the view that the nerve fibres are constricted by the contraction or thickening of concentric fibres can no longer be upheld. Indeed the degree of degeneration in many nerves is disproportionate to the overgrowth of connective tissue. It seems more probable that the nerve fibres are compressed, or their metabolism interfered with, by the accumulation of interstitial fluid within the perineurium. This view would be consistent with the remissions of the disease which are sometimes observed. The reason for the accumulation of this fluid and for the accompanying increase of interstitial connective tissue must lie in some hereditary metabolic dyscrasia the nature of which still remains obscure.

Infiltration of the peripheral nervous system in primary amyloidosis

De Navasquez and Treble (1938) described a case of weakness and wasting of the muscles without sensory loss, associated with diarrhoea, impotence and finally heart failure. Post-mortem examination revealed great enlargement of the heart from amyloid infiltration. The spleen and testes were also enlarged and diffusely infiltrated and there were minor degrees of infiltration, especially in the walls of the small arteries and arterioles, in the other organs of the body cavity. The *dorsal root ganglia* and *peripheral nerves* were infiltrated throughout their course with oval or rounded nodular deposits of amyloid in the perineurium and endoneurium. Some, but not all, of these deposits were related to small arteries. They referred to a similar, but apparently familial, case which was described as *atypical interstitial neuritis* by de Bruyn and Stern (1929) and to other cases of generalised amyloidosis with weakness of the limbs, in which the peripheral nerves were not so fully examined (Lubarsch 1929). Since then a number of similar isolated cases has been reported (Goetze and Kruecke 1941). Some cases are familial (Kantarjian and De Jong 1953). Andrade (1952), who has found the condition to be very common and known for many years in fishing villages in the Oporto region, examined 75 cases and reported two post-mortem examinations and several biopsies. The disease often affected several members of a family which might belong to any social grade. It ran a progressive course with gastro-intestinal disturbances (diarrhoea or obstinate constipation) and impotence as early symptoms. These were followed by loss of thermal and pain sensibility which might be the cause of trophic ulcers on the feet. Paraesthesiae and diffuse pains in the limbs were common symptoms. Loss of tactile and postural sense and weakness and wasting of the limbs usually followed signs of analgesia. The pupils were often unequal and reacted poorly to light. The tendon reflexes were lost, sometimes at an early stage. Death occurred in most cases from cardiac failure.

Pathology. The changes in the organs of the body cavity are those of generalised amyloidosis. In the testes diffuse and sometimes nodular deposits throughout the connective tissue and blood-vessels cause compression and atrophy of the parenchyma and loss of spermatogenesis. The pancreas is severely infiltrated and this may be an important factor in causing diarrhoea. Both the somatic and sympathetic nervous systems are infiltrated. In the dorsal root ganglia there may be both diffuse infiltration of the connective tissue and nodular deposits under the capsule of the nerve cells. In the peripheral nerves also the deposits are often nodular, separating and compressing the nerve fibres and causing degeneration of their myelin sheaths (Fig. 13.4). There is less destruction of axons, but in old-standing and severe cases very few nerve fibres may survive as far as the peripheral twigs (Blackwood 1952). To some extent also the damage to nerve fibres may be ischaemic, due to thickening of the walls and reduction of the lumen of the small vessels, as in the case of Kernohan and Woltman (1942).

In the case of Goetze and Kruecke there were small softenings in the cerebellar and cerebral cortex and areas of granular atrophy of the cerebral cortex associated with amyloid infiltration of the arteries supplying these areas. They also found amyloid infiltration of the interstitial tissues and of occasional muscle fibres in the voluntary muscles, as well as in the heart. In other cases (Lubarsch 1929) amyloid infiltration of the voluntary muscle has been so great as to cause rigidity.

It is evident from the clinical histories of cases of generalised primary amyloidosis that the peripheral nerves are commonly involved, but nervous symptoms are often over-shadowed by

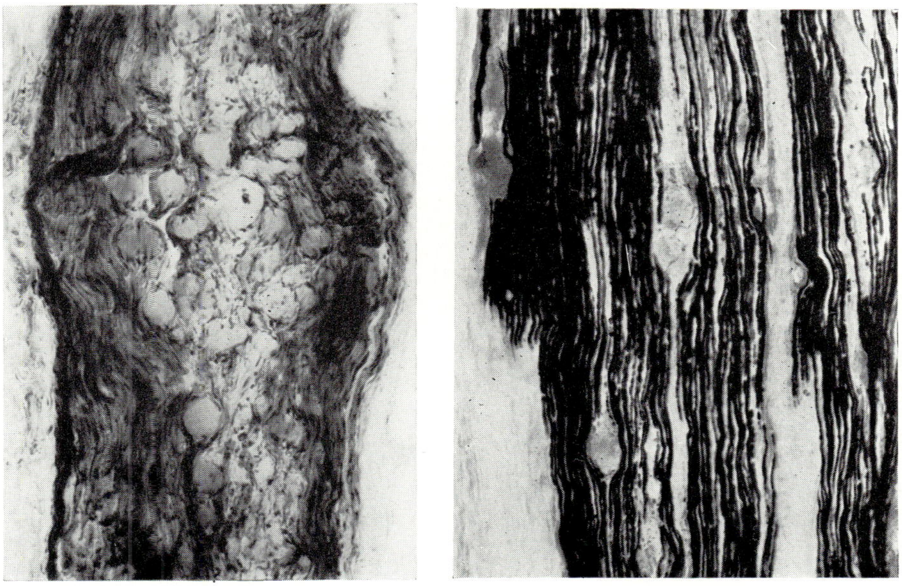

(*a*) (*b*)

FIG. 13.4. Infiltration of peripheral nerves in generalised amyloidosis.
(*a*) Haematoxylin van Gieson × 120. (*b*) Weigert-Pal alum carmine.

those of cardiac failure. In some cases with severe involvement of the heart and abdominal viscera the peripheral nerves appear to be quite free from deposits; in others, such as those described by Andrade in Portugal, peripheral nerve paralysis appears early and dominates the clinical picture. In western Tennesse also Jones and Frazier (1950), among 15 cases of primary amyloidosis in 600 consecutive autopsies, found symptoms of peripheral neuritis in 5. The high incidence of primary amyloidosis in this district is shown by these figures, and was still more evident in cases over the age of 50 years (3·5 per cent).

The local incidence of the disease, and the experimental production of amyloid infiltration in rats by diets rich in casein and deficient in vitamin C, suggest that in the human also the disease may be due to dietary conditions in association with hereditary predisposition, but Andrade was unable to discover any peculiarity of diet or of environmental conditions common to his cases.

Clinical pathology. In many cases the cerebrospinal fluid has shown an increase in protein to between 100 and 250 mg. per 100 ml. with a moderate mid-zone precipitation of gold sol. The Congo-red absorption test is usually positive in varying degree and biopsy of the gums may show deposits of amyloid in the subepithelial connective tissue.

(Revised by W. Blackwood.)

REFERENCES

Andrade, C. (1952) *Brain*, **75**, 408.

Baker, A. B. (1943) *Journal-Lancet*, **63**, 384.

Bielschowsky, M. (1922) *J. Psychol. Neurol.*, **29**, 182; (1924) *Arch. Neurol. Psychiat.* (Chicago), **9**, 91.

Biemond, A. (1951) *Folia Psychiat. Neurol. Neerland*, **54**, 216.

Blackwood, W. (1952) *Proc. 1st Internat. Cong. Neuropath.*, Rome, **3**, 421.

Bogaert, L. van (1953) *Acta Neurol. Psychiat. Belgica*, **53**, 37.

Bradford, J. R., Bashford, E. F. and Wilson, J. A. (1918–19) *Quart. J. Med.*, **12**, 88.

Brodal, A., Böyesen, S. and Frovig, A. C. (1953) *Arch. Neurol. Psychiat.* (Chicago), **70**, 1.

de Bruyn, R. S. and Stern, R. O. (1929) *Brain*, **52**, 84.

Cammermeyer, J. (1956) *J. Neuropath.*, **15**, 340.

Cammermeyer, J., Haymaker, W. and Refsum, S. (1954) *Amer. J. Path.*, **30**, 643.

Cathcart, C. W. (1896) *Edin. Med. J.*, **42**, 37.

Charcot, J. M. and Marie, P. (1886) *Rev. de Med.*, **6**, 97.

Claude, H. (1909) *Rev. Neurol.*, **17**, 1420.

Dejerine, J. and Sottas, I. (1893) *Contes rend. Soc. de Biol.*, **45**, 63.

Dejerine, J. and Thomas, A. (1906) *Nouv. Icon. de la Salpêt.*, **19**, 477.

Denny-Brown, D. (1951) *J. Neurol. Psychiat.*, **14**, 237.

Donath, J. (1905) *Wien. klin. Wschr.*, 1327.

Finean, J. B. and Woolf, A. L. (1962) *J. Neuropath. Exp. Neurol.*, **21**, 105.

Friedreich, N. (1873) Ueber progressive Muskelatrophie.

Getzowa, S., Stuart, G. and Krikorian, K. S. (1933) *J. Path. Bact.*, **37**, 483.

Goetze, W. and Kruecke, W. (1941) *Arch. f. Psychiat. Nervenkr.*, **114**, 183.

Gombault, A. and Mallet (1889) *Arch. de méd. expérim.*, **1**, 385.

Gordon, N. and Hudson, R. E. B. (1959) *Brain*, **82**, 41.

Greenfield, J. G. and Bosanquet, F. D. (1953) *J. Neurol. Psychiat.*, **16**, 213.

Guillain, G., Barré, J. A. and Strohl, A. (1916) *Bull. et mém. Soc. med. hôp. de Paris*, **40**, 1462.

Harris, W. and Newcomb, W. D. (1929) *Brain*, **52**, 108.

Haymaker, W. and Kernohan, J. W. (1949) *Medicine*, **28**, 59.

Herringham, W. (1888) *Brain*, **9**, 231.

Hicks, E. P. (1922) *Lancet* (i), 319.

Holmes, G. (1917) *Brit. Med. J.* (ii), 37.

Jackson, M. (1949) *Med. J. Australia* (i), 433.

Jéquier, M. (1948) *Rev. Oto-neuro-ophthal.*, **20**, 431.

Jones, R. S. and Frazier, D. B. (1950) *Arch. Path.*, **50**, 366.

Jughenn, H., Krücke, W. and Wadulla, H. (1949) *Arch. Psychiat. Nervenkr.*, **182**, 153.

Kantarjian, A. D. and de Jong, R. N. (1953) *Neurology*, **3**, 399.

Kennedy, F. (1919) *Arch. Neurol. Psychiat.* (Chicago), **2**, 621.

Kernohan, J. W. and Woltman, H. W. (1942) *Arch. Neurol. Psychiat.* (Chicago), **47**, 132.

Landry, O. (1859) *Gaz. hebd. de Med.*, **6**, 472, 486.

Lassen, H. C. A. and Fog. M. (1943) *Acta med. Scand.*, **115**, 117.

Lubarsch, O. (1929) *Virchows Archiv. path. Anat.*, **271**, 867.

Marinesco, G. (1894) *Arch. de Méd. expériment*, **6**, 921.

de Navesquez, S. and Treble, H. A. (1938) *Brain*, **61**, 116.

Osler, W. (1892) *The Principles and Practice of Medicine*, Appleton, New York.

Refsum, S. (1946) *Heredopathia atactica polyneuritiformis*, Grundt, Oslo; (1955) in *Clinical Neurology* (A. B. Baker), **3**, 1938.

Renon, L. and Monier-Vimard, D. (1909) *Bull. et Mém. Soc. med. hôp. de Paris*, **28**, 32.

Roemheld. (1908) *Dtsch. Z. Nervenheilk.*, **36**, 94.

Roseman, E. and Aring, C. D. (1941) *Medicine*, **20**, 463.

Russell, W. R. and Garland, H. G. (1930) *Brain*, **53**, 376.
Sabin, A. B. and Aring, C. D. (1941) *Amer. J. Path.*, **17**, 469.
Sainton, P. (1899) *Nouv. Icon. de la Salpêtrière*, **12**, 317.
Schob, F. (1912) *Münch. med. Wschr.*, **59**, 1831; (1923) *Z. ges. Neurol. Psychiat.*, **83**, 481.
Stuart, G. and Krikorian, K. S. (1933) *Brit. Med. J.* (i), 501.
Tocantins, L. M. and Reimann, H. A. (1939) *J. Amer. med. Ass.*, **112**, 2251.
Tooth, H. H. (1886) *Peroneal type of progressive muscular atrophy*, Lewis, London; (1888) *Brain*, **10**, 243.
Virchow, R. (1855) *Virchows Arch. f. path. Anat.*, **8**, 537.
Wolf, A., Rubinowitz, A. H. and Burchell, S. C. (1932) *Bull. N.Y. Inst. Neurol.*, **2**, 373.

CHAPTER 14

LESIONS OF THE NERVOUS SYSTEM ASSOCIATED WITH DISEASES OR MALFORMATIONS OF THE CRANIUM AND SPINAL COLUMN

By J. G. Greenfield

Although the skull and vertebral column normally protect the brain and spinal cord, disease or malformation of these bony envelopes may cause local or more widespread pressure either on the nervous parenchyma or on the blood-vessels which supply it, with effects which resemble those of tumours arising in these bones. But in some the pressure is more widely spread, in others is more sharply localised and in most cases is more chronic. The pathogenesis of these lesions has been somewhat neglected although many are common and some are severely disabling. Very few studies of the effects of diffuse, long-continued pressure on the brain have been made and even the simpler pathology of spinal cord compression is imperfectly understood. In many acute early cases the loss of function is greater than can easily be explained by the lesions found, but the reverse may be true in long-standing cases in which the lower limbs retain useful function in spite of very severe lesions in the cord. In some cases the pathogenesis of the functional disability may be suggested by the character of the minor lesions which are found, but in other cases it remains uncertain. Mechanical pressure would seem to be more likely to compress blood-vessels than solid tissue, and veins more than arteries. Many of the effects of pressure have therefore been attributed to venous stasis and oedema and others to compression or spasm of small arteries. Myelin seems to be more vulnerable both to mechanical pressure and to minor degrees of anoxia than nerve cells and axons. Certainly in the spinal cord the effects of pressure are usually greatest in the myelin of the white columns. Movement of the cord or lower medulla over bony prominences on the dorsal surface of the vertebral bodies may have a specially deleterious effect on nervous tissue. This effect may be secondary to ischaemic or vascular stasis, but McAlhany and Netsky (1955) found that the greatest demyelination often lay either immediately under a tumour or on the opposite side of the cord and attributed this to the direct effects of pressure.

The type of lesion which is found in the spinal cord under conditions of acute or more chronic compression is well established. The earliest lesion is usually a rounded or wedge-shaped area of vacuolar degeneration in the posterior part of the lateral columns. This may be unilateral or bilateral and consists of distended myelin sheaths many of which contain swollen axons. In more advanced cases these lesions become more extensive and similar areas often appear in the deeper parts of the dorsal columns. The ventral third of the white matter usually remains intact. Areas of more frank necrosis in which the neuroglial scaffolding also suffers may appear in the centre of the older areas and there may also be areas of softening in the grey matter, most often near the base of the ventral horns. Cavitation often appears in the deeper parts of the dorsal columns or in the region of the grey commissure. In chronic cases the myelin loss is replaced by overgrowth of neuroglial and connective tissue fibres, among which many axons still persist. There is usually shrinkage of the ventral horns associated with atrophy and loss of nerve cells, and hyaline thickening of the small intramedullary vessels.

Although this progressive type of degeneration is very common in cases of subacute or chronic compression of the cord, many cases of sudden paraplegia due to pressure are associated in their early stages with frankly necrotic changes in the cord which may involve all its transverse section or be confined to some part of this. In such cases a vascular causation is most probable but thrombosis of vessels is rarely found. It seems likely that they are due to compression of an important radicular vessel in or close to the intervertebral foramen.

The effects of compression of the brain have been less studied, but definite changes have been found in the cerebellar cortex by Scharenberg (1953) and others. These consist of atrophy, degeneration and loss of nerve cells, affecting first the Purkinje cells, and gliosis of the granular and molecular layers. These effects are greatest near the surface of the parts subjected to most direct pressure. In cases with tonsillar herniation atrophy and gliosis is often severe in the herniated parts.

Hyperostosis frontalis interna

(Stewart-Morel Syndrome. Metabolic craniopathy)

Morgagni (1765) described bossing of the inner table of the frontal bones in an obese woman with abnormal facial hirsutism. This triad was accepted in Great Britain towards the end of the nineteenth century as occurring not infrequently in mental patients (Bevan Lewis 1889, Clouston 1898). Stewart (1927–8), who made post-mortem examinations of 3 cases in insane middle-aged women, was the first to draw attention to the atrophy and sclerosis of the anterior lobe of the pituitary which often accompanies the bony changes. All his patients were obese, two had facial hirsutism, and one had polyuria. Morel (1930) described the condition independently and the association of bony overgrowth and endocrine disturbances has been called the Stewart-Morel syndrome.

The bony condition consists of sessile or more bossed symmetrical thickenings of the inner table of the frontal squames on either side of the groove for the sagittal sinus. They are formed of cancellous bone covered on its inner surface by compact bone. Although confined in most cases to the frontal squames a similar condition may be found also on the inner surface of the parietal bones. No alteration takes place in the outer table or in the external shape or size of the skull, but its internal capacity is reduced according to the amount of new bone formation. Radiological examination has shown that the condition is in most cases steadily progressive. When the bony overgrowth is considerable the convexity of the frontal lobes shows a corresponding depression, but in many cases no gross changes are found in the brain.

The condition is almost confined to females of middle age or over but not always past the climacteric. Of the few cases in which it has occurred in males, a considerable number have followed trauma.

Hemphill and Stengel (1940) examined a woman of 65 and her daughter, aged 32, both of whom had frontal and parietal hyperostosis interna. Both were paranoid but not demented. Towards the end of her life the mother suffered from intense headaches and tenderness of the skull. Post-mortem examination of the brain showed a moderate degree of flattening of the frontal lobes related to the areas of bony thickening. Histological examination of the cortex showed atrophy and loss of nerve cells in the 3rd and 5th layers, especially in the frontal and to a less degree in the parietal lobes. It was associated with degeneration and loss of fibres in the tangential and supraradial layers, hyperplasia of astrocytes and superficial fibrous gliosis.

Degenerative and atrophic changes were also found in the supra-optic nucleus. The pituitary showed considerable fibrous tissue overgrowth and a localised acidophilic adenoma.

Associated changes in the pituitary may consist, as in Stewart's cases, of atrophic sclerosis of the anterior lobe with some invasion of the pars nervosa by basophil cells. Compact masses of acidophil cells in the posterior part of the anterior lobe, basophilic adenomatous formations and, more rarely, hypophyseal tumours have been described. Henschen (1936) found a constant increase of basophil cells and loss of chromophobe cells in the anterior lobe. He found nothing unusual in the ovaries or other endocrine glands.

Henschen found it impossible to relate hyperostosis frontalis to any nervous or mental symptoms, although when severe it was almost always associated with obesity and hirsutism. In an examination of two hundred female skulls he found hyperostosis frontalis in nearly 40 per cent of all over the age of 47, but in 8 per cent it was slight and only in 9 per cent was it severe.

Petersen (1947) in a careful analysis found that hyperostosis of the cranium occurred in 20–32 per cent of women over the age of 40 who showed signs of endocrine disturbance as against 7–16 per cent of normal women. He recognised two forms of the abnormality, the classical hyperostosis frontalis interna and a diffuse sclerotic thickening of the cranial vault without bossing; these occurred with equal frequency in all the conditions that he investigated. They were especially common in elderly, obese diabetic women. He found a positive correlation between hyperostosis and hypertrichosis but none between hypertrichosis and obesity in women below the age of 40. However, the high incidence of elderly obese women in cases of hyperostosis made Morgagni's triad more common than could be expected from a chance combination of its constituent elements. Although hyperostosis was no more common in epileptics than in normal subjects, three-quarters of his patients with hyperostosis were epileptic. He concluded that both forms of hyperostosis cranii were evidence of hormonal disturbance and therefore likely to occur along with other endocrine symptoms, but he did not accept the association of either form with a definite clinical syndrome.

Osteitis deformans
(Paget's disease of bone)

The skull and spinal column are common sites of osteitis deformans, and this may produce lesions in the central nervous system or in the cranial or spinal nerve roots. The rarefaction of the bony trabeculae, which constitutes the early stage of the disease, makes the bone less able to resist the effects of gravity in spite of its increased thickness, so that, as it thickens, it becomes moulded to a new shape. The vault of the skull becomes wider, slightly longer in its antero-posterior diameter and reduced in height. But as there is no great change in its capacity the brain is not compressed. A similar change at the base of the skull, especially round the foramen magnum, is one of the causes of platybasia and basilar invagination (Bull *et al.* 1959). In such cases the inferior surface of the cerebellum may be compressed by flattening of the base of the posterior fossa.

In some cases optic atrophy results from narrowing of the optic foramina. Loss of hearing and nystagmus may be due either to changes in the bones of the cochlea and labyrinth or to narrowing of the internal auditory meatus. Involvement of other cranial nerves is rare.

In osteitis deformans of the spine there is usually some degree of kyphosis, and in some cases this may be a rather sharp curvature. But the paraplegia, which sometimes results, appears to be more often due to the general reduction in the lumen of the canal, or to more local pressure by bony prominences which may form on the dorsal surfaces of the vertebral bodies. In 2 cases reported by Wyllie (1923) laminectomy showed a loss of the space which normally exists between the cord and the bone, and absence of pulsation in the cord. In the more serious case, on which the present writer performed an autopsy, bony projections from the dorsal surfaces of the 6th and 8th thoracic vertebral bodies compressed the cord at these levels. The dura mater was everywhere in contact with the walls of the spinal canal and was abnormally adherent to them. The changes in the spinal cord are those already described as resulting from compression.

Bony abnormalities in the region of the foramen magnum

Abnormalities in the floor of the posterior fossa, or in the articulation of the skull with the atlas or of the atlas with the axis may be the cause of serious neurological symptoms. The most common of these are (1) *Occipitalisation or assimilation of the atlas*, that is partial or more complete bony fusion of the atlas with the ring of the foramen magnum, (2) *Basilar invagination* or *impression* and (3) *Anomalies* either in the *odontoid process* itself or in its relation to the atlas. In over 100 patients with bony abnormalities in the region of the foramen magnum McRae (1953) found 28 instances of the first type, 21 of the second and 17 of the third, and others with combinations of these. Since in most cases these are congenital abnormalities symptoms often begin in childhood or early adult life. In some cases they appear to follow an injury to the head or neck.

(1) Assimilation or fusion of the atlas with the margin of the foramen magnum does not of itself cause compression or abnormal angulation of the medulla, but it may be combined with other abnormalities, such as an odontoid process which is abnormally long, angulated backwards or placed unusually high or a reduction in size of the foramen magnum. In McRae's series neurological signs were always present if the anteroposterior diameter of the spinal canal behind the odontoid process were less than 20 mm. The lack of movement between the skull and atlas may also throw an abnormal strain on the atlanto-axial joint and produce abnormally free movement of the odontoid process in relation to the arch of the atlas or actual dislocation at this joint. This strain may be increased by fusion of the 2nd and 3rd cervical vertebrae as in List's case 3 (1941). Assimilation of the atlas may also be associated with platybasia or basilar invagination.

(2) Basilar invagination has been defined in relation to lateral radiographs of the skull as an abnormal protrusion of the tip of the odontoid process above Chamberlain's line, that is a line drawn from the back of the hard palate to the posterior margin of the foramen magnum. There is some uncertainty as to the limits of the normal in this respect. The tip of the dens not infrequently lies 5 mm. above Chamberlain's line in normal individuals and occasionally 1 or 2 mm. higher (Saunders 1943), but in basilar invagination it is often more than 10 mm. above this line. The condition has also been defined in anteroposterior views by the relation of the tip of the odontoid process to a line joining the tips of the mastoid processes. This line normally passes through the occipito-atlantal joints which lie at about the same level as the dens.

Basilar invagination is often associated with platybasia, that is flattening of the angle between the orbital plates and the clivus of the sphenoid. This angle, which normally is 135° or less, becomes 145° or more in platybasia. These malformations are usually developmental and Bull *et al.* (1955) have found evidence of hereditary transmission. In rare cases they result from softening of the base of the skull by osteitis deformans, rickets, osteomalacia or osteogenesis imperfecta. In most cases the atlas is tilted in relation to the skull, so that its anterior arch, carrying the odontoid process with it, may lie at a higher level than the spinous processes. Basilar invagination is not uncommonly associated with fusion of two or more cervical vertebrae. It may produce abnormal angulation of the lowest part of the medulla or the first cervical segment over the prominence formed by the odontoid process and transverse ligament. This angulation and pressure vary with the position of the head and some patients relate their symptoms to head movements. Thickening of the transverse ligament of the atlas and of the dural sheath are often present and increase the constriction of the cord and medulla. The effect on these structures is usually gradual but eventually there is degeneration of white matter and reduction in the size of the cord, especially in its anteroposterior diameter. In some cases the cord has been described as a fibrous ribbon and in a case of the writer's, associated with extensive fusion of cervical vertebrae (Klippel-Feil malformation, Fig. 14.4), it measured only 2 mm. in its anteroposterior diameter.

(3) Separation of the odontoid process from the axis may result either from fracture across the base of the odontoid or from tearing of a persistent cartilaginous union at this level. Fusion of the dens with the body of the axis normally occurs during the 3rd to 4th year, but in many normal subjects some hyaline cartilage persists here throughout life. In most cases this is no more than a small central disc, but in some it is larger and may cover most of the plane of junction. The writer has examined a case in which the lower surface of the separated odontoid process was covered by cartilage (Greenfield 1953). Separations which result from slight strains or injuries may be explained most easily on these lines. In these cases the inferior surface of the separated odontoid usually has a smooth horizontal line. Other congenital anomalies may be associated. In 2 of McRae's cases the tip of the odontoid was fused to the anterior lip of the foramen magnum. The separated odontoid process, which is often shorter and smaller than normal, retains its relation to the anterior arch of atlas, but the separation allows of abnormal anteroposterior movement of the atlas on the axis and in many cases there is permanent forward dislocation of the head and atlas at this level. In some such cases the appearance of nervous symptoms and signs may be delayed for weeks (Wallace and Bruce 1910) or even years (Bachs *et al.* 1955); 3 of McRae's cases were asymptomatic. But in most cases there is a gradual or more rapid onset of signs of compression of the spinal cord.

In atlanto-axial dislocation the atlas is displaced forward in relation to the axis and lower cervical spine and the odontoid process is separated from the anterior arch of the atlas. In these cases McRae found little or no gliding of the atlas on the axis and little anteroposterior movement of the skull on the atlas; flexion and extension movements occurred chiefly at lower levels of the cervical spine. In his cases the dens lay from 5 to 17 mm. behind the arch of the atlas and the anteroposterior diameter of the spinal canal at this level was correspondingly reduced, but in spite of this 4 of his 6 cases showed no signs of spinal compression.

The relationship of malformations in the region of the foramen magnum to syringomyelia is not altogether clear. McRae and others have found these anomalies common in cases with clinical evidence of syringomyelia, and it might be considered that obstruction to the venous drainage of the cord by bony pressure or dural constriction may produce oedema and eventual cavitation of the cervical cord. On the other hand List (1941) found the Arnold-Chiari or Chiari's Type I malformation in 3, and hydromyelia in another, of his 7 cases of bony malformations at this level. He concluded that these had no causal relationship to one another but were all equally the results of a developmental disturbance at about the 3rd week of intra-uterine life. The relationship of the Arnold-Chiari malformation to syringomyelia has already been referred to and List's theory appears all the more probable since cavitation of the cervical cord does not commonly occur in cases of acquired compression either by bony lesions or tumours at this level. It is, however, important to distinguish the Arnold-Chiari malformation from the tonsillar herniation, sometimes combined with transverse grooving on the dorsal surface of the medulla, which may result from reduction in size of the posterior fossa of the skull by acquired basilar invagination.

Degenerations and protrusions of intervertebral discs

Protrusion of intervertebral discs appears to have been first recognised by Luschka (1858) who also described the small neurocentral joints of the cervical vertebrae which play an important part in the pathology of cervical discs. Cases of spinal compression due to this cause were described by Walton and Paul (1905), Middleton and Teacher (1911) and by Goldthwaite (1911).

Anatomical considerations. The anatomy of intervertebral discs was studied by Luschka (1856), Schmorl (1929), Andrae (1929) and Beadle (1931). The central part of the disc consists of soft cellular fibrocartilage, with very fine collagenous fibres, the *nucleus pulposus.* This is surrounded by a ring of much firmer fibrocartilage, the *annulus fibrosus,* which is attached directly to the margin of the vertebral bodies. Between the nucleus pulposus and the spongiosa of the bone there is a thin layer of hyaline cartilage. These three forms of cartilage merge into one another without any abrupt transition. In the central part of the nucleus pulposus, in addition to numerous cartilage cells, there may be a few myxomatous or physaliphorous cells which are vestigial remains of the notochord. The ring of the annulus fibrosus is thicker anteriorly than posteriorly, so that the nucleus pulposus lies eccentrically. This may explain why herniations seldom take place in a forward direction. In the child the nucleus pulposus constitutes by far the greater part of the disc, but as age advances it becomes gradually encroached on by the annulus fibrosus, and after middle age becomes considerably dehydrated and shrinks in its vertical diameter. In children and young adults it is under considerable tension, so that on sawing through the vertebral bodies in a sagittal plane the nuclei bulge out from the surface. When bearing the weight of the body, this tension must be even greater. The normal disc has been compared to a fully inflated tyre; it allows rocking and, to a minor degree, torsion movements between the vertebral bodies, while at the same time it absorbs jars in the longitudinal direction. At the thoracic level the ribs and intercostal muscles limit the forward and backward flexion of the spine and very little rotation is possible. The thoracic intervertebral discs are thus protected from many of the stresses and strains to which those at higher and lower levels are subject and protrusions at this level are relatively rare.

Pathology. Three types of lesions of intervertebral discs may cause neurological symptoms: (1) Horizontal tearing. (2) Herniation of the nucleus pulposus. (3) Degeneration leading to osteophytosis. These are often combined.

(1) *Tearing* may occur at the lower thoracic and lumbar levels in severe lesions associated with dislocation. Spondylolisthesis at the lumbosacral or lower lumbar level is also probably associated with horizontal tearing of the disc and tearing or more gradual stretching of the anterior and posterior longitudinal ligaments. At the cervical level tearing, usually of a single disc, is found in the sudden traumatic subluxations which have already been described in Chapter 6. Such tears, without herniation of the nucleus, are most often seen in middle-aged or elderly subjects in whom the nucleus is less tense.

(2) *Herniation of the nucleus pulposus* occurs almost always in a backward direction, since the annulus fibrosus is thinner posteriorly. The nucleus may herniate through a weakened or torn part of the annulus, or between annulus and bone or, in rare cases, through the spongy bone to its posterior or posterolateral surface (Beadle). The herniations through the hyaline cartilage into the spongy tissue of the vertebral body, which may be seen near the centre of the disc in about 38 per cent of normal subjects (Schmorl), are of themselves of little importance, but by reducing tension in the nucleus pulposus they may lead to bulging of the annulus fibrosus and to osteophytosis. Their effects are therefore similar to those of degeneration of the nucleus pulposus. Herniation of the nucleus pulposus is most common in young

adults in whom the nucleus is more tense and the annulus thinner than in older subjects. They may be caused either by trauma or by sudden or severe muscular strain. Posterior or posterolateral herniations may burst through the annulus into the spinal canal either as a single mass or in several fragments, but more commonly they are checked by the outer fibres of the annulus and the posterior longitudinal ligament and so form a localised bulge into the spinal canal or intervertebral foramen. Owing to the firm central strands of the posterior longitudinal ligament in the lumbar region herniations here are usually posterolateral rather than posteromedian. They may be unilateral or bilateral.

(3) Degeneration of intervertebral discs is so common as to be almost physiological after the age of 50. As has been seen the nucleus pulposus loses water during life so that the percentage in its composition falls from 88 per cent at birth to 70 per cent at the age of 70. This desiccation of the nucleus is associated with shrinkage and increase in its fibrous tissue so that the transition from nucleus to annulus fibrosus becomes more gradual. There is also loss of tension which allows of some bulging of the annulus fibrosus in all directions when any pressure is put on the disc. The condition then resembles that of a partially deflated tyre. This is commonly followed by bony outgrowths from the margins of the upper and lower surfaces of the vertebral bodies, forming the *lipping* which is very commonly seen after middle age especially on the ventral surface of the lower thoracic and lumbar vertebral bodies. Schmorl found this condition in 10 per cent of young adults in the third decade, in 35 per cent in the fourth decade, in 70 per cent in the fifth decade and in 90 per cent of men over 50 and women over 60 years of age (Collins 1950). In most cases it remains slight at the cervical and upper thoracic levels where the pressure on the discs in the erect posture is less. But if for any reason, such as Schmorl's intra-osseous herniations, there is considerable loss of nuclear substance in a disc, lipping tends to occur above and below it. At the cervical level some loss of disc space associated with ventral lipping is recognised by radiologists as an early sign of degeneration of a disc. Schmorl recognised this process to be degenerative and distinguished it from rheumatic and inflammatory conditions by the term *spondylosis deformans*. Collins (1950) prefers the term *osteophytosis*, but it is probable that formation of osteophytes is secondary to the bulging of the annulus fibrosus which is itself secondary to loss of disc substance, and that bone formation follows the curve which the annulus assumes when pressure is applied to the disc. Anterior lipping causes no neurological symptoms and many cases with minor degrees of posterior lipping are also asymptomatic. But in a minority of cases bony transverse ridges on the dorsal surface of the cervical vertebrae associated with protrusions of disc substance are the cause of paraplegia or tetraplegia. Osteophytes in relation to the neurocentral joints of the lower cervical vertebrae also may cause signs of pressure on the roots of the brachial plexus. Degeneration of discs and osteophytosis is thus a common cause of neurological symptoms at the cervical level whereas herniation of nuclear substance is the usual cause of symptoms at the lumbar level. Since the causes and effects of protrusions of intervertebral discs differ in this and other ways according to the level at which they are situated, those at the cervical, thoracic and lumbar levels will be considered separately.

Cervical discs

Anatomical considerations. The lower 5 cervical vertebrae differ from all the others in the shape of their bodies. These are considerably wider in the transverse than in the anteroposterior direction and are saddle-shaped. When viewed from the front the lateral margins of the upper surface are seen to be curved sharply upwards, and the upper edges of these 'uncinate processes' come into contact through fibrocartilage with recesses on the outer margins of the inferior surface of the body of the upper vertebra, and thus form a joint in which there is usually a cavity (Frykholm 1951, Bull 1948). These *neurocentral joints* prevent lateral displacement of the vertebral bodies and also ensure that in flexion and extension movements of the neck the vertebral bodies rock on a pivot near their centre. The superior surfaces of the vertebral bodies are slightly convex in the anteroposterior direction, and the inferior surfaces correspondingly concave, with their anterior lips slightly overhanging the body of the subjacent bone. The shortness of the spinous processes at the cervical level allows more backward movement (extension) than at the thoracic level where the spines are imbricated. Forward flexion also is more free. Lateral flexion and rotation are limited by the neurocentral joints and articular processes, but the joint between the latter is rather lax and allows of some movement. These movements are associated with moulding of the intervertebral discs. Owing to the position of the neurocentral joints there is little difference between the tensions produced within the discs by full flexion and full (backward) extension of the neck.

Pathology. A few cases in which sudden flexion of the neck by external force has caused tearing of the annulus fibrosus and backward herniation of a large mass of nucleus pulposus have been verified by operation or post-mortem examination. These have usually been in young adults. The spinal cord is compressed by the herniated tissue and when this has been removed by operation there has sometimes been considerable or even apparently complete restoration of its function. Small central or posterolateral protrusions which encroach on the canal or the intervertebral foramina are more common. Many of these cases are caused by trauma such as blows by which the head is suddenly jerked backwards or forwards. When sudden pain in the arm, shoulder or trunk has been felt at the time of the injury it is probable that there has been a herniation of the nucleus pulposus through a torn or stretched part of the annulus. Operation or post-mortem examination shows a posteromedian or posterolateral protrusion of disc material which in the early stages may be fairly soft, but later becomes firmer and often fibrous or partly calcified or may be covered with a thin layer of bone. In the cervical region the posterior longitudinal ligament is rather weaker at its centre than more laterally and therefore herniations are likely to be either median or in close relation to the intervertebral foramina (Brain *et al.* 1952). The age of onset in such cases is usually below 40.

In cases of degeneration of discs symptoms come on more gradually. There may be no history of injury, or trauma, often of minor degree, may have occurred several months or years previously. X-ray examination in these cases may show loss of disc space at one or more levels, often associated with anterior and posterior osteophytosis and this may also be seen by oblique views in the intervertebral canals. In some cases paraplegia may come on suddenly after a degree of flexion or extension of the neck which is not very abnormal. For example, cases of paraplegia after tooth extraction and after tonsillectomy have occurred in the writer's experience. In such cases also there is often radiological evidence of previous degeneration of one or more discs. It is in fact doubtful whether paraplegia can follow such minor strains unless there is already degeneration of a disc. In patients over middle life the backward protrusion of the annulus fibrosus, which is the chief cause of pressure on the cord, may be visualised by myelography, but may not be visible at operation with the head in the normal position and the muscles relaxed. Surgeons therefore tend to stress the importance of the transverse bony ridges with which the bulging is associated. On post-mortem examination also no protrusion may be visible, but on flexion and extension of the neck there is abnormal mobility at one or more intervertebral joints.

Whereas nuclear herniations at the cervical level are most often found either between the 5th and 6th, or the 6th and 7th bodies, chronic degenerations are equally common in the two discs next above these (Brain *et al.* 1952). Their incidence at these levels may be partly explained by their tendency to occur immediately below congenitally fused vertebrae, usually the

2nd and 3rd or the 2nd, 3rd and 4th. The strong leverage which the fused segments exert on this disc is probably the cause of its premature degeneration. In cases of severe degeneration limited to one disc the vertebrae above it may tend to move forward out of line with those below it especially on flexion or extension of the neck. In other cases bony ridges may be seen at several levels, or in myelograms the column of myodil is seen to be indented opposite several discs (Figs. 14.1 and 14.2).

Protrusions of intervertebral discs, whether due to herniation or degeneration, give rise to hyperplasia of the fibrous tissue in their neighbourhood. The dura mater becomes thickened and adherent to the posterior longitudinal ligament and there is also thickening and fibrosis of the pia arachnoid especially round the roots. Narrowing of one or more intervertebral canals by cartilagenous protrusion and osteophytosis, along with thickening of the fibrous tissue of the dural sleeve (Frykholm 1951), may cause degeneration of the nerve roots that pass through them. This is most common between the 5th and 6th and 6th and 7th vertebrae and is usually bilateral but may be greater on one side. Although in most cases both ventral and dorsal components of the root are damaged, in some cases the position of the protrusion is such that it presses chiefly on the ventral root.

The effects of disc protrusion on the spinal cord vary in different cases according to variations in the causative factors.

(1) *Lesions of roots* in the intervertebral foramina show themselves by wedge-shaped areas of degeneration in the dorsal columns which pass medially and become narrower in successively higher segments (Fig. 14.5). When a ventral root is severely damaged there is an outgrowth of fresh neurites from the axons proximal to the level of damage and these may form a stump neuroma at the entrance to the intervertebral foramen or, more commonly, leashes of myelinated fibres which run in the meninges or pass along the walls of blood vessels into the tissues of the cord. Such regenerative phenomena are very common in chronic cases of lesion of cervical discs.

(2) Posteromesial or posterolateral protrusions may press on the ventral surface of the cord, and encroach on the restricted space of the spinal canal. Normally the antero-posterior diameter, as measured by radiographs, of the spinal canal from C3 to C7, with the neck in the neutral position, is 17 mm. (Wolf *et al.* 1956) but in cases of cervical spondylosis with myelopathy this measurement averages 14 mm. (Payne and Spillane 1957). When the neck is extended this distance, from the spur on the postero-inferior aspect of one vertebra to the base of the spinous process of the vertebra below, may be reduced by 2 mm., and if there is any posterior movement of one vertebra upon the other, as may occur (Penning 1962), the distance is even further reduced. Posteriorly, in hyperextension, the ligamentum flavum may be infolded and press upon the cord (Taylor 1956, Nugent 1960). The effects of pressure by the firm boss of cartilage on the anterior spinal artery are probably even more important than pressure on the substance of the cord, since at the cervical level this vessel supplies not only the ventro-lateral white columns and grey matter but also the ventral third or quarter of the dorsal columns (Bolton 1939). The tension of the ligamentum denticulatum aids this pressure since by its attachment to the dura mater, which is itself anchored by the root sleeves, it prevents the cord from moving backwards (Kahn). Allen (1952) observed that flexion of the neck during operations might produce blanching of the cord at the level of disc protrusion, and it is possible that the mechanical effects of compression are supplemented by spasm of the artery. To these effects may be added in some cases those of compression of the nutrient branches in their course through the intervertebral foramina. These branches are very variable both in position and importance, but a common arrangement is for a fairly large branch, which may be unilateral or bilateral, to enter along with the root of C6 or C7. The flow in the anterior spinal artery is caudalward and, as

14.1

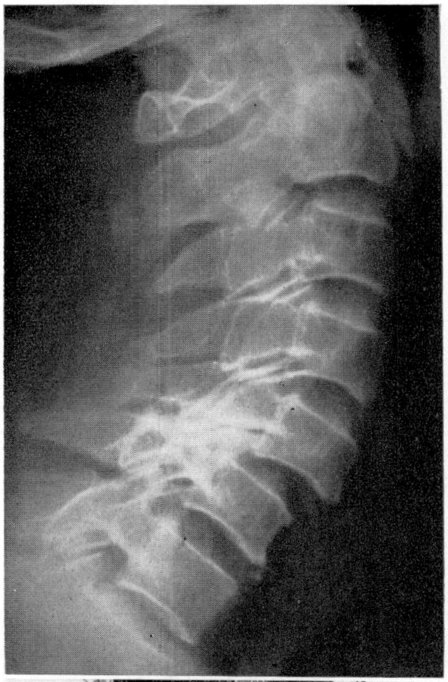

14.2

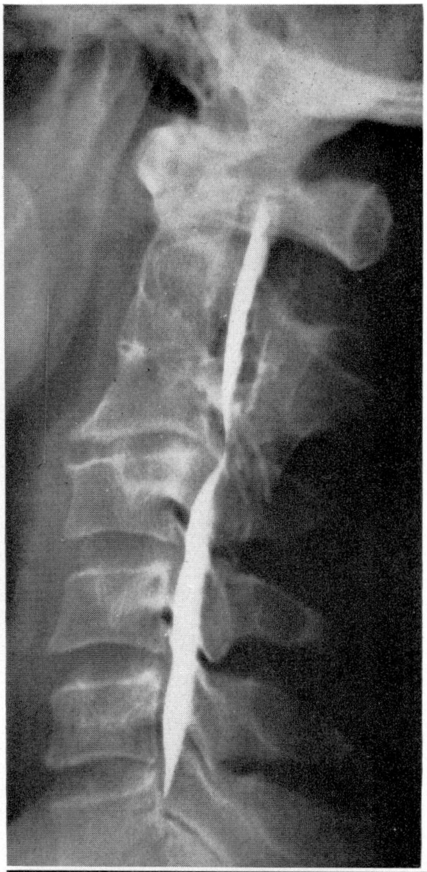

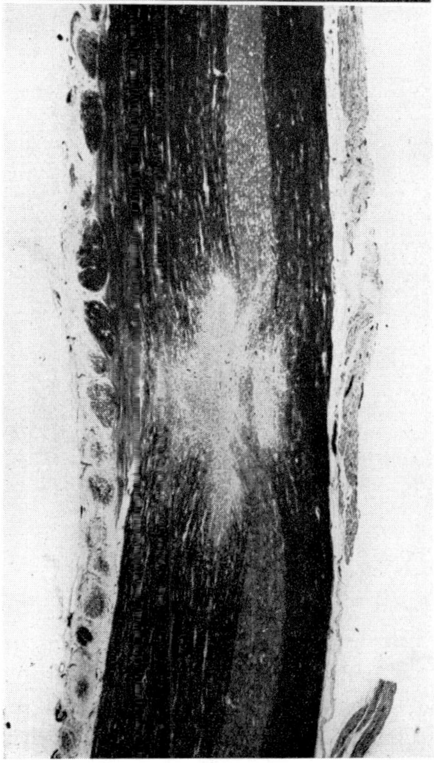

14.3

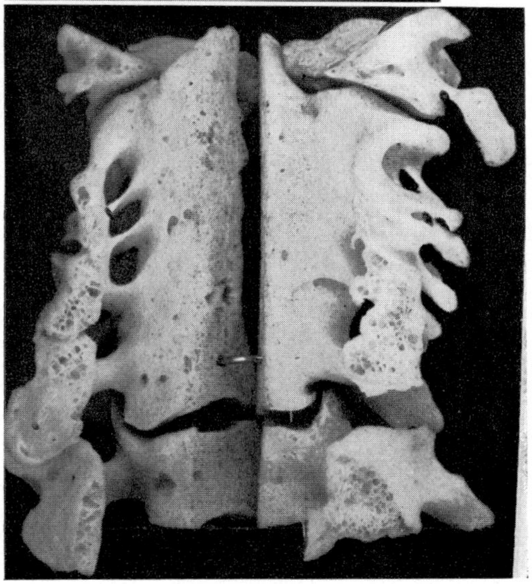

14.4

FIG. 14.1. X-ray photograph. Degeneration of the disc between C.5 and C.6 is made more evident by hyper-extension of the neck.

FIG. 14.2. Myelogram of cervical spine, showing narrowing of the disc space and backward protrusion of the disc between C.3 and C.4. Note the congenital fusion of C.2 and C.3. (Case 1 of Mair and Druckman 1953.)

FIG. 14.3. Longitudinal section of the cervical cord from a case with 18 years' history of slight paraplegia due to degeneration of the disc between C.7 and Th.1. (Myelin stain. Case 4 of Mair and Druckman 1953.)

FIG. 14.4. Klippel-Feil deformity. Congenital fusion of vertebrae from C.2 to C.6. This was associated with basilar impression. Severe paraplegia resulted from angulation of the cord over the protruding odontoid process.

Bolton (1939) showed, a valvular arrangement at the junction of branches with the main vessel prevents them from supplying the cord above the level at which they join it. These factors explain the ischaemic changes in the ventral horns which are frequently seen in one or two segments below the level of compression. For example, loss of nerve cells and ischaemic changes in those that remain may be found in the 1st thoracic segment when the cord has been compressed by protrusion of the disc between the 5th and 6th cervical vertebrae (7th cervical segment) (Mair and Druckman 1953).

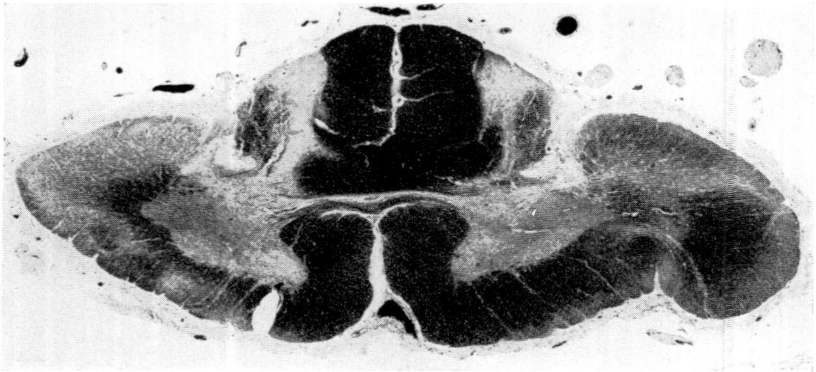

14.5

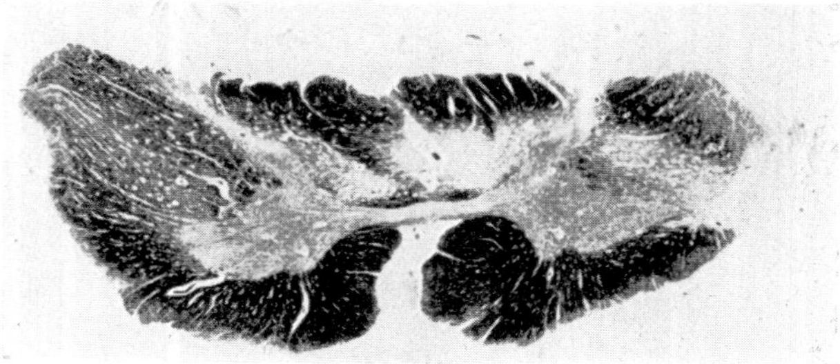

14.6

FIG. 14.5. Cervical disc protrusion. Section of the cord at the level of C.4–C.5 from a case with multiple disc protrusions involving chiefly the intervertebral foramina at the lower cervical level. The cord is flattened antero-posteriorly as a result of pressure and tension on the ligamentum denticulatum and shows degeneration in the dorsal columns due to lesions of the lower cervical nerve roots. (Myelin.)

FIG. 14.6. Section of the cord at the level of a disc protrusion (C.6–C.7) showing degeneration in the region of attachment of the ligamentum denticulatum on one side and degeneration in the ventral part of the dorsal columns chiefly on the same side. (Myelin.)

The greatest changes are seen in the spinal cord at the level of compression (Wilkinson 1960, Hook *et al.* 1960). Here the cord is flatter than normal from compression in its anteroposterior diameter. Not infrequently there is some demyelination of the white matter at the point of attachment of the thickened ligamentum denticulatum in a line passing inwards from this towards the base of the ventral horns, suggesting the lines of tension to which the cord has been subjected. Ill-defined areas of demyelination are also commonly found in the ventral parts of the dorsal columns either in the midline or at one or both sides (Fig. 14.6). These are not so easily explained. They may be due to ischaemia in the area of terminal supply of the anterior spinal artery or to venous stasis.

(3) In cases of severe disc lesions there is the further factor of abnormal mobility of the spine and consequent abnormal bending of the spinal cord. This is most likely to occur in cases with fusion of vertebrae. In all these cases the lesions of the nervous parenchyma are often associated with hyaline changes in the walls of the intramedullary vessels.

Thoracic discs

Protrusions of intervertebral discs at the thoracic level are, for the reasons stated, comparatively rare. Some are due to trauma, but in a few cases the spinal injury has been masked by fractures of the legs or has only begun to cause paraplegia after some weeks or months. On the available evidence the great majority of protrusions at this level begin as herniations of nuclear tissue which later becomes more fibrous and may undergo calcification or bone formation. The normal slight kyphosis at the thoracic level brings the spinal cord into constant contact with these firm or hard projections and in its slight upward and downward movements it is rubbed against them. This may cause necrosis and loss of tissue on the ventral surface of the cord, resulting in a cavity in which the nodule is embedded. In other respects the lesions in the cord are a combination of the effects of pressure, tension and ischaemia similar to that seen at the cervical level.

Logue (1952), from a review of the literature and his own experience, considered that protrusions at this level constituted only about 2–3 per cent of all disc protrusions. Most occurred in patients of middle or later age and few appeared to be related to trauma. They were only found in the lower 9 discs and seldom above the level of the 6th. In his cases the damage to the cord appeared to be disproportionate to the degree of protrusion, suggesting that it was due more to ischaemia than to pressure.

Lumbar discs

Although the lumbar spine is robust and well supported by muscles it has to withstand very heavy compressive strains, especially in athletic young adults. Lesions of lumbar discs are therefore very common under the age of 40. They may be caused by external violence, such as a fall on the sacrum, but many cases can be attributed to severe muscular strain, especially lifting heavy weights in a stooping position. As the majority of protrusions at this level occur between the lower lumbar vertebrae or between the lowest of these (4th, 5th or 6th) and the sacrum, they do not damage the spinal cord and their effects are those of compression or attrition of the roots of the cauda equina. Almost all are due to herniation of the nucleus pulposus, but spondylolisthesis due to tearing of the disc may occur between the lowest lumbar vertebra and the sacrum or between the two lowest lumbar vertebrae. Herniations are usually posterolateral. When they project chiefly into the intervertebral foramen they compress only the corresponding root, usually the 4th or 5th lumbar. They are usually associated with thickening of the connective tissue around the articular joints and this may contribute to the narrowing of the intervertebral foramina. When they project into the canal the roots which pass over them to a lower level are affected. Usually only a few roots are involved, but in a few cases there is severe damage to most of the lower roots of the cauda equina. In these cases flaccid paralysis and anaesthesia of the ankles and feet, and loss of sphincter control, may come on suddenly or progressively over a few days. In 17 cases of this kind Jennett (1956) found large herniations of nucleus pulposus which almost filled the spinal canal. In a further 8 cases the herniation was not so large but the nerve roots were bound together by thickened arachnoid.

Degeneration of lumbar discs with osteophytosis is also very common at the lumbar level, but prominent bony ridges on the dorsal surface of the vertebral bodies are proportionately rarer than at the cervical level. In severe cases osteophytes may occlude the intervertebral canal which contains the important *arteria radicis anterior magna* or other important vessel going to the lumbosacral segments of the cord. These vessels are usually unpaired and their occlusion may lead to partial or even complete necrosis of the tissues of the cord at this level. Suh and Alexander (1939) found that the arteria radicis magna most often entered along with the 2nd lumbar root, but in different subjects it ranged from the 8th thoracic to the 4th lumbar root. A fairly large posterior spinal artery usually enters the spinal canal along a different root.

Spillane (1952) drew attention to the frequency of severe protrusions at the lumbar level in achondroplasics, and related it to the dorsolumbar kyphosis which is common in these dwarfs.

Lumbar puncture and radiography

In cases of cervical disc protrusion there is very seldom any increase in the cell count in the cerebrospinal fluid but some excess of protein is found in about one third of the cases and partial or complete spinal block in a similar proportion. When no block can be demonstrated by the usual technique Clarke and Robinson (1956) recommend 'postural manometry', i.e. compressing the jugular veins with the neck fully flexed or fully extended. By using the latter position they could demonstrate spinal block in 10 cases in which none was found in the normal position.

When the site of the protruded disc is at the thoracic level protein increase and spinal block become more common. Protrusions in the lumbar region are most often below the usual level of puncture, through the third interspace, so that no spinal block is found unless there are considerable arachnoidal adhesions. But there is often a considerable rise in protein in the cerebrospinal fluid. In severe lesions of the cauda equina Jennett (1956) constantly found a complete spinal block and considerable excess of protein when the puncture was made below the level of the protrusion; in 2 of his cases the fluid was yellow and clotted spontaneously.

The diagnosis rests chiefly on radiography both by direct views and by myelograms with opaque media. At the cervical level anteroposterior views are of little value owing to the shape of the vertebral bodies but oblique views outlining the intervertebral foramina are useful especially in cases with root symptoms. As some degree of degeneration of cervical discs is very common in middle-aged patients slight indentation of the opaque medium, usually at several levels, may be seen in many normal cervical spines, especially when the myelogram is taken with the neck fully extended. This appearance may usually be discounted. Deeper indentations, especially if associated with posterior lipping, are more important. Protrusions at a single level are less common and are more often the result of trauma. Some, especially those between C3 and 4, may be secondary to fusion of vertebrae.

Pott's paraplegia

(Paraplegia associated with spinal caries)

The name *Pott's disease* should be reserved for the association of paraplegia with spinal curvature due to tuberculous caries, since Percival Pott (1779) was the first to draw attention to this association in English literature. But as the name is often used for the spinal disease alone (although this was described by Galen) the term *Pott's paraplegia* is here used to avoid ambiguity. A fuller account of the condition was published in France in the same year (1779) by David and indeed Pott did not recognise the tuberculous nature of the spinal disease until a later publication (1782).

Pott's paraplegia occurs in from 5 to 20 per cent of all cases of spinal caries involving the cervical and thoracic vertebrae. As is well known spinal caries is most common in the thoracic vertebrae and paraplegia is therefore most often due to lesions at this level, but caries of cervical vertebrae carry an equal risk of paraplegia (Butler 1935). This may precede obvious disease of the spine, especially in adults, but usually follows either very soon after its appearance or at a shorter or longer interval. In cases with angular kyphosis due to caries of one or more vertebral bodies three factors may combine to damage the spinal cord: (1) The presence of granulation tissue or a cold abscess in the epidural space, (2) bending of the cord, and (3) compression or disease of its nutrient vessels. The first of these factors is probably the most important and has received most attention, but either or both of the latter may contribute to cause the more severe and permanent forms of paraplegia.

(1) Whether the primary disease is in the vertebral bodies or, as rarely occurs, in the laminae, granulation tissue tends to reach the epidural space, where it spreads both up and down the canal and around the cord. It soon fills the space between cord and bone and becomes adherent to the dura mater; but this usually resists invasion and becomes thickened by the formation of new fibrous tissue on its outer surface. The granulation tissue compresses the cord and probably produces oedema in it by impeding the venous drainage. The formation of a cold abscess in the epidural space will probably have the same effect. This compression of the cord is the most probable cause of the minor degrees of paraplegia which improve after treatment. In some such cases improvement coincides with, and appears to be due to, the tracking of a cold abscess into the soft paravertebral tissues.

The most usual lesion in early cases is a vacuolar type of myelin degeneration in the latera or anterolateral columns. This is often more diffuse than that which is seen in ischaemic lesions and may be due to oedema secondary to venous obstruction. The myelin is often more damaged than the axons. In 3 cases of Pott's paraplegia, associated with a sharp kyphosis and epidural granulation tissue, Holmes (1906) could find no evidence of Wallerian degeneration of long tracts above or below the lesion in spite of considerable damage to myelin at this level. But in some cases there are more severe degenerative or necrotic lesions of the white or grey matter.

(2) Prolonged angulation of the cord over a sharp kyphosis usually results in thinning of the cord at that level, especially in its anteroposterior diameter. This may not be associated with much damage to the white columns of the cord, but there is evident loss of tissue, and in many cases, definite demyelination at this level. More acute and severe lesions of the cord may be produced in cases of rapid collapse of a vertebral body, or when the cord is bent over a relatively intact intervertebral disc between two diseased vertebrae, or is compressed by a sequestrum which is pushed backwards into the spinal canal by the angulation (Seddon 1935). Dislocation of the spine is also liable to produce severe damage to the cord.

(3) In all these cases an important radicular artery may be compressed in the intervertebral foramen or may be the seat of tuberculous arteritis before it enters the dural sheath. This may account for some cases of severe paraplegia of rapid onset in cases in which the vertebral and epidural disease is not unusually severe.

Compression of the spinal cord in other inflammatory diseases of the spine

A number of other micro-organisms may cause osteomyelitis of the vertebral bodies or laminae with spread of inflammatory granulation tissue into the epidural space. Of these the most common is staphylococcus pyogenes which may produce an epidural abscess which tracks down the spinal canal, or a more localised mass of granulomatous tissue which compresses the cord. Subacute cases of this kind may occur after one or more attacks of staphylococcal infection in other parts of the body. Sometimes, in the writer's experience, they contain little or no pus and their aetiology has only been proved by bacteriological examination. But more frankly purulent abscesses also may compress the spinal cord. In most cases the effects on the cord are reversible so that function returns after pressure is relieved.

Typhoid spine is another form of osteomyelitis or periostitis in which compression of the cord may occur. In such cases paraplegia may be the first, or an early symptom, but it is usually preceded by pain in the back, or round the body. The interval, sometimes of months or years, between the initial infection and the spinal disease may confuse the diagnosis in these cases.

Cerebrospinal fluid. In Pott's paraplegia, and other forms of epidural granuloma, a complete spinal block is almost always found. The protein is raised, often to very high levels, but there is rarely any increase in the cell count. In cases of *typhoid spine* the fluid usually contains a relatively high titre of antibodies to the causative organism.

(Revised by W. Blackwood.)

REFERENCES

Allen, K. L. (1952) *J. Neurol. Psychiat.*, **15**, 20.
Andrae, R. (1929) *Beit. pathol. Anat.*, **82**, 464.
Bachs, A., Barraquer-Bordas, L., Barraquer-Ferre, L., Canadell, J. M. and Modolell, A. (1955) *Brain*, **78**, 537.
Beadle, O. C. (1931) *M.R.C. Special Report Series*, 161, H.M. Stationery Office, London.
Bolton, B. (1939) *J. Neurol. Psychiat.*, **2**, 137.
Brain, W. R., Northfield, D. W. C. and Wilkinson, M. (1952) *Brain*, **75**, 187.
Bull, J. W. B. (1946) *Proc. Roy. Soc. Med.*, **40**, 85; (1948) ibid., **41**, 513.
Bull, J. W. B., Nixon, W. L. B. and Pratt, R. T. C. (1955) *Brain*, **78**, 229.
Bull, J. W. B., Nixon, W. L. B., Pratt, R. T. C. and Robinson, P. L. (1959) *Brain*, **82**, 10.
Butler, R. W. (1935) *Brit. J. Surg.*, **22**, 738.
Clarke, E. and Robinson, P. K. (1956) *Brain*, **79**, 483.
Clouston, T. S. (1898) *Clinical lectures on Mental Diseases*, 5th Edition.
Collins, D. H. (1950) *The pathology of articular and spinal diseases*, Arnold, London.
David, J. P. (1779) in *Medical Classics*, E. C. Kelly, 1936, **1**, 4.
Frykholm, R. (1951) *Acta chir. Scand.*, **101**, 345.
Goldthwaite, J. W. (1911) *Boston Med. Surg., J.*, **164**, 365.
Greenfield, J. G. (1953) *Rev. Méd. de la Suisse Romande*, **73**, 227.
Hemphill, R. E. and Stengel, E. (1940) *J. Ment. Sci.*, **86**, 341.
Henschen, F. (1936) *Ann. d'Anat. pathol. med. chir.*, **13**, 943.
Holmes, G. (1906) *Brain*, **29**, 514.
Hook, O., Lidvall, H. and Astrom, K. E. (1960) *Neurology*, **10**, 834.
Jennett, W. B. (1956) *J. Neurol. Psychiat.*, **19**, 109.
Kahn, E. A. (1947) *J. Neurosurg.*, **4**, 191.
Lewis, B. (1889) *Text book of Mental Disease.*
List, C. F. (1941) *Arch. Neurol. Psychiat.* (Chicago), **45**, 577.
Logue, V. (1952) *J. Neurol. Psychiat.*, **15**, 227.
Luschka, H. (1856) *Virchows Archiv.*, **9**, 311; (1858) *Die Halbgelenke des Menschlichen Korpers*, Berlin.
McAlhany, H. J. and Netsky, M. G. (1955) *J. Neuropathol. exper. Neurol.*, **14**, 276.
McRae, D. L. (1953) *Acta Radiol.*, **40**, 335.
Mair, W. G. P. and Druckman, R. (1953) *Brain*, **76**, 70.
Middleton, G. S. and Teacher, J. H. (1911) *Glasgow med. J.*, 139.
Morel, F. (1930) *Syndrome d'hyperostose frontale interne avec adipose et troubles cérébraux*, Doin, Paris.
Morgagni. (1765) *De sedibus et causis morborum*, Litt. II, Epist. 27, Padova.
Nugent, G. R. (1959) *Neurology*, **9**, 273.
Payne, E. E. and Spillane, J. D. (1957) *Brain*, **80**, 571.
Penning, L. (1962) *Neurology*, **12**, 513.
Petersen, J. (1947) *Acta med. Scand.*, **128**, 71.
Pott, P. (1779 and 1782) in *Medical Classics*, E. C. Kelly, 1936, **1**, 4.
Saunders, W. W. (1943) *Radiology*, **41**, 589.

Scharenberg, K. (1953) *J. Neuropath.*, **12**, 11.
Schmorl, G. (1929) *Klin. Wchnschr.*, **8**, 1, 243; (1929) *Fortschr. Geb. Röntgen*, **40**, 629.
Seddon, H. J. (1935) *Brit. J. Surg.*, **22**, 769.
Spillane, J. D. (1952) *J. Neurol. Psychiat.*, **15**, 246.
Stewart, R. M. (1927–8) *J. Neurol. Psychopath.*, **8**, 321.
Suh, T. H. and Alexander, L. (1939) *Arch. Neurol. Psychiat.*, **41**, 659.
Taylor, A. R. (1956) *Lancet* (i), 717.
Wallace, D. and Bruce, A. (1910) *Rev. Neurol. Psychiat.* (Edinburgh), **8**, 1.
Walton, G. L. and Paul, W. E. (1905) *Boston med. Surg. J.*, **153**, 114.
Wilkinson, M. (1960) *Brain*, **83**, 589.
Wolf, B. S., Khilani, M. and Malis, L. (1956) *J. Mt. Sinai Hosp.*, **23**, 283.
Wyllie, W. G. (1923) *Brain*, **46**, 336.

INDEX

Figures given in heavy type indicate principal references.